Pharmacology

Pharmacology

H. P. Rang
MB BS MA DPhil FRS
Director, Sandoz Institute for Medical Research;
Visiting Professor of Pharmacology, University College, London

M. M. Dale
MB BCh PhD
Senior Lecturer, Department of Pharmacology,
University College, London

CHURCHILL LIVINGSTONE
EDINBURGH LONDON MELBOURNE AND NEW YORK 1987

CHURCHILL LIVINGSTONE
Medical Division of Longman Group UK Limited

Distributed in the United States of America by Churchill
Livingstone Inc., 1560 Broadway, New York, N.Y. 10036, and
by associated companies, branches and representatives
throughout the world.

First published 1987

ISBN 0-443-03407-9

British Library Cataloguing in Publication Data

Rang, H. P.
  Pharmacology.
  1. Pharmacology
  I. Title   II. Dale, M. Maureen
  615'.1   RM300

Library of Congress Cataloging in Publication Data

Rang, H. P.
  Pharmacology.
  Includes index.
  1. Pharmacology.   I. Dale, M. Maureen.   II. Title.
[DNLM: 1. Pharmacology.   QV 4 R196p]
RM300.R35   1986   615'.1   86–12914

Produced by Longman Singapore Publishers (Pte) Ltd.
Printed in Singapore

Preface

This book is intended primarily for preclinical medical students and science students studying pharmacology, but clinicians who wish to brush up their basic science and scientists in other disciplines who want to get an overall grasp of pharmacology may find it useful.

It is the successor to '*Applied Pharmacology*' by H O Schild and has developed out of it. Both authors were students under Heinz Schild and in writing the present book we have had very much in mind his approach to pharmacology. However, because of the developments in the subject and in the biological sciences in general, we felt it apposite not just to update his text but to rewrite it. We have reduced somewhat the element of clinical pharmacology in view of the fact that this material is best dealt with when students have had some experience of clinical medicine and because there are now many excellent textbooks on clinical pharmacology. Consequently we have abandoned the title '*Applied Pharmacology*' in favour of '*Pharmacology*', the subject being defined as 'the study of the effects of chemical substances on living tissue'. Inherent in this definition is the fact that pharmacology is not synonymous with clinical pharmacology; it provides the clinician with the agents used in therapeutics and with the understanding of how they work, but it is concerned not only with drugs used in treatment but also with drugs used as investigatory tools. With this definition in mind we have concentrated on pharmacodynamics and pharmacokinetics, and in the context of the former we have stressed *mechanisms* of action, believing that if an individual understands more of *how* a drug works he or she will use it more intelligently in the clinic or laboratory. In addition to dealing with drugs as such, we have placed emphasis on 'mediators', since understanding the body's method of controlling its own functions is a route not only to the understanding of how exogenous chemical substances affect it but also to the rational development of new drugs. Descriptions of peripheral neurotransmitters such as acetylcholine and noradrenaline, of hormones such as hydrocortisone, and of inflammatory mediators such as histamine, have always formed part of pharmacology textbooks and it is well known that investigation of the actions and structure/activity relationships of these substances has led to the development of valuable drugs for the clinician. We have carried this approach a little further, with an eye on future developments. Thus, in the sections on the central nervous system we have included discussions of various CNS neurotransmitters and neuromodulators (GABA, glutamate, neuropeptides, etc), and their possible significance in some clinical disorders, even though useful drugs that are known to act by affecting the metabolism or actions of these mediators have yet to emerge. Similarly we have included brief descriptions of inflammatory mediators such as platelet activating factor and interleukin-I and their possible role in conditions such as asthma and rheumatoid arthritis. Drugs used in inflammation and as immunosuppressives form an important part of the therapeutic armamentarium and an appreciation of how they act and how new drugs in this area are likely to be developed requires some knowledge of what happens in inflammation. Since pathology and immunology generally come later in the medical course than pharmacology, and since pharmacology students generally do not study these subjects at all, we have included a brief outline of the main events in the inflammatory and immune responses.

While making it clear that any mistakes in the book are our own, we would like to acknowledge help and advice from the following people: Dr J G Blackman, Dr D G Haylett, Isobel Heyman, Dr D M James, Dr I F James, Prof. J Mandelstam, Dr R Pitt-Rivers and Dr G Robinson. In particular we wish to acknowledge the invaluable help of Janet Martin, who drew all the diagrams and Marie-Claire Stuart, Annabel Giles and Joyce Mancini who prepared the text.

London
1987

H P Rang
M M Dale

Contents

SECTION ONE: GENERAL PRINCIPLES

1: Mechanisms of drug action 3
  Systems of medicine 3
  The binding of drug molecules to cells 4
    Receptor classification 6
    Note on terminology 6
    Quantitative aspects 7
      Agonist dose-response curves 8
      Competitive antagonism 9
      Partial agonists and the concept of
        efficacy 10
    Direct measurement of drug binding to
      receptors 12
    Isolation and characterization of
      receptor molecules 14
    Receptor-effector linkage 16
      Direct regulation of ionic permeability 16
      Mechanisms involving a second
        messenger 19
      Regulation of DNA transcription 27
  Types of drug antagonism 28
    Chemical antagonism 28
    Pharmacokinetic antagonism 28
    Antagonism by receptor block 28
    Physiological antagonism 31
  Desensitization and tachyphylaxis 31
  Definition of terms 33

2: Measurement in pharmacology 35
  Bioassay 35
    General principles of bioassay 37
      Use of standards 37
      Design of bioassays 38
      Quantal and graded responses 41
    Bioassays in man 42
      Clinical trials 43
    Measurement of toxicity 46

  Therapeutic index 48
  Chemical assay methods 50
    Radioimmunoassay 50
    Chromatographic techniques 51
    Mass spectrometry 53
    Spectrophotometry and fluorimetry 55

3: Absorption, distribution and fate of drugs 57
  Translocation of drug molecules 57
    Movement of drug molecules across
      cellular barriers 58
      Diffusion through lipid 58
      Carrier-mediated transport 62
    Partion into body fat 62
    Binding of drugs to plasma proteins 63
  Phases of drug disposition 65
  Drug absorption 66
    Absorption from the alimentary canal 66
      Sublingual administration 66
      Oral administration 66
      Bioavailability 68
    Other routes of administration 69
      Rectal administration 69
      Cutaneous administration 69
      Eye-drops 69
      Administration by inhalation 70
      Administration by injection 70
  Distribution of drugs in the body 71
    Body fluid compartments 71
    Volume of distribution 72
  Removal of drugs from the body 72
    Drug metabolism 73
      Phase I reactions 74
      Phase II reactions 76
      Induction of microsomal enzymes 77
      First-pass metabolism 77
      Pharmacologically active drug
        metabolites 78

Renal excretion of drugs and drug
   metabolites   78
  Glomerular filtration   78
  Tubular secretion and reabsorption   78
  Diffusion across the renal tubule   79
  Drug excretion expressed as clearance   79
  Biliary excretion and enterohepatic
   circulation   81
Pharmacokinetics   81
  Single compartment model   81
  More complicated kinetic models   86
   Two compartment model   86
   Saturation kinetics   87
  Special drug delivery systems   89

4: Individual variation and drug interactions   90
Effects of age   90
Genetic factors   92
Drug interactions   94
  Pharmacodynamic interaction   94
  Pharmacokinetic interaction   95
   Absorption phase   95
   Effects on drug distribution   96
   Effects on drug metabolism   96
   Haemodynamic effects   97
   Effects on drug excretion   97

SECTION TWO: CHEMICAL MEDIATORS

**5: Chemical transmission and the autonomic
   nervous system   101**
Basic anatomy and physiology of the
  autonomic nervous system   103
  General principles of chemical
   transmission   106
   Denervation supersensitivity   106
   Dale's principle   106
  Recent developments   107
   Presynaptic interactions   108
  Transmitters other than acetylcholine
   and noradrenaline   110
  Basic steps in neurochemical
   transmission—sites of drug action   111

6: Cholinergic transmission   113
Muscarinic and nicotinic actions of
  acetylcholine   113
  Acetylcholine receptors   114
Physiology of cholinergic transmission   115
  Acetylcholine synthesis and release   116

Electrical events in transmission   116
  Depolarization block   117
Effects of drugs on cholinergic transmission   118
  Muscarinic agonists   119
  Muscarinic antagonists   121
  Ganglion stimulating drugs   124
  Ganglion blocking drugs   125
  Neuromuscular blocking drugs   129
   Drugs affecting acetylcholine synthesis   129
   Drugs that inhibit acetylcholine release   130
  Drugs that enhance cholinergic
   transmission   137
   Distribution and function of
    cholinesterase   137
   Drugs that inhibit cholinesterase   138
   Cholinesterase reactivation   142
   Myasthenia gravis   143
   Other drugs which enhance
    transmission   144

7: Adrenergic transmission   146
Classification of adrenergic receptors   146
Physiology of adrenergic transmission   148
  The adrenergic neuron   148
  Noradrenaline synthesis   150
  Noradrenaline storage   151
  Noradrenaline release   151
  Uptake and degradation of
   catecholamines   153
Drugs acting on adrenoceptors   156
  Structure-activity relationships   156
  Adrenoceptor agonists   158
  Adrenoceptor blocking agents   161
   α-receptor antagonists   161
   β-receptor antagonists   167
Drugs that affect adrenergic neurons   169
  Drugs that affect noradrenaline synthesis   170
  Drugs that affect noradrenaline storage   170
  Drugs that affect noradrenaline release   170
   Adrenergic neuron blocking drugs   171
   Indirectly-acting sympathomimetic
    amines   172
  Drugs that affect presynaptic receptors   173
  Inhibitors of noradrenaline uptake   174
Definition of terms   175

8: Local hormones, inflammation and allergy   177
The inflammatory reaction and the immune
  response   178
  Vascular events   178

Cellular events 181
The significance of the specific
immunological response 182
Mediators of inflammation and allergy 187
Histamine 187
Eicosanoids 192
Bradykinin 198
Platelet activating factor (PAF) 201
Interleukin-1 203
γ-Interferon 203

**9: Drugs used to suppress inflammatory and
immune reactions** 204
Non-steroidal anti-inflammatory drugs
(NSAIDs) 204
Pharmacological actions 204
Mechanism of action of NSAIDs 207
Anti-rheumatoid drugs 213
Drugs used in gout 216
Antagonists of histamine 218
Immunosuppressants 221

**SECTION THREE: DRUGS AFFECTING
MAJOR ORGAN SYSTEMS**

10: The heart 227
Physiology of cardiac function 227
Cardiac rate and rhythm 227
Disturbances of cardiac rhythm 229
Cardiac contraction 231
Myocardial oxygen consumption and
coronary blood flow 234
Coronary atherosclerosis and its
consequences 235
Drugs that affect cardiac function 236
Autonomic transmitters and related
drugs 236
Cardiac glycosides 239
Chemistry 239
Pharmacological actions 239
Effects on the heart in normal and
pathological states 240
Pharmacokinetic aspects 243
Adverse effects 244
Antidysrhythmic drugs 244
Class I antidysrhythmic drugs 245
Class II antidysrhythmic drugs 247
Class III antidysrhythmic drugs 247
Class IV antidysrhythmic drugs 248
Anti-anginal drugs 250

Organic nitrates 250
Dipyridamole 254
Other drugs that affect the heart 254
Methylxanthines 254
Purines 254
Other agents 255

11: The circulation 256
Vascular smooth muscle 256
Vasoconstrictor drugs 258
Sympathomimetic amines 258
Angiotensin 259
Vasopressin (Antidiuretic hormone) 259
Vasodilator drugs 260
Nitroprusside 260
Hydrallazine 260
Diazoxide 261
Papaverine 261
Endogenous mediators 261
Serotonin 261
Purines 265
Dopamine 266
Atrial peptides 268
Vasodilator drugs that act indirectly 269
The renin-angiotensin system 269
Angiotensin coverting enzyme
inhibitors 270
Angiotensin antagonists 270
Clinical use of vasodilator drugs 272
Hypertension 272
Cardiac failure 273
Shock and hypotensive states 273
Migraine 275

12: Haemostasis and thrombosis 281
Blood coagulation 281
Coagulation defects 283
Vitamin K 283
Unwanted coagulation 285
Oral anticoagulants 286
Injectable anticoagulants 287
Platelet adhesion and activation 289
Platelets and arachidonate metabolites 292
Antiplatelet agents 293
Fibrinolysis 294
Fibrinolytic drugs 294
Antifibrinolytic drugs 295
Therapeutic uses of anticoagulants, anti-
platelet agents and fibrinolytic drugs 295
Venous thromboembolism 295

Arterial thromboembolism 295
Miscellaneous conditions 296

13: The respiratory system **297**
The regulation of respiration 297
Drugs which affect respiration 298
Respiratory stimulants 298
Drugs causing respiratory depression 299
Functions of the lung unrelated to
respiration 299
The regulation of the musculature, blood
vessels and glands of the airways 299
Disorders of respiratory function 301
Drugs used to treat asthma 304
Drugs used for cough 307

14: The kidney **309**
The structure and function of the nephron 309
The control of extracellular fluid
osmolarity 315
Concentrating mechanisms: the
counter-current multiplier system
in the medulla 315
Acid-base balance 316
Potassium balance 317
Excretion of organic molecules 318
Arachidonic acid metabolites and renal
function 318
Drugs acting on the kidney 318
Diuretics 318
The development of diuretic drugs 319
Diuretics acting directly on the cells
of the nephron 321
Diuretics acting indirectly by modify-
ing the content of the filtrate 325
Obsolete or near obsolete diuretics 326
General aspects of the action of
diuretics 326
Drugs which alter the pH of the urine 327
Drugs which alter the excretion of
organic molecules 328

15: The gastrointestinal tract **330**
The innervation and hormones of the
gastrointestinal tract; gastric
secretion; the regulation of acid
secretion 330
Drugs used in the diagnosis and treatment
of gastric and duodenal disorders 335
Stimulants of gastric acid secretion 336

H_2-receptor antagonists 336
Anticholinergic agents 337
Antacids 338
Drugs which promote the healing of
ulcers 339
Vomiting 339
Emetic drugs 342
Anti-emetic drugs 342
The motility of the gastro-intestinal tract 346
Purgatives 347
Drugs which increase gastro-intestinal
motility 349
Antidiarrhoeal drugs 350
Pharmacology of bile 352

16: The endocrine system **358**
The pituitary 358
The anterior pituitary (adenohypophysis) 358
Hypothalamic hormones 359
Growth hormone-releasing factor
(GHRF) 359
Somatostatin 361
Thyrotropic-releasing hormone
(protirelin; TRH) 361
Corticotrophin-releasing factor (CRF) 362
Gonadotrophin-releasing factor 362
Anterior pituitary hormones 362
Growth hormone 362
Prolactin 363
Corticotrophin 366
Melanocyte-stimulating hormones
(MSH) 366
Gonadotrophic hormones 366
Posterior pituitary (neurohypophysis) 366
Antidiuretic hormone (ADH) 367
Oxytocin 369
Thyroid 369
Regulation of thyroid function 371
Actions of thyroid hormones 373
Abnormalities of thyroid function 374
Drugs used in hyperthyroidism 375
Drugs used in hypothyroidism 378
The endocrine pancreas 378
Insulin, glucagon, somatostatin and the
control of blood glucose 379
Diabetes mellitus and drugs used in the
treatment of diabetes mellitus 386
Insulin 388
Oral hypoglycaemic agents 390

ACTH and the adrenal steroids 393
  Glucocorticoids 394
  Corticotrophin 403
  Mineralocorticoids 404
Parathyroid hormone, vitamin D, and
  bone mineral homeostasis 405
  The structure of bone; calcium;
    phosphate and parathormone 405
  Vitamin D 408
  Calcitonin 410
  Other agents used in disorders of
    calcium and phosphate metabolism 410

17: The reproductive system **413**
Endocrine aspects 413
  Hormonal control of the female
    reproductive system 413
  The behavioural effects of sex hormones 415
  Oestrogens 415
  Anti-oestrogens 419
  Progestogens 419
  Anti-progestogens 421
  Hormonal control of the male
    reproductive system 421
  Androgens 422
  Anabolic steroids 423
  Anti-androgens 423
  Gonadotrophin releasing hormone 424
  Gonadotrophins 424
  Miscellaneous drugs affecting the
    reproductive system 424
  Drugs used for contraception 425
The uterus 426
  The motility of the uterus; innervation
    and action of sympathomimetic
    amines; the role of posterior
    pituitary hormones 426
  Oxytocic drugs 428

18: The haemopoietic system **433**
Types of anaemia 433
Iron 434
Vitamin B_{12} and folic acid 437
Vitamin C 443

**SECTION FOUR: THE CENTRAL NERVOUS
SYSTEM**

**19: Chemical transmission and drug action in
    the central nervous system** **447**
Individual neurotransmitters 448
  Noradrenaline 448

Central noradrenergic pathways 448
  Functional aspects 449
Dopamine 451
  Dopamine pathways in the CNS 451
  Dopamine receptors in the CNS 453
  Functional aspects 453
Serotonin 455
  Central serotonin pathways 455
  Functional aspects 455
Acetylcholine 457
  Central cholinergic pathways 458
  Functional aspects 459
Amino-acid transmitters 460
  GABA 461
  Glycine 462
  Excitatory amino-acids 463
Neuropeptides 464
  Opioid peptides 466
Purines 468
Histamine 468
The classification of psychotrophic drugs 469

20: General anaesthetic agents **471**
Physicochemcial theories of anaesthesia 472
  Lipid theory 472
  Hydrate theory 473
  Protein theory 473
The effects of anaesthetics on the nervous
  system 474
  Stages of anaesthesia 475
Effects on the cardiovascular and
  respiratory systems 475
Inhalation anaesthetics—
  pharmacokinetic aspects 476
  The solubility of anaesthetics 476
  Induction and recovery 478
  Metabolism of inhalation anaesthetics 480
Individual inhalation anaesthetics 480
  Diethyl ether 481
  Halothane 481
  Nitrous oxide 481
  Methoxyflurane 482
  Enflurane 482
Intravenous anaesthetic agents 482
  Thiopentone 483
  Althesin 484
  Ketamine 485

21: Anxiolytic and hypnotic drugs **486**
The measurement of anxiolytic activity 486

Tests on animals   486
Tests on humans   487
Classification of anxiolytic and hypnotic
    drugs   488
Benzodiazepines   488
    Chemistry and structure-activity
        relationships   488
    Pharmacological effects   488
    Mechanism of action   490
    Benzodiazepine antagonists   491
    Pharmacokinetic aspects   493
    Adverse effects   494
Other sedative and hypnotic drugs   496
    Barbiturates   496
    Meprobamate   497
    Chloral hydrate and trichlorethanol   498
    Glutethimide and methaqualone   498

22: Neuroleptic drugs   499
The nature of schizophrenia   499
    Theories of schizophrenia   499
Neuroleptic drugs   502
    Chemical aspects   502
    Mechanism of action   505
    Behavioural effects   506
    Other effects related to dopamine
        antagonism   507
    Actions unrelated to dopamine
        antagonism   508
    Side effects   509
    Pharmacokinetic aspects   509
    Clinical uses and clinical efficacy   510

23: Drugs used in affective disorders   513
The nature of affective disorders   513
    The monoamine theory of depression   513
    Animal models of depression   516
Antidepressant drugs   517
    Types of antidepressant drug   517
    Measurement of antidepressant activity   517
    Tricyclic antidepressants   518
        Chemical aspects   518
        Mechanism of action   519
        Actions and side effects   520
        Pharmacokinetic aspects   521
    Monoamine oxidase inhibitors
        (MAOI)   522
        Chemical aspects   522
        Pharmacological effects   523
        Side effects and toxicity   524

Interactions with drugs and foods   524
'Atypical antidepressants'   525
Electroconvulsive therapy (ECT)   526
Clinical effectiveness of antidepressant
    treatments   526
Lithium   528
    Pharmacological effects and
        mechanism of action   528
    Pharmacokinetic aspects and toxicity   529

**24: Drugs used in treating motor disorders:
    epilepsy, Parkinsonism and spasticity   530**
Epilepsy   530
    Types of epilepsy   531
    Cellular mechanisms underlying
        epilepsy   531
    Mechanism of action of anticonvulsant
        drugs   533
    Individual drugs   535
        Phenytoin   535
        Phenobarbitone   536
        Primidone   537
        Ethosuximide   537
        Trimethadione   538
        Valproate   538
        Carbamazepine   538
        Benzodiazepines   539
Parkinsonism   539
    Levodopa   541
    Other drugs used in Parkinsonism   543
Huntington's chorea   544
Muscle spasm and centrally-acting muscle
    relaxants   544
    Mephenesin   545
    Baclofen   545

25: Analgesic drugs   547
Neutral mechanisms of pain sensation   547
    Nociceptive afferent neurons   547
    The substantia gelatinosa and the gate
        control theory   548
    Descending inhibitory controls   549
    Chemical mediators and the nociceptive
        pathway   550
    Pain and nociception   553
Morphine-like drugs   553
    Chemical aspects   554
    Opioid receptors   555
    Cellular mechanism of action   557
    Pharmacological actions   558

Effects on the central nervous system   558
Effects on the gastrointestinal tract   560
Other actions   560
Tolerance and dependence   560
Metabolism and pharmacokinetic aspects   563
Unwanted effects   563
Other opioid analgesics   563
Opioid antagonists   565

26: Central nervous system stimulants and psychotomimetic drugs   **568**
Convulsants and respiratory stimulants   568
Psychomotor stimulants   571
Amphetamines and related drugs   571
Pharmacological effects   571
Tolerance and dependence   573
Pharmacokinetic aspects   573
Uses and unwanted effects   573
Cocaine   573
Methylxanthines   574
Pharmacological effects   574
Uses and unwanted effects   575
Psychotomimetic drugs   575
LSD, psilocin and mescaline   576
Phencyclidine   577

27: Local anaesthetics and other drugs that affect excitable membranes   **579**
Na^+ and K^+ channels of excitable membranes   579
Drugs that affect Na^+ channels   582
Local anaesthetics   583
Chemical aspects   584
Mechanism of action   584
Effects on other physiological systems   586
Unwanted effects   587
Pharmacokinetic aspects   587
Methods of administration   587
Tetrodotoxin and saxitoxin   588
Agents that affect Na^+ channel gating   589
Agents that affect K^+ channels   590

SECTION FIVE: CHEMOTHERAPY

28: Basic principles of chemotherapy   **595**
The molecular basis of chemotherapy   595
Biochemical reactions as potential targets   597

The formed structures of the cell and/or specialized cell types as potential targets   603
Resistance to antibiotics   604
Genetic determinants of antibiotic resistance   604
The transfer of resistance genes between genetic elements within the bacterium   605
The transfer of resistance genes between bacteria   605
Biochemical mechanisms of resistance to antibiotics   606

29: Cancer chemotherapy   **608**
General principles of action of anticancer drugs   609
Drugs used in cancer chemotherapy   610
Alkylating agents   610
Antimetabolites   614
Cytotoxic antibiotics   618
Vinca alkaloids   619
Cisplatin   619
Hormones   619
Radioactive isotopes   620
Miscellaneous agents   620
Drug resistance   620
Cell cycle: Drug effects and their possible clinical applications   621
Possible future strategies for cancer chemotherapy   622

30: Antibacterial agents   **626**
Sulphonamides   628
Penicillin   631
Cephalosporin and cephamycins   634
Tetracyclines   636
Chloramphenicol   637
Aminoglycosides   638
Other antibiotics   640
Antimycobacterial agents   643
Drugs used to treat tuberculosis   643
Drugs used to treat leprosy   645

31: Antiviral drugs   **647**
Inhibition of attachment to or penetration of host cells   647
Inhibition of nucleic acid synthesis   648
Interferon   650

32: Antifungal drugs   **652**
     Amphotericin; Nystatin   653
     Flucytosine   654
     Imidazoles   654
     Tolnaftate; Griseofulvin   656

33: Antiprotozoal drugs   **657**
   Malaria   657
     The life cycle of the malaria parasite   657
     Antimalarial drugs   660
       4-Aminoquinolines   660
       Drugs affecting the synthesis or
         utilization of folate   663
       Potential new antimalarial drugs   664
   Amoebiasis   665
     Metronidazole   665
     Diloxanide; Chloroquine etc.   666
   Leishmaniasis   667
   Trypanosomiasis   667
   Trichomoniasis   668

34: Anthelminthic drugs   **669**
     Actions of anthelminthic drugs   670

SECTION SIX: GENERAL TOPICS

**35: Non-therapeutic drugs: nicotine, alcohol
     and cannabis**   **677**
     Nicotine and tobacco   678
     Alcohol   683
     Cannabis   689

36: Harmful effects of drugs   **692**
     Types of drug toxicity   692
       Hepatotoxicity   693
       Mutagenesis and carcinogenicity   695
       Tetratogenesis   698
       Allergic reactions to drugs   702

Figure acknowledgement references   **706**

Index   **711**

General principles

1

Mechanisms of drug action

Pharmacology can be defined as the study of the manner in which the function of living systems is affected by chemical agents. It is a rather young science, having first achieved independent recognition at the end of the nineteenth century in Germany. Long before this, of course, medical remedies based on herbs were in widespread use, but there was a surprising reluctance to apply anything resembling scientific principles to therapeutics. Even Robert Boyle (1692), who laid the scientific foundations of chemistry in the middle of the seventeenth century, was content when dealing with therapeutics, to describe and recommend a hotchpotch of messes consisting of worms, dung, urine and the moss from a dead man's skull. It may be said, indeed, that therapeutics was scarcely influenced by science until the mid-nineteenth century, at which date Virchow dismissed the subject thus: 'Therapeutics is in an empirical stage cared for by practical doctors and clinicians, and it is by means of a combination with physiology that it must rise to be a science, which today it is not.' At that time the knowledge of the normal and abnormal functioning of the body were simply too incomplete to provide even a rough basis for understanding drug effects; at the same time there was a strong feeling that disease and death were semi-sacred subjects, appropriately dealt with by authoritarian, rather than scientific doctrines.

The history of malaria treatment shows how clinical practice could display an obedience to authority, and ignore what appear to be easily ascertainable facts. Cinchona bark was recognized as a specific and effective treatment, and a sound protocol for its use was laid down by Lind in 1765. In 1804, however, Johnson stated, on the basis of clinical practice in India, that cinchona bark was unsafe until the fever had subsided, and recommended instead the use of large doses of calomel in the early stages. This advice, though murderous in practice, was generally acted upon for the next 40 years.

SYSTEMS OF MEDICINE

Repeated attempts were made to construct systems of therapeutics, many of which produced even worse results than pure empiricism. One of these was **allopathy**, which was espoused by James Gregory (1735–1821). The favourite remedies were blood-letting, emetics and purgatives, and these were used until the dominant symptoms of the disease were suppressed. Many patients died from such treatment, and it was in reaction against it that Hahnemann introduced the practice of **homoeopathy** in the early nineteenth century. The guiding principles of homoeopathy are (a) that like cures like, and (b) that activity can be enhanced by dilution. The system rapidly drifted into absurdity: for example, Hahnemann recommended the use of drugs at dilutions of $1:10^{60}$, equivalent to one molecule in a sphere the size of the orbit of Neptune. Many other systems of therapeutics have come and gone, but the variety of dogmatic principles that they embodied has tended to hinder rather than advance scientific progress. Scientific understanding of drug action—the kind of understanding that enables us to predict what pharmacological effects a novel chemical substance is likely to produce, or to design a chemical that will produce a specified therapeutic effect—is still extremely patchy. To get to the root of how the intrusion of a particular chemical substance affects the functioning of any given cell or organ obviously requires a detailed knowledge of the normal biochemical and physiological machinery, and it must be remembered that physiology only began to be studied intensively about 100 years ago, and biochemistry only about 50 years ago. Even so, from the plethora of experimental data on drug action amassed in the last 50 years or so, certain generalizations emerge, and these are discussed in this chapter.

To begin with we should gratefully acknowledge Paul Ehrlich (1913) for insisting that drug action should be understood in terms of conventional chemical interactions between drugs and tissues, and for dispelling the idea that the remarkable potency and specificity of action of some drugs put them somehow out of reach of chemistry and physics and required the intervention of magical 'vital forces'. Although it is the case that many drugs produce actions in doses and concentrations so small that the dimensions assume an almost astronomical remoteness, low concentrations still involve very large numbers of molecules. Thus one drop of a solution of a drug at only 10^{-10} M still contains about 10^{10} drug molecules, so there is no mystery in the fact that it may produce an obvious pharmacological response. Some bacterial toxins (e.g. diphtheria toxin) act with such precision that a single molecule taken up by a target cell is sufficient to kill it.

THE BINDING OF DRUG MOLECULES TO CELLS

One of the basic tenets of pharmacology is that drug molecules must exert some chemical influence on one or more constituents of cells in order to produce a pharmacological response. In other words, drug molecules must approach the molecules of which cells are made sufficiently closely that the functioning of the cellular molecules is altered. Of course, the molecules in the organism vastly outnumber the drug molecules, and if the drug molecules were merely distributed at random, the chance of an interaction with any particular class of cellular molecule would be negligible. Pharmacological effects therefore require, in

general, the non-uniform distribution of the drug molecules within the body or tissue, which is the same as saying that drug molecules must be 'bound' to particular constituents of cells and tissues in order to produce an effect. Ehrlich summed it up thus: 'Corpora non agunt nisi fixata', (In this context, 'A drug will not work unless it is bound'). A consideration of the different types of drug binding leads us to a useful general classification of drug action which is valid, even though for most drugs we have little or no information about the molecular details of the binding process.

To get an appreciation of the range of possibilities in the binding of drug molecules, let us consider examples at two extremes, namely **ethanol** and **histamine** (an endogenous amine released locally from damaged tissues) which are about as different as two drugs can be, in four general respects:

1. *Potency.* Most effects of histamine are produced in concentrations ranging from about 10^{-8} to 10^{-5} M, whereas ethanol is effective at concentrations ranging from about 10^{-2} to 10^{-1} M in body fluids. The legal limit for driving a car (80 mg/100 ml blood) corresponds to about 18 mM ethanol. On a molar basis, the difference in potency between ethanol and histamine is thus about five or six orders of magnitude. The high potency of histamine is by no means exceptional in pharmacology: drugs which act at concentrations of about 10^{-9} M are quite common and there are reliable reports of effects produced at 10^{-11}–10^{-12} M (for example, the action of serotonin on mollusc hearts, and the action of peptides such as angiotensin on vascular smooth muscle).

2. *Biological specificity.* Histamine has a number of pharmacological actions, but it may produce opposite effects on apparently similar tissues, and it is without observable effects on many more. Thus it causes a powerful contraction of bronchial smooth muscle, but a relaxation of vascular smooth muscle, stimulating gastric secretion, but not salivary secretion. In contrast ethanol produces a more or less similar inhibitory effect on most cells and tissues. The physiological effects of alcohol may be highly complex but at a cellular level its actions are rather uniform, whereas those of histamine are highly selective, in the sense that its actions are confined to a few specific cell types.

3. *Chemical specificity.* Changes in the chemical

structure of a drug molecule may have a large or small effect on its pharmacological activity. With histamine small chemical modifications have drastic effects. For example an isomer in which one nitrogen and one carbon atom in the imidazole ring are transposed, giving a pyrrazole ring, has only about one thousandth of the potency of histamine on smooth muscle, whereas addition of a methyl group to the imidazole ring (4-methylhistamine) produces a compound which has a similar potency to histamine in some tissues, but lacks its action on other tissues.

Ethanol, on the other hand, is very similar in its pharmacological actions to a wide range of simple organic molecules, including most of the inhalation anaesthetics, such as diethyl ether, chloroform, halothane etc. In general, the spectrum of pharmacological activity among this wide range of simple substances is rather similar, and the potency is closely related to physicochemical properties (particularly lipid solubility; see Chapter 20) rather than to the conformation of the molecule. Halothane is unusual among such drugs in possessing an asymmetric carbon atom, and it has been found that there is no significant difference in the pharmacological activity of the two enantiomers.

Thus we have a contrast between drugs for which the shape and charge distribution of the molecule are the major determinants of its activity, and those for which the molecular shape is fairly unimportant and the potency is mainly dependent on physical properties.

4. *The existence of specific antagonists.* The actions of ethanol on cells and tissues cannot, in general, be prevented by the co-administration of any other drugs, unless those drugs themselves produce effects that are opposite to those of ethanol. For instance, the soporific effect of ethanol can be opposed only by drugs such as caffeine or amphetamine which by themselves produce an awakening effect. There is no known agent which prevents ethanol from producing its effects. Even though such an agent would undoubtedly make a fortune for the pharmaceutical company that produced it, the lack of a clearly-defined binding site for ethanol in tissues makes it highly unlikely that it will ever be found.

With histamine, in contrast, many specific antagonists are known—drugs which by themselves produce no evident effect on the tissue, but will abolish the effect of histamine. Several lines of evidence (see p. 28) show that these agents act by competition with histamine for binding to the tissue constituents (histamine receptors) through which histamine exerts its actions. There are many examples of this type of competitive drug antagonism, and, where it occurs, it provides the clearest evidence for the existence of specific receptor sites for the drugs concerned. There are, however, several examples (such as prostaglandins and many pharmacologically active peptides) which meet the first three criteria for actions dependent on specific receptor sites, but for which effective competitive antagonists have not so far been discovered.

The four criteria discussed—potency, biological specificity, chemical specificity and the existence of specific antagonists—distinguish very sharply between the two drugs chosen as examples, and other similarly contrasting examples could have been chosen. There are, however, many drugs whose basic mode of action cannot be so simply characterized. Many central nervous system depressants (e.g. barbiturates, see Chapter 21) act in a biologically non-specific way, but have a degree of potency and chemical specificity that suggest a more selective type of interaction with cell constituents than is the case for ethanol. Local anaesthetics (see Chapter 27), too, fall into this type of intermediate category. The main thrust of pharmacological research in recent years has been to try to characterize, in molecular terms, the primary site of action of many different types of drug. The success of this approach has led to many hitherto confusing drugs being shown to act quite specifically on a particular type of tissue component, such as an enzyme, carrier molecule or DNA molecule. There are several examples of drugs whose actions were until recently not understood at all, only described. Aspirin is one example where, thanks to the work of Vane and his colleagues on prostaglandins (see Chapter 8), a multitude of apparently unrelated effects can now be explained in terms of inhibition of a single enzyme (or perhaps a class of enzymes) responsible for converting arachidonic acid to prostanoids. Similarly a group of minor tranquillizers (benzodiazepines) has recently been shown to act on specific receptor sites in the brain, thereby potentiating the action of an inhibitory neurotransmitter (γ-aminobutyric acid; see Chapter 21); the action of morphine-like analgesics (see Chapter 25) has similarly been narrowed to specific receptor sites for these drugs, which had been described in exhaustive physiological detail many years previously without any real insight into mechanism having been achieved.

RECEPTOR CLASSIFICATION

Once the action of a drug can be interpreted in terms of its combination with a special type of receptor, this provides a valuable means for classification and refinement in drug design. For example, by the mid-1960s, analysis of the numerous actions of histamine (see Chapter 8) showed that some of its effects (the H_1 effects, such as smooth muscle contraction), were strongly antagonized by the competitive histamine antagonists then known. Black and his colleagues, in 1970, suggested that the remaining actions of histamine, which included its powerful stimulant effect on gastric secretion and its effects on the heart, might represent a second class of histamine *receptor*. They tested this by preparing histamine analogues, some of which showed selectivity in stimulating gastric secretion, while having only a weak effect on smooth muscle. By seeing which parts of the histamine molecule conferred this type of specificity, they were able to develop selective antagonists, and such antagonists proved to be equally potent in blocking all of the effects now classified as H_2 effects. It now appears that all of the diverse actions of histamine can be classified in terms of two distinct types of histamine receptor. Other examples of successful receptor classification appear repeatedly in this book, for the concept of categorizing drug action in terms of receptors is a central one in pharmacology. It may be going too far to say that receptor classification does for pharmacology what the periodic table does for chemistry, but it is certainly true that our understanding of drug effects has become, in recent years, both simpler and more comprehensive as result of the untiring efforts of receptor taxonomists. Though an unclassifiable drug action does not offend in quite the way that an unclassifiable chemical element would, it acts as a powerful irritant.

A NOTE ON TERMINOLOGY

'Receptor' can be used to mean any clearly-defined target molecule with which a drug molecule has to combine in order to elicit its specific effect. Thus the voltage-sensitive sodium channel of excitable membranes can be regarded as the 'receptor' for local anaesthetics (see Chapter 27), or the enzyme dihydrofolate reductase can be regarded as the 'receptor' for methotrexate (see Chapter 28). In each case the drug molecule combines with, and incapacitates, the protein molecule, thus producing its effect. This is rather different from the situation where, for example, adrenaline acts on a receptor in the heart (see Chapter 7). In this case, the receptor molecule does nothing until the complex is formed. When adrenaline binds to it, a process is initiated (see p. 20) leading to the activation of adenylate cyclase and thence a further train of reactions leading to an increase in force and rate of the heartbeat. The receptor produces an effect only when adrenaline is bound, and this, in general, is true of all hormone and neurotransmitter receptors. In this context, certain substances (agonists) can be said to 'activate' the receptors, and others (antagonists) may combine at the same site without causing activation. Receptors of this type form a key part of the system of chemical communication that all multicellular organisms use to coordinate the activities of their cells and organs. Without them we would be no better than a bucketful of amoebae. The distinction between agonists and antagonists only exists for receptors with this type of physiological regulatory role; we cannot speak of 'agonists' for the noradrenaline carrier or for the voltage-sensitive sodium channel or for dihydrofolate reductase. The distinction between these two types of drug binding site is almost equivalent to the distinction in enzymology between an allosteric regulatory site and the active site of an enzyme. In pharmacology it is best to reserve the term 'receptor' for interactions of the regulatory type, where the ligand may function either as an agonist or as an antagonist, which in practice limits it to receptors which have a physiological regulatory function, and this usage will be observed in this book.

QUANTITATIVE ASPECTS

The first step in drug action on specific receptors is the formation of a reversible **drug-receptor complex**, the reactions being governed by the Law of Mass Action. Let us suppose that a piece of tissue, such as heart muscle or smooth muscle, contains a total number of receptors, N_{tot}, for an agonist, such as adrenaline. When the tissue is exposed to adrenaline at concentration x_A and allowed to come to equilibrium, a certain number N_A of the receptors will become occupied, and the number of vacant receptors will be reduced to $N_{tot}–N_A$. Normally the number of adrenaline molecules applied to the tissue in solution greatly exceeds N_{tot}, so that the binding reaction does not appreciably reduce x_A. The magnitude of the response produced by the adrenaline will be related (even if we do not know exactly how) to the number of receptors occupied, so it is useful to consider what quantitative relationship is predicted between N_A and x_A.

The reaction can be represented by:

$$\begin{array}{ccccc} A & + & R & \underset{k_{-1}}{\overset{k_{+1}}{\rightleftarrows}} & AR \\ \text{drug} & & \text{free receptor} & & \text{complex} \\ (x_A) & & (N_{tot}-N_A) & & (N_A) \end{array}$$

The Law of Mass Action (which states that the rate of a chemical reaction is proportional to the product of the concentrations of reactants) can be applied to this reaction.

Rate of forward reaction $= k_{+1}x_A(N_{tot}-N_A)$ (1)
Rate of backward reaction $= k_{-1}N_A$ (2)
At equilibrium the two rates are equal:
$k_{+1}x_A(N_{tot}-N_A) = k_{-1}N_A$ (3)

The proportion of receptors occupied or **occupancy**, $p_A = N_A/N_{tot}$, which is independent of N_{tot}, is:

$$p_A = \frac{x_A}{x_A + k_{-1}/k_{+1}}. \tag{4}$$

Defining the **equilibrium constant** for the binding reaction, $K_A = k_{-1}/k_{+1}$, equation (4) can be written

$$p_A = \frac{x_A}{x_A + K_A} \quad \text{or} \quad p_A = \frac{x_A/K_A}{x_A/K_A + 1} \tag{5}$$

This important result is known as the **Langmuir equation**, after the physical chemist who derived it

to describe the adsorption of gases by metal surfaces*.

The equilibrium constant, K_A, is a characteristic of the drug and of the receptor; it has the dimensions of *concentration*, and is numerically equal to the concentration of drug required to occupy 50% of the sites at equilibrium (verify from equation (5) that when $x_A = K_A$, $p_A = 0.5$). The higher the **affinity** of the drug for the receptors, the lower will be K_A.

Equation (5) describes the relationship between occupancy and drug concentration, and generates a characteristic curve known as a **rectangular hyperbola**, as shown in Figure 1.1 (*top*). It is common in pharmacological work to use a logarithmic scale of concentration; this converts the hyperbola to a **symmetrical sigmoid** curve Fig. 1.1 (*bottom*).

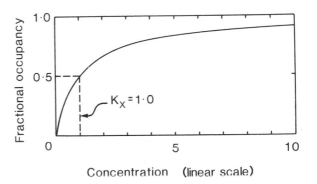

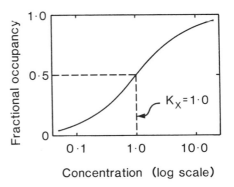

Fig. 1.1 Theoretical relationship between occupancy and ligand concentration, plotted according to equation (5). The upper curve plotted with a linear concentration scale, is a rectangular hyperbola. The lower curve with a logarithmic concentration scale, is a symmetrical sigmoid curve.

* It should actually have been named after A V Hill, the physiologist who derived it in 1909, but so many equations bear his name that it would be excessive to insist on adding another.

Agonist concentration-effect curves

It has only recently become possible to measure directly the binding of drugs to their receptors in tissues (see p. 12) and to show that equation (5) is obeyed. Much more often it is a *biological response*, such as a rise in blood pressure, contraction or relaxation of a strip of smooth muscle in an organ bath, or activation of an enzyme that is actually measured, and plotted as a **concentration-effect**, or **dose-response curve**, as in Figure 1.2. These look similar to the theoretical concentra-

response which modifies the primary response to the drug. It is obviously unrealistic to expect that the final effect will be directly proportional to occupancy in this instance, and the same is true of most drug-induced effects. A second difficulty in drawing inferences about agonist affinity from concentration-effect curves is that the concentration of the drug *at the receptors* is often not known, even though the concentration in the organ bath is simple to calculate. Thus agonists may be subject to rapid enzymic degradation, or uptake by cells, as they diffuse from the surface towards their site of

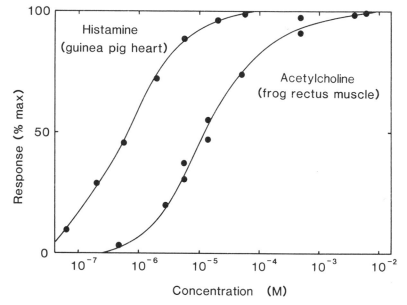

Fig. 1.2 Experimentally observed concentration-effect curves. Though the lines, drawn according to the binding equation (5), fit the points well, such curves do not give correct estimates of the affinity of drugs for receptors, because the relationship between receptor occupancy and response is usually non-linear.

tion-occupancy curves in Figure 1.1 (*bottom*), and it is tempting to try to use such experimental curves to measure the affinity of agonist drugs for their receptors, by making the assumption that the response produced is directly proportional to occupancy. This is, however, rarely valid, for in general the response is a complex, non-linear function of occupancy. For an integrated physiological response, such as a rise in arterial blood pressure produced by adrenaline, several different processes interact. Adrenaline increases cardiac output, constricts some blood vessels while dilating others, and the change in arterial pressure itself evokes a reflex

action, and a steady state can be reached in which the agonist concentration at the receptors is very much less than the concentration in the bath. In the case of acetylcholine, for example, which is hydrolysed by cholinesterase present in most tissues (see Chapter 6), the concentration reaching the receptors can be less than 1% of that in the bath, and an even bigger difference has been found with noradrenaline, which is avidly taken up by sympathetic nerve terminals in many tissues (see Chapter 7). Thus, even if, as in Figure 1.2, the concentration-effect curve looks just like a facsimile of the binding curve, it cannot be used directly to determine the affinity of the agonist for the receptors.

Competitive antagonism

Equation (5) describes the relationship between concentration and occupancy when a single drug is present. The treatment can easily be extended to describe the situation when two or more competing drugs are present. 'Competing' means that the receptor can bind only one drug molecule at a time. If the two drugs are designated A and B, the reactions can be represented as follows:

$$A \quad + \quad R \underset{k_{-1A}}{\overset{k_{+1A}}{\rightleftharpoons}} \quad AR$$

$$(x_A) \quad (N_{tot} - N_A - N_B) \qquad (N_A)$$

$$B \quad + \quad R \underset{k_{-1B}}{\overset{k_{+1B}}{\rightleftharpoons}} \quad BR$$

$$(x_B) \quad (N_{tot} - N_A - N_B) \qquad (N_B)$$

As before, at equilibrium, the forward and backward rates are equal:

$$k_{+1A}x_A(N_{tot} - N_A - N_B) = k_{-1A}N_A \quad (6)$$
$$k_{+1B}x_B(N_{tot} - N_A - N_B) = k_{-1B}N_B \quad (7)$$

Therefore:

$$p_A = \frac{x_A/K_A}{x_A/K_A + x_B/K_B + 1} \quad (8)$$

Comparing this result with equation (5) shows that adding drug B (the competitive antagonist), as expected, reduces the occupancy by drug A, if the concentration of A is kept the same. Alternatively, the concentration of A may be *increased* (to x'_A say), so as to restore p_A to the value reached in the absence of the antagonist; the ratio r ($= x'_A/x_A$) by which the concentration will need to be increased, is given (from equations 5 and 8) by:

$$r = \frac{x_B}{K_B} + 1 \quad (9)$$

If it is assumed that the response of the test system depends *only* on the agonist occupancy p_A, then it is predicted from the theory given above that the effect of the competitive antagonist on the response can also be overcome by increasing the agonist concentration r-fold. Equation (9) is therefore useful experimentally, because it should apply to measurements of biological responses as well as to direct measurements of agonist binding. Equation (9), which is often known as the **Schild equation**

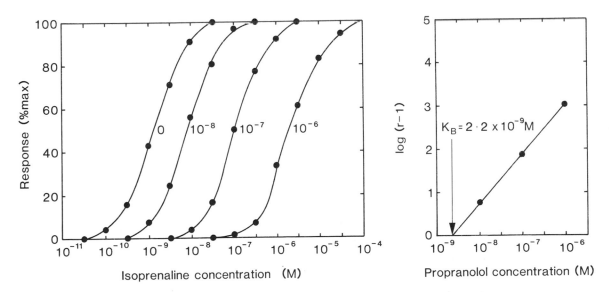

Fig. 1.3 Competitive antagonism of isoprenaline by propranolol measured on isolated guinea pig atria. *Left.* Concentration-effect curves at various propranolol concentrations (indicated on curves). Note progressive shift to right without change of slope or maximum. *Right.* Schild plot (equation 10). The equilibrium constant (K) for propranolol is given by the abscissal intercept (2.2×10^{-9} M). (Results from: Potter, 1967)

after its originator, predicts two characteristic properties of competitive antagonism:

1. The **dose ratio** r depends *only* on the concentration and equilibrium constant of the antagonist, and not on the size of response that is chosen as a reference point for the measurements, nor on the equilibrium constant for the agonist. On a semilogarithmic concentration-effect plot, therefore, the effect of the competitive antagonist will be to shift the curve to the right, without changing its slope or maximum, a characteristic that can easily be tested experimentally.

2. The dose ratio achieved should increase linearly with x_B, and the slope of a plot of $(r-1)$ against x_B is equal to $1/K_B^*$. This relationship, being independent of the characteristics of the agonist, should be the same for all agonists that act on the same population of receptors.

These relationships have been verified for many examples of competitive antagonism (Fig. 1.3). Equation (9) has often been shown to be accurately obeyed up to dose ratios as high as 10 000, making it one of the most precisely-obeyed relationships encountered in biology.

Partial agonists and the concept of efficacy

In the discussion so far, drugs have been regarded either as **agonists**, which in some way 'activate' the receptor when they occupy it, or as **antagonists**, which cause no activation. It has become clear, however, that the ability of a drug molecule to activate the receptor is a continuously graded, rather than an all-or-nothing, property. If a series of chemically related agonist drugs, acting on

the same receptors, is tested on a given biological system, it is often found that the *maximal* response (the largest response that can be produced by that drug in high concentration) differs from one drug to another. Generally there are several agonists whose maximal response corresponds to the full response of the tissue (the largest response that the tissue is capable of giving). These drugs are known as **full agonists**, and those whose maximal response falls short of the full response are known as **partial agonists** (Fig. 1.4). The difference between them lies in the relationship between occupancy and response. Figure 1.5 shows the relationship between occupancy and concentration for a drug whose equilibrium constant is 1.0 µM. If the drug is a full agonist it might produce a maximal response at about 0.2 µM, the relationship between response and occupancy being shown in the lower panel. The situation for a partial agonist with the same affinity

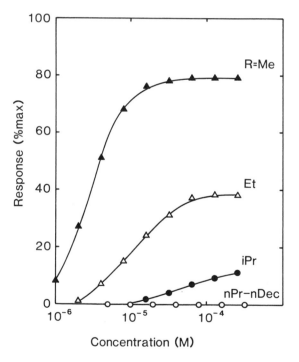

Fig. 1.4 Partial agonists. Concentration-effect curves for substituted methonium compounds on frog rectus abdominis muscle. The compounds were members of the decamethonium series (see Chapter 6), R Me$_2$ N (CH$_2$)$_{10}$ N Me$_2$ R. The maximum response obtainable decreases (i.e. efficacy decreases) as the size of R is increased. With R = nPr or larger, the compounds cause no response, and are pure antagonists. (Results from: Van Rossum, 1958)

---

* Equation (9) can be expressed logarithmically in the form:

$$\log_{10}(r-1) = \log_{10} x_B - \log_{10} K_B. \quad (10)$$

Thus a plot of $\log_{10}(r-1)$ against $\log_{10} x_B$, usually called a **Schild plot**, should give a straight line with unit slope and an abscissal intercept equal to $-\log_{10} K_B$. A commonly-used convention, analogous to the pH and pK notation, is to express antagonist potency as a pA_2 value; under conditions of competitive antagonism $pA_2 = -\log_{10} K_B$. Numerically, pA_2 is defined as **the negative logarithm of the molar concentration of antagonist required to produce an agonist dose ratio equal to 2**. As with pH notation its principal advantage is that it produces simple numbers, a pA_2 of 6.5 being equivalent to $K_B = 3.2 \times 10^{-7}$ M.

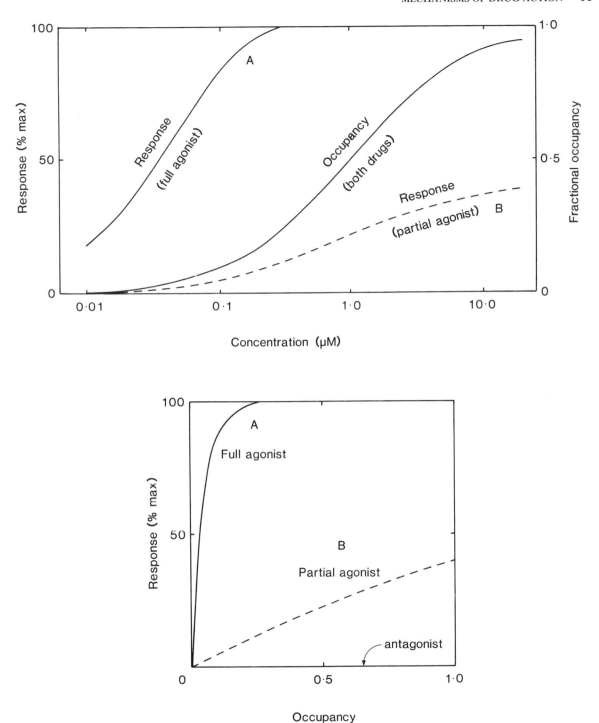

Fig. 1.5 Theoretical occupancy and response curves for full and partial agonists. *Top*. Occupancy curve for both drugs. Response curves A and B for full and partial agonist respectively. *Bottom*. Relationship between response and occupancy for full and partial agonist, corresponding to response curves above. Note that A produces maximal response at about 20% occupancy, while B produces only a submaximal response even at 100% occupancy.

is also shown, the essential difference being that the response at any given occupancy is much smaller, so that it cannot produce a maximal response even at 100% occupancy. This can be expressed quantitatively in terms of **efficacy**, a parameter defined by Stephenson (1956) which is a characteristic of a particular drug, and describes the 'strength' of a single drug-receptor complex in evoking a response of the tissue. Efficacy can only be measured in relative terms, and Stephenson arbitrarily defined a partial agonist capable of eliciting 50% of the full response of the tissue as having an efficacy equal to 1.0. A full agonist must therefore have an efficacy exceeding 1.0, and a pure competitive antagonist has zero efficacy. In his studies on the contraction of smooth muscle by a series of acetylcholine-like agonists, Stephenson found that many full agonists were capable of eliciting 50% responses at very low occupancies, often less than 1%, representing efficacies greater than 100. If a full response can occur when only a small fraction of the receptors is occupied, the system may be said to possess **spare receptors**, or a **receptor reserve**. This is often found among drugs that elicit smooth muscle contraction, but seems to be less important for other types of receptor-mediated response, such as secretion, smooth muscle relaxation or cardiac stimulation, where the effect is more nearly proportional to receptor occupancy. When we talk of spare receptors, this does not imply any actual subdivision of the receptor pool, but merely that the pool is larger than the number needed to evoke a full response. This surplus of receptors over the number actually needed might seem to be a somewhat profligate biological arrangement. In the context of the physiological role of receptors in mediating the actions of hormones and transmitters, however, it makes sense, because it means that a given *number* of hormone-receptor complexes, corresponding to a given level of biological response, can be reached with a lower concentration of hormone than would be the case if fewer receptors were provided. Economy of hormone secretion is thus achieved, at the expense of providing more receptors. The same condition exists at many chemically-transmitting synapses (see Chapter 5), where the number of receptors is large in relation to the number that have to be occupied by transmitter in order for the synapse to function; again we may speculate that the body's motive is to economise in the number of transmitter molecules that have to be released in order to make the synapse function.

DIRECT MEASUREMENT OF DRUG BINDING TO RECEPTORS

Though the basic principles governing the binding of drugs to receptors, and the mode of action of competitive antagonists were enunciated many years ago, by A J Clark and others, it was not until quite recently that the binding process was studied directly, by the use of radioactive drug molecules. In the early 1960s, the binding of atropine to muscarinic receptors in smooth muscle was measured in this way, and also the binding of oestrogens to specific receptors in uterine tissue; such methods now provide a very widely-used and direct approach for investigating receptors of many different kinds. The main requirement for the method is to find a compound (which may be an agonist or antagonist for the receptors that are being studied) which binds with sufficient affinity and specificity, is not metabolized, and can be labelled (usually with ^3H, ^{14}C or ^{125}I) to a sufficient specific radioactivity to enable minute amounts of binding to be measured. The usual procedure is to incubate samples of the tissue (or membrane fragments) with various concentrations of radioactive drug until equilibrium is reached. The tissue is then removed, or the membrane fragments separated by filtration or centrifugation, and dissolved in scintillation fluid for measurement of its radioactive content. In such experiments there is invariably a certain amount of 'non-specific binding' (i.e. drug taken up by structures other than receptors) and the success of the technique lies partly in selecting the ligand so that this component does not swamp out the specific binding. The amount of non-specific binding is estimated by repeating the experiment in the presence of a saturating concentration of a (non-radioactive) ligand that inhibits completely the binding of the radioactive drug to the receptors, leaving behind the non-specific component (Fig. 1.6).

If the specific binding follows the Langmuir equation (equation 5), the relationship between the

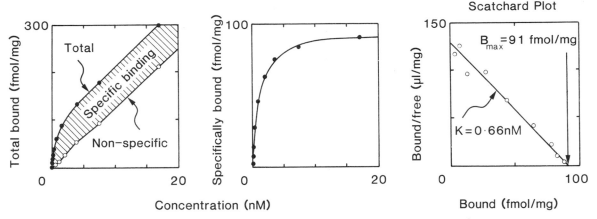

Fig. 1.6 Measurement of receptor binding (β-adrenoceptors in cardiac cell membranes). The ligand was ^{3}H-cyanopindolol, a derivative of pindolol (see Chapter 7). *Left.* Measurements of total and non-specific binding at equilibrium. Non-specific binding is measured in the presence of a saturating concentration of a non-radioactive β-receptor antagonist, which prevents the radioactive ligand from binding to β-receptors. The difference between the two lines (shaded) represents specific binding. *Centre.* Specific binding plotted against concentration. The curve is a rectangular hyperbola (equation 11). *Right.* Scatchard plot (equation 12). This gives a straight line from which the binding parameters K and B_{max} can be calculated.

amount bound (B) and ligand concentration (x) should be:

$$B = \frac{B_{max}x}{x+K} \qquad (11)$$

B_{max} is the total number of binding sites in the preparation (often expressed as pmol/mg protein) and K is the equilibrium constant (see equation 5). This relationship is, of course, non-linear and to make it easier to estimate B_{max} and K from experimental results, equation (11) may be rearranged to:

$$\frac{B}{x} = \frac{B_{max}}{K} - \frac{B}{K} \qquad (12)$$

A plot of B/x against B (known as a **Scatchard plot**; Fig. 1.6) gives a straight line from which both B_{max} and K can be estimated. Statistically, this procedure is not without problems, but it is widely used because of its convenience.

Such methods have been used to estimate the number of receptors in many different tissues. 20 years ago, the direct measurement of binding to receptors was an adventurous business, which gave a new dimension to research on receptor mechanisms. There is now a danger that as the measurement of binding has become easier in many instances than the measurement of pharmacological

effects, the 'receptors' that are identified on the basis of binding measurements will have no connection with pharmacological effects. When combined with pharmacological studies, however, binding measurements have proved very valuable. It has, for example, been confirmed that the spare receptor hypothesis for muscarinic receptors in smooth muscle is correct, for agonists are found to bind, in general, with rather low affinity, and a maximal biological effect occurs at low receptor occupancy. It has also been shown, in skeletal muscle and other tissues, that denervation leads to an increase in the number of receptors in the target cell, a finding that accounts, at least in part, for the phenomenon of denervation supersensitivity. More generally, it appears that receptors for many hormones and transmitters tend to increase in number, usually over the course of a few days, if the relevant hormone or transmitter is absent or scarce, and to decrease in number if it is in excess. The mechanism of these changes is not well understood, but the process represents an important cause of adaptation leading to gradual changes in responsiveness to drugs or hormones with continued administration (see p. 31).

Binding studies have also, in some instances, revealed an unsuspected heterogeneity among receptors. For example, agonist binding to muscarinic receptors (see Chapter 6), and also to β-

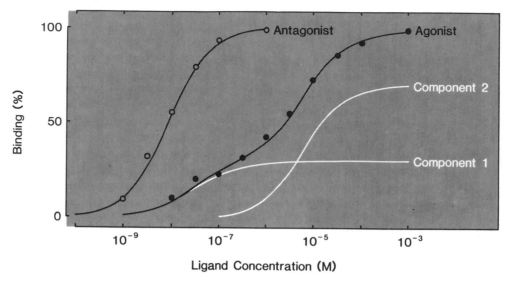

Fig. 1.7 Comparison of binding curves for muscarinic agonists and antagonists (brain membrane preparation). The antagonist binding curve (benzhexol) is well-fitted by a single component ($K = 8.3\,\mu M$). The agonist binding curve (oxotremorine-M) is fitted by the sum of two separate components. Component 1 ($K = 27\,\mu M$) comprises 30% of the total sites, and component 2 ($K = 5.9\,\mu M$) comprises 70%.

Such complex binding curves are common for agonists. (Results from: Birdsall et al, 1978)

adrenoceptors (see Chapter 7) reveals at least two populations of binding sites (Fig. 1.7). It is suggested that this may be due to the fact that receptors can exist either on their own or coupled within the membrane to another macromolecule (e.g. to adenylate cyclase in the case of β-adrenoceptors; see p. 19), which constitutes part of the effector system on which the receptor exerts its regulatory effect.

ISOLATION AND CHARACTERIZATION OF RECEPTOR MOLECULES

If a tightly-bound radioactive ligand is available, with which to label the receptor molecules selectively, it may be possible to extract and purify the radioactively-labelled receptor material—an essential pre-requisite to discovering how the receptor works in molecular terms. This approach has been used very successfully in the case of the nicotinic acetylcholine receptor (see Chapter 6), where advantage was taken of two natural curiosities. The first is that the electric organs of many fish, such as rays (*Torpedo sp.*) and electric eels (*Electrophorus sp.*) consist of modified muscle tissue in which the

acetylcholine-sensitive membrane is extremely abundant, and these organs contain much larger amounts of acetylcholine receptor than any other tissue. Secondly, the venom of many snakes of the cobra family contain polypeptides which bind with very high specificity to nicotinic acetylcholine receptors. These substances, known as α-toxins, can easily be labelled, and used to assay the receptor content of tissues and tissue extracts. The best-known is **α-bungarotoxin**, which is the main component of the venom of the Malayan banded krait (*Bungarus multicinctus*). It was first used to label acetylcholine receptors by Lee and his colleagues in 1970, and has been used in many subsequent studies.

Treatment of muscle or electric tissue with non-ionic detergents brings the membrane-bound receptor protein into solution, and it can be purified by the technique of affinity chromatography, in which a receptor ligand, bound covalently to the matrix of a chromatography column, is used to absorb the receptor and separate it from other substances in the extract. The receptor can then be eluted from the column by flushing it through with a solution containing an antagonist, such as gallamine (Fig. 1.8).

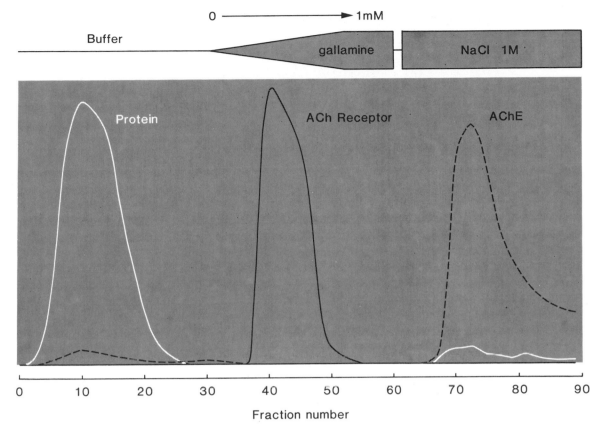

Fig. 1.8 Purification of acetylcholine receptor (AChR) by affinity chromatography. Membranes from *Torpedo* electric organ were solubilized in detergent and applied to an affinity column consisting of resin beads to which a gallamine derivative had been coupled. This retained AChR and cholinesterase on the column, allowing most of the protein to pass through (first peak). Elution with a gradient of gallamine displaced AChR from the column (second peak). Acetylcholinesterase (AChE) was retained until a high salt concentration was applied (third peak). This procedure results in a several thousand-fold purification of AChR in a single step. (From: Olsen et al, 1972)

The nicotinic acetylcholine receptor (Popot & Changeux, 1984) consists of four different types of subunit, one of which, the α-subunit of M_r 40 000, bears the acetylcholine binding site. It is interesting that the complete receptor oligomer (M_r 250 000) contains two of these subunits, and there is evidence that both must bind acetylcholine molecules in order for the receptor to be activated. This receptor is sufficiently large to be seen in electron micrographs, and Figure 1.9 shows a reconstruction of the way in which it is thought to be inserted into the membrane. Evidence that the material extracted by detergent treatment and purified by affinity chromatography as a M_r 250 000 oligomer comprises *both* the receptor *and* the associated ionic channel which it controls, comes from experiments in which the receptor protein has been

inserted into artificial lipid bilayers, which then show an increased ionic conductance in the presence of acetylcholine or a similar agonist.

Purification of the acetylcholine receptor subunits enabled stretches of their amino acid sequence to be determined, which has in turn enabled the gene for all four subunits to be isolated and separately cloned (Dolly & Barnard, 1984), so revealing their complete amino-acid sequences. Injection of the cloned DNA into toad oocytes causes the synthesis of the ACh receptor by this cell, and insertion of the receptor into its membrane, which then becomes sensitive to acetylcholine.

Progress in isolating and characterizing other receptors has not been nearly so rapid, mainly because of difficulty in extracting them from their membrane environment without irretrievably

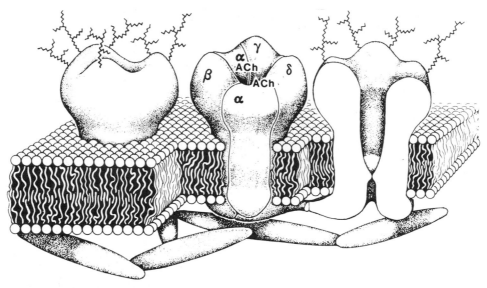

Fig. 1.9 Reconstruction of the nicotonic acetylcholine receptor (AChR), based on electron microscopy and neutron scattering data from Torpedo electric organ membranes. The receptor and associated ion channel consists of 5 protein subunits (α_2, β, γ, σ) all of which traverse the membrane, and surround a central pore. ACh binds to the α subunits, and two ACh molecules must bind in order to open the channel. (From: Kistler & Stroud, 1981)

losing their special characteristics. However, success has been reported with insulin receptors, as well as with β-adrenoceptors and muscarinic acetylcholine receptors, and no doubt many more will follow. The impact that knowledge of the molecular details of various receptor sites, and of their linkage with effector systems will have on the study of pharmacology, and on the design of new drugs, is not to be underestimated.

RECEPTOR-EFFECTOR LINKAGE

Receptors are clearly coupled to many different types of cellular effect, some of which may be very rapid such as those involved in synaptic transmission, which occupy, in general, a millisecond time scale. Other receptor-mediated effects, such as those produced by thyroid hormone or various steroid hormones, are very slow, and occur over hours or days. There are also many examples of intermediate time scales—catecholamines, for example, usually act in a matter of seconds, whereas many peptides take rather longer to produce their effects. Not surprisingly, very different types of linkage between the receptor occupation and the ensuing response are involved. Though the picture

is far from complete, three types of receptor-effector linkage can be recognized (Fig. 1.10) and these correlate well with the speed of response.

1. Direct regulation of membrane permeability to ions.
2. Regulation via an **intracellular second messenger**.
3. Regulation of DNA transcription, and hence of protein synthesis.

1. Direct regulation of ionic permeability

The fastest type of receptor-mediated response occurs when a neurotransmitter acts on the post-synaptic membrane of a nerve or muscle cell and transiently increases its permeability to particular ions. Most excitatory neurotransmitters such as acetylcholine at the neuromuscular junction (see Chapter 6) or glutamate in the central nervous system (see Chapter 19) cause an increase in sodium and potassium permeability. This results in a net inward current carried mainly by sodium ions, which depolarizes the cell and increases the probability that it will generate an action potential. The action of the transmitter reaches a peak in a fraction of a millisecond, and usually decays within a few milliseconds.

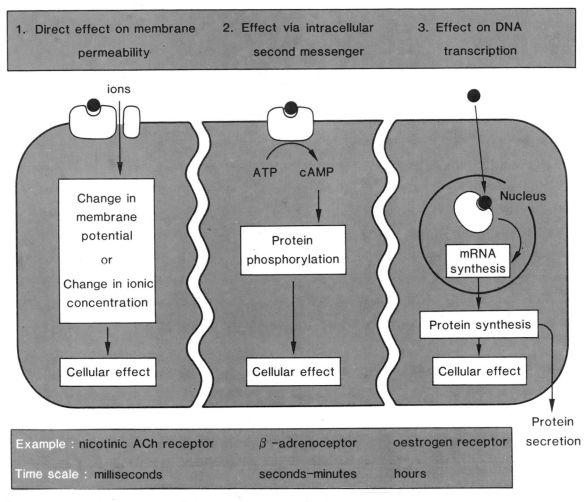

Fig. 1.10 Three types of receptor-controlled process.

The sheer speed of this response makes it likely that the coupling between the receptor and the ionic channel is a direct one, and there is now good evidence that this is so. It is possible to record a permeability response in minute fragments of membrane with artificial medium replacing the intracellular compartment; furthermore, as mentioned above, purified acetylcholine receptors can function as ionic gates in completely artificial membranes. These findings rule out the involvement of any biochemical intermediates, in the cell or within the membrane, in the transduction process.

A radically new experimental approach, which made it possible for the first time to study the properties of individual receptor-operated ionic channels, is the use of **noise analysis**, introduced by Katz & Miledi in 1972. Studying the action of acetylcholine at the motor endplate they observed that small random fluctuations of membrane potential were superimposed on the steady depolarization produced by acetylcholine (Fig. 1.11). These fluctuations arise because, in the presence of an agonist, there is a dynamic equilibrium between open and closed ionic channels. In the steady state the rate of opening balances the rate of closing, but from moment to moment the number of open channels will show random fluctuations about the mean. By measuring the amplitude of these fluctuations, the **conductance** of a single ionic channel can be calculated, and by measuring their frequency (usually in the form of a spectrum in which the noise power of the signal is plotted as a function

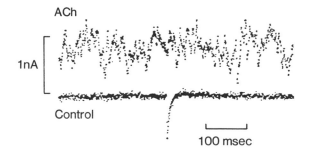

ACh

1nA

Control

100 msec

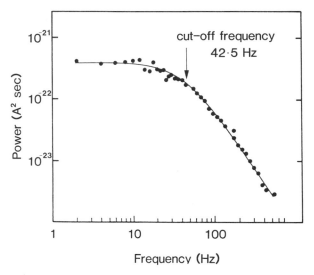

Power (A^2 sec)

10^{-21}

10^{-22}

10^{-23}

cut–off frequency
42·5 Hz

Frequency (Hz)

1   10   100

Fig. 1.11 Acetylcholine-induced noise at the frog motor
endplate. *Top.* Records of membrane current recorded at high
gain under voltage-clamp. The upper noise record was recorded
during the application of ACh from a micropipette. The lower
record was obtained in the absence of ACh, the blip in the
middle being caused by the spontaneous release of a packet of
ACh from the motor nerve. The steady (DC) component of the
ACh signal has been removed by electronic filtering, leaving the
high frequency noise signal.

Bottom. Power spectrum of ACh-induced noise recorded in a
similar experiment to that shown above. The spectrum is
calculated by Fourier analysis and fitted with a theoretical
(Lorentzian) curve, which corresponds to the expected
behaviour of a single population of channels whose lifetime
varies randomly. The cut-off frequency (at which the power is
half of its limiting low-frequency value) enables the mean
channel lifetime to be calculated.

(From: (Top) Anderson & Stevens, 1973; (Bottom) Ogden et
al, 1981)

of frequency) the average duration for which a
single channel stays open (**mean channel lifetime**)
can be calculated. In the case of acetylcholine
acting at the endplate, the channel conductance is
about 20 picosiemens (pS), which is equivalent to

an influx of about 10^7 ions per second through a
single channel under normal physiological conditions, and the mean life time is 1–2 milliseconds.
The magnitude of the single channel conductance
confirms that we must be dealing with a physical
pore through the membrane, since the rate of ionic
movement is too large to be compatible with a
carrier mechanism. In studies with different acetylcholine-like agonists it has usually been found that
the channel conductances are all about the same,
whereas the mean channel lifetime varies. A simple
scheme which accounts for these observations, and
also gives a physical explanation of **efficacy**, for this
type of drug response (see p. 10) is as follows:

$$A \ + \ R \underset{k_{-1}}{\overset{k_{+1}}{\rightleftharpoons}} AR \underset{\alpha}{\overset{\beta}{\rightleftharpoons}} AR^* \qquad (13)$$

channel closed   channel
open

The conformation R*, representing the open state
of the ion channel, is thought to be the same for all
agonists, to account for the finding that the channel
conductance does not vary. Kinetically, it appears
that the drug binding reaction $A + R \rightarrow AR$ is rapid
compared with the conformational change $AR \rightarrow$
AR^*, so that the mean channel lifetime is essentially
a measure of the closing rate constant, α, which
clearly varies from one drug to another. In this
scheme, an agonist of high efficacy, which activates
a large proportion of the receptors that it occupies,
will be characterized by $\beta > \alpha$ whereas a drug of
low efficacy will have the characteristic $\alpha > \beta$. For a
pure antagonist, $\beta = 0$.

Studies on other transmitters that mediate fast
synaptic responses show that although the ionic
selectivity of the channel varies according to the
nature of the synapse, as well as its conductance
and mean lifetime, the basic mechanism of scheme
(13) appears to be quite general.

Recording methods have now been refined,
mainly due to the work of Neher & Sakmann, to
the point where the very small current flowing
through a single ionic channel can be measured
directly (Fig. 1.12), and the results have fully confirmed the interpretation of channel properties
based on noise analysis. This remarkable technique
provides a view, unique in biology, of the physiological behaviour of individual protein molecules,

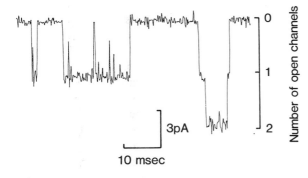

Fig. 1.12 Single acetylcholine-operated ion channels at the frog motor endplate recorded by the patch-clamp technique. The pipette, which was applied tightly to the surface of the membrane, contained $10\,\mu M$ ACh. The downward deflections show the currents flowing through single ion channels in the small patch of membrane under the pipette tip. Towards the end of the record two channels can be seen to open simultaneously. The conductance and mean lifetime of these channels agrees well with indirect estimates from noise analysis (see Fig. 1.11). (Figure courtesy of D Colquhoun & D C Ogden)

and can be expected to give a much clearer idea of how agonists and antagonists act on synaptic receptors.

2. Mechanisms involving a second messenger

The very direct linkage between receptor and effector discussed in the previous section, in which the ionic channel is part of the same macromolecule as the receptor, is not the only way in which receptors can regulate cellular function.

In many instances the effect of a drug, hormone or transmitter acting on extracellular receptors is transmitted to the interior of the cell through the involvement of a **second messenger**. Two substances that are known to serve this function are (a) **cyclic-adenosine-3',5'-monophosphate (cAMP)** and (b) **calcium ions** (Table 1.1). These two second messengers regulate many different kinds of cellular activity,

Table 1.1 Examples of drugs and hormones that act through second messengers

	Second messenger		
		cAMP	
Drug/hormone	Ca^{++}	Increase	Decrease
Drug/hormone			
Muscarinic agonists	smooth muscle	—	heart
β-agonists	—	heart liver fat cells	—
α_1-agonists	liver fat cells salivary gland	—	—
α_2-agonists	—	—	liver fat cell platelet
Histamine (H_1)	smooth muscle	—	—
Histamine (H_2)	—	heart gastric mucosa	—
Serotonin	blowfly sal. gland neurons	—	—
Prostaglandins	—	fat cells platelets	—
Thromboxanes	—	—	platelet
Dopamine	—	neurons	—
Peptides:			
Substance P	salivary gland	—	—
Vasopressin	liver	kidney	—
Glucagon		liver heart	—
ACTH	—	adrenal cortex	—
Opioids	—	—	neurons

including among others, muscle contraction and relaxation, secretion, changes in membrane permeability to various ions, transport mechanisms and cell division. In many cases, these cellular responses are due to changes in the state of **phosphorylation** of various intracellular proteins, usually enzymes whose catalytic activity is thereby regulated (Schulman, 1982; Nestler & Greengard, 1984).

Protein phosphorylation occurs by means of a series of specific **protein kinases**, enzymes which catalyse the transfer of phosphate groups from ATP to particular protein molecules (usually to serine or threonine residues). The phosphate groups are continuously removed by **phosphatases**.

The basic system of intracellular control through second messengers and protein phosphorylation is summarized in Figure 1.13, and some of the known protein kinases are listed in Table 1.2.

In the rest of this section we will consider how receptor occupation is linked to changes in the intracellular concentrations of cAMP and Ca^{++}, and how these second messengers act to regulate protein phosphorylation and other intracellular events.

Regulation of cAMP

The role of cAMP as a second messenger was first revealed by the work of Sutherland and his colleagues in the late 1950s.

This discovery demolished at a stroke the barriers that existed between biochemistry and pharmacology, to the great benefit of both disciplines. There are now complete journals devoted to cAMP, a rare honour for a molecule, (though calcium now shares the same dubious distinction).

Cyclic-AMP is a nucleotide synthesized within the cell from ATP by the action of a membrane-bound enzyme, adenylate cyclase (see Fig. 1.10). It

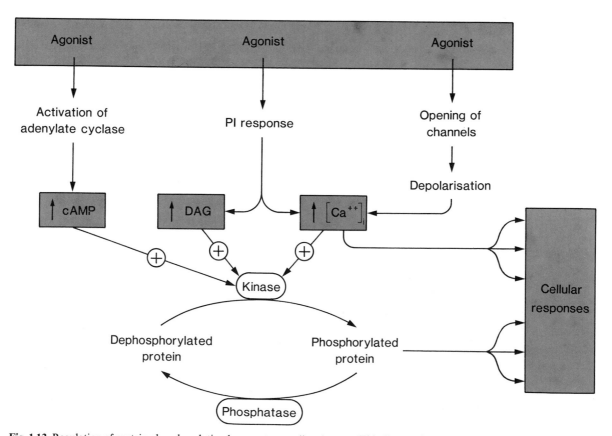

Fig. 1.13 Regulation of protein phosphorylation by receptor-mediated events. This diagram is greatly simplified. (For a more elaborate description see: Nestler et al, 1984)

Table 1.2 Functions of some kinase enzymes that are targets for drug and hormone actions

Kinase	Activated by	Cellular response
Ca^{++}-dependent protein kinase (membrane bound)	Ca/calmodulin	Exocytosis, ?Transmitter synthesis
Protein kinase C (membrane bound)	Ca/calmodulin, Membrane phospholipids, DAG	Numerous e.g. platelet aggregation, cell activation by lectins
Phosphorylase kinase	cAMP, Ca/calmodulin	Increased glycogenolysis
Glycogen synthase kinase	Ca/calmodulin	Decreased glycogen synthesis
Myosin light chain kinase	cAMP, Ca/calmodulin	Smooth muscle, contraction, ?Regulation of skeletal muscle contractility and motility of non-muscle cells
Insulin-like hormone receptors (e.g. insulin, epidermal growth factor)	Specific hormones	Metabolic responses, cell division, etc

Note: many insulin-like hormones appear to work by directly activating a specific kinase, without the intervention of a second messenger. (see Hollenberg, 1982)

is produced continuously and inactivated by hydrolysis to 5'-AMP, by the action of a family of enzymes known as phosphodiesterases. Many different drugs, hormones and neurotransmitters produce their effects by increasing or, in a few cases, decreasing the catalytic activity of adenylate cyclase (Table 1.1). The mechanism by which many different agents can regulate the activity of the same enzyme has been intensively studied, (Schramm & Selinger, 1984) as have the mechanisms by which cells respond in various ways to changes in cAMP concentration, and there is general agreement that the following components are required (Fig. 1.14):

1. *The receptor* (R). There may be several different receptor species (R_1, R_2 etc.) in the membrane of a single cell, through which different drugs and hormones can control the function of a single population of adenylate cyclase molecules. The receptors face outwards, and respond to changes in the extracellular concentration of hormones or transmitters.

2. *The nucleotide regulatory protein* (N). This also lies within the membrane, but facing the inside, which acts as the link between R and the adenylate cyclase molecule. Its name derives from the fact that this protein binds guanosine nucleotides, guanosine diphosphate (GDP) and guanosine triphosphate (GTP) which occur within cells. Through this mechanism the intracellular concentration of GDP and GTP exerts a secondary controlling influence on adenylate cyclase.

3. *Adenylate cyclase* (AC). This faces the inside of the membrane, and catalyses cAMP formation within the cell. AC is active only when associated with N.

4. *cAMP-dependent protein kinase*. This is an intracellular enzyme which is active only when complexed with cAMP. This protein kinase phosphorylates a variety of other enzymes, converting them from an inactive to an active form (or vice versa). The enzymes affected, and hence the nature of the cellular response, vary widely in different systems.

An ingenious series of experiments by Schramm and his colleagues have shown that the receptor and adenylate cyclase are separate membrane enti-

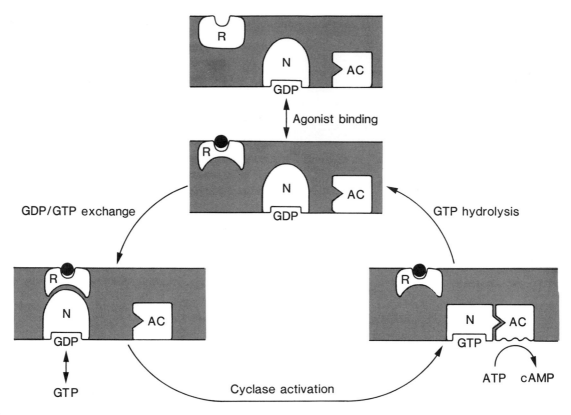

Fig. 1.14 Receptor regulation of adenylate cyclase. Occupation of the receptor (R) by agonist changes its conformation, causing it to bind to the N-protein. GDP bound to the N protein is then exchanged for GTP, causing the N protein to leave the receptor and bind to, thus activating, adenylate cyclase (AC). The N protein acts as a GTPase, and AC activation ceases as soon as GTP is hydrolysed. Cholera toxin inhibits GTP hydrolysis, causing persistent AC activation. (From: Abramson & Molinoff, 1984)

ties, and that both are quite mobile within the membrane. Turkey erythrocytes possess β-receptors, and respond to isoprenaline with an increase in adenylate cyclase activity. This response is abolished irreversibly by N-ethylmaleimide, an alkylating agent that inactivates adenylate cyclase. If the erythrocytes are then fused (by addition of Sendai virus) with tumour cells, which possess adenylate cyclase but no β-receptors, and therefore do not normally respond to isoprenaline, the hybrid cells now respond once again to isoprenaline (Fig. 1.15), showing that the receptor from the erythrocyte can regulate the adenylate cyclase from the tumour cell. This result also demonstrates that one or both of these proteins must be freely mobile within the membrane.

An interesting detail is that **Cholera toxin**, a protein secreted by the *Cholera* vibrio, which causes intense and prolonged secretion from the intestinal mucosa, also works by activating adenylate cyclase. It binds specifically to the G-protein, and prevents the enzymic hydrolysis of GTP, thus causing the adenylate cyclase to remain coupled to the G-protein, so that cAMP continues to be synthesized. The major physiological consequences of the disease are the result of an excess of cAMP within those cells which selectively take up the toxin.

A number of drugs and hormones appear to act by inhibiting adenylate cyclase, and reducing the intracellular concentration of cAMP (see Table 1.1). There is evidence that a mechanism similar to that shown in Figure 1.14 may be responsible, with the substitution of a different type of N protein, which inhibits rather than activates adenylate cyclase. There appears to be a single pool of adenylate cyclase molecules in the membrane and there are often several types of inhibitory and facilitatory

Cyclase inactivated

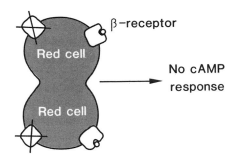

Cyclase

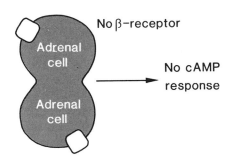

Cyclase

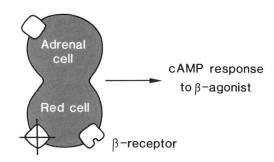

Cyclase inactivated

Fig. 1.15 Cell-fusion experiment to show coupling of β-adrenoceptor and adenylate cyclase (AC). *Top*: fusion of turkey red cells, after inactivation of AC. No response to β-agonist. *Middle*: fusion of adrenal cells, which have active AC but no β-receptors. No response to β-agonist. *Bottom*: fusion of AC-inactivated red cells with adrenal cells. AC from adrenal cell can now be activated by β-agonist binding to β-receptor from red cell. (From: Schramm et al, 1977)

receptors acting upon it, so that there is competition among the various receptors for the available cyclase molecules, just as drug molecules compete for common receptor sites. The fact that competition can occur at different stages of the process, and that GTP (the regulation of which is very poorly understood at present) plays a key role in the linkage are two of the factors that contribute to the bewildering complexity of many of the regulatory effects that have been described.

cAMP is hydrolysed within cells by **phosphodiesterase**, an enzyme which is inhibited by drugs such as methylxanthines (e.g. theophylline, caffeine; see Chapters 13 & 26). The similarity of some of the actions of these drugs to those of catecholamines probably reflects their common property of increasing the intracellular concentration of cAMP.

Regulation of intracellular calcium concentration by receptors

A rise in $[Ca^{++}]_i$ has often been demonstrated in response to hormones and transmitters (see Table 1.1 for examples). Sometimes this occurs by a net influx of Ca^{++} from outside the cell, but it may represent a release of sequestered Ca^{++} without any net transfer into the cell. The 'normal' $[Ca^{++}]_i$ is about 10^{-7} M and many intracellular processes are sensitive to $[Ca^{++}]_i$ in the range 10^{-7}–10^{-6} M. Normally about 99% of intracellular Ca^{++} is bound. The extracellular calcium concentration $[Ca^{++}]_o$ is about 2×10^{-3} M. Thus changes in intracellular Ca^{++} binding or in membrane permeability can readily control $[Ca^{++}]_i$. The normally low level is maintained by a balance between influx and active extrusion of Ca^{++} from the cell by an ATP-driven transport system similar to the Na–K-pump. For general reviews on intracellular Ca^{++} regulation, see Carafoli & Crompton (1978) and Racker (1980).

Studying the calcium response produced by a range of drugs and hormones, Michell noted in 1975 that in every case there was an accompanying increase in the rate of degradation of a class of minor membrane phospholipids, the **phosphatidylinositols** (Ptd Ins) (Fig. 1.16). Ptd Ins is split by phospholipase C to form diacylglycerol (DAG) and inositol 1-phosphate. The DAG is then phosphorylated to form phosphatidic acid (PA), while

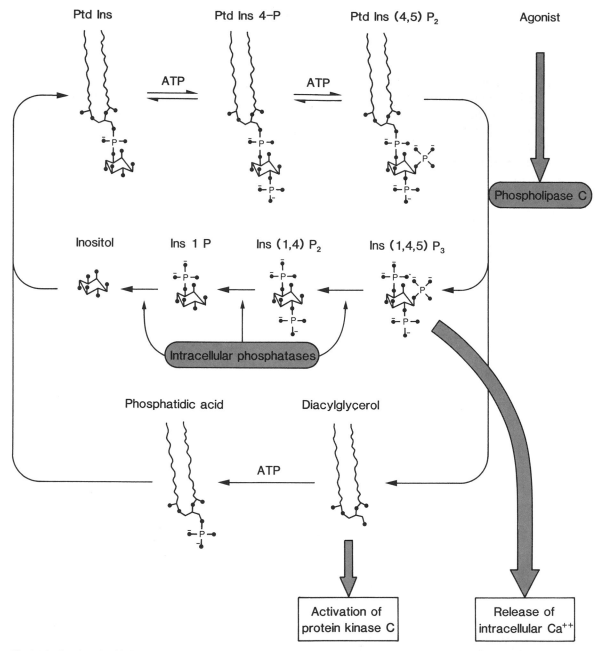

Fig. 1.16 The phosphatidylinositol cycle. Oxygen atoms (black dots) and phosphorus atoms (P) are shown attached to the carbon skeleton. The agonist-activated enzyme phospholipase C acts on Ptd Ins (4, 5) P_2 in the membrane to produce two second messengers: (1) triphosphoinositol (Ins (1, 4, 5) P_3) which is released into the cytosol; (2) diacylglycerol which remains in the membrane and activates protein kinase C, thus initiating various protein phosphorylation reactions.

the inositol phosphates are dephosphorylated and then recoupled with PA to form Ptd Ins once again. The resynthesis of Ptd Ins takes some time, because the enzymes required are in the cytosol rather than the membrane, so depletion of Ptd Ins may occur following an agonist response, leading to desensitization (see p. 31). Agonists accelerate this cycle by activating phospholipase C, a membrane enzyme which may be coupled to receptors in a similar way to adenylate cyclase, discussed above.

It has recently been found that phospholipase C acts mainly, not on Ptd Ins itself, but on a derivative which has two additional phosphate groups attached to the inositol residue. This compound, Ptd Ins 4,5 P_2, produces **triphosphoinositol** (1,4,5 Ins P_3) on hydrolysis, and this product has been shown to be very effective in releasing calcium from intracellular stores (Berridge et al, 1983; Putney et al, 1983). It is short-lived, being quickly dephosphorylated within the cell, giving rise to inactive di- and mono-phosphoinositol before being reincorporated in Ptd Ins in the membrane.

The Ptd Ins response is involved in other ways besides regulating $[Ca^{++}]_i$, for DAG directly affects the activity of a membrane bound protein kinase (**protein kinase C**) and thus controls protein phosphorylation (Nishizuka, 1984; Nestler et al, 1984).

Another possible mechanism to explain the linkage between the receptor and Ca^{++} translocation is the **transmethylation hypothesis** (Hirata & Axelrod, 1980). Phosphatidyl ethanolamine (PE) and phosphatidyl choline (PC; Fig. 1.17) are membrane phospholipids whose interconversion is catalysed by two **methyltransferase** enzymes which are constituents of the membrane. The methyl groups required to convert PE to PC come from a methyl donor, S-adenosylmethionine (SAM). Agonists cause an increase in activity of the methyltransferases, causing conversion of PE to PC. PE is located on the cytoplasmic surface of the membrane, and shifts to the outer surface (**phospholipid flip-flop**) when it is successively methylated. This apparently makes the membrane structure more fluid, and may enhance Ca^{++} permeability. It may also facilitate the lateral diffusion of other membrane constituents and thus enhance the coupling of other receptors with, for example, adenylate cyclase, thus acting as a regulator of various other receptor-controlled processes. Furthermore the PC produced is partly hydrolysed in the membrane to form arachidonic acid, a precursor in prostaglandin synthesis. According to Hirata & Axelrod, therefore, the transmethylation reaction controls at least three major cellular mechanisms, namely Ca^{++} entry, adenylate cyclase activation, and arachidonic acid metabolism.

Calmodulin and protein kinases

It is now known, mainly from the work of Cheung in the early 1970s, that nearly all of the intracellular effects produced by calcium involve a protein,

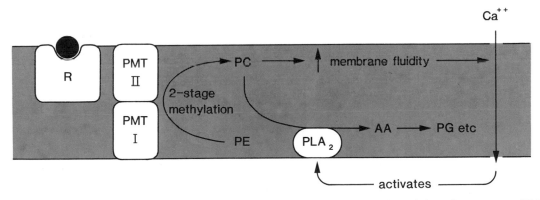

Fig. 1.17 Receptor-mediated phospholipid transmethylation pathway. The two phospholipid methyltransferase enzymes (PMT I and PMT II) are activated by agonist combining with the receptor. Phosphatidyl ethanolamine (PE) is then converted, by successive addition of two methyl groups, to phosphatidylcholine (PC) and in the process moves from the inner to the outer membrane surface. This is postulated to increase membrane fluidity and permeability to calcium. PC is also a substrate for phospholipase A_2, leading to production of arachidonic acid (AA) and mediators of the prostaglandin (PG) series. (From: Hirata & Axelrod, 1980)

calmodulin, which is found in all cells. Calmodulin consists of a single peptide chain containing 148 amino acid residues. It is a very stable protein, with an abundance of acidic amino acids, and it has many sequences in common with another calcium-binding protein, **troponin C**, which is the protein of skeletal and cardiac muscle responsible for mediating the effect of calcium on the contractile machinery. One molecule of calmodulin can bind four Ca^{++} ions, which induces in it a conformational change to a predominantly α-helical structure. In this form the Ca^{++}-calmodulin complex binds to, and activates, one of many different types of **acceptor protein**, most of which are enzymes that are inactive until combined with Ca^{++}-calmodulin. The concentration of ionized Ca^{++} needed to activate this system is usually between 10^{-7} and 10^{-6} M, and the 'resting' concentration in many cells is below 10^{-7} M, so the calmodulin mechanism operates only when the ionized calcium concentration has been increased by some means. There is evidence that calmodulin can activate some acceptor proteins when only two or three of its calcium sites are occupied, so the degree of saturation of the sites, which varies as a function of the intracellular ionized Ca^{++} concentration, affects the pattern, as well as the intensity of the effect produced. In many cases the acceptor protein is an enzyme, though calmodulin-sensitive membrane proteins are thought to mediate effects of intracellular Ca^{++} on membrane permeability to various ions, and on exocytosis (see Chapter 5). The number of calmodulin-activated enzymes reported is large and growing. They include various protein kinases, some of which are also regulated by cyclic-AMP, several of the enzymes involved in

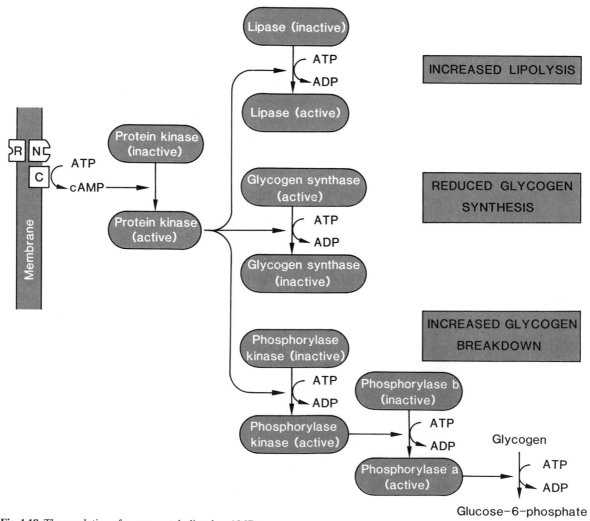

Fig. 1.18 The regulation of energy metabolism by cAMP.

cyclic-AMP metabolism, (see above), such as phosphodiesterase, adenylate cyclase and guanylate cyclase, as well as Ca^{++}-activated ATP-ase, which is the enzyme involved in the active transport system responsible for the normal low intracellular Ca^{++} concentration. **Phospholipase A_2**, the enzyme for generating arachidonic acid from membrane phospholipids, and thus providing the precursor for prostaglandin synthesis (see Chapter 8), is also calmodulin-activated. The effect of intracellular Ca^{++} in promoting cell division also requires calmodulin, which has been shown by immunohistochemical methods to bind to the protein of the microtubules, and promote aggregation to form the mitotic spindle. The biological activity of calmodulin is strongly inhibited by **trifluoperazine** (an antipsychotic drug of the penothiazine group; see Chapter 22) which appears to stop the Ca^{++}-calmodulin complex from binding to the acceptor protein. This provides a useful tool for studying calmodulin-mediated effects, but it is unlikely that the pharmacological actions of trifluoperazine depend on this action. Examples of some well-studied protein kinases, and the cellular reactions in which they are believed to be involved, are shown in Table 1.2. Figure 1.18 shows the way in which kinase controlled regulation of various enzymes involved in glycogenolysis and lipolysis accounts for the effects of β-adrenoceptor activation on liver muscle and fat cells. In these cells, cAMP binds to, and activates, a protein kinase, which in turn catalyses the phosphorylation of various other enzymes. In fat cells, phosphorylation of a lipase occurs; this activates the enzyme and initiates triglyceride hydrolysis, with the release of fatty acids from the cell. In liver and muscle, protein kinase catalyses the phosphorylation of two different enzymes. One is glycogen synthase, which is rendered *inactive* by phosphorylation, thus halting glycogen formation; the other is phosphorylase kinase, which is *activated*, and in turn activates (by phosphorylation) the phosphorylase that catalyses the cleavage of glycogen. The end result, in both liver and fat, is the mobilization of energy stores, in the form of glycogen or triglyceride, to usable fuels. The primary step—activation of protein kinase—seems to be common to most, if not all, of the many instances of regulation by cAMP that have been studied. In some cases the substrate for proteins

kinase appears to a membrane protein involved in the control of membrane permeability, and this mechanism may account for certain slow synaptic responses—lasting for seconds or minutes—that are produced by various transmitter substances.

3. Regulation of DNA transcription

This type of receptor-mediated effect is characteristic of steroid hormones, and is quite different from the mechanisms described so far. One of the important advances of the past 10–15 years, due largely to the work of Jensen in Chicago, has been the recognition that the highly varied effects of different steroid drugs and hormones (which include numerous effects on the reproductive system, effects on the kidney causing salt and water retention, anti-inflammatory actions etc) all operate through the same basic mechanism. The receptor for steroids is an intracellular protein which was until recently believed to exist as a soluble constituent of the cytosol. Studies with fluorescent antibody labelling (King & Greene, 1984) have recently shown, however, that the receptor protein is bound to the nuclear chromatin. The steroid molecule crosses the cell membrane readily, being highly lipid soluble, and binds to the receptor. Certain regions of the DNA sequence show a high affinity for particular steroid-receptor complexes, and the binding of the complex to DNA switches on the process of gene transcription at a region of the DNA molecule several hundred base residues away from the region that binds the steroid-receptor complex. An increase in RNA polymerase activity and the production of specific mRNA occur within a few minutes of adding the steroid. One steroid may result in the production of several different mRNA species within one cell, and hence lead to the production of several different proteins. For example, cells of the chicken oviduct are stimulated by progesterone to synthesize the various different protein constituents of egg-white, though there is no evidence for the existence of more than one type of progesterone receptor in this tissue. It is the ability of this regulatory system to switch on the synthesis of many different proteins that leads to the great diversity of steroid actions, which are discussed in more detail in Chapters 16 & 17.

TYPES OF DRUG ANTAGONISM

The situation commonly arises in pharmacology where the effect of one drug is diminished or completely abolished in the presence of another. The foregoing discussion of the ways in which drugs may act shows that several different points of attack are possible, and the following classification may be helpful.

1. Chemical antagonism
2. Pharmacokinetic antagonism
3. Antagonism by receptor block
   a. Reversible competitive antagonism
   b. Irreversible, or non-equilibrium, competitive antagonism
4. Non-competitive antagonism, i.e. block of receptor–effector linkage
5. Physiological antagonism.

Chemical antagonism

This refers to the uncommon situation where the two substances combine in solution, so that the effect of the active drug is lost. The most obvious example is the inactivation of heavy metals (lead, cadmium etc) whose toxicity is reduced by administration of a chelating agent (e.g. **dimercaprol**) which binds the metal ions tightly to form an inactive complex.

Pharmacokinetic antagonism

This describes the situation in which the 'antagonist' effectively reduces the concentration of the active drug at its site of action. This can happen in various ways. The rate of metabolic degradation of the active drug may be increased (e.g. the reduction of the anticoagulant effect of **warfarin** when an agent that accelerates its hepatic metabolism, such as **phenobarbitone**, is given; see Chapters 3 & 4). Alternatively the rate of absorption of the active drug from the gastrointestinal tract may be reduced, or the rate of renal excretion may be increased. A less obvious example is the antagonism of the action of adrenergic neurone blocking agents (see Chapter 6) which are actively taken up by adrenergic nerve terminals and act to prevent noradrenaline release, by agents such as tricyclic

antidepressant drugs (see Chapter 23) which block this uptake mechanism. Interactions of this sort are discussed in more detail in Chapter 4. They have a tendency to occur unexpectedly in clinical situations, and are a major preoccupation of clinical pharmacologists.

Antagonism by receptor block

Reversible competitive antagonism has been discussed in some detail earlier in this chapter. Its key features are **surmountability**, expressed in the parallel shift of the agonist log-concentration effect curve without any reduction in the maximal response, and the **linear Schild plot** (see p. 9). These characteristics reflect the fact that the rate of dissociation of the antagonist molecules is sufficiently high that, on addition of the agonist, a new equilibrium is rapidly established. The agonist is effectively able to displace the antagonist molecules from the receptors, although, of course, the agonist has no power to evict a bound antagonist molecule, or vice versa. What happens, in fact, is that by occupying a proportion of the vacant receptors, the agonist reduces the rate of association of the antagonist molecules, so that the rate of dissociation temporarily exceeds that of association, and the overall antagonist occupancy falls.

Irreversible or **non-equilibrium competitive antagonism** occurs when the antagonist dissociates very slowly, or not at all, from the receptors, with the result that no change in the antagonist occupancy takes place when the agonist is applied[*]. The fractional occupancy by the agonist is thus reduced in proportion to the proportion of receptors not occupied by the antagonist. Thus, if the fraction of receptors blocked by the antagonist is p_B, the agonist occupancy, p_A, is given by:

$$p_A = \frac{x_A}{x_A + K_A}(1 - p_B) \qquad (14)$$

This means that the antagonism is **non-surmountable** because, no matter how high the agonist concentration, the agonist occupancy cannot ex-

---

[*] Some authors refer to this type of antagonism as **non-competitive**, but this term is best reserved for antagonism that does not involve occupation of the receptor site (see p. 31).

a. Reversible competitive antagonism

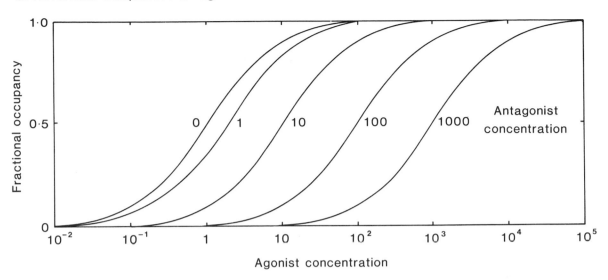

b. Irreversible competitive antagonism

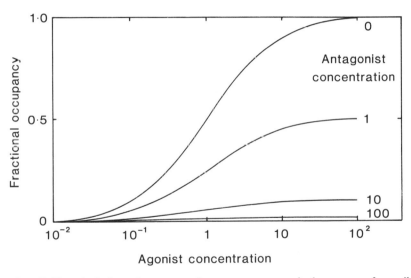

Fig. 1.19 Hypothetical agonist concentration-occupancy curves in the presence of reversible and irreversible competitive antagonists. The concentrations are normalized with respect to the equilibrium constants (i.e. 1.0 corresponds to a concentration equal to K, and results in 50% occupancy).

ceed $(1 - p_B)$. The effect of reversible and irreversible antagonists is compared in Figure 1.19. In some cases (Fig. 1.20 *left*) the theoretical effect is accurately reproduced, but the distinction between reversible and irreversible competitive antagonism (or even non-competitive antagonism; see below) is not always as obvious as the theoretical curves in Figure 1.19 would suggest. This is because of the phenomenon of spare receptors (see p. 12); if the agonist occupancy required to produce a maximal biological response is very small (say 1% of the total receptor pool), then it is possible to block irreversibly nearly 99% of the receptors without reducing the maximal response, and the effect of a lesser degree of antagonist occupancy will be to produce a parallel shift of the log-concentration effect curve

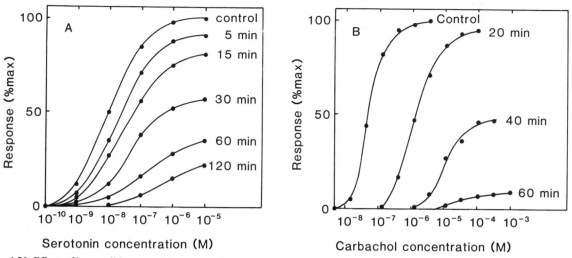

Fig. 1.20 Effects of irreversible competitive antagonists on agonist concentration-effect curves. *Left*. Rat stomach smooth muscle responding to serotonin at various times after addition of methysergide (10^{-9} M). *Right*. Rabbit stomach responding to carbachol at various times after addition of dibenamine (10^{-5} M).
  (After: (Left) Frankhuijsen & Bonta, 1974; (Right) Furchgott, 1965)

that is indistinguishable from reversible competitive antagonism (Fig. 1.20 *right*). In fact, it was the finding that an irreversible competitive antagonist of histamine was able to reduce the sensitivity of a smooth muscle preparation to histamine nearly 100-fold without reducing the maximal response that first gave rise to the spare receptor hypothesis.

Irreversible competitive antagonism occurs with

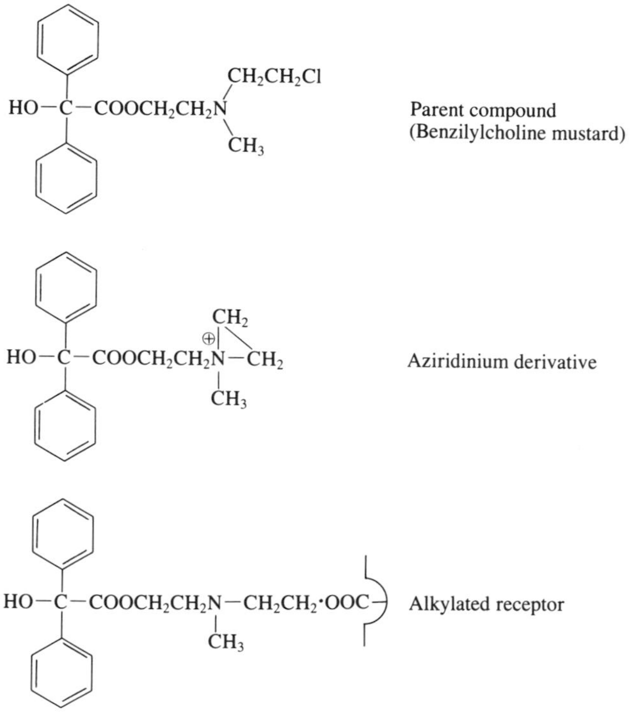

Fig. 1.21 Receptor alkylation as a mechanism of irreversible competitive antagonism. Formation of the reactive aziridinium ion occurs spontaneously in solution. This species has a high affinity for muscarinic acetylcholine receptors, which are alkylated and thus irreversibly blocked.

drugs that form covalent bonds with the receptor, such as haloalkylamines (Fig. 1.21). These agents are converted in solution to aziridinium ions which are highly reactive and readily alkylate groups such as—COOH or—SH in the receptor site, forming a bond that may be stable for hours or days. There are other examples where the antagonist, though not covalently bound, is still so firmly attached that dissociation is very slow, and produces a pattern of antagonism resembling Figure 1.19b.

With antagonists that dissociate very slowly or not at all from the receptors, no appreciable recovery occurs when the drug is washed out, and their effect can be studied by testing the responsiveness of the tissue after application of a low antagonist concentration for varying periods of time. An experiment of this kind is shown in Figure 1.19. Another example of an irreversible competitive antagonist is α-bungarotoxin (see p. 14) acting on acetylcholine receptors at the neuromuscular junction.

Non-competitive antagonism describes the situation where the antagonist blocks at some point the chain of events that leads to the production of a response by the agonist. For example, drugs such as **verapamil** and **nifedipine** prevent the influx of calcium ions through the cell membrane (see Chapter 11) and thus block, quite non-specifically, the contraction of smooth muscle produced by other drugs. As a rule, the effect will be to reduce the slope and maximum of the agonist log-concentration-response curve as in Figure 1.19b, though it is quite possible for some degree of rightward shift to occur as well.

Many drugs, some of them thought until recently to act as competitive acetylcholine antagonists, have been found to produce a non-competitive block of the effects of acetylcholine on nicotinic receptors. Their effect appears to result from block of the cation-selective ionic channels that are controlled by these receptors (see p. 37), and an interesting point is that in many instances the blocking agent can act on the channel only after it has been opened by acetylcholine. The degree of block therefore increases if the agonist concentration is increased—the exact opposite of competitive antagonism. Drugs that work in this way include **hexamethonium** (a ganglion-blocking drug; see Chapter 6) and **tubocurarine** (a neuromuscular

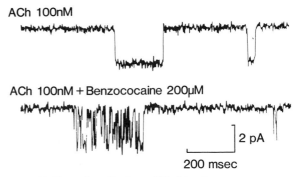

ACh 100nM

ACh 100nM + Benzococaine 200µM

2 pA

200 msec

Fig. 1.22 The action of a channel blocking drug on acetylcholine-operated channels at the frog motor endplate, recorded by the patch clamp technique (see Fig. 1.12). Addition of the local anaesthetic, benzocaine (see Chapter 27), causes the channel openings to be interrupted repeatedly as molecules of benzocaine block and escape from the open channel. (From: Ogden et al, 1981)

blocking drug which has both competitive and non-competitive actions; see Chapter 6). Local anaesthetics may have a similar effect on acetylcholine-mediated responses, though this is not their principle action. Figure 1.22 shows the way in which such a drug repeatedly blocks and dissociates from a single ion channel in the muscle membrane.

Physiological antagonism

This is a term used loosely to describe the interaction of two drugs whose opposing actions in the body tend to cancel each other. For example, noradrenaline raises arterial pressure by acting on the heart and peripheral vessels; histamine lowers arterial pressure by causing vasodilatation, and they can be said to act as physiological antagonists.

It can be seen that the distinction between physiological and non-competitive antagonism is not a sharp one. Thus, if one drug lowers intracellular cAMP by inhibiting adenylate cyclase and another has the opposite effect, the antagonism could be classified as either non-competitive or physiological. In practice, where two drugs act on separate cells or separate physiological systems to produce balancing actions, the term physiological antagonism is usually applied.

DESENSITIZATION AND TACHYPHYLAXIS

It is often found that the effect of a drug gradually

diminishes when it is given continuously or repeatedly. **Desensitization** and **tachyphylaxis** are synonymous terms used to describe this phenomenon, which often develops in the course of a few minutes. The term **tolerance** is conventionally used to describe a more gradual decrease in responsiveness to a drug, taking days or weeks to develop, but the distinction is not a sharp one. The term **refractoriness** is also sometimes used, mainly in

relation to a loss of therapeutic efficacy. **Drug resistance** is a term used to describe the loss of effectiveness of antimicrobial drugs.

Many different mechanisms can give rise to this type of phenomenon, and they are rather poorly understood.

1. *Change in receptors.* Among receptors directly coupled to ionic channels, desensitization is often rapid and pronounced. At the neuromuscular junction (Fig. 1.23 *top*) there is evidence that the desensitized state is caused by a slow conformational change in the receptor, resulting in tight binding of the agonist molecule without the opening of the ionic channel. A similar change has been described for the β-adrenoceptor (Fig. 1.23 *bottom*), which becomes, on desensitization, unable to activate adenylate cyclase, though it can still bind the agonist molecule.

2. *Loss of receptors* In some cases, prolonged exposure to agonists results in the gradual reduction in the number of receptors as measured by drug binding studies. This also occurs with β-adrenoceptors (Fig. 1.23 *bottom*), and appears to be a slower process than the 'uncoupling' from adenylate cyclase mentioned above.

In studies on cell cultures the number of β-adrenoceptors can fall to about 10% of normal in 8 hours in the presence of a low concentration of isoprenaline. Recovery to normal takes several days. Similar changes have been described for other types of receptor, including those for various peptides. The fate of the vanishing receptors is not certain, but there is some evidence that they are taken into the cell by endocytosis of patches of the membrane. This type of elaborate regulatory mechanism appears to be common for hormone receptors, and has obvious relevance to the effects produced when drugs are given for extended periods.

3. *Exhaustion of mediators.* In some cases desensitization is associated with depletion of essential intermediate substance. Drugs such as amphetamine, which acts by releasing noradrenaline and other amines from nerve terminals (see Chapters 7 & 19) show marked tachyphylaxis because the releasable stores of noradrenaline become depleted.

Desensitization to serotonin, in certain situations where it acts to cause calcium entry by stimulating

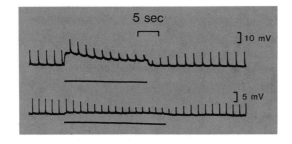

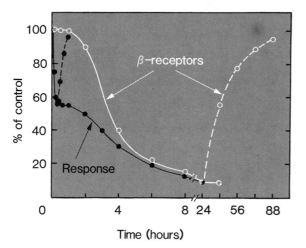

Fig. 1.23 Two kinds of receptor desensitization. *Top*: Acetylcholine at the frog motor endplate. Brief depolarizations (upward deflections) are produced by short pulses of ACh delivered from a micropipette. A long pulse (horizontal line) causes the response to decline with a time-course of about 20 seconds, due to desensitization, and it recovers with a similar time-course.

Bottom: β-adrenoceptors of rat glioma cells in tissue culture. Isoprenaline (1 μM) was added at time zero, and the adenylate cyclase response and β-adrenoceptor density measured at intervals. The response declined rapidly at first, with no change in the number of adrenoceptors (early uncoupling phase of desensitization); it then declined more slowly, concomitantly with a loss of receptors (late down-regulation phase). The dotted lines show the recovery of the response and receptor density after the isoprenaline is washed out during the early or late phase. (From: (Top) Katz & Thesleff, 1957; (Bottom) Perkins, 1981)

Ptd Ins breakdown (see p. 23) has been attributed to depletion of Ptd Ins. It is likely that many more examples of this type will come to light as more biochemical mechanisms of drug action become elucidated.

4. *Increased metabolic degradation.* Tolerance to some drugs, for example barbiturates (see Chapter 21), occurs partly because repeated administration of the same dose produces a progressively lower plasma concentration. This also happens to an appreciable extent with ethanol. In general, the degree of tolerance that results is rather slight, and in both of these examples other mechanisms contribute to the substantial tolerance that actually occurs.

5. *Physiological adaptation.* Disappearance of a drug's effect may occur because it is nullified by a homeostatic response. For example, diuretics which act by inhibiting carbonic anhydrase (see Chapter 14) produce only a transient diuresis because the acidosis that is produced reduces the loss of bicarbonate in the urine, and hence limits the diuresis. There are undoubtedly many more instances in which homeostatic responses operate in such a way as to modify or counteract drug effects, and if they occur slowly the result will be a gradually developing tolerance. It is a very common experience that many side effects of drugs, such as nausea or sleepiness, tend to subside even though drug administration is continued. We may assume that some kind of physiological adaptation is involved, though nothing is known of the mechanism of such changes.

RECEPTOR MECHANISMS

DEFINITIONS OF SOME COMMON TERMS

Receptor. A protein molecule which is capable of selectively binding a drug, hormone or neurotransmitter, thereby eliciting a physiological response.

Agonist. A drug, hormone or transmitter substance that elicits a cellular response when it combines with receptors.

A **full agonist** is a drug that is capable, at a sufficiently high concentration, of producing a maximal cellular response.

A **partial agonist** is an agonist whose maximum effect is less than the maximal response of which the tissue is capable.

Antagonist. A drug that prevents the effect of an agonist.

Competitive antagonists act by binding to agonist receptors.

Reversible competitive antagonist—a receptor antagonist that equilibrates sufficiently rapidly with the receptors that its occupancy is reduced (according to the Mass Action equation for competing ligands; p. 9) when the agonist concentration is increased. A reversible competitive antagonist causes the agonist log concentration-effect curve to shift to the right without change in slope or maximum.

Irreversible competitive antagonist—a receptor antagonist that dissociates from the receptors slowly or not at all. The slope and maximum of the agonist log concentration-effect curve are likely to be reduced.

Non-competitive antagonists do not bind to the same receptor sites as the agonist, but reduce its effect in some other way.

Ligand. Any substance that binds to a particular type of receptor.

Occupancy. The fraction of the receptors occupied by a ligand.

Dose ratio. The ratio by which the agonist concentration must be increased in the presence of an antagonist in order to elicit an equal biological response.

Equilibrium and rate constants. Quantitative parameters governing receptor-binding reactions

$$A + R \underset{k_{-1}}{\overset{k_{+1}}{\rightleftharpoons}} AR$$

Equilibrium constant (or equilibrium dissociation constant or dissociation constant), K

$$K = \frac{k_{-1}}{k_{+1}}$$

When the reaction is at equilibrium

$$K = \frac{[A] \cdot [R]}{[AR]}$$

K has the dimensions of concentration.

Affinity constant (or association constant) is the reciprocal of K and has the dimensions concentration^{-1}.

Association and dissociation rate constants, k_{+1} and k_{-1}, measure the rate at which association and dissociation occur.

Efficacy. A parameter that varies between different agonists and expresses the ability of the agonist-receptor complex to elicit a physiological response. Efficacy is high for full agonists, low for partial agonists and zero for competitive antagonists. Sometimes termed **intrinsic activity**.

Langmuir equation. The equation relating equilibrium occupancy (p_A) to ligand concentration (x_A) for a simple binding reaction where there is no interaction between sites.

$$p_A = \frac{x_A}{x_A + K_A}$$

The binding curve (p_A vs x_A) is hyperbolic.

Scatchard plot. A procedure for linearizing the Langmuir equation by plotting p_A/x_A against p_A (see p. 13).

Cooperativity. A deviation from the Langmuir binding equation that occurs if there is interaction between the sites (i.e. if binding of one ligand molecule to a receptor affects the probability of binding to adjacent receptors).

Positive cooperativity, which occurs when the binding of one molecule favours the binding of others, is quite common, and causes the binding curve to become sigmoid instead of hyperbolic.

Negative cooperativity, which occurs when the binding of one molecule discourages the binding of others, is uncommon.

Hill plot, Hill coefficient. The Hill plot is a logarithmic transformation of the Langmuir equation which provides a convenient test for the presence of cooperativity in a binding reaction.

$$\ln\left(\frac{p_A}{1-p_A}\right) = \ln x_A - \ln K_A$$

To construct a Hill plot, $\ln(p_A/1-p_A)$, or, for binding measurements, $\ln(B/B_{max} - B)$, is plotted against $\ln x_A$.

The slope of the line is the Hill coefficient. A Hill coefficient equal to 1.0 denotes lack of cooperativity, a larger value denoting positive cooperativity. A value less than 1.0 indicates either negative cooperativity or the presence of more than one class of binding site.

Spare receptors. The existence of more receptors in a tissue than require to be occupied by agonist in order to evoke a maximal response.

REFERENCES AND FURTHER READING

Berridge M J 1981 Phosphatidylinositol metabolism and calcium gating in a 5-HT receptor system. In: Birdsall N J M (ed) Drug receptors and their effectors. Macmillan, London

Berridge M J, Dawson R M C, Downes C P, Heslop J P, Irvine R F 1983 Changes in the levels of inositol phosphates after agonist-dependent hydrolysis of membrane phosphoinositides. Biochem J 212: 473–482

Carafoli E, Crompton M 1978 The regulation of intracellular calcium. Current Topics in Membrane Transport 10: 151–216

Dolly J O, Barnard E A 1984 Nicotinic acetylcholine receptors: an overview. Biochem Pharmacol 33: 841–858

Greengard P 1978 Phosphorylated proteins as physiological effectors. Science 199: 146–152

Hirata F, Axelrod J 1980 Phospholipid methylation and biological signal transmission. Science 209: 1082–1090

Hollenberg M D 1982 Receptor-mediated phosphorylation reactions. Trends in Pharmacological Sciences 3: 271–273

Jakobs K H, Schultz G 1981 Actions of hormones and transmitters at the plasma membrane: inhibition of adenylate cyclase. In: Lamble J W (ed) Towards understanding receptors. Elsevier, Amsterdam

King W J, Greene G L 1984 Monoclonal antibodies localize oestrogen receptor in the nuclei of target cells. Nature 307: 745–747

Nestler E J, Greengard P 1984 Protein phosphorylation in the nervous system. Wiley, New York

Nestler E J, Walaas S I, Greengard P 1984 Neuronal phosphoproteins: physiological and clinical implications. Science 225: 1357–1364

Nishizuka Y 1984 Turnover of inositol phospholipids and signal transduction. Science 225: 1365–1370

Popot J L, Changeux J-P 1984 Nicotinic receptor of acetylcholine: structure of an oligomeric integral receptor protein. Physiol Rev 64: 1162–1239

Putney J W, Burgess G M, Halenda S P, McKinney J S, Rubin R P 1983 Effects of secretagogues on [^{32}P] phosphatidylinositol 4,5-biphosphate metabolism in the exocrine pancreas. Biochem J 212: 483–488

Racker E 1980 Fluxes of Ca^{++} and concepts. Fed Proc 30: 2422–2425

Rodbell M 1980 The role of hormone receptors and GTP-regulatory proteins in membrane transduction. Nature 284: 17–21

Schramm M, Selinger Z 1984 Message transmission: receptor controlled adenylate cyclase system. Science 225: 1350–1356

Schulman H 1982 Calcium-dependent protein phosphorylation. Handbook of Experimental Pharmacology 58: 425–478

Stephenson R P 1956 A modification of receptor theory. Br J Pharmac 11: 379–393

Welshons M V, Lieberman M E, Gorski J 1984 Nuclear localization of unoccupied oestrogen receptors. Nature 307: 747–749

Measurement in pharmacology

It is necessary to have reliable methods for measuring drug effects, in order to be able to compare quantitatively the effects of different substances, or of the same substance under different circumstances. It is also necessary to be able to measure the concentration of drugs and other active substances in, say, the blood or other body fluids. The first of these requirements is met by the techniques of bioassay; the second requirement may be met by chemical techniques, but the needs for high sensitivity (since drug concentrations are often very low) and high selectivity (since innumerable other substances are present in any biological sample), are frequently better met by biological rather than chemical assay techniques. Impressive advances in sensitivity and specificity of chemical assay techniques have, however, been made in recent years, and the use of bioassay where the need is simply to measure the concentration of a known substance is now less important than it used to be. In this chapter the principles underlying the main types of bioassay are discussed, together with an account of some chemical methods that are particularly useful in pharmacological studies.

BIOASSAY

Bioassay is defined as the estimation of the concentration or potency of a substance by measurement of the biological response that it produces.

The uses of bioassay are:

1. To measure the pharmacological activity of new or chemically undefined substances.
2. To measure the concentration of known substances.
3. To investigate the function of endogenous mediators.
4. To measure the clinical effectiveness of a form of drug treatment.
5. To measure drug toxicity.

Bioassay is essential in the **development of new drugs**, for the first stage in assessment of a new compound will usually be to compare its biological activity in various test systems with that of known compounds. The choice of suitable test systems for this preliminary bioassay is important and not always easy. The tests must be sufficiently simple and economical to be used routinely on numerous compounds, and must also be as specific as possible for the type of biological activity that is being sought. This may be fairly obvious; local anaesthetic activity, for example, can be measured reliably by the ability of a substance to block action potential propagation in an isolated length of peripheral nerve, and the results obtained in this way correlate well with activity in clinical use. False negatives and false positives are unlikely, and the test has good predictive value. In other cases, appropriate test systems are not at all obvious. When, for example, antipsychotic drugs are being sought, there is no single reliable test system. Many assays, on whole animals and on isolated systems, have been devised that give some indication of antipsychotic activity, but each will throw up false positive or negative results. Assessment of a new compound usually consists of carrying out a battery of such assays, and constructing a profile of activity. Clinical effectiveness, it is hoped, may appear to be associated with a particular pattern of activity in such a profile, rather than with activity in one particular test system.

In general, the more complex and imperfectly

understood the mechanism of action of a drug the more difficult it is to predict clinical effectiveness from the results of assays based on laboratory test systems. In the case of antipsychotic drugs, for example, it may not be until the point of actual clinical trial that it can be reliably determined whether the drug even possesses therapeutic activity of the kind required.

For **measurement of the concentration of known substances**, bioassay is, as mentioned earlier, steadily being displaced by chemical assays, which are usually quicker and more accurate than bioassay. The British Pharmacopoeia (1980), however, still lays down bioassay as the official method for estimating the activity of a number of substances, such as **corticotrophin**, **insulin** and **heparin**. The activity of **digitalis** (in the form of a crude extract of foxglove leaves) also has to be assayed biologically, even though chemical methods exist for assaying the individual active constituents of the crude preparation. **Acetylcholine**, though identified chemically as a neurotransmitter in 1933 (see Chapter 5), has until recently been impossible to assay chemically at a sensitivity great enough to measure the minute amounts released by nerve terminals, and progress in studying its release depended for many years on highly sensitive, but extremely laborious, bioassays. Mass spectrometry (see p. 53) and radioenzymatic assays for acetylcholine have now, however, surpassed bioassay in sensitivity, and will doubtless replace it.

Bioassay is indispensible in the **study of new types of hormonal, or other chemically-mediated, control systems**. Mediators in such systems are recognized initially by the biological effects that they produce, and it is only later that their chemical identity, and hence the possibility of using more direct chemical assay methods, is established. Very exceptionally, things happen the other way about, and a mediator is first identified chemically and then shown to be functionally important. **Dopamine**, for example, was found in nervous tissue and assumed to function merely as a precursor for noradrenaline (see Chapter 7), before being shown to act as a transmitter in its own right. Much more often the first step is the finding that a tissue extract or some other biological sample produces an effect on an assay system. For example, the ability of extracts of the posterior lobe of the pituitary to produce a rise

in blood pressure and a contraction of the uterus was observed at the turn of the century. These actions were made the basis of quantitative assay procedures and a standard preparation of the extract was established by international agreement in 1935. By use of these assays it was shown that two distinct peptides were responsible, and they were eventually identified and synthesized in 1953. Biological assay had already revealed much about the synthesis, storage and release of the hormones, and was essential for their purification and identification. Though it is highly unlikely that future hormones and mediators will require 50 years of laborious bioassays before being chemically characterized, bioassay remains crucial to such studies.

The principle of **parallel assays** devised by Gaddum has sometimes been useful in identifying unknown mediators. If the biological activity of a sample is thought to be due, for example, to serotonin, then measurements of the relative potency of the sample, assayed against authentic serotonin, ought to give the same result, irrespective of what assay system is used. If a range of assay systems is used, and the relative potency of serotonin and the unknown substance is the same in all of them, then it is likely that the activity is due to serotonin. If, on the other hand, in one or more assay systems the relative potency is not found to be the same, it must be concluded that the biological activity is not wholly due to serotonin, but partly at least to other substances.

The use of parallel assays was developed to an almost baroque splendour in the work of Vane and his colleagues, who have studied the generation and destruction of many endogenous active substances, especially prostanoids (see Chapter 8) by the technique of cascade superfusion (Fig. 2.1) in which the sample is run sequentially over a series of test preparations chosen to differentiate between different active constituents of the sample. The pattern of responses produced effectively identifies the active material, and the use of such assay systems for 'on line' analysis of blood samples has been invaluable in studying the production and fate of short-lived mediators such as prostanoids.

Measurement of the **therapeutic effectiveness** of drugs is an important and highly specialized form of biological assay. The need to use man as an experimental animal (particularly when the indi-

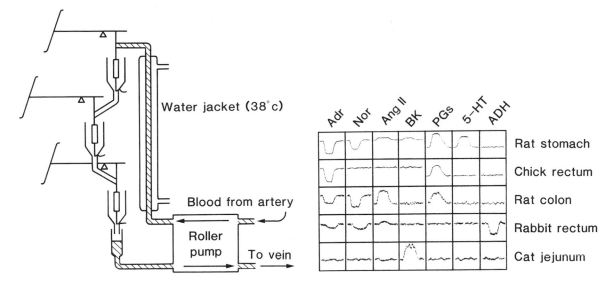

Fig. 2.1 Parallel assay by the cascade superfusion technique. Blood is pumped continuously from the test animal over a succession of test organs, whose responses are measured by a simple transducer system. The response of these organs to a variety of test substances (at 0.1–5 ng/ml) is shown on the right. Each active substance produces a distinct pattern of responses, enabling unknown materials present in the blood to be identified and assayed. (From: Vane, 1969)

Adr, adrenaline; Nor, noradrenaline; Ang II, angiotensin II; Bk, bradykinin; PG, prostaglandin; 5HT, 5-hydroxytryptamine; ADH, antidiuretic hormone.

viduals involved are patients seeking medical advice, rather than selected volunteers) imposes many restrictions. Some of the basic principles involved in clinical trials are discussed later in this chapter.

Drug toxicity is measured in two distinct ways. In one kind of test, the ability of experimental animals to withstand large doses of the drug is assessed, the simplest such measurement being the **LD_{50} test**, a bioassay designed to measure the lethal dose in animals (see below). The other kind of toxicity measurement takes the form of **monitoring**, and is designed to detect an increased incidence of harmful effects when the drug is given therapeutically to patients. For most practical purposes, the manifestation of drug toxicity in this form, as 'adverse reactions' in a proportion of patients, is of more importance than the acute toxicity as measured by the LD_{50} test.

GENERAL PRINCIPLES OF BIOASSAY

This section is concerned with laboratory-based assays rather than with clinical trials or monitoring, which are discussed later.

The use of standards

In 1950 J H Burn wrote: 'Pharmacologists today strain at the king's arm, but they swallow the frog, rat and mouse, not to mention the guinea pig and the pigeon'. He was referring to the fact that the king's arm was long since abandoned as a standard measure of length, whereas drug activity was constantly being defined in terms of dose needed to cause, say, vomiting of a pigeon or cardiac arrest in a mouse, and a plethora of 'pigeon units', 'mouse units' and the like, which no two laboratories could agree on, contaminated the literature*. Even if two laboratories cannot agree, because their pigeons differ, on the activity in pigeon units of the same sample of an active substance, they should nonetheless be able to agree that preparation X is, say, 3.5

---

* More picturesque examples of absolute units of the kind that Burn would have frowned upon are the PHI and the mHelen. PHI, cited by Colquhoun (1971), stands for 'purity in heart index' and measures the ability of a virgin pure-in-heart to transform, under appropriate conditions, a he-goat into a youth of surpassing beauty. The mHelen is a unit of beauty, 1 mHelen being sufficient to launch 1 ship.

times as active as standard preparation Y on the pigeon test. Biological assays are therefore designed to measure the relative potency of two preparations, usually a standard and an unknown.

The best kind of standard is, of course, the pure substance, but it is often necessary to establish standard preparations of various hormones, natural products and antisera against which laboratory samples can be calibrated, even though the standard preparations are not chemically pure.

The design of bioassays

Given the aim of comparing the activity of two preparations, a **standard (S)** and an **unknown (U)** on a particular preparation, what a bioassay must provide is an estimate of the dose of U that will produce the same biological effect as that of a known dose of S. As Figure 2.2 shows, provided

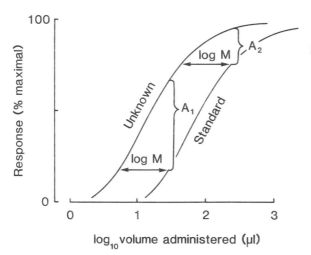

Fig. 2.2 Comparison of the potency of unknown and standard by bioassay. Note that comparing the magnitude of responses produced by the same dose (i.e. volume) of standard and unknown gives no quantitative estimate of their relative potency. (The differences, A_1 and A_2, depend on the dose chosen.) Comparison of equi-effective doses of standard and unknown gives a valid measure of their relative potencies. Since the lines are parallel, the magnitude of the effect chosen for the comparison is immaterial; i.e. log M is the same at all points on the curves.

that the log dose-effect curves for S and U are parallel, the ratio, M, of equiactive doses will not depend on the magnitude of response chosen. M thus provides an estimate of the potency ratio of the two preparations. It is worth noting that a comparison of the *magnitude* of the effects pro-

duced by *equal doses* of S and U does not provide an estimate of M, because the ratio of the effects produced by S and U will vary according to the dose chosen.

The main problem with all types of bioassay is that of **biological variation**, and the principles of design of bioassays are largely to do with (a) minimizing variation, (b) avoiding systematic errors resulting from variation, and (c) estimation of the limits of error of the assay result.

Examples of the extent of biological variation encountered in two fairly typical bioassays are shown in Figure 2.3; in each case there is about a three-fold range in the drug dose needed to produce a given biological response in the population of frogs or human subjects that was tested. In the examples shown in Figure 2.3 the distributions of individual effective doses (IED) are approximately symmetrical, and correspond roughly to the **normal distribution**. The potency of the drug in such an assay is usually expressed in terms of the **median value** of the IED (known as the ED_{50} because it corresponds to the dose required to produce a response in 50% of the subjects tested). The ED_{50} can be read off the cumulative frequency distribution curve as shown in Figure 2.3B. If, as in Figure 2.3A & B, the distribution of IED values is nearly symmetrical, the mean IED for the population will agree quite closely with the ED_{50} (Fig. 2.3B). Commonly, however, the distribution of IED values is skewed to the right, as in Figure 2.3C, and it may then be useful to plot the doses on a logarithmic scale (see Colquhoun (1971) for a more detailed discussion).

Direct bioassays

With a direct bioassay the aim is to determine the doses of standard and unknown that produce the same response. Thus, in the type of experiment shown in Figure 2.3A, a standard preparation of digitalis is injected slowly into each of a group of frogs, and the dose required to stop the heart is determined for each. A similar experiment on another group of frogs is carried out with the unknown. The potency ratio, M, of U to S, is then given by:

$$M = \frac{ED_{50} \text{ standard}}{ED_{50} \text{ unknown}}$$

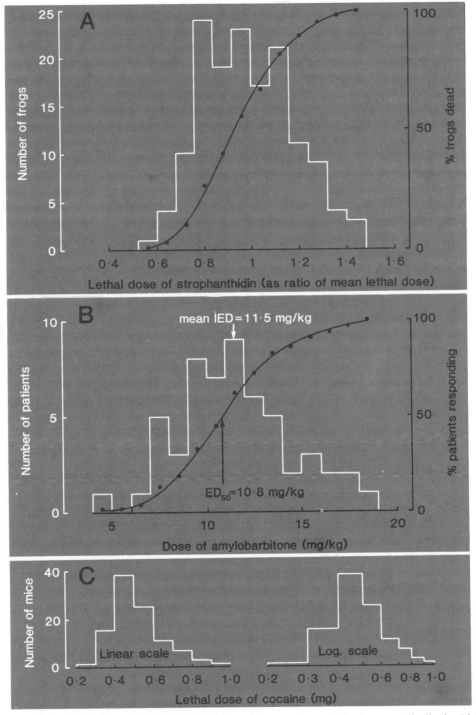

Fig. 2.3 Examples of biological variation. **A.** Histogram (left hand ordinate) and cumulative frequency distribution (right hand ordinate) of the lethal dose of a cardiac glycoside (strophanthidin) in frogs. The deviations extend roughly from 50% below the mean to 50% above. (Data from: Behrens, 1929). **B.** Histogram and cumulative frequency distribution of the intravenous dose of pentobarbitone needed to cause a standard degree of drowsiness in obstetric patients. The scatter is rather greater than in A, presumably because the endpoint is less clearly defined. Note that the ED_{50} is not identical with the mean IED. **C.** Histograms of the lethal dose of cocaine in mice, plotted on linear and logarithmic concentration scales. Note that the linear scale gives a skewed distribution, whereas on a logarithmic scale it is roughly symmetrical. (Data from: Colquhoun, 1971)

It must be remembered that the estimates of the ED_{50} values, and hence the estimates of M, are associated with an appreciable error, and it is important to be able to calculate this error, as a guide to the reliance that can be placed on the assay result. Statistical techniques for determining the error associated with an assay result are described in detail elsewhere (Finney, 1964; Colquhoun, 1971), and it is important that the design of a bioassay experiment should permit its error to be calculated efficiently. The limits of error are usually expressed as 5% confidence limits, which means the limits within which 95% of the results would be expected to fall if the assay were performed many times on samples from the same population of animals.

A much less laborious type of direct assay is the **matching assay**, in which a repeatable *graded* response, such as contraction of a length of smooth muscle, or rise in blood pressure of an anaesthetized animal is used. Doses of standard and unknown are adjusted until a good match is achieved and these doses are used to calculate the potency ratio. If the responses show little variation, this is quite straightforward, but if they vary markedly it is impossible to achieve a consistent match. A weakness of such assays is that they give no information about the confidence limits of the result.

Indirect bioassays

With an indirect assay, no attempt is made to achieve exactly matching responses to standard and unknown; instead, comparisons are based on analysis of dose-response curves, and the matching doses of standard and unknown are calculated rather than measured directly. Such calculations become much simpler if the dose-response curves are linear. In many cases this can be achieved (see Chapter 1) by using a logarithmic dose scale and restricting observations to the middle region of the log dose-effect curve, which is usually close to a straight line. The use of a logarithmic dose scale also means that the curves for standard and unknown will normally be parallel, and the potency of the unknown, relative to the standard, is determined by the horizontal distance between the two curves (see Fig. 2.2). Assays of this type are known as **parallel line assays**, and a convenient and simple design is the $2+2$ assay, in which two doses of

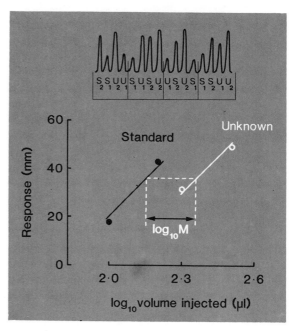

Fig. 2.4 Two-plus-two bioassay of an unknown versus a standard pituitary extract on an isolated rat uterus. Two doses of unknown (U_1 and U_2) and two standard (S_1 and S_2) were tested. They were chosen to give responses of similar magnitude, and with U_1/U_2 equal to S_1/S_2 for convenience in analysis. The four doses were tested in random order in each block (upper traces). The mean responses are shown below, with the calculated regression lines and potency ratio. In this assay $\log_{10} M = 0.20$; $M = 1.58$. Since the standard contained 400 mU/ml, the unknown was estimated as $400/1.58 = 252$ mU/ml. Analysis of variance was used to calculate the 5% confidence limits (± 24 mU/ml) from the individual assay responses. (From: Holton, 1948)

standard (S_1 and S_2) and two of unknown (U_1 and U_2) are used (Fig. 2.4). The doses are chosen to give responses lying on the linear part of the log-dose response curve, and to achieve overlap between the responses to the standard and unknown. For arithmetical convenience the ratio between the two doses (S_1/S_2) is the same for standard and unknown. With this rather formalized design, the doses are usually given in a series of **randomized blocks**, each consisting of the four doses, S_1, S_2, U_1, and U_2, but given random order as in the record shown in Figure 2.4. The fact that each dose is repeated several times means that an inherent measure of the variability of the test system is available from this type of assay, and this can be used, by means of straightforward statistical analysis, to estimate the confidence limits of the final result. It can be seen from Figure 2.5 that the precision of the assay

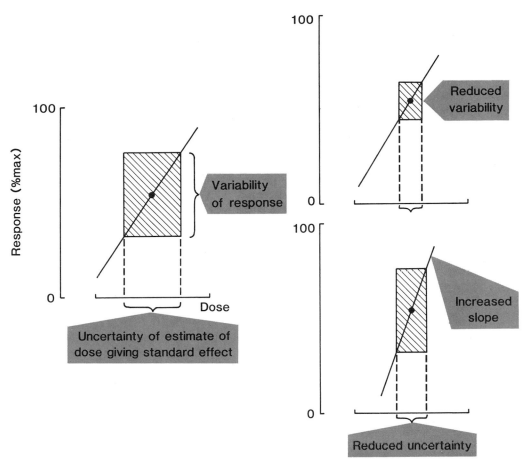

Fig. 2.5 Relationship between **variability** (i.e. variation of response to a given dose) and **discrimination** (i.e. the slope of the dose-response relationship) in determining the precision of a bioassay. Reducing variability or increasing discrimination are both ways of improving precision.

depends both on the inherent variability of the test system and on the steepness of the log dose-response curve; the steeper the curve and the less the variability, the more precise will the assay be. In practice, most bioassays will give results whose 5% confidence limits lie within ±20%, and many will do better than this.

The 2 + 2 assay also detects whether or not the two log-dose effect lines deviate significantly from parallelism. If the lines are not parallel, which may be the case if the assay is used to compare two drugs whose mechanism of action is not the same, it is not possible to define the relative potencies of S and U unambiguously in terms of a simple ratio. The experimenter must then face up to the fact that there are qualitative as well as quantitative differences between the two drugs, so that comparison

requires measurement of more than a single dimension of potency. An example of this kind of difficulty is met when diuretic drugs (see Chapter 14) are compared. Some ('low ceiling') diuretics are capable of producing only a small diuretic effect, no matter how much is given; others ('high ceiling') can produce a very intense diuresis (described as 'torrential' by authors with vivid imaginations). A comparison of two such drugs requires not only a measure of the doses needed to produce an equal low-level diuretic effect, but also a measure of the relative heights of the ceilings.

Quantal and graded responses

The measure of response used in an assay may be a **graded** phenomenon, such as a change in blood glucose concentration, or contraction of a strip of smooth muscle, or a change in the time taken for a rat to run a maze; or it may be **all-or-nothing**, such as death, loss of righting reflex or success in maze-running within a stipulated time. With the latter type of response, known as a **quantal response**, because it either happens or it doesn't, the proportion of animals responding will vary according to the dose used, and the relationship between log dose and proportion of animals responding generally looks like Figure 2.3. The shape and slope of such a curve is governed by the individual variation between animals; in principle, if the frogs used had been identical, the line relating percentage mortality to dose of digitalis would jump from 0 to 100% when the lethal dose was reached. The steepness of quantal dose-response curves, and, therefore, the precision of assays based on quantal responses can be improved by using a uniform population of animals. With graded responses, the steepness of the dose-response curve is a property of the test system and has nothing to do with biological variation.

Quantal responses can be used in essentially the same way as graded responses for the purposes of bioassay, though the appropriate statistical procedures are slightly different.

BIOASSAYS IN MAN

It is often useful to carry out bioassays in man when, for example, animal tests fail to predict human responses, or when the response is subjective and not measurable in animals. Thus, the human uterus differs markedly in its pharmacological responsiveness from other species, so it is often useful to test oxytocic drugs in human subjects. A non-invasive device can be used to record uterine activity through the abdominal wall, and the tests are carried out post-partum to avoid risk to the foetus. This technique was used by Myers-cough & Schild (1958) to compare the oxytocic activity of ergometrine and its methyl derivative. They used an ingenious adaptation of the $2 + 2$ design, in which any one subject received only two doses, in various combinations, out of the four that were used to complete the assay.

Measurement of analgesia (see Chapter 25) also

has to be carried out in man. Though many animal tests have been devised (for example, measuring the time taken for rats to jump off a surface heated to a mildly painful temperature) they often fail to predict accurately the subjective relief of pain in man. One method of measuring analgesia in man is to employ a graded stimulus, such as radiant heat, and determine the threshold at which pain is felt. It is generally agreed, however, that this type of artificial and superficial pain is quite different in quality and connotation from clinical pain and provides a relatively poor model. More useful assessments of analgesic drugs have, therefore, been developed on the basis of subjective reports of relief from persistent pain, such as that of malignant disease. Figure 2.6 shows a comparison of morphine and codeine in

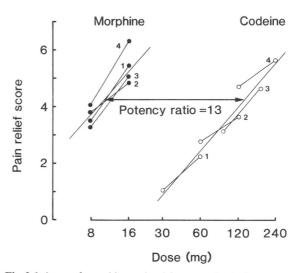

Fig. 2.6 Assay of morphine and codeine as analgesics in man. Each of four patients (numbered 1–4) was given, on successive occasions in random order, four different treatments (high and low morphine, and high and low codeine), by intramuscular injection and the subjective pain relief score calculated for each. The calculated regression lines gave a potency ratio estimate of 13 for the 2 drugs. (From: Houde et al, 1965)

which a modified $2 + 2$ design was used. Each of the four doses was given on different occasions to each of the four subjects, the order being randomized and both subject and observer being unaware of the dose given. Pain relief was assessed by questions from the trained observer, and the assay gave a remarkably precise comparison of the activities of the two drugs. Morphine turned out to be thirteen times as potent as codeine. This, of course, does not prove its superiority, but merely shows that a smaller dose is needed to produce the same effect. Such a measurement is, however, an essential preliminary to assessing the relative therapeutic merits of the two drugs, for any comparison of other factors such as side effects, duration of action, tolerance or dependence, needs to be done on the basis of doses that are equiactive so far as analgesia is concerned.

Clinical trials

A clinical trial is a method for comparing objectively the results of two or more therapeutic regimes. It is important to realize that, until about 30 years ago, methods of treatment were chosen largely on the basis of clinical impression and personal experience rather than objective testing. Though many drugs, whose effectiveness is not in doubt, remain in use without ever having been subjected to a controlled clinical trial, any new drug is nowadays required to have been tested in this way before being licensed for general clinical use*.

A clinical trial aims to compare the response to a new treatment (A) with that to an existing 'standard' treatment (B). Treatment A might be a new drug, or a new combination of existing drugs, or any other kind of therapeutic intervention such as a surgical operation, diet, physiotherapy etc. The standard against which it is judged (treatment B) might be a currently used drug treatment or a placebo or no treatment at all. Unlike the kind of bioassay that we have been considering up to this point, the clinical trial does not normally give any information about potency or the form of the dose-response curve, but merely compares the *response* produced by two stipulated therapeutic regimes.

---

*It is fashionable in some quarters to argue that to require evidence of efficacy of therapeutic procedures in the form of a controlled trial runs counter to the doctrines of 'holistic' medicine. This is a fundamentally anti-scientific view, for science advances only by generating predictions from hypotheses, and by subjecting the predictions to experimental test. If a system of medicine is set up whose hypotheses are deemed to be immune to experimental test, then, like a religious doctrine, it lies outside the realm of science. This does not, of course, make it wrong, but it makes it incompatible with scientific medicine, and one must view with great suspicion the suggestion that elements of both systems can be rationally combined without coming into fundamental conflict.

The investigator must decide in advance what dose to use and how often to give it, and the trial will only show him whether his chosen regime performed better or worse than the standard treatment; it will not tell him whether increasing or decreasing the dose would have improved the response and he would have to do another trial to ascertain that. The basic question posed by a clinical trial is thus less sophisticated than that addressed by conventional bioassays. The organization of clinical trials, and the problem of avoiding bias, is, however, immeasurably more complicated, time-consuming and expensive than with any laboratory-based assay.

Avoidance of bias

There are two main strategies that aim to minimize bias in clinical trials, namely **randomization** and the **double-blind technique**.

If two treatments are being compared on a series of selected patients, the simplest form of randomization is to allocate each patient to A or B by reference to a series of random numbers. If the number of patients is large enough, roughly equal numbers will be assigned to each group. In a small series, however, the groups could end up poorly matched, and a compromise solution is to split the series into blocks of, say, eight patients, each block consisting of four of A and four of B, arranged in random order. Another difficulty with simple randomization is that the treatment groups may turn out to be ill-matched with respect to a variable characteristic such as age or sex. The chance of serious mismatching of the groups obviously decreases as the size of the series increases. With small scale trials, **stratified randomization** is often used to avoid the difficulty. Thus the subjects might be divided into groups (strata) according to age, random allocation to A or B being used within each group. It is possible to treat two or more characteristics of the trial population in this way. Thus, if it were important to balance the groups with respect to age and sex, it might be necessary to define three age bands, each being split into males and females, making six strata in all. Severity of disease is another variable that is often incorporated into such stratification schemes. It will be appreciated that the number of strata can quickly become large, and the process is self-defeating when the number of subjects in each becomes too small. As well as avoiding error resulting from imbalance of groups assigned to A and B, stratification can also allow more sophisticated conclusions to be reached. B might, for example, prove to be better than A in a particular group of patients even if it is not significantly better overall.

The **double-blind technique**, which means that neither subject nor investigator is aware, at the time of the assessment, which treatment is being used, is intended to minimize subjective bias. It has been repeatedly shown that both participants, with the best will in the world, contribute to bias if they know which treatment is which, so the use of a double-blind technique is an important safeguard. It is not always possible, however. A dietary regime, or a surgical operation, for example, cannot be disguised, and even with drugs, their pharmacological effects may reveal to the patient what he is taking, and predispose him to report accordingly*. In general, however, the use of a double-blind procedure, with precautions if necessary to disguise such clues as the taste or appearance of the two drugs, is an important precaution.

The size of the sample

Both ethical and financial considerations dictate that the trial should involve the minimum number of subjects, and much statistical thought has gone into the problem of deciding in advance how many subjects will be required to produce a useful result. The results of a trial cannot, by their nature, be absolutely conclusive. This is because it is based on a sample of patients and there is always a chance that the sample was highly atypical. The chance of a 'freak' sample may be small but it is finite. Two types of erroneous conclusion are possible, referred to as **Type I** and **Type II errors**. A Type I error occurs if a difference is found between A and B when none actually exists. A Type II error occurs if

no difference is found though A and B do actually differ. A major factor that determines the size of sample needed is the degree of certainty of avoiding either type of error that the investigator seeks. The probability of incurring a Type I error is expressed as the **significance** of the result. To say that A and B are different at the 0.05 level of significance means that the probability of observing a difference as great as that actually observed, if A and B were not actually different (i.e. the chance of incurring a Type I error) is less than 1 in 20. For most purposes this level of significance is considered acceptable as a basis for drawing conclusions. The probability of avoiding a Type II error (i.e. failing to detect a real difference between A and B) is termed the **power** of the trial. We tend to regard Type II errors more leniently than Type I errors, and trials are often designed with a power of 0.8–0.9 (i.e. a 10–20% probability that a real difference between treatments will go undetected). To increase the significance and the power of a trial requires more patients.

The second factor that determines the sample size required is the *magnitude* of difference between A and B that is regarded as clinically significant. For example, to show that a given treatment reduces the mortality in a certain condition from 50% (in the control group) to 40% (in the treated group) within a given time would require 850 subjects, assuming that we wanted to achieve a 0.05 level of significance and a power of 0.9. If we were content to reveal a reduction to 30% (and very likely miss a reduction to 40%) only 210 subjects would be needed.

Sequential trials

The purpose of sequential trials is to minimize the number of subjects used, by computing the results continuously as the trial proceeds and stopping it as soon as a result (at a pre-determined level of significance) is achieved. The usual procedure, in this type of trial, is that the subjects are paired, one subject receiving each treatment (alternatively a cross-over design can be used in which each subject receives both treatments consecutively). The result of each individual comparison is scored as **A better than B**, **B better than A**, or **no discernible difference**, and the analysis is performed graphically (Fig. 2.7). The example shown is a three-way comparison of

---

* The distinction between a true pharmacological response, and a beneficial clinical effect produced by the knowledge, based on the pharmacological effects that the drug produces, that an active drug is being administered, is not easy to draw, and we should not expect a clinical trial to resolve such a fine semantic issue.

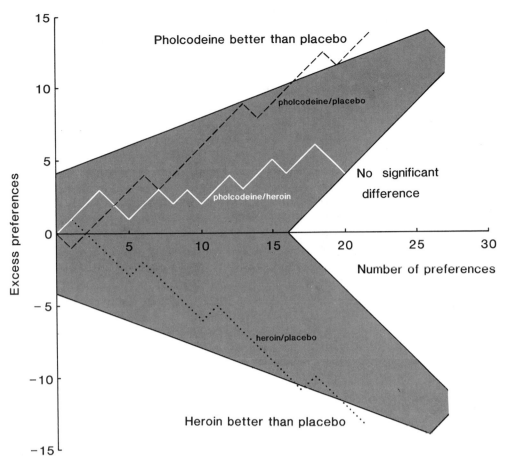

Fig. 2.7 Sequential clinical trial to compare pholcodeine, heroin and placebo as cough suppressants. Each of 27 patients was given, under double blind conditions, the three treatments on successive occasions and asked to rank them in order of effectiveness. The stated preferences were then plotted on the diagram. The lines comparing either drug with placebo crossed the 0.05 significance limit after about 20 preferences had been expressed, showing both drugs to be significantly better than placebo. The line comparing heroin and pholcodeine failed to show a significant difference. The right hand limit corresponds to a power of 0.85 (i.e. a 15% chance that a real difference exists). (From: Snell & Armitage, 1957)

heroin, pholcodeine and placebo used as cough suppressants in patients with chronic cough. Each patient was given all three treatments consecutively, in random order, and rated them in order of effectiveness. The solid line on the diagram represents the comparison between pholcodeine and heroin. If a subject preferred pholcodeine the line was extended upwards and to the right; if he preferred heroin the line was drawn downwards and to the right. Overall the line was nearly horizontal, and after 24 subjects it crossed the boundary indicating that no significant difference could be demonstrated. The other two lines progress fairly steadily towards the boundaries indicating that both heroin (lower boundary) and pholcodeine

(upper boundary) were better than the placebo. The position of the boundaries in such a diagram is calculated on the basis of the significance level and power required. In Figure 2.7 the significance was set at 0.05 and the power 0.85. Because of their simplicity and economy, sequential trials are widely used. They are not, as a rule, suitable where assessment of the result of treatment takes a long time (e.g. where death rates are being compared) since all the subjects will have been committed to the trial before any results are obtained.

The organization of clinical trials

The organization of a clinical trial is liable to be a

massive undertaking. A recent trial of the effectiveness of urokinase in the treatment of pulmonary embolism may be taken as an example. The aim of the trial was to answer the simple question whether patients with pulmonary embolism (a common and dangerous consequence of prolonged bed-rest, in which venous thrombi forming in the legs come free and impact in the pulmonary artery) do better if treated with the fibrinolytic agent, urokinase, than with heparin. The trial involved 14 hospitals in the United States and was organized by a six member Policy Board under which worked a dozen committees, panels and sub-committees concerned with different aspects of the study. As with all multi-centre trials, careful standardization of diagnostic and investigative procedures was essential. A committee was set up to achieve this, and a visiting team had to be sent to each centre to ensure the necessary uniformity. In the course of 2 years, 160 patients entered the trial, having been selected on the basis of rigid diagnostic and age criteria. They were assigned at random to the two treatment groups—heparin (H) 78 patients, urokinase (U) 82 patients—and were subjected to an extremely detailed investigative procedure to assess the severity and progress of the disease. The main results are summarized in Table 2.1, which shows that there were six deaths in the U group and seven in the H group, an insignificant difference. The incidence of bleeding complications and repeat emboli was also similar in the two groups.

This example gives an idea of the scale of organization needed to carry out a satisfactory clinical trial

Table 2.1 Trial of urokinase *versus* heparin in treatment of pulmonary embolism

	Urokinase	Heparin
Number of patients	82	78
Deaths:		
Day 1	1	2
Day 2–14	5	5
Total	6	7
Complications:		
Bleeding		
moderate	15	10
severe	22	11
Recurrent pulmonary embolism	14	18

From: Urokinase pulmonary embolism trial (1973). Circulation 47 (supp. II)

to answer a simple and clear cut question, and also demonstrates the problem of detecting an improvement in mortality over the already low figure of 9% (in the heparin group). Because of the small numbers, the probability of a Type II error is quite large.

MEASUREMENT OF TOXICITY

During the stages of drug development that are carried out before a new compound is tested in man, extensive toxicity testing is done in various animal species and with *in vitro* systems. The simplest type of toxicity test is the LD_{50} (Lethal Dose for 50% of a group of animals), in which various doses of the drug, estimated to cover the range from 0 to 100% lethality, are administered to groups of 10 animals. The mortality in each group within a fixed period of time (say 2 days) is determined and used to construct a curve relating fractional mortality to dose. Standard statistical procedures are available (Colquhoun, 1971) for estimating the LD_{50} from such data. It is a crude and relatively uninformative test for many reasons. It measures only mortality and not sublethal toxicity; the value obtained varies widely between species and cannot be safely extrapolated to man; it measures only acute toxicity following a single administration, and not long-term toxicity; it cannot measure **idiosyncratic** reactions (i.e. reactions occurring at low dosage in a small proportion of subjects) though such reactions may be more relevant in practice than 'high dose' toxicity (see Chapters 4 & 36). An example of the weakness of the LD_{50} test as a measure of toxicity is shown in Figure 2.8. A single oral dose of indomethacin was given to groups of rats and the percentage mortality noted 24 hours and 14 days later. There was a nearly 30-fold difference in the LD_{50} according to the time at which the assessment was made, and a dose of indomethacin that was 100% lethal within 14 days caused no deaths within 24 hours. This example shows strikingly that the arbitrary choice of experimental conditions for the LD_{50} test can drastically alter the results obtained. The LD_{50} test is particularly inappropriate when used to assess the safety of substances such as food additives or cosmetics, where there is negligible likelihood of accidental poisoning. It is more appropriate for assessing the toxicity of industrial chemicals, such

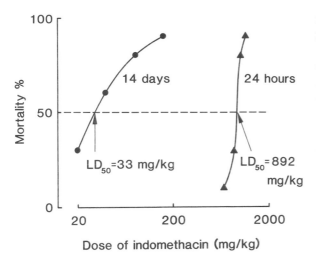

Fig. 2.8 Comparison of acute and chronic toxicity of indomethacin in mice. The LD_{50} measured 24 hours after dosing is 27 times larger than the LD_{50} measured at 14 days. Variability is also much less for the acute test, shown by the steeper curve. (From: Beyer, 1978)

as insecticides, or of drugs that are likely to be taken in large overdose, though species differences greatly limit its usefulness even in these applications. The continuing widespread use of the LD_{50} test is due mainly to the stringent requirements of national regulatory bodies. A recent Home Office report on the LD_{50} test concluded that although some rough measure of acute toxicity in animals was needed for many substances, a simple 'limit' test, aimed at determining the effect on animals of the largest dose likely to be administered to a human being, would often suffice. By dispensing with unnecessary precision, the report argued, the number of animals used for measurement of LD_{50} could be considerably reduced.

Toxicity takes many forms, and cannot be measured purely in terms of increased mortality. The battery of tests through which potential new drugs are put during their development is designed to reveal many types of toxicity that are known to occur in man, and regulatory authorities require extensive and detailed studies of animal toxicity before they will grant a licence for testing in man and eventual sale of a new drug. Public opinion is inclined to demand the unattainable, namely a *certainty* that a drug lacks toxicity when used under clinical conditions, before any drug is released for widespread use. But, as Witts has pointed out 'the

final test of the safety of a drug is in fact its release for general use'.

Two factors in particular make it unrealistic to expect studies on animals and human volunteers to serve as a complete safeguard against toxicity in clinical use. First, only such effects as are looked for are likely to be found. In 1960, when thalidomide was developed, the possibility of drug-induced foetal malformations (teratogenesis) had not yet been recognized, and the animal tests used at that time did not anticipate this form of toxicity; nor was there any likelihood of discovering it from studies on human volunteers. Discovery came only as a result of astute clinical detective work, about a year after the drug had been released and very successfully promoted. Once recognized, the effect can be tested for in animals, and future disasters on the thalidomide scale* are highly unlikely. However, unsuspected types of toxicity will continue to appear, and are exemplified by the syndrome of sclerosing peritonitis produced by practolol, and the increased incidence of thrombotic disorders in women taking oral contraceptives.

Secondly, toxic effects may occur only in a very small proportion of patients. Thus, an effect occurring in 1 in 1000 individuals will escape detection in a clinical trial on a few hundred patients, but may be of considerable clinical importance. For example, phenylbutazone (an anti-inflammatory drug: see Chapter 9) causes, as a rare side effect, aplastic anaemia, which has a high mortality. Phenylbutazone is estimated to kill 22 patients out of every million treated with the drug, and to be responsible for about 30 deaths annually in England and Wales. It is obvious that such an infrequent event could not be discovered by any kind of preliminary trial in man. In common with other types of idiosyncratic reaction, it does not seem to become any more frequent if the dose of the drug is increased, so would also escape detection in high-dose toxicity tests in animals. The recognition that animal studies and clinical trials cannot completely eliminate the risk of toxic effects when the drug is released for general clinical use has necessitated the

---

* An estimated 10 000 children born with severe malformations. (See: Sjostrom 1972)

development of various **monitoring** schemes, which are intended to facilitate detection of toxicity. In nearly all developed countries there is an official regulatory body (known in Britain as the Committee on the Safety of Medicines) which undertakes such monitoring, relying mainly on voluntary reporting by doctors of incidents that they think may be the result of adverse reactions to drugs. In Britain, about 3000 such reports are received annually and the aim is that classification of reported incidents by drug and by type of reaction will reveal rare forms of toxicity, such as the phenylbutazone example mentioned above. This type of surveillance was introduced in most countries shortly after the thalidomide tragedy and it has been instrumental in drawing attention to several important types of drug toxicity. The increased incidence of thrombosis in women taking high-oestrogen contraceptive pills, and the occurrence of sclerosing peritonitis and ocular damage caused by the practolol, were first detected in this way. The function of monitoring is to sound an alarm; because of the haphazard origin of the data, it cannot by itself provide convincing evidence of toxicity. The next stage is therefore an epidemiological study designed to discover whether or not the incidence of the suspected type of reaction is actually enhanced in patients treated with the drug.

THERAPEUTIC INDEX

Ehrlich recognized that a drug must be judged not only by its useful properties, but also by its toxic effects, and he expressed the therapeutic usefulness of a drug in terms of the ratio between the minimum effective dose and the maximum tolerated dose.

$$\text{i.e. Therapeutic index} = \frac{\text{Maximum non-toxic dose}}{\text{Minimum effective dose}}$$

Unfortunately the variability between individuals is not taken into account in this definition. Even if we could measure the maximum tolerated dose and minimum effective dose in one individual, others would give different results, and it is quite possible that the effective dose in some individuals will be toxic to others.

A widely-used definition which takes into account individual variation is:

$$\text{Therapeutic index} = \frac{LD_{50}}{ED_{50}}$$

This definition has the advantage that the relevant quantities are measurable (though LD_{50} can only be measured in animals) and it gives some idea of the margin of safety in use of a drug, by drawing attention to the importance of the *relative* toxic and effective doses of a drug. Therapeutic index is, however, very rarely quoted as a number, for it can be highly misleading as a guide to the safety of a drug in clinical use. There are several reasons for this:

1. LD_{50} is not a good guide to toxicity, since it is based only on mortality in animals. The kind of adverse effect that, in practice, limits the clinical usefulness of a drug, is likely to be overlooked in the LD_{50} test.
2. ED_{50} is often not definable, since it depends on what measure of effectiveness is used. Analgesic drugs, for example, may need to be given in different dosages according to the nature and severity of the pain. The ED_{50} for aspirin used for a mild headache would be much lower than the value for aspirin as an anti-rheumatic drug.
3. Some very important forms of toxicity are **idiosyncratic** (i.e. only a small proportion of individuals are susceptible; see Chapter 4). In other cases, toxicity depends greatly on the clinical state of the patient. Thus, propranolol is dangerous to an asthmatic patient in doses that are harmless to a normal individual. More generally, we can say that wide individual variation (see Chapter 4) in either the effective dose or the toxic dose of a drug make it inherently less predictable, and therefore less safe, though this is not reflected in the therapeutic index.

These shortcomings mean that therapeutic index is of little value as a measure of the clinical usefulness of a drug, and it has often been pointed out that digoxin is a most useful drug in spite of its unfavourable therapeutic index. Therapeutic index has rather more relevance as a measure of the impunity with which an overdose may be given. Thus, one reason why the benzodiazepines have replaced barbiturates as hypnotic drugs (see

Chapter 21) is that their therapeutic index is very large compared with barbiturates, so they are much less likely to kill when taken in accidental or deliberate overdose.

In summary, though the therapeutic index expresses a valid general concept, it provides no measure of the actual usefulness of a drug. It is well to be suspicious of mathematically defined quantities that cannot be enumerated.

CHEMICAL ASSAY METHODS

Until about 20 years ago chemical assay methods were generally too insensitive to be of much use in pharmacology, but there are now several analytical methods whose sensitivity and specificity match or exceed that of bioassay. The most important of these techniques are:

1. Radioimmunoassay (RIA) and related types of saturation analysis
2. Gas chromatography and mass-spectrometry (GCMS)
3. High performance liquid chromatography (HPLC)
4. Fluorimetry.

Radioimmunoassay (RIA)

RIA was first developed in 1960 for the assay of insulin. The principle is simple (Fig. 2.9). The requirements are: (a) an antibody which combines specifically and with high affinity with the substance to be assayed; (b) a radioactively labelled version of the substance to be assayed; and (c) a method for separating antibody-bound from free material in the solution.

The unknown sample is added to a tube containing a fixed amount of antibody and a fixed amount of the radioactive standard. If the sample has a high content of the test substance, the amount of radioactive standard bound to the antibody is reduced (Fig. 2.10). There is thus an inverse relationship between the amount of bound radioactivity and the amount of the test substance in the unknown sample. Construction of a standard curve with known amounts of the test substance allows the amount in the unknown samples to be calculated.

Obtaining a suitable antibody is the most problematical part. Most drug molecules are not antigenic, but can be made so by coupling them covalently to a protein such as serum albumin. When such a complex is injected many different antibodies are produced, only a few of which will react with the drug molecule on its own, and some of these may bind with too low affinity to be useful. Much trial and error is usually involved, though the growing use of monoclonal antibodies, which can be produced in large quantities *in vitro*, will greatly facilitate the process. It may not be necessary to use an antibody at all if another type of high affinity binding protein is available. Thus, thyroxine can be assayed with thyroglobulin as the binding protein, and steroids can be assayed by means of the high affinity cytoplasmic receptor (see Chapter 1) to which they bind in cells. In this case the method is referred to as 'radioreceptor assay'.

Producing a radioactively labelled version of the substance to be assayed is usually straightforward. Most proteins and peptides can be labelled by substitution of ^{125}I into tyrosine residues without much loss of biological activity, and small molecules can often be labelled by synthesis from radioactive starting materials.

Efficient separation of the bound and free radioactivity in the assay mixture is essential. Many methods have been devised, including gel filtration, addition of activated charcoal or finely divided silicates to extract the free ligand. Alternatively, the antibody may be precipitated by addition of a suitable anti-IgG (double antibody method) or it may be covalently attached to a solid support (such as the wall of the assay tube) thus obviating the need for a separation step.

Enzyme-linked immunoassay (EIA) is a variant of RIA in which the label used is an enzyme rather than a radioisotope (Fig. 2.9). In the simplest type of EIA the enzyme-coupled derivative (E–X) of the substance to be assayed is prepared, by a covalent coupling reaction, and a standard quantity is added to the assay mixture together with antibody and the sample to be assayed. The amount of E–X that combines with Ab will depend on the amount of X in the sample. Usually, the enzymic activity of E–X–Ab is much less than that of E–X, so that no separation step is required. All that is needed is a simple (usually photometric) measure of enzyme

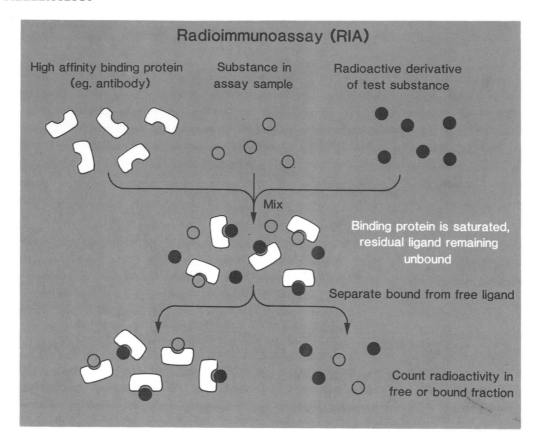

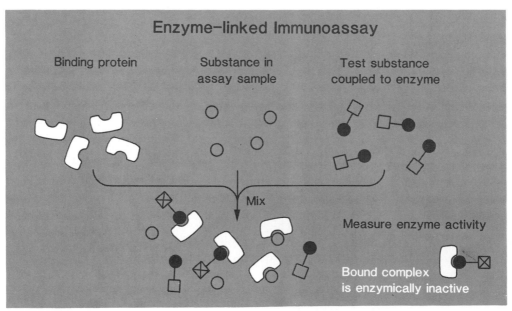

Fig. 2.9 The principle of immunoassay. With radioimmunoassay (top panel) separation of the bound and free ligand is necessary before the final measurement. With enzyme-linked immunoassay (bottom panel) separation is not needed, nor is any radioactive material used, so the technique is usually quicker and safer than radioimmunoassay.

activity in the mixture. The more X is present, the greater the amount of free E–X and the greater the enzymic activity. An assay of this type, known as EMIT (enzyme multiplied immunoassay technique) has been developed for the antiepileptic drug phenytoin (see Chapter 24). The drug can be coupled to glucose-6-phosphate dehydrogenase (G6PDH). Enzyme activity is lost when the complex binds to antibodies raised against phenytoin, and is very simply measured by a photometric technique. This type of assay is now in routine clinical use for monitoring phenytoin in plasma during anti-epileptic therapy.

Some examples of immunoassays that are useful in pharmacology are given in Table 2.2.

Table 2.2 Some clinically important drugs measurable by radioimmunoassay

Adriamycin	Morphine
Bleomycin	Nortryptiline
Carbamazepine	Pethidine
Chlorpromazine	Phenobarbitone
Cytosine arabinoside	Phenytoin
Diazepam	Prednisolone
Digitoxin	Procainamide
Digoxin	Propranolol
Ethosuximide	Quinidine
Imipramine	Tetrahydrocannabinol
Lignocaine	

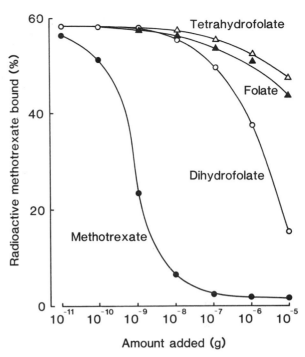

Fig. 2.10 Radioimmunoassay of the anti-tumour drug, methotrexate in plasma. The antibody used in this assay was raised against a methotrexate-protein conjugate. It binds methotrexate with very high affinity, enabling less than 1 ng to be assayed in a blood sample. Cross-reaction with folate derivatives, which occur endogenously and are chemically very similar to methotrexate, is slight. Dihydrofolate binds with less than 1/1000 the affinity of methotrexate, and the other two analogues even less. (Data from: Paxton J W, 1978)

As with any assay method, the most important characteristics by which immunoassays have to be judged are (a) **sensitivity** and (b) **specificity**. In general, the sensitivity of immunoassays is high, because antibody affinity is usually sufficiently high that effective competition between standard and sample occurs at very low concentrations, and also because radioactivity can be measured with very high sensitivity. In the case of enzyme-linked assays, the fact that one enzyme molecule gives rise to many molecules of product greatly enhances the overall sensitivity. Many immunoassays can work in the range 10^{-14}–10^{-12} moles, which makes them among the most sensitive assay methods currently available.

Where the technique is used for assay of blood or tissue concentrations of drugs at various times after systemic administration, it is important to ascertain that metabolites of the parent compound do not cross-react appreciably in the assay. If the likely metabolites are known, this can be checked directly, but difficulties can arise when the technique is used with drugs whose metabolic fate is not fully known. An example of an assay of very high specificity is shown in Figure 2.10. The assay was designed to measure the plasma concentration of methotrexate, a cytotoxic drug that very closely resembles the natural metabolite dihydrofolic acid (see Chapter 29). It was important to check that naturally-occurring folic acid derivatives did not cross-react, and Figure 2.10 shows that the assay was about 1000 times as sensitive to methotrexate as to di-hydrofolic acid, and even less sensitive to other folic acid derivatives.

Chromatographic techniques

Chromatography provides a versatile repertoire of techniques for achieving separation of different chemical substances. Coupled with a detector of sufficient sensitivity, chromatography provides the basis for many useful assay systems.

The basic principle by which chemical separation is achieved is common to all types of chromatography. The **stationary phase** consists of particles of a substance such as resin, cellulose or alumina packed into a tube through which the **mobile phase** flows. The mobile phase is a liquid (usually an aqueous solution) or a gas, into which is introduced the sample containing the substances to be separated. Separation occurs because the stationary phase either binds, or selectively excludes, substances present in the sample. If binding occurs, for example in **ion-exchange chromatography** when the stationary phase possesses fixed negatively charged groups and the sample contains a basic substance, the sample will be retarded relative to the solvent as the solution flows through the column. The more it is bound to the stationary phase the longer it will take to emerge. Many chemical factors, such as molecular size, pK_a, hydrophobicity etc, will affect the degree of binding, and hence separation of the different chemical species occurs as they pass through the column. A **gel filtration** column works the other way round, by partially or completely excluding the molecules of the test substance from the stationary phase, on the basis of their molecular size. The stationary phase consists of particles, usually of a crosslinked carbohydrate, whose water-filled interstices are sufficiently narrow that large molecules, such as proteins, are partly or completely excluded and remain confined to the mobile phase.

With such a column large molecules pass through quickly while small molecules, which are in diffusional equilibrium with the water-filled crevices of the gel particles, travel more slowly.

The main drawback of conventional liquid chromatography as a routine assay method is its slowness. The need for full equilibration of the distribution of the test substance between the mobile and the stationary phase to occur at each point in the column limits the rate of flow that can be used, and a single run usually takes several hours. Two technical advances, namely **gas chromatography** and **high performance liquid chromatography** have succeeded in overcoming this problem and reducing the run time from hours to minutes, thus greatly increasing the usefulness of the method for routine assays.

Gas chromatography (GC)

The diffusion rate of molecules in a gaseous as opposed to a liquid medium is so much higher, particularly if the temperature is increased, that the column flow rate can be greatly increased, allowing separation to be achieved in a few minutes. The obvious drawback is that the test substance must be volatile, and most drugs are not. They can, however, often be converted to volatile derivatives by reactions such as esterification, or sometimes simply by controlled thermal decomposition (pyrolysis), and GC is now very widely used to measure the concentration of drugs and drug metabolites in

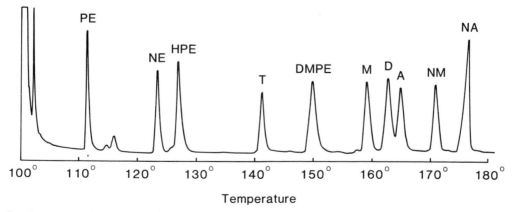

Fig. 2.11 Gas chromatography of catecholamine derivatives after conversion to volatile derivatives. The compounds are displaced from the column by gradually raising the temperature at 1.5°/min, so the whole run took about 60 minutes. PE = phenylethylamine; NE = norephedrine; HPE = hydroxyphenylethylamine; T = tyramine; DMPE = dimethoxyphenylethylamine; M = metanephrine; D = dopamine; A = adrenaline; NM = normetanephrine; NA = noradrenaline. (From: Capella & Horning, 1966)

body fluids for studies of drug metabolism and pharmacokinetics. It is also used as a preliminary separation procedure for samples that are to be analysed by mass spectrometry (see below). Its main limitations are that quite elaborate sample preparation may be needed to produce a suitable volatile derivative, and that it is unsuitable for substances, such as proteins, which cannot be rendered volatile, or for substances that are unstable at the temperatures (up to a few hundred degrees centigrade) at which GC columns operate efficiently. An example of the high resolution that can be achieved with GC is shown in Figure 2.11.

High performance liquid chromatography (HPLC)

In this modification of conventional liquid chromatography the improvement is brought about mainly by reducing the particle size of the stationary phase (to 5–20 µm), so as to reduce the diffusion distance, and hence speed up equilibration of the test molecules between the two phases. To achieve adequate flow rates through such tightly packed columns requires high pressures, and the plumbing, pumps and sample injection devices need to be engineered with great precision. HPLC overcomes many of the drawbacks of GC, however, and its greater range of applicability has led to its widespread use in pharmacology. The increase in speed and resolution compared with conventional liquid chromatography is impressive, and has meant that HPLC can be used for many routine analytical procedures. Figure 2.12 shows the analysis of a sample of 'heroin' from an illicit dealer. Heroin itself (diacetylmorphine, peak 6) amounts to only about 40%, the rest consisting partly of hydrolysis products (morphine and monoacetylmorphine) and partly of other contaminants (mainly caffeine). To calculate the amount of substances present from the peaks in UV absorption that are used for monitoring requires calibration based on the UV absorption coefficient of the substances that are present; in Figure 2.12 the proportion of heroin is actually greater than it looks because of its low absorbance at the monitoring wavelength used.

Mass spectrometry

In a mass spectrometer the substance is converted

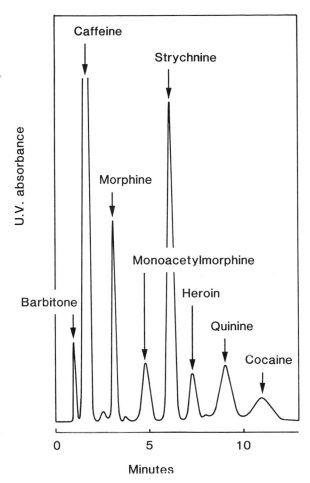

Fig. 2.12 HPLC analysis of materials found in illicit heroin samples. To obtain a quantitative estimate standards must be tested to give a conversion factor relating concentration to UV absorbance.

to a volatile form, introduced into an evacuated chamber, and then ionized. The resulting ions are accelerated in an electric field, as a beam, which is deflected, usually by applying a transverse magnetic field. The degree of deflection of individual ions depends on the ratio of their mass to their charge (m/e ratio), those with the largest m/e ratio being deflected least. At the end of the instrument is a narrow slit through which a slice of the ion beam passes to a detector which measures its intensity at any moment. The basic plan of the instrument is shown in Figure 2.13. In most instruments the strength of the magnetic field is varied in a scanning fashion, so that the beam of ions separated according to their m/e ratios sweeps across the detec-

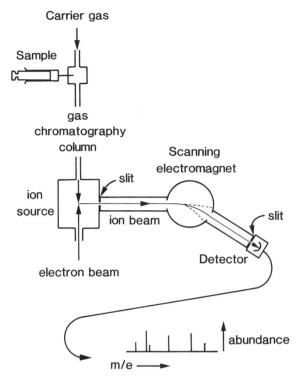

Fig. 2.13 Diagram of gas chromatography–mass spectrometry (GCMS) equipment. The sample emerges from the gas chromatography column, which achieves an initial fractionation, into the ionization chamber. The ion beam is continually scanned by a varying magnetic field which deflects individual particles according to their mass/charge (m/e) ratio, producing a pattern of peaks at the detector. The height of each peak is proportional to the abundance of each ion in the beam.

tor slit in sequence. Very precise scanning can be achieved, which enables the instrument to distinguish easily ions whose mass differs by much less than 1 dalton. Detectors can also be made extremely sensitive, allowing samples containing as little as 10^{-12}–10^{-15} mole of the test substance to be assayed, a sensitivity that very few bioassays can match.

For most biological applications the sample is first put through a GC column, the outlet of which is connected directly to the inlet of the mass spectrometer. This combined GCMS technique means that the sample is considerably purified before being subjected to MS analysis. Without this preliminary step, most biological samples would produce an uninterpretable forest of peaks because of the multitude of substances present. Even with the GC step it is usually necessary to carry out some preliminary

chemical purification before the sample is introduced, so GCMS, though uniquely powerful in its selectivity and sensitivity, is a technically demanding and expensive method.

A useful method for quantifying the output from a GCMS system, so that the amount of substance present in the original sample can be calculated from the size of the peak, involves the use of an **internal standard**. This is a pure sample of the substance being assayed, or of a closely related substance, labelled with an isotope such as deuterium or carbon-13. A known amount of the standard is added to the sample at the beginning of the analysis, and the mixture is carried through the whole preparative procedure. Because the standard is *chemically* the same as the test substance, though *isotopically* distinct, the proportion of the two will not change during the procedure, even though substantial preparative losses may occur. The isotopic difference means that the standard will produce a separate peak in the mass spectrometer, and the amount of the test substance in the original sample can be determined simply from the ratio of the test and standard peaks, knowing the amount of standard that was added.

An example of the use of GCMS to assay acetylcholine at very high sensitivity is shown in Figure 2.14. In this procedure, controlled heating is used to convert acetylcholine to a volatile tertiary amine, dimethylaminoethanol acetate. The GC stage separates this from other amines formed from substances, such as choline, which may also be present. Electron impact in the mass spectrometer breaks the amine into ionized fragments, the main one being $(CH_3)_2NCH_2^+$ (m/e ratio = 58). The fully deuterated internal standard undergoes the same reaction to produce a fragment $(CD_3)_2NCD_2^+$ of m/e ratio 66. The two traces in Figure 2.14 show the simultaneous monitoring of the appearance of peaks at m/e 58 and 66. The acetylcholine peak (B) at m/e 58 emerges from the gas chromatograph simultaneously with the internal standard (A) at m/e 66. The later peak (C) at m/e 58 represents contamination with propionylcholine. This produces the same ionized pyrolysis product as acetylcholine in the mass spectrometer, but is retarded more than acetylcholine on the gas chromatograph column, resulting in clear separation. The very high sensitivity of the method can be appreciated from the

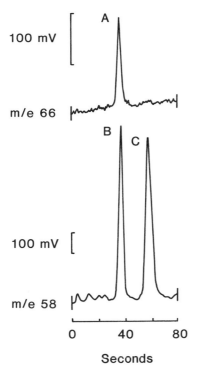

100 mV

m/e 66

A

B   C

100 mV

m/e 58

0   40   80

Seconds

Fig. 2.14 GCMS analysis of choline esters. The traces were obtained by monitoring the efflux from the GC column at two m/e ratios. The peak at m/e ratio 66 (A) is the product of the standard of deuterium labelled ACh. Unlabelled ACh (5 pmol) gives a product of m/e ratio 58 (peak B). The later peak (C) at this m/e ratio comes from propionylcholine (5 pmol) in the sample, which passes more slowly through the GC column, but gives rise on pyrolysis in the MS ionization chamber to the same ion (m/e ratio 58) as ACh. Assay of such small quantities of these closely similar compounds would be extremely difficult by any other technique. (From: Polak & Molenaar, 1979)

large acetylcholine peak, which represents only 5 pmol (about 1 ng).

GCMS methods have been applied to many different pharmacological problems with great success. Unfortunately the equipment is still too costly, and the procedures usually too complex and time-consuming, for the method to be widely available for routine assay work.

Spectrophotometry and fluorimetry

The fact that molecules can absorb energy from photons provides the basis for many analytical techniques that have found pharmacological application. In **absorption spectrophotometry** the amount of light emerging after passing through a standard sized cell containing a chemical solution is measured. The fraction of light absorbed, which is estimated by comparing the intensity of the emergent beam with that of the incident beam, depends on: (a) the nature of the absorbing compound; (b) its concentration and the length of the light-path through the solution; and (c) the wavelength of the light. Because of the wavelength specificity of particular chemical groups, substances may be distinguished by the differing shapes of their absorption spectrum, and this can be used to distinguish changes in a particular chemical component in a mixture. Where high sensitivity is not important, the simplicity of absorption spectroscopy is a great advantage, and the technique is widely used. For many drugs the concentration needed to give a satisfactory absorption signal for assay purposes is in the range 3–30 µM (roughly 1–10 µg/ml).

When a molecule absorbs a photon, the energy causes one of its electrons to move into an unstable higher energy state. This 'excited' state persists only for a very brief time (10^{-8}–10^{-7} sec) and the molecule recovers by releasing the energy in the form of another photon, of lower energy (i.e. longer wavelength) than the one that was absorbed. These emitted photons can be detected as fluorescence by a sensitive, wavelength-selective photomultiplier tube. **Fluorescence spectrophotometry** (fluorimetry) is both more sensitive and more selective than absorption spectrophotometry. It is more sensitive (Table 2.3) because only a minute fraction of the incident light needs to be absorbed. By using a strong enough incident beam a detectable fluorescence signal can be produced even though the large majority of incident photons pass straight through without being absorbed. It is somewhat more selective because both the absorption spectrum and the emission spectrum vary in shape (i.e. show maxima at different wavelengths) with different substances, so that discrimination between substances can be optimized by adjusting the wavelength of both the incident beam and the detector. Although all molecules, in principle, show the property of fluorescence, its strength varies greatly and in practice the molecule must possess a suitably substituted aromatic ring to provide a measurable signal. The solvent, pH, and the presence of other substances dissolved in it can all affect the fluorescence signal, but the technique is nevertheless a

Table 2.3 Sensitivity of absorbance and fluorescence assays. Data from: Richens & Marks (1981)

Drug	Approximate therapeutic plasma concentration (μM)	Approximate sensitivity limits	
		Absorbance (μM)	Fluorescence (μM)
Aspirin	250	10	0.05
Chloroquine	0.4	7	0.15
Desmethylimipramine	0.2	15	0.4
Isoniazid	30	15	0.7
Methotrexate	0.8	4	0.04
Procainamide	20	10	0.04
Quinine	15	12	0.006
Tetracycline	5	8	0.05

very versatile and sensitive one, with many pharmacological uses. Table 2.3 compares the sensitivities of absorption and fluorescence assays for some common drugs, and shows that therapeutic plasma concentrations are generally in the working range of fluorescence assays, but are often too low for absorption assays.

Fluorescence assays may be made even more sensitive by chemically modifying the assay substance in order to enhance its fluorescence. Noradrenaline, for example, is only weakly fluorescent, but can be reacted with ethylenediamine to give a highly fluorescent condensation product. This has formed the basis of a widely-used assay for measuring the catecholamine content of tissues and body fluids. Histamine is routinely assayed by a similar method, whereas serotonin is sufficiently fluorescent to be assayed without derivatization. With all of these endogenous amines the replacement of cumbersome bioassay methods by fluorimetric assays was essential before their tissue distribution and metabolism could be studied in detail.

REFERENCES AND FURTHER READING

Armitage P 1978 Sequential clinical trials. Blackwell, Oxford
Burn J H, Finney D J, Goodwin L G 1950 Biological standardization. Oxford University Press, Oxford
Colquhoun D 1971 Lecture notes on biostatistics. Oxford University Press, Oxford
Finney D J 1964 Statistical method in biological assay. Griffin, London
Harris E L, Fitzgerald J D (eds) 1970 The principles and practice of clinical trials. Churchill Livingstone, Edinburgh
Miller J N 1982 Developments in non-isotopic immunoassay. Nature 295: xiii
Myerscough P R, Schild H O 1958 Quantitative assays of oxytocic drugs on the human post-partum uterus. Br J Pharmacol 13: 207
Paxton J W 1981 Development of radioimmunoassays for drugs. Methods Find Exp Clin Pharmacol 3: 105–117
Richens A, Marks V 1981 Therapeutic drug monitoring. Churchill Livingstone, Edinburgh
Schwartz D, Flamant R, Lellouch J 1980 Clinical trials. Academic Press, London
Sjostrom N 1972 Thalidomide and the power of the drug companies. Penguin, London
Watson J T 1976 Introduction to mass spectrometry: biomedical, environmental and forensic applications. Raven Press, New York
Wisdom G B 1976 Enzyme-immunoassay. Clin Chem 22: 1243–1255
Yalow R S 1980 Radioimmunoassay. Ann Rev Biophys Bioeng 9: 327–345

Absorption, distribution and fate of drugs

The action of any drug requires the presence of an adequate concentration in the fluid bathing the target tissue. In most cases the time course of a drug's action simply reflects the time course of the rise and fall of its concentration at the target tissue. The exceptions to this are certain 'hit and run' drugs, which act irreversibly, or almost so, and whose effects remain after the concentration has dropped to zero. Examples are drugs which kill cells, or render them incapable of division, or inactivate an enzyme or receptor irreversibly. In this chapter the relationship between the administration of a drug, the time course of its distribution and the magnitude of the concentration attained in different regions of the body is discussed. This part of pharmacology is termed **pharmacokinetics** (what the body does to the drug), to distinguish it from **pharmacodynamics** (what the drug does to the body). The distinction is a useful one, though the words might cause dismay to an etymological purist.

The two fundamental processes which determine the concentration of a drug at any moment and in any region of the body are (a) **translocation of drug molecules** and (b) **chemical transformation of drug molecules**. It is only by the movement of molecules or by the formation or disappearance of molecules that the concentration of a drug in any given region can change.

In the first part of this chapter we discuss these two basic processes, and in the second part we consider particular tissues and organs in more detail with emphasis on the different routes of administration and the different patterns of drug distribution that are possible. The third part sets out some quantitative principles which are helpful in interpreting pharmacokinetic data and in predicting how different drugs will behave in practice.

TRANSLOCATION OF DRUG MOLECULES

Drug molecules move around the body in two ways:

1. By **bulk flow transfer** (i.e. in the bloodstream)
2. By **diffusional transfer** (i.e. molecule-by-molecule, over short distances).

With bulk flow transfer the chemical nature of the drug molecules makes no difference. The cardiovascular system provides a very fast long-distance distribution system for all solutes irrespective of their chemical nature. In general, what distinguishes one drug pharmacokinetically from another are its **diffusional** characteristics, in particular its ability to cross the non-aqueous diffusion barriers, composed of cell membranes that separate the various aqueous compartments of the body (i.e. plasma, interstitial fluid, intracellular fluid, and transcellular fluid: see Fig. 3.11). Aqueous diffusion must, of course, occur as part of the overall mechanism of drug transport, since it is this process which delivers drug molecules to and from the non-aqueous barriers. The rate of diffusion of a substance depends mainly on its molecular size, the diffusion coefficient for small molecules being inversely proportional to the square root of molecular weight. Thus, large molecules diffuse more slowly than small ones but the variation with molecular weight is relatively slight. The great majority of drugs fall within the molecular weight range 200–1000, and variations in aqueous diffusion rate have only a small effect on their overall pharmacokinetic properties. Thus, for most purposes we can regard the body as a series of interconnected **well-stirred compartments** within which the drug concentration remains uniform. It is the movement *between* compartments, which generally involves the penetration of non-aqueous diffusion barriers, that determines where, and for how long, a drug will be present in the body after it has been administered. The analysis of drug movements with the help of a simple compartmental model is discussed in a later section (see p. 81).

THE MOVEMENT OF DRUG MOLECULES ACROSS CELLULAR BARRIERS

The barriers between aqueous compartments in the body consist of cell membranes. A single layer of membrane separates the intracellular from the extracellular compartments. An epithelial barrier, such as that represented by the gastrointestinal mucosa or the renal tubule, consists of a layer of cells tightly connected to each other so that molecules must traverse two layers of membrane to pass from one side to the other. The vascular endothelium constitutes a slightly more complicated type of barrier. In most parts of the body there are gaps between the endothelial cells of the capillaries, which are large enough to permit small molecules to cross by aqueous diffusion, but too small to allow molecules exceeding about 30 000 molecular weight (i.e. most protein molecules) to pass through. In some vascular beds, especially those of the central nervous system and the placenta, the capillary endothelium is continuous, and penetration by drug molecules involves the crossing of the endothelial cell membrane, an important detail which makes these vascular beds quite distinct from those of other organs, with major pharmacokinetic consequences.

In general, there are four main ways by which small molecules cross cell membranes (Fig. 3.1)

(a) By diffusing through the **lipid**
(b) By diffusing through **aqueous pores** that traverse the lipid
(c) By combination with a **carrier molecule** which

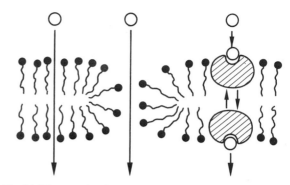

Fig. 3.1 Diagram showing routes by which solutes can traverse cell membranes.

acts as a ferry-boat across the lipid region of the membrane
(d) By **pinocytosis**.

Of these routes diffusion through lipid (a) and carrier-mediated transport (c) are particularly important in relation to pharmacokinetic mechanisms; diffusion through aqueous pores (b) is unimportant in this context. It is postulated that these pores, whose existence is somewhat controversial, account for the high permeability of most cell membranes to small polar molecules, such as water and urea. Their estimated diameter, about 0.4 nm, is too small for most drug molecules, whose minimum diameter is seldom less than about 1 nm. Pinocytosis (d) involves the invagination of a part of the cell membrane and the trapping within the cell of a small vesicle containing extracellular constituents. The vesicle contents can then be released within the cell, or extruded from the other side of the cell. This mechanism appears to be important for the transport of some macromolecules but there is no evidence that it contributes appreciably to movements of small molecules. Mechanisms (a) and (c) will now be discussed in more detail; mechanisms (b) and (d) will not be considered further.

Diffusion through lipid

Non-polar substances (i.e. substances within whose molecules the electrons are uniformly distributed, with the result that there is no separation of positive and negative charges within the molecule) dissolve

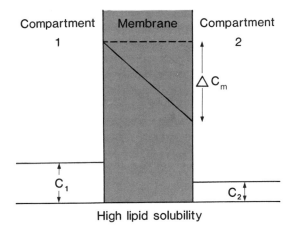

High lipid solubility

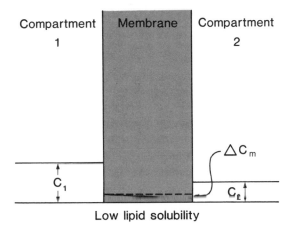

Low lipid solubility

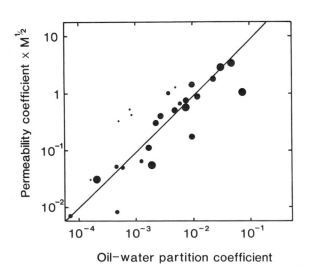

Oil−water partition coefficient

freely in non-polar solvents, such as lipids, and therefore penetrate cell membranes very freely, by diffusion. The **permeability coefficient, P,** for a substance diffusing passively through a membrane is given by the number of molecules crossing the membrane per unit area, per unit time and per unit concentration difference across the membrane. It is clear that permeant molecules must be present within the membrane in sufficient numbers, and that they must be mobile within the membrane if rapid permeation is to occur. Thus two chemical factors contribute to P, namely **solubility** in the membrane (which can be expressed as a **partition coefficient** for the substance distributed between the membrane phase and the aqueous environment), and **diffusivity**, which is a measure of the mobility of molecules within the lipid and is expressed as a **diffusion coefficient.** Among different drug molecules the diffusion coefficient varies only slightly, as noted above, so the most important variable is the partition coefficient (Fig. 3.2). There is thus a close correlation between lipid solubility and the permeability of the cell membrane to different substances. For this reason lipid solubility is one of the most important determinants of the pharmacokinetic characteristics of a drug, and many properties, such as rate of absorption from the gut, penetration into the brain and other tissues, and duration of action can be predicted from knowledge of a drug's lipid solubility.

pH and ionization

One important complicating factor in relation to membrane permeation is that many drugs are weak

Fig. 3.2 The importance of lipid solubility in membrane permeation. The upper and middle diagrams show the concentration profile in a lipid membrane separating two aqueous compartments. A lipid soluble drug (upper diagram) is subject to a much larger transmembrane concentration gradient (ΔC_m) than a lipid-insoluble drug (middle diagram). It therefore diffuses more rapidly even though the aqueous concentration gradient ($C_1 - C_2$) is the same in both cases. *Bottom.* Permeability of plant cells to organic non-electrolytes of varying molecular volume (indicated by size of points). There is a linear relationship between $P \times M^{\frac{1}{2}}$ and lipid solubility, which applies irrespective of the molecular volume. The $M^{\frac{1}{2}}$ term corrects approximately for the variation of the free diffusion coefficient with molecular size. This data shows that for organic non-electrolytes, permeation involves diffusion through lipid rather than traversing pores of a fixed size.

acids or bases, and can therefore exist in both unionized and ionized form, the ratio of the two forms varying with pH.

For a weak base, the ionization reaction is:

$$BH^+ \overset{K_a}{\rightleftharpoons} B + H^+$$

and the dissociation constant pK_a is given by the Henderson–Hasselbalch equation:

$$pK_a = pH + \log_{10}\frac{[BH^+]}{[B]}$$

For a weak acid:

$$AH \overset{K_a}{\rightleftharpoons} A^- + H^+$$

$$pK_a = pH + \log_{10}\frac{[AH]}{[A^-]}$$

In either case the ionized species, BH^+ or A^-, has very low lipid solubility and is virtually unable to permeate membranes except, rarely, where a specific transport mechanism exists. The lipid solubility of the uncharged species, B or AH, will depend on the chemical nature of the drug; for the majority of

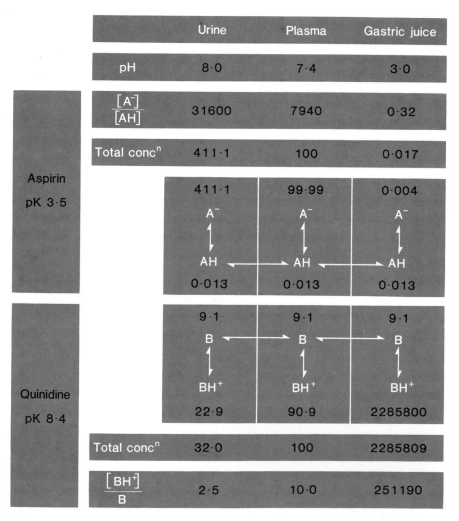

Fig. 3.3 Theoretical partition of a weak acid (aspirin) and a weak base (quinidine) between aqueous compartments (urine, plasma and gastric juice) according to the pH difference between them. Numbers represent relative concentrations (Total plasma concentration = 100). It is assumed that the uncharged species in each case can permeate the cellular barrier separating the compartments, and thus reaches the same concentration throughout. Variations in the fractional ionization as a function of pH give rise to the large total concentration differences with respect to the plasma.

drugs the uncharged species is sufficiently lipid-soluble to permit rapid membrane permeation, though there are exceptions (e.g. the group of antibiotics related to streptomycin) where even the uncharged molecule is insufficiently lipid soluble to cross membranes appreciably. This is usually due to a preponderance of hydrogen-bonding groups, such as hydroxyls, which render the uncharged molecule hydrophilic.

pH partition and ion trapping

Ionization affects not only the rate at which drugs permeate membranes, but also the steady state distribution of drug molecules between aqueous compartments if a pH difference exists between them. The diagram in Figure 3.3 shows the distribution of a weak acid (aspirin, $pK_a = 3.5$) and a weak base (quinine, $pK_a = 8.4$) between compartments buffered at different pH. Within each compartment the ratio of ionized to unionized drug is governed by the pK_a and the pH of that compartment, according to the Henderson–Hasselbalch equation. It is assumed that the unionized species can cross the membrane, and therefore reaches an equal concentration in each compartment. The ionized species is assumed not to cross at all. The result is that at equilibrium the total (ionized + unionized) concentration of the drug will be different in each compartment, with an acidic drug being concentrated in the compartment with high pH, and vice versa.

In Figure 3.3 the central compartment (pH 7.4) represents the plasma/extracellular fluid; the left hand compartment (pH 8) represents the renal tubular lumen under conditions when an alkaline urine is being produced; the right hand compartment (pH 3) represents the gastric lumen under conditions of acid secretion. It can be seen that the theoretical maximum effect of ion trapping can be very large indeed. Aspirin would be concentrated more than four-fold with respect to plasma in an alkaline renal tubule, and about 6000-fold in plasma with respect to the acidic gastric contents. The theoretical equilibrium state shown in Figure 3.3 is actually unlikely to be achieved in reality, for two main reasons. Firstly the assumption of total impermeability to the charged species is not realistic, and even a small permeability will considerably attenu-

ate the concentration difference that can be reached. Secondly, body compartments rarely approach equilibrium. Thus, neither the gastric contents nor the renal tubular fluid stands still. There is a continuous flow of glomerular fluid (in which the drug concentration will roughly equal that of plasma) into the tubule, and a flow of urine out of it. The flux of drug molecules into and out of the tubule as a result of this bulk flow is likely to exceed the transmural fluxes represented in Figure 3.3, and will have a considerable effect on the steady state drug concentrations reached. In the case of the stomach, an oral dose of 200 mg aspirin will result in a relatively high (say 1 mg/ml) concentration within the gastric lumen. The 'theoretical' plasma concentration from Figure 3.3 corresponding to this would be 6000 mg/ml, a figure which cannot even be approached because the drug, after diffusing into the stomach capillaries, is rapidly washed away by the blood flow and diluted in a large volume of

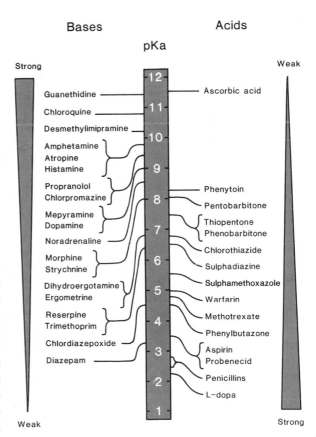

Fig. 3.4 pK_a values for some acidic and basic drugs.

circulating plasma. Thus the pH partition mechanism should not be interpreted in a too literally quantitative way. It does, however, correctly explain the qualitative effect of pH changes in different body compartments on the pharmacokinetics of weakly acidic or basic drugs, particularly in relation to their gastric absorption, renal excretion and penetration of the blood-brain barrier. Values of pK_a for some common drugs are shown in Figure 3.4.

The major predictions are:

1. Acidic, but not basic, drugs are likely to be absorbed from the stomach.
2. Urinary acidification will accelerate the excretion of weak bases, and retard that of weak acids, while urinary alkalinization will have the opposite effect.
3. Increasing the plasma pH will cause weakly acidic drugs to be extracted from the central nervous system into the plasma.

Carrier-mediated transport

Many cell membranes possess specialized transport mechanisms by which the entry and exit of physiologically important molecules, such as sugars, amino acids, neurotransmitters, metal ions, into and out of cells is regulated. In many cases the transport system achieves the necessary chemical specificity by employing a carrier molecule—i.e. a protein molecule incorporated in the membrane—which binds the transported molecule and ships it to the other side of the membrane either by a shuttling of the carrier from one side to the other, in the manner of a ferry, or by a 'turnstile' type of conformation change. Such systems may operate purely passively, without any energy source; in this case they merely facilitate the process of transmembrane equilibration of the transported species in the direction of its electrochemical gradient and the mechanism is called **facilitated diffusion**. Alternatively, they may be coupled to an energy source, either directly to ATP hydrolysis or indirectly to the electrochemical gradient of another species such as Na^+; in this case transport can occur against an electrochemical gradient and is called **active transport**. Carrier-mediated transport involves (a) binding and (b) translocation. It is thus similar in some ways to a receptor-mediated process (see Chapter 1) and has certain important features in common. Thus, the binding step shows the characteristic of **saturation**. With simple diffusion the rate of transport increases directly in proportion to the concentration gradient, whereas with carrier-mediated transport the carrier sites become saturated at high ligand concentrations and the rate of transport does not increase beyond this point. **Competitive inhibition** of transport also occurs if a second ligand is present which binds to the carrier. The competing ligand may itself be transported or it may not, but in either case the interaction is very similar to the interaction at a receptor between an agonist and a competitive antagonist.

Carriers of this type are ubiquitous in the body and many pharmacological effects are the result of interference with them. Thus nerve terminals usually have transport mechanisms for accumulating the specific neurotransmitter that they release, and there are many examples of drugs that act by inhibiting these transport mechanisms (see Chapters 5–7 & 14). From a pharmacokinetic point of view, though, there are only a few sites in the body where carrier-mediated drug transport is important, the main ones being:

1. the renal tubule
2. the biliary tract
3. the blood-brain barrier
4. the gastrointestinal tract.

The characteristics of these transport systems are discussed later, when patterns of distribution and elimination in the body as a whole are considered more fully.

In addition to the processes so far described which govern the transport of drug molecules across the barriers between different aqueous compartments, there are two additional factors which have a major influence on drug distribution and elimination. These are:

1. Partition into body fat and other tissues
2. Binding to plasma proteins.

PARTITION INTO BODY FAT

Fat represents a large, non-polar compartment in the body. On average, fat constitutes about 15% of body weight, and its volume is about 25% of that of the total body water, though these proportions are highly variable. Thus, if a non-polar drug molecule has a fat:water partition coefficient of 10, roughly 75% of the drug would, at equilibrium, be dissolved in the body fat, exerting no pharmacological action, but forming a large reservoir of drug in communication with the plasma compartment. In practice this is important for only a few drugs, mainly because the effective fat:water partition coefficient is relatively low for most drugs. In many cases drugs are largely ionized at physiological pH, which greatly reduces their lipid solubility, and in other cases lipid solubility is limited by the presence of hydrophilic groups in the molecule. **Morphine**, for example, though quite lipid-soluble enough to cross the blood-brain barrier, has a lipid:water partition coefficient of only 0.4, so sequestration of the drug by body fat is of little importance. With **thiopentone**, on the other hand (fat:water partition coefficient approximately 10), accumulation in body fat is considerable, and has important pharmacokinetic consequences when the drug is used as an intravenous anaesthetic agent (see Chapter 20).

The second factor that limits the accumulation of drugs in body fat is its low blood supply—less than 2% of the cardiac output—in relation to its mass—roughly 15% of body weight. Thus drugs are only delivered to body fat rather slowly, and can therefore only accumulate there slowly, so that the theoretical equilibrium distribution between fat and body water is never closely approached. For practical purposes, therefore, partition into body fat is important only for a few highly lipid-soluble anaesthetic drugs, as well as for some environmental contaminants, such as insecticides, which are taken in over a period of time and may slowly accumulate in high concentration in body fat.

Body fat is not the only tissue in which drugs can accumulate. Thus some drugs (e.g. **mepacrine**, an antimalarial drug; see Chapter 33) have a high affinity for cell nuclei, and are strongly taken up by the liver. **Tetracyclines** (see Chapter 30) accumulate slowly in bones and teeth, because they have a high affinity for calcium.

Table 3.1 Some drugs that bind to plasma albumin

Drug	% bound at therapeutic concentration	% binding sites occupied
Diazepam Chlordiazepoxide Warfarin	95–99	< 1
Phenylbutazone	98	20
Amitriptyline Nortriptyline Chlorpromazine Imipramine Desmethylimipramine Indomethacin	90–95	< 1
Sulphisoxazole Tolbutamide Valproic acid	90–95	50–60
Phenytoin	90	3
Alprenolol Digitoxin Hydrallazine	85–90	< 1
Quinidine	70	< 1
Lignocaine	50	< 1
Aspirin	50	50

Drugs with high % bound will be susceptible to displacement. Drugs that occupy 50% or more of sites may cause effects by displacement.

BINDING OF DRUGS TO PLASMA PROTEINS

At normal therapeutic plasma concentrations many drugs exist in the plasma mainly in the bound form. The fraction of drug that is free in aqueous solution can be as low as 1%, the remainder being associated with plasma protein. This binding can be demonstrated by various methods that enable free and bound drug to be separated. Thus, if the plasma is dialysed against a protein-free aqueous medium the drug concentration in the protein-free compartment will be much lower than that in the plasma compartment, because only the free drug molecules are able to cross the dialysis membrane. There are also spectroscopic and fluorescence techniques which distinguish between free and bound molecules on the basis of their optical properties.

The most important protein in relation to drug binding is **plasma albumin** which binds many acidic drugs, and a smaller number of basic drugs (see Table 3.1). Other plasma proteins, including **β-globulin** and an **acid glycoprotein**, which are present in much smaller amounts than albumin, have also been implicated in the binding of certain basic drugs, such as **tubocurarine** and **quinidine**.

The amount of a drug that is bound to protein will depend on three factors: (a) the free drug concentration; (b) its affinity for the binding sites; and (c) the protein concentration. As a first approximation, the binding reaction can be regarded as a simple association of the drug molecules with a finite population of binding sites, exactly analogous to drug receptor binding (see Chapter 1).

$$D + S \rightleftharpoons DS$$

free drug   binding site   complex

We would then expect a hyperbolic saturation curve if the amount bound is plotted against the free concentration (Fig. 3.5). Actually, the binding

the binding curve, where the amount bound varies nearly in direct proportion to the free concentration [D]. Under these conditions the *fraction* of the total drug in the plasma that is bound to plasma protein (given in Table 3.2) is independent of the drug concentration. However, some drugs (e.g. **tolbutamide** and some **sulfonamides**) work at plasma concentrations at which the binding to protein is approaching saturation (i.e. on the flat part of the binding curve). This means that addition of more drug to the plasma will increase the amount bound, [DS], relatively less than it increases the amount free, [D]. Doubling the dose of such a drug can therefore *more* than double the free (pharmacologically active) concentration. This is shown theoretically in Figure 3.5, and a real example, with the

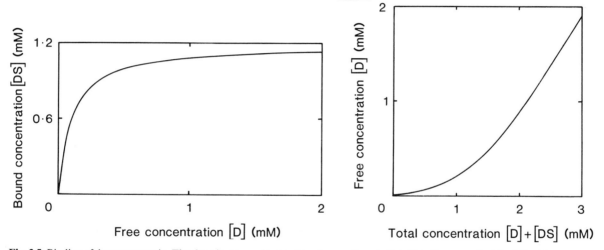

Fig. 3.5 Binding of drugs to protein. The drug is assumed to bind to plasma albumin (total binding capacity 1.2 mM) with an equilibrium constant of 0.1 mM. *Left*. Relationship between bound and free concentration, showing saturation of binding sites. *Right*. Relationship between free concentration and total concentration. The non-linearity, which results from binding-site saturation, means that progressive increments of the dose given can cause disproportionately large increments in the free concentration.

curve is usually more complex, because each albumin molecule has at least two binding sites for most drugs, but the general shape of the curve resembles Figure 3.5. The normal concentration of albumin in plasma is about 0.6 mM. With two sites per albumin molecule the drug binding capacity of plasma albumin would therefore be about 1.2 mM. For most drugs the total plasma concentration required for a clinical effect is much less than 1.2 mM (Table 3.2), so the albumin binding sites are far from saturation, corresponding to the left hand corner of

anti-inflammatory drug **phenylbutazone**, is shown in Figure 3.6. The existence of binding sites on plasma albumin for which many different drugs have an affinity means that competition can occur between them, so that administration of drug B can reduce the protein binding, and hence increase the free plasma concentration, of drug A. To do this drug B needs to occupy an appreciable fraction of the binding sites; most of the drugs in Table 3.1 will not affect the binding of other drugs because they occupy, at therapeutic plasma concentrations, only

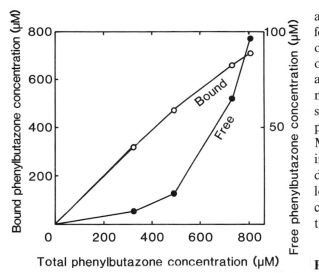

Fig. 3.6 Binding of phenylbutazone to plasma albumin, showing the disproportionate increase in free concentration as the total concentration increases (see Fig. 3.5). (Data from: Brodie & Hogben, 1957)

a tiny fraction of the available sites and it is only a few drugs (e.g. sulfonamides and aspirin, which occupy, at therapeutic concentrations, about 50% of the binding sites), that can displace other drugs and cause unexpected effects. The *displaced* drug need not occupy an appreciable fraction of the sites, so diazepam, for example, would be displaced from protein binding sites by aspirin, but not vice versa. Much has been made of the importance of binding interactions of this kind as a source of untoward drug interactions in clinical medicine, but a critical look at the evidence suggests that this type of competition is less important than was once thought (see Chapter 4).

PHASES OF DRUG DISPOSITION

We will now consider how the basic processes responsible for the translocation and distribution of

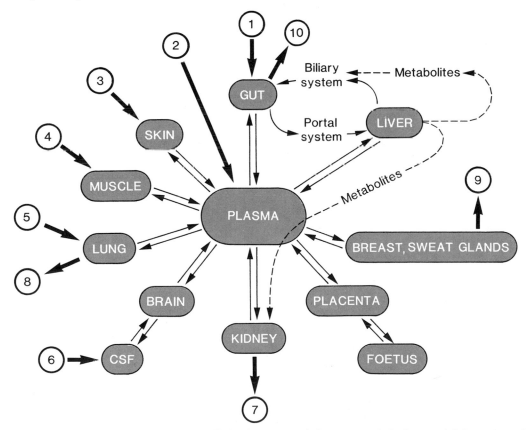

Fig. 3.7 The main routes of drug administration and elimination. *Routes of administration*: 1. Oral or rectal, 2. Intravenous, 3. Percutaneous, 4. Intramuscular, 5. Inhalation, 6. Intrathecal. *Routes of elimination*: 7. Urine, 8. Expired air, 9. Milk, sweat, 10. Faeces.

drug molecules—diffusion, penetration of membranes, partition, and binding to protein—influence the overall behaviour of drug molecules in the body. This can be divided into four phases:

1. Absorption from the site of administration
2. Distribution within the body
3. Metabolic alteration
4. Excretion.

The main pharmacokinetic pathways which will be considered are shown schematically in Figure 3.7.

DRUG ABSORPTION

Absorption is defined as the passage of a drug from its site of administration into the plasma. It must therefore be considered for all routes of administration, except for the intravenous route. There are instances, such as the inhalation of a bronchodilator aerosol to treat asthma, where absorption as just defined is not required for the drug to act, but in most cases the drug has to enter the plasma before it can reach its site of action and has first to be absorbed.

The main routes of administration are:

1. Sublingual
2. Oral
3. Rectal
4. Application to epithelial surfaces (e.g. skin, cornea, vagina, nasal mucosa)
5. Inhalation
6. Injection
   a. subcutaneous
   b. intramuscular
   c. intravenous
   d. intrathecal.

ABSORPTION OF DRUGS FROM THE ALIMENTARY CANAL

Sublingual administration

Absorption directly from the oral cavity is sometimes useful (provided the drug does not taste too horrible) when a rapid response is required, particularly when the drug is either unstable at gastric pH or rapidly metabolized by the liver. Examples of drugs that are often given sublingually include **glyceryl trinitrate** (see Chapter 10) and **isoprenaline** (see Chapter 13). Drugs absorbed from the mouth pass straight into the systemic circulation without entering the portal system, and so escape **first pass metabolism** (see below). Unfortunately high molecular weight substances are not well absorbed by this route, otherwise it would be extremely useful for administration of insulin and other peptides.

Oral administration

The great majority of drugs are taken by mouth, and swallowed. Some drugs (e.g. **alcohol** and **aspirin**) can be rapidly absorbed from the stomach, but in most cases little absorption occurs until the drug passes through the pyloric sphincter.

Drug absorption from the intestine

Measurements of drug absorption either *in vivo* or *in vitro* have shown that the basic mechanism is the same as for other epithelial barriers, namely passive transfer at a rate determined by the ionization and lipid solubility of the drug molecules. Figure 3.8

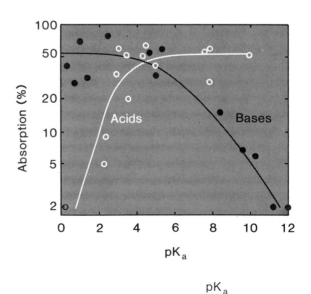

Fig. 3.8 Absorption of drugs from the intestine as a function of pK_a, for acids and bases. Weak acids and bases are well absorbed; strong acids and bases are poorly absorbed. (From: Schanker et al, 1957)

shows the rate of absorption of a series of weak acids and bases as a function of their pK_a values. As expected, strong bases of pK_a 10 or higher are poorly absorbed, as are strong acids of pK_a less than 3, because they are fully ionized. Several clinically important drugs are strong bases, including quaternary ammonium compounds, such as tubocurarine and the hypotensive drug **guanethidine**, which are poorly absorbed from the gastrointestinal tract. Tubocurarine is used as a muscle relaxant during anaesthesia (see Chapter 6) and is always given intravenously. Guanethidine, on the other hand is taken orally, for its absorption, though incomplete, is enough to produce the desired effect. Other highly polar molecules, such as the **aminoglycoside antibiotics** (see Chapter 30) are also very poorly absorbed, and they can be used orally to sterilize the gut in preparation for intestinal surgery, without causing systemic effects.

There are a few instances where intestinal absorption depends on carrier-mediated transport rather than simple lipid diffusion. Examples include **levodopa**, a drug used in treating Parkinsonism (see Chapter 24), which is taken up by the carrier that normally transports phenylalanine, and **fluorouracil** (see Chapter 29), a cytotoxic drug that is transported by the system that carries the natural pyrimidines, thymine and uracil. **Iron**, too, is absorbed in association with a specific carrier protein, known as transferrin, and calcium is similarly absorbed by means of a vitamin D-dependent carrier system.

Factors affecting gastrointestinal absorption

As a rule about 75% of a drug given orally will be absorbed in 1–3 hours, but numerous factors can alter this, some physiological and some to do with the formulation of the drug. The main factors are:

1. Gastrointestinal motility
2. Splanchnic blood flow

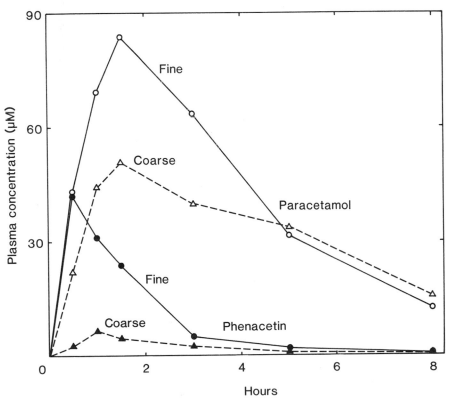

Fig. 3.9 Effect of particle size on absorption of drugs given by mouth. Note that with phenacetin, which is quickly metabolized, slow absorption reduces the peak plasma concentration by about 90%, rendering the drug ineffective. With paracetamol, the effect on peak plasma concentration is less marked. (Data from: Prescott et al, 1970)

3. Particle size and formulation
4. Chemical factors.

Gastrointestinal motility has a large effect. Many disease states reduce it, and slow down drug absorption. Drug treatment can also affect it, either reducing motility (e.g. drugs that block muscarinic receptors) or increasing it (e.g. **metoclopramide**, a drug that speeds up gastric emptying). Excessively rapid movement of the gut contents can also impair absorption. A drug taken after a meal is usually slowly absorbed because its progress to the small intestine is delayed.

Splanchnic blood flow is greatly reduced in hypovolaemic states, with a resultant slowing of drug absorption.

Particle size and formulation have major effects on absorption. An example with phenacetin is shown in Figure 3.9. Another example concerns the antibiotic penicillin. Oral **penicillin** (see Chapter 30) may be formulated as the free acid, which is rather insoluble, or as the potassium salt, which is very soluble. If the salt is given, the drug precipitates as free acid as soon as it reaches the stomach, where the pH is low, giving rise to a suspension of very fine particles, from which absorption is rapid. If the acid form of oral penicillin is ingested as such however, it fails to dissolve appreciably in the stomach and absorption is much slower, because of the larger particle size. Another example concerns **digoxin** (see Chapter 10). In 1971 certain patients treated in a New York hospital for cardiac failure were found to require unusually large maintenance doses of digoxin. In a study on normal volunteers it was found that standard oral digoxin tablets from different manufacturers resulted in grossly different plasma concentrations (Fig. 3.10) even though the digoxin content of the tablets was the same, because of differences in particle size. Because digoxin is rather poorly absorbed anyway, small differences in the pharmaceutical preparation can make a large difference to the extent of absorption.

Many pharmaceutical preparations are formulated to produce the desired absorption characteristics. Thus capsules may be designed to remain intact for some hours after ingestion in order to delay absorption, or tablets may have a resistant coating to give the same effect. In some cases, a

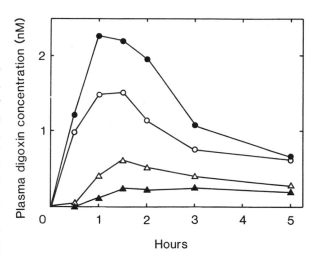

Fig. 3.10 Variation in oral absorption among different formulations of digoxin. The four curves show the mean plasma concentration attained for the four preparations, each of which was given on separate occasions to four subjects. The large variation has caused the formulation of digoxin tablets to be standardized since this study was published. (From: Lindenbaum et al, 1971)

mixture of slow and fast-release particles is included in a capsule to produce more sustained absorption.

Chemical factors affecting drug absorption do so by influencing the state of the drug in the intestine. Thus **tetracycline antibiotics** (see Chapter 30) bind strongly to calcium ions, and calcium-rich foods (especially milk) prevent their absorption. Similarly, the use of liquid paraffin as a laxative will retard the absorption of lipophilic substances, such as vitamin K.

Bioavailability

To get from the lumen of the small intestine into the systemic circulation a drug must not only penetrate the intestinal mucosa; it must also run the gauntlet of enzymes in the gut wall and in the liver which may inactivate it. The term **bioavailability** is used to indicate the overall proportion of the drug that passes into the systemic circulation after oral administration, taking into account both absorption and local metabolic degradation. It is a convenient term for making bland generalizations, but the concept creaks badly if attempts are made to use it with quantitative precision, or even to define it*. One problem is that it is not a characteristic solely of the drug preparation, since variations in enzyme activity of the gut wall or the liver, in gastric pH or intestinal motility will all affect it. Because of this, one cannot speak of the bioavailability of a particular preparation, but only of that preparation in a given individual on a particular occasion. Even with this caveat, the concept is not really helpful, because it relates only to the total *proportion* of the drug that reaches the systemic circulation, and ignores the time taken. Thus, if a drug is completely absorbed in 30 minutes, it will reach a much higher plasma concentration, and have a more dramatic effect, than the same drug absorbed over 6 hours. It is significant that one rarely sees a value assigned to 'bioavailability', and it is well to be wary of ostensibly measurable quantities which are used impressionistically, but not actually given values. These uncertainties do not prevent pharmaceutical companies emphasizing the high bioavailability of their preparations as a selling point. They understand impressionism well.

OTHER ROUTES OF ADMINISTRATION

Rectal administration

This is used either for drugs that are required to produce a local effect (e.g. anti-inflammatory drugs for use in ulcerative colitis; see Chapter 13), or to produce systemic effects. Substances absorbed from the rectum largely by-pass the liver en route to the systemic circulation. This can be an advantage for drugs that would otherwise be rapidly inactivated by the liver (e.g. **progesterone**, **testosterone**). Other possible reasons for preferring rectal to oral administration for systemic drugs are that the drug causes gastric irritation (common with anti-inflammatory drugs) or that the patient is vomiting or unable to swallow pills; often, though, the reasons appear to be more cultural than pharmacological.

*The definition of bioavailability offered by the US Food and Drugs Administration is: '*The rate and extent to which the therapeutic moiety is absorbed and becomes available to the site of drug action*'. The reader may be forgiven for finding this confusing. The double use of 'and' gives the definition four possible meanings, two of which are obfuscated by the uncertain meaning of the phrase 'becomes available to the site of drug action'.

Cutaneous administration

Most drugs are absorbed very poorly through unbroken skin, because their lipid solubility is too low. A number of organophosphate insecticides (see Chapter 7), which must be able to penetrate an insect's cuticle in order to work, are however absorbed through skin and accidental poisoning among farm workers who get in the way of the crop sprayer is not uncommon. A case is recounted of a 35-year-old florist in 1932. 'While engaged in doing a light electrical repair job at a work bench he sat down in a chair on the seat of which some "Nico-Fume liquid" (a 40% solution of free nicotine) had been spilled. He felt the solution wet through his clothes to the skin over the left buttock, an area about the size of the palm of his hand. He thought nothing further of it and continued at his work for about fifteen minutes, when he was suddenly seized with nausea and faintness... and found himself in a drenching sweat. On the way to hospital he lost consciousness'. He survived, just, and then, four days later: 'On discharge from the hospital he was given the same clothes that he had worn when he was brought in. The clothes had been kept in a paper bag and were still damp where they had been wet with the nicotine solution.' The sequel was predictable. He survived again, but felt thereafter 'unable to enter a greenhouse where nicotine was being sprayed.'

In clinical practice, cutaneous administration is used mainly when a local effect on the skin is required (e.g. topically-applied steroids). Appreciable absorption may nonetheless occur and lead to systemic effects. Occasionally drugs [such as **glyceryl trinitrate** (used in angina) or **hyoscine** (used to prevent seasickness)] intended for systemic use are given transcutaneously, in the form of a special stick-on plaster.

Eye-drops

Many drugs can be applied as eye-drops, relying on absorption through the epithelium of the conjunctival sac to produce their effects. Adequate lipid solubility is necessary for absorption to occur. Thus, in treating glaucoma, a tertiary amine or uncharged form of anticholinesterase (e.g. **eserine** or **dyflos**; see Chapter 6) works much better than a quaternary compound (e.g. **neostigmine**). Systemic absorption occurs when eye-drops are given, and can result in side effects. Some of the drug passes through the naso-lacrimal duct into the nasal cavity whence it may be absorbed or swallowed.

Administration by inhalation

This route is used for **volatile and gaseous anaesthetics** (see Chapter 20). For these agents the lung serves as the route of both administration and elimination, and the rapid exchange that is possible as a result of the large surface area and blood flow makes it possible to achieve rapid adjustments of plasma concentration. The pharmacokinetic behaviour of inhalation anaesthetics is discussed more fully in Chapter 20.

Drugs used for their effects on the lung are also given by inhalation. Bronchodilators, such as **isoprenaline** or **salbutamol** are given as aerosols, so as to achieve much higher concentrations in the lung than elsewhere in the body, thus minimizing side effects. Though intended to act locally, drugs given in this way are usually absorbed rapidly into the systemic circulation, and side effects, such as tachycardia following isoprenaline inhalation, can easily be detected. **Local anaesthetics** are sprayed into the bronchial tree in preparation for bronchoscopy, and systemic side effects (e.g. hypotension and convulsions; see Chapter 27) are one of the hazards of this procedure.

Inhalation is also used for administration of **cromoglycate**, an anti-asthma drug (see Chapter 13). This drug is insoluble in water, and is inhaled as a dry powder, which is dispersed as a fine cloud by means of a special type of inhaler.

Administration by injection

Intravenous injection is the fastest and most certain route of drug administration. If a single bolus injection is given it produces a very high concentration of drug which will first reach the lungs and then the systemic circulation. The actual peak concentration reaching the tissues depends critically on the rate of injection, which should be cautiously slow. Administration by steady intravenous infusion is useful when drugs have to be given to ill patients in hospital, as it avoids the uncertainties of absorption from other sites, and involves no disturbance to the patient. Drugs that are given intravenously include **heparin** (see Chapter 12), **lignocaine** (when it is used as an antidysrhythmic drug; see Chapter 10), certain **anaesthetic agents** (see Chapter 20), **ergometrine** (see Chapter 17) and **diazepam** (see Chapter 21).

Subcutaneous or intramuscular injection of drugs usually produces a faster effect than oral administration, but the rate of absorption depends greatly on the site of injection and on physiological factors, especially local blood flow. In general, subcutaneous injection results in rather faster absorption than intramuscular injection, but the difference is not large.

The rate-limiting factors in absorption from the injection site are (a) diffusion through the tissue, and (b) removal by local blood flow. The importance of the former is shown by the powerful effect of **hyaluronidase**, an enzyme which breaks down the intercellular matrix. Adding hyaluronidase to the injection fluid increases the rate of diffusion through the interstitial space, and greatly speeds up drug absorption.

Absorption from a site of injection may be increased by increasing local blood flow by the application of heat or massage. Local blood flow may be a critical factor if parenteral injections are given to patients with a failing peripheral circulation. Thus, if a patient is given a subcutaneous injection of morphine after severe trauma, absorption may be slow, resulting in inadequate analgesia, and further doses may be given. When the circulation is restored, however, a rapid and potentially dangerous absorption of morphine may occur.

Methods for delaying absorption

It may be desirable to delay absorption either to reduce the systemic actions of drugs that are being used to produce a local effect, or to increase the duration of action of a drug by causing it to be absorbed slowly over a long period. Thus, the addition of adrenaline or noradrenaline to a solution of local anaesthetic reduces the absorption of the local anaesthetic into the general circulation;

this usefully prolongs the anaesthetic effect, as well as reducing systemic toxicity. A more heroic procedure that is used to produce local anaesthesia of a whole limb (e.g. for the setting of a fracture) involves the application of an arterial pressure cuff to arrest the blood flow, followed by intravenous injection of the anaesthetic below the cuff. The anaesthetic diffuses gradually into the tissues and exerts its effect until the cuff is released. If the cuff is released too soon a potentially lethal dose of the drug may escape into the systemic circulation; thus, much depends on the integrity of the pneumatic cuff.

Another method of delaying absorption from intramuscular or subcutaneous sites is to administer the drug in a relatively insoluble 'slow release' form. This may be achieved by converting it into a poorly soluble salt, ester, or complex which is injected either as an aqueous suspension or an oily solution. **Procaine penicillin** (see Chapter 30) is a salt of penicillin which is only slightly water-soluble; when injected as an aqueous suspension it is slowly absorbed and exerts a prolonged action. Esterification of the steroid hormones, **oestradiol**, **testosterone** and **deoxycortone**, increases their solubility in oil and in this way slows down their rate of absorption when they are injected in an oily solution.

The physical characteristics of a preparation may also be changed so as to influence its rate of absorption. Examples of this are the **insulin zinc suspensions** (see Chapter 16); insulin forms a complex with zinc, the physical form of which can be altered by varying the pH at which the reaction occurs. One form consists of a fine amorphous suspension which is relatively rapidly absorbed, and another consists of a suspension of large crystals which are slowly absorbed. These two preparations can be mixed to produce an immediate, but sustained, effect.

Another method used to achieve slow and continuous absorption of certain steroid hormones is the **subcutaneous implantation** of solid pellets. The rate of absorption is proportional to the surface area of the implant, so a flat pellet gives a more uniform rate of absorption than a spherical one. Implants of **deoxycortone acetate** have been used in the treatment of Addison's disease and their effect may last for periods up to 6 months. **Testosterone** and **oestradiol** may also be administered in this way.

Intrathecal injection

Injection of a drug into the subarachnoid space via a lumbar puncture needle is used for some specialized purposes. Some antibiotic drugs cross the blood-brain barrier very slowly, and may be given intrathecally to treat meningitis. Regional anaesthesia can be produced by injecting a local anaesthetic (see Chapter 27) intrathecally, and recently opiate analgesics (see Chapter 25) have been used successfully in this way.

DISTRIBUTION OF DRUGS IN THE BODY

BODY FLUID COMPARTMENTS

Body water can be considered to be distributed into compartments as shown in Figure 3.11. The total

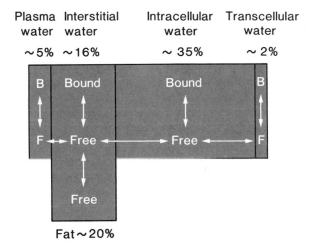

Fig. 3.11 The main body fluid compartments, expressed as % of body weight. Drug molecules exist in bound or free form in each aqueous compartment, but only the free drug is able to move between compartments.

body water as a percentage of body weight varies from 50 to 70%, being rather less in women than in men.

Extracellular fluid comprises the **blood plasma** (about 4.5% of body weight), **interstitial fluid** (16%) and **lymph** (1–2%). **Intracellular fluid** (30–40%) is the sum of the fluid contents of all cells in the body. **Transcellular fluid** (2.5%) includes the cerebrospinal, intraocular, peritoneal, pleural and synovial fluids and digestive secretions. The foetus may also be regarded as a special type of transcellular compartment. To enter any of these compartments from the extracellular compartment a drug must cross an epithelial barrier, which means that it has to be able to enter cells.

Within each of these aqueous compartments drug molecules will, in general exist both in free solution, and in bound form; and drugs that are weak acids or bases will exist as an equilibrium mixture of the charged and the uncharged form, the position of the equilibrium depending on the pH.

The equilibrium pattern of distribution between the various compartments will thus depend on:

1. Permeability across tissue barriers
2. Binding within compartments
3. pH partition
4. Fat: water partition.

Volume of distribution

The apparent volume of distribution, V_d, is defined as the volume of fluid required to contain the total amount, Q, of drug in the body at the same concentration as that present in the plasma, C_p.

$$V_d = \frac{Q}{C_p} \qquad 3.1$$

Values of V_d* have been measured for many drugs (Table 3.2), and some general patterns can be distinguished.

Drugs confined to the plasma compartment

The plasma volume is about 0.05 l/kg body weight. A few drugs, such as **heparin** (see Chapter 12) are confined to the plasma compartment because the molecule is too large to cross the capillary wall

---

*The experimental measurement of V_d is complicated by the fact that the amount of drug present in the body, Q, does not stay constant, because of metabolism and excretion of the drug, during the time that it takes for it to be distributed among the various body compartments that contribute to the overall V_d. It therefore has to be calculated indirectly from a series of measurements of plasma concentrations as a function of time. On the basis of a 2-compartment model (see p. 86) the distribution volume of each compartment can be calculated, but the validity of such estimates necessarily depends on the validity of the kinetic model used.

easily. More often, retention of a drug in the plasma reflects strong binding to plasma protein (see Table 3.1). For example, with **phenylbutazone** or **warfarin** only the small fraction (about 2%) that is free can equilibrate with other compartments and most of the drug is retained in the plasma; it is nevertheless the free drug in the interstitial fluid that exerts a pharmacological effect. Some dyes, such as Evans blue, bind even more strongly to plasma albumin, and the distribution volume of Evans blue is used experimentally to measure plasma volume.

Drugs distributed in the extracellular compartment

The total extracellular volume is about 0.2 l/kg, and this is the approximate distribution volume for many polar compounds, such as **tubocurarine**, **gentamicin** and **carbenicillin**. These drugs cannot easily enter cells because of their low lipid solubility, and, importantly, do not quickly cross the blood-brain barrier or the placental barrier. Distribution volumes in excess of the theoretical value of 0.2 l/kg result either from a limited degree of penetration into cells, or from binding of the drug in the extravascular compartment.

Distribution throughout the body water

Total body water represents about 0.55 l/kg, and this distribution volume is achieved by relatively lipid-soluble drugs that readily cross cell membranes (e.g. **pentobarbitone**, **phenytoin**, **ethanol**, **diazepam**). Binding of the drug anywhere outside the plasma compartment, as well as partitioning into body fat, can increase V_d beyond the theoretical value for total body water, and thus there are many drugs that give values well in excess even of the total body volume (e.g. **morphine**, **digoxin**, **haloperidol**). Drugs with a large distribution volume will almost invariably reach the brain and the foetus, as well as other transcellular compartments.

REMOVAL OF DRUGS FROM THE BODY

The main routes by which drug molecules leave the body are (a) the kidneys, (b) the lungs and (c) the biliary system. Excretion via the lungs occurs only with highly volatile or gaseous agents, so the great

Table 3.2 Distribution volumes for some drugs compared with volumes of body fluid compartments

Volume (litres/kg body weight)	Compartment	V_d (litres/kg body weight)	
0.05	Plasma	0.05–0.1	Heparin Insulin Phenylbutazone
		0.1–0.2	Warfarin Aspirin Sulphamethoxazole Tolbutamide
0.2	ECF	0.2–0.4	Methyldopa Methotrexate Glyceryl trinitrate Tubocurarine
		0.4–0.7	Hydrallazine Theophylline Atenolol
0.55	Total body water		Digitoxin Ethanol Neostigmine Phenytoin Phenobarbitone
		1–2	Hexobarbitone Indomethacin Paracetamol Diazepam Lignocaine
		2–5	Nitrazepam Morphine Propranolol Digoxin Chlorpromazine
		> 10	Nortriptyline Imipramine

majority of drugs leave the body in the urine. Some drugs are secreted into the bile, via the liver, but in most cases reabsorption occurs from the intestine. There are only a few examples where this process accounts for the elimination of an appreciable fraction of the unchanged drug (e.g. **rifampicin**, **cromoglycate**). Drugs may also be excreted in secretions such as milk or sweat, but these are quantitatively unimportant compared with renal excretion except insofar as excretion into milk can have effects on a suckling child.

Before being excreted in the urine most drugs undergo metabolic alteration, which occurs predominantly in the liver.

In this section we consider first the main pathways of drug metabolism, and then the factors that determine the rate of renal elimination.

DRUG METABOLISM

Enzymatic modification of drug molecules usually abolishes their pharmacological activity, but there are exceptions to this (see Table 3.3), which are discussed later in this chapter.

Metabolic alteration of drug molecules involves two kinds of biochemical reaction, which often occur sequentially, known as **Phase I** and **Phase II reactions**.

Phase I reactions usually consist of **oxidation**, **reduction** or **hydrolysis**, and the products are often more reactive, and sometimes more toxic than the parent drug.

Phase II reactions involve **conjugation**, which normally results in inactive compounds.

Phase I reactions often serve to introduce a

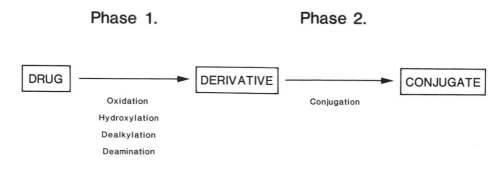

Fig. 3.12 The two phases of drug metabolism.

relatively reactive group, such as hydroxyl, into the molecule. This functional group then serves as the point of attack for the conjugating system which attaches a larger substituent to it, such as a glucuronyl, sulphate or acetyl group (Fig. 3.12).

Both stages normally decrease the lipid solubility of the substance, which has the effect of increasing the rate of renal elimination (see below), and the system of drug metabolizing enzymes may be regarded as a non-selective detoxification system for ridding the body of a wide range of foreign substances.

Phase I and Phase II reactions take place mainly in the liver, though there are some important exceptions of drugs that are metabolized in the plasma (e.g. hydrolysis of **suxamethonium** and **procaine** by plasma cholinesterase, see Chapters 6 & 27), in the lung (e.g. various **prostanoids**, see Chapter 8), or in the wall of the intestine (e.g. **tyramine**, see Chapter 7). Within the liver the enzymes involved are intracellular. Many are attached to the smooth endoplasmic reticulum and they are often called 'microsomal' enzymes because, on homogenization and differential centrifugation, the endoplasmic reticulum is broken into very small fragments that sediment only after prolonged high speed centrifugation. To reach these metabolizing enzymes a drug must cross the hepatocyte

membrane. Polar molecules do this very slowly compared with non-polar molecules except where specific transport mechanisms exist, so for these drugs hepatic metabolism is in general less important, and a greater proportion is excreted unchanged in the urine.

Phase I reactions

Oxidative reactions, which include **hydroxylation** of nitrogen and carbon atoms, N- and O-**dealkylation**, and **oxidative deamination** are catalysed by a complex enzyme system known as the **mixed function oxygenase** system, which resides on the smooth endoplasmic reticulum. At least four separate enzymes are involved, the most important being **cytochrome P-450**, a haem protein which binds molecular oxygen as well as the substrate molecule and forms part of the electron transfer chain. Though the chemical end result may appear to be very different (e.g. hydroxylation, O-dealkylation or deamination) with different drugs, these reactions all start with a hydroxylation step catalysed by the P-450 system. This produces a reactive intermediate from which the end-product is derived (Fig. 3.13).

The metabolism of **imipramine** (Fig. 3.14) provides a typical example of how these reactions can combine to give rise to a whole family of metabolites.

	Substrate		Transient intermediate		Product
N-dealkylation	R-NH-CH$_3$	$\xrightarrow{+O}$	(R-NH-CH$_2$OH)	$\longrightarrow$	R-NH$_2$+CH$_2$O
Deamination	R-CH-NH$_2$	$\xrightarrow{+O}$	(R-CHOH-NH$_2$)	$\longrightarrow$	R-CHO+NH$_3$
O-dealkylation	R-O-CH$_3$	$\xrightarrow{+O}$	(R-O-CH$_2$OH)	$\longrightarrow$	R-OH-CH$_2$O

Fig. 3.13 Examples of phase I reactions.

Not all drug oxidation reactions involve the mixed function oxygenase system. For example, ethanol is metabolized by a soluble cytoplasmic enzyme, alcohol dehydrogenase. Other exceptions include the non-microsomal enzyme **xanthine oxidase**, which is involved in uric acid synthesis and is also responsible for inactivation of the cytotoxic drug **6-mercaptopurine**, and **monoamine oxidase**

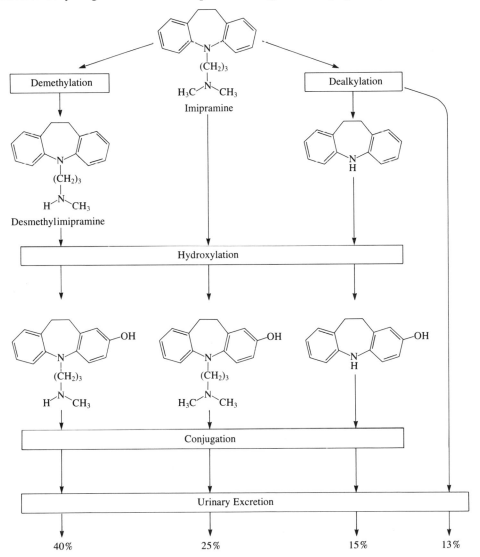

Fig. 3.14 The main routes of metabolism of imipramine. (From: Crammer et al, 1969)

which inactivates many biologically active amines (e.g. **noradrenaline, tyramine, serotonin**; see Chapters 7 & 19). These enzymes occur in many tissues besides the liver.

Reductive reactions are much less common than oxidative ones, but some are important. For example, the anticoagulant drug **warfarin** (see Chapter 12) is inactivated by conversion of a ketone to a hydroxyl group. Many steroids are administered as ketones (e.g. **cortisone** and **prednisone**; see Chapter 16) which must be reduced to the corresponding hydroxy-compounds in order to act (Table 3.3). These reductive reactions also involve microsomal enzymes.

Hydrolytic reactions occur in many tissues, and are not brought about by the hepatic microsomal enzymes. Both ester and amide bonds are susceptible to hydrolysis, the former more readily than the latter. Thus, the local anaesthetic **procaine**, which is

possess anyway, or which may result from a Phase I reaction, it is susceptible to conjugation, i.e. attachment of a substituent group. The conjugate, which is almost always pharmacologically inactive (unlike the products of Phase I reactions), and less lipid soluble than its precursor, is then excreted in the urine or in the bile.

The groups most often involved in conjugate formation are **glucuronyl, sulphate, methyl, acetyl, glycyl** (Fig. 3.15) and **glutamyl**. Glucuronide formation involves the formation of a high energy phosphate compound, uridine diphosphate glucuronic acid (UDPGA) from which the glucuronic acid part is transferred to an electron-rich atom (N, O or S) on the substrate, forming an amide, ester or thiol bond. This is catalysed by an enzyme, UDP glucuronyl transferase, which has a very broad substrate specificity, so the reaction occurs with a wide variety of drugs and other foreign molecules.

Acetylation and methylation reactions occur with

Table 3.3 Some drugs that produce active or toxic metabolites

Inactive	Active	Toxic
	Heroin ⎫ ⎬ → Morphine Codeine ⎭	
	Propranolol → 4-hydroxypropranolol	
	Phenacetin → Paracetamol →	Hydroxylated derivative
	Imipramine → Desmethylimipramine	
	Amitriptyline → Nortriptyline	
	Diazepam → Nordiazepam → Oxazepam	
Cortisone → Hydrocortisone		
Prednisone → Prednisolone		
Parathion → Paraoxon		
Cyclophosphamide → Ketocyclophosphamide		
Chloral hydrate → Trichloroethanol		
Azathioprine → Mercaptopurine		
	Halothane →	Trifluoroacetic acid
	Sulphonamides →	Acetylated derivatives
	Methoxyflurane →	Fluoride

an ester, is rapidly inactivated by plasma cholinesterase, whereas its amide analogue, **procainamide**, is not attacked by this enzyme, and is thus suitable for systemic use as an antidysrhythmic drug (Chapter 10).

Phase II reactions

If a drug molecule has a suitable 'handle' (e.g. a hydroxyl, thiol or amino group), which it may

acetyl-CoA and S-adenosyl methionine, respectively, acting as the donor compounds.

The enzymes involved in most of these conjugation reactions are associated, like the oxidase system, with the smooth endoplasmic reticulum of liver cells. There are exceptions, for example sulphate conjugation which is mediated by non-microsomal enzymes, and acetylation, which occurs mainly in the reticulo-endothelial cells. Other tissues, such as lung and kidney, are also sites of

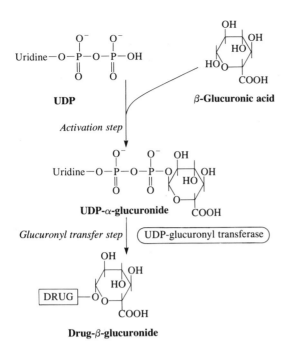

Fig. 3.15 The glucuronide conjugation reaction.

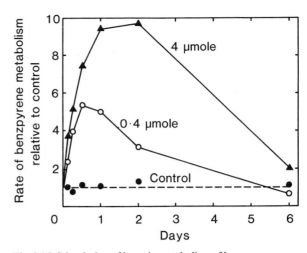

Fig. 3.16 Stimulation of hepatic metabolism of benzpyrene. Young rats were given benzpyrene (i.p.) in the doses shown, and the benzpyrene metabolizing activity of liver homogenates measured at the times up to 6 days. (From: Conney et al, 1957)

conjugation of some drugs. A number of important endogenous substances, such as bilirubin, and adrenal corticosteroids are conjugated by the same system. Glucuronide formation is the commonest conjugation reaction, reflecting the very broad substrate specificity of the enzyme, UDP-glucuronyl transferase. The highly polar nature of the glucuronic acid group means that the conjugates are usually pharmacologically inactive, and rapidly excreted.

Induction of microsomal enzymes

A number of drugs (e.g. **phenobarbitone, ethanol, phenylbutazone** and many others) have the property of increasing the activity of the microsomal oxidase and conjugating systems. Many carcinogenic chemicals (e.g. **benzpyrene**) also have this effect (see Chapter 36). The effect can be very large—Figure 3.16 shows a nearly ten-fold increase in the rate of benzpyrene metabolism 2 days after a single dose of the drug. The effect is referred to as **induction**, and it is the result of an increased synthesis of microsomal enzymes, rather than a change in the activity of existing enzyme molecules. In each case the rate of metabolism of the inducing agent itself is increased, and the metabolism of other compounds may be

increased also. Phenobarbitone is a particularly versatile inducer, and significantly increases the rate of degradation of many other drugs, to a clinically important degree (see Chapter 4). Some environmental contaminants, such as DDT, also have a strong inducing effect. The pattern of enzyme induction is not the same for all inducing agents. Thus phenobarbitone and many related substances cause a non-selective increase in many microsomal enzymes (including glucuronyl transferases) whereas polycyclic hydrocarbons such as benzpyrene and DDT produce a more selective effect, and cause an abnormal oxidase enzyme to appear. Enzyme induction, by accelerating Phase I metabolism can increase, as well as decrease, drug effects. There are many drugs, e.g. **paracetamol**, whose Phase I metabolites are mainly responsible for their toxicity (see Chapter 36), and in these cases toxicity is enhanced in the presence of inducing agents. The carcinogenic action of some polycyclic hydrocarbons is associated with the increased formation of highly reactive oxidative products (e.g. epoxides) in the liver, which cause secondary damage to DNA.

First-pass metabolism

Some drugs are removed from the portal circulation very efficiently by the liver, and metabolized, so that the amount reaching the systemic circulation is considerably less than the amount absorbed into the portal vein. This is known as the **first-pass effect**, and it is significant for several clinically important drugs, including **glyceryl trinitrate** (see Chapter 10), which is given sublingually so as to by-pass the portal circulation, **lignocaine** (Chapter 27), **morphine** (Chapter 25) and **propranolol** (Chapter 7). In the case of propranolol, the first-pass metabolite, 4-hydroxypropranolol, is itself pharmacologically active, so oral administration is not precluded.

Pharmacologically active drug metabolites

In some cases (see Table 3.3) the drug administered becomes biologically active only after it has been metabolized by the liver. Thus, some corticosteroids are given as inactive ketone derivatives (e.g. **cortisone**), which are activated by reduction in the liver. Similarly **azathioprine**, an immunosuppressant drug, is metabolized to the active form, **mercaptopurine**. These examples, in which the parent compound lacks activity of its own, are known as **pro-drugs** (see p. 89). In other instances, metabolites may have similar pharmacological actions to the parent compound (e.g. **phenacetin**, which is converted to **paracetamol**, with very similar analgesic properties; also **benzodiazepines**, many of which form active metabolites, which cause their effects to persist even when the parent drug has disappeared). There are also cases in which metabolites are reponsible for certain toxic effects. The liver toxicity of paracetamol is an example of this (see Chapter 36), as well as the nephrotoxicity of the anti-tumour drug, **cyclophosphamide** (see Chapter 29).

RENAL EXCRETION OF DRUGS AND DRUG METABOLITES

Drugs differ very greatly in the way in which they are handled by the kidney, ranging from **penicillin** (see Chapter 30), which is cleared from the blood almost completely on a single transit through the kidney, to **chlorpropamide** (see Chapter 16), which is cleared extremely slowly, so that the blood leaving the kidney contains almost as much drug as that entering it. The majority of drugs fall somewhere in between, and the products of Phase I and Phase II metabolism are nearly always cleared more quickly than the parent compound.

There are three basic processes that account for these wide differences in renal excretion:

1. Glomerular filtration
2. Active tubular secretion or reabsorption
3. Passive diffusion across tubular epithelium.

Glomerular filtration

The glomerular capillaries filter the plasma in such a way that any drug molecule can pass through irrespective of its charge, provided its molecular weight is below about 20 000. Plasma albumin (MW 68 000) is almost completely held back. So far as drugs are concerned, with the exception of a few macromolecular substances such as heparin or dextrans, all pass the glomerulus as readily as water, so that the concentration in the glomerular filtrate is the same as that of the free drug in the plasma. If a drug binds appreciably to plasma albumin, however, the concentration in the filtrate will be less than the total plasma concentration. If, like phenylbutazone, a drug is 98% bound to albumin, the concentration in the filtrate is only 1/50 of that in plasma and clearance by filtration is correspondingly reduced.

Tubular secretion and reabsorption

Glomerular filtration removes at most about 20% of the drug from the blood reaching the kidney. The remaining 80% passes on to the peritubular capillaries of the proximal tubule, where there are two independent and relatively non-selective carrier systems, which transport drug molecules into the tubular lumen; one of these transports acidic drugs (as well as various endogenous substances, such as uric acid); the other system handles basic substances. Some of the more important drug molecules that are transported by these two carrier systems are shown in Table 3.4. The carriers can transport drug molecules against an electrochemical gradient and can, therefore, reduce the plasma concentration nearly to zero. Since at least 80% of the drug delivered to the kidney is presented to the carrier, tubular secretion is potentially the most rapid mechanism for drug elimination available to the kidney. Unlike glomerular filtration, carrier-mediated transport can achieve maximal drug clearance even when most of the drug is bound to

Table 3.4 Some drugs and related substances that are actively secreted into the proximal renal tubule

Acids	Bases
Acetazoleamide	Amiloride
p-Aminohippuric acid	Dopamine
Aminosalicylic acid	Histamine
Cephaloridine	Mecamylamine
Chlorpropamide	Mepacrine
Chlorothiazide	Morphine
Ethacrynic acid	Pethidine
Frusemide	Procaine
Glucuronic acid conjugates	Quaternary ammonium
Glycine conjugates	compounds
5-Hydroxyindole acetic	Quinine
acid	Serotonin
Indomethacin	Tolazoline
Mersalyl	Triamterene
Penicillins	
Phenylbutazone	
Probenecid	
Renal radiocontrast media	
Salicylic acid	
Sulphate conjugates	
Sulphathiazole	
Sulphinpyrazone	
Thiazide diuretics	
Uric acid	

plasma protein*. **Penicillin**, for example, though about 80% bound, and therefore cleared only slowly by filtration, is almost completely removed by proximal tubular secretion, and its overall rate of elimination is very high.

Table 3.4 shows that many different drugs share the same transport system, and competition can occur between them. The most important example is the drug **probenecid**, which was developed for the purpose of prolonging the action of penicillin, by retarding its excretion. Probenecid is itself only slowly transported, but competitively inhibits the

transport of other drugs. It also inhibits uric acid *reabsorption* (which relies on the same carrier), and, though no longer much used to enhance the action of penicillin, is useful in treating gout (see Chapter 9).

Diffusion across the renal tubule

As the glomerular filtrate passes through the renal tubule, water is progressively reabsorbed, the volume of urine emerging being only about 1% of that of the filtrate. If the tubule is freely permeable to drug molecules the drug concentration in the filtrate will remain close to that in the plasma, and some 99% of the filtered drug will be reabsorbed passively. Drugs with high lipid solubility, and hence high tubular permeability are therefore slowly excreted. If the drug is highly polar, and therefore of low tubular permeability, the filtered drug will not be able to leave the tubule, and its concentration will rise steadily, until it is about 100 times as high in the urine as in the plasma. Drugs handled in this way include **gallamine**, and antibiotics such as **streptomycin**. Many drugs, being weak acids or weak bases, change their ionization when the pH is changed (see p. 59), and this can markedly affect renal excretion. The **ion-trapping** effect means that a basic drug will be more rapidly excreted in an acid urine, because the low pH within the tubule will favour ionization and thus inhibit reabsorption. An acidic drug will similarly be most rapidly excreted if the urine is made alkaline (see Fig. 3.17).

This effect can be made use of clinically. **Forced alkaline diuresis**, in which a diuretic drug (see Chapter 14) is combined with an infusion of sodium bicarbonate to increase urinary pH is an effective way of accelerating the excretion of certain acidic drugs such as barbiturates or aspirin. Acidification of the urine can be similarly used to accelerate the excretion of basic drugs such as **amphetamine** (Fig. 3.17).

Drug excretion expressed as clearance

Renal clearance, CL_r, is defined as the notional volume of plasma from which a substance is completely removed by the kidney in unit time, and is calculated from the plasma concentration, C_p, the urinary concentration, C_u, and the rate of flow of urine, V, by the equation:

$$CL_r = \frac{C_u \cdot V}{C_p} \qquad 3.2$$

---

* Because filtration involves isosmotic movement of both water and solutes, it will not affect the free concentration of drug in the plasma. Thus the equilibrium between free and bound drug will not be disturbed, and there will be no tendency for the bound drug to dissociate as the blood traverses the glomerular capillary. The rate of clearance of the drug by filtration is therefore reduced directly in proportion to the fraction that is bound. In the case of active tubular secretion, this is not so; secretion may be retarded very little even though the drug is mostly bound. This is because the carrier transports drug molecules unaccompanied by water. As free drug molecules are taken from the plasma, therefore, the free plasma concentration tends to fall. This causes a net dissociation of bound drug from the protein, so that effectively all of the drug, bound and free, is available to the carrier.

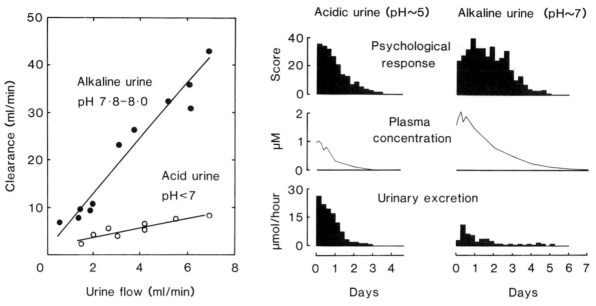

Fig. 3.17 The effect of urinary pH on drug excretion. **A.** Phenobarbitone clearance in the dog as a function of urine flow. Alkalinizing the urine increased clearance about 5-fold. **B.** Amphetamine excretion in man. Acidifying the urine increases the rate of renal elimination of amphetamine, reducing its plasma concentration and its effect on the subject's mental state. (Data from: Gunne & Anggard, 1974)

The clearance of a substance depends, of course, on how it is handled by the processes of filtration, active secretion and passive diffusion; in relation to drug excretion three special cases are relevant:

1. A drug (e.g. **gallamine**) that is completely filtered (i.e. not protein bound) but neither reabsorbed nor secreted. This is the pharmacological equivalent of **inulin**, and its clearance will correspond to the glomerular filtration rate—about 120 ml/min.
2. A drug that is completely removed (by active tubular secretion) during a single transit through the kidney. This is the pharmacological equivalent of **p-aminohippuric acid** (PAH) and its clearance will correspond to the renal plasma flow—about 700 ml/min. The nearest familiar example is **penicillin**, though its clearance is lower than that of PAH because not all of it is removed during a single passage.
3. A drug that reaches equilibrium between plasma and urine by passive diffusion. If the drug is not ionized, or if the urinary pH is the same as that of

plasma, the urinary concentration will equal the free plasma concentration, and if the drug is not protein-bound the clearance will simply equal the rate of urine formation—normally about 1 ml/min, but highly variable. For weak acids and bases this value will be multiplied by the pH partition factor (see Fig. 3.3), and it will also be reduced in proportion to the fraction of drug bound to plasma albumin. **Barbiturates** are an example of a group of drugs that are handled in this way.

Thus the rate of renal clearance of drugs can vary very greatly, from less than 1 ml/min to the theoretical maximum of about 700 ml/min. The interpretation of these values in terms of the rate at which drugs are removed from the body, expressed as **plasma half-life**, is discussed in a later section.

As well as varying markedly from drug to drug, renal elimination varies considerably amongst individuals, and from time to time in the same individual, for reasons that are discussed in more detail in Chapter 4. For a small, but important, group of

Table 3.5 Drugs that are largely excreted unchanged in the urine

100%–75%	Amiloride, Frusemide, Hexamethonium Gallamine, Chlorothiazide Gentamicin, Practolol, Methotrexate Atenolol, Ampicillin Digoxin, Pyridostigmine
75%–50%	Amphetamine, Carbenicillin Benzylpenicillin, Cimetidine Cephaloridine, Oxytetracycline Frusemide Procainamide, Neostigmine, Methyldopa Clonidine
~ 50%	Ampicillin, Propantheline, Tubocurarine

drugs (Table 3.5), which are not inactivated by metabolism, the rate of renal elimination is the main factor that determines their duration of action. These drugs have to be used with special care in individuals whose renal function may be impaired.

The clearance concept is also useful in quantifying the rate of metabolic degradation of drugs, since this can be expressed in terms of the notional volume of plasma from which the drug is completely removed by metabolism in unit time. Thus the rate of hepatic metabolism can be denoted by CL_{hep}. More generally, CL_{met} can be used to define the overall metabolic clearance, including sites other than the liver.

Biliary excretion and enterohepatic circulation

Liver cells possess transport systems, rather similar to those of the renal tubule, which transfer various substances from plasma to bile. In addition to acid and base handling systems, hepatocytes have a third mechanism which transports various uncharged molecules. Various hydrophilic drug conjugates (particularly **glucuronides**) are concentrated in bile and delivered to the intestine, where the glucuronide is usually hydrolysed, releasing the active drug once more; the drug can then be reabsorbed and go round the cycle repeatedly.

The effect of this is to create a 'reservoir' of recirculating drug, which can amount to about 20% of the drug in the body, and which tends to prolong the duration of action. There are only a few examples where this effect is significant, e.g. **digoxin**, which is excreted in the bile in an unconjugated form; **morphine**, **chloramphenicol** and **stilboestrol**, which are transported as glucuronides.

There are also a few drugs that are excreted to an appreciable extent in the bile. **Cromoglycate**, which is administered by inhalation in the treatment of asthma is excreted mainly unchanged in the bile. **Rifampicin** is absorbed from the gut and gradually deacetylated, retaining its biological activity. Both forms are secreted in the bile but the deacetylated form is not reabsorbed, so eventually most of the drug leaves the body in this form, in the faeces.

PHARMACOKINETICS

We have now discussed the various processes of absorption, distribution, metabolism and elimination of drugs that determine their overall kinetic behaviour. In this section a simple quantitative model is presented which provides a view of how the system will behave when these processes are operating simultaneously, and in particular enables us to predict the **time-course** of drug action (an extremely important characteristic from a clinical point of view).

SINGLE COMPARTMENT MODEL

Consider first a highly over-simplified model of a human being, which consists only of a single compartment into which a quantity of drug is introduced rapidly by intravenous injection, and from which it can escape either by being metabolized or by being excreted (Fig. 3.18). If the volume of the compartment is V_d, and an amount Q of drug is introduced

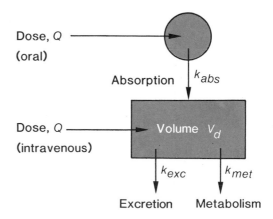

Fig. 3.18 Single compartment pharmacokinetic model.

at time zero, the initial concentration, $C(0)$, will be given by:

$$C(0) = \frac{Q}{V_d}. \qquad 3.3$$

We will assume (realistically for most drugs) that the rate of elimination by both metabolism and renal excretion is directly proportional to the drug concentration. Thus:

Rate of loss by metabolism $\quad = CL_{met}.C$
Rate of loss by renal excretion $= CL_{exc}.C$
Overall rate of loss $\qquad\qquad = CL_s.C$

where CL_s denotes the **systemic clearance** ($= CL_{met} + CL_{exc}$).

The total rate of loss of drug from the compartment, $-dQ/dt$, at any moment is equal to the sum of the rates of metabolism and excretion:

$$-\frac{dQ}{dt} = \frac{CL_s.Q(t)}{V_d} \qquad 3.4$$

Expressing this equation in terms of concentration, $C(t)$, gives:

$$-\frac{dC}{dt} = \frac{CL_s.C(t)}{V_d}. \qquad 3.5$$

Integration of this differential equation gives an **exponential** curve (Fig. 3.19) described by the equation:

$$C(t) = C(0)\exp\frac{-CL_s}{V_d}.t \qquad 3.6$$

Taking logarithms:

$$\ln C(t) = \ln C(0) - \frac{CL_s}{V_d}.t \qquad 3.7$$

Thus, plotting $C(t)$ logarithmically against t gives a straight line whose slope gives the **rate constant for elimination, k_{el}**:

$$k_{el} = \frac{CL_s}{V_d} \qquad 3.8$$

Substituting this value in equation 3.7:

$$\ln C(t) = \ln C(0) - k_{el}.t \qquad 3.9$$

Rearranging:

$$k_{el} = \frac{1}{t}.\ln\frac{C(0)}{C(t)} \qquad 3.10$$

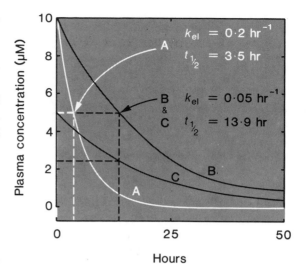

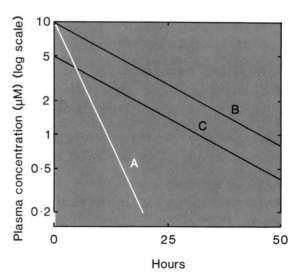

Fig. 3.19 Predicted behaviour of single compartment model following intravenous drug administration at time 0. Drugs A and B differ only in their elimination rate constant, k_{el}. Curve C shows the plasma concentration time course for a smaller dose of B. Note that $t_{\frac{1}{2}}$ (indicated by broken lines) does not depend on the dose. *Top.* linear concentration scale. *Bottom.* logarithmic concentration scale.

Thus, the rate constant k_{el} has the units time^{-1} and equation 3.8 shows that it varies directly with CL_s, and inversely with V_d.

Rearrangement of equation 3.9 gives:

$$t = \frac{1}{k_{el}}.\ln\frac{C(0)}{C(t)} \qquad 3.11$$

An easily conceptualized parameter is the **half-**

time for elimination, or **half-life, $t_{\frac{1}{2}}$**, which is equal to the time taken for $C(t)$ to decrease by 50%. At this time $C(0)/C(t) = 2$, so from equation 3.11 it can be seen that $t_{\frac{1}{2}}$ is related to k_{el} by:

$$t_{\frac{1}{2}} = \frac{\ln 2}{k_{el}} = \frac{0.693}{k_{el}} \qquad 3.12$$

The important points are (a) that the duration for which the drug persists, of which $t_{\frac{1}{2}}$ provides a measure, is short if k_{el} is high, and if V_d is low; and (b) that the plasma concentration falls exponentially, which follows from the assumption that the rate of elimination is directly proportional to the plasma concentration.

The discussion of distribution volumes (p. 72) and renal clearances (p. 79) for drugs of different kinds enables us to predict plasma half-times on the basis of renal elimination (Table 3.6) for drugs of

Table 3.6 Expected pharmacokinetic characteristics of drugs with different properties in a standard 70 kg subject

Drug type	CL_r $l\,min^{-1}$	V_d litres	$t_{\frac{1}{2}}$
Lipid soluble No pH partition	0.001	42	20 days
Lipid soluble Excretion favoured by pH partition	0.03	42	16 hours
Non-lipid soluble No tubular transport	0.120	12	69 min
Non-lipid soluble Complete tubular secretion	0.70	12	12 min

high and low lipid solubility that are, or are not, actively secreted. Actual rates of drug elimination do not show such an extreme variation as the examples in Table 3.6, for various reasons:

(1) Drug metabolism is not taken into account in these examples. For most lipid soluble drugs this is more important than renal clearance, so half-times are generally much shorter than the hypothetical value of 20 days based on renal clearance alone.

(2) The single compartment model is unrealistic as a description of rapidly eliminated drugs, because exchanges between plasma and tissue compartments (which the model ignores) can be slow compared with the 'theoretical' plasma half-time, and

are likely to be rate-limiting in controlling elimination from the plasma compartment.

Effect of varying dosage schedules

So far we have considered the time course of the plasma concentration following a single intravenous injection. What happens if the drug is given repeatedly at regular intervals, or as a continuous infusion? In either case the plasma concentration will increase up to a point where a steady state is reached, such that the *mean* rate of drug elimination is equal to the *mean* rate of administration. Thus if the drug is infused continuously at a rate of X moles/min, then once a steady state is reached, with plasma concentration $C(steady\ state)$, the rate of elimination must equal X:

$$X = CL_s \cdot C(steady\ state)$$

Therefore: $C(steady\ state) = X/CL_s.$ 3.13

The drug concentration approaches this steady-state value exponentially, with a half-time equal to that for elimination of the drug (Fig. 3.20). When the infusion is stopped the plasma concentration declines to zero with the same time course.

Repeated injections give a more complicated pattern (Fig. 3.21), but the principle is the same: in the steady state the mean plasma concentration, $C(steady\ state)$, is such that the mean rate of elimination is equal to the mean rate of administration. Thus if dose Q is given every T hours (the mean rate of administration being Q/T), then:

$$C(steady\ state) = \frac{Q}{T \cdot CL_s} \qquad 3.14$$

The mean steady state concentration is thus the same as for a continuous infusion at the same rate, but the concentration will oscillate about the mean through a range Q/V_d, which is the increment in concentration produced by each dose. The steady state is reached, as with continuous infusion, with an approximately exponential time course. Using smaller doses at shorter intervals (keeping Q/T constant) reduces the amplitude of the swings in concentration, but affects neither the steady state concentration nor the rate at which it is approached.

In practice a steady state is effectively reached

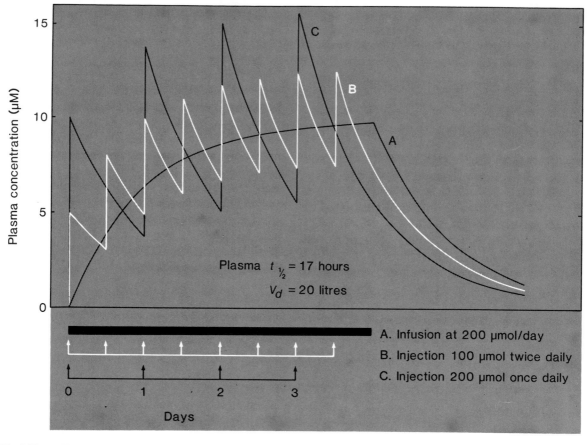

Fig. 3.20 Predicted behaviour of single compartment model with continuous or intermittent drug administration. **A.** Smooth curve showing effect of continuous infusion for 4 days. **B.** The same total amount of drug given in 8 equal doses. **C.** The same total amount of drug given in 4 equal doses. Note that in each case a steady state is effectively reached after about 2 days (about $3 \times t_{\frac{1}{2}}$), and that the mean concentration reached in the steady state is the same for all 3 schedules.

after an interval of about three plasma half-times has elapsed. Speedier attainment of the steady state can be achieved by starting with a larger **loading dose**. This is often done, for example, at the start of a course of treatment with digoxin for cardiac failure (see Chapter 10).

It must again be emphasized that the simple behaviour predicted for the single compartment model only roughly corresponds to real life. Inclusion of other body compartments, particularly slowly-equilibrating ones such as body fat, will result in additional exponential components in the overall kinetic behaviour. Pharmacokinetic studies in man show that to produce a realistic simulation the inclusion of two or three compartments is necessary for most drugs.

Effect of variation in rate of absorption

If a drug is absorbed slowly, from the gut or from an injection site, into the plasma, it is (in terms of a compartmental model) as though it was being injected slowly into the bloodstream. For the purpose of kinetic modelling the transfer of drug from the site of administration to the central compartment can be represented approximately by a rate constant, k_{abs} (see Fig. 3.18). This assumes that the rate of absorption is directly proportional, at any moment, to the amount of drug still unabsorbed, which is at best a rough approximation to reality. The effect of slow absorption on the time-course of the rise and fall of the plasma concentration is shown in Figure 3.21. The curves show the effect of

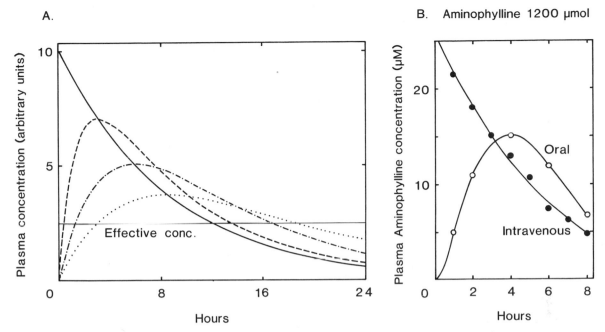

Fig. 3.21 A. Predicted behaviour of single compartment model with drug absorbed at different rates from the gut or an injection site. The elimination half-time, $t_{\frac{1}{2}el}$ is 6 hours.

——————— $t_{\frac{1}{2}abs} = 0$ (equivalent to intravenous administration)
— — — — $t_{\frac{1}{2}abs} = 1\,\text{hr}$
—·—·—·— $t_{\frac{1}{2}abs} = 3\,\text{hr}$
············· $t_{\frac{1}{2}abs} = 6\,\text{hr}.$

Note that the peak plasma concentration is reduced and delayed by slow absorption, and the duration of action somewhat increased. **B.** Measurements of plasma aminophylline concentration in man following equal oral and intravenous doses. (Data from: Swintowsky, 1956)

spreading out the absorption of the same total amount of drug over different periods of time. In each case, all of the drug is absorbed, but the peak concentration appears later and becomes lower and less sharp if absorption is slow. Once absorption is complete, the plasma concentration declines with the same half-time, irrespective of the rate of absorption. It can be shown that, for the kind of pharmacokinetic model discussed here, the *area* under the plasma concentration-time curve, (Fig. 3.21), is directly proportional to the total amount of drug introduced into the plasma compartment, irrespective of the rate at which it enters. Measurements of this area (unpleasantly abbreviated to **AUC**, for **Area under the curve**) following oral administration can therefore be used to determine the fraction of the oral dose that enters the bloodstream, and thus to measure **bioavailability** (see p. 68). Incomplete absorption, or destruction by first-pass metabolism before the drug reaches the plasma

compartment, will reduce the area under the curve, whereas changes in the rate of absorption will not affect it.

Again it is worth noting that provided absorption is complete the relation between the rate of administration and the steady-state plasma concentration (equation 3.14) is unaffected by k_{abs}, though the size of the oscillation of plasma concentration with each dose will be reduced if absorption is slow.

The effect of protein binding

The effect of protein binding on drug elimination is not straightforward. It is often stated that, because the bound fraction is unavailable for elimination (since it is excluded from glomerular filtration, and cannot enter hepatocytes), binding necessarily prolongs the action of a drug. However, binding also reduces V_d, by retaining part of the drug in the plasma, and may not greatly reduce CL_{exc} and

CL_{met}, since active transport systems can work efficiently even though the drug is reversibly bound. The overall effect on the rate of drug elimination is therefore unpredictable and usually not very large. Curry (1980) advises 'dismiss the idea that protein binding is a major influence on elimination' and suggests instead that it 'is a magnificently efficient mass transit system, collecting drug molecules at their sites of absorption and depositing them at their sites of storage, action and elimination, with breathtaking efficiency'. Breathless or not, let us agree with him and pass on.

MORE COMPLICATED KINETIC MODELS

So far we have considered a single compartment pharmacokinetic model, in which the rates of absorption, metabolism and excretion are all assumed to be directly proportional to the concentration of drug in the compartment from which the transfer is occurring. This is a useful way to illustrate some basic principles, but it is clearly a physiological over-simplification. The characteristics of different parts of the body, such as brain, body fat and muscle, are quite different in terms of their blood supply, partition coefficient for drugs, and the permeability of their capillaries to drugs. These differences, which the single compartment model ignores, can considerably affect the time-course of drug distribution and drug action, and much theoretical work has gone into the mathematical analysis of more complex models. Discussions can be found in specialized texts (e.g. Notari, 1980). They are beyond the scope of this book, and perhaps also beyond the limit of what is actually useful, for the experimental data on pharmacokinetic properties of drugs is seldom accurate or reproducible enough to enable complex models to be critically tested.

We shall now discuss briefly two modifications of the simple single-compartment model, both of which bring it nearer to reality without involving excessive complications. The first is the two-compartment model, which introduces a separate 'peripheral' compartment to represent the tissues, in communication with the 'central' plasma compartment. The second allows for the possibility that drug metabolizing enzymes may show 'saturation', so that the rate of metabolic degradation does not increase indefinitely in proportion to the drug concentration.

Two-compartment model

This is a widely-used approximation, in which the tissues are lumped together as a peripheral compartment, which drug molecules can enter and leave only via the central compartment (Fig. 3.22)

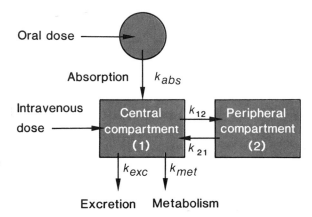

Fig. 3.22 Two compartment pharmacokinetic model.

which normally represents the plasma. For some drugs, however, which equilibrate particularly rapidly with extravascular compartments, some of these compartments may also be included in the central compartment. The effect of adding a second compartment to the model is to introduce a second exponential component into the predicted time-course of the plasma concentration, so that it comprises a fast and a slow phase. This pattern is often found experimentally, and is most clearly revealed when the concentration data are plotted semi-logarithmically (Fig. 3.23). If, as is often the case, the transfer of drug between the central and peripheral compartments is relatively fast compared with the rate of elimination, then the fast phase (often called the **α-phase**) can be taken to represent the *redistribution* of the drug (i.e. drug molecules passing from plasma to tissues, thereby rapidly lowering the plasma concentration). The plasma concentration reached when the fast phase is complete, but before any elimination has occurred allows a measure of the combined distribution volumes of the two compartments; and the half-time for the slow phase (the **β-phase**), provides

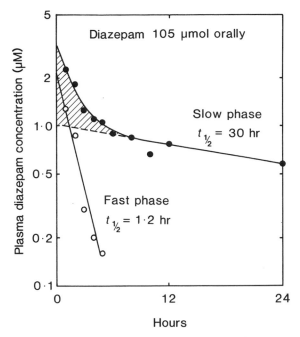

Fig. 3.23 Kinetics of diazepam elimination in man following a single oral dose (semilogarithmic plot of plasma concentration versus time). The experimental data (closed symbols) follows a curve that becomes linear after about 8 hours (slow phase). Plotting the deviation of the early points (shaded area) from this line on the same coordinates (open symbols) reveals the fast phase. This type of two-component decay is consistent with the two-compartment model (Fig. 3.22) and is obtained with many drugs. (Data from: Curry, 1980)

an estimate of the rate constant for elimination, k_{el}. If a drug is rapidly metabolized the α- and β-phases are not well separated, and the calculation of V_d and k_{el} is not straightforward. Problems also arise with drugs (e.g. very fat-soluble drugs) for which it is unrealistic to lump all the peripheral tissues together, so caution is needed in the interpretation of such pharmacokinetic data.

It is important to realize that the addition of extra compartments to the basic model affects only the predicted time-course of drug action, and not the steady-state. Thus the relation between plasma concentration and dose derived for the single-compartment model (equation 3.10) still applies.

Saturation kinetics

In a few cases where drugs are inactivated by metabolic degradation, e.g. **ethanol**, **phenytoin**, **salicylate**, **hydralazine**, the time-course of dis-

appearance of drug from the plasma does not follow the exponential or biexponential pattern shown in Figures 3.19 & 3.23, but is initially linear (i.e. the drug is removed at a constant rate, that is *independent* of plasma concentration). This is often called **zero-order kinetics** to distinguish it from the usual **first-order kinetics** which we have considered so far (terms which have their origin in chemical kinetic theory), though **saturation kinetics** is a better term. Figure 3.24 shows the example of ethanol. It

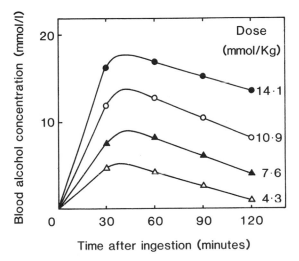

Fig. 3.24 Saturating kinetics of alcohol elimination in man. The blood alcohol concentration falls *linearly* rather than exponentially, and the rate of fall does not vary with dose. (From: Drew et al, 1958)

can be seen that the rate of disappearance of ethanol from the plasma is constant at about $0.2 \, \text{mmol} \, l^{-1}$ per hour irrespective of its plasma concentration. The explanation for this is that the rate of oxidation by the enzyme alcohol dehydrogenase reaches a maximum at low ethanol concentrations, because of limited availability of the co-factor, NAD^+ (see Chapter 35).

Saturation kinetics can have several important consequences (see Fig. 3.25). One is that the duration of action is more strongly dependent on dose than is the case with drugs that do not show metabolic saturation. Another consequence is that the relationship between dose and steady state plasma concentration is steep and unpredictable, and does not obey the proportionality rule implicit in equation 3.14 for non-saturating drugs. The maximum rate of metabolism sets a limit to the rate at which

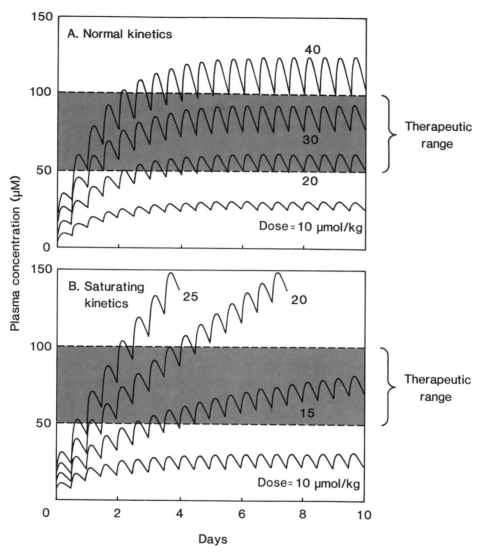

Fig. 3.25 Comparison of non-saturating and saturating kinetics for drugs given orally every 12 hours. The curves for saturating kinetics (bottom panel) are calculated from the known pharmacokinetic parameters of the anti-epileptic drug phenytoin (see Chapter 24).

The top panel shows an imaginary drug, similar to phenytoin at the lowest dose, but with normal kinetics.

Note: (a) that no steady state is reached with higher doses of phenytoin; (b) that a small increment in dose results after a time in a disproportionately large effect on plasma concentration. With normal kinetics the steady state plasma concentration is directly proportional to dose. Curves were calculated with the 'Sympak' pharmacokinetic modelling program written by Dr J G Blackman, University of Otago, NZ.

the drug can be administered, and if this rate is exceeded the amount of drug in the body will, in principle, increase indefinitely, and never reach a steady state (Fig. 3.25). This does not actually happen, because there is always some dependence of the rate of elimination on the plasma concentration (usually because other, non-saturating metabolic pathways, or renal excretion, contribute significantly at high concentrations). Nevertheless, the steady state plasma concentration of drugs of this kind varies with dose more widely and less predictably than it does with non-saturating drugs. Similarly, variations in the rate of metabolism (e.g. through enzyme induction) also produce disproportionately large changes in the plasma concentration. These problems are well recognized for drugs such as phenytoin, an antiepileptic drug (see Chapter 24) whose plasma concentration needs to be closely controlled to achieve an optimal clinical effect. The dose of phenytoin needed to achieve the optimal plasma concentration varies widely from individual to individual, mainly because it shows saturating kinetics, and it is usual to measure the plasma concentration at regular intervals.

Special drug delivery systems

Several new approaches are being actively explored at present which attempt to improve certain aspects of drug delivery (see Vaizoglu & Speiser, 1982; Gregoriadis, 1981, 1982 for reviews).

1. **Sustained release preparations** to avoid the need for frequent dosage. Depot preparations of esterified phenothiazines (e.g. **fluphenazine undecanoate**) which are slowly hydrolysed, and whose antipsychotic action lasts for weeks after a single injection, are one example.
2. **Pro-drugs** (see p. 78). Examples are given in Table 3.3. Most of the examples in clinical practice confer no obvious benefits, and have been found to be pro-drugs only retrospectively, not having been designed with this in mind. Some do, however, have advantages. Thus, the cytotoxic drug **cyclophosphamide** (see Chapter 29) becomes active only after it has been metabolized in the liver, and can therefore be taken orally without causing serious damage to the gastrointestinal epithelium. Other problems could

theoretically be overcome by the use of suitable pro-drugs; for example, instability of drugs at gastric pH, strong gastric irritation, poor absorbability, failure of drug to cross blood-brain barrier, etc, but in practice the usefulness of this approach has so far been limited. Albert (1965) warns the optimistic pro-drug designer '.... he will have to bear in mind that an organism's normal reaction to a foreign substance is to burn it up for food.'

3. **Antibody-drug conjugates**. One of the aims of cancer chemotherapy is to improve the selectivity of cytotoxic drugs. An interesting possibility is to attach the drug to an antibody directed against a tumour-specific antigen, which will bind selectively to tumour cells. Such approaches look promising in experimental animals, but it is too early to say whether they will succeed in man.
4. **Packaging in liposomes**. Liposomes are minute vesicles, produced by sonication of an aqueous suspension of certain phospholipids. They can be filled with non lipid-soluble drugs, which are retained until the liposome is disrupted. When injected, liposomes are mainly taken up by reticulo-endothelial cells, especially in the liver, and there is a possibility of achieving selective delivery of drugs (e.g. in hepatic amoebiasis or hepatic tumours) in this way. In the future, it may also be possible to direct drugs selectively by incorporating antibody molecules, against specific tissue antigens, into the surface layer of the liposome (Gregoriadis, 1981).

REFERENCES AND FURTHER READING

Bundgaard H, Hansen A B, Kofod H 1982 Optimization of drug delivery. Munskgaard, Copenhagen
Caldwell J, Jakoby W B 1983 Biological basis of detoxification. Academic Press, London
Curry S H 1980 Drug disposition and pharmacokinetics. Blackwell, Oxford
de Leve L D, Piafsky K M 1983 Clinical significance of plasma binding of basic drugs. In: Lamble J W (ed) Drug metabolism and distribution. Elsevier, London
Gibaldi M 1984 Biopharmaceutics and clinical pharmacokinetics. Lea & Febiger, Philadelphia
Gibaldi M, Perrier D 1975 Pharmacokinetics. Dekker, New York
Gibaldi M, Prescott L 1983 Handbook of clinical pharmacokinetics. ADIS Health Service Press, Sydney
Gorrod J W, Beckett A H 1978 Drug metabolism in man. Taylor & Francis, London
Gregoriadis G 1981 Targetting of drugs: implications in medicine. Lancet 2: 241–246

Gregoriadis G 1982 Use of monoclonal antibodies and liposomes to improve drug delivery. Drugs 24: 261–266
Juliano R L 1980 Drug delivery systems: characteristics and biomedical applications. Oxford University Press, Oxford
Jusko W J, Gretch M 1976 Plasma and tissue protein binding of drugs in pharmacokinetics. Drug Metab Rev 5: 43–140
Lamble J W (ed) 1983 Drug metabolism and distribution. Elsevier, Amsterdam
Notari R E 1980 Biopharmaceutics and clinical pharmacokinetics. Dekker, New York
Richens A, Marks V 1981 Therapeutic drug monitoring. Churchill Livingstone, Edinburgh
Theorell P, Dedrick R L, Condliffe P G 1974 Pharmacology and pharmacokinetics. Plenum, London
Vaizoglu O, Speiser P 1982 'Intelligent' drug delivery systems. Trends in Pharmacological Sciences 3: 28–30
Wagner J G 1975 Do you need a pharmacokinetics model and, if so, which one? J Pharmacokin Biopharm 3: 457

Individual variation and drug interactions

Variability in the effect of a drug, given either to different individuals, or to the same individual on different occasions, results from either (a) differing concentrations of the drug at the site of action, or (b) differing physiological responses to the same drug concentration. Variation of the first kind is often called **pharmacokinetic**, and may occur because of differences in absorption, distribution, metabolism or excretion of the drug; variation of the second kind is called **pharmacodynamic**, and its possible causes are legion. In most cases, the variation is *quantitative*, in the sense that the drug may produce a larger or smaller effect, or may act for a longer or shorter time, while still exerting qualitatively the same effect. In other cases, the action is qualitatively different (e.g. the haemolytic reaction that drugs such as primaquine may cause in certain susceptible individuals). Such instances are known as **idiosyncratic** reactions.

In the last chapter the effect of various factors, such as bioavailability, food intake, gastric and urinary pH etc on the absorption and elimination of drugs were discussed, all of which contribute substantially to quantitative variations in drug responses. In this chapter some other important factors responsible for variation in drug response are presented under three headings:

1. **Age**
2. **Genetic factors**
3. **Drug interactions**.

The influence of a fourth factor, namely the existence of **disease states**, is also important as a cause of individual variation, but it is beyond the scope of this book. General accounts can be found elsewhere (e.g. Curry, 1980; Gorrod & Beckett, 1978; Smith & Rawlins, 1973; Gibaldi & Prescott, 1983).

EFFECTS OF AGE

The main reason that age affects drug action is that drug metabolism and renal function are less efficient in very young, as well as in old individuals, so that with some exceptions drugs tend to produce greater and more prolonged effects at the extremes of life. Variations in **tissue sensitivity** with age, so that a given plasma concentration produces a different effect, are also important with some drugs.

Renal excretion

Renal function in the newborn, measured either as glomerular filtration rate or as maximal tubular secretory rate, is only about 20% of the adult value (normalized to body surface area). It develops rapidly to adult level, in less than a week. In premature infants, development of full renal function is rather slower. From the age of about 20,

Table 4.1 Plasma half-lives for antibiotics that are mainly excreted unchanged in the urine, as a function of age

Drug	1st week	4th week	Adult
Ampicillin	4.0	1.7	1–2
Methicillin	2.4	1.4	0.5
Oxacillin	> 1.5	1.2	0.5
Neomycin	5.4	3.7	2.0
Colistin	2.6	2.3	3–5
Kanamycin	8.9		2.0
Streptomycin	7.0		2–3

(Data from: Reidenberg, 1971 Renal function and drug action. W B Saunders, Philadelphia)

renal function begins to decline slowly falling by about 25% at 50 and by 50% at 75. There is a corresponding change in the rate of renal elimination of drugs. Table 4.1 shows the plasma half-life of various antibiotics that are mainly eliminated by the kidney, as a function of age. Figure 4.1 shows

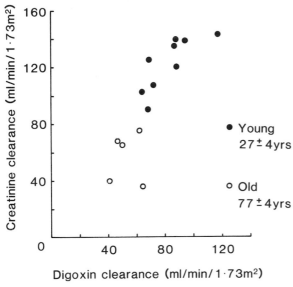

Fig. 4.1 Relationships between renal function (measured as creatinine clearance) and digoxin clearance in young and old subjects. (From: Ewy et al, 1969)

the renal clearance of **digoxin**, which is closely correlated with creatinine clearance, in young and old subjects. The tendency for the plasma digoxin concentration to increase steadily with age, even though the dose is not changed, is a well-recognized cause of glycoside toxicity (see Chapter 10). Renal immaturity in premature infants can have a very large effect on drug elimination. Thus in newborn premature babies the antibiotic **gentamicin** has a plasma half-life of 18 hours, compared with about 2 hours for adults. In full-term newborn babies the value is about 6 hours. It is therefore necessary to reduce and space out doses to avoid toxicity in the newborn.

Drug metabolism

In the neonate, and particularly in premature babies, the hepatic microsomal oxidase, glucuronyl transferase, and acetyl transferase, and also the

plasma esterases, are poorly developed compared with the adult, taking about 8 weeks to reach the adult level of activity. In children up to about 10 years old the liver weight is greater in proportion to body weight than in the adult, and drug metabolism can be more rapid than in the adult, though the difference is not large.

The relative lack of conjugating activity in the newborn can have serious consequences, as in the 'grey baby' syndrome caused by the antibiotic **chloramphenicol** (see Chapter 30). At first thought to be a specific biochemical sensitivity to the drug in young babies, this sometimes fatal condition was shown to result simply from accumulation of very high tissue concentrations of chloramphenicol because of very slow hepatic conjugation. If allowance is made for this, chloramphenicol is no more toxic to babies than to adults. Slow conjugation is also one reason why **morphine** (which is excreted mainly as the glucuronide) is not used as an analgesic in labour. Any drug transferred to the newborn baby will have a long plasma half-life ($t_{\frac{1}{2}}$), and can cause prolonged respiratory depression.

The activity of hepatic microsomal enzymes declines slowly (and very variably) with age. The steadily increasing plasma $t_{\frac{1}{2}}$ of the anxiolytic drug, **diazepam** (Fig. 4.2) is one example of this. As can be seen the effect is large, amounting to a roughly four-fold change between the ages of 20 and 70, and requires a considerable adjustment of dosage to compensate for it. In other instances, the effect of age is less marked. With **antipyrine**, for example,

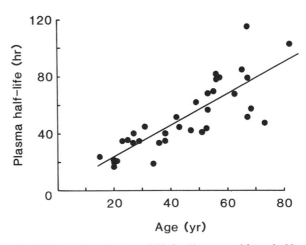

Fig. 4.2 Increasing plasma half-life for diazepam with age in 33 normal subjects. (From: Klotz U et al, 1975)

plasma $t_\frac{1}{2}$ increases only about 50% between the ages of 26 and 78, while with **phenylbutazone** the change is even smaller, about 30%. Even though the mean $t_\frac{1}{2}$ does not change much, there is a striking increase in the *variability* of $t_\frac{1}{2}$ between individuals with age, a fact of some clinical importance. Thus a population of old people will contain some individuals with grossly reduced rates of drug metabolism whereas a young population will not show such extremes.

Variations in sensitivity

There are many examples where the same plasma concentration of a drug will cause different effects in young and old subjects. Thus anxiolytic and hypnotic drugs such as **benzodiazepines** and **barbiturates** produce more confusion and less sedation in elderly than in young subjects. Hypotensive drugs tend to cause a larger fall in arterial pressure, together with giddiness, in old patients.

Amphetamine, which causes excitement and sleeplessness in adults, tends to have the opposite effect in hyperactive children.

GENETIC FACTORS

Drug metabolism

It has been established from studies on identical and non-identical twins that much of the individual variability in plasma $t_\frac{1}{2}$ for various drugs is genetically determined. Thus $t_\frac{1}{2}$ values for **phenylbutazone** and **coumarin** anticoagulants in pairs of identical twins are 6–22 times less variable than in fraternal twins, and it has been estimated that genetic factors account for two-thirds of the observed phenotypic variation of $t_\frac{1}{2}$ values for phenylbutazone in man (Vessell & Page, 1968). The effect of this kind of variation is to produce a continuous, or roughly Gaussian, distribution of pharmacokinetic characteristics within a population of subjects. Figure 4.3 (*left*) shows the distribution of plasma concentrations achieved 3 hours after a fixed dose of salicylate in 100 subjects; genetic factors will contribute only a part of the variation seen, the rest being due to physiological factors affecting absorption (e.g. gastric pH and gastrointestinal motility), or elimination of the drug (e.g. urine flow and urinary pH).

In some special cases the population can be clearly seen to consist of two distinct subclasses. A well-known example concerns the rate of acetylation of the anti-tuberculosis drug, **isoniazid** (Fig. 4.3 *right*). Given the same oral dose, about half the population shows a plasma concentration of less than 1.5 µmol/l whereas in the other half it is 2–5 µmol/l. The elimination of isoniazid depends mainly on acetylation, involving acetyl-CoA and an

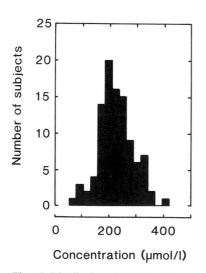
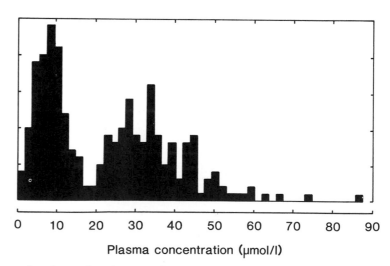

Fig. 4.3 Distribution of individual plasma concentrations for two drugs in man. *Left*: Plasma salicylate concentration 3 hours after oral dosage with sodium salicylate at 0.19 mmol/kg. *Right*: Plasma isoniazid concentration 6 hours after oral dosage at 71 µmol/kg. Note the normally distributed values for salicylate, compared with the bimodal distribution with isoniazid. (From: (*left*) Curry, 1980; (*right*) Price Evans, 1963)

acetyltransferase enzyme. The population contains roughly equal numbers of 'fast acetylators' and 'slow acetylators' and family studies have shown that this characteristic is controlled by a single recessive gene, associated with low hepatic acetyltransferase activity. Isoniazid used clinically gives rise to two main forms of toxicity. One is a peripheral neuropathy, produced by isoniazid itself, whose incidence is greater in slow than in fast acetylators. The other is hepatotoxicity, produced by degradation of the acetylated metabolite to acetylhydrazine; its incidence is greater in fast acetylators. This type of genetic variation thus produces a qualitative change in the pattern of toxicity seen with the drug. The same enzyme is important in the degradation of other drugs, such as **hydrallazine** (see Chapter 11), **procainamide** (Chapter 10) and various **sulphonamides** (Chapter 30). The clinical significance of acetylator polymorphism is discussed in detail by du Sonich & Lambert (1983).

Another well-studied example of genetic variation in the rate of drug metabolism is that of **suxamethonium** hydrolysis (Kalow, 1962). Suxamethonium (see Chapter 6) is a short-acting neuromuscular blocking drug, widely used in anaesthesia, which is inactivated in a few minutes by hydrolysis, catalysed by plasma cholinesterase. About 1 in 3000 individuals fail to inactivate suxamethonium rapidly, and show a neuromuscular block that can last several hours. This is due to a recessive gene that gives rise, in homozygotes, to an abnormal type of plasma cholinesterase. The abnormal enzyme has a modified pattern of substrate and inhibitor specificity; it handles many substrates quite normally, but not suxamethonium. It is most easily detected by measuring the inhibition of plasma cholinesterase activity, using benzoylcholine as substrate, by **dibucaine**, which inhibits the abnormal enzyme less effectively than the normal enzyme (see Chapter 6). The enzyme in the heterozygote, which hydrolyses suxamethonium at a more or less normal rate, shows a reduced sensitivity to dibucaine which is intermediate between the normal and the homozygous enzyme (Fig. 4.4). There are other, nongenetic, reasons why suxamethonium hydrolysis may be impaired in an individual patient (see later) so in a patient who shows prolonged paralysis with this drug it is important to discover whether this genetic abnormality is present, and to test members of the family who may be similarly abnormal.

New examples of polymorphic variations of drug metabolism are being discovered all the time, and the list is now quite long (see Lamble, 1983). Drugs for which such variation is important include **phenytoin**, an antiepileptic drug (see Chapter 34); **debrisoquin**, a hypotensive drug (Chapter 11); **paraoxon**, an anticholinesterase used as an insecticide; and **mercaptopurine**, an anti-tumour drug (Chapter 29).

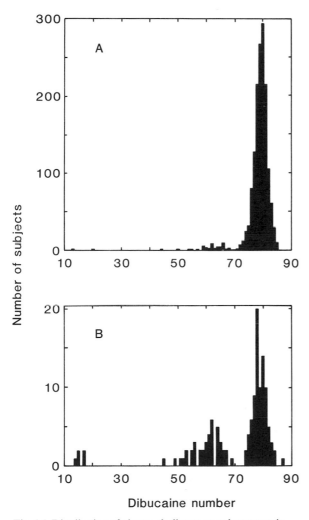

Fig. 4.4 Distribution of plasma cholinesterase phenotypes in man. Dibucaine number is a measure of the percentage inhibition of plasma cholinesterase by 10^{-5} M dibucaine. The abnormal enzyme has, in addition to low enzymic activity, a low dibucaine number. **A**. Normal population; **B**. Families of subjects with low or intermediate dibucaine numbers. (From: Kalow, 1962)

Idiosyncratic reactions

An idiosyncratic reaction is a qualitatively different type of drug effect (usually harmful) that occurs in a small proportion of individuals. In some cases such reactions are immunological in origin (see Chapter 36), but there are several instances where genetic anomalies are responsible.

An interesting example concerns the antimalarial drug **primaquine** (Chapter 33) which is well tolerated in most individuals. In 5–10% of black males, however, the drug causes haemolysis of red cells leading to severe anaemia. This reaction, in sensitive individuals, also occurs with other aniline derivatives, including some sulphonamide drugs. The underlying abnormality consists of a deficiency of the enzyme glucose-6-phosphate dehydrogenase (G6PD) from the red cells, a trait that is inherited as a sex-linked recessive. This enzyme is necessary to maintain the content of reduced glutathione (GSH) in red cells, GSH being necessary to prevent haemolysis. Aniline derivatives cause GSH to drop, harmlessly in normal cells, but enough to cause haemolysis in G6PD-deficient cells. Interestingly, the heterozygotic females, who show no tendency to haemolysis, have an increased resistance to malaria infection, a fact which accounts for the persistence of the gene in malaria-endemic regions.

Another clinically important example of an idiosyncratic reaction is the effect of **barbiturates** and some other drugs in precipitating attacks of acute porphyria in susceptible individuals. Hepatic porphyria is an inherited disorder in which one of the enzymes required for haem synthesis is lacking, with the result that various porphyrin-containing haem precursors accumulate, giving rise to acute attacks of gastrointestinal, neurological and behavioural disturbances. The synthesis of these porphyrins is from a precursor, δ-amino laevulinic acid (ALA), which is formed in the liver by the action of an enzyme, ALA synthetase. This enzyme is induced, like various other hepatic enzymes, by drugs such as barbiturates, and is also regulated by a complex feedback mechanism which is affected by a range of porphyrogenic drugs which have no direct inducing effect on other enzymes. The result is an increase in ALA production, and hence increased porphyrin accumulation.

There are various other examples of genetically-determined idiosyncratic reactions. They include the condition of malignant hyperpyrexia, a dangerous metabolic reaction to drugs such as **halothane** and **suxamethonium**, which is known to be an inherited trait though its biochemical basis is not well understood; and alcohol-induced flushing and nausea that occurs in a proportion of subjects treated for diabetes with **sulfonylurea drugs** (see Chapter 16).

DRUG INTERACTIONS

The administration of one drug (A) can alter the action of another (drug B) by one of two general mechanisms, namely modification of the pharmacological action of B without altering its concentration in the tissue fluid (i.e. pharmacodynamic interaction) or alteration of the concentration of B that reaches its site of action (i.e. pharmacokinetic interactions).*

PHARMACODYNAMIC INTERACTION

Pharmacodynamic interaction can occur in many different ways, and can result in either reduction or enhancement of the action of B in the presence of A. There are many mechanisms, and some examples of practical importance are probably more useful than attempts at classification.

1. **β-receptor antagonists** diminish the effectiveness of bronchodilators, such as salbutamol, that are β-receptor agonists (see Chapter 7).

2. Many **diuretics** lower plasma potassium concentration (see Chapter 14), and thereby enhance some actions of cardiac glycosides and predispose to glycoside toxicity.

3. **Monoamine oxidase inhibitors** increase the amount of noradrenaline stored in adrenergic nerve terminals and thereby enhance the actions of drugs such as ephedrine and tyramine, which work by releasing stored noradrenaline.

---

*A third category of *pharmaceutical* interactions should be mentioned, in which drugs interact *in vitro* so that one or both are inactivated. No pharmacological principles are involved, just chemistry. An example is the formation of a complex between thiopentone and suxamethonium, which may not be mixed in the same syringe.

4. **Sulphonamides** produce their antibacterial action by inhibiting competitively the incorporation of p-aminobenzoic acid (PABA) into folate by bacterial cells (see Chapter 30). Administration of procaine, which is metabolized to PABA, opposes the antibacterial effect of sulphonamides.

5. **Adrenergic neurone blocking drugs,** such as guanethidine (see Chapter 7), have to be taken up by adrenergic nerve terminals in order to act. Drugs which prevent this uptake, such as the tricyclic antidepressant drugs, oppose the antihypertensive action of these agents (Fig. 4.5).

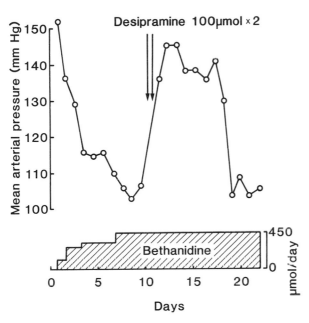

Fig. 4.5 Interaction of desipramine and bethanidine in a hypertensive patient. After the arterial pressure has been lowered by bethanidine, the effect is temporarily reversed by two doses of desipramine. This occurs because desipramine blocks the uptake of bethanidine by sympathetic nerve terminals. (From: Mitchell et al, 1970)

6. **Coumarin anticoagulants** work by competition with vitamin K, preventing hepatic synthesis of various blood clotting factors (see Chapter 12). If vitamin K production in the intestine is inhibited (e.g. by locally-acting antibacterial drugs) or its absorption is inhibited (e.g. by administration of liquid paraffin), the anticoagulant action of coumarins may be increased.

7. **Sulphonamides** prevent the synthesis of di-hydrofolic acid by bacteria; **trimethoprim** inhibits its reduction to tetrahydrofolate. Given together the drugs have a strongly synergistic action (see Chapter 30).

8. **Bacteriostatic antibacterial drugs** (e.g. chloramphenicol, sulphonamides) prevent bacterial cell division. Most bactericidal drugs (e.g. penicillins) kill organisms when they are in the process of dividing, and thus become relatively ineffective when given simultaneously with bacteriostatic drugs (see Chapter 30).

PHARMACOKINETIC INTERACTION

All of the four major processes that determine the pharmacokinetic behaviour of a drug—absorption, distribution, metabolism and excretion—are capable of being affected by co-administration of other drugs. Such interactions have received a great deal of attention in recent years, and examples, both theoretical and actual, have sprouted in the literature like mushrooms. Extensive catalogues of such effects are now available (e.g. Stockley, 1981; Griffin & D'Arcy, 1984; Hansten, 1985). Some of the more important mechanisms are given here, with examples.

Absorption phase

Gastrointestinal absorption may be slowed by drugs that inhibit gastrointestinal motility, such as **atropine** or **opiates,** or accelerated by drugs (e.g. **metoclopramide**; see Chapter 15) which hasten gastric emptying. Alternatively, drug A may interact with drug B in the gut in such a way as to inhibit absorption of B. Thus calcium, and also iron, forms an insoluble complex with **tetracycline** antibiotics and retards their absorption; **liquid paraffin**, given as a laxative will retain some highly lipid-soluble drugs in the intestine. Other mechanisms include the effect, produced by antidepressant drugs which inhibit monoamine oxidase (see Chapter 23), of preventing destruction of various dietary monoamines, especially tyramine, in the wall of the gut and in the liver. Tyramine is then absorbed and can produce a strong pressor effect. This is the basis of the 'cheese reaction' (see Chapter 23). Another simple example is the addition of **adrenaline** to local anaesthetic injections for infiltration anaesthesia (see Chapter 27). The vasoconstrictor effect of adrenaline slows down the absorption of the anaesthetic, thus prolonging its local effect.

Effects on drug distribution

The main type of interaction in this category occurs when one drug competes with another for binding to plasma protein (see Chapter 3). For a significant degree of interaction to occur it is necessary (a) that drug A should be given in sufficient dosage that an appreciable fraction of the protein binding sites are occupied (This generally means attaining a plasma concentration approaching 1 mM—see Chapter 3) and (b) that a large proportion of drug B should normally be bound to protein, so that inhibition of protein binding will substantially affect its distribution. Though many drugs have an appreciable affinity for plasma albumin and therefore might potentially be expected to interact, there are rather few instances where these conditions are met. Protein-bound drugs that are given in large enough dosage to act as 'displacing agents' include **phenylbutazone**, **aspirin** and various **sulphonamides**, as well as **chloral hydrate** whose metabolite, trichloracetic acid, binds very strongly to plasma albumin. Drugs that are likely to show effects as a result of a reduction of protein building include the anticoagulant **warfarin**, the hypoglycaemic drug **tolbutamide**, and the cytotoxic agent **methotrexate**.

The effect of displacing a drug from plasma albumin can be complex. On the one hand the *free* plasma concentration, and hence the effect of the drug, will increase, but the rate of metabolism and excretion may also be increased, leading to a shorter action. The *total* plasma concentration decreases as a result of reduced binding. An example is shown in Figure 4.6 where administration of chloral hydrate (a hypnotic) to a patient taking warfarin at regular intervals causes a decrease in total plasma warfarin, but an increase in its action, expressed as a prolongation of the prothrombin time. The plasma $t_{\frac{1}{2}}$ of warfarin was reduced. In the newborn, binding of unconjugated bilirubin to plasma albumin is an important way of keeping it out of the brain. This is important because a high concentration of unconjugated bilirubin seriously impairs brain development, producing a form of brain damage known as **kernicterus**. Administration of displacing drugs is therefore ill-advised in jaundiced neonates.

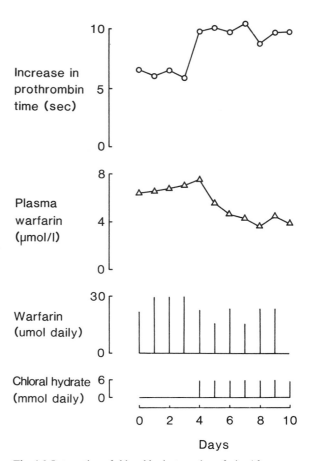

Fig. 4.6 Interaction of chloral hydrate and warfarin. After a steady anticoagulant effect (measured by increased prothrombin time) had been attained, administration of the hypnotic, chloral hydrate, increased the anticoagulant effect while reducing the total plasma warfarin concentration. This effect is due to displacement of warfarin from binding to plasma protein. (From: Sellers & Koch-Weser, 1970)

Effects on drug metabolism

The most important type of interaction results from **enzyme induction** (see Chapter 3). At least 200 drugs are known to be capable of producing this effect and thereby causing a decrease in the pharmacological activity of a range of other drugs. Since the inducing agent is normally itself a substrate for the induced enzymes, the process results in slowly-developing **tolerance**. This is important for drugs such as **barbiturates** and **ethanol**, as well as for the antituberculosis drug, **rifampicin**.

There are many examples of clinically important drug interactions resulting from enzyme induction, a few of which are listed in Table 4.2. A well-known

Table 4.2 Examples of drugs that induce or inhibit drug-metabolizing enzymes

Drugs modifying enzyme action	Drugs whose metabolism is affected
ENZYME INDUCTION	
Phenobarbitone and other barbiturates Rifampicin Griseofulvin Phenytoin Ethanol Phenylbutazone	Warfarin Oral contraceptives Corticosteroids Tolbutamide Digitoxin (as well as drugs listed in left hand column)
ENZYME INHIBITION	
Disulfiram	Coumarin anticoagulants
Allopurinol	Mercaptopurine, azathioprine
Ecothiopate and other anticholinesterases	Suxamethonium, procaine, propanidid
Chloramphenicol	Phenytoin

Corticosteroids	Various drugs e.g.
	    tricyclic antidepressants,
	    cyclophosphamide

MAO inhibitors	Pethidine

example is effect of **phenobarbitone** which reduces the steady state plasma concentration, and the pharmacological effect, of the warfarin-like anticoagulant **dicoumarol**. It is likely that part of the variability in rates of drug metabolism between individuals results from varying exposure to environmental contaminants such as DDT which are strong enzyme inducers.

Enzyme induction can serve a useful purpose. Excessive neonatal jaundice can cause brain damage because inconjugated bilirubin penetrates the blood-brain barrier. Administration of phenobarbitone to induce glucuronyl transferase increases bilirubin conjugation and reduces this risk.

Enzyme inhibition occurs with a number of drugs and this can slow down the metabolism, and hence increase the action, of various others. Some drugs that have this effect owe their own pharmacological actions to enzyme inhibition, and it is coincidental that their target enzymes also play a role in the metabolism of other drugs. Thus **allopurinol** is a drug used to treat gout (see Chapter 10), and it acts by inhibiting xanthine oxidase, an enzyme which converts purines to uric acid (overproduction of which leads to gout). Xanthine oxidase also metabolizes certain cytotoxic purine analogues, such as **mercaptopurine** and **azathioprine**, whose action is thus potentiated and prolonged by allopurinol. **Di-**

sulfiram is an inhibitor of aldehyde dehydrogenase; it causes ethanol ingestion to produce an unpleasant feeling of flushing and nausea resulting from accumulation of acetaldehyde. Disulfiram also inhibits metabolism of other drugs, such as **warfarin** and some **benzodiazepines**, and consequently prolongs their action. **Anticholinesterases**, such as ecothiopate will inhibit the metabolism, by plasma cholinesterase, of drugs such as **suxamethonium**, **procaine** and **propanidid**, with potentially serious consequences. In other cases the inhibition of drug metabolism is rather unexpected, since the offending agents are not recognized as enzyme inhibitors. Thus steroids can enhance by this mechanism the actions of a range of drugs including some antidepressants and some cytotoxic drugs. The only rule is: if in doubt about the existence of a possible interaction, look it up. Some examples are given in Table 4.2.

Haemodynamic effects

If a drug (e.g. **lignocaine** or **propranolol**) is rapidly metabolized by the liver so that its hepatic clearance approaches the hepatic blood flow (i.e. it shows extensive first-pass metabolism), then variations in hepatic blood flow will significantly affect the rate at which it is inactivated. A reduction in cardiac output will reduce hepatic blood flow, and it has been found that propranolol, for example, reduces the rate of metabolism of lignocaine by this mechanism.

Effects of drug excretion

The main mechanisms by which one drug can affect the rate of renal excretion of another are:

1. By altering protein binding, and hence rate of filtration
2. By inhibiting tubular secretion
3. By altering urine flow and/or urine pH.

Effects on protein binding have been discussed already (see Chapter 3). In general, reduction of protein binding has only a small effect on renal excretion, and it can be in either direction.

Inhibition of tubular secretion. The clearest example is **probenecid** (see Chapter 14), which was

Table 4.3 Examples of drugs that inhibit renal tubular secretion

Drugs causing inhibition	Drugs whose $t_{\frac{1}{2}}$ is affected
Probenecid Phenylbutazone Sulphonamides Aspirin Thiazide diuretics Indomethacin Dicoumarol	Penicillin Chlorpropamide Indomethacin

developed expressly to inhibit penicillin secretion and thus prolong its action. Other drugs have an incidental probenecid-like effect which can result in enhancement of the actions of substances which

rely on tubular secretion for their elimination. Table 4.3 gives some examples.

Alteration of urine flow and pH. Not surprisingly, diuretic drugs tend to increase the urinary excretion of other drugs. Thus **frusemide** (see Chapter 14) increases the rate of excretion of **indomethacin** and lowers its plasma concentration. There are not many reported examples of accidental interactions based on this mechanism, but the use of diuretics in the treatment of drug poisoning is well-established. Similarly the effect of urinary pH on the excretion of weak acids and bases (see Chapter 3) is put to use in the treatment of poisoning, though it does not seem to be much involved in producing accidental interactions.

REFERENCES AND FURTHER READING

Caldwell J, Jakoby W B 1983 Biological basis of detoxication. Academic Press, London

Curry S H 1980 Drug disposition and metabolism. Blackwell, Oxford

du Sonich P, Lambert C 1983 What is the clinical meaning of the acetylator phenotype? In: Lamble J W (ed) Drug metabolism and distribution. Elsevier, Amsterdam

Gibaldi M, Prescott L 1983 Handbook of clinical pharmacokinetics. ADIS Health Science Press, Sydney

Gorrod J W, Beckett A H 1978 Drug metabolism in man. Taylor & Francis, London

Griffin J P, D'Arcy P F 1984 A manual of adverse drug interactions. Wright, Bristol

Hansten P D 1985 Drug interactions. Lea & Febiger, Philadelphia

Kalow W 1962 Pharmacogenetics. W B Saunders, Philadelphia

Lamble J W (ed) 1983 Drug metabolism and distribution. Elsevier, Amsterdam

Smith S E, Rawlins M D 1973 Variability in human drug response. Butterworth, London

Stockley I H 1981 Drug interactions. Blackwell, Oxford

Vessell E S 1977 Genetic and environmental factors affecting drug disposition in man. Clin Pharm Ther 22: 659–679

Vessell E S, Page J G 1968 Genetic control of drug levels in man: phenylbutazone. Science 189: 1479–1480

Chemical mediators

Chemical transmission and the autonomic nervous system

It is the profusion of chemical signals by which cells in the body communicate with one another that provides many opportunities for specific drug effects. In this chapter we consider the process of chemical transmission in the peripheral nervous system, and discuss the various ways in which the process can be pharmacologically subverted. It is clear that the central nervous system uses very similar mechanisms to those described here, and that the same general principles apply, but the relative anatomical and physiological simplicity of the peripheral nervous system have made it the proving ground for most of the important discoveries about chemical transmission. Because these discoveries have led directly to the categorization of many major types of drug action, it is apt to recount briefly how the subject first developed. An excellent account is given by Bacq (1975).

In the latter half of the nineteenth century, when experimental physiology became established as an approach to the understanding of living organisms, the peripheral nervous system and particularly the autonomic nervous system received a great deal of attention. The fact that electrical stimulation of nerves could elicit a whole variety of physiological effects, from blanching of the skin to arrest of the heart, presented a real challenge to comprehension, particularly of the way in which the signal was passed from the nerve to the effector tissue. Du Bois Reymond in 1877 was the first to put the alternatives clearly: 'Of known natural processes that might pass on excitation, only two are, in my opinion, worth talking about; either there exists at the boundary of the contractile substance a stimulatory secretion...; or the phenomenon is electrical in nature.' The latter view was more generally believed. It was shown in 1869 that an exogenous substance, muscarine, could mimic the effects of stimulating the vagus nerve, and that atropine could inhibit the actions of both muscarine and nerve stimulation. J N Langley in 1905 showed the same for the actions of nicotine and curare at the neuromuscular junction. These phenomena were generally ascribed to stimulation and inhibition respectively, of the nerve endings, rather than to interference with a chemical transmitter.

Credit for suggesting, in 1904, that adrenaline might be the transmitter substance mediating the actions of the sympathetic nervous system goes to T R Elliot; the suggestion was coolly received, until Langley, the highly authoritarian Professor of Physiology at Cambridge at that time, suggested a year later that transmission to skeletal muscle involved the secretion by the nerve terminals of a substance related to nicotine.

One of the key observations for Elliot was that degeneration of sympathetic nerve terminals did not abolish the sensitivity of smooth muscle preparations to adrenaline (which the electrical theory predicted) but actually enhanced it. The hypothesis of chemical transmission was put to direct test by Dixon in 1907, who tried to show that vagus nerve stimulation released from a dog's heart into the blood a substance capable of inhibiting another heart. The experiment failed, and the atmosphere of scepticism discouraged Dixon from pursuing it. It was thus not until 1921 that Loewi, in Germany, showed that stimulation of the vago-sympathetic trunk to an isolated and cannulated frog's heart could cause the release into the cannula of a substance ('Vagusstoff') that would inhibit another heart if the cannula fluid was transferred from the first heart to the second—a classic and much-quoted experiment that proved extremely difficult for even Loewi to repeat reproducibly. In an autobiographical sketch, Loewi tells us that the idea of chemical transmission arose in a discussion that he had in 1903, but no way of testing it experimentally occurred to him until he dreamed of the appropriate experiment one night in 1920. He wrote some notes of this very important dream in the middle of the night, but in the morning could not read them. The dream obligingly returned the next night, and, taking no chances, he went to the laboratory at 3 a.m. and carried out the experiment successfully. Loewi's experiment may be, and was, criticized on numerous grounds (it could, for example, have been potassium rather than a neurotransmitter which was acting on the recipient heart), but a series of further experiments proved him to be right. His findings can be summarized as follows:

1. Stimulation of the vagus caused the appearance of a substance in the perfusate of the frog heart capable of producing in a second heart an inhibitory effect resembling that of vagus stimulation.
2. Stimulation of the sympathetic caused the appearance of a substance capable of accelerating a second heart. Loewi concluded later, from fluorescence measurements, that this substance was adrenaline. (In the frog heart adrenaline, not noradrenaline, acts as adrenergic transmitter.)
3. Atropine prevented the inhibitory action of the vagus on the heart but did not prevent release of 'Vagusstoff'. Atropine thus prevented the effects, rather than the release, of the transmitter.
4. When 'Vagusstoff' was incubated with ground-up frog heart muscle it became inactivated. This effect is due to enzymatic destruction of acetylcholine by cholinesterase.
5. Physostigmine (eserine), which potentiated the effect of vagus stimulation on the heart, prevented destruction of 'Vagusstoff' by heart muscle, providing evidence that the potentiation is due to inhibition of cholinesterase which normally destroys the transmitter substance acetylcholine.

A few years later, in the early 1930s, Dale, working in London with a succession of gifted colleagues, many of them fugitives from Nazi Germany, showed convincingly that acetylcholine was also the transmitter substance at the neuro-muscular junction of striated muscle, and at auto-nomic ganglia. One of the keys to Dale's success lay in the use of very highly sensitive bioassays, especially the leech dorsal muscle, for measuring acetylcholine release. Figure 5.1 shows the way in which these assays could be used to measure and identify the active substance released on stimulation of parasympathetic nerves to the heart and stomach.

Chemical transmission at sympathetic nerve terminals was demonstrated at about the same time as

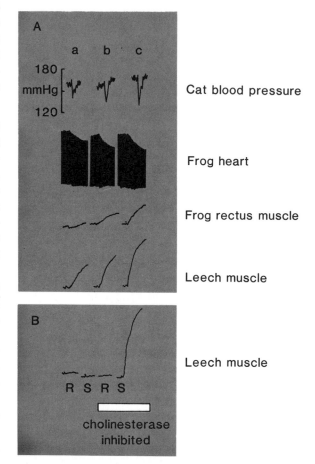

Fig. 5.1 Use of bioassay to demonstrate acetylcholine release from autonomic nerves. **A.** Assay of perfusate from dog stomach, collected during vagal stimulation. In each panel, response (b) is produced by the perfusate. Responses (a) and (c) are two standard doses of acetylcholine. Note that on all four test preparations the perfusate gave a response midway between the acetylcholine standards, suggesting strongly that the active substance in the perfusate was acetylcholine itself. **B.** Assay of blood from dog coronary vein, collected during vagal stimulation (S) and at rest (R). Activity on the leech muscle was detectable only after the dog was treated with a cholinesterase inhibitor to prevent destruction of acetylcholine in the blood. (From: **(A)** Dale & Feldberg, 1934; **(B)** Feldberg & Krayer 1933)

cholinergic transmission and by very similar methods. One of the difficulties of Loewi's experiments on the frog heart was that the sympathetic and parasympathetic nerves to the heart run very close together, and were usually stimulated simultaneously. Whether the heart accelerated or slowed depended on many things, including the time of year, a fact which gave his critics some good ammunition. He usually found, though, that whatever response the donor heart produced also occurred in the recipient and he coined the term 'Acceleranstoff' for the mediator of the excitatory effect. It was the work of Cannon and his colleagues at Harvard in the 1930s that showed the phenomenon of chemical transmission at sympathetic nerve endings unequivocally, by experiments *in vivo* in which tissues made supersensitive to adrenaline by prior sympathetic denervation were shown to respond after a delay to the transmitter released by stimulation of the sympathetic nerves to other parts of the body. The chemical identity of the transmitter, tantalizingly like adrenaline, but not identical with it, caused a good deal of confusion for some years, until von Euler in 1946 showed it to be the non-methylated derivative, **noradrenaline**.

BASIC ANATOMY AND PHYSIOLOGY OF THE AUTONOMIC NERVOUS SYSTEM

The autonomic nervous system conveys all of the outputs from central nervous system to the rest of the body except for the motor innervation of skeletal muscle. The autonomic nervous system is largely outside the influence of voluntary control and the main processes that it regulates are:

1. Contraction and relaxation of smooth muscle
2. All exocrine and certain endocrine secretions
3. The heart beat
4. Certain steps in intermediary metabolism.

There is some argument about whether the term 'autonomic nervous system' should be taken to include the many afferent fibres which run in the same nerve bundles as the efferent fibres. From a pharmacological point of view it is the efferent pathways that have special properties, and the afferent fibres will not be discussed in this section.

The main difference between the autonomic and the somatic efferent pathways is that the former consists of *two* neurons arranged in series, whereas the latter uses a *single* neuron to connect the central nervous system to the skeletal muscle fibre (see Fig. 5.2). The two neurons in the autonomic pathway are known respectively as **pre-ganglionic** and **post-ganglionic** and they synapse in an **autonomic ganglion**, which lies outside the central nervous system, and which contains the endings of a group of pre-ganglionic fibres and the cell bodies of a group of post-ganglionic fibres.

The autonomic nervous system consists of two anatomical divisions, **sympathetic** and **parasympathetic** (see Fig. 5.3). The sympathetic pre-ganglionic neurons have their cell bodies in the lateral horn of the grey matter of the thoracic and lumbar segments of the spinal cord, and the fibres leave the spinal cord in the spinal nerves. Just outside the spinal cord they leave the spinal nerve as a fine *ramus communicans* which runs to the **paravertebral sympathetic chain,** an interconnected longitudinal string of sympathetic ganglia which is found bilaterally on either side of the spinal column. These ganglia contain the cell bodies of the post-ganglionic sympathetic neurons, whose axons form a second *ramus communicans* which rejoins the somatic spinal nerve. Many of the post-ganglionic sympathetic fibres reach their peripheral destinations in the various branches of the spinal nerves. Others, destined for abdominal and pelvic viscera, have their cell bodies in a group of unpaired **prevertebral ganglia** which are found in the abdominal cavity. The only exception to the two-neuron arrangement is the innervation of the adrenal medulla, which secretes catecholamines in response to sympathetic nerve activity. The cells of the adrenal medulla are, in effect, modified post-ganglionic sympathetic neurons, and the nerves supplying the gland are equivalent to pre-ganglionic fibres, there being no ganglionic relay between the spinal cord and the adrenal gland.

The parasympathetic nerves emerge from two separate regions of the central nervous system. The **cranial outflow** consists of pre-ganglionic fibres in four of the cranial nerves, namely the oculomotor nerve, (carrying parasympathetic fibres destined for the eye), the facial and glossopharyngeal nerves (carrying fibres to the salivary glands and the nasopharynx), and the vagus (carrying fibres to the thoracic and abdominal viscera). The ganglia lie scattered in close relation to the target organs, and the post-ganglionic neurons are much shorter than in the sympathetic system. Parasympathetic fibres destined for the pelvic and abdominal viscera emerge from the sacral region of the spinal cord as a bundle of nerves known as the *nervi erigentes* (since stimulation of these nerves evokes erection of genital organs—a fact of some importance to those responsible for artificial insemination of livestock). These fibres synapse in a group of scattered **pelvic ganglia**, whence the short post-ganglionic fibres run to target tissues such as the bladder, rectum and genitalia.

The two main neurotransmitters that operate in the autonomic system are **acetylcholine** and **noradrenaline**, whose sites of action are shown diagrammatically in Figure 5.2. This diagram also shows the type of postsynaptic receptor with which the

transmitters interact at the different sites. This receptor classification is discussed more fully in Chapters 6 and 7. Certain generalizations are valid:

1. All motor nerve fibres leaving the central nervous system use acetylcholine as their transmitter, and it acts on nicotinic receptors. There is one partial exception to this generalization. Though transmission through autonomic ganglia relies mainly on the activation of nicotinic receptors by acetylcholine released from the pre-ganglionic neurone, some excitation is due to activation of muscarinic receptors (see Chapter 6).

2. All post-ganglionic parasympathetic fibres release acetylcholine, and it acts on muscarinic receptors.

3. All post-ganglionic sympathetic fibres *with two important exceptions*, release noradrenaline, which may act on either α- or β-adrenoceptors (see Chapter 7). The two exceptions, where acetylcholine is the transmitter and acts on muscarinic

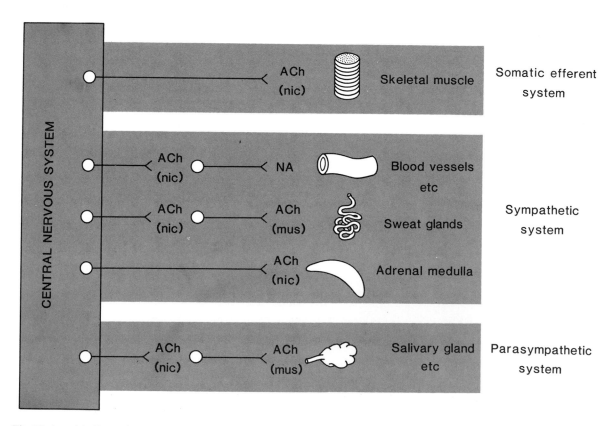

Fig. 5.2 Acetylcholine and noradrenaline as transmitters in the peripheral nervous system. The two types of acetylcholine receptor, nicotinic and muscarinic (see Chapter 6) are indicated.

Table 5.1 The main effects of the autonomic nervous system

Organ	Receptor type	Sympathetic	Parasympathetic
Heart			
SA node	β_1	Rate ↑	Rate ↓
Atrial muscle	β_1	Force ↑	Force ↓
AV node	β_1	Automaticity ↑	Cond. vel. ↓
			AV block
Ventricular muscle	β_1	Automaticity ↑	No effect
		Force ↑	
Blood vessels			
Arterioles			
Coronary	α	Constriction	
Muscle	β_2	Dilatation (mainly cholinergic)	No effect
Viscera			
Skin	α	Constriction	No effect
Brain			
Erectile tissue	α	Constriction	Dilatation
Salivary gland	α		
Veins	α	Constriction	No effect
	β_2	Dilatation	
Viscera			
Bronchi			
Smooth muscle	β_2	Dilatation	Constriction
Glands		No effect	Secretion
GI tract			
Smooth muscle	α_2, β_2	Motility ↓	Motility ↑
Sphincters	α_2, β_2	Constriction	Dilatation
Glands		No effect	Secretion
Uterus			
pregnant	α	Contraction	Variable
non-pregnant	β_2	Relaxation	
Male sex organs	α	Ejaculation	Erection
Eye			
Pupil	α	Dilatation	Constriction
Ciliary muscle	β	Relaxation (slight)	Contraction
Skin			
Sweat glands	α	Secretion (mainly cholinergic)	No effect
Pilomotor	α	Piloerection	No effect
Salivary glands	α, β	Secretion	Secretion
Lacrimal glands		No effect	Secretion
Kidney	β_2	Renin secretion	No effect
Liver	α, β_2	Glycogenolysis	No effect
		Gluconeogenesis	

Note: The receptor types given for the sympathetically-mediated responses are discussed more fully in Chapter 7. The parasympathetic responses are all mediated by muscarinic acetylcholine receptors (see Chapter 6).

receptors, are: (a) fibres supplying **sweat glands** and **piloerector muscles**; and (b) some **vasodilator fibres** in skeletal muscle.

In some situations, e.g. the visceral smooth muscle of the gut, bladder and bronchial system, and the heart, the sympathetic and the parasympathetic systems produce opposite effects, but there are others where only one division of the autonomic system operates. The sweat glands and most blood vessels, for example, have only a sympathetic innervation, whereas the ciliary muscle of the eye has only a parasympathetic innervation. There are other examples, such as the salivary glands, where the two systems produce similar, rather than opposing, effects. It is a mistake to think of the sympathetic and parasympathetic systems as physiological opponents. Each serves its own physiological function and can be more or less active in a particular organ or tissue according to the need of the moment. Cannon rightly emphasized the general role of the sympathetic system in evoking 'fight or flight' reactions, but this state of affairs is not the usual one for most animals, who make more subtle physiological use of their autonomic systems.

Table 5.1 lists some of the more important autonomic responses in man.

TWO GENERAL PRINCIPLES OF CHEMICAL TRANSMISSION

Denervation supersensitivity

It is known, mainly from the work of Cannon on the sympathetic system, that if a nerve is cut and its terminals allowed to degenerate the structure supplied by it becomes supersensitive to the transmitter substance released by the terminals. Thus skeletal muscle, which normally responds to injected acetylcholine only if a large dose is given directly into the arterial supply, will, after denervation, respond by contracture to much smaller amounts. Other organs, such as salivary glands and blood vessels show similar supersensitivity to acetylcholine and noradrenaline when the postganglionic nerves degenerate, and there is evidence that pathways in the central nervous system show the same phenomenon.

Several mechanisms are known to contribute to denervation supersensitivity. The extent and mechanism of the phenomenon varies from organ to organ. Reported mechanisms include:

1. *Proliferation of receptors.* This is particularly marked in skeletal muscle, where the number of acetylcholine receptors increases 20-fold or more after denervation and they are no longer localized to the endplate region of the fibres. Elsewhere much smaller increases in receptor number (about twofold) have often been reported, but there are examples where no change occurs.

2. *Loss of mechanisms for transmitter removal.* At adrenergic synapses the loss of neuronal uptake of noradrenaline contributes substantially to denerva-

tion supersensitivity. At cholinergic synapses a partial loss of cholinesterase occurs.

3. *Increased postjunctional responsiveness.* In some cases the postsynaptic cells become supersensitive without a corresponding increase in the number of receptors. Thus, smooth muscle cells become partly depolarized and hyperexcitable and this phenomenon contributes appreciably to their supersensitivity. The mechanism of this change, and its importance for other synapses is not known.

Supersensitivity can occur, but is less marked, when transmission is interrupted by processes other than nerve section. Pharmacological block of ganglionic transmission, for example, if sustained for a few days, causes some degree of supersensitivity of the target organs, and long-term blockade of postsynaptic receptors also causes receptors to proliferate, leaving the cell supersensitive when the blocking agent is removed. Phenomena such as this are of importance in the central nervous system, where such supersensitivity can cause 'rebound' effects when drugs are given for some time and then stopped.

Dale's principle

This principle, advanced rather tentatively by Dale in 1934, states, in its modern form: 'a mature neuron makes use of the same transmitter at all of its synapses.' Dale considered it unlikely that a single neuron could store and release different transmitters at different nerve terminals, and his view has been substantiated by physiological and neurochemical evidence. It is known, for example, that the axons of motor neurons have branches that synapse on interneurons in the spinal cord, as well as the main branch that innervates skeletal muscle fibres in the periphery. The transmitter at both the central and the peripheral nerve endings is acetylcholine, in accordance with Dale's principle. The enzymes involved in transmitter synthesis are produced in the cell body and transported to the terminals by axonal transport. The enzymes, and the transmitter itself, are present throughout the cell, and not just at the terminals, and it is rather unlikely that different sets of enzymes, corresponding to different transmitters, could be directed selectively to particular terminals.

Various pieces of recent evidence have been held

to refute the generality of Dale's principle (Burnstock, 1976, 1981). Thus it has been shown that sympathetic neurons, during development, switch from being cholinergic to being adrenergic. It has also been shown that nerves can synthesize, and probably release, more than one transmitter at a time. There are numerous examples of neurons that have been shown by fluorescence histochemistry to contain both a monoamine such as serotonin and a peptide such as somatostatin, and it is likely, but not proven, that both substances have a transmitter role. Though Dale's principle was framed before these complexities were discovered, it is not seriously undermined by them—there is still no example of a neuron known to release different transmitters at different terminals (Segal, 1983).

RECENT DEVELOPMENTS

Though the representation of the autonomic system in Figures 5.2 & 5.3 remains basically correct and

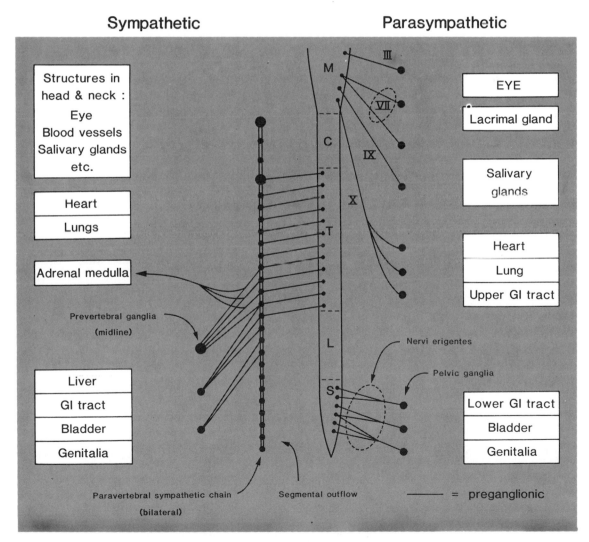

Fig. 5.3 Basic plan of the mammalian autonomic nervous system.

serviceable, recent work has shown that it is over-simplified, particularly in two respects:

1. Pre-synaptic interactions occur to an important extent
2. Transmitters other than acetylcholine and noradrenaline are involved.

PRE-SYNAPTIC INTERACTIONS

The diagram in Figure 5.2 suggests that transmitters act only on post-synaptic structures, but it is now clear that the pre-synaptic terminals which synthesize and release transmitter in response to electrical activity in the nerve fibre, are themselves sensitive to transmitter substances, and to other substances which may be produced locally in tissues, known loosely as **neuromodulators** (for review see Vizi, 1980). Such pre-synaptic effects can act either to enhance or to inhibit transmitter release.

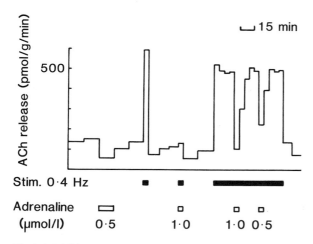

Stim. 0·4 Hz

Adrenaline
(μmol/l)   0·5   1·0   1·0 0·5

Fig. 5.4 Inhibitory effect of adrenaline on acetylcholine release from post-ganglionic parasympathetic nerves in the guinea-pig ileum. The intramural nerves were stimulated electrically where indicated, and the acetylcholine released into the bathing fluid determined by bioassay. Adrenaline strongly inhibits acetylcholine release. (From: Vizi, 1979)

Figure 5.4 shows the inhibitory effect of adrenaline on the release of acetylcholine (evoked by electrical stimulation) from the post-ganglionic parasympathetic nerve terminals of the intestine. It is now known that these nerve terminals are sensitive to noradrenaline as well as adrenaline, and that release of noradrenaline from nearby sympathetic nerve terminals can also inhibit acetylcholine release. There is anatomical evidence showing that adrenergic and cholinergic nerve terminals often lie close together in the myenteric plexus, so it is likely that the opposing effects of the sympathetic and parasympathetic systems result not only from the opposite effects of the two transmitters on the smooth muscle cells, but also from the inhibition of acetylcholine release by noradrenaline acting on the parasympathetic nerve terminals.

A similar situation exists in the heart, where a mutual pre-synaptic inhibition has been demonstrated; noradrenaline inhibits acetylcholine release, as in the myenteric plexus, and acetylcholine also inhibits noradrenaline release.

The importance of these pre-synaptic interactions has become increasingly apparent over the last 10-15 years, and there is good evidence, not only for the type of **heterotropic** interaction described above, where one neurotransmitter affects the release of another, but also for **homotropic** interaction, where the transmitter affects the nerve terminals from which it is being released. There is evidence (Rand *et al*, 1982), though it is not universally accepted (Kalsner, 1982), that this type of **auto-inhibitory feedback** acts powerfully at noradrenergic nerve terminals. One of the strongest pieces of evidence is that the amount of noradrenaline released from tissues in response to repetitive stimulation of sympathetic nerves is increased ten-fold or more in the presence of an antagonist that blocks the pre-synaptic noradrenaline receptors (see Chapter 7), which suggests that the released noradrenaline can inhibit further release by at least 90%.

A similar state of affairs seems to exist at cholinergic nerve terminals as well, where transmitter release can be increased considerably by antagonists that block the inhibitory action of acetylcholine on its own nerve terminals.

The main difference between the adrenergic and cholinergic control of transmitter release is that the receptors for noradrenaline on nerve terminals are pharmacologically distinct from the post-synaptic receptors (see Chapter 7), so that it has been possible to develop drugs that act selectively, as agonists or antagonists, on the pre- or post-synaptic receptors. The acetylcholine receptors that mediate pre- and post-synaptic effects do not, however, appear to be pharmacologically distinguishable, and it has not yet been possible to develop selective drugs.

Not only do cholinergic and adrenergic nerve terminals respond to acetylcholine and noradrenaline, as described above, but they are also affected by many other substances that may be present in tissues, including prostaglandins, purines (such as adenosine and ATP), dopamine, serotonin, gamma-aminobutyric acid (GABA), opioid peptides and many other substances. Evidence as to the physiological role and pharmacological significance of these multifarious interactions is at present very patchy, and the field is changing rapidly. There is no doubt, though, that the simple description of the autonomic nervous system represented in Figure 5.2 is now a misleading oversimplification. Figure 5.5 shows some of the main pre-synaptic interactions that have been described between adrenergic and cholinergic neurons of the autonomic nervous

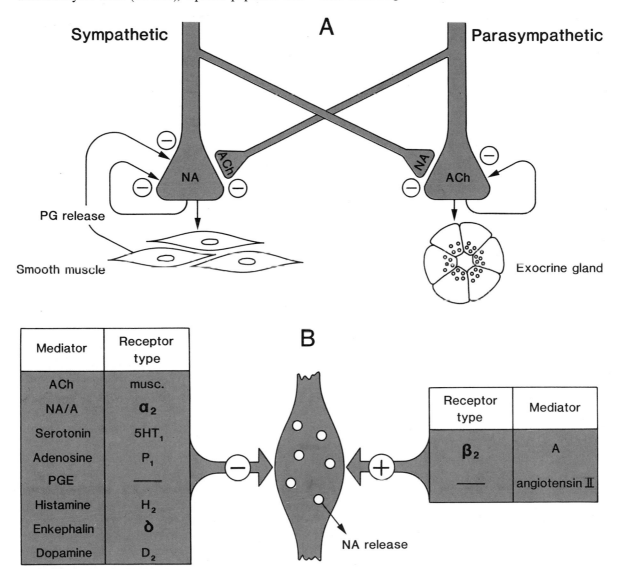

Fig. 5.5 Pre-synaptic regulation of transmitter release from adrenergic and cholinergic nerve terminals. **A**. Postulated homotropic and heterotropic interactions between sympathetic and parasympathetic nerves. **B**. Some of the known inhibitory and facilitatory influences on noradrenaline release from sympathetic nerve endings. Abbreviations: ACh, acetylcholine; NA, noradrenaline; PG, prostaglandin.

system, as well as showing some of the many chemical influences that are believed to regulate transmitter release from adrenergic neurons.

TRANSMITTERS OTHER THAN ACETYLCHOLINE AND NORADRENALINE

There is now strong evidence that substances other than the two classical peripheral neurotransmitters also act as transmitters in the peripheral nervous system. The evidence comes partly from morphological studies based on selective labelling of putative transmitter substances within neurons. Fluorescence microscopy has revealed, for example, that particular neurons in the myenteric plexus are aglow with **serotonin** (5-hydroxytryptamine) while in sympathetic ganglia there is a population of interneurons (small intensely fluorescent, or SIF cells) that are rich in **dopamine**. Immunofluorescent staining has also revealed many neurons in the periphery that contain particular peptides, such as **thyrotrophin releasing hormone (TRH)**, **enkephalins**, **substance P**, **vasoactive intestinal polypeptide (VIP)**, **somatostatin** and many others. The sheer abundance of such putative transmitter substances, which in a few cases have been shown to be released and to exert physiological effects in response to nerve stimulation, is somewhat bewildering, and it will be some time before the importance, as distinct from the existence, of all of these substances can be assessed.

Functional evidence that stimulation of autonomic nerves produces effects that are not due to acetylcholine or noradrenaline comes from the finding that the contraction of organs such as the colon or bladder in response to parasympathetic nerve stimulation is almost unaffected by acetylcholine antagonists such as atropine (see Chapter 6), in contrast to parasympathetic responses elsewhere (e.g. the heart or the eye), which are effectively blocked by atropine. Similarly, it is found that stimulation of the nerve supply to the stomach, after cholinergic and adrenergic transmission has been fully blocked with appropriate drugs, causes a relaxation of the muscle. In nearly all cases where this non-adrenergic, non-cholinergic (NANC) transmission has been discovered, it seems to be mediated by local interneurons, such as those of the myen-

teric plexus, in the wall of the organ, which are activated by acetylcholine released from the preganglionic autonomic fibres.

There have been many attempts to identify the transmitter substance(s) released by NANC nerves, and Burnstock (1972, 1985) has produced considerable evidence that **adenosine triphospate (ATP)** may function in this role. ATP release in response to nerve stimulation has been shown, and application of ATP to different tissues very often mimics the effect, whether excitatory or inhibitory, of stimulation of NANC nerves. Unfortunately there are so far no specific antagonists of the actions of ATP, so the crucial test of whether such a drug will block NANC transmission cannot be performed, and the transmitter role of ATP remains controversial. The pharmacology of responses to ATP and other purines is discussed in Chapter 11.

There is also very strong evidence, summarized by Gershon (1981) that **serotonin** is a transmitter at interneurons of the myenteric plexus, and that those 'serotonergic' neurons are important in the regulation of peristalsis. Other effects of serotonin and its antagonists are discussed in Chapter 11.

A third substance recently elevated to the status of a peripheral neutransmitter is **dopamine** (Bell, 1982). It is well-known to be a precursor of noradrenaline (see Chapter 7), and to function as a central neurotransmitter (see Chapter 19), but its peripheral transmitter role has only recently become evident. Stimulation of sympathetic nerves to the kidney, if noradrenergic responses are blocked pharmacologically, causes a pronounced vasodilatation, which can be produced by injecting dopamine, and is blocked by dopamine antagonists. There is also evidence of dopamine-containing neurons in the nerve supply to the kidney. Similar phenomena have now been described in other vascular beds, such as the skin and coronary vessels, so the system may have rather widespread functions. The actions of dopamine and other drugs that act on dopamine receptors are described in Chapters 11 and 19.

The role of peptides as neurotransmitters in the peripheral nervous system has only just begun to be explored. Among the convincing stories so far are: (a) The decapeptide **LHRH (luteinizing hormone releasing hormone**, originally described as a hypothalamic factor regulating LH release; see Chapter 17) functions as a transmitter in sympathetic ganglia producing a very slow post-synaptic depolarization (slow epsp) lasting for several minutes after a period of pre-ganglionic nerve stimulation. It is probably released from the same nerve terminals as acetylcholine, which is responsible for the fast epsp (Jan & Jan, 1983); (b) **Vasoactive intestinal polypeptide (VIP)** is released along with acetylcholine, and possibly from the same nerve terminals, when the parasympathetic nerve supply to the salivary gland is stimulated (Lundberg & Hokfelt, 1983). Acetylcholine is responsible for the secretory response from the gland cells, while VIP causes the vasodilatation necessary to sustain fluid secretion from the gland. Other exocrine glands, and also the wall of the intestine where VIP is fairly abundant, seem to have a similar vasodilator control; (c) **Substance P** has been shown to mediate the slow epsp in sympathetic ganglion cells produced by repetitive stimulation of the pre-ganglionic nerve (Otsuka & Konishi, 1983). The list of putative neurotransmitter roles for peptides is long and growing, and the advice given by Cooper et al (1982) in a section called 'A readers guide to peptide poaching' cannot be bettered: Stay tuned, the data flow fast.

Coexistence of amines and peptides in the same cell has long been recognized in endocrine glands, and it has been suggested (see Pearse, 1983 for a short review) that there is a specific class of endocrine cell (of which the enterochromaffin cell is an example) derived from the embryonic neural crest ectoderm, which displays this dual biochemical function. Pearse called these endocrine cells **APUD (amine-precursor-uptake-decarboxylation) cells**, and suggests that they represent a system of neuroendocrine cells whose functions are intermediate between those of the nervous and endocrine systems. It now seems clear that such cells are also abundant in the nervous system itself, where peptides appear to be the mediators of a variety of slow, long-range interactions between nerve cells, such interactions being more reminiscent of an endocrine than a conventional neurotransmitter mechanism.

BASIC STEPS IN NEUROCHEMICAL TRANSMISSION—SITES OF DRUG ACTION

The following processes take place at chemically-transmitting synapses (see Fig. 5.6.)

1. Uptake of transmitter precursors by nerve terminals.*
2. Synthesis of transmitter in nerve terminals.*
3. Storage of transmitter in releasable form.
4. Degradation of surplus transmitter within nerve terminals.
5. Depolarization of nerve terminal by propagated action potential.
6. Influx of Ca^{++} ions in response to depolarization.
7. Release of transmitter in quantal packets.*
8. Diffusion of transmitter to post-synaptic receptors.
9. Interaction with receptors and production of post-synaptic effect.
10. Inactivation of transmitter within synaptic cleft.*

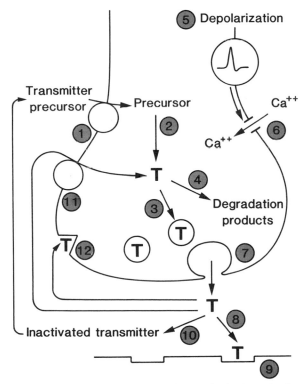

Fig. 5.6 The main processes involved in synthesis, storage and release of amine transmitters. The numbering corresponds with the text (see opposite). These processes are well characterized for several monoamine transmitters (e.g. acetylcholine, noradrenaline, dopamine, serotonin), but may well differ significantly with other transmitters (e.g. amino acids, purines, peptides).

11. Reuptake of transmitter or of degradation product by nerve terminals.*
12. Interaction of transmitter with pre-synaptic receptors.

Depending on the particular synapse, some of these steps may be absent, or have at least not been clearly shown to occur. Thus at peptide-releasing synapses the steps marked with an asterisk have not so far been demonstrated. It is likely that most peptides are produced by cleavage of fragments from precursor proteins that are made in the Golgi apparatus in the cell body, being then conveyed to the terminals by axonal transport, and there is no evidence that peptides are (as amine transmitters are known to be) released in quantal packets.

At adrenergic synapses, step 10 is unimportant as a mechanism for terminating transmitter action, the noradrenaline being recaptured intact by the nerve terminals, whereas at cholinergic synapses, acetylcholine is rapidly inactivated by hydrolysis, and only the choline moiety is recaptured. Step 12 is also of variable importance at different synapses.

The mechanism by which amine transmitters are stored and released is generally believed to involve the numerous synaptic vesicles that are found within the nerve terminals, which are known to contain a relatively high concentration of transmitter. The fact that transmitters are released in discrete multi-molecular packets, and that electron microscopic images consistent with the extrusion of the vesicular contents by fusion of the vesicle membrane with the terminal membrane have been seen, strongly suggests that exocytosis is the process responsible for release. Also consistent with this hypothesis is the fact that other vesicular constituents, such as proteins and ATP, are released along with the transmitter. There is however, biochemical evidence that does not favour the vesicle hypothesis (Cooper et al, 1982) and the matter is not finally settled.

Figure 5.6 provides a useful framework for considering the ways in which drugs can influence the process of neurochemical transmission, for all of the steps shown (except for transmitter diffusion, step 8) can be influenced by drugs. In many cases the process can be changed either way. Thus, invasion of the nerve terminal by an action potential can be prevented by drugs such as local anaesthetics (Chapter 27), or enhanced by drugs such as 4-aminopyridine (see Chapter 6). Similarly the receptors can be blocked or activated by exogenously applied drugs. The actions of the great majority of drugs that act on both the peripheral nervous system (see Chapters 6 & 7) and the central nervous system (Chapters 22–25) are explicable in terms of this general scheme.

REFERENCES AND FURTHER READING

Bacq Z M 1975 Chemical transmission of nerve impulses: a historical sketch. Pergamon Press, Oxford
Bell C 1982 Dopamine as a postganglionic autonomic neurotransmitter. Neuroscience 7: 1–8
Burnstock G 1972 Purinergic nerves. Pharm Rev 24: 509–581
Burnstock G 1976 Do some nerve cells release more than one transmitter? Neuroscience 1: 239–248
Burnstock G 1981 Review lecture. Neurotransmitters and trophic factors in the autonomic nervous system. J Physiol 313: 1–36
Burnstock G 1985 Purinergic mechanisms broaden their sphere of influence. Trends in Neurosciences 8: 5–6
Cooper J C, Bloom F E, Roth R H 1982 The biochemical basis of neuropharmacology. Oxford University Press, New York
Gershon M D 1981 The enteric nervous system. Ann Rev Neurosci 4: 227–272
Jan Y N, Jan L Y 1983 A LHRH-like peptidergic neurotransmitter capable of 'action at a distance' in autonomic ganglia. Trends in Neurosciences 6: 320–325

Kalsner S 1982 The presynaptic receptor controversy. Trends in Pharmacological Sciences 8: 11–16
Kuffler S W, Nicholls J G, Martin A R 1984 From neuron to brain. Sinauer, New York
Lundberg J M, Hokfelt T 1983 Coexistence of peptides and conventional neurotransmitters. Trends in Neurosciences 6: 325–333
Otsuka M, Konishi S 1983 Substance P—the first peptide neurotransmitter? Trends in Neurosciences 6: 317–320
Pearse A G E 1983 The neuroendocrine division of the nervous system: APUD cells as neurones or paraneurones. In: Osborne N E (ed) Dale's principle and communication between neurones. Pergamon Press, Oxford
Rand M J, McCulloch M W, Story D F 1982 Feedback modulation of noradrenergic transmission. Trends in Pharmacological Sciences 3: 8–11
Segal M 1983 Specification of synaptic action. Trends in Neurosciences 6: 118–121
Vizi E S 1980 Presynaptic modulation of neurochemical transmission. Prog Neurobiol 12: 181–290

Cholinergic transmission

The discovery of the pharmacological action of acetylcholine arose from work on adrenal glands. Adrenal extracts were known to produce a rise of blood pressure owing to their content of adrenaline. In 1900 Reid Hunt found that after such extracts had been freed of adrenaline they produced a fall of blood pressure instead of a rise. He attributed the fall to their content of choline but at a later stage concluded that a more potent derivative of choline must be responsible. With Taveau he tested a number of choline derivatives and discovered that **acetylcholine** was some 100 000 times more active than choline in lowering a rabbit's blood pressure.

Although Hunt's studies suggested that acetylcholine may be a normal constituent of tissues, its physiological function was not apparent at that time and it remained for many years an interesting pharmacological curiosity.

MUSCARINIC AND NICOTINIC ACTIONS OF ACETYLCHOLINE

In a study of the pharmacological actions of acetylcholine carried out in 1914 Dale distinguished two types of activity which he designated as **muscarinic** and **nicotinic**. Muscarinic actions are those which can be reproduced by the injection of muscarine, the active principle of the poisonous mushroom *Amanita muscaria*, and they are characterized by the fact that they can be abolished by small doses of atropine.

On the whole, muscarinic actions correspond to those of parasympathetic stimulation as shown in Table 5.1. After the muscarinic effects have been blocked by atropine, larger doses of acetylcholine produce another set of effects, closely similar to those of **nicotine**. They include **stimulation of all autonomic ganglia, stimulation of voluntary muscle**, and **secretion of adrenaline** by the medulla of the suprarenal gland.

The muscarinic and nicotinic actions of acetylcholine are demonstrated in Figure 6.1 in an experiment on the blood pressure of an anaesthetized cat. Small and medium doses of acetylcholine produce a transient fall in blood pressure due to arteriolar vasodilatation and slowing of the heart. Atropine abolishes these effects. A large dose of acetylcholine given after atropine produces nicotinic effects: an initial rise in blood pressure due to a stimulation of sympathetic ganglia and consequent vasoconstriction, and a secondary rise resulting from stimulation of secretion of adrenaline from the adrenal glands.

Dale's classification was originally made on pharmacological grounds, but it has proved to correspond closely to the main physiological functions of acetylcholine in the body. The muscarinic actions correspond to those of acetylcholine released at post-ganglionic parasympathetic nerve endings, with two significant exceptions. (1) Acetylcholine causes generalized vasodilatation, even though most blood vessels have no parasympathetic innervation. It has recently been shown that this action is an indirect one; acetylcholine acts on endothelial cells, which respond by releasing a short-lived and still unidentified mediator, which relaxes the smooth muscle cells (Furchgott, 1981). The physiological function of this is uncertain, since acetylcholine is not normally present in circulating blood. (2) Acetylcholine evokes secretion from sweat glands, which are innervated by cholinergic fibres of the sympathetic nervous system (see Table 5.1). The nicotinic actions correspond to those of acetylcholine released at the ganglionic synapses of the sympathetic

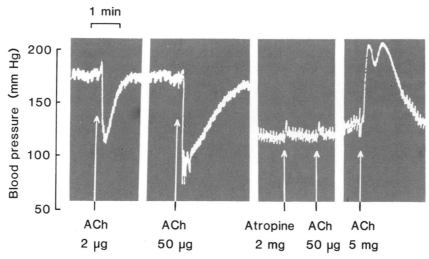

Fig. 6.1 Dale's experiment showing that acetylcholine produces two kinds of effect on the cat's blood pressure. Arterial pressure was recorded with a mercury manometer from a spinal cat. *Panel 1*: ACh causes a fall in blood pressure due to vasodilatation; *Panel 2*: A larger dose also produces bradycardia. These are both muscarinic effects; *Panel 3*: After atropine (muscarinic antagonist) the same dose of ACh has no effect; *Panel 4*: Still under the influence of atropine, a much larger dose of ACh causes a rise in blood pressure (due to stimulation of sympathetic ganglia), accompanied by tachycardia, followed by a secondary rise (due to release of adrenaline from the adrenal gland). These effects result from its action on nicotinic receptors. (From: Burn, 1963)

and parasympathetic systems, the motor endplate of voluntary muscle and the endings of the splanchnic nerves around the secretory cells of the suprarenal medulla.

ACETYLCHOLINE RECEPTORS

Dale's classification provides the basis for distinguishing the two major classes of acetylcholine receptor. Within each class, however, there are further subdivisions. In the case of nicotinic receptors it has long been recognized that there are considerable pharmacological differences between the receptors of striated muscle fibres and those of autonomic ganglia. Muscarinic receptors seemed, until recently, to be much more homogeneous, but it is now clear that more than one type exists.

Nicotinic receptors

In general, agonists show rather little selectivity between ganglionic and neuromuscular receptors. One exception is **decamethonium** (see below), which is a potent depolarizing agent (i.e. agonist) at the neuromuscular junction, but a weak antagonist on autonomic ganglia. Among antagonists there is

strong selectivity. For example, **α-bungarotoxin** (see Chapter 1) blocks acetylcholine receptors at the neuromuscular junction at very low concentrations, but has no effect on autonomic ganglia. On the other hand, agents such as **mecamylamine** (see below) block ganglionic, but not neuromuscular, acetylcholine receptors.

Muscarinic receptors

It now appears that there are at least two subclasses (M_1 and M_2 respectively) of muscarinic receptor (Hirschowitz et al, 1984), though most of the well-known muscarinic antagonists show little specificity between them. M_1 receptors mediate the muscarinic effects of acetylcholine on sympathetic ganglia (slow depolarizing response, see below) and on the gastric parietal cells, which are responsible for vagally-induced gastric acid secretion. Drugs that act selectively on M_1 receptors include the antagonist **pirenzepine**, and an agonist known as McN A 343.

M_2 receptors, for which there are so far no highly selective agonists or antagonists, mediate most of the peripheral muscarinic effects of acetylcholine, including those on smooth muscle, cardiac muscle and most glands (excluding the gastric mucosa). It now appears that a further subdivision of M_2 receptors may be required, since many drugs are proving to have significant selectivity among these tissues, particularly between the smooth muscle and cardiac responses.

The tendency of receptor subtypes to proliferate rapidly, and to acquire a string of Greek and numerical suffixes, is apt to be distinctly bewildering, and poses the question of what actual molecular and functional variations of the receptor underly the observed differences. Work on this subject is now proceeding rapidly, as more receptor proteins are being characterized biochemically. In the case of the nicotinic receptor, small variations in the primary amino acid sequence occur between receptors from different sources (e.g. muscle and electroplax), but information on the ganglionic receptor is still lacking. Muscarinic receptors have not yet been fully analysed, but it is possible that differences in their interaction with membrane lipids, or in their state of glycosylation, may account for the functional variations.

PHYSIOLOGY OF CHOLINERGIC TRANSMISSION

This subject is well reviewed by, for example, Ginsborg & Jenkinson (1976) and Kuffler *et al* (1984).

The ways in which drugs can affect cholinergic transmission fit into the general pattern shown in Figure 5.6. The events that occur in a typical cholinergic nerve terminal are shown in Figure 6.2.

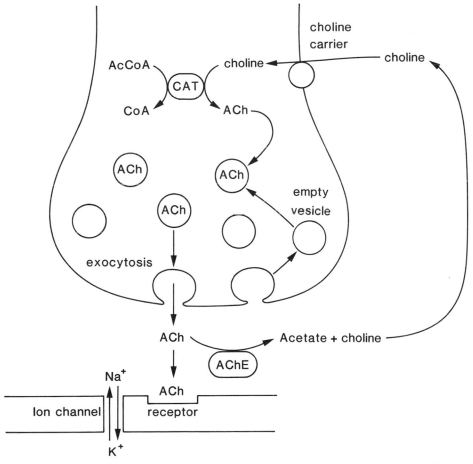

Fig. 6.2 Events at a cholinergic synapse. ACh is shown acting post-synaptically on a nicotinic receptor controlling a cation channel (e.g. at the neuromuscular or ganglionic synapse). Elsewhere (e.g. heart, smooth muscle) ACh acts on muscarinic receptors, which act indirectly to regulate the target cell (see Chapter 1). CAT = choline acetyl transferase; AChE = acetylcholinesterase.

ACETYLCHOLINE SYNTHESIS AND RELEASE

Excellent reviews on acetylcholine metabolism may be found in Marchbanks (1975), MacIntosh & Collier (1976) and Blusztajn & Wurtman (1983).

Acetylcholine is synthesized within the nerve terminal from choline, most of which is taken up into the nerve terminal by a special choline transport system. The concentration of choline in the blood and body fluids is normally about 10^{-5} M, but in the immediate vicinity of cholinergic nerve terminals it increases, probably to about 1 mM, when the released acetylcholine is hydrolysed, and it appears that more than 50% of this choline is normally recaptured by the nerve terminals. Free choline within the nerve terminal is acetylated by a cytosolic enzyme, **choline acetyltransferase (CAT)**, the source of the acetyl groups being acetyl-CoA. The rate limiting process in acetylcholine synthesis appears to be choline transport, the activity of which is regulated according to the rate at which acetylcholine is being released. Cholinesterase is present in the pre-synaptic nerve terminals and acetylcholine is continuously hydrolysed and resynthesized. Inhibition of the nerve terminal cholinesterase causes the accumulation of 'surplus' acetylcholine in the cytosol, from which it is not immediately available for release. Most of the acetylcholine synthesized, however, is packaged into synaptic vesicles, in which its concentration is very high (about 100 mM), and from which, according to most authorities, release occurs by exocytosis. Nothing is known about the mechanism of packaging of acetylcholine; in contrast to adrenergic transmission (see Chapter 7) no drugs are known that specifically affect this process. As at other chemically transmitting synapses, exocytosis occurs in response to calcium entry, which normally results from the depolarization that occurs when an action potential arrives at the terminal. Following its release, the acetylcholine diffuses across the synaptic cleft* to combine with receptors on the post-synaptic cell. Some of it succumbs on the way to

---

* At post-synaptic parasympathetic nerve terminals (e.g. those supplying intestinal smooth muscle) there is often no clearly defined 'synaptic cleft', such as exists at the neuromuscular or ganglionic synapse, and the transmitter may have to diffuse tens of microns to its site of action.

hydrolysis by cholinesterase, an enzyme that is bound to the basement membrane of the nerve terminal, which lies between the pre- and post-synaptic membranes. At fast cholinergic synapses (e.g. the neuromuscular and ganglionic synapses) but not at slow ones (smooth muscle, gland cells, heart etc) the released acetylcholine is hydrolysed very rapidly (within 1 ms), so that it acts only very briefly. At the neuromuscular junction which has been studied more fully than any other cholinergic synapse, a single nerve impulse releases about 300 synaptic vesicles (altogether about 3 million acetylcholine molecules) from the nerve terminals supplying a single muscle fibre, containing altogether about 3 million synaptic vesicles. Approximately 2 million acetylcholine molecules combine with receptors, of which there are about 30 million on each muscle fibre, the rest being hydrolysed without reaching a receptor. The acetylcholine molecules remain bound to receptors for, on average, about 2 ms, and are quickly hydrolysed after dissociating, so that they cannot combine with a second receptor. The result is that transmitter action is very rapid and very brief, which is important for a synapse that has to initiate speedy muscular responses, and which may have to transmit signals at high frequency.

ELECTRICAL EVENTS IN TRANSMISSION AT CHOLINERGIC SYNAPSES

The effect of acetylcholine on the post-synaptic membrane is to cause a large increase in its permeability to small cations, particularly to sodium and potassium ions, and to a less extent, calcium ions. Because of the large inwardly-directed electrochemical gradient for sodium ions across the cell membrane, an inflow of sodium ions occurs, causing depolarization of the post-synaptic membrane. This transmitter-mediated depolarization is called an **endplate potential (epp)** in a skeletal muscle fibre (Ginsborg & Jenkinson, 1976), or a **fast excitatory post-synaptic potential (fast epsp)** if it occurs in an autonomic neuron (Skok, 1980). In a muscle fibre the localized epp spreads to adjacent, electrically excitable parts of the muscle fibre; if its amplitude is sufficient to reach the threshold for excitation an action potential is initiated, which propagates to the rest of the fibre and evokes a contraction.

In a nerve cell, depolarization of the cell body or a dendrite by the fast epsp causes local currents to flow. This depolarizes the axon hillock region of the cell, from which, if the epsp is large enough, an action potential is initiated. Figure 6.3 shows

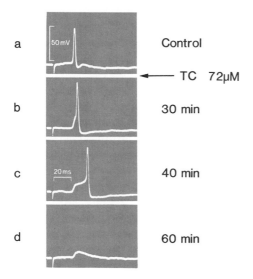

Fig. 6.3 Cholinergic transmission in an autonomic ganglion cell. Records were obtained with an intracellular microelectrode from a guinea-pig parasympathetic ganglion cell. The artefact at the beginning of each trace shows the moment of stimulation of the pre-ganglionic nerve.

Tubocurarine, an acetylcholine antagonist, causes the epsp to become smaller. In record (c) it only just succeeds in triggering the action potential, and in (d) it has fallen below the threshold. Following complete block antidromic stimulation (not shown) will still produce an action potential (cf. depolarization block, Fig. 6.4). (From Blackman et al, 1969)

that **tubocurarine**, a drug that blocks the action of acetylcholine on the post-synaptic membrane of the ganglion cell (see p. 128) reduces the amplitude of the fast epsp until it no longer initiates an action potential, though the cell is still capable of responding when it is stimulated directly. Most ganglion cells are supplied by several pre-synaptic axons, and it requires simultaneous activity in more than one to make the post-ganglionic cell fire. At the neuromuscular junction, where there is only one nerve fibre supplying each muscle fibre, the amplitude of the epp is normally more than enough to initiate an action potential—indeed transmission still occurs when the epp is reduced by 70–80%, and is said to show a large **margin of safety**—which means that fluctuations in transmitter release (e.g.

during repetitive stimulation) do not affect transmission.

Transmission through autonomic ganglia is more complex than at the neuromuscular junction. Though the primary event at both is the occurrence of an epp or fast epsp resulting from the action of acetylcholine on nicotinic receptors, this is followed in the ganglion by a succession of much slower post-synaptic potential changes, whose physiological significance is not clear. These comprise, according to most authors:

1. A slow epsp, which lasts for 2–5 s. This is produced by acetylcholine acting on muscarinic receptors, and thereby closing potassium channels. These muscarinic receptors are pharmacologically distinct from those subserving most other muscarinic responses (see p. 114).

2. A slow inhibitory post-synaptic potential (slow ipsp), which consists of a hyperpolarization of the membrane lasting about 10 s. The transmitter is not known, though it has been suggested that the response is mediated by dopamine released from an interneuron. It has also been suggested that adenosine or ATP may be the transmitter (see Chapter 5).

3. A late slow epsp, lasting for 1–2 minutes. This is thought to be mediated by a peptide, which may be substance P in some ganglia, and a LHRH-like peptide in others (see Chapter 5). Like the slow epsp, it is produced by a decrease in potassium conductance.

Depolarization block

Depolarization block occurs at cholinergic synapses when the excitatory nicotinic receptors are *persistently* activated by nicotinic agonists, and it results from a decrease in the electrical excitability of the post-synaptic cell. This is shown in Figure 6.4. Application of nicotine to a sympathetic ganglion causes a depolarization of the cell, which at first initiates action potential discharge. After a few seconds this discharge ceases, and transmission is blocked. The loss of electrical excitability at this time is shown by the fact that antidromic stimuli also fail to produce an action potential. The main reason for the loss of electrical excitability during a period of maintained depolarization is that the voltage-sensitive sodium channels become **inactivated (i.e. refractory)** and no longer able to open in

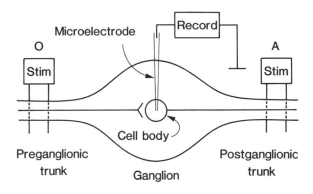

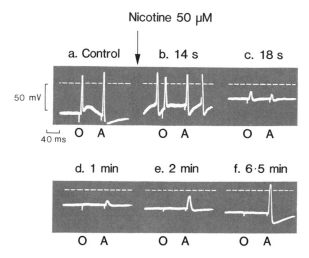

Fig. 6.4 Depolarization block of ganglionic transmission by nicotine.

Top. System used for intracellular recording from sympathetic ganglion cells of the frog, showing the location of orthodromic (O) and antidromic (A) stimulating electrodes. Stimulation at O excites the cell via the cholinergic synapse, whereas stimulation at A excites it by electrical propagation of the action potential.

Bottom. The effect of nicotine. **a.** Control records. The membrane potential is $-55\,\text{mV}$ (dotted line $= 0\,\text{mV}$) and the cell responds to both O and A. **b.** Shortly after adding nicotine the cell is slightly depolarized, but still responsive to O and A. **c, d.** The cell is further depolarized, to $-25\,\text{mV}$, and produces only a vestigial action potential. The fact that it does not respond to A shows that it is electrically inexcitable. **e, f.** In the continued presence of nicotine, the cell repolarizes, and regains its responsiveness to A, but is still unresponsive to O, because the ACh receptors are desensitized by nicotine. (From: Ginsborg & Guerrero, 1964)

response to a brief depolarizing stimulus. The work of Burns & Paton (1951), on the neuromuscular blocking action of decamethonium (see p. 132), elegantly demonstrated that it is membrane depolar-ization *per se* that causcs thc transmission block, by showing that depolarization induced electrically rather than pharmacologically also caused block, and that restoration of the membrane potential (by passing current through the endplate region of the muscle fibres) was able to restore neuromuscular transmission in the presence of decamethonium.

A second type of effect is also seen in the experiment shown in Figure 6.4. After nicotine has acted for several minutes, the cell partially repolarizes, and its electrical excitability returns, but, in spite of this, transmission remains blocked. This type of secondary, non-depolarizing block occurs also at the neuromuscular junction, where it is often referred to as **Phase II block**, the initial phase of block caused by depolarization being called **Phase I**. The main factor responsible for Phase II block appears to be **receptor desensitization** (see Chapter 1). This causes the depolarizing action of the blocking drug to subside, but at the same time the receptors become desensitized to acetylcholine, so that transmission fails for this reason.

EFFECTS OF DRUGS ON CHOLINERGIC TRANSMISSION

Drugs can influence cholinergic transmission either by acting on acetylcholine receptors or by affecting the release or destruction of endogenous acetylcholine.

Drugs that act on acetylcholine receptors may:

1. Mimic the action of acetylcholine (e.g. cholinergic agonists, such as **muscarine**, **nicotine** and various synthetic analogues of acetylcholine).
2. Block the action of acetylcholine (e.g. cholinergic antagonists, such as **atropine**, **tubocurarine** and other agents that are specific for different types of acetylcholine receptor).

Drugs that affect the release or destruction of acetylcholine may:

1. Enhance the evoked release of acetylcholine (e.g. **4-aminopyridine** and related drugs which affect the electrical properties of the pre-synaptic nerve terminals).
2. Inhibit cholinesterase, thereby increasing and prolonging the action of acetylcholine (e.g. **neostigmine**).

3. Inhibit acetylcholine release, either by inhibiting synthesis (e.g. **hemicholinium**, which blocks choline uptake) or by inhibiting the release mechanism itself (e.g. **botulinum toxin, magnesium ion, aminoglycoside antibiotics**).

In the rest of this chapter we will consider the following groups of drugs, which are subdivided according to their physiological site of action.

1. Muscarinic agonists.
2. Muscarinic antagonists.
3. Ganglion stimulating drugs.
4. Ganglion blocking drugs.
5. Neuromuscular blocking drugs.
6. Anticholinesterases and other drugs that enhance cholinergic transmission.

MUSCARINIC AGONISTS

Structure-activity relationships

This group of drugs is often referred to as **parasympathomimetic** because the main effects that they produce in the whole animal resemble those of parasympathetic stimulation. The structures of the most important compounds are given in Table 6.1. In this group is included acetylcholine itself and a number of closely related choline esters which are agonists at both muscarinic and nicotinic receptors. The reason for classifying them as muscarinic agonists is that they produce muscarinic responses at much lower concentrations than are needed to elicit nicotinic responses (see Fig. 6.1), and their limited therapeutic usefulness reflects their action on muscarinic receptors.

Table 6.1 Muscarinic agonists

Drug	Structure	Receptor specificity Musc	Nic	Hydrolysis by AChE
Acetylcholine		+++	+++	+++
Carbachol		++	+++	−
Methacholine		+++	+	++
Bethanechol		+++	−	−
Muscarine		+++	−	−
Pilocarpine		++	−	−
Oxotremorine		++	−	−

Acetylcholine itself (Table 6.1) is among the most potent agonists at both muscarinic and nicotinic receptors. The key features of the molecule that are important for its activity are: (a) the quaternary ammonium group, which is strongly basic and bears a positive charge; (b) the ester group which bears a partial negative charge. Compounds such as choline, which possess the quaternary ammonium group but lack an ester bond have only very weak activity, and tertiary amines in which one of the N-methyl groups is replaced by —H are also very weak. Enlargement of the quaternary ammonium group by substitution of ethyl or larger groups for the methyl groups almost abolishes activity, and increasing or decreasing the length of the chain separating the ester and quaternary groups also greatly reduces activity. The presence of the ester group makes the molecule susceptible to hydrolysis by cholinesterase. Some modifications that can be made to the acetylcholine molecule without drastic loss of activity are shown in Table 6.1. The effects of these modifications are: (a) to reduce the susceptibility of the compound to hydrolysis by cholinesterase; and (b) to alter the relative activity on muscarinic and nicotinic receptors. Substitution of the acetyl group by a carbamyl group yields **carbachol**, which has a similar potency to acetylcholine on both nicotinic and muscarinic receptors, but is not readily hydrolysed. Addition of a side chain methyl group on the β carbon atom produces **methacholine**, which acts selectively on muscarinic receptors but is rapidly hydrolysed. Combining these two modifications results in **bethanechol**, which is selective for muscarinic receptors and stable to hydrolysis.

Muscarine and pilocarpine are naturally occurring compounds which act as cholinergic agonists. The structure of muscarine can be seen to be close to that of acetylcholine, though that of pilocarpine is not. It is a tertiary amine and a weak base, so that a substantial fraction remains unionized at physiological pH. It differs from the other drugs mentioned in being a partial agonist for many muscarinic responses, and it is also said to have a selective action in stimulating secretion from sweat, salivary, lacrimal and bronchial glands with relatively less effect on gastrointestinal smooth muscle and the heart compared with other muscarinic agonists.

Oxotremorine is a synthetic tertiary amine that strongly stimulates muscarinic receptors. It has similar peripheral actions to that of other muscarinic agonists, but is relatively more active on the muscarinic receptors of central neurons, which has made it a useful experimental drug, though it is not used therapeutically.

Effects of muscarinic agonists

The main actions of muscarinic agonists are readily understood in terms of the parasympathetic nervous system.

Cardiovascular effects include cardiac slowing and a decrease in cardiac output. The latter action is due mainly to a decreased force of contraction of the atria, since the ventricles have only a sparse parasympathetic innervation and a low sensitivity to muscarinic agonists (see Table 5.1). Generalized vasodilatation also occurs (a muscarinic effect that is not associated with a cholinergic innervation) and these two effects combine to produce a sharp fall in arterial pressure (see Fig. 6.1). The mechanism of action of muscarinic agonists on the heart is discussed in Chapter 10.

Smooth muscle, other than vascular smooth muscle, contracts in response to muscarinic agonists. Tested *in vitro*, vascular smooth muscle usually contracts also, but *in vivo* the endothelium-dependent relaxant effect (see p. 113) predominates. Peristaltic activity of the gastrointestinal tract is increased, which can cause colicky pain, and the bladder and bronchial smooth muscle also contract.

Exocrine glands are caused to secrete, leading to sweating, lacrimation, salivation and bronchial secretion. The combined effect of bronchial secretion and constriction can interfere with breathing.

Effects on the eye are of some importance. The parasympathetic nerves to the eye supply the **constrictor pupillae** muscle which runs circumferentially in the iris, and the **ciliary muscle** which adjusts the position of the ciliary body within the anterior chamber of the eye, and hence the curvature of the lens (Fig. 6.5). Contraction of the ciliary muscle in response to activation of muscarinic receptors pulls the ciliary body forwards and inwards, thus relaxing the tension on the suspensory ligament of the lens, allowing the lens to bulge more and reducing its

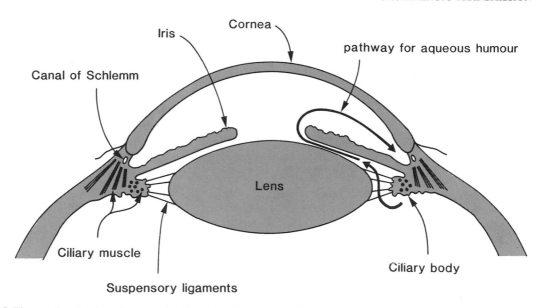

Fig. 6.5 The anterior chamber of the eye, showing the pathway for secretion and drainage of the aqueous humour.

focal length. This parasympathetic reflex is thus necessary to accommodate the eye for near vision.

The constrictor pupillae is important not only for adjusting the pupil in response to changes in light intensity, but also in regulating the intraocular pressure. Aqueous humour is secreted slowly and continuously by the cells of the epithelium covering the ciliary body and it is removed continuously by drainage into the **canal of Schlemm** (Fig. 6.5) which runs around the eye close to the outer margin of the iris. The intraocular pressure is normally 10–15 mmHg above atmospheric, which keeps the eye slightly distended. Abnormally raised intraocular pressure can damage the eye irreversibly, for example by stretching the scleral layer and causing the retina to become detached. In some individuals drainage of aqueous humour becomes impeded when the iris is dilated because folding of the iris tissue occludes the drainage angle, and the intraocular pressure rises for this reason. Activation of the constrictor pupillae muscle by muscarinic agonists will, in these circumstances, lower the intraocular pressure, though in a normal individual it will have little effect. The increased tension in the ciliary muscle produced by these drugs may also play a part in improving drainage by realigning the connective tissue trabeculae through which the canal of Schlemm passes.

Uses and side effects of muscarinic agonists

The main use of muscarinic agonists is in treating glaucoma (raised intraocular pressure) by local instillation in the form of eye drops. Pilocarpine is the most effective as, being a tertiary amine, it can cross the conjunctival membrane. It is a stable compound whose action lasts for about 1 day.

Minor uses include the suppression of atrial tachycardias (see Chapter 10), which relies on the inhibition of pacemaker activity in the atrium; the stimulation of gastrointestinal activity, for example after abdominal surgery when intestinal paralysis may be troublesome; and the stimulation of bladder emptying, when a neurological lesion has disturbed the normal emptying mechanism.

The side effects of these drugs are considerable, and they are generally poorly absorbed from the gastrointestinal tract, so they are now seldom used except in glaucoma. When a drug of this kind is needed for systemic use, bethanechol, which combines selectivity for muscarinic receptors with resistenace to hydrolysis, is most often used.

MUSCARINIC ANTAGONISTS

Structure-activity relationships

These drugs are often referred to as **parasympatho-**

Table 6.2 Muscarinic antagonists, with acetylcholine for comparison

Drug	Structure
Acetylcholine (agonist)	
Atropine	
Homatropine	
Atropine methonitrate	
Hyoscine	
Propantheline	
Lachesine	
Cyclopentolate	
Pirenzepine	

lytic because they selectively reduce or abolish the effects of parasympathetic stimulation. All of them are competitive antagonists of acetylcholine at muscarinic receptors. The structures of some of the most important compounds are shown in Table

6.2, in which the structure of acetylcholine is also shown for comparison.

The two naturally occurring compounds, **atropine** and **hyoscine**, are alkaloids found in solanaceous plants. The deadly nightshade (*Atropa belladonna*) contains mainly atropine, whereas the thorn apple (*Datura stramonium*) contains mainly hyoscine. The plants produce the biologically active L-isomer in each case, but racemization occurs readily and the official drug names refer to the racemic mixture. **Homatropine** is synthesized from atropine and is pharmacologically very similar. These three compounds are all tertiary ammonium compounds, largely ionized at physiological pH but sufficiently lipid soluble (on account of the small proportion that is unionized) to be readily absorbed from the gut or conjunctival sac, and, importantly, to penetrate the blood-brain barrier.

Among synthetic muscarinic antagonists, the quaternary derivative of atropine, **atropine methonitrate**, has peripheral actions very similar to those of atropine but, because of its exclusion from the brain, lacks central actions. Others include **lachesine** and **propantheline**. In general these drugs retain the cationic nitrogen atom and the ester group in a similar steric relationship as in acetylcholine, conversion of agonist to blocking activity being produced by the addition of bulky substituents at either end of the molecule.

Pirenzepine is a recently introduced selective muscarinic antagonist, which acts mainly at M_1 receptors (Hammer & Giachetti, 1984; see p. 114).

Effects of muscarinic antagonists

All of these drugs produce basically similar peripheral effects, though some show a degree of selectivity, e.g. for the heart or the gastrointestinal tract, probably reflecting heterogeneity among muscarinic receptors (see p. 115).

The main effects of atropine are:

Inhibition of secretions. Salivary, lacrimal, bronchial and sweat glands are inhibited by very low doses of atropine, producing an uncomfortably dry mouth and skin. Gastric secretion is only slightly reduced.

Effects on heart rate. The first effect produced is, paradoxically, **bradycardia**, which results from a central action, increasing vagal activity. Slightly larger doses produce the expected **tachycardia**, due to block of cardiac muscarinic receptors. The tachycardia is modest, up to 80–90 beats/min in man. This is because there is no effect on the sympathetic system, but only inhibition of the existing parasympathetic tone. The response of the heart to exercise is unaffected. Arterial blood pressure is unaffected, since most resistance vessels have no cholinergic innervation.

Effects on the eye. The pupil is dilated (mydriasis)* and becomes unresponsive to light. Relaxation of the ciliary muscle causes paralysis of accommodation (cycloplegia), so that near vision is impaired. Intraocular pressure may rise; though this is unimportant in normal individuals, it can be dangerous in patients suffering from glaucoma.

Effects on the gastrointestinal tract. Gastrointestinal motility is inhibited, though this requires larger doses than the other effects listed, and is not complete. This is because excitatory transmitters other than acetylcholine are important in normal function of the myenteric plexus (see Chapters 5 & 15). In pathological conditions in which there is increased gastrointestinal motility, atropine is rather more effective in causing inhibition.

Effects on other smooth muscle. Bronchial, biliary and urinary tract smooth muscle are all relaxed by atropine. Reflex bronchoconstriction (e.g. during anaesthesia) is prevented by atropine, whereas bronchoconstriction caused by local mediators, such as histamine (e.g. in asthma) is unaffected (see Chapter 13). Biliary and urinary tract smooth muscle are only slightly affected, probably because transmitters other than acetylcholine (see Chapter 5) are important in these organs.

Effects on the central nervous system. Atropine produces mainly excitatory effects on the central nervous system. At low doses this causes mild restlessness; higher doses cause agitation and disorientation. In **atropine poisoning** which occurs mainly in young children who eat deadly nightshade berries, marked excitement and irritability result in hyperactivity and a considerable rise in body temperature, which is accentuated by the

loss of sweating. These central effects are evidently the result of blocking muscarinic receptors in the brain since they are opposed by anticholinesterase drugs, such as **physostigmine**, which is an effective antidote to atropine poisoning. It is thus surprising that hyoscine has different central actions, causing marked sedation in low doses, though similar effects in high dosage. Hyoscine also has a useful anti-emetic effect (see below).

Atropine, and other antimuscarinic drugs, also affect the extrapyramidal system, reducing the involuntary movement and rigidity of patients with Parkinson's disease (see Chapter 24).

The actions of pirenzepine differ from those of most muscarinic antagonists, since it selectively inhibits gastric secretion at doses which have little effect on other systems, such as the heart, salivary gland, bladder or eye (see Chapter 15).

Uses of antimuscarinic drugs

The main uses are:

1. As premedication for anaesthesia. Inhibition of bronchial and salivary secretion, and of reflex bronchoconstriction are all valuable effects since they reduce the risk of airway obstruction and of postoperative pneumonia resulting from inhaled secretions. In addition, the block of muscarinic receptors in the heart reduces the bradycardia that occurs with some anaesthetics (see Chapter 20) and with neuromuscular blocking drugs such as suxamethonium. **Atropine** and **hyoscine** are the agents used, the latter having the advantage of causing sedation.

2. Gastrointestinal disorders. Muscarinic antagonists were once widely used to reduce gastric acid secretion in peptic ulcer, but selective histamine antagonists (see Chapter 15) have now largely replaced them. Some agents (e.g. **propantheline**, which is a quaternary ammonium compound and therefore lacks central actions) are used to reduce gastrointestinal motility. They are more effective where the hypermotility is drug-induced (e.g. by anticholinesterase drugs or sympathetic neuron blocking drugs) than when it has a pathological cause. Quaternary derivatives such as **atropine methonitrate** are sometimes used to inhibit gastrointestinal motility, as they do not act centrally. They have the disadvantage of poor absorption,

---

*The alluring quality of dilated pupils was well understood by Greek and Roman courtesans, whose cosmetic use of eyedrops made from deadly nightshade berries led to the plant being called *belladonna*. Inability to see properly was evidently considered a price worth paying.

however, and have appreciable ganglionic and neuromuscular blocking actions in addition to blocking muscarinic receptors. **Pirenzepine** is currently under test in the treatment of peptic ulceration.

3. In ophthalmology. Pupillary dilatation and paralysis of accommodation are useful in the treatment of various inflammatory conditions of the eye, and also as an aid to thorough ophthalmoscopic examination. Atropine given as eyedrops produces an effect that lasts for several days. Various synthetic drugs produce a shorter action, and some are claimed to cause relatively less cycloplegia and hence cause less visual disturbance. **Homatropine**, **cyclopentolate** and **tropicamide** are examples of drugs developed specifically for ophthalmic use.

4. For motion sickness. **Hyoscine** is useful for its central action in preventing motion sickness, though drowsiness and dry mouth are troublesome side effects.

GANGLION STIMULATING DRUGS

In addition to the agonists listed in Table 6.1 that act on both muscarinic and nicotinic receptors there are a few drugs that act selectively on nicotinic receptors; some of these affect both ganglionic and motor endplate receptors, but some show selectivity (Kharkevich, 1980).

Nicotine, **lobeline** and **dimethylphenylpiperazinium (DMPP)** are three drugs that affect ganglionic nicotinic receptors preferentially (Table 6.3). Nicotine and lobeline are tertiary amines found in the leaves of tobacco and lobelia plants respectively. Nicotine has a well-established place in pharmacological folk-lore as it was the substance on the tip of Langley's paint-brush which he found to stimulate muscle fibres when applied to the endplate region, and which caused him to postulate in 1905 the existence of a 'receptive substance' on the surface of the fibres. Both of these substances

Table 6.3 Nicotinic agonists

Drug	Structure	Main site & type of action	
Nicotine		Autonomic ganglia	Stimulation then block
		CNS	Stimulation
Lobeline		Autonomic ganglia	Stimulation
		Sensory terminals	Stimulation
Dimethylphenyl-piperazinium		Autonomic ganglia	Stimulation
Suxamethonium		NMJ	Depolarization block
Decamethonium		NMJ	Depolarization block
Acetylcholine Carbachol	See Table 6.1		

affect the neuromuscular junction in concentrations only slightly greater than those that affect ganglia. DMPP is a synthetic quaternary ammonium compound that is more selective for ganglionic receptors. Being quaternary it lacks the central actions of nicotine.

These substances are of no therapeutic value. They are useful for experimental purposes, and nicotine is, of course, important in relation to smoking and snuff-taking (see Chapter 35). They produce a generalized stimulation of autonomic ganglia and a complex pattern of mixed sympathetic and parasympathetic responses. A rise in arterial blood pressure occurs partly as a result of stimulation of sympathetic ganglia, causing vasoconstriction, and partly because of adrenaline release from the adrenal medulla, where the nicotinic receptors resemble those of the ganglia. Gut motility may be either increased or decreased; cigarette smoking usually inhibits gastric motility and diminishes hunger. Secretion of saliva, bronchial mucus and sweat are increased. In larger doses, ganglionic stimulants produce, paradoxically, a block of transmission. This is a manifestation of **depolarization block** (see p. 117), but it does not normally occur when nicotine is taken by smoking.

The stimulant effect of nicotinic agonists is not confined to cholinergic synapses, but can also occur at certain nerve endings and axons, where acetylcholine has no known function. Non-myelinated axons are depolarized by nicotinic agonists, and so are many sensory nerve endings, particularly those in the lungs and heart. When these are stimulated by drugs such as lobeline, a variety of respiratory and cardiovascular reflex responses is produced. Adrenergic nerve terminals, also, are depolarized by nicotinic agonists and caused to release transmitter. All of these effects are blocked by antagonists that affect nicotinic receptors, but as far as is known they are pharmacological curiosities with no physiological importance.

GANGLION BLOCKING DRUGS

Ganglion block can occur by several mechanisms (Brown, 1980):

1. By interference with acetylcholine release. The mechanisms involved are the same as at the neuromuscular junction (see p. 130 and Chapter 5), and the same substances, namely botulinum toxin, hemicholinium, and magnesium ion, are effective in causing block. Skeletal muscle paralysis occurs at the same time as ganglion block, the latter being of little practical importance.

2. By interference with the post-synaptic action of acetylcholine. Ganglion blocking drugs of practical importance all act by this mechanism, and are discussed in more detail below.

3. By prolonged depolarization. Nicotine (see Fig. 6.4) can block ganglia, after initial stimulation, in this way, and so can acetylcholine itself if cholinesterase is inhibited so that it can exert a continuing action on the post-synaptic membrane. This type of block is much less important at the ganglionic synapse than at the neuromuscular junction (see p. 132).

Inhibitors of acetylcholine action

The major ganglion blocking drugs all act by inhibiting the post-synaptic action of acetylcholine; they do not themselves cause depolarization, and hence block transmission without causing initial stimulation.

Tetraethylammonium (Table 6.4) was the first ganglion blocking drug to be characterized. It was shown in 1915 to block the effect of nicotinic agonists on ganglia. Unfortunately it is a drug with numerous other pharmacological effects and was unsuitable for use in man.

Hexamethonium (Table 6.4) was discovered by Paton & Zaimis in 1948. They investigated a series of methonium compounds of the same basic structure in which the length of the polymethylene chain was varied systematically, and found that the pharmacological actions of members of this series vary according to chain length (Fig. 6.6). Compounds with five or six carbon atoms in the methylene chain linking the two quaternary groups produce *ganglionic* block and when the chain contained nine or ten carbon atoms they produce *neuromuscular* block. Pharmacological activity varies sharply with chain length; alteration of the length by one carbon atom may change the activity by a factor of 20 as shown in Figure 6.6. The action of hexamethonium is similar to that of tetraethylammonium, but is considerably more potent and specific.

Table 6.4 Nicotinic antagonists

Drug	Structure	Main site	Mechanism
Hexamethonium		Ganglia	Mainly channel block
Tetraethyl ammonium		Ganglia	
Mecamylamine		Ganglia	Receptor block
Trimetaphan		Ganglia	Receptor block
Tubocurarine		NMJ	Receptor block (Some channel block) Channel block in ganglia)
Gallamine		NMJ	Receptor block (Some channel block)
Pancuronium		NMJ	Receptor block

Table 6.4 Nicotinic antagonists (*contd.*)

Drug	Structure	Main site	Mechanism
Atracurium	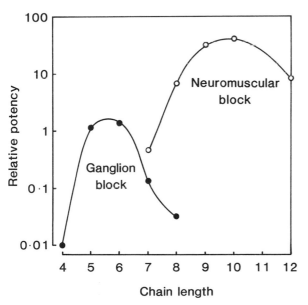 point of spontaneous cleavage	NMJ	Receptor block

Other ganglion blocking drugs which have little or no effect on the neuromuscular junction include **mecamylamine**, **pempidine** and **trimetaphan**. The first two are non-quaternary bases that were developed to give better absorption and a longer duration of action than hexamethonium. Trimetaphan is a strongly basic compound whose plasma half-life is so short that it can be administered as a slow intravenous infusion for certain types of anaesthetic procedure that require controlled hypotension.

Mechanism of action of non-depolarizing ganglion blocking drugs

Hexamethonium blocks the response of the ganglion to acetylcholine or other ganglionic stimulants, but does not itself stimulate or depolarize the ganglion. Mainly because of the structural similarity of the methonium series of compounds to acetylcholine it has generally been believed that they act as competitive antagonists at the receptor sites. Recently, however, the action of many ganglion blocking agents has been shown to result from a block, not of the receptor, but of the associated ionic channel (Fig. 6.7) (see Chapter 1).

Fig. 6.6 The ganglionic and neuromuscular blocking activity of the homologous series of methonium compounds, measured in an anaesthetized cat. Ganglion blocking activity is maximal at C6 (hexamethonium) and neuromuscular blocking activity at C10 (decamethonium). (From: Paton & Zaimis, 1949)

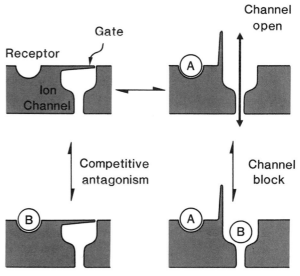

Fig. 6.7 Acetylcholine antagonism by competitive receptor block (left) and channel block (right). Recent evidence favours the latter mechanism of action for many ganglion blocking drugs. A = ACh molecule; B = blocking molecule.

Of the agents listed above, hexamethonium and pempidine appear to act mainly by channel block, whereas trimetaphan and mecamylamine act on the receptor. Tubocurarine (see p. 131) blocks ganglionic as well as neuromuscular transmission; however, on the ganglion its action is on the ionic channel whereas at the neuromuscular junction it binds mainly to the receptor, though also to the channel.

The chief characteristics that distinguish a competitive receptor blocking action from a non-competitive channel blocking action are:

1. Most channel blocking drugs can block the channel only after it has been opened. Thus the block *increases* in intensity when the agonist concentration is increased—the reverse of what happens with competitive block (see Chapter 1), where the block becomes *less* at high agonist concentration (i.e. it is surmountable). This property gives rise to the phenomenon of **use-dependent block** (described also for local anaesthetic drugs, see Chapter 27), which means that synapses that transmit at high frequency are blocked more readily than synapses that transmit only occasionally.

2. Channel blocking drugs (if they are cationic) become more effective when the membrane is hyperpolarized whereas competitive blocking agents do not. This is because the site within the channel to which the blocking drug binds lies within the transmembrane electric field, in contrast to the superficial location of the receptor site. Hyperpolarizing the cell will thus make the potential at the channel binding site more negative with respect to the outside and cationic drug molecules will bind to it more strongly.

Effects of ganglion blocking drugs

The effects of ganglion blocking drugs are numerous and complex, as would be expected, since both divisions of the autonomic nervous system are blocked indiscriminately. Even large doses do not totally abolish transmission, because the excitatory action of the muscarinic receptors remains. The description by Paton (1954) of 'hexamethonium man' cannot be bettered:

'He is a pink complexioned person, except when he has stood in a queue for a long time, when he may get pale and faint. His handshake is warm and dry. He is a placid and relaxed companion; for instance he may laugh but he can't cry because the tears cannot come. Your rudest story will not make him blush, and the most unpleasant circumstances will fail to make him turn pale. His collars and socks stay very clean and sweet. He wears corsets and may, if you meet him out, be rather fidgety (corsets to compress his splanchnic vascular pool, fidgety to keep the venous return going from his legs). He dislikes speaking much unless helped with something to moisten his dry mouth and throat. He is long-sighted and easily blinded by bright light. The redness of his eyeballs may suggest irregular habits and in fact his head is rather weak. But he always behaves like a gentleman and never belches or hiccups. He tends to get cold and keeps well wrapped up. But his health is good; he does not have chilblains and those diseases of modern civilization, hypertension and peptic ulcer, pass him by. He gets thin because his appetite is modest; he never feels hunger pains and his stomach never rumbles. He gets rather constipated so that his intake of liquid paraffin is high. As old age comes on, he will suffer from retention of urine and impotence, but frequency, precipitancy and strangury will not worry him. One is uncertain how he will end, but perhaps if he is not careful, by eating less and less and getting colder and colder, he will sink into a symptomless, hypoglycaemic coma and die, as was proposed for the universe, a sort of entropy death.'

The most important effects are on the cardiovascular system and on visceral smooth muscle.

Cardiovascular system. A marked fall in arterial blood pressure results mainly from block of sympathetic ganglia, which causes arteriolar vasodilatation. Cardiac output falls slightly, but effects of the sympathetic and parasympathetic systems tend to oppose each other. The loss of certain cardiovascular reflexes has important effects. In particular, the venoconstriction, which occurs normally when a subject stands up from a sitting or lying position and which is necessary if the central venous pressure is to be prevented from falling sharply, is reduced. Standing thus causes a sudden fall in cardiac output and in arterial pressure (postural hypotension) which can cause fainting. Similarly, the vasodilatation of skeletal muscle during exercise is normally accompanied by vasoconstriction elsewhere (e.g. splanchnic area) produced by sympathetic activity. If this adjustment is prevented, the overall peripheral resistance falls and the blood pressure also falls (post-exercise hypotension).

Visceral smooth muscle. There is an inhibition of secretion and motility of all parts of the gastrointestinal tract, which leads to severe constipation. The peristaltic reflex, which can be elicited by raising the pressure within an isolated length of intestine, is inhibited by ganglion block. Bladder emptying is also inhibited, resulting in urinary retention, and the loss of autonomic reflexes causes impotence and failure of ejaculation.

Uses of ganglion blocking drugs

Ganglion blocking drugs were the first really effective antihypertensive drugs (see Chapter 11). They had many disadvantages but their success in reducing the mortality of hypertensive patients paved the way for the development of more selective compounds. Attempts to use ganglion blocking drugs to inhibit gastric acid secretion were unsuccessful because of their many side effects. They are now clinically obsolete, with the exception of trimetaphan, a very short-acting drug that is used in anaesthesia, in conjunction with a tilting operating table, to produce controlled hypotension, with the aim of minimizing bleeding during certain kinds of surgery. The short action of trimetaphan

means that it can be given as an intravenous infusion to produce minute-to-minute control of blood pressure.

NEUROMUSCULAR BLOCKING DRUGS

The pharmacology of neuromuscular function is well reviewed by Bowman (1980) and Zaimis (1976).

Drugs can block neuromuscular transmission in three main ways:
1. By interfering with acetylcholine synthesis
2. By interfering with acetylcholine release
3. By interfering with the post-synaptic action of acetylcholine. This category includes all of the clinically useful drugs and may be further subdivided into:
   a. Non-depolarizing blocking agents, which act by blocking acetylcholine receptors (and, in some cases, also by blocking ion channels)
   b. Depolarizing blocking agents, which are agonists at acetylcholine receptors (see p. 114).

DRUGS AFFECTING ACETYLCHOLINE SYNTHESIS

The steps in the synthesis of acetylcholine in the pre-synaptic nerve terminals are shown in Figure 6.2. The rate-limiting process appears to be the transport of choline into the nerve terminal, and the only important drugs that inhibit acetylcholine synthesis do so by blocking this step. A few com-

Table 6.5 Comparison of effects of different types of neuromuscular block

	Type of block		
	Non-depolarizing	*Depolarizing*	*Choline uptake inhibition*
Effect of anticholinesterase	Block reversed	Block enhanced	No effect
Response to tetanus	Rapid fade	Sustained	Slow fade
Initial fasciculations	Absent	Present	Absent
Rate of onset	Fast (c. 1 min)	Fast (c. 30 sec)	Slow
Effect of depolarizing drugs*	Block reversed	Block enhanced	No effect
Effect of competitive antagonist*	Block enhanced	Block reduced	Block enhanced
Effect of choline	No effect	No effect	Block reversed
Effect of increased stimulation frequency	No effect	No effect	Block enhanced
Effect in myasthenic patients	Blocking potency increased	Blocking potency reduced	Blocking potency increased

* In doses too small to affect transmission in normal muscle

pounds that inhibit choline acetylase have been reported, but they are of low potency and specificity. Two drugs that inhibit choline transport are **hemicholinium** and *triethylcholine*, which are useful as experimental tools, but have no clinical applications. Both of these compounds are chemically related to choline. Hemicholinium acts as a competitive inhibitor of choline uptake, but is not appreciably taken up itself. Triethylcholine, as well as inhibiting choline uptake, is itself transported and acetylated within the terminals, forming acetyltriethylcholine. This is stored in place of acetylcholine, and released as a false transmitter, but has no depolarizing effect on the post-synaptic membrane. These drugs affect all peripheral cholinergic synapses, but because of their quaternary ammonium structure, they do not cross the blood-brain barrier.

The type of transmission block that they produce is characterized by a **slow onset** (because of the time taken for the acetylcholine stores to run down), **frequency dependence** (because the more acetylcholine is being released the more the store will be depleted), and **reversal by addition of choline** (see Table 6.5). Their slow, frequency-dependent blocking action makes these drugs unsuitable for use in anaesthesia. It was thought that they might be useful in selectively reducing the tone of hyperactive muscles in spasticity, but the margin of safety before respiratory paralysis occurred proved to be too narrow.

DRUGS THAT INHIBIT ACETYLCHOLINE RELEASE

Acetylcholine release by a nerve impulse involves the entry of calcium ions into the nerve terminal; the increase in $[Ca]_i$ increases the rate of quantal release, probably by increasing the frequency of exocytotic events within the terminal (see Fig. 6.2). Agents that inhibit the impulse itself (e.g. local anaesthetics; see Chapter 27) will obviously cause neuromuscular block, though they are not used for this purpose. Agents that inhibit calcium entry have a similar effect. These include **magnesium ion**, and various **aminoglycoside antibiotics** (e.g. streptomycin and neomycin; see Chapter 30). Intravenous magnesium salts were once used as anaesthetic agents, for the effect on transmitter release is a general one that affects central as well as peripheral synapses. Aminoglycoside antibiotics occasionally produce muscle paralysis as an unwanted side effect when used clinically. The paralysis can be reversed by administration of calcium salts. Surprisingly, **calcium antagonists** (see Chapter 10), which block calcium entry into many cells, have little effect on the release of neurotransmitters. The reason for this is not known.

Two potent neurotoxins, namely **botulinum toxin** and **β-bungarotoxin**, act specifically to inhibit acetylcholine release. **Botulinum toxin** is a protein produced by the anaerobic bacillus *Clostridium botulinum*, an organism that can multiply in preserved food, and is responsible for an extremely serious type of food poisoning. The potency of botulinum toxin is extraordinary. It is estimated that the minimum lethal dose in a mouse is less than 10^{-12} g, amounting to only a few million molecules. It binds tightly to cholinergic nerve terminals and it is calculated that no more than a few molecules need to be bound by each nerve terminal in order to inhibit acetylcholine release. It is presumed that, in common with other extremely potent toxins, such as cholera and diptheria toxins, botulinum toxin must possess enzymic activity which allows a few molecules entering a cell to initiate a reaction in which many substrate molecules are affected. With botulinum toxin no details have yet been discovered, but it may well be an important key to understanding how transmitter release occurs.

Botulinum poisoning causes progressive parasympathetic and motor paralysis, with dry mouth, blurred vision and difficulty in swallowing, followed by progressive respiratory paralysis. Treatment with antitoxin is effective only if given before symptoms appear, for once the toxin is bound its action cannot be reversed. Mortality is high, and recovery, in non-fatal cases, takes several weeks. Anticholinesterases and drugs that increase transmitter release (see p. 144) are ineffective in restoring transmission. Among the more spectacular outbreaks of botulinum poisoning was an incident on Loch Maree in Scotland in 1922 when all eight members of a fishing party died after eating duck paté for their lunch. Their ghillies, consuming humbler fare no doubt, survived.

β-bungarotoxin is a protein contained in the venom of various snakes of the cobra family, and has a similar action to botulinum toxin. The same venoms also contain **α-bungarotoxin** (see p. 14) which blocks post-synaptic acetylcholine receptors, so these snakes evidently cover all eventualities as far as causing paralysis of their victims is concerned.

DRUGS THAT ACT POST-SYNAPTICALLY

Non-depolarizing blocking agents

Claude Bernard showed in 1856 that 'curare' causes paralysis by blocking neuromuscular transmission, rather than by abolishing nerve conduction or muscle contractility, and J N Langley suggested in 1905 that it acts by combining with a 'receptive substance' at the motor endplate.

Chemistry and structure-activity relationships

'**Curare**' is a mixture of naturally occurring alkaloids found in various South American plants and used as arrow poisons by South American Indians. Many of these substances have neuromuscular blocking activity, but the most important is **tubocurarine** (see Table 6.4) whose structure was elucidated in 1935. Tubocurarine is still widely used in clinical medicine, but a number of synthetic drugs with very similar actions have been developed, the most important ones being **gallamine** and **pancuronium**. Recently a new drug, **atracurium** (Stenlake et al, 1983), with a particularly short duration of action, has been introduced. These substances are all quaternary ammonium compounds, which means that they are poorly absorbed and generally rapidly excreted. They also fail to cross the placenta, which is important in relation to their use in obstetric anaesthesia. The failure of tubocurarine to be absorbed when taken orally means that it can be used safely in the hunting of animals for food.

By comparison with the depolarizing drugs (see

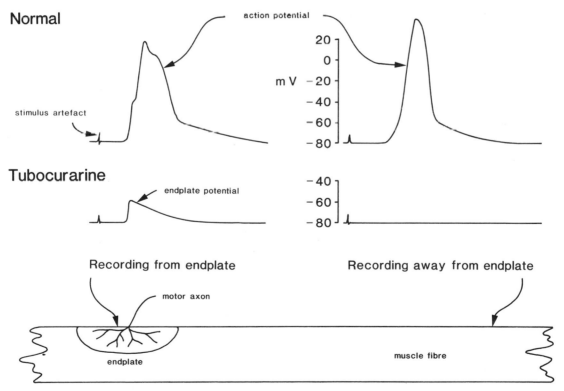

Fig. 6.8 The effect of tubocurarine on neuromuscular transmission. *Top.* Microelectrode recording at the endplate (left) normally shows a complex response to nerve stimulation, consisting of an endplate potential (epp), from the peak of which the action potential is initiated. The action potential is distorted by the local increase in conductance produced by the transmitter. Away from the endplate a simple propagated action potential is recorded (right). *Bottom.* Tubocurarine reduces the epp amplitude, so that no action potential is generated.

Table 6.5), non-depolarizing drugs are generally bulkier and more rigid molecules. In both groups most of the highly active compounds have two cationic groups (three in the case of gallamine). The interaction with the acetylcholine receptor site appears to be one-to-one so the significance of the additional basic groups is not clear at present.

Mechanism of action

These drugs have all been shown to act as competitive antagonists (see Chapter 1) at the acetylcholine receptors of the endplate, and this largely accounts for their actions. The amount of acetylcholine released by a nerve impulse normally exceeds by several-fold what is needed to elicit an action potential in the muscle fibre. It is therefore necessary to block 80–90% of the receptor sites before transmission actually fails. When this happens it is still possible to record a small endplate potential in the muscle fibre though its amplitude fails to reach threshold (Fig. 6.8). In any individual muscle fibre transmission is all-or-nothing, so graded degrees of block represent a varying proportion of muscle fibres failing to respond. In this situation, where the endplate potential amplitude in all of the fibres is close to threshold—just above in some, just below in others—small variations in the amount of transmitter released, or in the rate at which it is destroyed will have a large effect on the proportion of fibres contracting, so the degree of block is liable to vary according to various physiological circumstances (e.g. stimulation frequency, temperature, cholinesterase inhibition, etc) which normally have relatively little effect on the efficiency of transmission.

In addition to blocking receptors some of these drugs also block ion channels in a manner similar to the ganglion blocking drugs. Though it can be clearly shown experimentally, this action is probably of little importance in practice. It has also been claimed, though the evidence is equivocal, that tubocurarine and some other drugs act pre-synaptically as well as post-synaptically, and inhibit the release of acetylcholine during repetitive stimulation of the motor nerve. This may play a part in causing the 'tetanic fade' seen with these drugs (see p. 134).

Effects of non-depolarizing blocking drugs

The effects of non-depolarizing neuromuscular blocking agents are mainly due to motor paralysis, though some of the drugs also produce clinically significant autonomic effects. The first muscles to be affected are the extrinsic eye muscles (causing double vision) and the small muscles of the face, limbs and pharynx (causing difficulty in swallowing). Respiratory muscles are the last to be affected and the first to recover. A heroic experiment in 1947 in which a volunteer was fully curarised under artificial ventilation established this orderly paralytic march, and showed that consciousness and awareness of pain were quite normal even when paralysis was complete. The special characteristics of non-depolarizing block, and the ways in which it differs from depolarization block are described on page 133.

Side effects of non-depolarizing blocking drugs

The main side effect of tubocurarine is a fall in arterial pressure, which is produced mainly by ganglion block. An additional cause is the release of histamine from mast cells (see Chapter 8), which can also give rise to bronchospasm in sensitive individuals. The other non-depolarizing blocking drugs cause less ganglion block and histamine release than tubocurarine, and hence less hypotension. Gallamine appears to block muscarinic receptors, particularly in the heart, which results in tachycardia.

Depolarizing blocking agents

This class of neuromuscular blocking drugs was discovered by Paton & Zaimis in their study of the effects of symmetrical bisquaternary ammonium compounds (see Fig. 6.6). **Decamethonium** (see Table 6.3), the 10-carbon compound, was found to cause paralysis without appreciable ganglion blocking activity. Several features of its action showed it to be different from competitive blocking drugs such as tubocurarine. In particular it was found to produce a transient twitching of skeletal muscle (fasciculation) before causing block, and when it was injected into chicks it caused a powerful extensor spasm, whereas tubocurarine simply caused flaccid paralysis. Burns & Paton showed in 1951 that its action was to cause a maintained depolarization at the endplate region of the muscle fibre, which led to a loss of electrical excitability (see p. 117), and they coined the term 'depolarization block'. The reason for the curious extensor spasm produced in birds is that they possess a special type of skeletal muscle, rare in mammals, that has many endplates scattered over the surface of each muscle fibre. A drug that causes endplate depolarization produces a widespread depolarization in such muscles, resulting in a maintained contracture. In normal skeletal muscle, with only one endplate per fibre, endplate depolarization is too localized to cause contracture on its own. Fasciculation occurs because the developing endplate depolarization initially causes a discharge of action potentials in the muscle fibre. This subsides after a few seconds as the electrical excitability of the endplate region of the fibre is lost.

Decamethonium itself was used clinically but has the disadvantage of too long a duration of action. **Suxamethonium** (see Table 6.4) is closely related in structure to both decamethonium and acetylcholine (consisting of two acetylcholine molecules linked by their acetyl groups). Its action is shorter than that of decamethonium because it is quickly hydrolysed by plasma cholinesterase. Suxamethonium and decamethonium act on the motor endplate just like acetylcholine (i.e. they are agonists which increase the cation permeability of the endplate). The difference is that decamethonium and suxamethonium, when given as drugs, diffuse slowly to the endplate and the concentration at the endplate persists for long enough to cause loss of electrical excitability. Acetylcholine, in contrast, when released from the nerve, reaches the endplate in very brief spurts and is rapidly hydrolysed *in situ*, so it never causes sufficiently prolonged depolarization to result in block. If cholinesterase is inhibited, however, (see p. 142) it is possible for the circulating acetylcholine concentration to reach a level sufficient to cause depolarization block.

Comparison of non-depolarizing and depolarizing blocking drugs

The neuromuscular block produced by these two mechanisms differs in many characteristics, which are set out in Table 6.5. The most important distinction is that anticholinesterase drugs are very effective in overcoming the blocking action of competitive agents (Fig. 6.9). This is mainly because the released acetylcholine, protected from hydrolysis, can diffuse further within the synaptic cleft, and so gains access to a wider area of post-synaptic membrane than it normally would. The chances of an acetylcholine molecule finding an unoccupied receptor are thus increased. This diffusional effect seems to be of more importance than a truly competitive interaction, for it is unlikely that appreciable dissociation of the antagonist can occur in the short time for which the acetylcholine is present. With depolarization block no reversal occurs with anticholinesterase drugs; indeed prolongation of the endplate potential can cause the block to be deepened slightly.

A mutual antagonism between competitive and depolarizing drugs can be demonstrated (Fig. 6.9). Addition of tubocurarine to a muscle partly paralysed with suxamethonium will reduce the depolarization, and, provided the tubocurarine concentration is not high enough to cause block in its own right, transmission will be restored. Similarly in a tubocurarine-blocked muscle the small depolarizing effect of suxamethonium can bring the membrane potential closer to threshold so that previously subthreshold endplate potentials exceed the threshold, and transmission is restored (Fig. 6.9). Though such dramatic effects are not likely in anaesthetic practice, the mutual antagonism means that combining the two types of blocking agent is likely to give unpredictable results.

The fasciculations seen with depolarizing agents as a prelude to paralysis do not occur with competitive drugs. There appears to be a correlation between the amount of fasciculation and the severity of the **postoperative muscle pain** that is often produced by depolarizing drugs, the mechanism of which is not clear.

Depolarizing blocking agents are strikingly *ineffective* in patients with **myasthenia gravis**. In this disease (see p. 143) there are fewer receptors than normal at the endplate, so less depolarization occurs. In contrast these patients are *hypersensitive* to competitive blocking agents, because their margin of safety for transmission is reduced or absent.

'Tetanic fade' is a term used to describe the

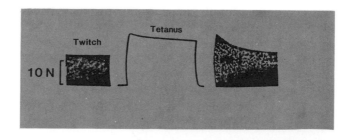

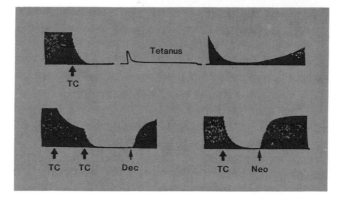

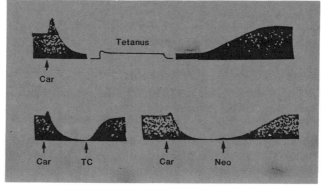

Fig. 6.9 Comparison of depolarizing and non-depolarizing (competitive) neuromuscular block. Contractions of the cat *tibialis* muscle were recorded in response to motor nerve stimulation. Twitches were produced by single stimuli delivered every 10 seconds (slow chart speed); tetani consisted of a 10 second train at 50 Hz (fast chart speed).

Top. Control records. The tetanus is well sustained, and is followed by slight post-tetanic potentiation of the twitch. This is due to a change in the contractile machinery of the muscle, not to facilitated neuromuscular transmission.

Middle. Tubocurarine (0.6 μmol/kg) blocks the twitch completely. The tetanus is not sustained, and is followed by exaggerated post-tetanic potentiation. This is due to a post-tetanic increase in ACh release, which transiently overcomes the block. Tubocurarine block can be reversed by a depolarizing drug (decamethonium) or an anticholinesterase (neostigmine).

Bottom. Depolarization block produced by carbolonium (35 nmol/kg), a drug very similar to suxamethonium or decamethonium. There is initial enhancement of the twitch, associated with repetitive firing of the muscle fibres, and then block. The tetanus is reduced, but well sustained, and is not followed by post-tetanic potentiation. This is because increased ACh release is ineffective in overcoming depolarization block. The block can be reversed by tubocurarine, but not by neostigmine. (Modified from: Bowman, 1980)

failure of muscle tension to be maintained during a brief period of nerve stimulation at a frequency high enough to produce a fused tetanus (about 50 Hz). In normal muscle tetanic fade is very slight, but in a muscle blocked with a non-depolarizing drug it becomes very marked (Fig. 6.9). This is because the acetylcholine released per impulse decreases during such a tetanus; normally this will not cause transmission failure, but if the margin of safety is lost, failure will occur as soon as transmitter release decreases. It is possible that a presynaptic action of the blocking drug contributes to this phenomenon. Fade does not occur with depolarization block, where muscle fibres that have not lost their electrical excitability will continue to respond during the tetanus. This difference forms the basis of a simple test used by anaesthetists to discover which type of block is present. Electrodes are used to stimulate a peripheral nerve, such as the ulnar nerve, through the skin, and muscle contraction is observed during a short period of tetanic stimulation.

Phase I and Phase II block

With repeated or continuous administration the action of depolarizing drugs tends to change. Initially the block shows the physiological characteristics of depolarization block, as described above (Phase I), but later it takes on some of the properties associated with non-depolarizing block (Phase II). Thus the block becomes partially reversible by anticholinesterase drugs, and begins to show tetanic fade. The mechanism of this change is not very clear, but it probably results from **receptor desensitization** produced by the continued presence of the depolarizing drug. When this happens the membrane potential is partially restored (see Fig. 6.4), but at the same time the endplate sensitivity to acetylcholine will be reduced—as with tubocurarine—accounting for the change in mechanism of the block. The transition from Phase I to Phase II block has often been reported when large or repeated doses of suxamethonium are used clinically.

Side effects and dangers of depolarizing drugs

Suxamethonium, the only drug of current clinical importance in this group, can produce a number of important adverse effects:

1. *Bradycardia.* This is preventable by atropine and probably due to a direct muscarinic action.

2. *Potassium release.* The increase in cation permeability of the motor endplates causes a net loss of potassium from muscle leading to a small rise in plasma potassium concentration (Fig. 6.10). In normal individuals this is not important, but in cases of

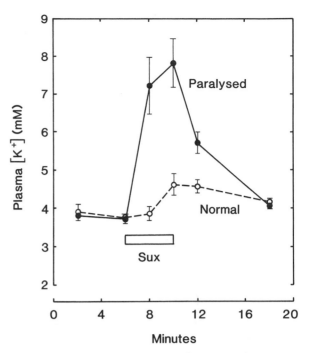

Fig. 6.10 Effect of suxamethonium on plasma potassium concentration in man. Blood was collected from veins draining paralysed and non-paralysed limbs of 7 injured patients undergoing surgery. The injuries had resulted in motor nerve degeneration, and hence denervation supersensitivity of the affected muscles. (From: Tobey et al, 1972)

trauma it may be. Figure 6.10 shows the greatly increased potassium release from muscles that have been paralysed by nerve injury. This increase occurs because of post-denervation spread of acetylcholine sensitivity to regions of the muscle fibre away from the endplates (see Chapter 5), so that a much larger area of membrane is sensitive to suxamethonium, and the resulting hyperkalaemia can be enough to cause serious ventricular dysrhythmia or even cardiac arrest.

3. *Increased intraocular pressure.* This results from contracture of extraocular muscles, which are physiologically similar to avian muscles (see p. 133), causing the eye to be squeezed from the outside. It is particularly important to avoid this if the eyeball has been damaged by injury.

4. *Prolonged paralysis.* The action of suxamethonium given intravenously normally lasts for less than 5 minutes because the drug is hydrolysed to succinylmonocholine, which is only weakly active, by plasma cholinesterase. Its action is prolonged by

various factors that reduce the activity of this enzyme:

a. Genetic variants in which plasma cholinesterase is abnormal (see Chapter 4). Severe deficiency, enough to increase the duration of action to 2 hours or more, occurs in only about 1 in 2000 individuals. In a very few individuals, the enzyme is completely absent and the drug's effect lasts for many hours.

b. Anticholinesterase drugs. The use of organo-phosphates to treat glaucoma (see p. 142) can inhibit plasma cholinesterase. Also, competing substrates for plasma cholinesterase (e.g. **pro-caine**, **propanidid**) can slow down suxamethonium hydrolysis.

c. Neonates, and patients with liver disease, may have low plasma cholinesterase activity, and show prolonged paralysis with suxamethonium.

5. *Malignant hyperthermia*. This is a rare con-genital condition, carried as an autosomal dominant gene (see Chapter 4), which results in intense muscle spasm and a very sudden rise in body temperature when certain drugs are given. The most commonly implicated drugs are suxamethonium and halo-thane, though it can be precipitated by a variety of other drugs. The biochemical cause is uncertain. The condition carries a very high mortality (about 65%), and is usually treated by administration of **dantrolene**, a drug which inhibits muscle contrac-tion by acting on the myofibrils.

Pharmacokinetic aspects

Neuromuscular blocking agents are used mainly in anaesthesia, to produce muscle relaxation. Though complete relaxation can be produced by anaes-thetic drugs alone, the concentrations needed to obliterate spinal reflexes are high and it is much more satisfactory to produce paralysis by blocking neuromuscular transmission. The drugs are given intravenously, and act within about 30 seconds. Their duration of action varies considerably (Fig. 6.11).

Suxamethonium acts normally for about 3 minutes, being hydrolysed by plasma cholinester-ase. It is used to produce transient paralysis for tracheal intubation or very brief procedures. Suxa-methonium is also used to produce short-lasting

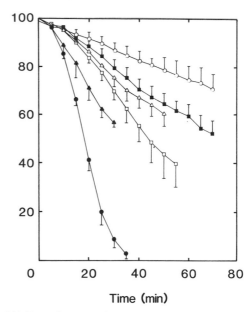

Fig. 6.11 Rate of recovery from various non-depolarizing neuromuscular blocking drugs in man. Drugs were given intravenously to patients undergoing surgery, in doses just sufficient to cause 100% block of the tetanic tension of the indirectly-stimulated *adductor pollicis* muscle. Recovery of tension was then followed as a function of time.
○ Dimethyltubocurarine
■ Tubocurarine
△ Pancuronium
□ Fazadinium
▲ Gallamine
● Atracurium
(From: Payne & Hughes, 1981)

paralysis in patients undergoing electroconvulsive therapy for depression (see Chapter 23). Avoidance of powerful muscle contractions reduces the risk of physical injury without diminishing the effective-ness of the treatment.

Tubocurarine is mainly metabolized by the liver, but 30–40% is excreted unchanged in the urine. Its action lasts for about 30 minutes, but some weak-ness is detectable for several hours.

Gallamine is rather shorter acting, and is elimin-ated entirely by the kidney. If renal clearance is low, therefore, its action is considerably prolonged.

Pancuronium has a similar duration of action to tubocurarine, and is mainly excreted unchanged in the urine.

Atracurium is an interesting development (Stenlake et al, 1983). It is a bisquaternary com-pound that was designed to be chemically unstable at physiological pH (splitting into two inactive fragments by cleavage at one of the quaternary nitrogen atoms; see Table 6.4), though indefinitely stable when stored at an acid pH. It has a shorter action than any of the other non-depolarizing drugs, and may prove to be less variable in this respect because its inactivation relies on chemical rather than biological factors. Because of the marked pH dependence of its degradation, however, its action becomes considerably briefer during respiratory alkalosis caused by hyperventilation.

The time course of recovery from various non-depolarizing drugs in man is shown in Figure 6.11.

DRUGS THAT ENHANCE CHOLINERGIC TRANSMISSION

The most important drugs in this category act either by inhibiting cholinesterase or by increasing acetylcholine release.

Distribution and function of cholinesterase

There are two distinct types of cholinesterase. **Acetylcholinesterase (AChE)**, otherwise known as **true cholinesterase**, is found in the synaptic cleft at cholinergic synapses, where its function is to hydrolyse the released transmitter. It is a membrane-bound enzyme, apparently incorporated into the basement membrane rather than the plasma membrane, since it can be extracted by treatment with certain proteolytic enzymes that disrupt the basement membrane. AChE has been purified and characterized as a protein; its molecular weight is about 250 000 and it consists of four major subunits. The enzyme is easily demonstrated histochemically (Fig. 6.12) by a technique in which acetylthiocholine is used as substrate and the resulting thiocholine used to form a sulphide precipitate with copper. AChE is also present in cholinergic nerve terminals, where it seems to have a role in regulating the free acetylcholine concentration, and in unexpected places such as the erythrocyte where its function is unknown. AChE is relatively specific for acetylcholine; other closely related esters such as methacholine and acetylthiocholine are also good substrates, but most esters are not.

Butyrylcholinesterase (BuChE) or **pseudocholinesterase**, actually consists of a family of enzymes

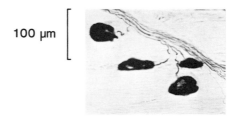

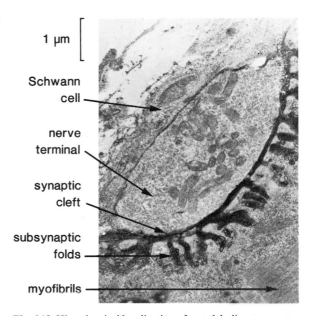

Fig. 6.12 Histochemical localization of acetylcholinesterase at the mouse neuromuscular junction. *Top*. Whole mount preparation showing individual motor axons (silver stained) terminating on AChE-stained endplates on separate muscle fibres. *Bottom*. Electron micrograph showing staining of AChE in synaptic cleft. (Micrographs kindly provided by Prof L W Duchen)

that have a widespread distribution, being found in tissues such as liver, skin and gastrointestinal smooth muscle, as well as in the plasma, where BuChE is soluble enzyme. It is not particularly associated with cholinergic synapses, and has a broader substrate specificity than AChE. It hydrolyses butyrylcholine more rapidly than acetylcholine, and many other esters, including **benzoylcholine**, **procaine**, **suxamethonium** and **propanidid** (a short acting anaesthetic agent; see Chapter 20), are also substrates. The function of this enzyme is not known, but the plasma enzyme is important in relation to the inactivation of the drugs listed above. Genetic variants of BuChE occur (see Chapter 4), which partly accounts for the variability in the duration of action of these drugs. The very short duration of action of acetylcholine given intravenously (see Fig. 6.1) results from its rapid hydrolysis in the plasma. Normally the activity of AChE and BuChE keep the plasma acetylcholine at an undetectably low level, so acetylcholine (un-

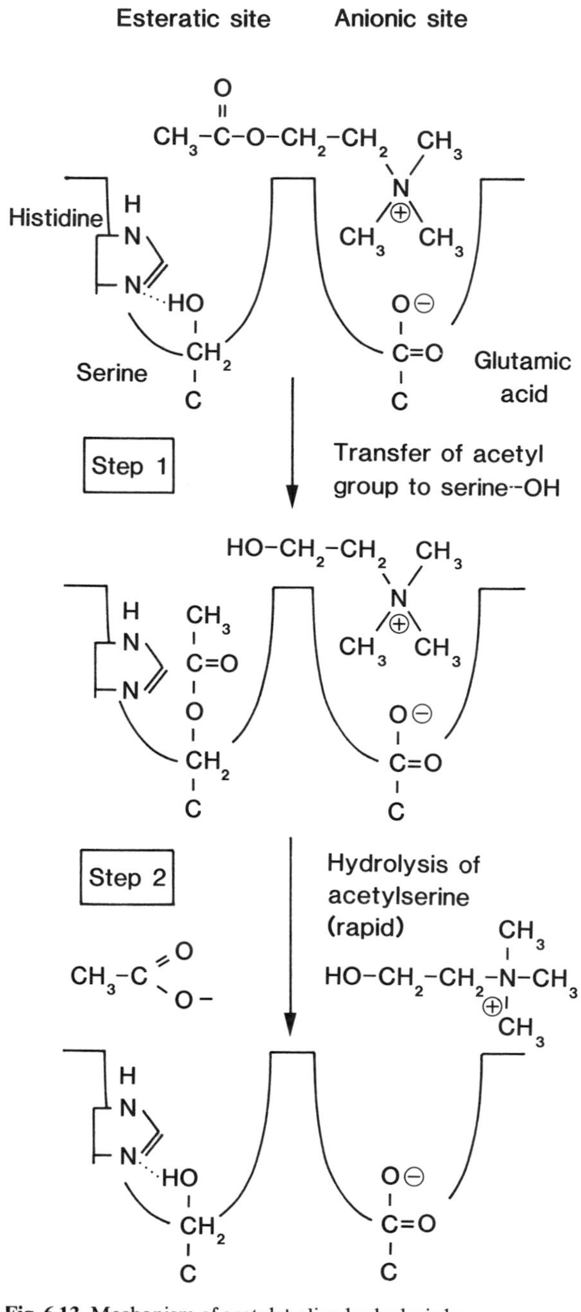

Fig. 6.13 Mechanism of acetylcholine hydrolysis by acetylcholinesterase.

like noradrenaline) is strictly a neurotransmitter and not a hormone.

The active site of AChE has been mapped in some detail. There are two distinct regions (Fig. 6.13), an anionic site which possesses a glutamate residue, and an esteratic site in which a histidine imidazole ring and a serine −OH group are particularly important. Catalytic hydrolysis occurs by a mechanism common to other serine hydrolases, whereby the acetyl group is transferred to the serine −OH group, leaving (transiently) an acetylated enzyme molecule and a molecule of free choline. Spontaneous hydrolysis of the serine acetyl group occurs rapidly, and the overall turnover number of AChE is extremely high (over 10 000 molecules of acetylcholine hydrolysed per second by a single active site).

Drugs that inhibit cholinesterase

Anticholinesterase drugs fall into three main groups according to the nature of their interaction with the active site, which determines their duration of action. Most of the clinically important drugs inhibit AChE and BuChE about equally.

Short-acting anticholinesterases

The only important drug in this group is **edrophonium** (Table 6.6), a quaternary ammonium compound which binds only to the anionic site of the enzyme. The ionic bond formed is readily reversible and the action of the drug is very brief. It is used mainly for diagnostic purposes, since improvement of muscle strength by an anticholinesterase is characteristic of myasthenia gravis (see p. 143), but does not occur when muscle weakness is due to other causes.

Medium duration anticholinesterases

This group (Table 6.6) includes **neostigmine** and **pyridostigmine**, which are quaternary ammonium compounds of clinical importance, and **physostigmine (eserine)**, a naturally-occurring tertiary amine whose effects on the autonomic nervous system were described many years before cholinergic transmission was understood. Physostigmine occurs

Table 6.6 Anticholinesterase drugs

Drug	Structure	Duration of action Long/med/short	Notes
Edrophonium		S	Used mainly in diagnosis of myasthenia gravis. Too short-acting for therapeutic use.
Neostigmine		M	Used i.v. to reverse competitive n–m block. Used orally in treatment of myasthenia gravis. Visceral side effects.
Physostigmine		M	Used as eye drops in treatment of glaucoma.
Pyridostigmine		M	Used orally in treatment of myasthenia gravis. Better absorbed than neostigmine, and has longer duration of action.
Dyflos		L	Highly toxic organophosphate, with very prolonged action.
Ecothiopate		L	Used as eye-drops in treatment of glaucoma. Prolonged action; may cause systemic effects.
Parathion		L	Converted to active metabolite by replacement of sulphur by oxygen. Used as insecticide, but commonly causes poisoning in man.

naturally in the Calabar bean, extracts of which were once used as ordeal poisons to assess the guilt or innocence of suspected criminals and heretics; death implied guilt.

These drugs all possess basic nitrogen atoms which combine with the anionic site, but are carbamyl, as opposed to acetyl, esters. Transfer of the carbamyl group to the serine −OH of the esteratic site occurs as with acetylcholine, but the carbamylated enzyme is very much slower to hydrolyse (Fig. 6.14a), taking minutes rather than microseconds. The anticholinesterase drug is therefore hydrolysed, but at a negligible rate compared to acetylcholine, and the slow recovery of the carbamylated enzyme means that the action of these drugs is quite long-lasting.

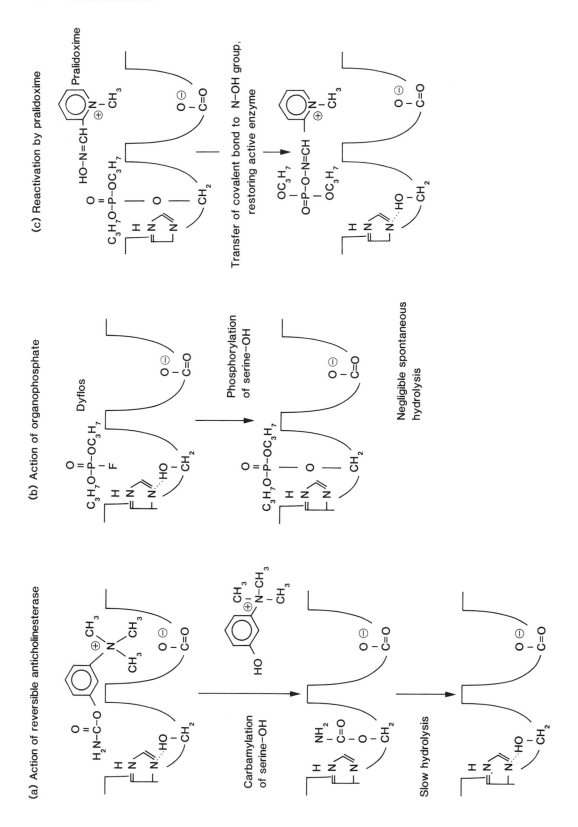

Fig. 6.14 Action of anticholinesterase drugs. **(a)** Reversible anticholinesterase (neostigmine). Recovery of activity by hydrolysis of the carbamylated enzyme takes many minutes. **(b)** Irreversible anticholinesterase (dyflos). **(c)** Reactivation of phosphorylated enzyme by pralidoxime.

Irreversible anticholinesterases

These drugs (Fig. 6.14b) are pentavalent phosphorus compounds containing a labile group such as fluoride (in **dyflos**) or an organic group (in **parathion** and **ecothiopate**). This group is released, leaving the residue of the molecule attached covalently through the phosphorus atom to the serine −OH group of the enzyme. Most of these organophosphate compounds, of which there are many, developed as war gases and pesticides as well as for clinical use, interact only with the esteratic site of the enzyme and have no cationic group. Ecothiopate is an exception in having a quaternary nitrogen group designed to bind also to the anionic site.

The inactive phosphorylated enzyme is usually very stable. With drugs such as dyflos, no appreciable hydrolysis occurs, and recovery of enzymic activity depends on the synthesis of new enzyme molecules, a process that may take weeks. With other drugs such as ecothiopate, slow hydrolysis occurs over the course of a few days, so that their action is not strictly-speaking irreversible.

Dyflos and parathion are volatile non-polar substances of very high lipid solubility, and are rapidly absorbed through mucous membranes and even through unbroken skin and insect cuticles, the use of these agents as war gases or insecticides relying on this property. The lack of a specificity-conferring quaternary group means that most of these drugs block other serine hydrolases (e.g. trypsin, thrombin) though their pharmacological effects result mainly from cholinesterase inhibition.

Effects of anticholinesterase drugs

The effects of cholinesterase inhibition are of three main types:

1. Effects on autonomic cholinergic synapses
2. Effects on the neuromuscular junction
3. Central effects.

Some organophosphate compounds can produce, in addition, a form of neurotoxicity not associated with cholinesterase inhibition.

Autonomic effects. These mainly reflect enhancement of acetylcholine activity at parasympathetic post-ganglionic synapses (i.e. increased secretions from salivary, lacrimal, bronchial and gastrointestinal glands, increased peristaltic activity, bronchoconstriction, bradycardia and hypotension, pupillary constriction, fixation of accommodation for near vision, fall in intraocular pressure). Large doses can stimulate, and later block autonomic ganglia, producing complex autonomic effects. The block, if it occurs, is a depolarization block and is associated with a build-up of acetylcholine in the plasma and body fluids. Neostigmine and pyridostigmine tend to affect neuromuscular transmission more than the autonomic system, whereas physostigmine and organophosphates show the reverse pattern. The reason is not clear, but therapeutic usage takes advantage of this partial selectivity.

Anticholinesterase poisoning (e.g. from contact with insecticides or war gases) causes severe bradycardia, hypotension and difficulty in breathing. Combined with a depolarizing neuromuscular block, and central effects (see below), the result may be life-threatening.

Effects on neuromuscular transmission. The twitch tension of a muscle stimulated *via* its motor nerve is increased by anticholinesterases. Electrophysiological recording shows that this is associated with **repetitive firing** in the muscle fibre. Normally, the acetylcholine is hydrolysed so quickly that each stimulus initiates only one action potential in the muscle fibre. When cholinesterase is inhibited a single endplate potential lasts for long enough to produce a short train of action potentials in the muscle fibre, and hence greater tension. Much more important is the effect produced when transmission has been blocked by a competitive blocking agent, such as tubocurarine. In this case, addition of an anticholinesterase can dramatically restore transmission (see Fig. 6.9). If a large proportion of the receptors is blocked, the majority of acetylcholine molecules will normally encounter, and be destroyed by, an AChE molecule, before reaching a vacant receptor; inhibiting AChE will thus increase the number of acetylcholine molecules that will find their way to a vacant receptor, and thus increase the endplate potential so that it reaches threshold. In **myasthenia gravis**, discussed in more detail below, transmission fails because there are too few acetylcholine receptors, and cholinesterase inhibition improves transmission just as it does in curarized muscle.

In large doses, such as can occur in poisoning,

anticholinesterases initially cause twitching of muscles, because spontaneous acetylcholine release can give rise to endplate potentials that reach the firing threshold, and may later cause a paralysis due to depolarization block, which is associated with the build-up of acetylcholine in the plasma and tissue fluids.

Effects on the central nervous system. Tertiary compounds, such as physostigmine, and the non-polar organophosphates penetrate the blood-brain barrier freely and affect the brain. The result is an initial excitation, which can result in convulsions, followed by depression which can cause uncon-sciousness and respiratory failure. These central effects are antagonized by atropine, so it is reason-able to suppose that they result from the activation of muscarinic receptors.

Neurotoxicity of organophosphates. Many organophosphates can cause a severe type of peri-pheral nerve demyelination, leading to slowly-developing weakness and sensory loss. This is not a problem with clinically used anticholinesterases, but occasionally occurs with accidental poisoning. In 1931 an estimated 20 000 Americans were af-fected, some fatally, by contamination of fruit juice with an organophosphate insecticide, and other similar outbreaks have been recorded. The mech-anism of this reaction is only partly understood, but it seems to result from inhibition of an esterase (not cholinesterase itself) specific to myelin.

Uses of anticholinesterases

The main clinical uses of these drugs are:

1. To reverse the action of non-depolarizing neuromuscular blocking drugs used during anaes-thesia. Neostigmine is most commonly used, as it lacks central effects, and also appears to cause rather less parasympathetic action in relation to its neuromuscular effect than other drugs. Atropine is, in any case, used routinely to block the muscarinic effects.

2. In the treatment of myasthenia gravis (see below). Neostigmine and pyridostigmine are used for this purpose, and are in most cases the most effective treatment available at present. Both are quaternary ammonium compounds, and hence rather poorly absorbed, but their lack of central effects is an advantage. Pyridostigmine acts for

slightly longer (3–6 hours) than neostigmine (2 4 hours). Both drugs produce side effects resulting from muscarinic actions, but these tend to wear off with continued use. Their use in excess can produce a cholinergic crisis consisting of muscarinic effects (salivation, gastrointestinal cramps, lacrima-tion, poor vision etc) together with muscle weak-ness, resulting presumably from depolarization block. It may be difficult to distinguish between this drug-induced weakness and the weakness of myas-thenia itself and a dose of edrophonium may be given to clarify the mechanism. If the weakness transiently improves it is due to myasthenia and more anticholinesterase is indicated; if it gets worse the anticholinesterase dose should be reduced.

3. In the treatment of glaucoma. Physostigmine or ecothiopate are used as eye drops to cause constriction of the pupil and contraction of the ciliary muscle, thus improving the drainage of aqueous humour. Systemic side effects may occur, and plasma cholinesterase activity may be reduced, which can cause prolongation of the action of suxamethonium, if this is given concurrently.

Cholinesterase reactivation

Spontaneous hydrolysis of phosphorylated cholin-esterase is extremely slow, a fact which makes poisoning with organophosphates very dangerous. Wilson, in 1955, developed a compound that can reactivate the enzyme by bringing into close prox-imity with the phosphorylated esteratic site an

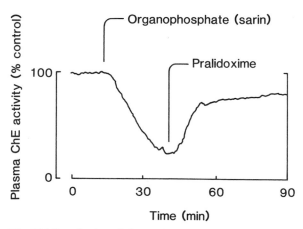

Fig. 6.15 Reactivation of plasma cholinesterase in a volunteer subject by intravenous injection of pralidoxime. (From: Sim, 1965)

oxime group which is a sufficiently strong nucleophile for the covalent bond to be transferred to it from the serine −OH of the enzyme. This compound, **pralidoxime** (Fig. 6.14c), also possesses a quaternary nitrogen atom so that it can bind to the anionic site. Its effectiveness in restoring cholinesterase activity in the plasma of a poisoned subject is shown in Figure 6.15. There are two drawbacks to its use as an antidote to organophosphate poisoning. The first is that the phosphorylated enzyme, undergoes within a few hours a change ('aging') that renders it no longer susceptible to reactivation, so that pralidoxime must be given early in order to work. Secondly, pralidoxime does not enter the brain, so cannot reverse the central effects of organophosphate poisoning.

Myasthenia gravis

The neuromuscular junction is a remarkably robust structure which very rarely fails, myasthenia gravis being one of the very few disorders that specifically affects it (see review by Drachman, 1981). This disease affects about 1 in 2000 individuals, who show muscle weakness and increased fatiguability resulting from a failure of neuromuscular transmission. Electrophysiological studies have shown that transmitter release is normal, but that the amplitude of the endplate potential is greatly reduced, so that it often fails to reach threshold. The tendency for transmission to fail during repetitive activity can be seen in Figure 6.16. Functionally, it results in the inability of muscles to produce sustained contractions, of which the characteristic drooping eyelids of myasthenic patients are a sign. The effectiveness of anticholinesterase drugs in improving muscle strength in myasthenia was discovered in 1931, long before the cause of the disease was known. In 1973 Fambrough used the technique of labelling the endplate receptors with radioactive α-bungarotoxin followed by autoradiography, and found that in myasthenic muscle the number of receptors per endplate was, on average, only about one-third of normal. Prior to this it had been suspected that myasthenia had an immunological basis, for removal of the thymus gland (which often shows pathological changes in this disease) was frequently of benefit. An immunological explanation for the disappearance of receptors from the

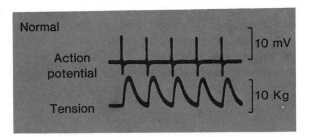

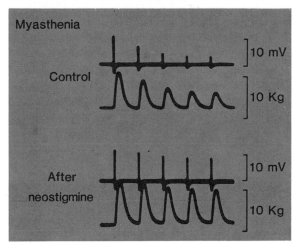

Fig. 6.16 Neuromuscular transmission in a normal and a myasthenic human subject. Electrical activity was recorded with a needle electrode in the *adductor pollicis* muscle, in response to ulnar nerve stimulation (3 Hz) at the wrist. *Top.* In normal subject, electrical and mechanical response is well sustained. *Middle.* In myasthenic patient, transmission fails rapidly when nerve is stimulated. *Bottom.* Treatment with neostigmine improves transmission. (From: Desmedt, 1962)

neuromuscular junction emerged in 1974, when the presence of antibody directed against the acetylcholine receptor protein was discovered in the serum of myasthenic patients (see Lindstrom et al, 1976; Vincent, 1980). It had earlier been found that immunization of rabbits with purified acetylcholine receptor caused, after a delay, symptoms very similar to human myasthenia gravis, and the availability of the pure receptor protein made it possible to detect the circulating antibody in the human patients. Myasthenia gravis can therefore be classified as an autoimmune disease, though the reason for the development of the immune response is still unknown. It is interesting that the antibodies found in myasthenic serum, though they bind strongly to receptors at the neuromuscular junction, do not directly affect their physiological function very much. The loss of receptors in myasthenic patients or immunized animals seems to occur because the antibody-receptor complex is more rapidly degraded by the muscle cell than the native receptor, and thus the membrane becomes depleted of receptors.

The improvement of neuromuscular function by anticholinesterase treatment (shown in Fig. 6.16) can be dramatic. It occurs because an acetylcholine molecule released into the synaptic cleft is less likely to be destroyed by an encounter with cholinesterase, and therefore more likely to reach one of the few remaining receptors. If the disease progresses too far the number of receptors remaining may become too few to produce an adequate endplate potential, and anticholinesterase drugs will then cease to be effective.

Alternative approaches to the treatment of myasthenia are to remove circulating antibody by plasma exchange which has recently been successfully tried, or, less drastically, to inhibit antibody production with steroids (e.g. **prednisolone**; see Chapter 16) or immunosuppressant drugs (e.g. **azathioprine**; see Chapter 9). Alternatively, drugs such as **4-aminopyridine** (see below), which increase transmitter release, may be effective.

Other drugs which enhance cholinergic transmission

It was observed many years ago that **tetraethylammonium**, better known as a ganglion blocking drug (see p. 125) could reverse the neuromuscular blocking action of tubocurarine, and this was shown to be because it increases the release of transmitter evoked by nerve stimulation. About 10 years ago compounds of the **aminopyridine** group were found to act similarly, and to be considerably more potent and selective in their actions than tetraethylammonium.

These drugs increase the evoked release of many different transmitters, and are not at all selective for cholinergic nerves. They work mainly by blocking voltage-sensitive potassium channels in the nerve membrane. These channels normally open during the passage of an action potential, and contribute to the rapid repolarization of the membrane. Blocking them therefore causes prolongation of the action potential, which allows more calcium to enter the nerve terminal and causes more transmitter to be released. They may also increase calcium entry by a mechanism independent of action potential duration, but this is not certain.

The compound most thoroughly studied is 4-aminopyridine (Fig. 6.17), but 3,4-diaminopyridine

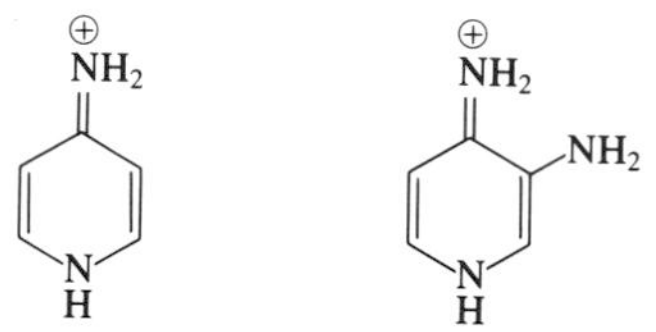

Fig. 6.17 Structures of aminopyridines.

acts very similarly. These compounds have been tried as agents for reversing the action of neuromuscular blocking drugs in myasthenia gravis and related neuromuscular disorders, and also in multiple sclerosis. In this latter condition action potential propagation may fail because of local patches of demyelination in the central nervous system. Blocking the outward potassium current across the nerve membrane, thus delaying repolarization, improves the chance of propagation of the action potential through a demyelinated stretch of nerve membrane, giving clinical improvement. The drawback with the aminopyridines is that they have powerful central effects, causing excitement and convulsions (presumably by blocking potassium channels of central neurons) and it is difficult to get a useful effect without excessive side effects. Compounds with greater selectivity would, however, be of great value.

REFERENCES AND FURTHER READING

Blusztajn J K, Wurtman R J 1983 Choline and cholinergic neurons. Science 221: 614–620
Bowman W C 1980 Pharmacology of neuromuscular function. Wright, Bristol

Brown D A 1980 Locus and mechanism of action of ganglion blocking agents. In: Kharkevich D A (ed) Pharmacology of ganglionic transmission. Handbook of Experimental Pharmacology 53: 185–235

Burns B D, Paton W D M 1951 Depolarisation of the motor end-plate by decamethonium and acetylcholine. J Physiol 115: 41–73

Drachman D B 1981 The biology of myasthenia gravis. Ann Rev Neurosci 4: 195–225

Furchgott R F 1981 The requirement for endothelial cells in the relaxation of arteries by acetylcholine and some other vasodilators. Trends in Pharmacological Sciences 2: 173–176

Ginsborg B L, Jenkinson D H 1976 Transmission of impulses from nerve to muscle. In: Zaimis E (ed) Neuromuscular Junction. Handbook of Experimental Pharmacology 42: 229–364

Hammer R, Giachetti A 1984 Selective muscarinic receptor antagonists. Trends in Pharmacological Sciences 5: 18–20

Hirschowitz B I, Hammer R, Giachetti A, Kierns J J, Levine R R (eds) 1984 Subtypes of muscarinic receptors. Trends in Pharmacological Sciences (Supplement)

Kharkevich D A (ed) 1980 Pharmacology of ganglionic transmission. Handbook of Experimental Pharmacology Vol 53

Kuffler S W, Nicholls J G, Martin A R 1984 From neuron to brain. Sinauer, New York

Lindstrom J M, Seybold M E, Lennon V M, Whittingham S, Duane D D 1976 Antibody to acetylcholine receptor in myasthenia gravis. Neurology 26: 1054–1059

MacIntosh F C, Collier B 1976 Neurochemistry of cholinergic terminals. In: Zaimis E J (ed) Neuromuscular junction. Handbook of Experimental Pharmacology 42: 99–228

Marchbanks R M 1975 Biochemistry of cholinergic neurons. Handbook of Experimental Psychopharmacology 3: 147–326

Skok V I 1980 Ganglionic transmission: morphology and physiology. In: Kharkevich D A (ed) Pharmacology of ganglionic transmission. Handbook of Experimental Pharmacology 53: 9–39

Stenlake J B, Waigh R D, Urwin J H, Dewar G H, Coker G G 1983 Atracurium: conception and inception. Br J Anaesth 55 (Supp): 35–45

Vincent A 1980 Immunology of acetylcholine receptors in relation to myasthenia gravis. Physiol Rev 60: 756–824

Zaimis E 1976 Neuromuscular function. Handbook of Experimental Pharmacology, Vol 42. Springer, Berlin

Adrenergic transmission

The adrenergic neuron has proved to be particularly important as a target for drug action, both as an object for investigation in its own right, and as a point of attack for many clinically useful drugs. For convenience a table summarizing much of the pharmacological information is given at the end of the chapter (see Table 7.5), together with a short glossary of special terms relating to adrenergic transmission.

CLASSIFICATION OF ADRENERGIC RECEPTORS

Oliver & Schafer demonstrated in 1896 that injection of extracts of adrenal gland caused a rise in arterial pressure. Following the subsequent isolation of adrenaline as the active principle, it was shown by Dale in 1913 that adrenaline causes two distinct types of effect, namely vasoconstriction in certain vascular beds (which normally predominates and causes the rise in arterial pressure) and vasodilatation in others. Dale showed that the vasoconstrictor component disappeared if the animal was first injected with an ergot derivative (see below), and noticed that adrenaline then caused a fall, instead of a rise, in arterial pressure. Dale, partly because of a disagreement with J N Langley, studiously avoided interpreting this result (which closely parallels his demonstration of the separate muscarinic and nicotinic components of the action of acetylcholine; see Chapter 6) in terms of a distinction between categories of receptor. Later pharmacological work, however, beginning with that of Ahlquist (1948) has shown clearly that several subclasses of adrenoceptor exist in the body. Ahlquist found that the rank order of the potencies

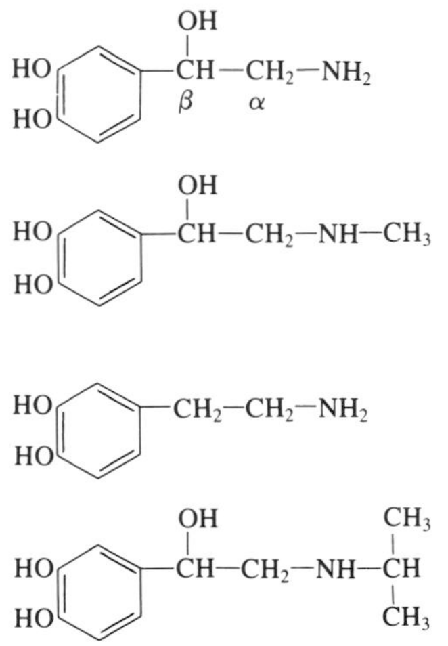

Fig. 7.1 Structures of the major catecholamines.

of various catecholamines, including adrenaline, noradrenaline and isoprenaline (a synthetic catecholamine; Fig. 7.1), fell into two distinct patterns, depending on what response was being measured. He postulated the existence of two kinds of receptor, α and β, defined in terms of agonist potencies as follows:

Receptor	Order of agonist potency
α	noradrenaline → adrenaline → isoprenaline
β	isoprenaline → adrenaline → noradrenaline

It was then recognized that certain ergot alkaloids, which Dale had studied, act as selective α-receptor antagonists, and that Dale's adrenaline reversal experiment reflected the unmasking of the β effects of adrenaline by α-receptor blockade. Various other α-receptor antagonists were known at that time, but selective β-receptor antagonists were not devel-

Table 7.1 Effects mediated by adrenoceptor subtypes

Tissue	Adrenoceptor			
	α_1	α_2	β_1	β_2
Smooth muscle				
Blood vessels	Constrict	Constrict		Dilate
Bronchi	Constrict			Dilate
GI tract				
Non-sphincter	Relax (hyperpolarization)		Relax (no hyperpolarization)	
Sphincter	Contract			
Uterus	Contract			Relax
Bladder				
Detrusor				Relax
Sphincter	Contract			
Seminal tract	Contract			Relax
Iris (radial)	Contract			
Ciliary muscle				Relax
Heart			Incr rate Incr force	
Skeletal muscle				Tremor
Liver	Glycogenolysis K^+ release			Glycogenolysis
Fat			Lipolysis	
Nerve terminals				
Adrenergic		Decr release	Incr release	
Cholinergic (some)		Decr release		
Salivary gland	K^+ release		Amylase secretion	
Platelets		Aggregation		
Mast cells				Inhibition of histamine release

oped until 1955. The use of these selective antagonists confirmed Ahlquist's original classification, but also suggested the existence of further subdivisions of both α- and β-receptors. It was first shown by Lands and his colleagues that different β-adrenoceptor agonists differ in their relative potency in eliciting different types of β-receptor mediated effects in different tissues, and subsequent studies with antagonists have confirmed the existence of two β-receptor subtypes, termed β_1 and β_2 (Table 7.1). A similar degree of selectivity among drugs acting on α-adrenoceptors has now been recognized, and both α- and β-adrenoceptors are generally divided into two distinct subclasses. Not surprisingly, since biological systems seldom submit meekly to our attempts to classify them, anomalies have arisen, which have prompted some bolder receptor taxonomists to propose various extensions to this classification. However, there seems little reason at present to go beyond the basic scheme.

The major effects that are produced by these receptors, and the pattern of specificity among various agonists and antagonists, are shown in Tables 7.1 & 7.2.

The distinction between β_1- and β_2-receptors is an important one, for β_1-receptors are found mainly in the heart, where they are responsible for the positive inotropic and chronotropic effects of catecholamines (see Chapter 10). β_2-receptors, on the other hand, are responsible for causing smooth muscle relaxation in many organs. The latter is often a useful therapeutic effect, while the former is more often harmful; consequently, considerable efforts have been made to find selective β_2 agonists, which would relax smooth muscle without affecting the heart, and selective β_1 antagonists, which would exert a useful blocking effect on the heart without at the same time blocking β-receptors in bronchial smooth muscle. The compounds listed in Table 7.2 are some of the results of these searches. It is

Table 7.2 Receptor specificity of adrenoceptor agonists and antagonists

	α_1	α_2	β_1	β_2
Agonists				
Noradrenaline	+++	+++	++	+
Adrenaline	++	++	+++	+++
Isoprenaline	—	—	+++	+++
Phenylephrine	++	—	—	—
Methylnoradrenaline	+	+++	—	—
Clonidine	—	+++	—	—
Salbutamol	—	—	+	+++
Dobutamine	—	—	+++	+
Antagonists				
Phentolamine	+++	+++	—	—
Phenoxybenzamine	+++	+++	—	—
Ergotamine	++PA	++	—	—
Dihydroergotamine	++	++	—	—
Yohimbine	+	+++	—	—
Prazosin	+++	+	—	—
Indoramin	+++	+	—	—
Propranolol	—	—	+++	+++
Oxprenolol	—	—	+++PA	+++
Practolol	—	—	+++	+
Atenolol	—	—	+++	+
Butoxamine	—	—	+	+++
Labetalol	+++	+	++	++

PA = partial agonist

important to realize that the selectivity of these drugs is relative rather than absolute, and that the compounds listed, for example, as selective β_1 antagonists invariably have some action on β_2-receptors as well. Unfortunately, there are appreciable species differences, and the high degree of receptor specificity found for some agonists and antagonists in experiments on guinea pig tissues *in vitro* has often not been borne out fully in measurements made on human subjects. Furthermore, recent studies have suggested that both types of β-receptor contribute to some effects, such as the chronotropic action, with the relative contribution of each varying from species to species.

The need to subdivide α-receptors arose when it was discovered in 1972 that catecholamines exert a pre-synaptic inhibitory effect (see Chapter 5), which is mediated by an α-receptor whose pharmacological specificity is different from that of the receptors responsible for the well-known effects of catecholamines. It was found, for example, that some agonists, such as **methylnoradrenaline** and **clonidine**, act selectively on the pre-synaptic (α_2) receptors, as do certain antagonists, such as **yohimbine**, while other antagonists (e.g. **prazosin**) do not affect the pre-synaptic receptors.

It was originally thought that the α_1/α_2 classification corresponded directly with the pre- or post-synaptic location of the receptors, but several exceptions to this rule are now known. Thus α_2-receptors occur on liver cells, platelets and smooth muscle cells of blood vessels, as well as on pre-synaptic nerve terminals.

Certain generalizations can be made about the cellular mechanisms through which the different types of adrenoceptor mediate their effects. β-receptors of both subtypes are linked to membrane-bound adenylate cyclase (see Chapter 1), and work by increasing the production of cAMP, whereas α_1-receptors have been shown, in many cases, to cause an increase in intracellular calcium concentration, either by increasing the permeability of the membrane to calcium or by releasing it from intracellular storage sites. The response of the cell (e.g. contraction or secretion) is secondary to the rise in free intracellular calcium. α_2-receptors, like β-receptors, act on adenylate cyclase, but they inhibit the enzyme and reduce the intracellular concentration of cAMP, thus producing effects opposite to those of β-receptor activation

Partial agonist effects

Several drugs that act on adrenoceptors have the characteristics of partial agonists (see Chapter 1), i.e. they block receptors, and thus antagonize the actions of full agonists, but also have a weak agonist effect of their own. Examples (see Table 7.2) include **ergotamine**, which has a substantial pressor effect when given alone (produced by α_1 receptor-mediated vasoconstriction), but also blocks the vasoconstrictor effect of noradrenaline, by occupying α-receptors. Several β-adrenoceptor blocking drugs (e.g. **alprenolol**, **oxprenolol**) cause, under resting conditions, an increase of heart rate, but at the same time oppose the tachycardia produced by sympathetic stimulation. This has been interpreted as a partial agonist effect, though there is evidence that mechanisms other than β-receptor activation may contribute to the tachycardia.

Clonidine is another example of a partial agonist. Its pharmacological actions are the result of activation of α_2-receptors, but the maximum degree of activation that it can produce is considerably less than that of other agonists. The possible clinical significance of partial agonists is discussed under the heading of individual drugs later in this chapter.

PHYSIOLOGY OF ADRENERGIC TRANSMISSION

THE ADRENERGIC NEURON

Adrenergic neurons in the periphery are post-ganglionic sympathetic neurons whose cell bodies lie in sympathetic ganglia. They generally have long axons which end, not in a discrete cluster of *boutons terminaux*, but in a series of varicosities strung along the branching terminal network (Fig. 7.2). These varicosities contain numerous synaptic vesicles, which are absent from other parts of the neuron, and there is good evidence that they represent the sites of synthesis and release of noradrenaline. The synaptic vesicles of adrenergic neurons are larger and more granular than in other neurons,

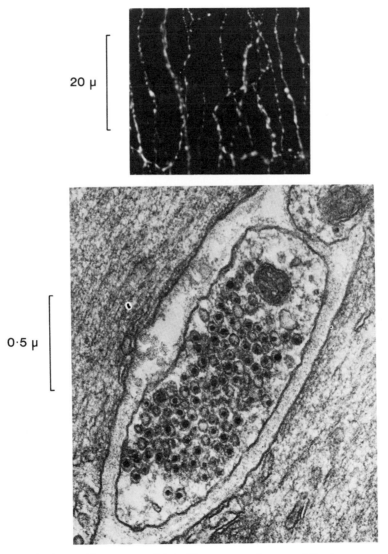

20 μ

0·5 μ

Fig. 7.2 Adrenergic nerve terminals. *Top.* Sheep mesenteric vein. Fluorescence microscopy following exposure to formaldehyde vapour. Varicosities containing NA can be seen along the path of individual nerve fibres. *Bottom.* Transmission electronmicrograph of adrenergic nerve terminal in mouse vas deferens, showing NA-containing vesicles with electron-dense core. (From: (Top) Burnstock, 1970; (Bottom) Furness et al, 1970)

and there is evidence that these large vesicles with an electron-dense core are the storage organelles for noradrenaline, which is released by exocytosis. Fluorescence histochemistry, in which formaldehyde treatment is used to convert catecholamines to fluorescent quinone derivatives, shows clearly that noradrenaline is present at high concentration in these varicosities (Fig. 7.2). In most peripheral tissues, and also in the brain, the tissue content of noradrenaline closely parallels the density of the sympathetic innervation. With the exception of the adrenal medulla and sympathetic ganglia, in which the cell bodies contain noradrenaline, there is very little noradrenaline in tissues other than that associated with sympathetic nerve terminals. Organs such as the heart, spleen, vas deferens and some blood vessels are particularly rich in noradrenaline (5–50 nmol/g tissue) and have been widely used for studies of adrenergic transmission. Except for the adrenal medulla, tissues contain very little adrenaline, and what there is probably resides in scattered chromaffin cells.

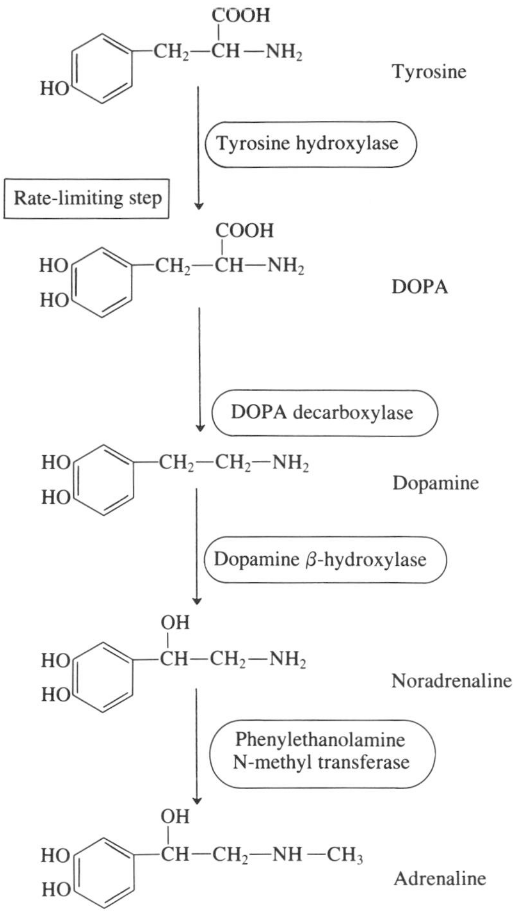

NORADRENALINE SYNTHESIS

The biosynthetic pathway for noradrenaline synthesis is shown in Figure 7.3. The metabolic precursor for noradrenaline is **L-tyrosine**, an aromatic amino-acid present in the body fluids, which is taken up (probably by a specific transport system) by adrenergic neurons. **Tyrosine hydroxylase**, the enzyme which catalyses the conversion of tyrosine to **dihydroxyphenylalanine (DOPA)** is found only in catecholamine-containing cells, probably free in the cytosol. It is a rather selective enzyme; unlike other enzymes involved in catecholamine metabolism, it does not accept indole derivatives as substrates, and so is not involved in serotonin metabolism. This first hydroxylation step is the main control point for noradrenaline synthesis. Tyrosine hydroxylase is inhibited by the end-product of the biosynthetic pathway, noradrenaline, and this provides the mechanism for the moment-to-moment regulation of the rate of synthesis; much slower regulation, taking hours or days, occurs by changes in the rate of production of the enzyme.

The tyrosine analogue **α-methyltyrosine**

Fig. 7.3 Biosynthesis of catecholamines

strongly inhibits tyrosine hydroxylase, and is used experimentally to block noradrenaline synthesis.

The next step, conversion of DOPA to dopamine, is catalysed by **DOPA decarboxylase**, an enzyme that is also found in the cytosol, but is by no means confined to catecholamine-synthesizing cells. It is a relatively non-specific enzyme, and catalyses the decarboxylation of various other L-aromatic amino acids as well as L-DOPA, such as L-histidine and L-tryptophan, which are precursors in the synthesis of histamine and serotonin, respectively. So far as noradrenaline synthesis is concerned, DOPA decarboxylase activity is not rate-limiting, and the DOPA content of neurons is normally very low. Though various factors, including certain drugs, affect the enzyme, it is not an effective means of regulating noradrenaline synthesis.

Dopamine-β-hydroxylase (DBH) is also a relatively non-specific enzyme, but its distribution is restricted to catecholamine-synthesizing cells. It is located in synaptic vesicles, probably in membrane bound form. A small amount of the enzyme is released from adrenergic nerve terminals in company with noradrenaline; this presumably represents enzyme that is in a soluble form within the vesicle, since there is evidence that the membrane proteins of the vesicle are retained when the vesicle discharges its contents by exocytosis. Unlike noradrenaline, the released DBH is not subject to rapid degradation or uptake, so its concentration in plasma and body fluids can be used as an index of overall sympathetic nerve activity.

Many drugs inhibit DBH, including copper-chelating agents and **disulfiram** (a drug whose main effect is to modify ethanol metabolism; see Chapters 3 & 35). Such drugs can cause a partial depletion of noradrenaline stores and interference with sympathetic transmission.

Phenylethanolamine N-methyl transferase (PNMT) catalyses the N-methylation of noradrenaline to adrenaline. The main location of this enzyme is in the adrenal medulla, which contains a population of adrenaline-releasing (A) cells separate from the smaller proportion of noradrenaline-releasing (N) cells. The A cells, which appear only after birth, lie adjacent to the adrenal cortex, and there is evidence that the production of PNMT is induced by an action of the steroid secreted by the adrenal cortex (see Chapters 1 & 16). PNMT is also found in certain parts of the brain, where there is some evidence that adrenaline may function as a transmitter. In these sites, also, PNMT formation is sensitive to steroid hormones, providing a possible mechanism whereby these hormones can affect brain function.

Noradrenaline turnover can be measured under steady-state conditions by measuring the rate at which labelled noradrenaline accumulates when a labelled precursor, such as tyrosine or DOPA, is administered. The turnover time is defined as the time taken for an amount of noradrenaline equal to the total tissue content to be degraded and resynthesized. In peripheral tissues the turnover time is generally about 5–15 hours, but it becomes much shorter if sympathetic nerve activity is increased. Under normal circumstances the rate of synthesis closely matches the rate of release, so that the noradrenaline content of tissues is constant, regardless of how fast it is being released.

NORADRENALINE STORAGE

Most of the noradrenaline in nerve terminals or chromaffin cells is contained in vesicles; only a little is free in the cytoplasm under normal circumstances. The concentration in the vesicles is very high (0.3–1.0 M), and it requires a special active carrier system to transport noradrenaline across the vesicle membrane.

Studies on isolated vesicles (chromaffin granules) have confirmed that they take up noradrenaline by an active transport mechanism fuelled by ATP. Certain drugs, such as **reserpine** (see below) interfere with this process and cause nerve terminals to become depleted of their noradrenaline stores. The vesicles contain two major constituents besides noradrenaline, namely ATP (about four molecules per molecule of noradrenaline) and a protein, called **chromogranin A**. These substances are released along with noradrenaline, and it is generally assumed that a reversible complex, depending partly on the opposite charges on the molecules of noradrenaline and ATP, is formed within the vesicle. This would serve both to reduce the osmolarity of the vesicle contents and also to reduce the tendency of noradrenaline to leak out of the vesicles within the nerve terminal.

NORADRENALINE RELEASE

There is good evidence that the steps linking the arrival of a nerve impulse at an adrenergic nerve terminal to the release of noradrenaline are basically the same as those at other chemically transmitting synapses (see Chapter 5). Depolarization of the nerve terminal membrane, which can be achieved experimentally by increasing the extracellular potassium concentration (showing that propagation of an action potential is not essential for release), causes an increased calcium permeability of the nerve terminal. Calcium enters the nerve terminal, and, by mechanisms that are not well understood, promotes the fusion and discharge of synaptic vesicles. Though there is dispute about whether exocytosis is a universal mechanism for transmitter release, studies on adrenergic neurons and on the adrenal medulla have provided strong evidence in favour of this mechanism. One convincing piece of evidence is that the proportion of chromogranin, ATP and noradrenaline released is the same as that present in the vesicle (which would not occur if the vesicles were, as postulated by some authors, merely a reservoir of transmitter and not the immediate vehicle of release). It has also been found that immunologically distinctive constituents of the vesicle membrane appear on the outer cell membrane when release is evoked, as would be expected of an exocytotic mechanism. A surprising feature of the release mechanism at the varicosities of adrenergic nerves is that the probability of release, even of a single vesicle, when a nerve impulse arrives at a varicosity, is very low (less than 1 in 50; Cunnane, 1984). This contrasts sharply with the cholinergic synapse, where a single impulse usually causes 100 or more vesicles to be discharged from each nerve terminal.

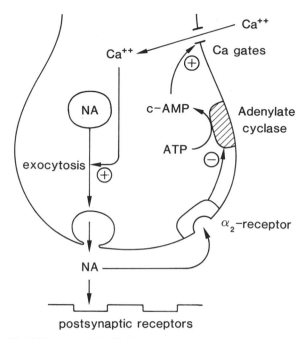

Fig. 7.4 Postulated feedback control of noradrenaline release. The pre-synaptic α_2-receptor inhibits adenylate cyclase, thereby reducing intracellular cAMP. cAMP acts to promote Ca^{++} influx in response to membrane depolarization, and hence to promote noradrenaline release.

Regulation of noradrenaline release

It has recently been shown, by the work of Langer, Starke and others, that transmitter release can be controlled by a variety of substances that act on **pre-synaptic receptors** (see reviews by Starke, 1977; Langer, 1980; and debate between Rand *et al* and Kalsner, 1982). Many different types of nerve terminal (cholinergic, adrenergic, dopaminergic, serotonergic, etc) are subject to this type of control, and many different mediators (e.g. acetylcholine, acting through muscarinic receptors, catecholamines acting through α_2-receptors, prostaglandins, purine nucleotides, etc) can act on pre-synaptic terminals. It is now recognized that pre-synaptic interactions, such as the inhibition of acetylcholine release from parasympathetic nerve terminals by noradrenaline released from sympathetic neurons, represent an important physiological control mechanism.

Of particular interest is the evidence suggesting that noradrenaline, by acting on pre-synaptic receptors, can regulate its own release (see Chapter 5). There is evidence that this occurs physiologically, and that released noradrenaline exerts a local inhi-

bitory effect on the terminals from which it came— the so-called **auto-inhibitory feedback mechanism** (Fig. 7.4). The main evidence comes from studies of noradrenaline overflow (Fig. 7.5), in which the amount of radioactivity is measured in the effluent from an organ whose stores of noradrenaline have been previously labelled by infusion of tritiated noradrenaline. It was shown many years ago that α-receptor blocking drugs increase (by 10-fold or more in some tissues) the amount of noradrenaline overflow that occurs in response to sympathetic nerve stimulation. Overflow is also markedly affected by drugs (including many α-receptor antagonists) that inhibit the *reuptake* of noradrenaline by nerve terminals (see below), and it is necessary to exclude this as a cause of the increased overflow seen in experiments such as that shown in Figure 7.5. Even when this is allowed for, however, it seems that most of the increase in overflow is due to an increase in noradrenaline release, representing the loss of the normal feedback regulation. The magnitude of the change in noradrenaline overflow implies that this regulatory mechanism can, in some

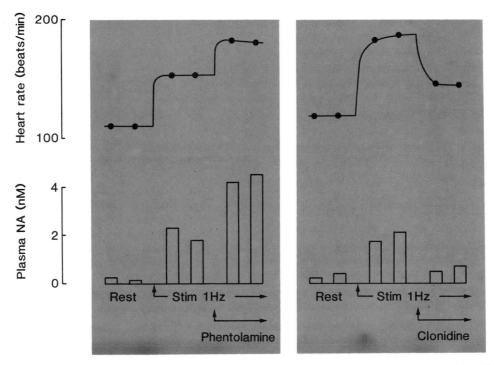

Fig. 7.5 Evidence for α-receptor mediated feedback regulation of noradrenaline release. The heart rate and noradrenaline content of coronary venous blood was measured in dogs during periods of stimulation of the cardioaccelerator (sympathetic) nerve. *Left.* Phentolamine, a α-adrenoceptor antagonist, increases the cardiac response and the noradrenaline release during nerve stimulation. *Right.* Clonidine, a selective α₂-adrenoceptor agonist, inhibits noradrenaline release. (Data from: Cavero I et al, 1979)

tissues, act to damp down noradrenaline release by 90% or more. Agonists or antagonists affecting these pre-synaptic receptors can, therefore, have large effects on sympathetic transmission. The physiological function of pre-synaptic receptors is still somewhat contentious, and there is evidence that, in most tissues, it is less influential than measurements of transmitter overflow would imply; thus, although large changes in noradrenaline overflow occur when the feedback mechanism is interfered with pharmacologically, the associated changes in the *tissue response* to sympathetic nerve activity are often rather small, suggesting that what is measured in overflow experiments may not be the physiologically important component of transmitter release.

The inhibitory feedback mechanism operates through α₂-receptors, and probably depends on inhibition of adenylate cyclase. It is interesting that sympathetic nerve terminals also possess β-receptors, coupled to activation of adenylate cyclase, which cause an increased noradrenaline release.

Whether they have any physiological function is not yet clear.

UPTAKE AND DEGRADATION OF CATECHOLAMINES

Catecholamines differ markedly from acetylcholine in the way in which their action is terminated following release at the synapse. There is no synaptically located enzyme, comparable with cholinesterase, which rapidly degrades catecholamines. Instead, reuptake of noradrenaline by adrenergic nerve terminals, and by other cells, is the main mechanism by which the released transmitter is inactivated. Circulating adrenaline and noradrenaline are degraded enzymically, but much more slowly than acetylcholine. The two main enzymes responsible are both located intracellularly, so uptake into cells necessarily precedes metabolic degradation.

Uptake of catecholamines

Indirect evidence that sympathetic nerves can take up amines from the circulation and release them again as transmitter came originally from the work of Burn and his colleagues. Burn found in 1932 that the pressor effect of indirectly-acting sympathomimetics (e.g. tyramine; see below) in whole animals was increased if the injection was preceded by injection of adrenaline, and he showed that this was because adrenaline was able to replenish the releasable amine stores of the nerve terminals. When tritiated noradrenaline became available, it was demonstrated that many tissues took it up rapidly from the circulation. Part of this uptake was shown to be by sympathetic neurons (for it disappeared when sympathetic nerves were allowed to degenerate) and the amine could be released again by sympathetic nerve stimulation. Iversen, in a detailed study of noradrenaline uptake by isolated rat hearts, found that two distinct uptake mechanisms were involved, each of them having the characteristics of a saturable active transport system capable of accumulating catecholamines against a large concentration gradient. These two mechanisms, called **Uptake 1** and **Uptake 2**, correspond to **neuronal** and **extraneuronal** uptake respectively. They have different kinetic properties as well as different substrate and inhibitor specificity, as summarized in Table 7.3.

The main differences are that Uptake 1 is a high affinity system with a relatively low maximum rate of uptake, whereas Uptake 2 has low affinity for noradrenaline, but a much higher maximum rate. The substrate specificity is also different, Uptake 1 being relatively selective for noradrenaline, whereas Uptake 2 also accumulates adrenaline and isoprenaline. The effects of several important drugs that act on adrenergic neurons depend on their ability to inhibit Uptake 1 or to enter the nerve terminal with its help (Table 7.3).

Metabolic degradation of catecholamines

Endogenous and exogenous catecholamines are metabolized mainly by two enzymes, **monoamine oxidase (MAO)** and **catechol-O-methyl transferase (COMT)**.

MAO occurs within cells, bound to the surface membrane of mitochondria. It is abundant in adrenergic nerve terminals, but is also present in many other places, such as liver and intestinal epithelium. MAO converts catecholamines to their

Table 7.3 Characteristics of Uptake 1 and Uptake 2

	Uptake 1	Uptake 2
Transport of noradrenaline (rat heart)		
V_{max} (nmol/g per min)	1.2	100
K_m (μM)	0.3	250
Specificity	NA > A > ISO	A > NA > ISO
Location	Neuronal	Non-neuronal (smooth muscle, cardiac muscle, endothelium)
Other substrates	Methylnoradrenaline Dopamine Serotonin Tyramine Adrenergic neuron-blocking drugs (e.g. guanethidine)	(+)-noradrenaline Dopamine Serotonin Histamine
Inhibitors	Cocaine Tricyclic antidepressants (e.g. desipramine) Phenoxybenzamine Amphetamine	Normetanephrine Steroid hormones (e.g. corticosterone) Phenoxybenzamine

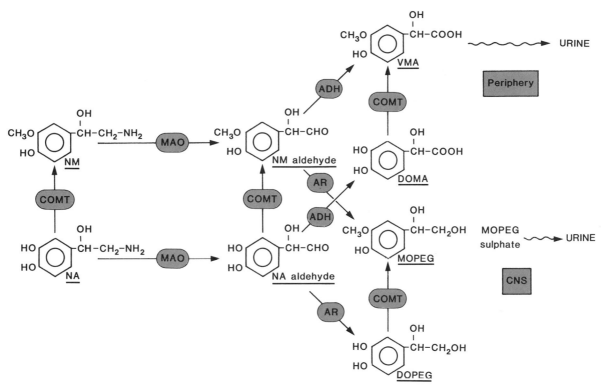

Fig. 7.6 The main pathways of noradrenaline metabolism in the brain and in the periphery. In the periphery, the oxidative branch (catalysed by ADH) predominates, giving VMA as the main urinary metabolite. In the brain, the reductive branch (catalysed by AR) predominates, producing MOPEG, which is conjugated to MOPEG sulphate before being excreted.

Abbreviations: Metabolites: NA, noradrenaline; NM, normetanephrine; VMA, vanillylmandelic acid; DOMA, 3,4-dihydroxy-mandelic acid; MOPEG, 3-methoxy, 4-hydroxyphenylglycol; DOPEG, 3,4-dihydroxyphenylglycol. Enzymes: MAO, monoamine oxidase; COMT, catechol-O-methyl transferase; ADH, aldehyde dehydrogenase; AR, aldehyde reductase.

corresponding aldehydes, which, in the periphery, are rapidly metabolized by **aldehyde dehydrogenase** to the corresponding carboxylic acid (Fig. 7.6). In the case of noradrenaline this yields **dihydroxymandelic acid (DOMA)**. MAO can also oxidize other mono-amines, important ones being dopamine and sero-tonin. It is inhibited by various drugs (Table 7.4), which are used mainly for their effects on the central nervous system, where these three amines all have transmitter functions (see Chapter 19). These drugs have important side effects that are related to disturbances of peripheral adrenergic transmission. Within sympathetic neurons MAO controls the content of dopamine and noradren-aline, and the releasable store of noradrenaline increases if the enzyme is inhibited. There is evidence that two types of MAO (A and B) exist, but little is known at present about their functions, MAO

Table 7.4 Actions of ergot alkaloids

Drug	α-adrenoceptor	Dopamine receptor	Serotonin receptor	Uterine contraction
Ergotamine	**PA**	— (emetic)	**PA**	+ +
Dihydroergotamine	**Agonist**	—	**PA**	+
Bromocriptine	Weak antag	**Agonist/PA**	—	
Ergometine	Weak agonist	Weak antag	PA/antag	+ + +
Methysergide	—	—	**Antag/PA**	—

Important effects indicated in **bold** type. PA denotes partial agonist

inhibitors are discussed in more detail in Chapter 23.

The second major pathway for catecholamine metabolism involves methylation of one of the catechol −OH groups to give a methoxy-derivative. COMT is a widespread enzyme which occurs in both neuronal and non-neuronal tissues. It acts on many different catechol-containing substrates, including the catecholamines themselves and the deaminated products, such as DOMA, that are produced by the action of MAO. O-methylation of noradrenaline gives rise to the metabolite **normetanephrine** (Fig. 7.6). When this product is acted on by MAO, or when DOMA is acted on by COMT, the product formed is **3-methoxy-4-hydroxy-mandelic acid (VMA)**, which is the main final metabolite of adrenaline and noradrenaline. In patients with tumours of chromaffin tissue which secrete these amines (a rare cause of high blood pressure), the urinary excretion of VMA is markedly increased (Fig. 7.7). This increase forms the basis of a diagnostic test for this condition.

In the periphery, neither MAO nor COMT is primarily responsible for the termination of transmitter action, most of the released noradrenaline being quickly recaptured by Uptake 1. Circulating catecholamines are usually inactivated by a combination of Uptake 1, Uptake 2 and COMT, the relative importance of these processes varying according to the agent concerned. Thus, circulating noradrenaline is removed mainly by Uptake 1, whereas adrenaline is more dependent on Uptake 2. Isoprenaline, on the other hand, is not a substrate for Uptake 1, and is removed by a combination of Uptake 2 and COMT.

The metabolism of noradrenaline in the central nervous system follows a different course (see Chapter 19 & Fig. 7.6). MAO is more important as a means of terminating transmitter action than it is in the periphery, and the resulting aldehydes are mainly reduced to the corresponding alcohols. The main excretory product of noradrenaline released in the brain is an ethyleneglycol derivative (MOPEG; see Chapter 19). Thus measurement of urinary VMA and MOPEG enables the central and peripheral release of noradrenaline to be quantified.

DRUGS ACTING ON ADRENOCEPTORS

STRUCTURE-ACTIVITY RELATIONSHIPS

The overall potency and receptor specificity for particular receptor types, of drugs that exert their effects by combining with adrenoceptors, depends on several factors:

1. Affinity and efficacy for adrenoceptors
2. Interaction with neuronal uptake systems
3. Interaction with MAO
4. Interaction with COMT.

The relationship of these different factors with chemical structure is, not surprisingly, complex, but there are certain useful generalizations which can be made. The noradrenaline molecule can be modified in several different ways to yield compounds that interact with adrenoceptors. Some of these are shown in Figure 7.8.

1. Increasing the bulkiness of substituents on the N-atom produces compounds (**adrenaline, isopren-**

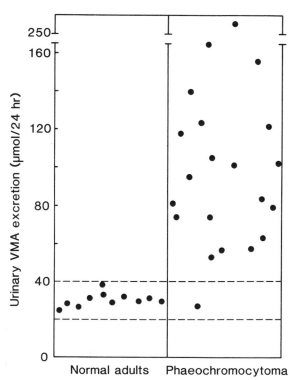

Fig. 7.7 Urinary excretion of VMA in normal subjects and patients with phaeochromocytoma. (From: Sandler & Ruthven, 1960)

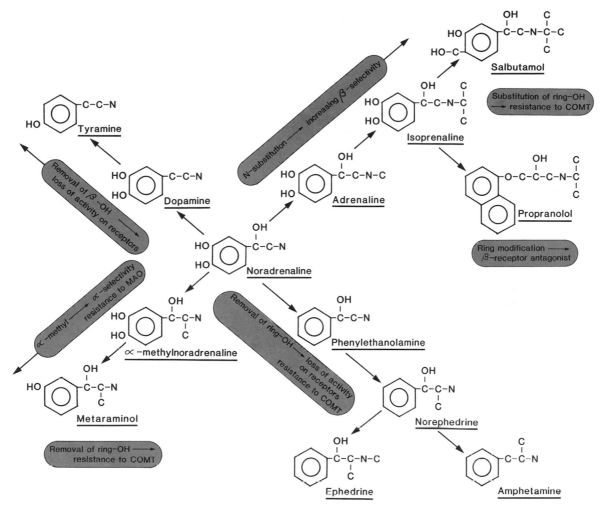

Fig. 7.8 Structure-activity relationships among catecholamines and related compounds.

aline and **salbutamol**) of relatively greater potency as β-agonists, and less susceptible to Uptake 1 and MAO.

2. Addition of an α-methyl group (**α-methylnoradrenaline, metaraminol**) increases α-receptor selectivity and also renders compounds resistant to MAO, though they remain susceptible to Uptake 1.

3. Removal of the β−OH group (**dopamine**) greatly reduces interaction with adrenoceptors. Most of the directly acting sympathomimetic amines, and the β-receptor antagonists (though not all α-receptor antagonists) retain this critical OH group.

4. Substitution of the catechol −OH groups by similar electron-withdrawing groups, or their transfer to different ring positions (**salbutamol** and many β-receptor antagonists) render compounds resistant to COMT, but usually retaining their receptor activity. Substitution of catechol −OH groups generally yields compounds that are not substrates for Uptake 1. Removal of one or both −OH groups (**phenylethylamine, tyramine**) abolishes affinity for receptors, though such compounds may still be indirectly-acting sympathomimetic amines, provided they are substrates for Uptake 1.

5. Extension of the alkyl side chain, with isopropyl substitution on the N-atom, and modification of catechol −OH groups (**propranolol, oxprenolol**, etc) produces potent β-receptor antagonists.

These general rules account fairly well for the

properties of many directly and indirectly acting sympathomimetric drugs and for β-receptor antagonists. α-receptor antagonists are much more heterogeneous, however, and defy such generalizations.

ADRENOCEPTOR AGONISTS

Examples of the main types of adrenoceptor agonist are given in Table 7.2 and the characteristics of individual drugs are summarized in Table 7.5.

Effects of adrenoceptor agonists

The major physiological effects mediated by different types of adrenoceptor are summarized in Table 7.1, and the more important ones are elaborated in this section.

Smooth muscle. All types of smooth muscle, except that of the gastrointestinal tract, contract in response to stimulation of α_1-adrenoceptors. Smooth muscle contraction caused by α-receptor stimulation results from an effect on the cell membrane, leading to an increase in calcium permeability, and also to a release of calcium from binding sites on the inner surface of the membrane (see Chapter 11). The resulting rise in the free intracellular calcium concentration activates the contractile mechanism. When α_1-agonists are given systemically to experimental animals or man the most important action is on vascular smooth muscle, particularly in the skin and splanchnic vascular beds, which are strongly constricted. Large arteries and veins, as well as arterioles, are constricted, resulting in decreased vascular compliance, increased central venous pressure and increased peripheral resistance, all of which contribute to an increase in systolic and diastolic arterial pressure. Some vascular beds (e.g. brain, coronary circulation, pulmonary circulation) are relatively little affected.

In the whole animal, baroreceptor reflexes are activated by the rise in arterial pressure produced by α-agonists, causing reflex bradycardia and inhibition of respiration.

Smooth muscle in the vas deferens, spleen capsule and eyelid retractor muscles (or nictitating membrane, in some species) is also stimulated by α-agonists and these organs are often used for pharmacological studies.

The α-receptors involved in smooth muscle contraction are mainly α_1 in type, though vascular smooth muscle possesses both α_1 and α_2-receptors. Since α_1-antagonists block the vascular response to sympathetic nerve stimulation more effectively than they block the response to applied noradrenaline, it has been suggested that the α_1-receptors lie close to the sites of release (and are mainly responsible for neurally-mediated vasoconstriction) while α_2-receptors lie elsewhere on the muscle fibre surface, and are activated by circulating catecholamines. The situation is probably not as simple as this, however (McGrath, 1983).

Stimulation of β-receptors causes relaxation of most kinds of smooth muscle by a mechanism involving an increase in intracellular cAMP concentration (see Chapter 1). There is evidence that cAMP works by activating a protein kinase, which then phosphorylates one or more proteins. It is not clear whether the relaxant effect in smooth muscle is produced mainly by an effect on one of the contractile proteins or on calcium binding within the cell. Relaxation is usually produced by β_2-receptors, though the receptor that is responsible for this effect in gastrointestinal smooth muscle is not clearly β_1 or β_2. In the vascular system, β-mediated vasodilatation is particularly marked in skeletal muscle, but it can be demonstrated also in many other vascular beds.

The powerful inhibitory effect of the sympathetic system on gastrointestinal smooth muscle is produced by both α- and β-receptors, this tissue being unusual in that α-receptors cause relaxation in most regions. Part of the effect is due to stimulation of pre-synaptic α_2-receptors (see below), which inhibit the release of excitatory transmitters (e.g. acetylcholine) from intramural nerves, but there are also α-receptors on the muscle cells, stimulation of which hyperpolarizes the cell (by increasing the membrane permeability to potassium), and inhibits action potential discharge. The sphincters of the gastrointestinal tract are contracted by α-receptor activation.

Bronchial smooth muscle is strongly dilated by activation of β_2-adrenoceptors, and selective β_2-agonists are important in the treatment of asthma (see Chapter 13). Uterine smooth muscle responds similarly, and these drugs are also used to delay premature labour.

Nerve terminals. Pre-synaptic adrenoceptors are present on both cholinergic and adrenergic nerve terminals (see Chapter 5). The main effect is inhibitory, and is mediated through α_2-receptors, but a weaker facilitatory action of β-receptors on adrenergic nerve terminals has also been described.

Heart. Catecholamines, acting on β_1-receptors exert a powerful stimulant effect on the heart (see Chapter 10). Both the **heart rate (chronotropic effect)** and the **force of contraction (inotropic effect)** are increased, resulting in a markedly increased cardiac output and cardiac oxygen consumption. The **cardiac efficiency** (see Chapter 10) is reduced. Catecholamines can also cause **disturbance of the cardiac rhythm**, culminating in ventricular fibrillation. In normal hearts the dose required to cause marked dysrhythmia is greater than that which produces the chronotropic and inotropic effects, but in ischaemic conditions dysrhythmias are produced much more readily. Figure 7.9 shows the overall pattern of cardiovascular responses to catecholamine infusions in man, reflecting their actions on both the heart and vascular system.

Metabolism. Catecholamines encourage the conversion of energy stores (glycogen and fat) to freely available fuels (glucose and free fatty acids), and cause an increase in the plasma concentration of the latter substances (see Chapter 16). An increased production of gluconeogenic substrates (e.g. lactic acid, amino acids) from various peripheral tissues also occurs. The detailed biochemical mechanisms vary from species to species, but in most cases the effects on carbohydrate metabolism of liver and muscle (Fig. 7.10) are mediated through β_2-receptors (though hepatic glucose release can also be produced by α-agonists), and the stimulation of lipolysis is produced by β_1-receptors. Adrenaline-induced hyperglycaemia in man is blocked completely by a combination of α- and β-antagonists but not by either on its own.

Skeletal muscle is affected by adrenaline, acting on β_2-receptors, though the effect is far less dramatic than that on the heart. The twitch tension of fast-contracting fibres (white muscle) is increased by adrenaline, particularly if the muscle is fatigued, whereas the twitch of slow (red) muscle is reduced. These effects depend on an action on the contractile proteins, rather than on the membrane, and the mechanism is poorly understood.

In man, adrenaline and other β_2-agonists cause a

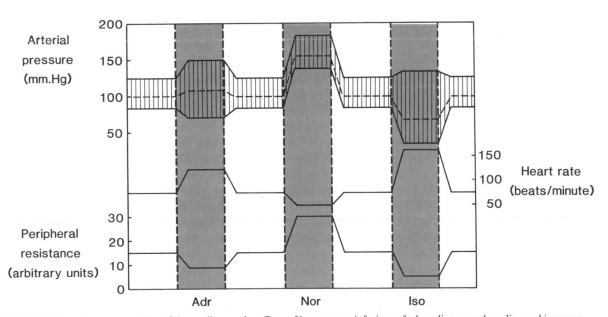

Fig. 7.9 Schematic representation of the cardiovascular effects of intravenous infusions of adrenaline, noradrenaline and isoprenaline in man. Noradrenaline (predominantly α-agonist) causes vasoconstriction and increased systolic and distolic pressure, with a reflex bradycardia. Isoprenaline (β-agonist) is a vasodilator, but strongly increases cardiac force and rate. Mean arterial pressure falls. Adrenaline combines both actions.

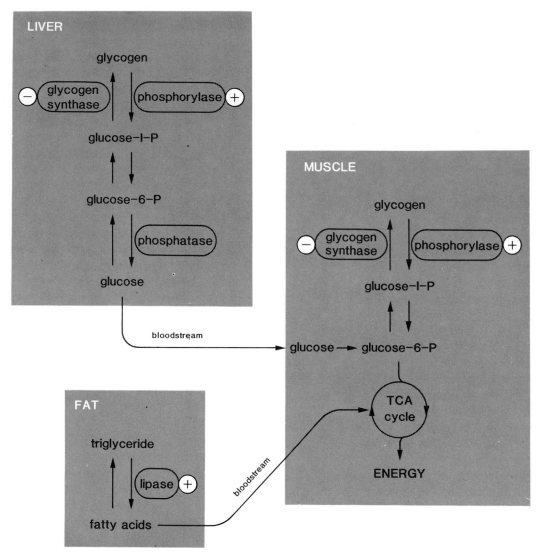

Fig. 7.10 Regulation of energy metabolism by catecholamines. The main enzymic steps that are affected by β-adrenoceptor activation are indicated by $+$ and $-$ signs, denoting stimulation and inhibition respectively.

marked tremor, the shakiness that accompanies fear or excitement being an example of this. It probably results from an increase in muscle spindle discharge, coupled with an effect on the contraction kinetics of the fibres, these effects combining to produce an instability in the reflex control of muscle length. β_2-agonists can improve motor function in spasticity, probably by a related mechanism. β-receptor antagonists, conversely, are sometimes used to control pathological tremor.

Histamine release by human and guinea pig lung tissue in response to anaphylactic challenge (see Chapter 8) is inhibited by catecholamines, acting apparently on β_2-receptors.

Lymphocytes are also sensitive to β-receptor agonists, both proliferation and lymphocyte-mediated cell killing being inhibited. The physiological and clinical importance of these effects has not yet been established.

Uses of adrenoceptor agonists

The main clinical uses of adrenoceptor agonists are:
  Treatment of asthma. The aim is to produce

bronchodilatation, which requires activation of β_2-receptors. **Isoprenaline**, given sublingually, or as an aerosol, produces a rapid effect, but is liable to cause tachycardia or ventricular dysrhythmias because of its β_1-actions. Isoprenaline is short-lasting because it is taken up by Uptake 2 and degraded by COMT. **Salbutamol** does not have these drawbacks, and is probably the most widely-used anti-asthmatic drug. The inhibitory effect of β-agonists on histamine release (see above) is probably not of great clinical importance. Asthma is discussed further in Chapter 13.

Prolongation of local anaesthetic action. **Adrenaline**, or a selective α-agonist, is very often added to local anaesthetic injections so as to cause vasoconstriction and delay absorption from the injection site. This can prolong the anaesthetic effect several-fold, though undesirable effects may occur from the systemic absorption of the adrenaline.

Nasal decongestion. Nose drops containing α-agonists, such as **phenylephrine**, are effective in unblocking stuffy noses, because of their vasoconstrictor and anti-secretory effects. Systemic preparations are also available. At one time amphetamine inhalers were used for this purpose, but were withdrawn when people began to use them for their central stimulant effect (see Chapter 26).

Acute anaphylactic (or Type 1 hypersensitivity) reactions. These are sudden and sometimes life-threatening immunological reactions (see Chapter 9) which can be caused by bee stings, or by hypersensitivity reactions to drugs (especially penicillin; see Chapter 36). The main effects are gross swelling of the skin and mucous membranes, which can obstruct breathing, and cardiovascular collapse due to vasodilatation. Subcutaneous adrenaline is effective as an emergency measure, and longer-acting α-agonists (e.g. methoxamine) can be used when the acute reaction is controlled.

Circulatory shock. The use of α-agonists to maintain blood pressure in circulatory shock is now obsolete, and probably does more harm than good (see Chapter 11) by further reducing perfusion to organs such as the kidney and brain, which are already in jeopardy.

Heart block. Isoprenaline, or other β_1-agonists, can be used to maintain the heart-beat when atrio-ventricular conduction is impaired (see Chapter 10). This can lead to sudden loss of consciousness, if the ventricular rate falls so low that the cardiac output becomes inadequate. The long-term solution is usually to implant an electrical pacemaker, but ventricular beating can be kept going in the interim by isoprenaline.

Hypertension. Clonidine, a selective α_2-agonist, is an effective hypotensive drug, whose action is partly central, and partly exerted on the pre-synaptic adrenergic nerve terminals (see Chapter 11).

ADRENOCEPTOR-BLOCKING DRUGS

The main drugs in this category are listed in Table 7.2 and further information is given in Table 7.6. In contrast to the situation with agonists, most adrenoceptor antagonists act selectively on α or β-adrenoceptors, very few drugs acting on both types. The subclassification of antagonists into α_1- and α_2-selective, or β_1- and β_2-selective compounds is less clear-cut, and many drugs show mixed effects.

α-receptor antagonists

The main groups are

1. Ergot derivatives (e.g. **ergotamine**)
2. Haloalkylamines (e.g. **phenoxybenzamine**)
3. **Yohimbine**
4. Miscellaneous synthetic compounds (e.g. **phentolamine, prazosin, indoramin**).

Ergot alkaloids

These compounds occur naturally in a fungus (*Claviceps purpurea*) that infests cereal crops. Epidemics of ergot poisoning have occurred, and still occur, when contaminated grain is used for food. The symptoms produced include mental disturbances and intensely painful peripheral vasoconstriction, leading to gangrene, which came to be known in the Middle Ages as **St Anthony's fire**, because it was normally cured by a visit to the shrine of St Anthony (which happened to be in an ergot-free region of France). Ergot contains many active substances, and it was a preoccupation with their complex pharmacological properties that led Dale to many important discoveries concerning acetylcholine, histamine and catecholamines.

Ergot alkaloids (Fig. 7.11) are molecules based on a complex aromatic acid, **lysergic acid**, and the

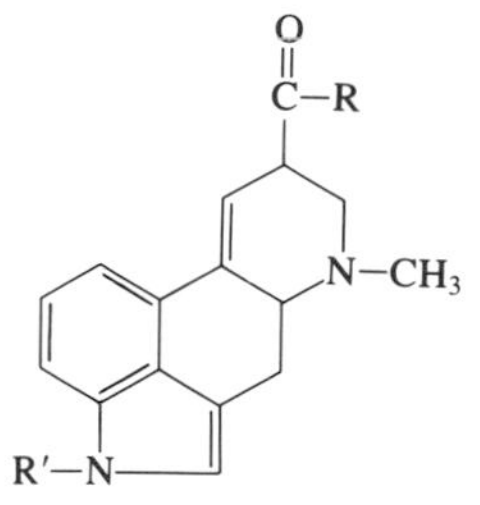

Fig. 7.11 Structures of ergot alkaloids.

	R	R'
Amine alkaloids		
Lysergic acid diethylamide (LSD)	N(C₂H₅)₂	H
Ergometrine	NH.CH(CH₃)CH₂OH	H
Methysergide	NH.CH(CH₃)CH₂OH	CH₃

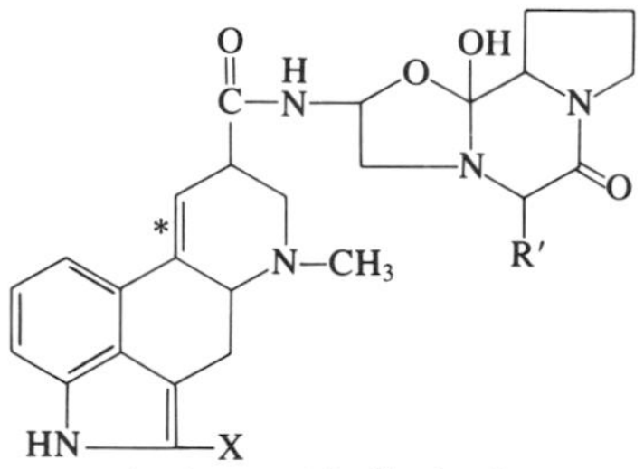

	R	R'
Amino acid alkaloids		
Ergotamine	CH₃	CH₂-phenyl
Dihydroergotamine	CH₃	CH₂-phenyl (double bond* saturated)
Bromocriptine	CH(CH₃)₂	CH₂.CH(CH₃)₂ (Br at X)

different compounds in this group display many different types of pharmacological action. Chemically they fall into two major categories, according to whether they possess an amine, or an amino-acid side-chain. Compounds with an amine side-chain include **lysergic acid diethylamide (LSD**; see Chapter 26), **methysergide** (Chapter 11) and **ergometrine** (Chapter 17). Compounds with an amino-acid side-chain include **ergotamine**, which acts on α-adrenoceptors, **dihydroergotamine**, and a semisynthetic compound, **bromocriptine**, which acts selectively on dopamine receptors (see Chapter 19). **Ergometrine**, which has a simple aliphatic side-chain, acts selectively on the smooth muscle of the uterus.

Actions of ergot alkaloids

These drugs all cause stimulation of smooth muscle, some being relatively selective for vascular smooth muscle, and others acting mainly on the uterus. In addition, the amino-acid alkaloids affect catecholamine and serotonin receptors in various ways. **Ergotamine** has the characteristics of a partial agonist on α-adrenoceptors, **dihydroergotamine** is a pure antagonist on α-adrenoceptors, and **bromocriptine** acts as an agonist on dopamine receptors, particularly in the central nervous system. **Methysergide** is relatively selective as an antagonist of serotonin, and this is also a property of some of the other amino-acid alkaloids. The pharmacological actions of these drugs are summarized in Table 7.4. As one would expect of drugs with so many actions, their physiological effects are complex, and rather poorly understood. In this chapter we concentrate on ergotamine, which acts mainly on α-receptors.

Further information on ergometrine, methysergide and bromocriptine, all of which have clinical uses based on other pharmacological actions, is presented elsewhere. The main physiological effects of ergotamine are as follows:

Vascular effects. When injected into an anaesthetized animal ergotamine causes a sustained rise in blood pressure, caused by vasoconstriction. This effect is blocked by pure α-receptor antagonists such as phentolamine. At the same time as causing a rise in blood pressure, ergotamine reverses the pressor effect of adrenaline. This **adrenaline reversal** was discovered by Dale accidentally when, at the end of a long day, he tried to carry out a bioassay of an adrenal gland extract by measuring its pressor effect on a cat into which he had previously injected ergot. It occurs because the α-receptors with which adrenaline normally combines are occupied, leaving the β-receptor-mediated vasodilatation unopposed. The same effect can be produced by any α-receptor antagonist. The vasoconstrictor effect of ergotamine is responsible for the peripheral gangrene of St Anthony's fire, and probably also for some of the effects of ergot on the central nervous system.

Other actions. Ergotamine causes uterine contraction, similar to the effect of ergometrine (see Chapter 17), and may also produce nausea and vomiting (an action shared with bromocriptine, and probably caused by stimulation of central dopamine receptors). It is also a partial agonist on certain serotonin receptors (see Chapter 11), an effect which may contribute to its vascular actions.

Uses. The main use of ergotamine is in the treatment of migraine, for which it is effective as a prophylactic, as is methysergide. It is unclear at present whether this effect is due to an interaction with α-adrenoceptors, or with serotonin receptors, or both. The question is discussed further in Chapter 11.

Side effects. Nausea and vomiting are troublesome side effects, and ergotamine must be avoided in patients with peripheral vascular disease, because of its vasoconstrictor action. An analogue, dihydroergotamine, produces an equal beneficial effect with fewer side effects.

Haloalkylamines

The most important member of this class of α-receptor antagonists is **phenyoxybenzamine**. The interesting feature of the chemistry of these compounds is that they possess an unstable N-chloroethyl group, also found in the nitrogen mustards that are used in cancer chemotherapy (see Chapter 29). This group enables the drug to bind *covalently* to a part of the receptor site (probably a carboxyl or sulphydryl group). Dissociation is therefore extremely slow, since it requires cleavage of this covalent bond. The half-time for recovery from the action of phenoxybenzamine is about 24 hours. Because of this very slow dissociation, the pattern of antagonism produced is of the **irreversible competitive type** (see Chapter 1) in which the slope and maximum of the log concentration-effect curve for noradrenaline are reduced, in contrast to the effect of a reversible competitive antagonist. Phenoxybenzamine is not highly specific for α-receptors, and also antagonizes the actions of acetylcholine, histamine and serotonin.

Phenoxybenzamine causes in man a **fall in arterial pressure** (because of block of α-receptor mediated vasoconstriction) and **postural hypotension**. The cardiac output and heart rate are increased. This is a reflex response to the fall in arterial pressure, mediated through β-receptors. Phenoxybenzamine blocks pre-synaptic $α_2$-receptors, as well as $α_1$-receptors, and this may enhance noradrenaline release, thus exaggerating the reflex tachycardia. Blood flow through cutaneous and splanchnic vascular beds is increased. Effects on non-vascular smooth muscle are slight, though pupillary constriction and failure of ejaculation sometimes occur. The uses of phenoxybenzamine and other α-receptor antagonists are described below.

Yohimbine

This is a naturally occurring alkaloid whose interest lies in its specificity for $α_2$-receptors. By blocking these receptors, while sparing $α_1$-receptors, it increases noradrenaline release, and produces sympathomimetic effects in some organs. Elsewhere, blockade of post-synaptic $α_2$-receptors causes a block of sympathetic responses, so the overall effects are complex. Vasodilatation, and a fall in blood pressure usually predominate, and its vasodilator effect has given it undeserved fame as an aphrodisiac (Dahl, 1980). It is not employed therapeutically, but has proved useful in the experimental analysis of α-receptor subtypes.

Other α-adrenoceptor antagonists

Phentolamine is a reversible competitive antagonist of noradrenaline, acting on both $α_1$- and $α_2$-receptors. Its actions are very similar to, but briefer than, those of phenoxybenzamine. Like many drugs that block the effects of sympathetic nerves, phentolamine causes an increase in gastrointestinal motility, resulting in diarrhoea and abdominal pain.

Prazosin and **indoramin** are recently-introduced drugs that are selective antagonists of $α_1$-receptors. They cause vasodilatation and fall in arterial pressure, but less tachycardia than occurs with non-selective α-receptor antagonists, presumably because they do not increase noradrenaline release from sympathetic nerve terminals. Cardiac output tends to decrease, as a result of the fall in central venous pressure due to dilatation of capacitance vessels, and the hypotensive effect is more dramatic than with non-selective α-receptor antagonists. Indoramin has some direct depressant effects on the myocardium, which may partly account for the lack of tachycardia with this drug. This is a worthwhile advantage in clinical use.

Labetalol is a mixed α- and β-receptor blocking drug. Much has been made of the fact that it combines the properties of α- and β-blocking drugs in one molecule. To a pharmacologist, accustomed to putting specificity of action high on the list of pharmacological saintly virtues, labetalol may seem like a step backwards rather than forwards.

Uses and side effects of α-receptor antagonists

The main uses of these drugs are related to their

Table 7.5 Summary of drugs that affect adrenergic transmission

Type	Drug	Main action	Uses/function	Side effects, toxicity	Pharmacokinetic aspects	Notes
SYMPATHOMIMETIC (directly-acting)	Noradrenaline	α/β-agonist	Not used clinically. Transmitter at post-ganglionic sympathetic neurons, and in CNS. Hormone of adrenal medulla.	Hypertension, vasoconstriction, tachycardia (or reflex bradycardia), ventricular dysrhythmias.	Poorly absorbed by mouth. Rapid removal by tissues. Metabolized by MAO & COMT. Plasma $t_{\frac{1}{2}} \sim 2$ min.	
	Adrenaline	α/β-agonist	Asthma (emergency treatment), anaphylactic shock cardiac arrest. Added to local anaesthetic solutions. Hormone of adrenal medulla.	As noradrenaline.	Given i.m. or s.c. As noradrenaline.	See Chapter 13.
	Isoprenaline	β-agonist (non-selective)	Asthma (obsolete), heart block. Not an endogenous substance.	Tachycardia, dysrhythmias.	Given sublingually, or as aerosol. Some tissue uptake, followed by inactivation (COMT). Plasma $t_{\frac{1}{2}} \sim 2$ h.	See Chapter 11. Now replaced by salbutamol in treatment of asthma (see Chapter 13).
	α-methyl-noradrenaline	α_2-agonist	Formed as false transmitter from methyldopa.	See methyldopa.	See methyldopa.	
	Salbutamol	β_2-agonist	Asthma, premature labour.	Tachycardia, dysrhythmias, tremor peripheral vasodilatation.	Given orally or by aerosol. Mainly excreted unchanged. Plasma $t_{\frac{1}{2}} \sim 4$ h.	See Chapter 13.
	Terbutaline	β_2-agonist	Asthma.	As salbutamol.	Poorly absorbed orally. Given by aerosol. Mainly excreted unchanged. Plasma $t_{\frac{1}{2}} \sim 4$ h.	
	Phenylephrine	α-agonist (non-selective)	Hypotensive states, nasal decongestion.	Hypertension, reflex bradycardia.	Given i.m. or intranasally. Metabolized by MAO. Short plasma $t_{\frac{1}{2}}$.	
	Methoxamine	α-agonist (non-selective)	Hypotensive states.	As phenylephrine.	Given i.v. or i.m. Plasma $t_{\frac{1}{2}} \sim 1$ h.	
	Clonidine	α_2-partial agonist	Hypertension, migraine.	Drowsiness, orthostatic hypotension, oedema and weight gain, rebound hypertension.	Well absorbed orally. Excreted unchanged and as conjugate. Plasma $t_{\frac{1}{2}} \sim 12$ h.	See Chapter 11.

Category	Drug	Action	Clinical uses	Unwanted effects	Pharmacokinetics	Notes
SYMPATHOMIMETIC (indirectly acting)	Tyramine	NA release	No clinical uses. Present in various foods.	As noradrenaline.	Normally destroyed by MAO in gut. Does not enter brain.	See Chapter 3.
	Amphetamine	NA release, MAO inhibitor, uptake 1 inhibitor, CNS stimulant	Used as CNS stimulant in narcolepsy, also (paradoxically) in hyperactive children. Appetite suppressant.	Hypertension, tachycardia, insomnia. Acute pshychosis with overdose. Dependence.	Well absorbed orally, penetrates freely into brain. Excreted unchanged in urine. Plasma $t_{\frac{1}{2}} \sim 12$ h, depending on urine flow and pH.	See Chapter 26.
	Ephedrine	NA release, β-agonist, weak CNS stimulant.	Asthma, nasal decongestion.	Similar to amphetamine.	As amphetamine, but less pronounced.	Contraindicated if MAO inhibitors are given.
ADRENOCEPTOR ANTAGONISTS	Phenoxybenz-amine	α-antagonist (non-selective, irreversible), Uptake 1 inhibitor	Peripheral vasospasm (e.g. Raynaud's *disease*), phaeochromocytoma.	Hypotension, flushing, tachycardia, nasal congestion, impotence.	Absorbed orally. Plasma $t_{\frac{1}{2}} \sim 12$ h.	Action outlasts presence of drug in plasma, because of covalent binding to receptor.
	Phentolamine	α-antagonist (non-selective), vasodilator	Rarely used	As phenoxybenzamine.	Usually given i.v. Metabolized by liver. Plasma $t_{\frac{1}{2}} \sim 2$ h.	
	Tolazoline	As phentolamine	Peripheral vasospasm.	As phenoxybenzamine.	As amphetamine.	Thymoxamine is similar. Indoramin is similar, but causes less tachycardia. See Chapter 11.
	Prazosin	α₁-antagonist	Hypertension.	As phenoxybenzamine, also drowsiness.	Absorbed orally. Metabolized by liver. Plasma $t_{\frac{1}{2}} \sim 4$ h.	See Chapter 11.
	Ergotamine	α-partial agonist, contracts uterus	Migraine.	Vomiting, diarrhoea, gangrene, drowsiness, mental disturbances.		
	Yohimbine	α₂-antagonist	Not used clinically. Claimed to be aphrodisiac.	Excitement, hypertension.		
	Propranolol	β-antagonist (non-selective)	Angina, hypertension, cardiac dysrhythmias, anxiety tremor, glaucoma.	Bronchoconstriction, cardiac failure, cold extremities, fatigue and depression, hypoglycaemia.	Absorbed orally. Extensive first-pass metabolism. About 90% bound to plasma protein. Plasma $t_{\frac{1}{2}} \sim 4$ h.	Timolol is similar, and used mainly to treat glaucoma. See Chapter 10.
	Alprenolol	β-antagonist (non-selective) (partial agonist)	As propranolol.	As propranolol.	Absorbed orally. Metabolized by liver. Plasma $t_{\frac{1}{2}} \sim 4$ h.	Oxprenolol and pindolol are similar. See Chapter 10.
	Practolol	β₁-antagonist	Hypertension, angina, dysrhythmias	As propranolol, also oculomucocutaneous syndrome.	Absorbed orally. Excreted unchanged in urine. Plasma $t_{\frac{1}{2}} \sim 4$ h.	Withdrawn from clinical use.
	Metoprolol	β₁-antagonist	Angina, hypertension, dysrhythmias	As propranolol, less risk of bronchoconstriction.	As practolol.	Acebutolol and atenolol are similar. See Chapter 10.

Table 7.5 (continued)

Type	Drug	Main Action	Uses/function	Side effects, toxicity	Pharmacokinetic aspects	Notes
ADRENOCEPTOR ANTAGONISTS (cont.)	Butoxamine	β_2-antagonist, weak α-agonist	No clinical uses.	—	—	—
	Labetalol	α/β-antagonist	Hypertension, phaeochromocytoma.	Postural hypotension, bronchoconstriction.	Absorbed orally. Conjugated in liver. Plasma $t_{\frac{1}{2}} \sim 4$ h.	See Chapters 10 & 11.
DRUGS AFFECTING NORADRENALINE SYNTHESIS	α-methyl-p-tyrosine	Inhibits tyrosine hydroxylase	Occasionally used in phaeochromocytoma.	Hypotension, sedation.	—	—
	Carbidopa	Inhibits dopa decarboxylase	Used as adjunct to L-dopa, to prevent peripheral effects.	—	Absorbed orally. Does not enter brain.	See Chapter 24.
	Methyldopa	False transmitter precursor	Hypertension.	Hypotension, drowsiness, diarrhoea, impotence, hypersensitivity reactions.	Absorbed slowly by mouth. Excreted unchanged or as conjugate. Plasma $t_{\frac{1}{2}} \sim 6$ h.	See Chapter 11.
	Reserpine	Depletes NA stores by inhibiting vesicular uptake of NA	Hypertension (obsolete).	As methyldopa. Also depression, Parkinsonism, gynaecomastia.	Poorly absorbed orally. Slowly metabolized. Plasma $t_{\frac{1}{2}} \sim 100$ h. Excreted in milk.	Antihypertensive effect develops slowly, and persists when drug is stopped.
DRUGS AFFECTING NORADRENALINE RELEASE	Guanethidine	Inhibits NA release Also causes NA depletion, and can damage NA neurons irreversibly	Hypertension.	As methyldopa. Hypertension on first administration.	Poorly absorbed orally. Mainly excreted unchanged in urine. Plasma $t_{\frac{1}{2}} \sim 100$ h.	Action prevented by Uptake 1 inhibitors (see Chapter 3). Bethanidine and debrisoquin are similar.
DRUGS AFFECTING NORADRENALINE UPTAKE	Imipramine	Blocks Uptake 1 Also has atropine-like action	Depression.	Atropine-like side effects. Cardiac dysrhythmias in overdose.	Well absorbed orally. 95% bound to plasma protein. Converted to active metabolite (desmethylimipramine). Plasma $t_{\frac{1}{2}} \sim 4$ h.	See Chapter 11. Desipramine and amitriptyline are similar. See Chapter 23.
	Cocaine	Local anaesthetic Blocks Uptake 1 CNS stimulant	Rarely used local anaesthetic. Major drug of abuse.	Hypertension, excitement, convulsions.	Well absorbed orally.	See Chapters 26 & 27.
MAO INHIBITORS	Phenelzine	Inhibits MAO	Depression.	Cheese reaction. Can cause hypotension.	Well absorbed orally. Acetylated in liver.	See Chapter 23.

cardiovascular actions. They have been tried for many purposes, but have only limited therapeutic applications.

In **hypertension**, non-selective α-blocking drugs are not very useful, because of their tendency to produce tachycardia and cardiac dysrhythmias, and increased gastrointestinal activity. Prazosin and indoramin are more effective and do not affect cardiac function appreciably. Certain side effects, however, are troublesome with all α-receptor antagonists, namely **postural hypotension**, **failure of ejaculation** and **drowsiness**.

Phaeochromocytoma is a catecholamine-secreting tumour of chromaffin tissue, and one of the effects is to cause episodes of severe hypertension. A combination of α- and β-receptor antagonists is the most effective way of controlling the blood pressure. The tumour may be surgically removable, and it is essential to block α- and β-receptors before surgery is begun, to avoid the effects of a sudden release of catecholamines when the tumour is disturbed mechanically. Labetalol, or a combination of α- and β-blocking drugs (e.g. phenoxybenzamine and propranolol), are effective for this purpose.

Peripheral vascular disease. Many types of peripheral vascular disease are caused by occlusion of relatively large arteries by atherosclerotic deposits, and drugs that block sympathetic transmission are ineffective, because the block has nothing to do with vasoconstriction. **Raynaud's disease** is a condition in which bouts of intense sympathetically-mediated arteriolar vasoconstriction occur in the hands and feet, usually in response to cold or vibration. Phenoxybenzamine and other α-antagonists may be used to reduce the vasoconstriction.

β-receptor antagonists

Drugs in this important category were first developed in 1958 by Black and his colleagues, ten years after Ahlquist had postulated the existence of the α- and β-subclasses of adrenoceptors. The first compound, **dichloroisoprenaline**, was a simple derivative of isoprenaline in which both ring −OH groups were placed by chlorine atoms. It has fairly low potency, and is also a partial agonist.

Further development led to **propranolol**, a much more potent drug that is a pure antagonist, and is the most widely used drug of this class. Propranolol has an equal blocking effect on β_1- and β_2-receptors. The potential clinical advantages of drugs with some partial agonist activity and with selectivity for β_1-receptors, led to the development of practolol (selective for β_2-receptors and a very weak partial agonist, but no longer used clinically because of its toxicity), **oxprenolol** and **alprenolol** (non-selective with considerable partial agonist activity), and **atenolol** (β_1-selective with no agonist activity). Many very similar drugs have been developed, and the characteristics of the most important compounds are set out in Tables 7.2 & 7.5.

Effects of β-receptor antagonists

The pharmacological actions of β-receptor antagonists can be deduced from Table 7.1. The effects produced in man depend on the degree of sympathetic activity, and are slight in subjects at rest. The most important effects are on the cardiovascular system and on bronchial smooth muscle.

In a subject at rest, propranolol causes little change in heart rate, cardiac output or arterial pressure, but reduces the effect of exercise or excitement on these variables (Fig. 7.12). Drugs with partial agonist activity, such as oxprenolol, increase the heart rate at rest, but reduce it during exercise. Maximum exercise tolerance is considerably reduced in normal subjects, partly because of the limitation of the cardiac response, and partly because the β-mediated vasodilatation in skeletal muscle is reduced. Coronary flow is reduced, but relatively less than the myocardial oxygen consumption, so oxygenation of the myocardium is improved, an effect of importance in the treatment of **angina pectoris** (see Chapter 10). In normal subjects, the reduction of the force of contraction of the heart is of no importance, but it may have serious consequences for patients with heart disease (see below).

An important, and somewhat unexpected, effect of β-receptor antagonists is their **antihypertensive action** (see Chapter 11). Patients with hypertension (though not normotensive subjects) show a gradual fall in arterial pressure that takes several days to develop fully. The mechanism is complex, and involves: (a) reduction in cardiac output; (b) reduction of renin release from the juxtaglomerular cells of the kidney; and (c) a central action, reducing

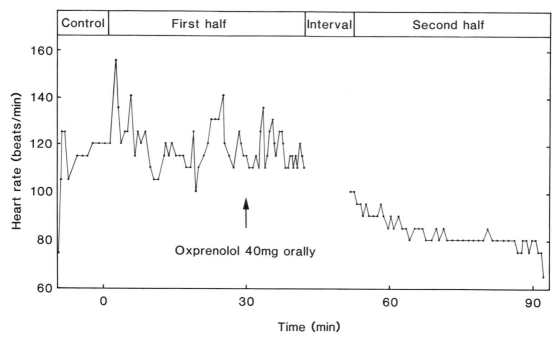

Fig. 7.12 Heart rate recorded continuously in a spectator watching a live football match, showing the effect of the β-adrenoceptor antagonist, oxprenolol. (From: Taylor & Meeran, 1973)

sympathetic activity. Blockade of the facilitatory effect of pre-synaptic β-receptors on noradrenaline release (see p. 153) may also contribute to the anti-hypertensive effect. The antihypertensive effect of β-receptor antagonists is clinically very useful. Because reflex vasoconstriction is preserved, postural and exercise-induced hypotension (see Chapter 11) are much less troublesome than with many other antihypertensive drugs.

β-receptor antagonists have an **antidysrhythmic effect** on the heart, which is of clinical importance (see Chapter 10).

Airways resistance in normal subjects is only slightly increased by β-receptor antagonists, and this is of no consequence. In asthmatic subjects, however, non-selective β-receptor antagonists such as propranolol, can cause severe bronchoconstriction, which does not, of course, respond to drugs such as salbutamol or adrenaline. This danger is less with β_1-selective antagonists, but none are so selective that this danger can be ignored.

In spite of the involvement of β-receptors in the lipolytic and hyperglycaemic actions of adrenaline, β-receptor antagonists cause only minor metabolic changes in normal subjects. They do not affect the onset of hypoglycaemia following an injection of insulin, but somewhat delay the recovery of blood glucose concentration. In diabetic patients, the use of β-receptor antagonists increases the likelihood of exercise-induced hypoglycaemia because the normal adrenaline-induced release of glucose from the liver is diminished.

Uses of β-receptor antagonists

The main uses of β-receptor antagonists are connected with their effects on the cardiovascular system, and are discussed in Chapters 10 & 11. They are:

Hypertension. In mild or moderate hypertension, β-receptor antagonists are now the most frequently used drugs, and are often combined with other hypotensive drugs (see Chapter 11). Their main advantage is that, unlike most antihypertensive drugs, they do not cause postural, or exercise-induced hypotension, nor do they cause side effects such as impotence or diarrhoea, which occur with drugs that cause a less selective inhibition of the sympathetic nervous system.

Cardiac dysrhythmias (see Chapter 10). Increased

sympathetic activity is a factor in many types of cardiac dysrhythmia, including the potentially fatal ventricular dysrhythmias that occur following a coronary thrombosis. β-receptor antagonists are effective in many types of dysrhythmia, and have been shown to reduce the incidence of death from ventricular fibrillation in patients suffering heart attacks.

Angina pectoris (see Chapter 10). β-receptor antagonists reduce cardiac work, particularly in exercise, by reducing the rate and force of contraction of the ventricle. The resulting reduction in cardiac oxygen consumption is effective in relieving anginal pain.

Other uses of β-receptor antagonists include:

Anxiety states. Symptoms of anxiety, such as tremor and palpitations, that are mediated by increased sympathetic activity, can be relieved by β-receptor antagonists.

Glaucoma. The production of aqueous humour is inhibited by β-receptor antagonists, thus lowering intraocular pressure. The mechanism of this effect is not well understood, but the advantage of this form of treatment compared with cholinergic agonists (see Chapter 6) is that accommodation and pupillary reactions are unaffected, so that vision is not impaired. Some β-receptor antagonists (e.g. **timolol**) can be used as eyedrops for this purpose.

Side effects of β-receptor antagonists

The main side effects of β-receptor antagonists are simply a consequence of their blocking action, namely:

Bronchoconstriction. This is normally of little importance, though it can be detected by measurement of forced expiratory rate. In asthmatic patients, this effect can be dramatic and life-threatening.

Cardiac failure. Patients with heart disease may rely on a degree of sympathetic drive to the heart to maintain an adequate cardiac output, and removal of this by blocking β-receptors will produce a degree of cardiac failure. In theory, drugs with partial agonist activity (e.g. oxprenolol, alprenolol) offer an advantage since they can, by their own action, maintain a degree of β-receptor activation, while at the same time blunting the cardiac response to increased sympathetic nerve activity or to circu-

lating adrenaline. Clinical trials so far, however, have not shown a clear advantage of these drugs measurable as a reduced incidence of cardiac failure.

Hypoglycaemia. Glucose release in response to adrenaline is a safety device that may be important to diabetic patients and to other individuals prone to hypoglycaemic attacks. The use of β-receptor antagonists can be hazardous in these patients. There is a theoretical advantage in using β_1-selective agents, since glucose release from the liver is controlled by β_2-receptors.

Fatigue and depression. These are often complained of by patients taking β-receptor blocking drugs. The physical fatigue is probably due to reduced cardiac output and reduced muscle perfusion in exercise.

Cold extremities. This results presumably from a loss of β-receptor-mediated vasodilatation in cutaneous vessels, and is a common side effect. Again, β_1-selective drugs ought to be less likely to produce this effect, but it is not clear that this is so in practice.

Other side effects associated with β-receptor antagonists are not obviously the result of β-receptor blockade. One is the occurrence of bad dreams, which occur mainly with highly lipid-soluble drugs such as propranolol, which enter the brain easily. A second is the serious **oculomucocutaneous syndrome** produced by practolol. This comprises lacrimal gland damage, leading to dryness of the cornea and sometimes blindness, together with sclerosing peritonitis, leading to digestive tract malfunction, and a skin rash. The cause of this reaction, which has led to the withdrawal of practolol from clinical use, is not known. It may well be immunological in origin, but this has not been conclusively shown.

DRUGS THAT AFFECT ADRENERGIC NEURONS

Emphasis in this chapter is placed on peripheral sympathetic transmission. The same principles, however, are applicable to the central nervous system (see Chapters 19 & 23), where many of the drugs mentioned here also act.

DRUGS THAT AFFECT NORADRENALINE SYNTHESIS

Only a few clinically important drugs affect noradrenaline synthesis directly. Examples are **α-methyltyrosine**, which inhibits tyrosine hydroxylase and has been used in the treatment of phaeochromocytoma, and **carbidopa**, a hydrazine derivative of dopa, which inhibits dopa decarboxylase. Its main use is as an adjunct to treatment of Parkinsonism with L-dopa (see Chapter 24). The peripheral side effects of L-dopa, which result from its conversion to dopamine and noradrenaline, are reduced by carbidopa, but, because the drug does not enter the brain, formation of dopamine in the brain, on which the therapeutic effectiveness of L-dopa depends, is not impaired.

An important indirect effect on noradrenaline synthesis is produced by **methyldopa**, a drug that is widely used in the treatment of hypertension (see Chapter 11). Methyldopa (see Fig. 7.8) is taken up by adrenergic neurons, where it is decarboxylated and hydroxylated to form the false transmitter **α-methylnoradrenaline**. This substance is not deaminated within the neuron by MAO and therefore tends to accumulate in larger quantities than noradrenaline, displacing noradrenaline from its storage sites in the vesicles. The false transmitter is released in the same way as noradrenaline, but differs in two important respects in its action on adrenoceptors. α-methylnoradrenaline is somewhat less active than noradrenaline on α_1-receptors and thus is less effective in causing vasoconstriction. But it is more active on pre-synaptic α_2-receptors, so the auto-inhibitory feedback mechanism operates more strongly than normal, thus reducing transmitter release below the normal levels. Both of these effects (as well as a central effect, probably caused by the same cellular mechanism) contribute to the hypotensive action. Other aspects of the pharmacology of methyldopa are discussed in Chapter 11.

A drug that subverts the machinery of the adrenergic neuron in a particularly dramatic way is **6-hydroxydopamine**, which is identical with dopamine except that it possesses an extra ring —OH group. It is taken up selectively by adrenergic nerve terminals, where it is converted to a reactive quinone which destroys the nerve terminal, producing a 'chemical sympathectomy'. The cell bodies survive, and eventually the sympathetic innervation recovers. The drug is useful for experimental purposes, but has no clinical uses. If injected directly into the brain it selectively destroys those nerve terminals (i.e. dopaminergic and noradrenergic) which take it up, but it does not reach the brain if given systemically.

DRUGS THAT AFFECT NORADRENALINE STORAGE

The main drug in this category is **reserpine**, an alkaloid of complex chemical structure, bearing no obvious relationship to catecholamines. It comes from a shrub, *Rauwolfia*, which has been widely used in India for centuries as a medicine for the treatment of mental disorders. Reserpine, at very low concentration, blocks the accumulation of noradrenaline, and other amines, by synaptic vesicles. The transmitter content of the vesicles leaks into the cytoplasm where it is degraded by MAO. The noradrenaline content of tissues thus drops to a low level, and sympathetic transmission is blocked. This effect is not confined to the periphery, nor to noradrenaline, for reserpine causes depletion of serotonin and dopamine from neurons in the brain in which these amines are transmitters (see Chapter 19). Reserpine, through its action on sympathetic nerve terminals, has some use as an antihypertensive drug (see Chapter 11), but its central effects, especially **depression**, which probably result from impairment of adrenergic and serotonin-mediated transmission in the brain (see Chapter 19) are a serious disadvantage.

Reserpine is a useful experimental drug, which can be used to test whether various physiological processes and drug effects require the presence of functional sympathetic nerve terminals.

DRUGS THAT AFFECT NORADRENALINE RELEASE

Drugs can affect noradrenaline release in four main ways:

1. By preventing exocytosis from occurring in response to depolarization of the nerve terminal (**adrenergic neuron blocking drugs**).

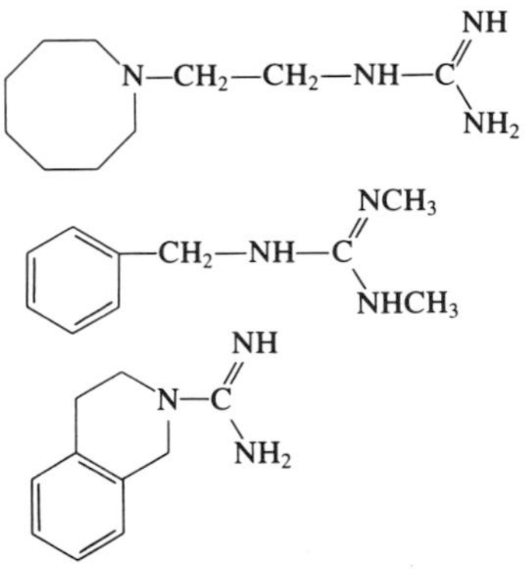

Fig. 7.13 Adrenergic neuron blocking drugs.

2. By causing noradrenaline release in the absence of nerve terminal depolarization (**indirectly-acting sympathomimetic drugs**).
3. By interacting with pre-synaptic receptors that inhibit or enhance depolarization-evoked release (e.g. **α_2-agonists**, **dopamine**, **prostaglandins**, etc). Effects mediated through α_2-adrenoceptors are discussed elsewhere in this chapter; the importance of the numerous other endogenous substances known to affect sympathetic nerve terminals is not clear at present. It is likely that these mechanisms are more important in the central than the peripheral nervous systems.
4. By increasing or decreasing available stores of noradrenaline (e.g. **reserpine**, see above; **monoamine oxidase inhibitors**). These drugs are discussed elsewhere in this chapter, and in Chapter 23, and are not considered further in this section.

Adrenergic neuron blocking drugs

These drugs (Fig. 7.13), of which **guanethidine** is the most important, were first discovered in the mid-1950s when alternatives to ganglion blocking drugs, for use in the treatment of hypertension, were being sought.

The main effect of guanethidine is to inhibit the release of noradrenaline from sympathetic nerve terminals. It has little effect on the adrenal medulla, and none on nerve terminals that release transmitters other than noradrenaline. Guanethidine, and drugs similar to it, such as **bretylium**, **bethanidine**, and **debrisoquin** (Fig. 7.13), are highly polar compounds with either a quaternary N^+ atom or a basic guanidinium group, so they do not enter the brain.

Effects of adrenergic neuron blocking drugs

Drugs of this class reduce or abolish the response of tissues to sympathetic nerve stimulation, but do not affect (or may potentiate) the effects of injected noradrenaline. Their ability to block noradrenaline release can be demonstrated by measurement, for example, of the release of radioactivity from organs such as the spleen or vas deferens, in response to stimulation of the sympathetic nerves after the transmitter stores have been labelled by infusion of radioactive noradrenaline.

The mechanism of action of guanethidine is somewhat complex, but the following facts are known:

1. Guanethidine is selectively accumulated by adrenergic nerve terminals. This occurs by means of Uptake 1, and is prevented by inhibitors of Uptake 1 (e.g. tricyclic antidepressant drugs), which also prevent the pharmacological action of guanethidine.

2. Guanethidine is itself stored in synaptic vesicles, and released by nerve stimulation.

3. Guanethidine and related drugs have some local anaesthetic activity. It is possible that the selective intraneuronal accumulation by Uptake 1 leads to a block of impulse propagation in the adrenergic nerve terminal, but direct evidence for this is so far lacking.

4. Guanethidine causes an initial release of noradrenaline, which can cause a paradoxical sympathomimetic effect before the block ensues.

5. Guanethidine causes a slowly-developing and long-lasting depletion of noradrenaline in sympathetic nerve endings, similar to the effect of reserpine. Inhibition of noradrenaline release occurs before this depletion has developed, but the depletion may have the effect of prolonging the blocking effect.

6. The action of guanethidine is opposed by indirectly-acting sympathomimetic drugs, such as amphetamine (see below). This may be because many of these drugs block Uptake 1, or it may occur because they displace guanethidine, as well as noradrenaline, from storage sites in the synaptic vesicles.

Overall it seems most likely that the principal action of guanethidine involves its accumulation by the synaptic vesicles, which are then unable to fuse with the cell membrane in the normal way, so that exocytosis is prevented. It is clear however, that the drug has other effects, leading to transmitter depletion. Given in large doses it causes structural damage to adrenergic neurons, which is probably due to the fact that the terminals accumulate the drug in high concentration.

Uses and side effects

The only important use of adrenergic neuron blocking drugs is in the treatment of hypertension (see Chapter 11). They are extremely effective in lowering blood pressure, but have severe side effects associated with the loss of sympathetic reflexes. The most troublesome are **postural hypotension**, **diarrhoea**, **nasal congestion** and **failure of ejaculation**.

Indirectly-acting sympathomimetic amines

Mechanism of action and structure-activity relationships

The most important drugs in this category are **tyramine**, **amphetamine** and **ephedrine**, all of which are structurally related to noradrenaline (Fig. 7.14). They each lack one or both of the catechol −OH

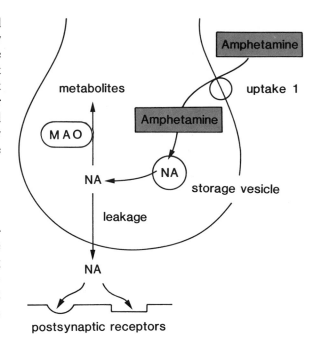

Fig. 7.15 The mode of action of an indirectly-acting sympathomimetic amine, amphetamine. Amphetamine enters the nerve terminal via the NA carrier (Uptake 1) and displaces NA from storage vesicles. Some of the NA is degraded by MAO within the nerve terminal and some escapes to act on post-synaptic receptors. Amphetamine also reduces NA reuptake via Uptake 1, so enhancing the action of the released NA.

groups, and thus have only weak actions on adrenoceptors, but sufficiently resemble noradrenaline to be transported into nerve terminals by Uptake 1. Once inside the nerve terminals they cause displacement of noradrenaline from the vesicles into the cytosol, where some of it is degraded by MAO, while the rest escapes to act on post-synaptic receptors (Fig. 7.15). Exocytosis is not involved in the release process, so their actions do not require the presence of calcium. They are not completely specific in their actions, and act partly by a direct effect on adrenoceptors, partly by inhibiting Uptake 1 (thereby enhancing the effect of the released noradrenaline), and partly by inhibiting MAO.

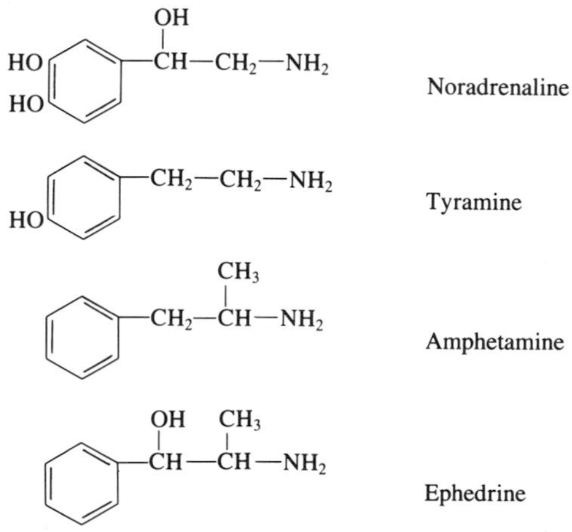

As would be expected, the effects of these drugs are strongly influenced by other drugs that modify adrenergic transmission. Thus, reserpine or 6-hydroxydopamine abolish their effects by depleting the terminals of noradrenaline. MAO inhibitors, on the other hand, strongly potentiate their effects

Fig. 7.14 Indirectly-acting sympathomimetic amines, with noradrenaline shown for comparison.

by preventing breakdown within the terminals of the transmitter displaced from the vesicles. MAO inhibition particularly enhances the action of tyramine because this substance is itself a substrate for MAO. Normally, dietary tyramine is destroyed by MAO in the gut wall and liver before reaching the systemic circulation. This is prevented when MAO is inhibited, and ingestion of tyramine-rich foods, such as cheese (see Chapter 4) can then provoke a sudden and dangerous rise in blood pressure. Inhibitors of Uptake 1, such as **imipramine** (see below) interfere with the effects of indirectly-acting sympathomimetic amines by preventing their uptake into the nerve terminals.

These drugs, especially amphetamine, have important effects on the central nervous system (see Chapter 26), which depend on their ability to release, not only noradrenaline, but also serotonin and dopamine from nerve terminals in the brain.

An important characteristic of the effects of indirectly-acting sympathomimetic amines is that marked tolerance (tachyphylaxis) develops. Repeated doses of amphetamine or tyramine, for example, produce progressively smaller pressor responses. This is probably caused by a depletion of the releasable store of noradrenaline, since the response can be restored, in experimental animals, by infusion of noradrenaline, which has the effect of replenishing the releasable store. A similar tolerance to the central effects also develops with repeated administration, which partly accounts for the liability of amphetamine and related drugs to cause dependence (see Chapter 26).

Effects and uses

The peripheral actions of these drugs closely resemble those of noradrenaline, namely **bronchodilatation**, **raised arterial pressure**, **peripheral vasoconstriction**, **tachycardia**, **increased force of myocardial contraction** and **inhibition of gut motility**, though they are longer lasting. The main central effects that occur, particularly with amphetamine, are:

1. Euphoria and excitement
2. Wakefulness and increased attentiveness
3. Loss of appetite
4. In large doses, a schizophrenia-like syndrome with hallucinations and stereotyped behaviour.

These central actions are discussed further in Chapter 26. Because of them, amphetamine is no longer used as a peripheral sympathomimetic substance. Ephedrine has much less central action, though it can cause excitement and insomnia, and is still sometimes used in the treatment of asthma (see Chapter 13), on account of its bronchodilator action.

Drugs that affect pre-synaptic receptors on adrenergic nerve terminals

Many kinds of pre-synaptic receptors have now been described on adrenergic nerve terminals, including autoreceptors which respond to the released noradrenaline itself, and receptors to various other endogenous substances, such as dopamine, prostaglandins, opioid peptides, acetylcholine, etc. The importance of these receptors in the overall pharmacological effects produced by these substances is not easy to establish, for in most cases the pre-synaptic receptors do not appear to differ in their specificity from receptors elsewhere, and so their effects cannot easily be studied in isolation. The α_2-receptor is an exception, since selective agonists and antagonists are known, though it is no longer believed that α_2-receptors are confined to pre-synaptic sites.

The main α_2-selective agonists that are of importance in medicine are **clonidine** and **α-methylnoradrenaline** (see Table 7.2), though several others are known. Clonidine is used in the treatment of **hypertension** and **migraine** (see Chapter 11), but in neither case is it firmly established that its useful effects result from an effect of pre-synaptic α_2-receptors. There is evidence that the antihypertensive action of clonidine is mainly central in origin, and that the α_2-receptors on which it acts in the brainstem are post-synaptic rather than pre-synaptic. Thus, although an inhibitory action on peripheral adrenergic nerve terminals is an attractive explanation for its hypotensive action, this mechanism may be only of minor importance. Similar evidence suggests that the action of methyldopa, which works through the release of α-methylnoradrenaline (see above), results partly from an effect on central, rather than peripheral α_2-receptors.

INHIBITORS OF NORADRENALINE UPTAKE

Neuronal reuptake of released noradrenaline (Uptake 1) is the most important mechanism by which its action is brought to an end. Many drugs inhibit this mechanism, presumably by blocking the carrier site, and thereby enhance the effects of both sympathetic nerve activity and injected noradrenaline. Uptake 1 is not responsible for clearing circulating adrenaline so these drugs do not affect responses to this amine.

The main class of drugs whose primary action is inhibition of Uptake 1 are the **tricyclic antidepressants** (see Chapter 23), for example **desipramine**. These drugs have their major effect on the central nervous system, but also cause tachycardia and cardiac dysrhythmias which are a reflection of their peripheral effect on sympathetic transmission. **Cocaine**, a well-known local anaesthetic (see

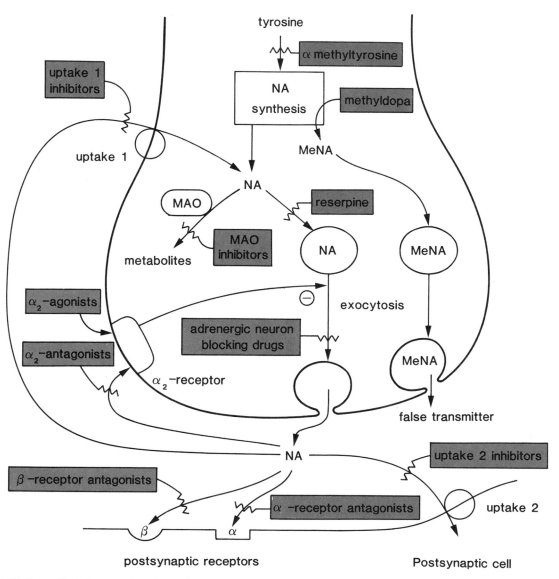

Fig. 7.16 Generalized diagram of an adrenergic nerve terminal showing sites of drug action (square boxes).
MeNA = α-methylnoradrenaline

Chapter 27), enhances sympathetic transmission, causing tachycardia and increased arterial pressure, by inhibiting Uptake 1. Its central effects of euphoria and excitement (see Chapter 24) are probably a manifestation of the same mechanism acting in the brain. It strongly potentiates the actions of noradrenaline in experimental animals or in isolated tissues, provided the sympathetic nerve terminals are intact.

Many drugs that act mainly on other steps in sympathetic transmission also inhibit Uptake 1 to some extent, presumably because the carrier molecule bears a steric relationship to other noradrenaline recognition sites, such as receptors and degradative enzymes. Examples include amphetamine, phenoxybenzamine and guanethidine. These effects are clearly demonstrated by measurements of ^{3}H-noradrenaline uptake by perfused tissues but it is not certain how important they are when the drugs are used in man.

Extraneuronal uptake (Uptake 2), which is important in clearing circulating adrenaline from the bloodstream, is not affected by most of the drugs that block Uptake 1. It is inhibited by phenoxybenzamine, however, and also by various corticosteroids (see Chapter 16). This action of corticosteroids may have some relevance to their therapeutic effect in conditions such as asthma, but it is not thought to be a major component of their effects.

The main sites of action of drugs that affect adrenergic transmission are summarized in Figure 7.16.

DEFINITION OF TERMS RELATING TO ADRENERGIC TRANSMISSION

Adrenergic. Term applied to a pre-synaptic neuron that releases noradrenaline as a transmitter. The term was coined by Dale 50 years ago. Purists (Dale among them) have always insisted that the term should be applied only to the pre-synaptic neuron, and deplore the tendency to use the word in other contexts (e.g. adrenergic synapse, adrenergic receptor, adrenergic excitation, etc). Other purists feel that it should be replaced by 'noradrenergic', but the original term seems likely to endure.

Adrenoceptors. Receptors for adrenaline and nor-

adrenaline. They are divided into α- and β-types, each of which has two further subtypes.

Adrenergic neuron blocking agent. A distinct class of drugs which block adrenergic transmission by inhibiting the release of noradrenaline from the nerve terminals. This group is quite distinct from adrenoceptor antagonists.

Catecholamine. A compound possessing a catechol nucleus (i.e. a benzene ring with two adjacent hydroxyl groups) and an amine-containing side chain. From a pharmacological point of view the most important catecholamines (see Fig. 7.1) are:

1. **Noradrenaline,** the transmitter substance released by the majority of post-ganglionic sympathetic neurons (i.e. adrenergic neurons), as well as certain neurons in the central nervous system. It is also stored and released by chromaffin cells of the adrenal medulla.
2. **Adrenaline,** a hormone secreted, along with noradrenaline, by the adrenal medulla. In mammals adrenaline probably has no peripheral neurotransmitter role (though it does in amphibia), though there is some evidence that it serves as a transmitter in the brain.
3. **Dopamine,** the metabolic precursor of noradrenaline and adrenaline. It functions as a neurotransmitter in its own right in many parts of the brain (see Chapter 19), and may also do so in certain peripheral neurons, producing vasodilatation in particular vascular beds (see Chapter 11).
4. **Isoprenaline,** a synthetic derivative of noradrenaline which is not found in the body. It acts selectively on β-adrenoceptors.

Chromaffin cells. Catecholamine-containing non-neuronal cells derived from neural crest ectoderm. They are so-called because they stain readily with various reagents that oxidize catecholamines to green or brown products. The largest group of chromaffin cells is in the adrenal medulla, but scattered cells are found in various tissues, including sympathetic ganglia, carotid and aortic bodies, and the wall of the intestine. **Phaeochromocytoma** and **carcinoid tumour** are examples of chromaffin cell tumours.

Sympathomimetic drug. A drug whose effects resemble those of activity in the sympathetic nervous system. The term includes drugs that act directly on adrenoceptors in tissues, as well as those that act indirectly by evoking the release of noradrenaline from sympathetic nerve terminals. Some sympathomimetic amines are catecholamines, but by no means all.

REFERENCES AND FURTHER READING

Angus J A, Korner P I 1980 Evidence against presynaptic α-adrenoreceptor modulation of cardiac sympathetic transmission. Nature 286: 288–291

Ariens E J, Simonis A M 1983 Physiological and pharmacological aspects of adrenergic receptor classification. Biochem Pharmacol 32: 1539–1545

Burnstock G, Costa M 1975 Adrenergic neurons. Chapman & Hall, London

Cooper J R, Bloom F E, Roth R H 1982 The biochemical basis of neuropharmacology. Oxford University Press, New York

Cunnane T C 1984 The mechanism of neurotransmitter release from sympathetic nerves. Trends in Neurosciences 7: 248–253

Dahl R 1980 My Uncle Oswald. Penguin, London

Green A R, Costain D W 1981 Pharmacology and biochemistry of psychiatric disorders. Wiley, New York

Kalsner S 1982 The presynaptic receptor controversy. Trends in Pharmacological Sciences 8: 11–16

Langer S Z 1981 Presynaptic regulation of the release of catecholamines. Pharmacol Rev 32: 337–362

McGrath J C 1983 The variety of vascular α-adrenoceptors. Trends in Pharmacological Sciences 4: 14–18

Molinoff P B 1984 α- and β-adrenergic receptor subtypes; properties, distribution and regulation. Drugs 28 (supp 2): 1–15

Rand M J, McCulloch M W, Story D F 1982 Feedback modulation of noradrenergic transmission. Trends in Pharmacological Sciences 3: 8–11

Starke K 1977 Regulation of noradrenaline release through presynaptic receptor systems. Rev Physiol Biochem Pharmacol 77: 1–124

Story D F, McCulloch M W, Rand M J, Standford-Starr C A 1981 Conditions required for the inhibitory feedback loop in noradrenergic transmission. Nature 293: 62–65

Local hormones, inflammation and allergy

The word 'hormone', as introduced by Bayliss & Starling, referred to a chemical substance which was secreted, without benefit of duct, directly into the blood stream and which acted at long range, often slowly, on a distant organ or tissue. When the role of some chemical substances in nervous transmission was established, **neurotransmitters** were held to be different from hormones in that they were released by neurons, not endocrine glands, and acted rapidly, briefly and at short range on an adjacent neuron or target cell. The fact that noradrenaline was released peripherally from the adrenal medulla as well as from sympathetic neurons, and thus could function as either hormone or neurotransmitter, indicated that the categories were not mutually exclusive and presaged a change in the conceptual framework within which chemical mediators were considered. Subsequently it was realized that some substances which were not neurotransmitters nevertheless acted briefly at short range on adjacent target cells (e.g. histamine from mast cells) and these were classed as **local hormones**. However, it has become clear that some of these 'local hormones' whose site, occurrence and locus of action had been considered to be peripheral (e.g. serotonin in platelets) were also neurotransmitters in the CNS. In addition it has been realized that neurons in what is indubitably a part of the CNS—the hypothalamus—release peptides and possibly amino acids into the blood stream for action on 'distant' target cells. Some of these peptides have turned out to be very similar to, or in some cases identical with, substances secreted by non-nervous tissues in peripheral organs such as the pancreas and the gastrointestinal tract. Furthermore, some of the peptides previously considered only as peripheral hormones, such as insulin

or glucagon, are now known to occur in neurons in both the central and autonomic nervous system. (In the absence of clear evidence of a direct role in synaptic transmission some peptides found in neurons are referred to as **neuromodulators** rather than neurotransmitters; see Chapter 19.) More recently it has been proposed that in the anterior pituitary, an endocrine gland, the cells may communicate with, and influence each other at short range in a manner reminiscent of the interaction of neurons.

Further complexity has been added to the problem of defining these terms by the finding that many of the substances usually considered as being hormones (insulin, glucagon, corticotrophin, chorionic gonadotrophin, somatostatin), as well as several regarded as neurotransmitters (acetylcholine, catecholamines) are found in unicellular organisms such as protozoa and bacteria. Many of these agents do not only occur in lower forms of life, they are also known to have biological effects in them. For example, adrenaline stimulates adenylate cyclase in protozoa—an effect blocked by propranolol; and opioid peptides alter the behaviour of amoebae—an effect blocked by naloxone.

It seems to be the case that the basic biochemical mechanisms involved in cell-to-cell communication arose very early in evolution and have been highly conserved; and that in higher organisms these basic elements have been adapted for more complex communication requirements. Clearly there is a variety of different ways in which the cells in the mammalian organism 'communicate' with each other by means of chemical messengers or mediators. Whether a cell responds to a chemical message will depend partly on whether it expresses the appropriate receptor and partly on the cell's situation, i.e. on whether it is easily accessible to the perfusing plasma or in close apposition to a neuron or a secreting cell. The chemical messengers themselves may be used differently in different circumstances.

It is evident that in classifying the physiologically active chemical substances in man, the original concept of separate categories of hormones and transmitters, as defined originally, must now be abandoned in favour of the idea of a spectrum of agents in which there are substances which are predominantly neurotransmitters at one end (e.g. acetylcholine) and substances which are predominantly hormones at the other (e.g. the sex steroids) and a range of substances in between, in which these characteristics may overlap. Many of these intermediate substances may be considered to be **local hormones** or **paracrine** secretions.

In the first part of this chapter consideration will be given to the ways in which cells and chemical messengers may interact when the body is under threat from an invading pathogen (disease-causing organism; see Chapter 28) or other type of injury. The process to be considered is **the inflammatory reaction**. When the process has been outlined, the chemical substances, which are thought to act as local hormones in this context will be dealt with in more detail. It should be noted that some mediators which are important in the context of inflammation, (e.g. histamine or the prostaglandins) also have other functions in the body and these functions will be mentioned separately. Drugs which modify the action of both the cells and mediators involved in these reactions are dealt with in the succeeding chapter.

THE INFLAMMATORY REACTION AND THE IMMUNE RESPONSE

A mammalian organism which has to deal with an invasion by a pathogen can call on an extensive array of powerful defensive reactions. That these reactions are normally successful is shown by the fact that when they are lacking or are suppressed by drugs, organisms not normally regarded as pathogens can, and often do cause disease. However, in some circumstances these reactions may be brought into play, inappropriately, against innocuous substances from outside the body (e.g. pollen) or against the tissues of the body itself, and the defensive reactions themselves may then produce damage and may indeed constitute part of the disease process (e.g. in asthma or rheumatoid arthritis). It is for these sorts of conditions that anti-inflammatory or in some cases, immunosuppressive drugs, may be required. Chemical mediators control or modulate these defensive reactions of the host, and an understanding of the action of drugs which affect inflammation and also the development of further anti-inflammatory agents, depends on an appreciation of the way in which the cells and the mediators of inflammation interact with each other. An outline of these interactions is given below. The outline will of necessity be a very general one, but a specific example to which most of the events described will apply, is a local staphylococcal infection causing an acute inflammatory reaction, i.e. a boil. The reactions which do not involve an immunological mechanism will be described first and then consideration will be given to how these reactions are sharpened and made more selective by the **specific immunological response**.

At the macroscopic level the characteristics of the inflammatory response are that the area is reddened, swollen, hot and painful and that there is interference with, or alteration of function. Examples of this latter characteristic are the spasm of bronchiolar smooth muscle which occurs in asthma or the restriction of movement in an inflamed joint.

In terms of what is happening within the tissues, the changes can be divided into vascular and cellular events.

VASCULAR EVENTS

The vascular events involve an initial dilatation of the blood vessels with increased blood flow, followed by slowing and then stasis of the blood, an increase in the permeability of the postcapillary venules and exudation of fluid. The vasodilatation is brought about by various mediators produced by the interaction of the microorganism with tissue cells (histamine, prostaglandins E_2 and I_2, platelet-activating factor etc). Some of these mediators (e.g. histamine, platelet-activating factor) are also responsible for the initial phase of increased vascular permeability. Neutrophil association with the walls of the post-capillary venules contributes to the later more prolonged phase of increased vascular permeability (see below).

The fluid exudate contains a variety of mediators which influence the cells in the vicinity and the blood vessels themselves. These include the components for three enzyme cascades; the complement system, the kinin system and the coagulation system.

The **complement system** is an enzyme cascade consisting of nine major components designated C1 to C9 (see: Roitt, 1984 for more detailed treatment of this topic). Activation of the cascade can be initiated by substances derived from microorganisms such as yeast cell walls, endotoxins, etc. This pathway of activation is termed 'the alternate pathway'. (The 'classical pathway' involves antibody and will be dealt with below.) One of the main events is the enzymic splitting of C3 which gives rise to various peptides, one of which, C3a (termed an 'anaphylatoxin'), can stimulate mast cells to secrete chemical mediators, and can also directly stimulate the smooth muscle of the bronchi or gastrointestinal tract, while another, C3b (termed an 'opsonin'), can attach to the surface of a microorganism and facilitate its ingestion by white blood cells. Enzymic action on a later component, C5, releases C5a which, in addition to causing release of

mediators from mast cells, is powerfully chemotactic (i.e. acts as a chemical attractant) for white blood cells and activates them. The actions of these complement-derived mediators is considered below and is dealt with in more detail by Roitt (1984). Assembly of the last components in the sequence (C5 to C9) on the cell membranes of certain bacteria or cells leads to the lysis of these bacteria or cells (see Chapter 28). Thus complement can mediate the destruction of invading bacteria or damage multicellular parasites, but it may sometimes cause injury to the host's own cells. The main event in the complement cascade—the splitting of C3—can also be brought about directly, by the principal enzymes of the coagulation and fibrinolytic cascades, thrombin and plasmin, respectively, and by enzymes released from white blood cells.

The **coagulation system** is described in Chapter 12. The end product is fibrin. When fibrin formation occurs in the tissues during a host/pathogen interaction it may serve to limit the extension of the infection. Furthermore, as explained above, the main enzyme of the coagulation system, thrombin, can activate the complement system, and the first enzyme in the extrinsic pathway of the coagulation system—Hageman factor or Factor XII—is also involved in the activation of both the kinin system (Fig. 8.1) and the fibrinolytic system.

The **kinin system** is another enzyme cascade which results in the production of potential medi-

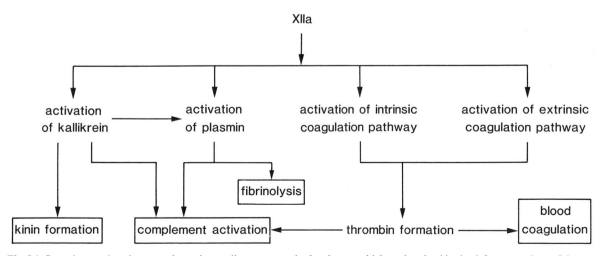

Fig. 8.1 Some interactions between the major mediator systems in the plasma, which are involved in the defence reactions of the host. XIIa is 'activated Hageman Factor' and is the initial plasma factor in the coagulation cascade (see Chapter 12). When plasma leaks out into the tissues as a result of increased vascular permeability, Factor XII is activated by contact with a negatively charged surface such as is provided by collagen, bacterial lipopolysaccharides (see Chapter 30), urate crystals etc.

ators of inflammation—the kinins—which have potent effects on blood vessels causing dilatation and increased vascular permeability. This system is dealt with in more detail below (see 'bradykinin' p. 198).

CELLULAR EVENTS

Some of the cells involved in the inflammatory reaction are already present in the tissues—the mast cells and tissue mononuclear phagocytes—while others gain access to the site from the blood. These latter, the **leucocytes** or white cells of the blood, are actively motile cells and are of two classes:

1. The **polymorphonuclear cells** (cells with many-lobed nuclei) which are subdivided into **neutrophils**, **eosinophils** and **basophils** on the basis of the staining properties of the granules in their cytoplasm. (These cells are also referred to as granulocytes.)
2. The **mononuclear** cells (or cells with single-bodied nuclei) which are subdivided into **monocytes** and **lymphocytes**.

Mast cells

These cells are capable of secreting or generating mediators which have the capacity to modify vascular and cellular reactions as well as to affect some of the plasma factors. Mast cells have, as constituents of the cell membrane, receptors both for a special class of antibody (IgE) and for complement components C3a and C5a. They can be activated to secrete mediators through these receptors and also by direct physical damage.

The main substance released by the mast cells is **histamine**, a paracrine secretion or local hormone (see p. 187). Through receptors which are termed H_1 receptors, histamine can dilate blood vessels, increase vascular permeability and contract smooth muscle such as that in the bronchioles and the gut. Histamine may, in addition, modulate the responses of other cells, possibly through other receptors—H_2 receptors. The mast cells also release **heparan** or **heparin** which has anticoagulant properties (see Chapter 12).

The polymorphonuclear leucocytes (polymorphs)

These are the first of the blood leucocytes to enter

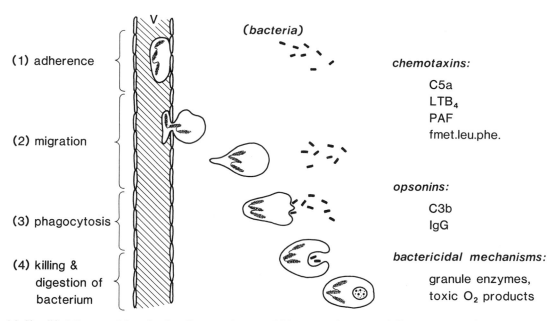

Fig. 8.2 Simplified diagram of the role of mediators and neutrophil leucocytes in an acute inflammatory reaction. V = post-capillary venule; LTB_4 = leukotriene B_4; PAF = platelet activating factor; C5a and C3b are complement components; f met.leu.phe is a bacterial peptide; IgG = immunoglobulin G. For details, see text.

the area of the inflammatory reaction (Fig. 8.2). They actively migrate through the wall of the vessel to the site of the invading pathogen, attracted by chemicals ('chemotaxins') released by the microorganism (e.g. the tripeptide formyl-met-leu-phe) or produced locally e.g. C5a (see above), or leukotriene B_4 (see p. 196). The chemotaxins may stimulate the cell to produce its own leukotriene B_4 which augments chemotaxis. Neutrophils, especially, are capable of engulfing, killing and digesting microorganisms. They, and the eosinophils, have receptors on their membranes for the complement product, C3b, which acts as an 'opsonin', ie it forms a link between polymorph and invading bacterium. (A further link may be made by antibody; see below.) The microbicidal process involves activation of the 'respiratory burst' of the leucocyte, during which there is a marked increase in O_2 consumption and the generation of superoxide, hydrogen peroxide and other toxic oxygen products. Neutrophils contain within their granules, a variety of digestive enzymes which can break down virtually all the components of most microorganisms. Some of these enzymes work optimally at the low pH found in lysosomes. Neutrophils may in some circumstances actively secrete the contents of their granules, among which are different enzymes (e.g. neutral proteases) which work optimally at the neutral pH of body fluids and which may be involved in the microbicidal process. These enzymes, when released extracellularly, can cleave complement components and start the kinin cascade. Thus the participation of the neutrophils provides another method for activating these powerful systems of mediator production. When exocytosis is inappropriately triggered, these enzymes may cause unwanted damage to the host's own tissues.

There is interesting new evidence that in certain types of inflammation, neutrophils play an important part in increasing vascular permeability in the postcapillary venules. The mechanism by which they do this is not yet understood.

Stimulus/activation coupling in the neutrophil involves the turnover of polyphosphoinositides and an increase in cytosolic calcium (see Chapter 1).

Eosinophils have capacities which are more important in the defence against helminths than against microorganisms. Basophils are very similar in many respects to mast cells.

Monocytes

The monocytes enter the area at a later stage of the reaction, several hours after the polymorphs. In the tissues they become transformed into macrophages (literally 'big eaters', as compared to the polymorphs which were originally called microphages or 'little eaters'). Similar cells, all belonging to the mononuclear phagocyte system, are present in various tissues, probably all derived originally from blood-borne monocytes. In some tissues they have a role in presenting antigenic material to lymphocytes in the initiation of an immune response. In the area of inflammation they engulf tissue debris and dead cells as well as microorganisms. They can secrete not only lysosomal enzymes, but complement components, eicosanoids (see below), the 'tissue factor' which starts the extrinsic pathway of the coagulation cascade (see page 282), interferon, a fibroblast-stimulating factor, pyrogens and factors such as interleukin-1 which modify the activities of lymphocytes. They are important in repair processes and when stimulated by glucocorticoids they secrete macrocortin, a polypeptide which inhibits the inflammatory response (see Chapter 16).

Platelets

Platelets are involved primarily in coagulation and thrombotic phenomena (see Chapter 12) but may play a part in inflammation. They secrete a variety of mediators, one of which, **platelet-derived growth factor**, is thought to be important in the repair processes which follow damage to blood vessels or an inflammatory response and which may be important in some cancers (p. 624).

MEDIATORS DERIVED FROM CELLS

Eicosanoids

When inflammatory cells are stimulated or damaged, another major mediator system is generated—the eicosanoids. These substances, which have a variety of different effects in an area of inflammation, are derived from arachidonic acid liberated from the phospholipids in the cell membrane. Arachidonic acid is metabolized by several pathways, the significance of which differs in different cell types. Most of the current anti-inflammatory drugs act, at least in part, by interfering with synthesis of the eicosanoids. Details of the synthesis and actions of the eicosanoids are given below (p. 192).

Platelet activating factor (PAF)

This is a lipid and is another very potent mediator derived from the phospholipids in the membranes of various cells by phospholipase A_2. Although called platelet activating factor (PAF), it has a variety of actions on other cell types, which are outlined below (p. 201).

Other inflammatory mediators derived from cells are *histamine* (p. 187) and *interleukin*-1 (p. 202).

THE SIGNIFICANCE OF THE SPECIFIC IMMUNOLOGICAL RESPONSE

The specific immunological response to an invading organism makes the host's defensive response very

much more specific and more efficient. It is a complex response, detailed consideration of which is beyond the scope of this book. A simplified version of the immune response will be given here, stressing only those aspects which are relevant for an understanding of anti-inflammatory and immunosuppressant drugs. (For more detailed coverage see Roitt, 1984.)

The key cells are the **lymphocytes** and the effector phase of the immune response consists of two components: a humoral (antibody-mediated) compotent and a cell-mediated component. Lymphocytes may be divided into two main groups: B cells which are responsible for antibody production, and T cells, which are responsible for cell-mediated reactions. T cells are also involved in complex ways with B cells and other T cells. They may assist these cells ('helper T cells' or 'T_h cells') or inhibit them ('suppressor T cells'). B lymphocytes tend to concentrate in quite different areas of the spleen and lymph nodes.

On first contact with an antigen (foreign protein

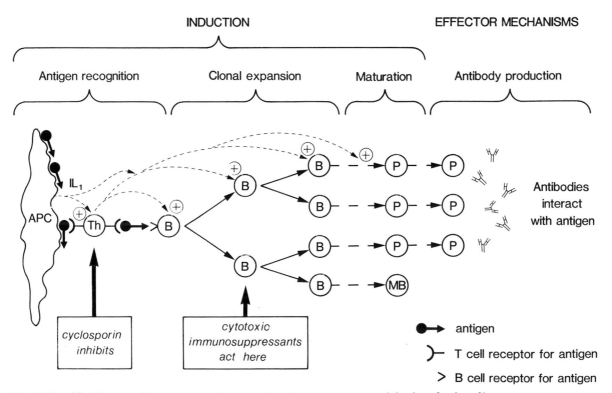

Fig. 8.3 Simplified diagram of induction of antibody-mediated immune response and the sites of action of immunosuppressant drugs. APC = antigen presenting cell; B = B lymphocyte; Th = T helper lymphocyte; IL_1 = Interleukin-1; P = plasma cell; MB = memory B cell. T cell factors induce proliferation and maturation of B cells.

or polysaccharide) the lymphocytes which 'recognize' it start to divide, giving rise to a large clone of cells which all have the capacity to recognize and respond to that antigen. These will either differentiate into plasma cells which will go on to produce antibodies (if they are B cells) or they will be involved in cell-mediated immune responses (if they are T cells). Others will form an increased population of antigen-sensitive *memory* cells and a second exposure to the antigen will then result in a much multiplied response.

The induction and regulation of the immune response

The events involved in the induction and regulation of the immune response are very complex and are not yet entirely understood. The interactions between cells and mediators are shown in simplified form in Figures 8.3 & 8.4.

Antigenic molecules introduced into the body reach the local lymph nodes via the lymphatics. In the nodes the antigen is presented to lymphocytes on the surface of large nonphagocytic dendritic cells called *antigen presenting cells* (APC). (Macrophages are also able to present antigen to lymphocytes, which they do after phagocytosing and processing these substances.) Dendritic cells and macrophages not only present antigen to lymphocytes but also release a peptide, **interleukin-1**, which facilitates the response of these cells. Interleukin-1 is an important mediator in certain sorts of chronic inflammation and drugs which modify its action are being vigorously sought in research programmes. Interleukin-1 is described in more detail below (p. 202).

The **induction of antibody-mediated responses** varies with the type of antigen. Some types of antigen are presented directly to B cells by antigen presenting cells. However, with most antigens, a complex cooperative process between T helper cells

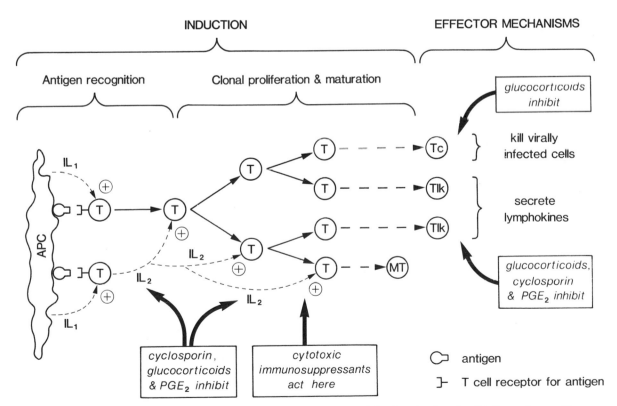

Fig. 8.4 Simplified diagram of induction of cell mediated immune response and the sites of action of anti-inflammatory and immunosuppressant drugs. APC = antigen presenting cell; T = T cell; Tc = cytotoxic T cell; Tlk = lymphokine-secreting T cell; IL_1 = interleukin-1; IL_2 = interleukin-2; MT = memory T cell; PG = prostaglandin.

and B cells is necessary. This latter process, which is illustrated in Figure 8.3, involves simultaneous recognition by T helper cells and B cells of different parts of the antigen molecule, by means of specific receptors, accompanied by the release of soluble factors from the T helper cell. These factors enable the B cells to proliferate and subsequently to mature into antibody-producing cells. Interleukin-1 is involved in both the direct B cell response and the T helper/B cell response to antigen.

In the **induction of cell-mediated immune responses**, T cells with specific receptors for antigen are activated, as described above, by the antigen presented on antigen presenting cells, plus the action of interleukin-1 (Fig. 8.4). These T cells then release a soluble factor, **interleukin-2**, which is a growth factor for T cells and causes proliferation of T cells, on which interleukin-2 receptors have been induced. The resulting effector T cells may be cytotoxic cells or lymphokine-producing cells (see below). Interleukin-2 may also be involved in B cell proliferation.

The **anti-inflammatory steroids** (see Chapter 16) and the immunosuppressive drug, **cyclosporin**, (see Chapter 9) act at the stage of interleukin-2 production and action. The cytotoxic **immunosuppressive drugs** (see Chapters 9 & 29) inhibit the proliferative phase of both B and T cells. Eicosanoids, which are described in detail below, are believed to play a part in controlling these processes. Thus prostaglandins of the E series inhibit lymphocyte proliferation, probably by inhibiting the release of interleukin-2. Leukotriene B_4 (see p. 196) may also be implicated in the regulation of T cell activation.

The effector phase of the immune response

The humoral immune response: antibodies and B lymphocytes

Antibodies are γ-globulins (immunoglobulins) which have two functions: (1) to 'recognize' and interact specifically with particular antigens, i.e. proteins or polysaccharides foreign to the host; and (2) to activate one or more of the host's defence systems. The foreign substances may be part of an invading organism (the coat of a bacterium) or may be released by such an organism (a bacterial toxin) or they may be materials introduced experimentally in the laboratory in studies of the immune response (e.g. the injection of egg albumin into the guinea pig).

In simple terms, an antibody is a Y-shaped molecule in which the arms of the Y (the 'Fab' portions) are the recognition sites for specific antigens and the stem of the Y (the 'Fc' portion) activates host defence mechanisms. B lymphocytes, the cells which are responsible for antibody production, 'recognize' foreign molecules by means of receptors on their surfaces. The mammalian organism possesses a vast number of different antibodies with recognition sites for different antigens. Thus antibodies can recognize and react with virtually all foreign molecules which the host is likely to encounter.

That the ability to make antibodies has survival value is evident if one considers what happens when this ability is absent. Some children are born without this ability and they suffer repeated infections—pneumonia, skin infections, tonsillitis, etc. Before the days of antibiotics they died in early childhood.

There are five classes of antibodies—IgG, IgM, IgE, IgA and IgD—which differ from each other in certain structural respects.

Antibodies markedly improve the host's response to an invading pathogen. Apart from their ability to interact *directly* with invading pathogens or with the toxins they liberate, thus impairing their capacity for damage, antibodies can multiply many-fold the effectiveness and specificity of the host's defence reactions in several ways:

1. *Antibodies and the complement sequence.* Antibodies may react with antigenic material on the pathogen and the antigen-antibody reaction leads to the exposure on the Fc portion of a binding site for complement which results in activation of the complement sequence with its biological repercussions—production of anaphylatoxin (C3a), chemotactic factor (C5a) and opsonin (C3b) and eventually the development of lytic potential. This route to C3 activation is referred to as 'the classical pathway' because it was investigated first. (The route outlined on page 179, initiated by microbial products such as endotoxin, is referred to as the 'alternate pathway' and was very probably developed much earlier in evolution.) The classical pathway provides an especially selective way of activating complement in response to a particular

pathogen—the antigen/antibody reaction which initiates it constituting a highly specific recognition event. The lytic property of complement may be used therapeutically: monoclonal antibodies and complement together may be used to cleanse bone marrow of cancer cells as an adjunct to chemotherapy or radiotherapy (see Chapter 29).

2. *Antibodies and the ingestion of bacteria.* Antibodies may attach to the particular antigenic moieties on the surface of microorganisms 'recognized' by their Fab portions, leaving the Fc part of the molecule projecting. Phagocytic cells (neutrophils and macrophages) have receptors on their membranes for these projecting Fc portions of antibody. Antibody thus forms a very specific link between microorganism and phagocyte and in addition is even more effective as an opsonin in facilitating ingestion (phagocytosis) than C3b (see Fig. 8.2).

3. *Antibodies and cellular cytotoxicity.* In some cases, e.g. in the case of parasitic worms, the invader may be too big to be ingested by phagocytes. *In vitro* studies show that antibody may still form a link between parasite and the host's white cells (in this case, eosinophils), which are then able to damage or kill the parasite by surface or extracellular actions. Something similar can be shown to occur *in vitro* with tumour cells as the targets and lymphocytes or neutrophils as the killer cells. Lymphocytes which are active in this type of effect do not seem to be typical B or T cells and are referred to as 'K' cells ('killer' cells).

4. *Antibodies and mast cells or basophils.* Mast cells and basophils have receptors for certain sorts of antibody (IgE), which can thus become attached to the cell membrane. When antigen reacts with this cell-fixed antibody, the whole panoply of pharmacologically active mediators is secreted. A complex reaction such as this, found widely throughout the animal kingdom, is unlikely to have been developed and retained during evolution unless it had survival value for the host. However, its precise biological significance in defence is not clear, though it may be of importance in association with responses involving the eosinophils, in reactions against parasitic worms. When inappropriately triggered by substances not inherently damaging to the host, it is implicated in certain types of allergic reactions (see below).

The cell-mediated immune response: T lymphocytes

The lymphocytes involved in cell-mediated responses are cytotoxic T cells (Tc) and T lymphocytes which generate and release lymphokines (Tlk cells) (see Fig. 8.4). Tc cells are killer cells, killing virally-infected host cells and thus limiting the proliferation of the viruses. The Tlk cells produce lymphokines which are complex protein mediators that have a number of different actions. Some lymphokines are chemotactic for neutrophils and macrophages, others cause proliferation of other lymphocytes (interleukin-2 is one of these), while some produce increased vascular permeability. One can 'activate' macrophages, i.e. render them more effective in killing certain microorganisms, such as the tubercle bacillus, which would otherwise survive within these cells—this is 'macrophage activating factor' or MAF which may be identical with γ-interferon (see below).

Individuals with T cell deficiencies are particularly susceptible to viral infections and infections with those bacteria, such as the tubercle bacillus, which can survive within the host's cells.

The specific immunological response, cell-mediated or humoral, is thus superimposed on the immunologically non-specific vascular and cellular reactions described previously, making them not only more effective but much more selective for particular invading organisms. An important aspect of the specific immunological response is that the clone of lymphocytes which are programmed to respond to the antigens of the invading organism is greatly expanded after the first contact with the organism. Thus subsequent exposure results in a greatly accelerated and more effective response. In some cases the response becomes so prompt and so efficient that, after the first exposure which initiates the specific immune response, some microorganisms can virtually never gain a foothold in the host's tissues again. Immunization procedures make use of this fact.

Unwanted inflammatory and immune responses

The very effective and complex responses described above may, in some circumstances, be inappropriately triggered by substances which are innocuous. When this happens it becomes necessary to use anti-inflammatory or immunosuppressive drugs. Unwanted immune responses are termed *allergic* or *hypersensitivity reactions* and have been classified into four types:

Type I. Immediate or anaphylactic hypersensitivity

This occurs when material which is not, in itself noxious (such as grass pollen, products from dead house dust mites, certain food stuffs, or some drugs) evokes the production of antibodies of the IgE type, which fix to mast cells. Subsequent contact(s) with the material causes the release of histamine from mast cells. In addition spasmogenic eicosanoids (see p. 192) may be produced. Eosinophils are thought to play an important part in this type of hypersensitivity. Other cells, polymorphs, macrophages or platelets may be involved and other mediators such as platelet activating factor may be produced. The effects may be localized to the bronchial tree (the initial phase of asthma), the nose (hay fever), the skin (urticaria) or sometimes the gastrointestinal tract. The reaction may be more generalized and produce anaphylactic shock.

Roughly speaking, this type of hypersensitivity represents mainly inappropriate deployment of the processes outlined above in section 4 of 'the humoral immune response' (see p. 185). Some important unwanted effects of drugs are due to anaphylactic hypersensitivity responses (see Chapter 36).

Type II. Antibody-dependent cytotoxic hypersensitivity

This occurs when the mechanisms outlined above [in section 3 of 'the humoral immune response'] are directed against cells within the host, which are or which appear to be foreign, e.g. after incompatible blood transfusions or the alteration of the host's cells by drugs. Examples of this latter class are the alteration by drugs of polymorphs which may lead to agranulocytosis (see Chapter 36) and of platelets which may lead to thrombocytopoenic purpura. The antigens form part of the surfaces of these cells and evoke antibodies. The antigen-antibody reaction may start the complement sequence (with its repercussions) or may provide a basis for the attack by killer cells.

Type III. Complex-mediated hypersensitivity

This may occur in certain circumstances when antibody reacts with *soluble* antigen. The antigen/antibody complexes can activate complement (see above) or attach to mast cells and stimulate the release of mediators (see above). An experimental example of a type III reaction is the Arthus reaction, which occurs if a foreign protein is injected subcutaneously into a rabbit or guinea pig which has a high concentration of circulating antibody against that protein. The area becomes red and swollen 3–8 hours later. This is because the antigen-antibody complexes settle in the small blood vessels, complement is activated, neutrophils are attracted and activated (by C5a), generating toxic O_2 products and secreting enzymes. Mast cells are also stimulated by C3a to release mediators. Something of this sort may be involved in late asthmatic reactions occurring 7–8 hours after contact with antigen. Damage caused by this process may be involved in certain types of kidney and arterial disease. Serum sickness is another example of a type III reaction.

Type IV. Cell-mediated hypersensitivity

The prototype of this reaction is the tuberculin reaction—the reaction seen when proteins derived from cultures of the tubercle bacillus are injected into the skin of a person who is sensitized to the bacillus. After 24 hours the area becomes reddened and thickened. An 'inappropriate' cell-mediated immune response (see above) has been stimulated and there has been an infiltration of mononuclear cells. Lymphokines are thought to be important mediators of this reaction. Cell-mediated hypersensitivity is the basis of the reaction seen with certain insect bites (ticks, mosquitoes) and is implicated in some rashes (e.g. in mumps and measles). It is thought to be involved in rheumatoid arthritis, possibly in the late phase of asthma and is very important in the skin reactions to drugs or industrial chemicals (see Chapter 36). In this latter case, the chemical combines with proteins in the skin to form the 'foreign' substance which evokes the cell-mediated immune response. A substance acting in this way is called a *hapten*.

Many **autoimmune** diseases (diseases caused by the host's immune system attacking his own tissue) are due to inappropriately deployed cell-mediated immune responses and immunosuppressive drugs may be used as part of the treatment.

The outcome of the inflammatory response

After this outline of the specific immune response one needs to return to a consideration of the host-pathogen interaction—the local acute inflammatory response. It should be clear that this may consist of the immunologically non-specific vascular and cellular events described initially, together with a varying degree of participation of the specific immunological response (either humoral or cell-mediated), the degree depending on several factors such as the nature of the pathogen and the organ or tissue involved. What is the result of the interaction? If the pathogen has been dealt with adequately there may be complete healing and the tissue may be virtually normal thereafter. If there has been damage (death of cells, pus formation, ulceration) repair may be necessary and may result in scarring. If the pathogen persists, the condition may proceed to *chronic* inflammation—a slow smouldering reaction which continues for months or even years and involves both destruction of tissue as well as local proliferation of cells and connective tissue. The principal cell types found in areas of chronic inflammation are **mononuclear** cells and abnormal cells derived from macrophages. There is usually also greatly increased activity of **fibroblasts** which lay down fibrous tissue. The response to some microorganisms has the characteristic of chronicity from the start. Examples are syphilis, tuberculosis and leprosy. In some chronic inflammatory conditions of great clinical importance, such as rheumatoid arthritis, the exact cause is not known, but inappropriately deployed immune responses are considered to be implicated.

How important are the chemical mediators in the inflammatory reaction?

In the above simplified outline of inflammation the role of the various chemical mediators has been stated as fact. This must now be qualified. In the highly complex repertoire of reactions which constitutes the host response to invading pathogen, the precise role of the different mediators has not been completely clarified. Adequate assessment of the role of a putative mediator requires that the substance considered should fulfil certain criteria, modified from those outlined by Dale in 1933 for neurotransmitters:

1. The substance should be generated or released in appropriate amounts during the response.
2. The substance should produce the effect specified both *in vivo* and *in vitro*. (It is clear that when multiple mediators are involved in a response it will be difficult to establish that a substance has fulfilled this criterion *in vivo*).
3. The enzymes necessary for synthesis should be present at the appropriate site.
4. A mechanism for stopping the action of the substance should exist.
5. Drugs which interfere with the action or with the synthesis, storage, release or breakdown of the substance should produce the predicted alteration of the response.
6. Receptors for the substance should be demonstrable on or in the relevant cells.
7. Experimental techniques or clinical conditions which result in deficiencies of the substance or of the synthesizing or metabolizing enzymes involved, should result in the appropriate increase or decrease of the response.

The mediators of pharmacological significance will be described below with a brief assessment of the extent to which they fulfil the above criteria. Drugs which affect the inflammatory and immune responses will be considered in the context of this approach.

MEDIATORS OF INFLAMMATION AND ALLERGY

HISTAMINE

Most of the early studies on the biological actions of this amine were carried out by Sir Henry Dale and his colleagues. Dale had shown that a local anaphylactic reaction (a Type I or 'immediate hypersensitivity reaction' see above) was the result of an antigen/antibody reaction in sensitized tissue and he subsequently demonstrated that histamine could largely mimic both the *in vitro* and *in vivo* anaphylactic responses. Feldberg and his co-workers showed that histamine was indeed released when antigen interacted with sensitized tissues, and later Riley and West identified the tissue mast cell as the main store of body histamine. After the first generation of antihistamine drugs was produced, following the work of Bovet and his co-workers, it became clear, as a result of careful quantitative studies by Schild, that there were two types of histamine receptor in the body and that this first generation of antihistamine drugs affected only one type—the H_1 receptors—while the second type, termed H_2 receptors, important particularly in gastric acid secretion, were unaffected. Black and his colleagues, following up this classification proposed by Schild, developed the second generation of antihistamine drugs—the H_2 receptor antagonists.

Synthesis and storage

Histamine is a basic amine, 2-(4-imidazolyl)-ethylamine, and is formed from histidine by histidine decarboxylase (Fig. 8.5). It is found in most tissues of the body but is present in high concentrations in the lungs and the skin and in particularly high concentration in the gastrointestinal tract. At the cellular level it is found largely in mast cells and basophils, but non-mast cell histamine occurs in the brain where it may be implicated in the activity of histaminergic neurons (see Chapter 19). The high histamine content of the gastrointestinal tract is due partly to the large number of mast cells in that tissue and partly due to the presence of histamine in mast-cell-like histaminocytes in acid-secreting glands in the stomach (see Chapter 15). In some species, such as the rabbit, histamine occurs in platelets.

The basophil content of the tissues is negligible and basophils form only 0.5% of circulating white blood cells. But in certain types of delayed hypersensitivity reaction (e.g. with contact allergens, tick bites, skin allografts, vaccinia virus) basophils may constitute 20–60% of infiltrating cells.

In mast cells and basophils, histamine is held in intracellular granules in a complex with an acidic protein and a glycosaminoglycan. In most tissues the mast cell glycosaminoglycan is a heparin of high molecular weight, termed macroheparin. As explained in Chapter 12, heparin has a strong electronegative charge. The metachromatic staining of mast cell granules is due to the interaction of

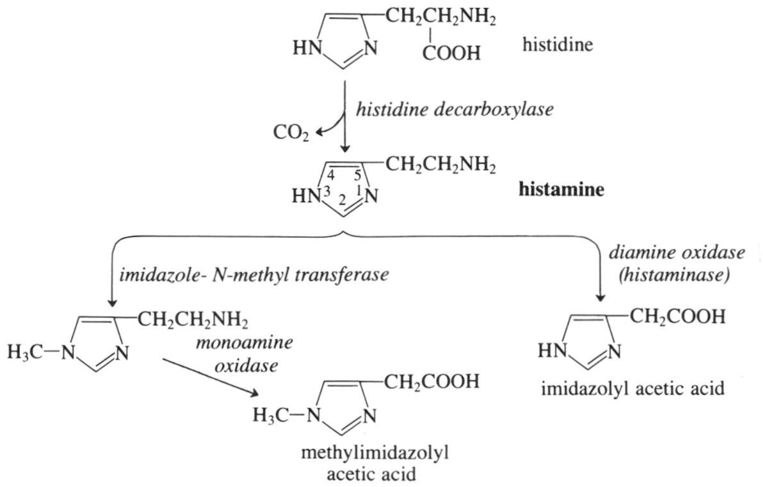

Fig. 8.5 Structure, biosynthesis and metabolism of histamine.

heparin with basic dyes. The acidic protein and the glycosaminoglycan comprise the matrix of the granule in which the basic molecule histamine is held by ionic forces and from which it can be released in exchange for sodium ions when the granule is exposed to the extracellular environment. The molar ratio for histamine, heparin and protein in mast cells is $1:3:6$ and the histamine content is approximately $0.1–0.2$ pmol per mast cell and 0.01 pmol per basophil.

Histamine release

Histamine is released from mast cells by a secretory process during inflammatory or allergic reactions. As explained earlier in this chapter, stimuli include the interaction of complement components C3a and C5a with specific receptors on the cell surface or the interaction of antigen with cell-fixed IgE antibodies. The secretory process is initiated by a rise in intracellular calcium. This follows cross-linking of receptors which causes an increase in calcium permeability and a release of calcium from intracellular stores. Some peptides, such as substance P, release histamine, though the concentrations required are fairly high. Various basic drugs such as morphine and tubocurarine and polybasic substances such as compound 48/80 (used in laboratory experiments) are effective histamine-releasers.

Agents which increase cAMP formation (e.g. β-adrenoceptor agonists; see Chapter 7) inhibit histamine secretion, so it is possible that cAMP-dependent protein kinase is an intra-cellular 'braking' mechanism. Glucocorticoids have very little effect on secretion of histamine for mast cells but inhibit basophil secretion (see Chapter 16).

After secretion, the concentration of histamine in the immediate vicinity of a mast cell may be as high as $10^{-4}–10^{-3}$ M though this concentration will decrease rapidly as a result of diffusion. There is evidence that released histamine exerts a negative feedback control on basophil secretion, by an action on H_2 receptors—the ED_{50} for this effect being approximately 10^{-6} M. Replenishment of the histamine content of mast cell or basophil is a slow process which may take days or weeks whereas turnover of histamine in the gastric 'histaminocyte' is very rapid.

Histamine may be metabolized by histaminase (which is a diamine oxidase) or by the methylating enzyme imidazole-N-methyltransferase (Fig. 8.5).

Sensitivity to the effects of histamine varies between tissues and between species. The guinea pig is very sensitive and the mouse very insensitive to this agent. Human sensitivity lies between these two extremes.

Mechanism of action of histamine

Histamine produces its action by an effect on specific histamine receptors which are of two types, distinguished by means of specific antagonist drugs.

H_1 receptors are found in human and guinea pig bronchial muscle and in guinea pig ileum, and stimulation causes contraction of the muscle. The histamine receptors in these different tissues can be shown to have the same affinity for H_1 antagonists such as mepyramine, the antagonism being competitive and specific (see Chapter 1 and below). A range of compounds have stimulant actions on H_1 receptors, the order of potency being histamine > 2 thiazolylethylamine > 2 methyl histamine > betahistine > 2-pyridylethylamine (Fig. 8.6).

H_2 receptors are found in the stomach, in rat uterus and in the heart and stimulation causes respectively, gastric acid secretion, relaxation of the uterus and increased activity of the heart. The receptors involved have a common affinity for the H_2 antagonists, such as cimetidine (see below) and antagonism by these compounds is competitive and specific. H_2 agonists produce the expected dose/response effects, the order of potency being impromidine > histamine > dimaprit or 4-methylhistamine > 2-methyl-histamine > betazole (Fig. 8.6).

Activation of H_1 receptors causes an increase in cytosolic calcium while activation of H_2 receptors causes stimulation of adenylate cyclase (see Chapter 1).

Actions of histamine

1. *Smooth muscle effects*. Histamine causes contractions of the smooth muscle of the ileum, the bronchi and bronchioles, and the uterus. The effect on the ileum is not as marked in man as it is in the guinea pig and the response of this latter tissue to hist-

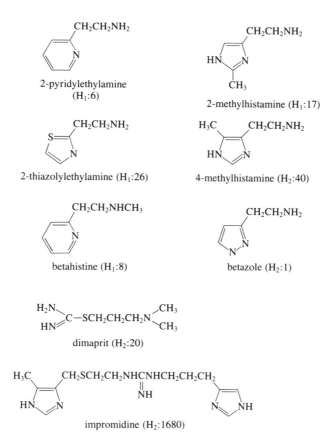

Fig. 8.6 Structures of some H_1 and H_2 agonists. The figures in brackets give approximate potency on guinea pig ileum for H_1 agonists, and on rat gastric acid secretion for H_2 agonists, taking histamine as 100 in each case.

amine is the basis of the standard bioassay for histamine, familiar to all students of experimental pharmacology. Bronchiolar constriction by histamine is also more marked in guinea pigs than in man, though histamine may be one of many factors causing reduction of air-flow in bronchial asthma (see Chapter 13). Uterine muscle in most species is contracted. In humans this is only significant if a massive release of histamine is produced by anaphylaxis during pregnancy, since this may lead to abortion.

2. *Cardiovascular effects.* The action of histamine on the cardiovascular system depends not only on the species but also on the way it is given. If infused slowly intravenously or injected subcutaneously it causes flushing of the skin and a rise in skin temperature; there is increased blood flow to the limbs, a rise in heart rate and cardiac output, but not necessarily any fall in blood pressure. A single rapid intravenous bolus injection, on the other hand, causes a fall in blood pressure due to vasodilatation and a rise in CSF pressure accompanied by an intense headache. The vasodilatation and fall in blood pressure is due to stimulation of both H_1 and H_2 receptors in resistance vessels, the contribution of each receptor type varying in different species; H_1 receptor effects predominate in man. Vasodilatation in some species (e.g. the rat) may be endothelium-dependent (p. 258).

The cardiac effects are due to a combination of a direct action on H_2 receptors in the heart, resulting in positive inotropic and chronotropic effects, and an indirect, reflex consequence of the fall in blood pressure.

If injected intradermally, histamine causes a reddening of the skin and a wheal, with a surrounding flare. This combination of effects was described by

Sir Thomas Lewis over 50 years ago and was termed 'the triple response'. The reddening is due to vasodilatation of the small arterioles and pre-capillary sphincters and the wheal due to increased permeability of the post-capillary venules. These effects are mainly H_1 receptor effects. (Contrary to popular belief, histamine does not increase capillary permeability. Its locus of action in increasing permeability is on the venules, as was demonstrated in careful, detailed experiments carried out by Majno & Palade and their colleagues in 1961.) The flare is due to an 'axon reflex'. This involves stimulation of sensory fibres and the passage of antidromic impulses through neighbouring branches of the same nerve with release of a vasodilator mediator, probably substance P (p. 552).

3. *Itching and pain*. These phenomena can be seen if histamine is injected into the skin or applied to a blister base and are due to stimulation of sensory nerve endings (p. 551).

4. *Gastric secretion*. Histamine stimulates the secretion of gastric acid by action on H_2 receptors. This topic is dealt with in Chapter 15.

It will be clear from the above that histamine is capable of producing many of the effects of inflammation and hypersensitivity—vasodilatation, increased vascular permeability, pain and the spasm of smooth muscle, and it has long been thought to be one of the major mediators of acute inflammation. It is surprising therefore that histamine H_1 antagonists do not have much effect on the acute inflammatory response per se; nor are they effective in a condition which has been con-

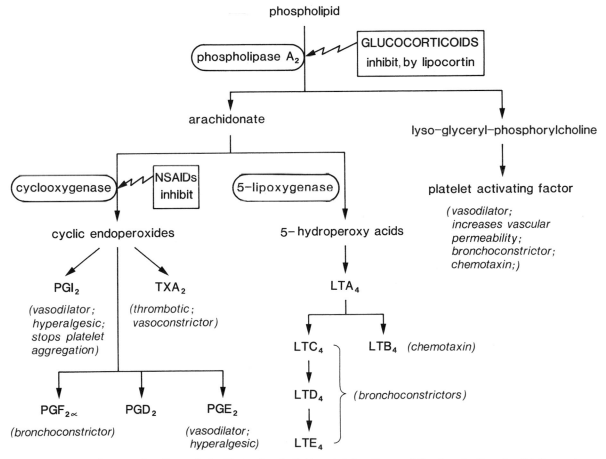

Fig. 8.7 Summary diagram of mediators derived from phospholipids and their actions, and the sites of action of anti-inflammatory drugs. The arachidonate metabolites are 'eicosanoids'. PG = prostaglandin; PGI_2 = prostacyclin; TX = thromboxane; LT = leukotriene; NSAIDs = non-steroidal anti-inflammatory drugs.

sidered to be a typical type 1 hypersensitivity reaction—the first phase of allergic bronchial asthma. On the basis of the criteria outlined earlier in this chapter it would appear that histamine is a mediator of critical importance only in some sorts of Type 1 hypersensitivity reaction such as allergic rhinitis and urticaria. The use of H_1 antagonists in these and other conditions is dealt with in Chapter 9. The use of H_2 antagonists is dealt with in Chapter 15.

EICOSANOIDS

These substances, unlike histamine, are not found preformed in the tissues. They are generated de novo from phospholipids in response to a surprisingly wide range of different stimuli and their presence has been detected in virtually every tissue in the body. They are implicated in the control of many physiological processes and they are among the most important mediators and modulators of the inflammatory reaction (Fig. 8.7). The non-steroidal anti-inflammatory drugs owe their actions largely if not entirely to inhibition of the biosynthesis of the eicosanoids. Anti-inflammatory steroids inhibit the synthesis of both the eicosanoids and platelet activating factor.

Interest in eicosanoids arose in the 1930s after reports that semen contained a substance which contracted uterine smooth muscle. The substance was believed to originate in the prostate and was named 'prostaglandin'. More than two decades later it became clear that prostaglandin was not just one substance but a whole family of compounds. In the 1960s two prostaglandins (**PGE & PGF$_{2\alpha}$**) were isolated in crystalline form and their structures elucidated by Bergstrom & Samuelsson. Subsequently several more prostaglandins were found to be generated in tissue and it was shown that these compounds were derived from **arachidonate**. In the early 1970s Vane advanced the hypothesis that inhibition of prostaglandin synthesis was the mechanism of action of aspirin-like drugs. Later intermediate substances in the synthetic pathway, two unstable cyclic endoperoxides, were isolated and identified and two rather different compounds derived from these intermediates were discovered—**thromboxane A$_2$** by Hamberg et al and

prostacyclin by Moncada & Vane and their colleagues. Later, the elucidation by Hamberg et al of a different pathway of arachidonate metabolism resulting in the production of the **leukotrienes** led to a further understanding of the role of arachidonate metabolites in physiological and pathological processes and eventually facilitated the solution to the long-standing problem of the chemical structure of the '**slow reacting substances**' produced during anaphylaxis (SRS-A). In 1982 Bergstrom, Samuelsson and Vane received the Nobel prize for Medicine for their work in this area.

The structure and biosynthesis of the eicosanoids

The principal eicosanoids are the prostaglandins, the thromboxanes and the leukotrienes. The term eicosanoid is derived from *eicosa*, indicating that there are 20 carbon atoms, and *enoic* meaning 'containing double bonds', because the main source of the eicosanoids is arachidonic acid, a 20-carbon unsaturated fatty acid containing four double bonds. However, a small proportion of these compounds may be derived from either dihomolinolenic acid or eicosapentaenoic acid. Arachidonic acid is found esterfied in the phospholipids

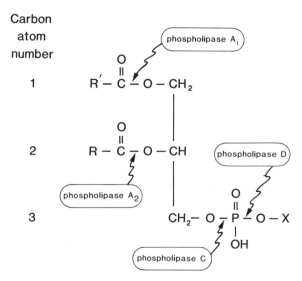

Fig. 8.8 Outline of structure of phospholipids and site of action of phospholipases. The numbering of the carbon atoms in the glycerol 'backbone' is given on the left. Unsaturated fatty acids, such as arachidonic acid, are usually located on the 2nd carbon. X = choline, ethanolamine, serine, inositol or hydrogen. This figure shows O-acyl residues on carbon atoms 1 and 2, but O-alkyl residues may occur (see Fig. 8.15).

(and to a lesser extent in the glycerides) of cell membranes and, as shown in Figure 8.8, within the phospholipids the arachidonic acid is usually located in the 2 position. The initial and rate-limiting step in eicosanoid synthesis is the liberation of arachidonate either in a one-step process involving phospholipase A_2, or in a two-step process involving first phospholipase C and then diacylglycerol lipase (Fig. 8.9). Note that phospholipase A_2 action can

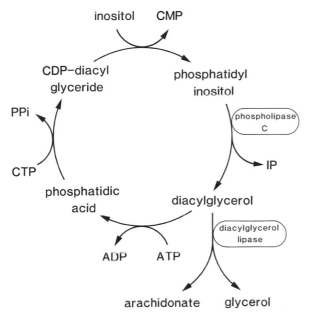

Fig. 8.9 Pathway of release of arachidonate from phosphatidylinositol (or polyphosphoinositides) by a two step mechanism involving pholipase C, then diacylglycerol lipase. IP = inositol phosphate.

give rise not only to arachidonic acid and thus the eicosanoids but also to lyso-glyceryl-phosphorylcholine (lyso-PAF) which is the precursor of another powerful mediator of inflammation—**platelet activating factor** (see Fig. 8.7 and below).

Stimuli which activate the enzymes which liberate arachidonic acid are many and diverse and vary with the cell type. Specific ligands for particular cells (thrombin in platelets, or C5a in neutrophils) may start the process, as may inflammatory mediators (bradykinin in fibroblasts, antigen-antibody reactions on mast cells) as well as general cell damage.

The anti-inflammatory action of the **glucocorticoids** is due mainly to the fact that they stimu-

late the production of a peptide mediator lipocortin, which inhibits phospholipase A_2 (p. 399).

The free arachidonic acid is metabolized by two main pathways—by a fatty acid cyclo-oxygenase which initiates the biosynthesis of the prostaglandins (together referred to as 'prostanoids') and thromboxanes, and by various lipoxygenases which initiate the synthesis of the leukotrienes (Figs. 8.10 & 8.11).

An autocatalytic mechanism is involved in the action of the cyclo-oxygenase enzyme. The enzyme first produces a lipid peroxide—the formation of a peroxy radical at C11 (compound 1, Fig. 8.10). This is followed by isomerization and introduction of a hydroperoxy group at C15, to give PGG_2 (compound 2, Fig. 8.10). It has been said that the lipid peroxide enhances the subsequent reactions of the enzyme and that its continued presence is needed to sustain cyclo-oxygenase activity. Thus, in the absence of sufficient lipid peroxide, little prostaglandin synthesis occurs, even if large amounts of substrate and enzyme are available. In normal conditions cellular peroxidases continuously reduce the lipid peroxide levels, ensuring that only moderate amounts of prostanoids are synthesized. In inflammatory reactions, stimulated phagocytic cells generate superoxide and hydrogen peroxide (see above) and these agents are believed to create an environment in which prostaglandin biosynthesis is favoured. (Reviewed by Lands 1981).

The anti-inflammatory action of the **nonsteroidal anti-inflammatory drugs** is due mainly to the fact that they inhibit the action of the fatty acid cyclo-oxygenase.

The products of the cyclo-oxygenase pathway: the prostanoids and thromboxanes

Cyclo-oxygenase is found bound to the endoplasmic reticulum and it catalyses the formation of **cyclic endoperoxides**, PGG_2 and PGH_2 (see Fig. 8.10). This reaction occurs in virtually every cell type in the body, but subsequent steps in arachidonate metabolism differ in different cells. In platelets the pathway leads to **thromboxane A_2** synthesis, in vascular endothelium it leads to **prostacyclin** synthesis and in macrophages mainly to synthesis of **prostaglandin E_2**.

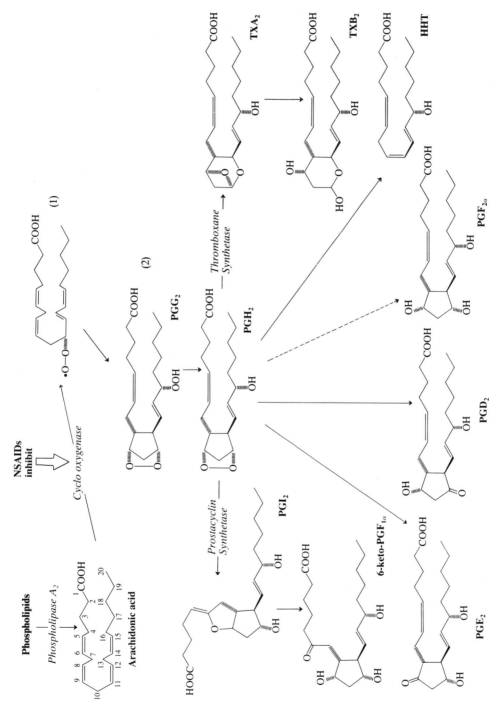

Fig. 8.10 The biosynthesis of prostaglandin, prostacyclin and thromboxane from arachidonate. Solid lines indicate known enzymic reactions and dotted lines, transformations not known to be enzymic. PG = prostaglandin; TX = thromboxane; NSAIDs = nonsteroidal anti-inflammatory drugs. (See text for details.)

The confusing nomenclature of the eicosanoids derives from the fact that the names of the first two prostaglandins were based on the separation procedure—**PGE** partitioned into **E**ther & **PGF** into the phosphate buffer (**F**osfat in Swedish). **PGA & PGB** (which may be artefacts) were so called because of their stability or otherwise in **acids** and **bases**. Thereafter other letters of the alphabet were filled in.

The subscript refers to the number of double bonds; thus PGE_2 has two double bonds. The Greek letter subscript, as in $PGF_{2\alpha}$ refers to the orientation of the hydroxyl on the ring. PGE_2, PGI_2, TXA_2 and $PGF_{2\alpha}$ are probably the most important products of the cyclo-oxygenase pathway.

is known to be released from mast cells by antigen/IgE interaction and to be a potent vasodilator.

The products of the lipoxygenase pathway

The lipoxygenases, which are found in lung, platelets and white blood cells, are soluble enzymes and are located in the cytosol. The biologically important products of their action are called leukotrienes: 'leuko' because they were found in white cells and 'trienes' because they contained a conjugated triene system of double bonds. The most important of this group of enzymes is the 5-lipoxygenase, which adds a hydroperoxy group to C5 in arachidonic acid (Fig. 8.11). The next step in the pathway is the

Table 8.1 The main actions of prostanoids and thromboxane*

Site	PGE_2	PGE_1	$PGF_{2\alpha}$	TXA_2
Blood vessels	Vasodilatation of arterioles, precapillary sphincters and venules.	Vasodilatation (as PGE_2)	Variable effects	Constriction
Platelets	Variable effect	Inhibition of aggregation		Aggregation
Kidney**	Vasodilatation, natriuresis and diuresis.			
Stomach	Inhibition of acid secretion. Increase mucous secretion.	As for PGE_2		
Intestine	Mainly spasmogenic. Increase secretions.	Mainly spasmogenic Increase secretions		
Lung	Vasoconstriction, bronchodilatation.	Vasodilatation, bronchodilatation	Vasoconstriction, bronchoconstriction	Bronchoconstriction
Heart	Positive inotropic.	Negative chronotropic		
Uterus (pregnant)†	Spasmogenic.	Spasmogenic	Spasmogenic	
Endocrine system	Release of GH, ACTH, LH and TSH from pituitary, steroids from adrenal cortex, insulin from pancreas. Causes luteolysis (see under $PGF_{2\alpha}$).		Release of gonadotrophins and prolactin. Causes luteolysis: i.e. inhibition of progesterone secretion and regression of *corpus luteum*.	
Hypothalamus	Pyretic	Pyretic		

* For PGI_2 see Chapter 12
** See Chapter 14
† See Chapter 17 for detail

Table 8.1 gives a general summary of the effects of the main prostaglandins. PGD_2 is not included in the table. It is found in the brain and in mast cells in various tissues. The full details of its functions and activities have not been elucidated, although it

synthesis of **leukotriene A_4 (LTA_4)**. This compound may be converted enzymically to LTB_4 and is also the precursor for an important class of cysteinyl-containing leukotrienes—LTC_4, LTD_4, LTE_4 and LTF_4. The first three of this latter group together

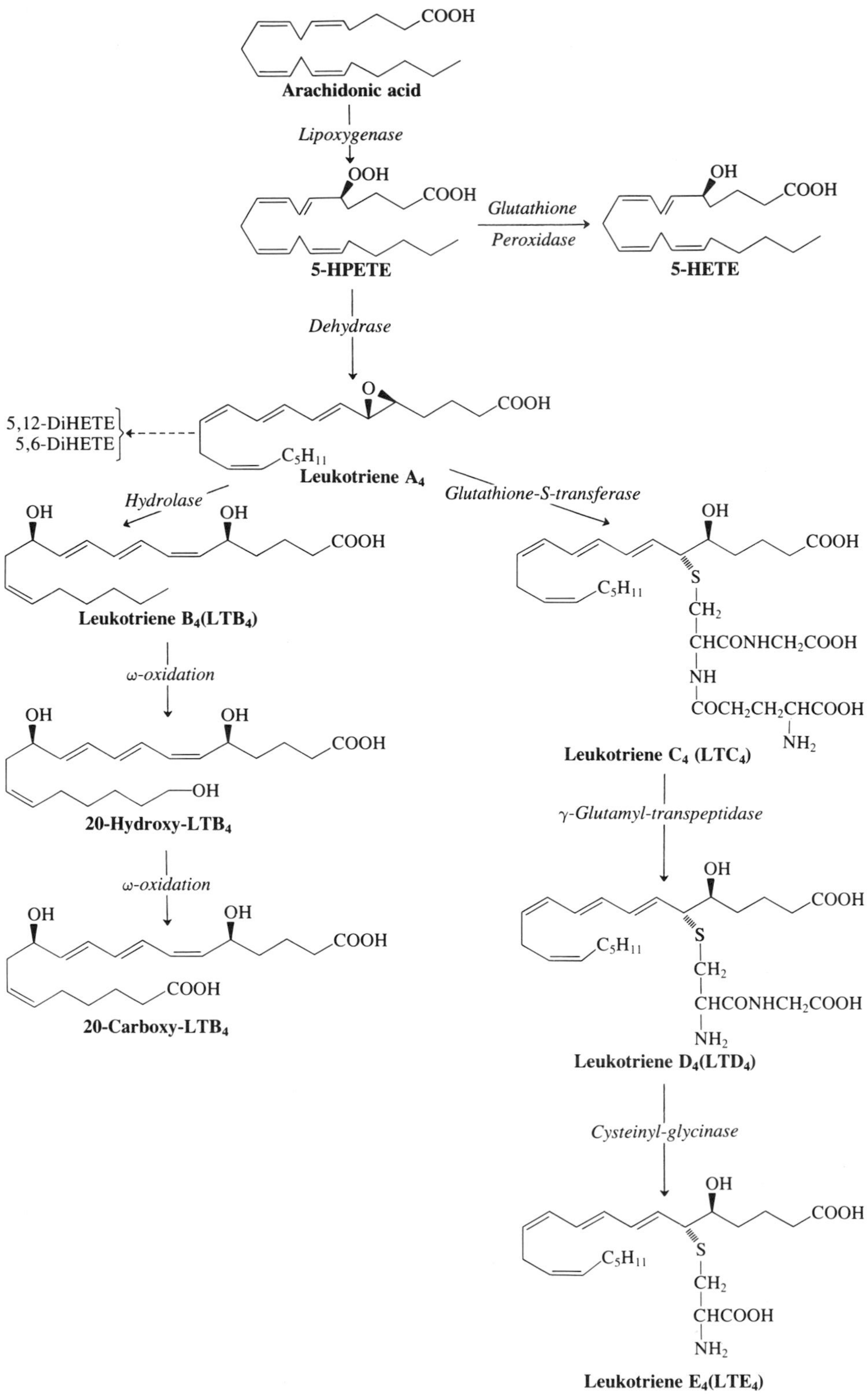

Fig. 8.11 The biosynthesis of leukotrienes from arachidonic acid.

constitute the substance shown many years ago to be generated in guinea pig lung during anaphylaxis—slow reacting substance of anaphylaxis (SRS-A). LTB_4 is produced mainly by neutrophils and the cysteinyl-leukotrienes mainly by macrophages and possibly by other cells.

The actions of the leukotrienes are listed in Table 8.2 and those actions which are relevant for inflammation are considered below.

rapidly to the biologically inactive TXB_2.

The catabolism of LTB_4 is illustrated in Figure 8.11.

The role of eicosanoids in inflammation

PGE_2 and PGI_2 are powerful *vasodilators* in their own right and also synergize with other vasodilators such as histamine and bradykinin. As re-

Table 8.2 Biological actions of leukotrienes (LTs)

Dihydroxy acid (LTB$_4$)	C-6 amino-acid-substituted LTs (LTC$_4$, LTD$_4$, LTE$_4$, LTF$_4$)
Aggregation of p.m.n.s.	Contraction of smooth muscle
Chemotaxis (p.m.n.s.)	Constriction of small airways
Chemokinesis of p.m.n.s.	Contraction of guinea pig parenchyma
Exudation of plasma	Secretion of mucus
Stimulation of phospholipase A$_2$ (in guinea pig lung)	Leakage from post-capillary venules
	Oedema formation
	Vasonconstriction
	Coronary arterial constriction
	Stimulation of phospholipase A$_2$ (in guinea pig lung)
	Antagonism by FPL-55712

(From: Piper P J 1983 Pharmacology of leukotrienes. Brit Med Bull 39: 255)

Catabolism of the eicosanoids

Several intracellular enzymes are involved in inactivation of the prostaglandins. This is exemplified by the degradation of PGE_2. There is an initial highly specific carrier-mediated uptake into cells followed by two main inactivating steps, an initial rapid phase catalysed by 'prostaglandin-specific' enzymes and a second, slower phase catalysed by general fatty acid-oxidizing enzymes. The prostaglandin-specific enzymes are present in high concentration in the lung, and 95% of infused prostaglandin E_2 is inactivated on first passage. The $t_{\frac{1}{2}}$ of prostaglandin E_2 in the circulation is less than one minute. (The first enzyme which acts in the initial phase, a prostaglandin dehydrogenase, increases markedly during pregnancy, which may serve to protect the uterus from the abortifacient effects of circulating prostaglandins.)

PGI_2 is not taken up into cells by the transport system in the lung and thus survives passage through the lung. It is metabolized mainly by the kidney.

The metabolites of the prostaglandins are excreted in the urine. Thromboxane A_2 decays

gards the *increase in vascular permeability*, they do not themselves have this action but they potentiate the effect of histamine and bradykinin. There is also interesting new evidence that their vasodilator effect facilitates the action of other agents such as C5a and LTB_4 which attract neutrophils, and that the neutrophils in turn produce *increased venular permeability* by an as yet unknown mechanism. As regards their role in production of *pain* in an area of inflammation, the prostaglandins do not themselves produce pain, but have been shown to potentiate the effect of subthreshold concentrations of other pain-producing mediators such as histamine and bradykinin (see Chapter 24). The balance between thromboxane A_2 and PGI_2 is believed to be important in the interaction of platelets and vascular endothelium (see Chapter 12) and may also be of importance in influencing *neutrophil adhesion* to the venular endothelium in that a decreased PGI_2 synthesis will facilitate this. LTB_4 is a powerful *chemotaxin* acting in picogram amounts, and when generated (in response to stimulation by C5a and the bacterial peptide fmet-leu-phe) by the first neutrophils arriving at the site of inflammation will amplify the mechanisms of *cellular accumulation* (see Fig. 8.2).

The cysteinyl-leukotrienes are powerful *spasmogens* being considerably more potent on *ileal* and *bronchial smooth muscle* than histamine. They also have a slower action. They can be shown to produce *wheezing* similar to that seen in asthmatic subjects and to cause *mucous secretion*, especially in inflamed airways and they are present in the sputum of chronic bronchitis in amounts which are biologically active. They may well be important mediators in asthma. Drugs which inhibit the synthesis of these agents or which antagonize their effects could be of great therapeutic importance in asthma. There is active research in this area and new compounds are likely to be available in the near future. Eicosanoids may have a role not only in the local inflammatory process but in one of the systemic manifestations of inflammation—*fever*. Various pyrogens (fever-producing agents) may be generated in inflammatory conditions. These include the lipopolysaccharide endotoxin of Gram-negative organisms (see Chapter 30), which causes fever by releasing 'endogenous pyrogen' from macrophages. Phagocytosis of bacteria or immune complexes has a similar effect in releasing 'endogenous pyrogen'. The endogenous pyrogen, which is thought to be similar, if not identical to, interleukin 1 (p. 202), enters the circulation and acts on receptors in the hypothalamus, resulting in an increase in the set-point for temperature regulation. There is evidence that PGE_1 may be implicated, linking the receptor activation to the subsequent events, which result in a rise in temperature. The antipyretic action of the non-steroidal inflammatory drugs is believed to be due largely due to their inhibition of the synthesis of PGE_1 in the hypothalamus, by virtue of their inhibition of cyclo-oxygenase.

In addition to the *mediator* function mentioned above, prostaglandins have been shown to have a significant *modulator* role on inflammatory cells, decreasing their activities. Thus PGE_2 decreases lysosomal enzyme release and the generation of toxic oxygen metabolites from neutrophils. It also inhibits lymphocyte activation and the generation and secretion of some effector lymphokines.

These modulator actions of the prostaglandins and their role in pyrogenesis are produced largely through a stimulant action on adenylate cyclase resulting in an increased intracellular cyclic AMP.

The role of eicosanoids in physiological reactions

Some physiological functions of prostanoids are outlined in Table 8.1. Other aspects of the role of prostanoids are dealt with in Chapters 14 & 17. The physiological role of leukotrienes is not yet clear though they are known to exert modulatory effects on the immune response, facilitating T cell activation by increasing cyclic GMP.

Therapeutic use of the eicosanoids

PGE_2 and $PGF_{2\alpha}$ are effective abortifacients. They are best given intravaginally to avoid their effects on other tissues. The main preparations are **dinoprost** ($PGF_{2\alpha}$) and **dinoprostone** (PGE_2). Dinoprost and dinoprostone can be given by the extra-amniotic route in the early stages of pregnancy and by the intra-amniotic route after 14–16 weeks gestation. Tablets for insertion into the vagina and preparations for intravenous injection are also available.

PGE_1 is used in treatment of congenital malformations of the heart in neonates, the purpose being to maintain the patency of the *ductus arteriosus* prior to surgical correction of the congenital defect. The preparation available is **alprostodil** which is given by intravenous infusion.

BRADYKININ

Bradykinin and the closely related peptide **kallidin** are vasoactive peptides formed by the action of enzymes on protein substrates termed **kininogens**. Information on these peptides derived originally from two separate lines of research. Werle and his colleagues described **kallikrein**, an enzyme in urine, which acts on serine proteins to liberate kallidin, which causes a fall in blood pressure. Independently, Rocha e Silva and his co-workers showed that certain snake venoms, when incubated with serum, gave rise to a hypotensive substance which also caused a slow contraction of certain smooth muscle preparations. Because of this slow action it was called *bradykinin*. The two substances are now known to be virtually identical. Bradykinin is a nonapeptide: arg-pro-pro-gly-phe-ser-pro-phe-arg. Kallidin is a decapeptide having the same structure as bradykinin but with an extra lysine on the N-terminal end.

Source and formation of bradykinin

An outline of the formation of bradykinin is given in Figure 8.12. Prekallikrein is present in plasma as

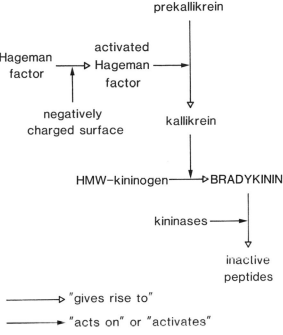

Fig. 8.12 The generation and breakdown of bradykinin. HMW-kininogen = high molecular weight kininogen. This substance probably acts both as a substrate for kallikrein and as a cofactor in the activation of prekallikrein (not shown).

the inactive precursor of the enzyme kallikrein. The substrate is *kininogen*. There are two forms of kininogen in plasma—high molecular weight kininogen (M_r 110 000) and low molecular weight kininogen (M_r 70 000). Prekallikrein can be converted to the active enzyme (which is a serine protease) in a variety of ways. One of the physiological activators, particularly in the context of inflammation, is Hageman factor (Factor XII of the blood clotting sequence; see Chapter 12 and Fig. 8.1). Hageman factor is normally in inactive form in the plasma and is activated by contact with surfaces having a negative charge, such as collagen, base-

ment membrane, bacterial lipopolysaccharides, urate crystals etc. As a result of the increased vascular permeability which occurs in inflammation, Hageman factor, prekallikrein and the kininogens leak out of the vessels with the plasma. Contact with the negatively charged surfaces promotes the interaction of prekallikrein and Hageman factor and this leads to kinin generation, bradykinin being clipped out of the high molecular weight kininogen molecule by the enzyme, which acts at two sites to release the nonapeptide (Fig. 8.13). Kallikrein can

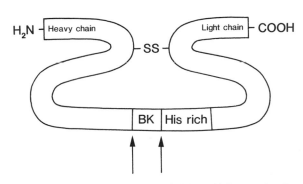

Fig. 8.13 Diagrammatic structure of high M_r kininogen showing the position of bradykinin adjacent to the histidine-rich area of the light chain of the cleaved molecule.

also activate the complement system, and can convert plasminogen to plasmin (see Fig. 8.1 and Chapter 12).

In addition to the plasma kallikrein described above, there are other kinin-generating kallikreins found in pancreas, salivary glands, colon and skin. Tissue kallikreins act on both high and low molecular weight kininogens and generate mainly kallidin.

A further kinin-generating serine protease may be released from mast cells and basophils when antigen interacts with IgE molecules bound to the surface of these cells.

Inactivation of bradykinin

The enzymes which inactivate bradykinin and related kinins are called **kininases** and there are two sorts (Figs. 8.12 & 8.14). The more specific enzyme is **kininase II** which is in fact the same as **angiotensin-converting enzyme** (see Chapter 11). This is a peptidyl dipeptidase which removes the two C-terminal

Sites of cleavage for Kinin formation

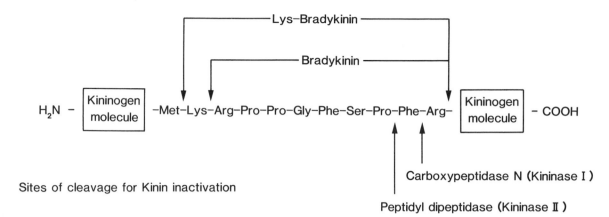

Fig. 8.14 Amino acid sequence of bradykinin. The site of proteolytic cleavage for formation of bradykinin are shown in the upper half of the figure. The sites of cleavage for bradykinin inactivation are shown in the lower half of the figure.

aminoacids from the kinin (Fig. 8.14). The enzyme is bound to the luminal surface of endothelial cells and is found mostly in the lung. It also cleaves the two C-terminal aminoacids from the inactive peptide, angiotensin I, converting it to the active vasoconstrictor peptide, angiotensin II (see Chapters 11 & 14). Thus the enzyme inactivates a vasodilator and activates a vasoconstrictor. The affinity of kinins for the enzyme (dissociation constant 10^{-7} M) is two orders of magnitude higher than the affinity of angiotensin for the enzyme (dissociation constant 10^{-5} M).

Kinins are also inactivated by the less specific **kininase 1**, a carboxypeptidase present in serum (Fig. 8.14). It removes the C-terminal arginine from bradykinin and also from complement components C3a, C5a, and C4a.

Pharmacological actions of bradykinin

Bradykinin is a very potent *vasodilator* and lowers blood pressure in all animals tested. Injected locally it produces arteriolar vasodilatation and increases the permeability of the post-capillary venules. Its vasodilator action is endothelium-dependent in most vascular beds; in some vessels, in some species, it is mediated by the vasodilator prostaglandins. Furthermore its vasodilator effect is potentiated by these prostaglandins. Bradykinin can be shown to activate phospholipase A_2 and liberate arachidonate, not only from vascular endothelium and

fibroblasts but also from the lung. The effect of bradykinin on vascular permeability is by a direct action and, unlike that of the prostaglandins PGE_2 and PGI_2, is independent of neutrophils.

Bradykinin is *spasmogenic* for several types of smooth muscle including that of the intestine, the uterus and the bronchial system. The contraction is slow and sustained in comparison with that produced by histamine. It causes *pain* if applied to a blister base and this effect is potentiated by prostaglandins (see Chapter 24).

The physiological role of bradykinin is still a matter of conjecture. Its release by tissue kallikrein may be of importance in controlling blood flow to certain exocrine glands and thus influencing the secretions of the glands. It is known to stimulate short circuit current (which reflects chloride secretion) in the intestine. Fluid secretion into the intestine is stimulated by this mechanism, and excessive bradykinin production is probably a factor in causing diarrhoea in many gastrointestinal disorders.

The role of bradykinin in inflammation and allergic reactions is also not entirely clear. It fulfils many of the Dale criteria and is capable of producing many of the phenomena of inflammation—pain, vasodilation, increased vascular permeability and spasm of smooth muscle. The enzymes necessary for both production and inactivation are known to be present and bradykinin itself has been shown to be present in nasal secretions after challenge with ragweed pollen in individuals allergic to this antigen. However, a full assessment of their possible role awaits the development of the relevant competitive antagonists. Such drugs could well prove to be of value therapeutically, possibly in allergic conditions, but certainly in acute pancreatitis, in which kinins released by pancreatic kallikrein are believed to be the cause of the severe pain and the fluid exudation into the peritoneal activity. There have been reports that bradykinin analogues containing D-amino acids in one or more positions have antagonist properties, and these may lead to valuable new drugs.

PLATELET ACTIVATING FACTOR (PAF)

Platelet activating factor, which is also variously termed **PAF-acether** and **AGEPC** (acetyl-glyceryl-ether-phosphorylcholine) is a member of a newly defined class of biologically active lipids which can produce effects at exceedingly low concentrations (less than 10^{-10} M). The name *platelet* activating factor, is misleading since PAF has actions on a variety of different target cells and is believed to be an important mediator in both acute and persisting allergic and inflammatory phenomena.

In structure it is 1-O-alkyl-2-acetyl-glyceryl-3-phosphorylcholine (Fig. 8.15). It is derived from 1-O-alkyl-2-acyl-glyceryl-3-phosphorylcholine (acyl-

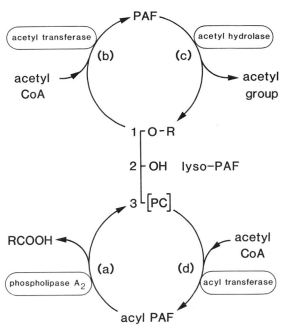

Fig. 8.16 The synthesis and breakdown of platelet activating factor (PAF) which is 1-O-alkyl-2-acetyl-glycero-3-phosphorylcholine.
LysoPAF is 1-O-alkyl-glycero-3-phosphorylcholine.
AcylPAF is 1-O-alkyl-2-acyl-glycero-3-phosphorylcholine.
The numbering of the carbon atom is given for lysoPAF.
PC = phosphorylcholine. The fatty acid removed from acyl PAF in reaction (a) may be arachidonic acid.

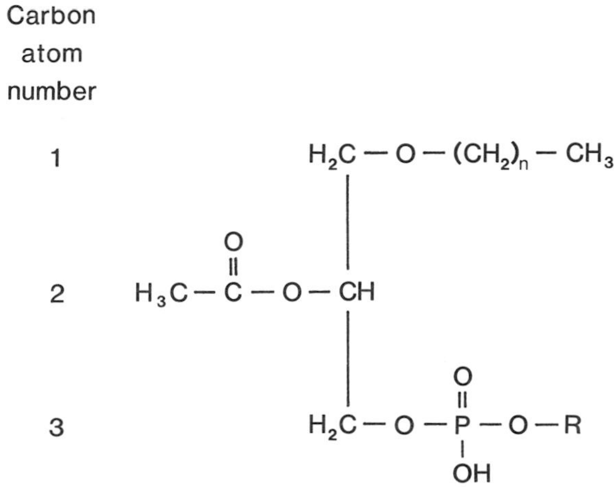

PAF) by phospholipase A_2 activity, resulting in 'lyso-PAF' which is then acetylated to give PAF, and is subsequently deacetylated to lyso-PAF (Fig. 8.16). PAF is generated and released from most inflammatory cells when these are stimulated. Thus it is released from polymorphs on phagocytosis of opsonized particles, from sensitized macrophages and basophils on interaction with antigen and from platelets on stimulation with thrombin. Inflammatory cells are known to have all the enzymes necessary both for the synthesis and inactivation of PAF and an increase in cytosolic calcium in these cells is involved in stimulation of the synthesis and subsequent breakdown of this agent.

Actions of PAF

This substance has a wide range of pharmacological actions and is capable of producing most of the phenomena of inflammation. In doses of 0.02–200 pmol injected locally it produces not only local *vasodilatation* and thus erythema but also

Carbon atom number

1    $H_2C - O - (CH_2)_n - CH_3$

2    $H_3C - \overset{\overset{\displaystyle O}{\|}}{C} - O - CH$

3    $H_2C - O - \overset{\overset{\displaystyle O}{\|}}{\underset{\underset{\displaystyle OH}{|}}{P}} - O - R$

Fig. 8.15 The structure of PAF (platelet activating factor). R = choline. The numbering of the carbon atoms in the glycerol backbone is given on the left. An 0-alkyl residue is attached to carbon atom 1 (c.f. Figure 8.8). This may be hexadecyl or octadecyl; compounds containing either of these have PAF activity.

increased vascular permeability and wheal formation. Unlike that produced by the prostaglandins, the increased vascular permeability caused by PAF is independent of neutrophils. Higher doses produce *hyperalgesia*. It induces local *platelet aggregation* and a pronounced *accumulation of leucocytes*—initially involving *neutrophils* and subsequently *mononuclear* cells. Tested *in vitro* PAF has powerful effects on neutrophils over a concentration range of $10^{-12}\,M–10^{-6}\,M$. It is a potent *chemotaxin* and also stimulates both polyphosphoinositide turnover and activation of phospholipase A_2 with generation of eicosanoids. On platelets it is active *in vitro* over a concentration range of $10^{-15}\,M–10^{-6}\,M$, causing *shape change*, and the release of the contents of dense granules and of α_1 and α_2 granules (p. 291). This effect is associated with polyphosphoinositide turnover and a rise in cytosolic calcium concentration; arachidonate metabolism is stimulated and thromboxane A_2 is generated. PAF is also a *spasmogen* on both bronchial and ileal smooth muscle.

If injected intravenously in doses of 1–100 nmol per kg it causes, in most experimental animals, bronchoconstriction (associated with platelet sequestration and aggregation in the lungs), pulmonary oedema, neutropenia and marked loss of plasma protein. Higher doses result in coronary vasoconstriction and circulatory collapse. The cellular and vascular changes are very similar to those of classical anaphylaxis and—with higher doses—to those of endotoxic shock.

All the enzymes necessary for its synthesis and degradation are present at inflammatory sites and the substrate necessary for its synthesis, alkyl-acyl-glycerophorylcholine, is a constituent of cell membranes. It is known to be generated by stimulated inflammatory cells.

In general, therefore, PAF fulfils a great many of the Dale criteria necessary for acceptance as a mediator of inflammation, many more, in fact, than any other single agent. Furthermore its effects are produced in very low concentrations. It is considered to be an important mediator in asthma (p. 303).

The anti-inflammatory actions of the glucocorticoids are almost certainly due, at least in part, to inhibition of PAF synthesis by virtue of the inhibitory effect of lipocortin on phospholipase A_2.

Competitive antagonists of the actions of PAF and/or more specific inhibitors of lyso-PAF acetyl transferase could well be extremely useful anti-inflammatory drugs.

INTERLEUKIN-1

Interleukin-1 is a glycoprotein of M_r 35 000. It is secreted by macrophages and by antigen-presenting dendritic cells as explained above (p. 183). Its synthesis and release is stimulated by exposure of the cell to bacterial, viral or fungal products, antigen/antibody complexes, adjuvants and, in the case of the macrophage, to the T cell lymphokine—macrophage activating factor (MAF)—which may be the same as γ-interferon. Other cells such as keratinocytes, endothelial cells, kidney cells etc, may generate small amounts of interleukin-1 (IL-1).

Actions

IL-1 has a wide range of different actions on different cell types.

1. It is of prime importance in the induction of the immune responses, as outlined above, facilitating the responses of both B & T cells to antigen.
2. It is a chemoattractant for neutrophils, and stimulates release of granule enzymes and activation of the respiratory burst with generation of toxic oxygen products.
3. It stimulates fibroblasts to proliferate and to synthesize collagen, and to generate collagenase and release prostaglandins.
4. It stimulates the synthesis of 'acute phase proteins'—a group of serum proteins formed in the liver during the inflammatory response.
5. It stimulates catabolism of certain tissues—wasting of muscle, bone resorption, degradation of cartilage. It can be shown *in vitro* to cause loss of amino acids from muscle and loss of proteoglycon from cartilage. Bone resorption probably involves activation of osteoclasts.
6. It causes fever. It is probably identical with the substance termed 'leucocyte endogenous pyrogen' which acts on receptors in the hypothalamus to alter the set-point of temperature regulation.

The detailed physiological role of IL-1 *in vivo* is not fully understood although clearly it is necessary for the induction of the immune response. The other actions cited above are thought to play a part in chronic inflammation. In particular it is considered to be of importance in rheumatoid arthritis. This troublesome and often crippling condition affects large numbers of people and constitutes a challenge to immunologists, pharmacologists and clinicians. Its cause is unknown though it is considered that whatever the initial stimulus might be (? injury, microbial products, B cell defect resulting in production of abnormal immunoglobulin) the joint damage is probably due to an inappropriate immune reaction. One of the main currently held hypotheses is that substances in the joint, perhaps cartilage derivatives, function as auto-antigens. Immune complexes consisting of antibody + immunoglobulin ('rheumatoid factor') may be implicated, activating complement, and thus causing attraction and activation of neutrophils and macrophages, which damage the cartilage. The cartilage auto-antigens are thought to stimulate local T cells, which release factors that activate synovial macrophages, which release interleukin-1. This substance has been shown to be present in the synovial fluid of rheumatoid joints. The actions of interleukin-1 outlined above would cause the tissue damage which occurs in these joints and, together with cartilage products released by its action, would stimulate local T cells. The cycle would thus begin again, resulting in chronic progressive pathology. Interleukin-1 is thus held to be a mediator of crucial importance in chronic inflammatory conditions such as rheumatoid arthritis, and the development of drugs which modify its release or its actions on target cells is a prime target for many pharmaceutical companies in the search for anti-arthritic drugs. A gene for human interleukin-1 has been cloned. Recent work suggests that there may be more than one interleukin-1.

γ-INTERFERON

Interferons are a group of inducible proteins secreted by a number eukaryotic cells (p. 650). There are three main families of interferons—α, β, and γ; these are antigenically distinct. γ-Interferon (also called Type II interferon) is produced by T lymphocytes during an immune response. It is a lymphokine and has been shown to be identical with 'macrophage-activating factor' (MAF). The other two families, α- and β-interferons (Type II interferons), have antiviral activity (see Chapter 31) and are reported to have anti-tumour effects (see Chapter 29).

REFERENCES AND FURTHER READING

Dale M M, Foreman J C (eds) 1984 Textbook of immunopharmacology. Blackwell Scientific Publications, Oxford
  Chapter 8. Dale M M, Foreman J C Histamine, p115–125
  Chapter 11. Mongar J L Complement, p147–157
  Chapter 12. Wiggins R C, Cochrane C G Kinins and kinin-forming systems, p158–169
  Chapter 13. Morley J, Hanson J M, Rumjanek U M Lymphokines, p170–186
  Chapter 14. Henson P Platelet activating factor, p187–195
  Chapter 16. Williams T J Mediators of inflammatory oedema formation, p210–216
  Chapter 28. Moore M Interferons, p347–370
Dinarello C A 1984 Interleukin-1: an important mediator of inflammation. Trends in Pharmacological Sciences 5: 420–422
Duff G 1985 Many roles for interleukin-1. Nature 313: 352–353
Feldman M 1985 Lymphokines and interleukins emerge from the primeval soup. Nature 313: 351–352
Ganellin C R, Parsons M E (eds) 1982 Pharmacology of histamine receptors. Wright, Bristol
  Chapter 6. Levi R, Owen D A A, Trzeciakowski J Actions of histamine on the heart and vasculature, p236–297
  Chapter 8. Parsons M E Histamine receptors in alimentary and genito-urinary smooth muscle, p323–350
  Chapter 11. Burland W L, Mills J G The pathophysiological role of histamine and potential therapeutic uses of H_1 and H_2 antihistamines p436–481
  Chapter 2. Ganellin C R Chemistry and structure-activity relationships of drugs acting at histamine receptors p10–102
Lands W E 1981 Actions of anti-inflammatory drugs. Trends in Pharmacological Sciences 2: 78–80
Lewis R A, Drazen J M, Figueredo J C, Copley E J, Austen K F 1982 A review of recent contributions on biologically active products of arachidonate conversion. Int J Immunopharmac 4: 85–90
Moncada S, Flower R J, Vane J R 1985 Prostaglandins, prostacyclin and thromboxane A_2. In: Gilman A G, Goodman L S, Rall T W, Murad F (eds) The pharmacological basis of therapeutics. Macmillan, New York, ch. 28
Piper P J (ed) 1983 Leukotrienes and other lipoxygenase products. John Wiley, Bristol
Roitt I 1984 Essential Immunology, 5th Ed. Blackwell Scientific Publications, Oxford
Salmon J A, Higgs G A 1987 Eicosanoids. In: Dale M M, Foreman J C Textbook of Immunopharmacology. Blackwell Scientific, Oxford, 2nd edition
Samuelsson B 1983 Leukotrienes: mediators of immediate hypersensitivity reactions and inflammation. Science 220: 568–575

Drugs used to suppress inflammatory and immune reactions

The main anti-inflammatory agents are the gluco-corticoids and the non-steroidal anti-inflammatory drugs. The glucocorticoids, which are also used as immunosuppressants, are dealt with in detail in Chapter 16 and the non-steroidal anti-inflammatory drugs (NSAIDs) are dealt with below.

Included in the category of anti-inflammatory agents are the anti-rheumatoid agents and drugs used in gout, descriptions of which follow the section on NSAIDs. Some of the anti-histamine drugs are also considered in this context. Finally the drugs used for immunosuppression are described at the end of this chapter.

NON-STEROIDAL ANTI-INFLAMMATORY DRUGS (NSAIDs)

The drugs in this group are among the most widely used of all therapeutic agents. The most important examples are listed in Table 9.1 and their chemical formulae are given in Figures 9.1–9.6. They are frequently prescribed for 'rheumatic' musculo-skeletal complaints; it is estimated that more than 20 million people in the United Kingdom experience this type of disorder and 8 million of these consult their doctors in the course of a year, constituting 23% of all consultations. In addition, very large quantities of these drugs are bought over the pharmacist's counter by the general public, without prescription, for treatment of headaches, tooth-aches and a variety of other minor complaints. It is probable that most bathroom medicine cupboards in the UK harbour a bottle containing aspirin or paracetamol or some other NSAID.

There are now more than 50 different NSAIDs on the market and there is a continuing flow of new preparations. The fact that so many new com-pounds have been produced and are still being produced is a reflection of the fact that none is ideal in controlling or modifying the signs and symptoms of inflammation, particularly in the common in-flammatory joint diseases.

PHARMACOLOGICAL ACTIONS

NSAIDs include a variety of different agents of different chemical classes. Most of these drugs have three major types of effect—they modify the in-flammatory reaction (*anti-inflammatory effects*), they reduce certain sorts of pain (*analgesic effect*) and they lower a raised temperature (*antipyretic effect*). In general, all of these effects are related to the primary action of the drugs—inhibition of ara-chidonate cyclo-oxygenase and thus inhibition of the production of prostaglandins and thrombox-anes. However some aspects of the action of indiv-idual drugs may occur by a different mechanism.

Not all NSAIDs manifest the three actions men-tioned to the same extent. Most are analgesic, but the degree of anti-inflammatory activity varies, some (such as **aspirin** and **indomethacin**) being strongly anti-inflammatory, some (such as **nap-roxen**, **meclofenamate** and **fenclofenac**) being mode-rately anti-inflammatory, while some (such as **paracetamol**) have essentially no anti-inflammatory activity at all (see Figs. 9.1–9.6 for structures).

In addition to these three categories of action, one of the NSAIDs, aspirin, has particularly pro-nounced actions on platelets (see Chapter 12).

Table 9.1 Comparison of some commonly used NSAIDs

Drug	Plasma t½ hours	Action Analg	Action Antipyr	Action Anti-infl	Comments
Salicylic acids (see Fig. 9.4)					
Aspirin	3–5	+	+	+	Fairly marked GIT upsets and haemorrhage. Tinnitus. Hypersensitivity reactions. Cheap & effective. A drug of first choice for mild analgesia. An encephalitis may occur in children with viral infections.
Diflunisal	8–13	+	−	+	10 × more potent in anti-inflammatory & analgesic effect than aspirin but only 1.5 × more potent in antipyresis. Less GIT irritation than aspirin.
Propionic acids (see Fig. 9.2)					
Naproxen	13	+	+	+	Drugs of first choice for inflammatory joint disease because they have the lowest incidence of side effects. Naproxen marginally superior. Fenbufen is a pro-drug, activated in the liver; less likely to cause bleeding in in GIT.
Ibuprofen	2	+	+	+	
Flurbiprofen	4	+	+	+	
Fenbufen	10	+	+	−	
Ketoprofen	2	+	+	+	
Acetic acids (see Fig. 9.1)					
Indomethacin	2	+	+	+ +	One of the most potent inhibitors of cyclo-oxygenase in *in vitro* test. Clinically effective but high incidence of side effects. Headache common.
Sulindac	7(18*)	+	+	+	A pro-drug manifesting reversible activation i.e. inter-convertible with its active sulphide metabolite; long duration of action. About half the potency of indomethacin.
Fenclofenac	12	+	+	+	Few GIT upsets. Rashes fairly common (25%). May have direct anti-rheumatic action.
Fenamates (see Fig. 9.6)					
Meclofenamic acid	2	+	+	+	Moderate anti-inflammatory actions. GIT upsets. Diarrhoea likely. Haemolytic anaemia has been reported.
Mefenamic acid	4	+	+	±	
Oxicam (see Fig. 9.3)					
Piroxicam	45	+	+	+ +	The most widely used NSAID world-wide for chronic inflammatory conditions. GIT irritation in 20% patients. Tinnitus. Rashes. Metabolized in the liver. Is given once daily. Multiple peaks in plasma suggests enterohepatic recycling. No accumulation in the elderly or in patients with renal impairment.
Pyrazolones (see Fig. 9.3)					
Phenylbutazone	50–100	±	+	+ +	Very potent. Retarded conjugation, thus long duration of action. More toxic than other NSAID. Renal & hepatic damage may occur, also bone marrow dysplasia. Use restricted to ankylosing spondylitis.
Azapropazone	20	+	+	+	Moderate efficacy. Mild GIT irritation.
Paracetamol (see Fig. 9.5)	2–4	+	+	−	Safe and effective mild analgesic in therapeutic doses. Overdose causes serious hepatotoxicity.

*Half-life of active metabolite
Analg = analgesic; Antipyr = antipyretic; Anti-infl = antiinflammatory; GIT = gastrointestinal tract

The main pharmacological actions and the common side effects of this group of drugs are outlined below, followed by a more detailed coverage of the salicylates and paracetamol. A comparison of some aspects of the pharmacology of some commonly used NSAIDs is given in Table 9.1. Finally the clinical application of the group as a whole is considered.

Antipyretic effect

Normal body temperature is regulated by a centre in the hypothalamus and involves a sensitive control of the balance between heat loss and heat production. Fever occurs when there is a disturbance of this hypothalamic 'thermostat', such that the set-point of body temperature is raised. As explained in Chapter 8, during an inflammatory reaction bacterial endotoxins cause the release from macrophages of a pyrogen (which is probably interleukin-1). There is a hypothesis, for which there is a reasonable amount of evidence, that this pyrogen causes the generation in the hypothalamus of PGE_1 and PGE_2 and that these prostaglandins cause the elevation of the set-point for temperature. If this is so, the action of the NSAIDs in promoting a return to the normal set-point for temperature could be explained as being due to inhibition of prostaglandin synthesis. Once there has been a return to the normal set-point of temperature the temperature-regulating mechanisms (dilatation of superficial blood vessels, sweating) then operate to reduce temperature. Normal temperature is not affected by NSAIDs. (For a discussion of this topic see Rainsford, 1984.)

Analgesic effect

As explained in Chapter 8, prostaglandins sensitize nocioceptive afferent nerve terminals to mediators such as bradykinin (see also Chapter 25). Thus in the presence of PGE_1 or PGE_2 pain will be felt even with subthreshold concentrations of inflammatory mediators such as histamine, serotonin or bradykinin—concentrations which on their own do not cause any pain at all. Also, intravenous infusions of prostaglandins result in headache, an effect which may be related to their vasodilator action on the cerebral vasculature.

NSAIDs are mainly effective against certain types of pain—those in which prostaglandin-induced hyperalgesia is amplifying the basic pain mechanisms. Thus they will be effective principally in pain associated with inflammatory processes and are usually considered to be effective against pain of mild to moderate intensity, particularly that due to bursitis or arthritis and pain of muscular or vascular origin. Some types of headache are relieved by NSAIDs, an effect which may be related to the inhibition of the vasodilator effect of prostaglandins. NSAIDs are usually effective in toothache. They also reduce the pain of postpartum states and dysmenorrhea and the pain of cancer metastases in bone—conditions which may be associated with increased prostaglandin synthesis.

Recent clinical data indicate that some NSAIDs (e.g. indomethacin, diflunisal, naproxen) may also be effective in the control of severe pain unrelated to inflammation (Shen, 1984; Rainsford, 1984).

Anti-inflammatory action

As has been described in Chapter 8, there are many chemical mediators of the inflammatory and allergic response. Each facet of the response—vasodilatation, increased vascular permeability, cell accumulation etc—can be produced by several different mechanisms and, furthermore, different mediators may be of particular importance in different inflammatory and allergic conditions. Drugs such as the NSAIDs, which inhibit cyclo-oxygenase and thus the synthesis of prostaglandins and thromboxanes, will affect mainly, possibly only, those aspects of inflammation in which these agents play a significant part. Thus they will reduce in particular the vasodilatation and erythema. The reduction in vasodilatation will also have an indirect effect on local oedema formation because of the synergistic effect which prostaglandin-induced vasodilatation has on other mechanisms of increased vascular permeability. These effects on the vessels, along with the analgesic effect produced in areas of inflammation (see above) mean that NSAIDs can reduce many of the local signs and symptoms of inflammation—the redness, the heat, the pain and the swelling.

However, drugs whose only action is inhibition of cyclo-oxygenase do not have any significant effect on *cellular accumulation* either in acute or chronic inflammation. Indeed there is even the possibility that by directing arachidonate metabolism from the cyclo-oxygenase pathway to the lipoxygenase pathway they may increase the production of the chemotaxin LTB_4 (and thus *increase* the influx of neutrophils and mononuclear phagocytes) and the generation of the spasmogens, LTC_4, LTD_4 and LTE_4. Furthermore cyclo-oxygenase inhibitors will have no effect on those processes which are responsible for tissue damage in, for example, rheumatoid arthritis, vasculitis and nephritis —processes such as the release of lysosomal enzymes and the production of the toxic products of O_2. In fact, in view of the evidence that prostaglandins such as PGE_2 and PGI_2 have modulatory effects on some of these phenomena (resulting in a *decrease* of lysosomal enzyme release, a *reduction* in the generation of toxic O_2 products, an *inhibition* of lymphocyte activation, etc) it is possible that administration of cyclo-oxygenase inhibitors in some chronic conditions such as rheumatoid arthritis, could actually exacerbate tissue damage in the long-term.

Other actions of NSAIDs

Aspirin has been reported to reduce the diarrhoea which may occur after radiation therapy for cervical cancer and which is thought to be due to prostaglandin production in the intestinal wall. A similar production of prostaglandins may be the basis for the effect of aspirin in reducing fluid loss in experimental cholera (see Chapter 15).

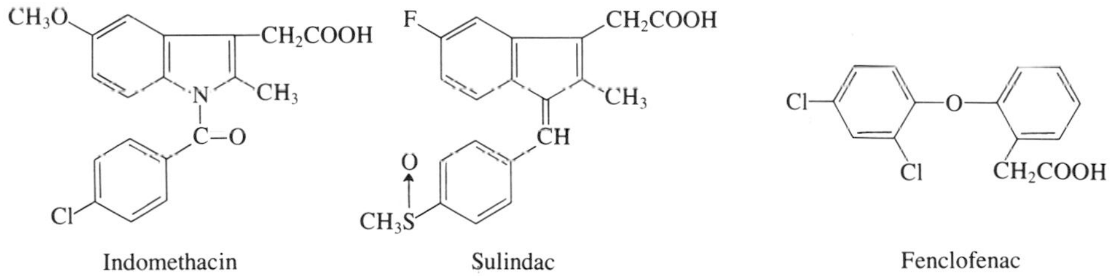

(see Figs. 8.7 & 8.10). Some types of inhibition involve binding of the drug to the enzyme and there is evidence that there are two binding sites. Interaction with the catalytic site determines the potency of the drugs but interaction with a supplementary site is also necessary. Weak cyclo-oxygenase inhibitors may interact mainly with the supplementary site.

Inhibition can occur by different mechanisms (as discussed by Lands 1981):

1. An irreversible time-dependent inactivation of the enzyme. **Aspirin** is the main example of a drug acting in this way. It acetylates the α-amino group of the terminal serine of the enzyme, forming a covalent bond. Further synthesis of prostanoids necessitates synthesis of new enzyme. This means that the effect of the drug continues after the drug itself has apparently been cleared from the tissue. Other NSAIDs, such as **indomethacin** (Fig. 9.1), also manifest a time-dependent inactivation of cyclo-oxygenase but the exact mechanism of action is not clear.

2. A rapid, reversible competitive inhibition. This action is manifested by the propionic acid NSAIDs, such as **ibuprofen** (Fig. 9.2), which binds reversibly

Fig. 9.1 Structures of acetic acid NSAIDs.

One NSAID, **sulindac** (Fig. 9.1), is a potent inhibitor of aldose reductase in the lens of the eye. This enzyme, which reduces glucose to sorbitol, is believed to be involved in the development of cataract and peripheral neuropathy in diabetes and sulindac has a role in the treatment of these diabetic sequelae.

MECHANISM OF ACTION OF NSAIDs

The main action of this group of drugs is, as stated above, *inhibition of arachidonate cyclo-oxygenase*

to the enzyme (K_d 5×10^{-6} M) competing with the natural substrate, arachidonic acid (K_d 2×10^{-6} M). Hydrophobic forces are important in this interaction. The oxicams, such as **piroxicam** (see Fig. 9.3), have a similar mechanism of action.

3. A rapid, reversible non-competitive inhibition. This effect involves antioxidant or free radical trapping properties which would inhibit or reduce the lipid peroxide-induced free radical chain reaction mechanism (reactions 1 & 2 in Fig. 8.10). An example of a drug with this mechanism of action is **paracetamol** (see Fig. 9.5). This drug is a relatively weak inhibitor of purified cyclo-oxygenase when

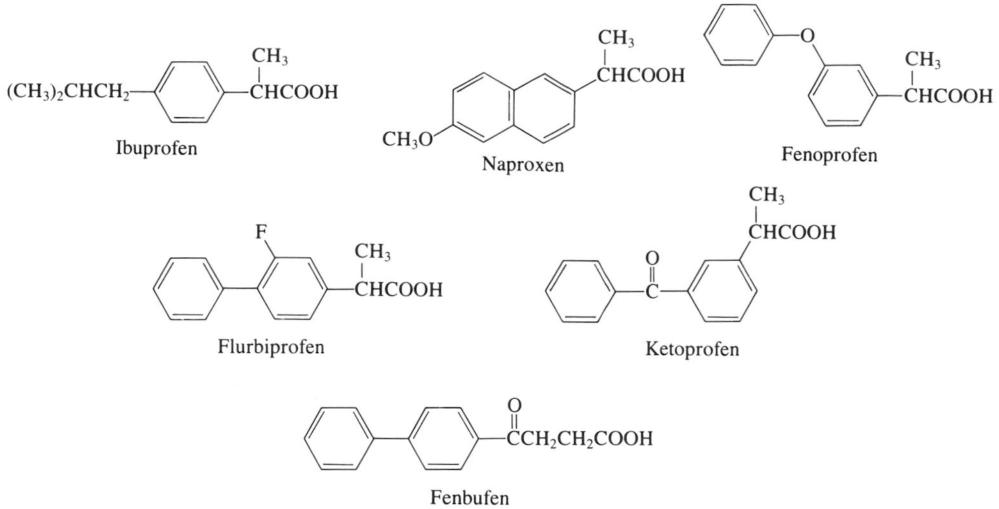

Fig. 9.2 Structures of propionic acid NSAIDs.

tested under standard assay conditions, in which the peroxide concentration may rise to a high level. If the peroxide concentration is reduced to levels found intracellularly *in vivo*, paracetamol's potency against cyclo-oxygenase is correspondingly increased (see Lands, 1981). This drug has analgesic actions but only very weak anti-inflammatory effects. This may well be a reflection of the fact that in areas of inflammation, the concentration of peroxides is high as a result of the presence of phagocytic cells, which generate these substances when activated (p. 181). Paracetamol is an effective analgesic in headaches and other pains associated with vascular changes, and is also an effective antipyretic in fever—conditions in which leucocyte infiltration is not a major factor. Another reason for the differential effects of paracetamol on pain and inflammation may be that paracetamol is more effective against the cyclo-oxygenase in the CNS than the cyclo-oxygenase in other tissues.

Other actions besides inhibition of cyclo-oxygenase may contribute to the anti-inflammatory effects of some NSAIDs. Reactive oxygen radicals produced by neutrophils and macrophages are thought to be implicated not only in eicosanoid production but in tissue damage in some conditions and NSAIDs which have a strong O_2 radical scavenging effect as well as cyclo-oxygenase-inhibitory activity (such as **phenylbutazone** and **sulindac**) may decrease tissue damage. Furthermore, since many NSAIDs are highly hydrophobic molecules,

they may interfere with the binding of hydrophobic mediators (such as the chemotactic peptides derived from bacteria) to their receptors on inflammatory cells. Certainly some of the pyrazolones (Fig. 9.3) have been shown to have this effect in experiments *in vitro*. This hydrophobicity probably also explains the binding of NSAIDs to serum albumin which has lipophilic pockets. The existence of similar lipophilic peptide sequences in other enzymes may explain the fact that several NSAIDs have inhibitory effects on these enzymes, albeit at concentrations much higher than that at which cyclo-oxygenase is inhibited.

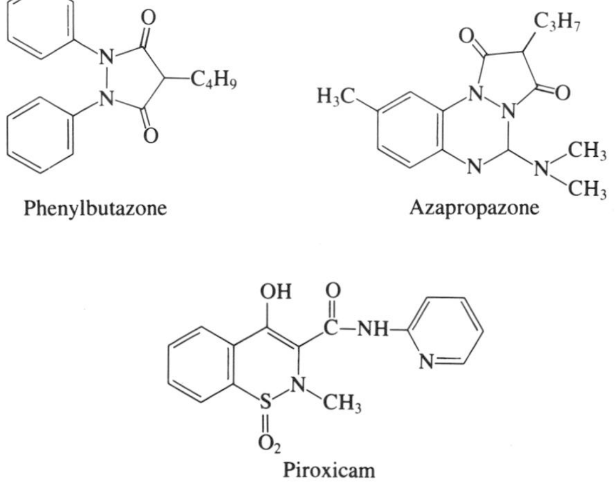

Fig. 9.3 Structures of pyrazolone NSAIDs and piroxicam.

GENERAL ASPECTS OF THE UNWANTED ACTIONS OF NSAIDs

Nearly a quarter of the adverse drug reactions reported to the Committee on the Safety of Medicines (CSM) in the UK are due to NSAIDs. These agents have also featured in the reports of deaths in which drugs have been implicated. Although this may be partly because NSAIDs are used extensively in the elderly who will obviously have a high mortality from natural causes, the inherent toxicity of these drugs is clearly a contributory factor. When NSAIDs are used in joint diseases there is a high incidence of side effects—more particularly in the gastrointestinal tract but also in liver, kidney, spleen, blood and bone marrow (see Rainsford and Velo, 1983).

The common *gastrointestinal side effects* are dyspepsia, nausea and vomiting. Diarrhoea also occurs fairly frequently, though some patients complain of constipation. A more hazardous side effect is mucosal damage which can lead to life-threatening haemorrhage, though fortunately this is fairly rare.

There are probably several reasons for the gastric damage. A direct irritant effect on the mucosa is probably important. The pharmacological effect of the drugs also plays a part, since they inhibit the synthesis of prostaglandins which, according to experimental evidence, normally exert some sort of protective action on the mucosa as well as inhibiting acid secretion. Certainly oral administration of prostaglandins, not only in experimental animals but in man, can be shown to diminish gastric damage.

The dosage form in which the NSAID is given is relevant. Tablets are more likely to result in damage than capsules, solutions or suspensions. 'Slow release' and 'enteric-coated' preparations also cause less damage. Some newer preparations are inactive 'pro-drugs' which release the active agent only after absorption, when they undergo metabolism in the liver and thus the possibility of gastric damage is circumvented.

In 1953 an association between NSAID consumption and *renal disease* was noticed, and mounting evidence that chronic NSAID consumption (mainly in the form of over-the-counter remedies for minor aches and pains) could cause chronic nephritis and renal papillary necrosis was published in the next 10 years, leading to the recognition of 'analgesic nephropathy' (Kerr & Ward, 1981). It is still not certain which NSAID is responsible for this condition, though **phenacetin** (see Fig. 9.5) is regarded as the most likely since this drug was used in all the reported cases of analgesic nephropathy up to 1975 and it is known to cause renal damage in animals. Because of this evidence, phenacetin was withdrawn from over-the-counter preparations in the 1970s and there now appears to be a fall in the incidence of analgesic nephropathy.

The mechanism by which phenacetin damages the kidney is not well understood. It is rapidly metabolized to another NSAID, **paracetamol** (see below) but paracetamol has no appreciable renal toxicity in animals and has not been implicated as a cause of analgesic nephropathy in man. It is therefore likely that an alternative metabolite of phenacetin is responsible for the effect.

Aspirin and **phenylbutazone** have also been suggested as a cause of analgesic nephropathy, but the evidence is hard to assess because most long-term users of NSAIDs take several different drugs.

The salicylates

Natural products which contain precursors of salicylic acid, such as willow bark (which contains the glycoside salicin) and oil of wintergreen (which contains methylsalicylate) have long been used for the treatment of rheumatism. Salicylic acid and acetylsalicyclic acid (**aspirin**) were amongst the earliest drugs synthesized. Aspirin is a simple organic acid (Fig. 9.4) with a pKa of 3.5. **Sodium salicylate** is a salt of acetylsalicylic acid which has two-

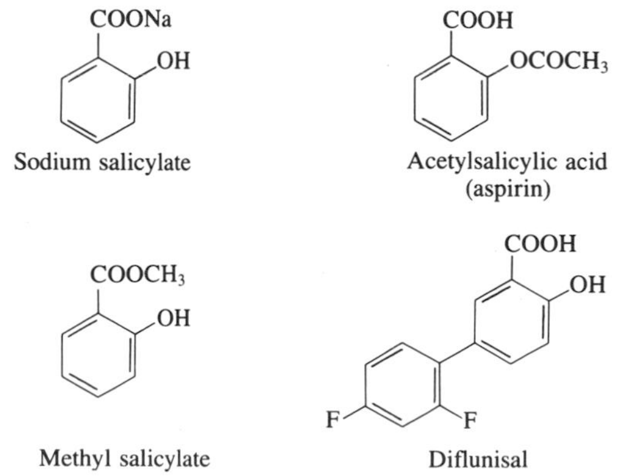

Fig. 9.4 Structures of salicylate NSAIDs

thirds of the potency of aspirin. Aspirin itself is relatively insoluble but its sodium and calcium salts are readily soluble. **Methylsalicylate** is used only in topical application. A newer member of this group is **diflunisal** (Fig. 9.4).

Pharmacokinetic aspects

As these drugs are weak acids they are largely unionized in the acid environment of the stomach and their absorption is thus facilitated. Aspirin is hydrolyzed by esterases in the plasma and the tissues, yielding salicylate. With low therapeutic doses most of the salicylate in the plasma is protein-bound. With high concentrations however, relatively less is bound and more is available for action in the tissues. Approximately 25% of the salicylate is oxidized, some is conjugated to glucuronic or sulphuric acid before excretion and about 25% is excreted unchanged. The rate of urinary excretion is higher in alkaline than in acid urine since more of the unchanged salicylate will be ionized and therefore less will be reabsorbed in the tubules.

Because of the possibility of saturation of the hepatic enzymes, the plasma half-life of aspirin will depend on the dose. With low dosage the $t_{\frac{1}{2}}$ is approximately 4 hours and elimination follows first-order kinetics. With high doses (more than 4 g per day) elimination follows saturation kinetics and the plasma half-life is more than 15 hours.

Unwanted effects

Salicylate may produce local and systemic toxic effects.

Locally, in the stomach, aspirin can give rise to a gastritis with focal erosions and bleeding. A study in a group of over 200 individuals with normal digestive tracts, who were given aspirin, showed that the majority lost between 2 and 6 ml of blood per day in the faeces. A small proportion of the individuals lost a good deal more. The basis of this is the direct irritant action on the mucosa of the aspirin itself, plus its pharmacological effect in inhibiting the synthesis of prostaglandins, which are thought to exert a protective action on the mucosa, as explained above. An inhibitory effect of aspirin on platelet aggregation (see Chapter 12) may contribute to the bleeding, and a decrease in the formation of PGI_2 (which inhibits gastric acid secretion

and affects blood flow) may also play a part.

Aspirin tablets are more likely to cause gastric damage than are suspensions or solutions, or slow-release and enteric-coated preparations.

Systemic effects depend on the dose. 'Salicylism' is a condition of chronic moderate toxicity which may occur with repeated ingestion of fairly large doses of salicylate. This is a syndrome consisting of tinnitus (noises in the head), dizziness and decreased hearing. Nausea and vomiting may also occur. Other unwanted effects include hypersensitivity reactions such as skin rashes and occasionally a type of asthma.

Salicylates can cause various metabolic changes, the nature of which depends on the dose. Large therapeutic doses of salicylate *alter the acid-base balance and the electrolyte balance* and toxic doses have serious effects on these functions. The sequence of events with toxic doses is as follows: salicylates uncouple oxidative phosphorylation (mainly in skeletal muscle) leading to increased O_2 consumption and thus increased production of CO_2. This stimulates respiration. Salicylates also stimulate respiration by a direct action on the respiratory centre. The resulting hyperventilation causes a respiratory alkalosis. Renal mechanisms, involving increased bicarbonate excretion normally compensate for this, and this condition of compensated respiratory alkalosis may occur in patients on high *therapeutic* doses of salicylates. Larger doses can cause a depression of the respiratory centre which leads eventually to retention of CO_2 and thus an increase in plasma CO_2. Since this is superimposed on a reduction in plasma bicarbonate, an uncompensated respiratory acidosis will occur. This may be complicated by factors leading to a metabolic acidosis, namely, the accumulation of metabolites of pyruvic, lactic and aceto-acetic acids, which is an indirect consequence of interference with carbohydrate metabolism, and the acid load associated with the salicylate itself.

Hyperpyrexia is likely to occur, and dehydration may follow from excessive vomiting.

With toxic doses of salicylates, disturbance of haemostasis may also occur, mainly as a result of the effect on platelet aggregation. The effect of these doses on the CNS is, initially, stimulation with excitement but eventually coma and respiratory depression.

Salicylate poisoning, with the signs and symptoms outlined above, is seen more commonly, and is more serious in children than in adults. The acid-base disturbance in children is usually a metabolic acidosis whereas that in adults is a respiratory alkalosis. Salicylate poisoning constitutes a medical emergency and the necessary treatment includes correction of the acid-base disturbance, therapy for the dehydration and hyperthermia and maintenance of kidney function. Gastric lavage and forced alkaline diuresis may be used for removal of the drug (the latter procedure only if there is adequate circulatory and renal function).

Some important interactions with other drugs

Aspirin causes a potentially hazardous increase in the effect of oral anticoagulants partly by displacing

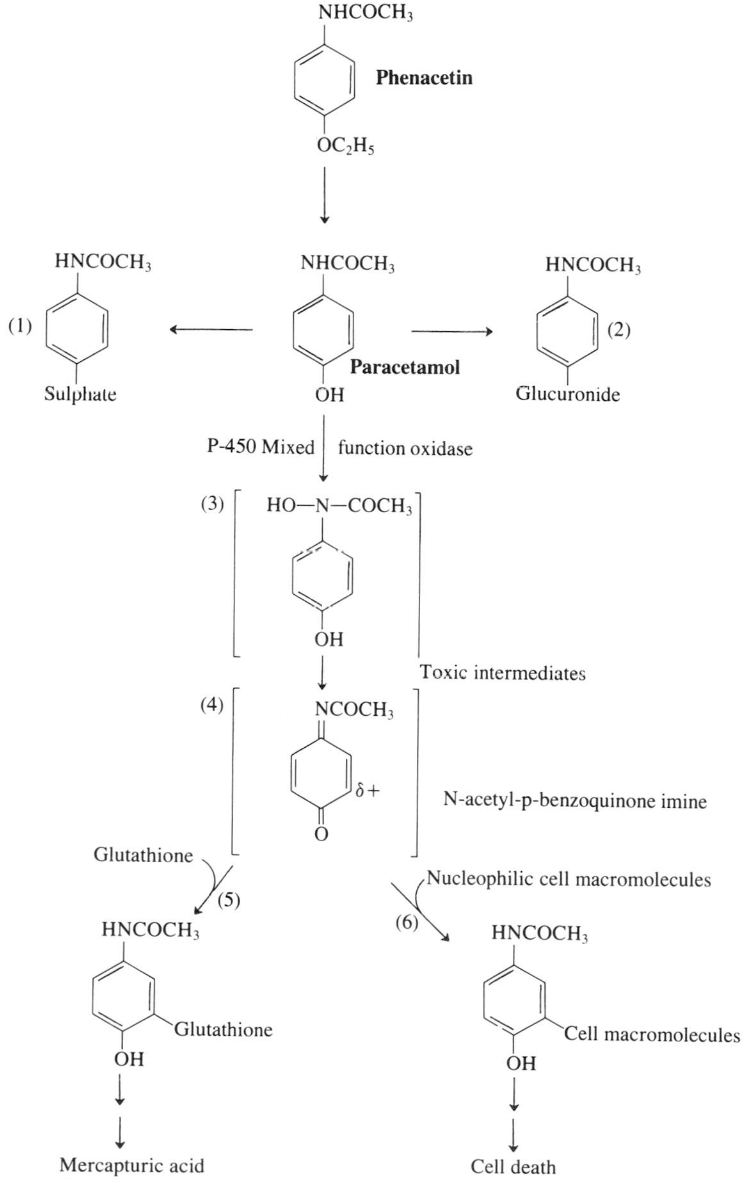

Fig. 9.5 The metabolism of phenacetin and paracetamol. With normal therapeutic doses paracetamol is metabolized by pathways 1 and 2, and with higher doses, by pathways 3, 4 and 5. When glutathione is depleted, the toxic intermediate interacts with proteins and there is cell damage (reaction 6).

them from plasma proteins and partly because its effect on platelets interferes with haemostatic mechanisms (see Chapter 12). Sodium salicylate does not have this effect. Aspirin interferes with the effect of uricosuric agents such as probenecid and sulphinpyrazone and since low doses of aspirin may, on their own, reduce urate excretion, aspirin should not be used in gout.

Paracetamol

This drug (called acetaminophen in the USA) is one of the most commonly used non-narcotic analgesic-antipyretic agents. It has only weak anti-inflammatory activity. Its mechanism of action and the possible explanation of its differential actions on pain and inflammation are discussed above. In structure it is a para-aminophenol derivative (Fig. 9.5).

Pharmacokinetic aspects

Paracetamol is given orally, is well absorbed and peak plasma concentrations are reached in 30–60 mins. A variable proportion is bound to plasma proteins and the drug is inactivated in the liver, being conjugated with glucuronic or sulphuric acids (reactions 1 and 2 in Fig. 9.5). The plasma half-life of paracetamol with therapeutic doses is 2–4 hours but with toxic doses the half-life may be extended to 4–8 hours.

Unwanted effects

With therapeutic doses side effects are few and uncommon, though allergic skin reactions may sometimes occur.

When toxic doses are ingested, a serious, potentially fatal hepatotoxicity is likely to occur. Renal toxicity and hypoglycaemia are also reported. The toxic effects on the liver are a result of saturation of the enzymes catalysing the normal conjugation reactions. The drug is then metabolized by the mixed function oxidases (reactions 3 and 4 in Fig. 9.5), the resulting toxic metabolite, N-acetyl-p-benzoquinone being inactivated by conjugation with glutathione (reaction 5 in Fig. 9.5). When glutathione is depleted the toxic intermediate accumulates and reacts with nucleophilic constituents in the cell

resulting in necrosis in the liver and also in the kidney tubules (reaction 6 in Fig. 9.5).

The initial symptoms of acute paracetamol poisoning are nausea and vomiting, the hepatotoxicity being a delayed manifestation which occurs 24–48 hours later. Treatment involves gastric lavage followed by oral activated charcoal. If the patient is seen sufficiently soon after ingestion liver damage can be prevented by giving: (a) agents which increase glutathione formation in the liver (e.g. **acetylcysteine**, which can be given orally or intravenously); and (b) agents which increase the conjugation reactions (**methionine**, **cysteamine**). The time since the taking of the drug and the plasma paracetamol level are the main guides as to whether the above agents should be given, bearing in mind that if more than 12 hours have passed since the ingestion of a large dose, the antidotes are not likely to be useful and may even make the situation worse, since these compounds have been reported to precipitate hepatic coma.

Benorylate is an aspirin-paracetamol ester. It is metabolized in the liver to give both active constituents. There is less gastrointestinal disturbance and blood loss than with aspirin itself and as it is more slowly absorbed than paracetamol, overdosage may not cause as much hepatotoxicity.

CLINICAL USE OF THE NSAIDs

There is considerable individual variation in response to NSAIDs and considerable unpredictable patient preference for one drug rather than another.

For analgesia

Most NSAIDs have analgesic actions; the types of pain for which they are effective are outlined in the section on pharmacological actions above. Single doses of aspirin (approx 600 mg) usually start to have an effect within a few minutes and reach peak action after 1–2 hours. The effect wears off after about 6 hours. Tolerance does not develop and subsequent doses will produce exactly the same pattern of response. Other NSAIDs which have this same pattern of effect are fenoprofen, ibuprofen and mefenamic acid. All of these drugs require thrice daily administration to control continuous pain.

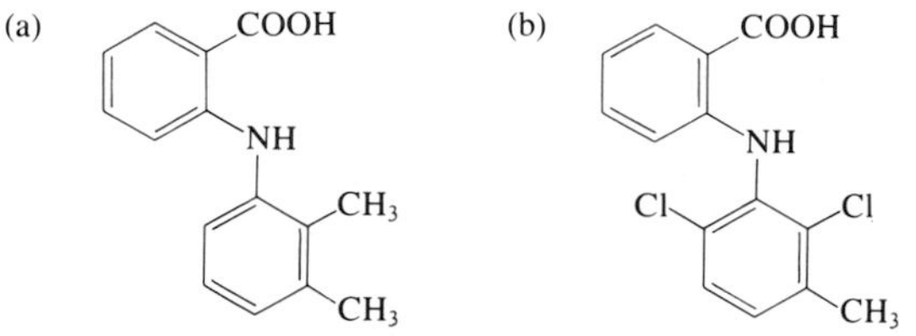

Fig. 9.6 Structures of fenamate NSAIDs. (a) Mefenamic acid, (b) Meclofenamic acid.

Drugs with longer half-lives, such as diflunisal or naproxen (which are given twice daily) and piroxicam (given once daily) have analgesic activity equal to the compounds specified above. Because of their long half-lives they may be more convenient for chronic pain but are less so for 'on demand' analgesia. Some pyrazalone derivatives (phenylbutazone) and some fenamates (e.g. flufenamic acid; Fig. 9.6) have little action in pain (such as headache) in which the inflammatory component is absent.

In general, aspirin is not only as effective an analgesic as any other NSAID, but is considerably cheaper and is the drug of choice for short-term therapy.

For anti-inflammatory effects

The main inflammatory conditions in which NSAIDs are used are rheumatoid arthritis and related connective tissue diseases, such as osteo-arthritis, gout, and soft tissue rheumatism.

With many NSAIDs, the dosage required for control of the signs and symptoms of inflammatory disease is considerably greater than for simple analgesia. Thus for anti-inflammatory actions, aspirin needs to be given in a daily (divided) dosage of 3–4 g, though with diflunisal the analgesic and anti-inflammatory dosage is similar. As therapy may need to be continued for long periods, side effects and toxic effects are likely to be seen. Side effects such as dyspepsia and rashes may become apparent within 2 weeks; more serious toxic effects such as peptic ulcer, bone marrow dysplasia and kidney and liver damage are less frequent but become commoner as treatment is prolonged.

The conditions specified are chronic diseases, often with intermittent acute exacerbations, and NSAIDs are the main drugs used for relieving symptoms such as pain, stiffness and swelling. Therapy usually needs to be continuous. Variation in response to NSAIDs is greater between patients than between drugs and it may be necessary to try a range of different preparations. Treatment should be initiated with an agent known to have a low incidence of side effects such as a propionic acid derivative or diflunisal or sulindac. If, after 2–3 weeks this proves unsatisfactory, another agent from this same group should be tried. If this also proves unsatisfactory the stronger but potentially more toxic agents such as indomethacin should be used.

Other uses

Aspirin has been used to treat radiation-induced diarrhoea.

ANTI-RHEUMATOID DRUGS

Some agents such as gold, penicillamine and some 4-aminoquinoline drugs are believed to have a specific action in modifying the disease process in rheumatoid conditions. The effects of these agents are slow in onset and some (e.g. penicillamine) are not thought to have a general anti-inflammatory action.

They are used in patients in whom therapy with NSAIDs has been ineffective and in patients in whom the disease is progressing and causing deformities. Glucocorticoids (see Chapter 16) may also be used in these conditions, as may immunosuppressant drugs (see below) and sulphasalazine.

Gold is probably the drug of first choice, with penicillamine as next choice. But these two agents should not be given simultaneously because penicillamine is a metal chelator. Intra-articular glucocorticoids should be tried before systemic glucocorticoids since this latter form of therapy needs to be continuous and continued and will usually result in iatrogenic Cushing's syndrome (p. 394).

Gold

First used in 1929 for rheumatoid arthritis, gold was shown to be efficacious in double-blind clinical trials in the 1960s. The preparations used are **sodium aurothiomalate**, **aurothioglucose** and **auranofin** (Fig. 9.7).

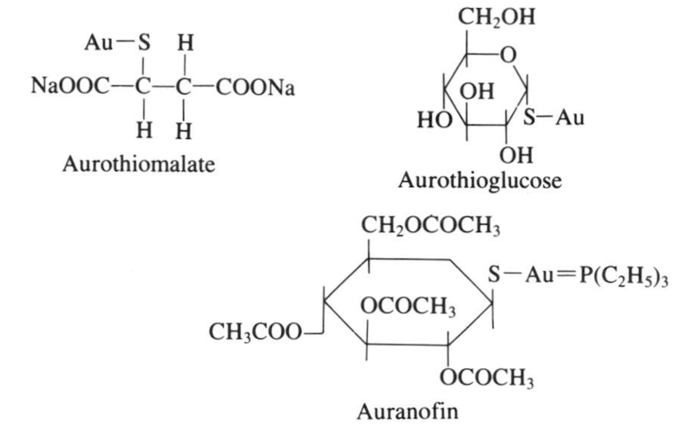

Fig. 9.7 Gold compounds used in rheumatoid arthritis.

Actions and mechanism of action

Gold salts are relatively effective in stopping the progression of bone and joint damage in rheumatoid arthritis. The action develops slowly, the maximum effect occurring after 3–4 months. Pain and joint swelling subside and the concentration of rheumatoid factor (an IgM antibody against host IgG) falls.

The precise *mechanism of action* is not fully understood. In experimental studies gold salts inhibit mitogen-induced lymphocyte proliferation, reduce both the release and the activity of lysosomal enzymes, decrease the production of toxic O_2 metabolites from phagocytes, inhibit chemotaxis of neutrophils and reduce the release of mast cell mediators. They may decrease production of interleukin-1. Any or all of these effects could be involved in their beneficial effects in rheumatoid disease.

Pharmacokinetic aspects

Sodium aurothiomalate is given by deep intramuscular injection and auranofin is given orally. Peak plasma concentrations of aurothiomalate are reached in 2–6 hours, most being bound to plasma protein. However, the salts gradually become concentrated in the tissues, not only in synovial cells in joints (where the concentration is 50% of the plasma concentration) but also in macrophages throughout the body, and in liver cells, kidney tubules and the adrenal cortex. The gold may remain for some time after treatment is stopped. Excretion is mostly renal, but some is excreted in the gastrointestinal tract. The half-life in the plasma is approximately 1 week in the initial stages but increases with treatment, thus it must be given with lengthening intervals between doses.

Unwanted effects

These are seen in about one-third of patients treated, and serious toxic effects in about 1 patient in 10. Toxicity appears to be related not to the plasma concentration but to the total amount of gold in the tissues.

Toxic effects are seen first in the skin (dermatitis occurs in 15–20% of patients) and in mucous membranes. The skin reactions have the characteristics of anaphylactic hypersensitivity reactions (see Chapter 8). Proteinuria may occur but often resolves. Blood dyscrasias are reported (leucopenia, thrombocytopenia, aplastic anaemia) as are toxic effects affecting the nervous system (encephalitis and peripheral neuritis). Hepatitis may occur. If care is exercised over dosage regimes, taking into account the problem of accumulation, and if therapy is stopped when the earlier symptoms appear, the incidence of serious toxic effects is relatively low. In patients in whom toxic effects do not occur, gold therapy can be continued for years.

Penicillamine

Abraham and his co-workers found dimethylcysteine (Fig. 9.8) among the substances produced by acid hydrolysis of penicillin and named it penicillamine. The D-isomer is used in therapy.

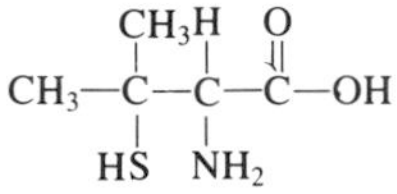

Fig. 9.8 Penicillamine (dimethyl cysteine).

Pharmacological actions and mechanism of action

About 75% of patients with rheumatoid arthritis respond to penicillamine. The effects take weeks to start and the main response is not seen for several months. The swelling of joints gradually subsides and nodules disappear. The progressive destruction of bone and joint surfaces may be retarded. The plasma concentration of rheumatoid factor falls in most patients as does the concentration of acute phase proteins and thus the erythrocyte sedimentation rate (which is increased as a result of the raised concentration of acute phase proteins). The concentration of IgA, often abnormally high in rheumatoid patients, is also decreased and there is a fall in the high levels of complexes —IgG/rheumatoid factor complexes and disulphide-bonded complexes between IgA and α_1-anti-trypsin—which occur in the serum and in the synovial fluid of such patients. (These complexes can stimulate the release of enzymes and the generation of toxic O_2 metabolites from phagocytic cells and are thus thought to be implicated in the production of tissue damage, as is explained in Chapter 8).

Evidence from studies in experimental animals suggests that there is an effect on T lymphocytes. Delayed hypersensitivity responses are decreased and from the kinetics of the responses it appears that the maintenance of a population of memory cells may be affected. The results of some studies suggest that the drug may interfere with macrophage function. It may thus decrease release of interleukin-1.

Penicillamine is also thought to modify rheumatoid disease by an effect on collagen synthesis, preventing the maturation of newly synthesized collagen. It acts at a late stage of collagen crosslinking.

The *mechanism of action* is still a matter of conjecture. The drug is known to have metal-chelating properties—an effect which is made use of in the treatment of hepatolenticular degeneration (Wilson's disease) in which there is copper accumulation in liver, kidneys and brain. In rheumatoid disease, a penicillamine-copper complex may act like superoxide dismutase and prevent formation of the toxic O_2 metabolites which are formed subsequent to superoxide generation in phagocytes.

Penicillamine is a highly reactive thiol compound, and in addition to chelating metals, substitutes for cysteine in cysteine-disulphide renal stones forming penicillamine-cysteine disulphide, which is very much more soluble; it therefore has a use in cystinuria.

Pharmacokinetic aspects

Penicillamine is given orally and only half the dose administered is absorbed. It reaches peak plasma concentrations in 1–2 hours, is 80% bound to plasma protein and excreted in the urine.

Unwanted effects

These occur in about 40% of patients and may necessitate cessation of therapy. Anorexia, nausea and vomiting are seen but often disappear with continued treatment, as is usually also the case with disturbances of taste, which are related to the chelation of zinc. Rashes and effects on the mucous membrane (e.g. mouth ulcers) are the most common unwanted effects and may resolve if the dosage is lowered. In 20% of patients proteinuria occurs; if renal function is otherwise normal it is possible to continue the drug. Bone marrow disorders (leucopenia, thrombocytopenia, aplastic anaemia) are absolute indications for stopping therapy as are the various autoimmune conditions (e.g. thyroiditis, myasthenia gravis) which sometimes supervene.

Chloroquine

Chloroquine is a 4-aminoquinoline drug used mainly to treat malaria (p. 660). It has been shown to cause remission of rheumatoid arthritis but it does not retard the progression of bone damage. It is also used in both systemic and discoid lupus erythematosis.

Pharmacological effects

These do not come on until a month or more after the drug is started, and about half the patients treated respond. Joint swelling subsides and the concentration of rheumatoid factor is reduced.

Mechanism of action

This is not fully understood. Chloroquine inhibits mitogen-induced lymphocyte proliferation and decreases leucocyte chemotaxis, lysosomal enzyme release and generation of toxic oxygen metabolites. It also reduces the generation of interleukin-1. Some of these effects may follow from the fact that it has a lysosomotrophic action, being concentrated in, and raising the pH of lysosomes, particularly in phagocytic cells such as macrophages, and thus interfering with the action of the acid hydrolases.

Some effects may follow from the fact that it inhibits phospholipase A_2 and therefore reduces the formation of the eicosanoids and also PAF (p. 191). It may also intercalate in the DNA and inhibit DNA and RNA synthesis, as it does in microorganisms (p. 603 & p. 661).

Pharmacokinetic aspects and unwanted effects

These are dealt with in Chapter 33.

Sulphasalazine

Sulphasalazine was introduced for use in rheumatoid arthritis but fell into disuse for this condition and has been used recently mainly for chronic inflammatory bowel disease. Recent controlled trials have indicated that it might after all be of value in producing remissions in active rheumatoid arthritis.

This drug is a combination of a sulphonamide (sulphapyridine) with a salicylate (Fig. 9.9) which is

Fig. 9.9 Sulphasalazine.

specifically concentrated in connective tissue. It is poorly absorbed after oral administration. Unwanted effects are usually not serious. The common side effects are gastrointestinal upsets, malaise and

headache. An interference with the absorption of folic acid has been seen and can be countered by giving folic acid supplements. As with other sulphonamides, there is a possibility that blood dyscrasias and anaphylactic-type reactions may occur in a few patients.

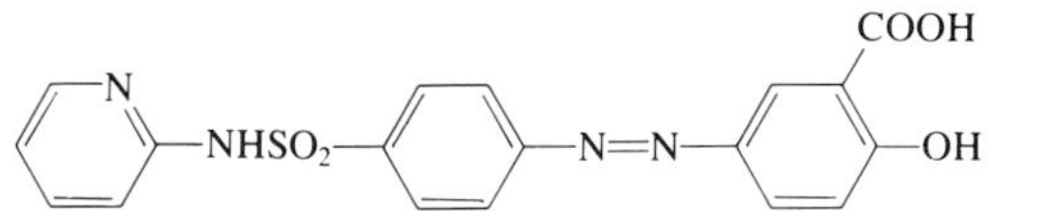

DRUGS USED IN GOUT

Gout is a genetically-determined metabolic disease in which there is overproduction of purines. It is characterized by intermittent attacks of acute arthritis produced by the deposition in the synovial tissue of joints of crystals of sodium urate—a product of purine metabolism. An inflammatory response occurs, involving activation of the kinin, complement and plasmin systems (see Chapter 8 & Fig. 8.1), generation of lipoxygenase products such as LTB_4 and local accumulation of neutrophil granulocytes. These engulf the crystals by phagocytosis, which causes generation of toxic oxygen metabolites and subsequently lysis of the cells with release of enzymes. Urate crystals also induce the production of interleukin-1 (p. 202).

Drugs used to treat gout may act in the following ways:

1. By inhibiting uric acid synthesis (allopurinol)
2. By increasing uric acid excretion (uricosuric agents: probenecid, sulphinyrazone)
3. By inhibiting leucocyte migration into the joint (colchicine)
4. By general anti-inflammatory and analgesic effects (NSAIDs: see p. 204).

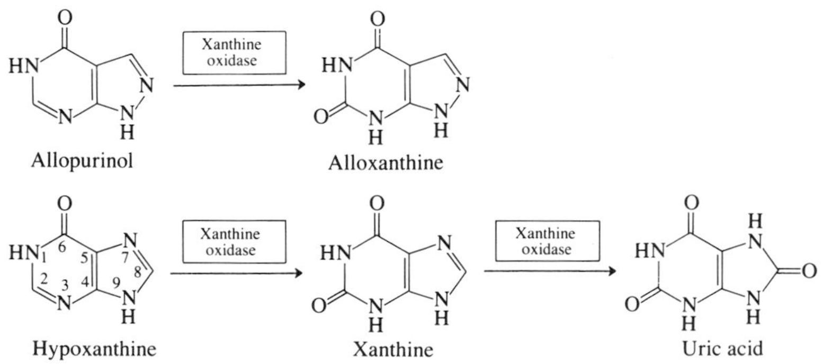

Fig. 9.10 Inhibition of uric acid synthesis by allopurinol (see text for details).

Allopurinol

This drug reduces the synthesis of uric acid by inhibiting xanthine oxidase (Fig. 9.10). It is an analogue of hypoxanthine and inhibits the enzyme mainly by substrate competition, although at high concentrations an element of non-competitive inhibition is introduced. Some degree of inhibition of *de novo* purine synthesis also occurs. Allopurinol is converted to alloxanthine by xanthine oxidase and this metabolite, which remains in the tissue for a considerable time, is an effective non-competitive inhibitor of the enzyme. The pharmacological action of allopurinol is largely due to alloxanthine.

The result of the action of the drug is that the concentration of the relatively insoluble urates and uric acid in tissues, plasma and urine decreases while that of the more soluble xanthines and hypoxanthines increases. The deposition of urate crystals in tissues ('tophi') is reversed and the formation of renal stones is inhibited.

Allopurinol is the drug of choice in the long-term treatment of gout, but it is ineffective in the treatment of the acute attack.

Pharmacokinetic aspects

Allopurinol is given orally, is well absorbed in the gastrointestinal tract, reaches peak plasma concentrations in 30–60 mins and is distributed throughout the body water. Its half-life is 2–3 hours, largely because it is converted to alloxanthine (Fig. 9.10).

This latter compound has a half-life of 18–30 hours. Neither allopurinol nor its metabolite are bound to plasma protein. Only a small proportion of allopurinol or its metabolite is excreted as such in the urine, renal excretion being a balance between glomerular filtration and probenecid-sensitive tubular reabsorption.

Unwanted effects

These are few. Gastrointestinal disturbances, allergic reactions (mainly skin rashes) may occur, but disappear if the drug is stopped. Acute attacks of gout may occur during the early stages of therapy.

Some important drug interactions

Allopurinol increases the effect of mercaptopurine, an antimetabolite which may be used in cancer chemotherapy, and also enhances the effect of cyclophosphamide. The effect of oral anticoagulants is increased due to inhibition of their metabolism.

Uricosuric agents

These are drugs which increase uric acid excretion by a direct action on the renal tubule. The two main agents are **probenecid** and **sulphinpyrazone** (Fig. 9.11). These are dealt with in Chapters 12 and 14.

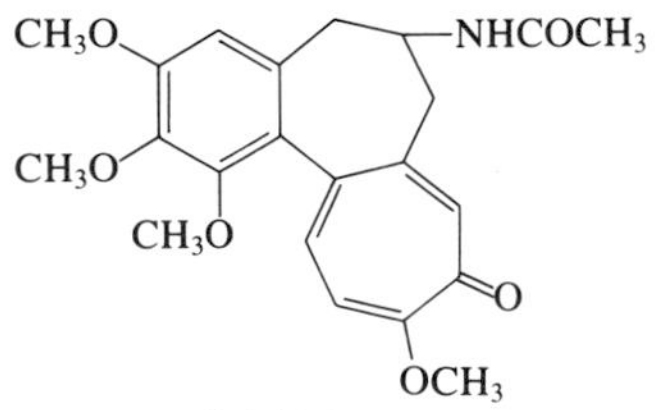

Colchicine

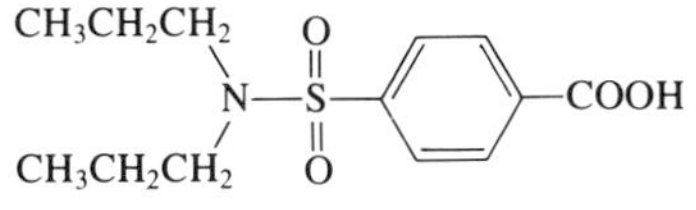

Probenicid

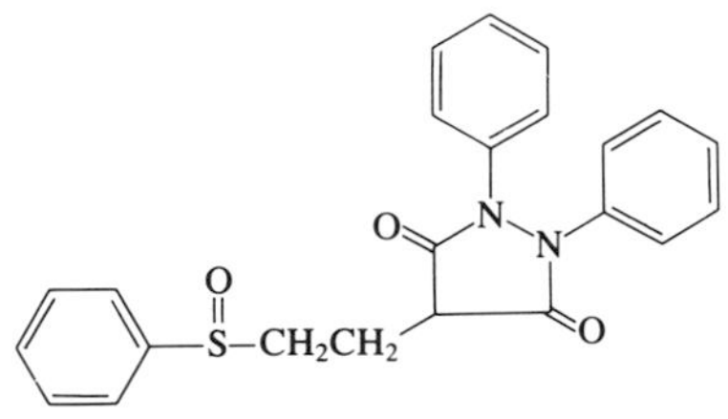

Sulphinpyrazone

Fig. 9.11 Structures of some drugs used in gout.

Colchicine

Colchicine (Fig. 9.11) has a specific effect in gouty arthritis and can be used both to prevent and to relieve acute attacks. Its main effect is to prevent the migration of neutrophils into the joint. Its mechanism of action is thought to be by binding to tubulin, the protein of the microtubules, resulting in their depolymerization. In cells such as neutrophils this effect of colchicine interferes with motility; when observed *in vitro*, colchicine-treated cells can be seen to have a 'drunken walk'. There is also evidence that colchicine prevents the production of an inflammatory glycoprotein by neutrophils which have phagocytosed urate crystals.

Pharmacokinetic aspects

Colchicine is given orally, is well absorbed and reaches peak concentrations in about an hour. It is excreted partly in the gastrointestinal tract and partly in the urine.

Unwanted effects

These are largely gastrointestinal—nausea, vomiting and abdominal pain. Severe diarrhoea may be a problem and with large doses may be associated with gastrointestinal haemorrhage and kidney damage. Rashes may occur, as may peripheral neuritis. Long courses of treatment have occasionally resulted in blood dyscrasias.

ANTAGONISTS OF HISTAMINE

There are two classes of histamine antagonists—H_1 receptor antagonists and H_2 receptor antagonists. The former group was discovered first by Bovet and his colleagues in the 1930s, at a time when the classification of the histamine receptors had not been elucidated. (Indeed the elucidation was possible only because these agents were available.) The term 'antihistamine' conventionally refers to the H_1 receptor antagonists, which affect various inflammatory and allergic mechanisms. These drugs are discussed in this section. The more recently discovered H_2 receptor antagonists, whose effect is mainly on gastric secretion, are discussed in Chapter 15 (p. 336).

H_1 receptors antagonists (H_1-antihistamines)

Mepyramine and **tripelennamine** were among the first H_1-antihistamines produced and they are still in use. As a result of further research in this area two important groups of drugs were developed—tricyclic antidepressants and the neuroleptic phenothiazines (see Chapters 22 & 23).

Some characteristic H_1-antihistamines are shown in Figure 9.12. All are lipid soluble and all contain a substituted ethylamine moiety.

Pharmacological actions

Many of these follow from the actions of histamine outlined in Chapter 8 (p. 187). Thus *in vitro* they inhibit histamine-induced contraction of the smooth muscle of the bronchi, the intestine and the uterus. They inhibit histamine-induced bronchospasm in the guinea pig *in vivo* but are of little value in allergic bronchospasm in man. They inhibit the increased vascular permeability caused by histamine.

Many of the actions of these drugs do not appear to be related to blockade of H_1 receptors and may well be due to antagonist effects at other receptors such as those for serotonin, α_1-agonists and muscarinic agonists.

Some H_1-antihistamines have pronounced effects in the CNS. These are usually listed as 'side effects' but often they are more clinically useful than the peripheral H_1 antagonist effects and should be recognised as such. Some are fairly strong sedatives and may be used for this action (e.g. **promethazine**; Table 9.2). Several are anti-emetic and are used to prevent motion sickness (e.g. **cyclizine**). This is dealt with in Chapter 15. Many H_1-antihistamines (e.g. **diphenhydramine**) also show significant competitive antagonism against the muscarinic effects of acetylcholine though their affinity is much lower for muscarinic than for histamine receptors. Thus, as measured on the guinea pig ileum, the pA_2 of mepyramine for the H_1 receptors is 9.2 and for the muscarinic receptors is 5. Two recently introduced H_1-antihistamines, **terfenadine** and **astemizole** have virtually no sedative or anticholinergic effects.

Several H_1-antihistamines show weak blockade at α_1-adrenoceptors (an example is the phenothiazine, **promethazine**) and some have local anaesthetic activity (diphenhydramine, pro-

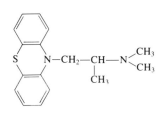

Fig. 9.12 Histamine H_1-antagonist drugs. The general structure is given at the top and consists of aromatic groups (Ar_1, Ar_2) linked by a short chain to a tertiary amino group.

methazine). **Cyproheptadine** (see Chapter 11) is a serotonin antagonist as well as being an H_1-antihistamine.

Unwanted effects

What is defined as 'unwanted' will depend to a certain extent on what the drugs are used for. When used for purely antihistamine actions, all the CNS effects are unwanted. When used for their sedative or anti-emetic actions, some of the CNS effects such as dizziness, tinnitus and fatigue are unwanted. The peripheral anti-muscarinic actions are always unwanted. The commonest of these is dryness of the mouth but blurred vision, constipation and retention of urine may occur. Unwanted effects not re-lated to the drugs' pharmacological actions are also seen; thus gastrointestinal disturbances are fairly common while allergic dermatitis can follow topical application of these drugs.

Pharmacokinetic aspects

The drugs are usually given orally, are well absorbed, reach their peak effect in 1–2 hours and are effective for 3–6 hours. **Meclozine** has a longer duration of action. Most appear to be widely distributed throughout the body though some do not penetrate the blood-brain barrier (e.g. terfenadine). They are metabolized in the liver and excreted in the urine. Astemizole has a slow onset of action and a long half-life (19 days).

Table 9.2 Some commonly used antihistamine drugs (see Fig. 9.12)

Class	Drug	Comment
Ethylenediamines	mepyramine (pyrilamine in USA)	Prototype antihistamine. Moderate degree of sedation. Some local anaesthetic activity. GIT side effects may occur. A useful general purpose H_1-histamine.
Oxyethylamines	diphenhydramine	Antimuscarinic activity. Markedly sedative. Effective in motion sickness. Used in Parkinsonism. Has some local anaesthetic activity. Few GIT side effects.
	dimenhydrinate	The 8-chlorotheophylline salt of di-phenhydramine. Markedly sedative. Used for motion sickness.
Arylalkylamines	chlorpheniramine	Less likely to be sedative. (CNS stimulation may occur as a side effect.)
Phenothiazines	promethazine	Markedly sedative. Strong anti-emetic effect and marked antimuscarinic activity. Local anaesthetic action. Effects longer lasting than with mepyramine.
Piperazines	cyclizine	Less likely to be sedative. Rather less antimuscarinic activity. Anti-emetic.
	meclozine	Minimal sedation. Marked antimuscarinic and anti-emetic activity. Long duration of action: 12–24 hours.
Butyrophenones	terfenadine	Little penetration of blood-brain barrier and thus less sedation. Little anti-muscarinic action.

GIT = gastrointestinal tract

Clinical uses

1. Allergic reactions: this group of drugs is useful for the prevention and treatment of some Type I hypersensitivity reactions—allergic rhinitis and urticaria. Replacement of one agent by another may be necessary during a course of treatment, sometimes because of the side effects, sometimes because the effects of a particular drug decreases.

2. Motion sickness: promethazine and diphen-hydramine are used (see Chapter 15).

3. Vertigo not associated with motion sickness: dizziness which may be accompanied by nausea

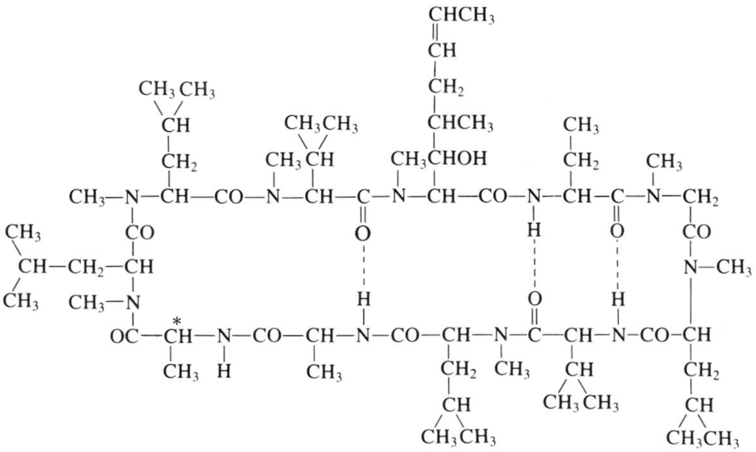

Fig. 9.13 Cyclosporin. The amino acid marked with asterisk is the D-isomer; all others are L-isomers.

and vomiting may have many causes—labyrinthine disorders, Meniere's disease, central neurological disorders etc. Vestibular disease may be iatrogenic, and follow therapy with aminoglycoside antibiotics (see Chapter 30), or with diuretics such as frusemide and ethacrynic acid (see Chapter 14). H_1-antihistamine drugs such as **dimenhydrinate** and **cyclizine**, or a phenothiazine may provide some relief from this condition (see Chapter 15). Dimenhydrinate can be given by injection.

IMMUNOSUPPRESSANTS

The drugs used for immunosuppression are cyclosporin, glucocorticoids, cytotoxic agents such as azathioprine and cyclophosphamide, and antilymphocyte serum.

Cyclosporin

Cyclosporin is a fungal peptide with powerful immunosuppressive activity, unique in that it has selective effects on lymphocytes. It was discovered by Borel and his co-workers in 1976 in the course of screening fungal products for anti-fungal activity. Cyclosporin was found to have only weak anti-fungal activity but during the concomitant toxicity testing was shown to have a markedly inhibitory effect on lymphocyte proliferation.

It is a cyclic peptide of 11 amino acids, several of which are N-methylated and one of which was previously unknown. Its structure is shown in Figure 9.13. The peptide has a M_r of 1203, is neutral and is unusually rich in hydrophobic amino acids, which makes it insoluble in water but soluble in lipids, in alcohol and in other organic solvents.

Pharmacological actions

Cyclosporin has been shown to prolong allograft survival in man and in experimental animals. In laboratory experiments it can be shown to suppress reversibly both cell-mediated and antibody-mediated responses (p. 182 & 183), and the therapeutic ratio for most effects is significantly greater than that of other immunosuppressive agents. It has no effect on the acute inflammatory response per se.

Cyclosporin is effective in a variety of reactions in which *cell-mediated responses* play a major part. Thus it results in *prolonged survival* of both *allografts* (grafts between members of the same species) and *xenografts* (grafts between different species). It has substantial action in preventing *graft versus host* reactions in rats. *Contact sensitivity reactions* in guinea pigs such as the skin reaction to oxazolone, are suppressed by cyclosporin if it is administered during sensitization. Cyclosporin prevents the expression of the *delayed hypersensitivity* response to tuberculin, in guinea pigs, if given at the time of challenge. It is also effective in several animal models of *autoimmune disease* in which the animals mount damaging immune responses against their own tissue. These include experimental allergic encephalomyelitis in guinea pigs (which has some similarity to human multiple sclerosis), adjuvant arthritis in rats (which has some similarities to human rheumatoid arthritis), autoimmune haemolytic anaemia in mice and autoimmune damage to the retina in rats.

Cyclosporin has a marked suppressive action on some *antibody-mediated responses*, notably those which involve T helper cells, but has little effect on antibody production against antigens which stimulate B cells directly.

In general it is effective mainly at the *induction phase* of the immune response—at the phase of antigen recognition and clonal proliferation (see Figs. 8.3 & 8.4) though some T cell *effector mechanisms* may also be affected.

Mechanism of action

Cyclosporin has a *selective* action on lymphocytes and within this group of cells appears to affect mainly, if not only, T lymphocytes. In antibody-production, cyclosporin inhibits the action of the T helper cell (see Fig. 8.3). In cell-mediated immune responses the drug has a more complex action. It acts on the induction stage and stops clonal proliferation of T cells by an effect at 2 different sites. There is good evidence that the main effect is inhibition of the synthesis of interleukin-2 (IL-2) by the IL-2-producing T cell (see Fig. 8.4). Cyclosporin not only blocks induction of the secretion of IL-2 but stops on-going IL-2 generation. There is also some evidence that cyclosporin may inhibit the expression of IL-2 receptors by the cells which respond to IL-2. In addition the drug also has some effects on the effector stage of the cell-mediated response. Thus it appears to inhibit the secretion of some effector lymphokines such as colony-stimulating factor and γ-interferon. As regards the effect on cytotoxic lymphocytes (Tc lymphocytes), the induction of these cells is inhibited but not the action of already formed Tc cells.

Recent work has provided some clues as to the biochemical mechanism of action of cyclosporin on lymphocytes. The inhibitory effect on interleukin-2 production appears to be due to a relatively selective action on IL-2 gene transcription. Cyclosporin has been shown to inhibit the synthesis of IL-2 transcripts and IL-2 mRNA accumulation. It has been suggested that cyclosporin may interfere with the mechanism by which the interaction of antigen with the T cell receptor is translated into an effect on the DNA. There is evidence that two pathways are involved in the response to interaction of antigen and receptor—protein kinase C activation and a rise in cytosolic calcium (see Chapter 1). It is this latter pathway which appears to be inhibited by cyclosporin since cyclosporin inhibits lymphocyte activation by a calcium ionophore but not by a protein kinase C activator.

Pharmacokinetic aspects

Cyclosporin can be given orally or by intravenous infusion. The degree of absorption from the gastro-intestinal tract may be different in different individuals but peak plasma concentrations are usually attained in about 3–4 hours. The plasma half-life is between 17 and 40 hours and there are two phases, the first phase having a half-life of approximately 1 hour and the second a half-life of approximately 25–30 hours. The plasma level can be determined by radioimmunoassay. Metabolism occurs in the liver and most of the metabolites (of which 14 have been recognized) are excreted via the kidney. It is possible that some of the drug remains in fat depots and cell membranes for some time after administration has stopped.

Unwanted effects

Unlike most other immunosuppressive agents, cyclosporin has no depressant effects on the bone marrow. Its most serious toxic effect is on the proximal tubule of the kidney which is reflected in increased blood urea and creatinine concentrations. This is the commonest unwanted effect and it may be a limiting factor in the use of the drug in some patients. Less important unwanted effects are mild hepatoxicity, anorexia, lethargy, hirsutism, tremor, gum hypertrophy, nausea and diarrhoea.

Lymphomata have been reported in patients on cyclosporin. However, according to a recent review, the incidence of lymphomata in renal and cardiac allograft patients on conventional immuno-suppressants was 2–13%, while in those on cyclosporin it was 3%. The development of lymphomata may be related to activation of latent Epstein-Barr viruses, leading to virus-induced B-cell proliferation. This could result from a diminution of the normal T cell control of virus-infected cells.

Glucocorticoids

The action of glucocorticoids as immunosuppressants involves both their anti-inflammatory effects and their effects on the immune response. These are described in Chapter 16 and the sites of action of the agents on cell-mediated immune reactions are indicated in Figures 8.3 & 8.4.

Cytotoxic agents

Azathioprine (Fig. 9.14) is the main cytotoxic agent used for immunosuppression and is widely used to control tissue rejection in transplant surgery. This drug is metabolized to give **mercaptopurine**, a purine analogue which inhibits DNA synthesis (see Chapter 29).

Both cell-mediated and antibody-mediated im-

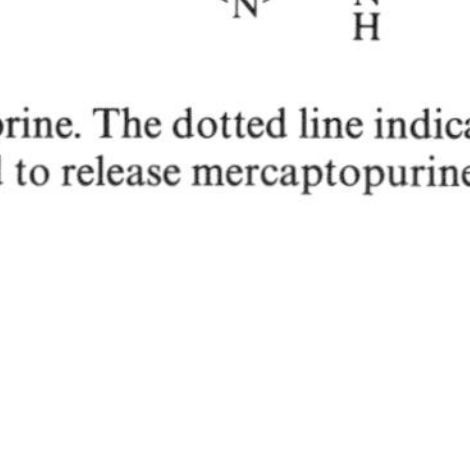

Fig. 9.14 Azathioprine. The dotted line indicates where the molecule is cleaved to release mercaptopurine.

mune reactions will be depressed by this drug since it inhibits the clonal proliferation phase of the induction of the immune response (see Figs. 8.3 & 8.4) by a cytotoxic action on mitosing cells.

As is the case with mercaptopurine itself the main unwanted effect is depression of the bone marrow. Other toxic effects which have been reported are nausea and vomiting, skin eruptions and a mild hepatotoxicity.

Cyclophosphamide is another cytotoxic agent with powerful immunosuppressive effects. It is an alkylating agent and its structure is given and its mechanism of action described in Chapter 29. As an immunosuppressant it affects the clonal proliferative phase of the immune response and reduces both antibody-mediated and cell-mediated immune reactions.

Chlorambucil, another alkylating cytotoxic agent, may also be used for immunosuppression and has effects similar to those of cyclophosphamide.

Antilymphocyte immunoglobulin

This agent is obtained by immunizing horses with human lymphocytes or with foetal thymic tissue. (It may also be produced in future by the hybridoma technique.) The IgG fraction of the horse antiserum is separated off and tested for potency by *in vitro* tests involving lymphocyte cytotoxicity. These tests give some idea of the potential clinical efficacy of the preparation but adequate methods of measuring the potency and thus for standardizing antilymphocyte immunoglobulin have yet to be devised.

Actions and mechanism of action

The lymphocytes affected by antilymphocyte immunoglobulin are the long-lived recirculating T cells. The immunoglobulin 'recognizes' and binds to protein on the lymphocyte surface and this antigen-antibody reaction results in the exposure of the complement binding site on the Fc portion of the immunoglobulin. The complement system is thus activated leading to the lysis of the lymphocyte (p. 179).

Antilymphocyte immunoglobulin affects mainly T cells and cell-mediated immune reactions, leaving B cells and antibody-mediated reactions relatively unaffected.

After organ transplantation it is given by intramuscular injection, initially on a daily basis but subsequently less frequently.

Unwanted effects

These are mainly those to be expected with injection of foreign protein. Antibodies against the horse immunoglobulin may be produced, anaphylactic reactions may occur and the complexes formed from the horse protein with the human antibody may localize in the glomerulus of the kidney. There may be local inflammation at the injection sites. Lymphomata have been reported.

If antilymphocyte immunoglobulin produced by the hybridoma technique becomes available, the reactions to foreign protein cited above should be substantially reduced.

CLINICAL USAGE OF IMMUNOSUPPRESSANTS

These drugs are used for three main purposes:

1. To suppress the host's response to organ allografts
2. To suppress the response of lymphocytes in the graft to host antigens, in bone marrow transplants
3. To treat a variety of conditions in which the immune response has been inappropriately stimulated. Autoimmune conditions such as idiopathic thrombocytopoenic purpura, haemolytic anaemia, and some types of glomerulonephritis often respond well. Immunosuppressants may also be used with effect in systemic lupus erythematosus, polyarteritis nodosa, psoriasis, ulcerative colitis and in some cases of rheumatoid arthritis.

The conventional therapy for this third category involves a combination of glucocorticoid and cytotoxic agents. For transplantation of organs or bone marrow and for haemolytic anaemia of the newborn, cyclosporin seems to be superior to other agents but is usually combined with a glucocorticoid, cytotoxic drugs, and antilymphocyte immunoglobulin.

REFERENCES AND FURTHER READING

Dale M M, Foreman J C (eds) 1984 Textbook of immunopharmacology. Blackwell Scientific, Oxford

Dinarello C A 1984 Interleukin-1: an important mediator of inflammation. Trends in Pharmacological Sciences 5: 420–422

Ganellin C R, Parsons M E (eds) 1982 Pharmacology of histamine receptors. Wright, Bristol

Kerr D N S, Ward M K 1981 In Chapter 12: Davies D M (ed) Textbook of adverse drug reactions. Oxford University Press, Oxford

Lands W E 1981 Actions of anti-inflammatory drugs. Trends in Pharmacological Sciences 2: 78–80

Nuki G 1983 Non-steroidal analgesic and anti-inflammatory agents. Br Med J 287: 39–43

Rainsford K D, Velo G P (eds) 1983 Side-effects of anti-inflammatory/analgesic drugs. Raven Press, New York

Rainsford K D 1984 Aspirin and the salicylates. Butterworth & Co., London

Shen T Y 1984 The proliferation of non-steroidal anti-inflammatory drugs (NSAIDs). In: Parnham M J, Bruinvels J (eds) Discoveries in pharmacology, Vol. 2: Haemodynamics, hormones and inflammation 523–553

Drugs affecting major organ systems

The heart

The effects of drugs on the heart will be considered under three main headings:

1. Effects on rate and rhythm
2. Effects on myocardial contraction
3. Effects on metabolism and blood flow.

Effects of drugs on these three aspects of cardiac function are, of course, not independent of each other. Thus if a drug affects the electrical properties of the myocardial cell membrane, it is likely to affect both the rate and rhythm of the heart, and its contraction; also a drug that affects contraction will inevitably alter metabolism and blood flow as well. Nevertheless, from a therapeutic point of view, these three classes of effect represent distinct clinical objectives in relation to the treatment, respectively, of cardiac dysrhythmias, cardiac failure and coronary insufficiency. We will now consider certain aspects of the pathophysiology of these functions of the heart, which provide the basis for understanding the effects of drugs upon them.

PHYSIOLOGY OF CARDIAC FUNCTION

CARDIAC RATE AND RHYTHM

Cardiac muscle cells are electrically excitable, like most other nerve and muscle cells, and the same underlying mechanism, namely a transient increase in membrane permeability to sodium ions in response to a depolarization of the membrane, is responsible. The main differences between cardiac muscle and most other kinds of excitable cell are:

1. The spontaneous, intrinsic rhythm generated by some specialized cells of the sino-arterial (SA) and atrio-ventricular (AV) nodes

2. The long duration of the action potential and long refractory period
3. A large influx of calcium ions (the 'slow inward current') during the plateau of the action potential.

The action potential of an idealized cardiac muscle cell is shown in Figure 10.1A, and is divided into four phases:

Phase 0, the fast upstroke, occurs when the membrane potential is depolarized to the critical firing threshold (about $-60\,mV$) at which point the inward current of sodium ions flowing through the voltage-dependent sodium channels becomes large enough to produce a regenerative ('all-or-nothing') depolarization. This mechanism is the same as that responsible for action potential generation by the membrane of nerve cells. The activation of these sodium channels by membrane depolarization is transient, and if the membrane remains depolarized for more than a few milliseconds, they close again (inactivation). They are therefore closed during the plateau of the action potential, and remain unavailable for the initiation of another action potential until the membrane repolarizes.

Phase 1, partial repolarization. This phase varies markedly in prominence in different parts of the heart, and occurs as the Na current is inactivated. There may also be a transient voltage-sensitive outward current.

Phase 2, the plateau, results from an inward calcium current, the **slow inward current**. The calcium channels show a pattern of voltage-sensitive activation and inactivation similar to the fast sodium channels, but with a much slower time course. Activation of the contractile machinery is due partly to the increase in intracellular calcium

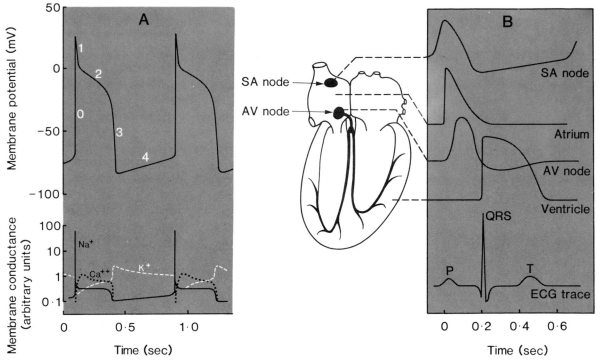

Fig. 10.1 The cardiac action potential.
A. Phases of the action potential (as recorded from a cardiac Purkinje fibre):
0—rapid depolarization
1—partial repolarization
2—plateau
3—repolarization
4—pacemaker depolarization.
The lower panel shows the accompanying changes in membrane conductance for Na^+, K^+ and Ca^{++} ions.
B. Conduction of the impulse through the heart, with the corresponding ECG trace. Note that the longest delay occurs at the AV node, where the action potential has a characteristically slow waveform.
(From: (A) Noble, 1975)

concentration that results directly from this influx and partly from the release of calcium from the sarcoplasmic reticulum, as in skeletal muscle. In certain parts of the heart, namely the SA and AV nodes, the fast sodium current is weak or absent, and the slow inward current is responsible for initiation and propagation of the action potential.

The plateau is assisted by a special property of cardiac muscle known as **inward-going rectification**, which means that the potassium conductance falls to a low level when the membrane is depolarized. Because of this there is, during the plateau, little tendency for outward potassium current to restore the resting membrane potential, so a relatively small inward calcium current suffices to maintain the plateau.

Phase 3, repolarization, occurs as the calcium

current inactivates. It happens abruptly because the inward-going rectification causes the potassium permeability to increase as soon as the membrane begins to repolarize, and the membrane potential 'flips' abruptly back to its resting level, close to the potassium equilibrium potential.

Phase 4, the pacemaker potential, is a gradual depolarization. This has been ascribed to a slowly-inactivating potassium permeability, but more recent evidence suggests that it may be due to a gradual increase of sodium permeability. When the membrane potential reaches threshold, the fast sodium current is activated again (phase 0).

Pacemaker activity is normally found only in the nodal and conducting tissue, other parts of the heart showing no inherent rhythmicity. The SA node normally discharges at a higher frequency than any other region, and so acts as pacemaker for the whole heart.

Figure 10.1B shows the action potential configuration in different parts of the heart. Phase 0 is absent in the nodal regions, and the conduction velocity is correspondingly slow in these regions (~ 5 cm/s) compared with other regions such as the Purkinje fibres (conduction velocity ~ 200 cm/s) which have the function of propagating the action potential simultaneously to the whole of the ventricular chambers. Regions which lack a fast inward current have a much longer refractory period than the fast-conducting regions. This is because the recovery of the slow inward current following its inactivation during the action potential takes a considerable time (a few hundred milliseconds), and the refractory period outlasts the action potential. With fast-conducting fibres, recovery from inactivation of the sodium current is quick, and the cell becomes excitable again as soon as it is repolarized. In normal operation, the cardiac action potential is conducted in an orderly sequence—SA-node, atrium, AV node, bundle of His, ventricle—timed by the SA node. This pattern can become disrupted either by heart disease, or by the action of drugs or circulating hormones, and an important therapeutic use of drugs is to restore a normal cardiac rhythm where it has become disturbed. The commonest cause of cardiac dysrhythmia is ischaemic heart disease, and it is now recognized that the majority of deaths following acute myocardial infarction result from ventricular fibrillation, and not directly from failure of contraction of the ischaemic muscle.

Disturbances of cardiac rhythm

Four basic mechanisms underlie pathological or drug-induced disturbances of cardiac rhythm:

1. Delayed after-depolarization
2. Re-entry
3. Abnormal pacemaker activity
4. Heart block.

These will now be described in more detail.

Delayed after-depolarization

Normal pacemaker activity, as described above, involves a spontaneous diastolic depolarization, which initiates an action potential when it reaches threshold. Non-pacemaker cells, therefore, normally remain quiescent if not excited by the arrival of an impulse from elsewhere in the heart. Under certain circumstances, however, the phenomenon of delayed after-depolarization occurs, which can lead to a repetitive discharge that does not depend on the arrival of an impulse from elsewhere (Fig. 10.2).

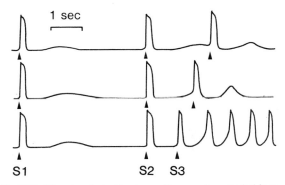

Fig. 10.2 After-depolarization in cardiac muscle recorded from dog coronary sinus in the presence of noradrenaline. The first stimulus (S1) causes an action potential followed by a small after-depolarization. As the interval S2–S3 is decreased the after-depolarization gets larger until it triggers an indefinite train of action potentials. (From: Wit & Cranefield, 1977)

The after-depolarization immediately follows the action potential, and there is good evidence that it occurs when intracellular calcium concentration increases beyond the normal range. Thus, it is accentuated if the extracellular calcium concentration (and hence the amount of calcium entering the cell during the plateau) is increased, and also by agents such as noradrenaline or cardiac glycosides (see below) which increase intracellular calcium; it is diminished by drugs that reduce the slow inward current (see below).

The after-depolarization is the result of a net inward current (known as the **transient inward current**) which occurs when the intracellular calcium concentration increases. Exactly how the current is generated is not known for certain. One possibility is that it results from activation of a **sodium–calcium exchange** mechanism across the cell membrane (see Fig. 10.4). This counter-transport system is thought to transfer one Ca^{2+} ion out of the cell in exchange for three Na^+ ions, resulting in a net influx of one positive charge, which acts to depolarize the cell. Increasing the intracellular calcium concentration will thus produce an increase in net inward current, and therefore membrane depolarization. Alternatively, there may be a direct effect of calcium on the membrane permeability to sodium and other ions, which could also lead to an inward current.

Whatever its mechanism, the importance of the transient inward current in the genesis of dysrhythmias, and its close relation to intracellular calcium concentration, is now well established.

Re-entry

In a normal cardiac rhythm, the conducted impulse dies out after it has activated the ventricles because it is surrounded by refractory tissue which it has just traversed. Re-entry describes the situation in which the impulse succeeds in re-exciting regions of the myocardium after the refractory period has subsided. A simple ring of tissue can give rise to a re-entrant rhythm if a **transient or unidirectional conduction block** is present (Fig. 10.3). Normally, an impulse originating at any point in the ring will propagate in both directions and die out when the two impulses meet, but if a damaged area shows either a transient block (so that one impulse is blocked but the second can get through; Fig. 10.3), or a unidirectional block, continuous circulation of

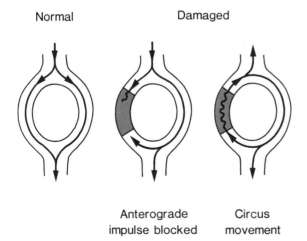

Normal   Damaged

Anterograde   Circus
impulse blocked   movement

Fig. 10.3 Generation of a re-entrant rhythm by a damaged area of myocardium. The damaged area (grey) conducts in one direction only. This disturbs the normal pattern of conduction, in which the impulse in the atria dies out as it converges on the AV node, and permits continuous circulation of the impulse to occur.

the impulse can occur; this phenomenon is known as circus movement, and was first demonstrated on rings of jellyfish tissue more than 75 years ago.

The 'ring' of tissue need not be anatomically distinct in the heart, but only functionally separate. If it retains a connection with the rest of the heart it can act as a focus for high frequency re-excitation of the whole atrium or ventricle. The re-entrant rhythm will persist only if the time taken for propagation round the ring exceeds the refractory period, and so may be halted by drugs which prolong the refractory period (see below). On the other hand, damaged myocardium may show extreme slowing of action potential propagation (from a normal value of about 1 m/s) which will tend to favour re-entry. This slowing is often associated with the attenuation or disappearance of the normal fast sodium current responsible for the fast upstroke of the action potential (see Fig. 10.1). This current is reduced because the damaged cells are somewhat depolarized during diastole compared with normal cells, so the fast sodium channels remain partly or completely inactivated, leaving only the slow inward current to support propagation of the action potential.

Studies on the properties of these 'slow responses' in damaged regions of the heart have confirmed the occurrence of transient or unidirectional conduction block necessary to initiate a re-entrant rhythm (Cranefield, 1975).

Re-entry is thought to be the mechanism of many types of dysrhythmia, the pattern depending on the site of the re-entrant circuit, which may be in the atria, ventricles or nodal tissue.

Abnormal pacemaker activity

Pacemaker activity in a normal heart is confined to the nodal and conducting tissue, which show slow depolarization during phase 4. It can occur in other parts of the heart, however, particularly under pathological conditions, the main predisposing factors being: (a) catecholamine action; and (b) partial depolarization, such as may occur in ischaemic damage.

Catecholamines, acting on β_1 receptors (see below) increase the rate of depolarization during phase 4, and can cause normally quiescent parts of the heart to take on a spontaneous rhythm. Myocardial ischaemia is known to cause an increase in sympathetic discharge to the heart, and can also cause release of adrenaline from the adrenal gland, both of which encourage the appearance of abnormal pacemakers. Partial depolarization resulting from ischaemic damage is probably due to a decrease in the activity of the electrogenic sodium pump, and has an effect on pacemaker activity similar to that of catecholamines.

Heart block

Nodal tissue may become damaged (e.g. by infarction) so that it fails to conduct at all. If this happens to the AV node or a major branch of the conducting system, the atria and ventricles beat independently (complete AV block) at rates determined by their own pacemakers. AV block may be partial, in which case a proportion of the sinus beats are transmitted to the ventricle. This may appear in a regular pattern (e.g. 2:1 or 3:1 block) in which every second or third impulse is transmitted. The ventricular rate, and cardiac output will then be low; if AV conduction fails completely in a sporadic fashion, sudden periods of unconsciousness may result (Stokes-Adams attacks).

These different mechanisms interact in complicated ways to give rise to pathological dysrhythmias, and it is often difficult to sort out the contributions of the four processes described above in any particular instance. They do, however, provide a starting point for understanding how drugs affect the rate and rhythm of the heart, which is a topic of great clinical importance.

CARDIAC CONTRACTION

The force with which a myocardial cell contracts when invaded by an action potential depends on both intrinsic and extrinsic factors. The **intrinsic** factors include those factors which regulate the intracellular ionized calcium concentration, as well as various biochemical factors, such as availability of ATP within the myocardial cell. Together these intrinsic factors, which are sensitive to a variety of drugs and pathological processes, may be said to regulate the myocardial **contractility**. The mechanical output of the heart in situ is determined, not

only by contractility, but also by **extrinsic** circulatory factors, such as the state of the arterioles and veins, blood volume, viscosity, etc, which can also be affected by drugs and/or disease.

Myocardial contractility

The contractile machinery of the myocardial cell is basically the same as in striated muscle. The interaction betwen actin and myosin filaments is normally suppressed by the presence of **tropomyosin** bound to the actin filament, which is associated with the **troponin complex**. One component of the troponin complex, troponin C, binds three or four calcium ions; when this happens, the conformation of the troponin complex changes, with the result that tropomyosin shifts out of the way, and binding of the myosin cross-bridge to the actin filament is permitted, thus initiating the contractile process. These changes are produced when the intracellular ionized calcium concentration $[Ca^{++}]_i$ exceeds about 10^{-7} M, and the system is fully activated at about 10^{-6} M ionized calcium.

The main mechanisms responsible for controlling $[Ca^{++}]_i$ are summarized in Figure 10.4. The major route of entry of calcium is the voltage-sensitive calcium channels in the surface membrane, whose activation by depolarization gives rise to the slow inward current (see previous section). Calcium enters the cell by this route with each action potential, and causes an immediate rise in $[Ca^{++}]_i$. Depolarization also, as in striated muscle, causes release of calcium from the sarcoplasmic reticulum, which adds further to the increase in $[Ca^{++}]_i$. Calcium entry is balanced by removal of calcium from the cell, the main agency for this being the **calcium–sodium exchange pump** (Fig. 10.4). This mechanism extrudes calcium ions in exchange for sodium ions (which are in turn extruded, electrogenically or in exchange for potassium ions, by the sodium–potassium pump). This interconnection between sodium and calcium movements across the membrane means that changes in $[Na^{+}]_i$, whether produced physiologically or pharmacologically, will affect $[Ca^{++}]_i$ as well, in the same direction. Thus inhibition of the sodium–potassium pump (e.g. by cardiac glycosides; see below) will tend to raise $[Na^{+}]_i$, slow down Ca–Na exchange, and secondarily raise $[Ca^{++}]_i$, thus facilitating con-

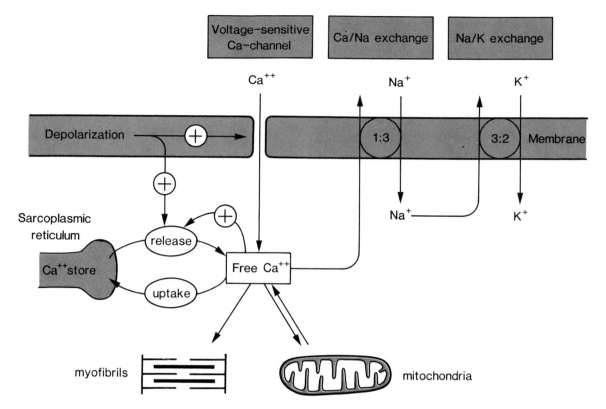

Fig. 10.4 The control of intracellular calcium in the myocardium. The phasic increase in $[Ca^{++}]_i$ associated with the action potential results from: (1) Ca^{++} entry through voltage-sensitive Ca^{++} channels; (2) release of Ca^{++} from sacroplasmic reticulum (SR) which involves (a) depolarization-induced release, and (b) Ca^{++} induced Ca^{++} release.

Ca^{++} entering the cell eventually leaves via the Ca^{++}/Na^+ exchange system so that a steady state is maintained. This process is much slower than the exchanges between SR and free cytosolic Ca^{++}. It functions electrogenically, because of the 1:3 coupling ratio, and is controlled by $[Na^+]_i$ as well as $[Ca^{++}]_i$ (see also Fig. 10.11).

traction. Conversely, inhibition of sodium entry (e.g. by lignocaine; see below) has the opposite effect.

Calcium is also exchanged between the cytosol and the sarcoplasmic reticulum, and between the cytosol and the mitochondria (Fig. 10.4). At any moment, more than 99% of the total cell calcium is sequestered by these intracellular organelles, so a small shift of calcium between these stores and the cytosol can cause a large change in $[Ca^{++}]_i$.

Many of the effects of drugs on cardiac contractility can be explained in terms of their effects on $[Ca^{++}]_i$, resulting from interactions with the voltage-sensitive calcium channels, the sarcoplasmic reticulum, or the sodium–potassium pump. Other factors that affect the force of contraction are the availability of oxygen and glucose. Cells de-

prived of oxygen quickly cease to contract, though it has recently been shown by Allen and his colleagues that their electrical activity, and the transient increase in $[Ca^{++}]_i$ associated with the action potential, is still normal even when the contraction has disappeared. The contractile proteins appear to be highly sensitive to intracellular pH, which drops rapidly when the cells undergo anaerobic glycolysis. If glycolysis is also impaired, which must happen in ischaemia because the cells are deprived of glucose as well as oxygen, the resulting fall in intracellular ATP concentration causes the sarcoplasmic reticulum to be unable to accumulate calcium, and the mechanical failure is probably due to the loss of this store of releasable calcium within the cell, rather than to a direct effect of ATP depletion on the contractile proteins.

Ventricular function curves and heart failure

The force of contraction of the heart is determined partly by its **contractility** (which, as described above, depends on the availability of intracellular calcium and ATP), and partly by the **resting length** of the muscle fibres, or **end-diastolic volume**. The end-diastolic volume is determined largely by the end-diastolic pressure (which is in turn a function of the **central venous pressure**), and its effect on the stroke work of the heart is expressed in the **Frank–Starling Law of the Heart,** which reflects an inherent property of the contractile system. The Frank–Starling Law can be represented as a **ventricular function curve** (Fig. 10.5).

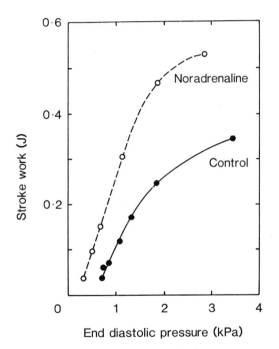

Fig. 10.5 The ventricular function curve in the dog. *Intrinsic control* (in this case increased myocardial contractility) is exemplified by the effect of noradrenaline infusion. *Extrinsic control* (the effect of external circulatory factors on the force of contraction of the heart) is shown by the relationship between stroke work and diastolic pressure. (From: Sarnoff S J et al, 1960)

The **stroke work** of the ventricle is measured by the area enclosed by the pressure-volume curve ($\int P.dV$) during the cardiac cycle. Roughly speaking, it is given by the product of stroke-volume and mean arterial pressure. As Starling showed, factors extrinsic to the heart can affect its performance in

various ways, and two patterns of response are particularly important:

1. An increase in central venous pressure (increased **pre-load**), without any change in peripheral resistance will increase the cardiac filling pressure, and hence the end-diastolic volume of the ventricles. This will increase the stroke volume, and thus increase both the cardiac output and the mean arterial pressure. The cardiac work and cardiac oxygen consumption both increase.

2. Peripheral arteriolar vasoconstriction may occur without any change in venous tone (increased **after-load**). Initially the end-diastolic volume and hence the stroke work, will be unchanged; constancy of stroke work in the face of an increased vascular resistance means that stroke volume must decrease. As this happens, the end-diastolic volume increases, which in turn increases the stroke work, until a steady state is established with an increased end-diastolic volume and the same cardiac output as before. As in the previous example, the cardiac work and cardiac oxygen consumption both increase.

The steep part of the ventricular function curve represents the normal operating range, where the central venous pressure is only a few centimetres of water above zero, and a large increase in stroke work can be achieved with only a small increase in the filling pressure. In fact, under normal circumstances, the Starling mechanism seems to play little part in controlling the cardiac output, for changes in contractility, mainly due to changes in sympathetic activity, achieve the necessary regulation without any substantial change in the ventricular filling pressure (Fig. 10.5). Thus, in a normal individual, exercise causes the central venous pressure, and end-diastolic volume to *decrease* rather than increase, because of the overriding influence of the autonomic nervous system.

Under various pathological conditions the heart may be unable to deliver as much blood as the tissues require, a condition known as **heart-failure**, even when its contractility is increased by sympathetic activity. This may happen because the myocardium is damaged (e.g. by ischaemia), because narrowing or incompetence of the valves has made its pumping action inefficient, or because excessive peripheral vascular resistance has increased the work required to maintain an adequate tissue blood flow (as in hypertension). Under these conditions the basal ventricular function curve is greatly depressed and there is insufficient reserve, in the sense of extra contractility that can be achieved by sympathetic activity, to enable the cardiac output to be maintained without a large increase in central venous pressure occurring (Fig. 10.5). An important consequence of cardiac failure is **oedema**, which affects both the peripheral tissues (causing swelling of the legs) and the lungs (causing breathlessness). Oedema is caused by the increase in venous pressure, and retention of sodium (see Chapter 11), rather than by the inadequate cardiac output per se.

MYOCARDIAL OXYGEN CONSUMPTION AND CORONARY BLOOD FLOW

In a normal human being at rest, the myocardium uses about 11% of the total body oxygen consumption, but receives as coronary blood flow only about 4% of the cardiac output, so it is, relative to its metabolic needs, one of the most poorly-perfused tissues in the body. The frequency with which coronary ischaemia occurs as a result of pathological disturbances is presumably related to this fact.

The coronary flow is, under normal circumstances, closely related to myocardial oxygen consumption, and both variables can change over a nearly ten-fold range between conditions of rest and maximal exercise.

The main physiological factors that regulate coronary flow are:

1. Physical factors
2. Vascular control by metabolites
3. Neural and humoral control.

Physical factors are mainly related to the fact that during systole the lateral pressure exerted by the myocardium on the vessels that pass through it equals or exceeds the perfusion pressure, so that flow only occurs during diastole. Thus tachycardia, in which diastole is shortened more than systole, tends to impair coronary flow unless coronary dilatation can compensate (Fig. 10.6). During diastole, the effective perfusion pressure is equal to the

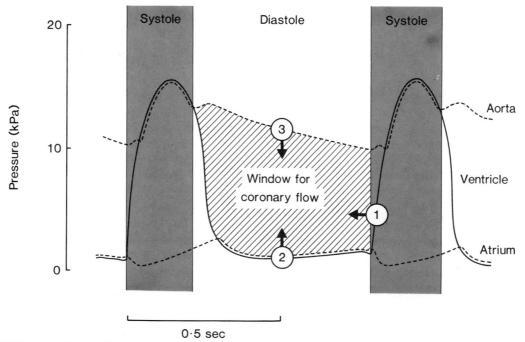

Fig. 10.6 Mechanical factors affecting coronary blood flow. The 'window' for coronary flow may be encroached upon by: (1) a shortening of diastole, which occurs when the heart rate increases; (2) increased atrial filling pressure; and (3) reduced diastolic arterial pressure.

difference between the aortic pressure and the ventricular pressure. Thus, if a reduction of diastolic aortic pressure occurs, or an increase in diastolic ventricular pressure, the perfusion pressure falls and so (unless other control mechanisms can compensate) does the coronary flow. Aortic incompetence is an example of a disorder that produces both of these effects.

Vascular control by metabolites is the most important mechanism by which coronary flow is regulated. A reduction in arterial Po_2 causes a marked vasodilatation of coronary vessels in situ, but has little effect on isolated strips of coronary artery. This suggests that it may be a change in the pattern in metabolites produced by the myocardial cells, rather than the change in Po_2 per se that controls the state of the coronary vessels. Substances produced when the myocardium functions under hypoxic conditions include **lactic acid**, but this substance is relatively ineffective as a coronary dilator. A **fall in pH** also occurs, and this has some dilator effect. The most popular candidate for the dilator metabolite is **adenosine**. This substance is produced continuously by myocardial cells, and the rate of production increases if the tissue is hypoxic. It has been suggested that this occurs because in hypoxia ATP splitting does not stop at ADP but continues all the way to adenosine. However, considerable coronary dilatation occurs at levels of hypoxia that cause the ATP content of myocardial cells to fall by only about 20%, so it seems unlikely that the adenosine is coming from that source. The effects of adenosine and other purine nucleotides on the myocardium and coronary vessels may be of importance in relation to the effects of some drugs that are used clinically, and are discussed more fully in a later section (p. 254).

There may also be a role for **prostaglandins** (see Chapter 8) in the regulation of coronary blood flow. Prostaglandins of the E series, as well as **prostacyclin**, are potent coronary dilators, and are released when the heart is made ischaemic. However inhibitors of prostaglandin synthesis have only a small effect of coronary blood flow, so it is unlikely that this system has a major physiological function.

Neural and humoral control. Coronary vessels have a dense sympathetic innervation, but the sympathetic nerves (like circulating catecholamines) exert only a small direct effect on the coronary circulation. The large coronary vessels possess α-adrenoceptors which mediate vasoconstriction, whereas the smaller vessels have β_2-receptors that have a dilator effect. Normally both effects are overshadowed by the vascular response to altered mechanical and metabolic activity, and these receptors are not of much pharmacological significance.

CORONARY ATHEROSCLEROSIS AND ITS CONSEQUENCES

Partial occlusion of coronary vessels by atheromatous deposits occurs in at least 75% of the adult population of developed countries, and the diseases which result are the major cause of illness and death in regions where malnutrition and the major microbial diseases have been eliminated.

Important consequences of coronary obstruction are: (1) development of collateral vessels; (2) anginal pain; and (3) myocardial infarction.

Collateral circulation

Normally, separate branches of the main coronary arteries supply the outer (epicardial) and inner (subendocardial) layers of muscle. Collateral channels between these branches are sparse and narrow, and occlusion of one of the supply vessels reduces blood flow to the affected part of the myocardium by up to 75%. The endocardial circulation appears to be more vulnerable than the epicardial, because the vessels reaching it must traverse the full thickness of the myocardium.

One consequence of a gradually developing occlusion of a major coronary artery is that the collateral channels widen and proliferate, and this may sustain an adequate myocardial flow even when the major vessel is fully blocked. These collateral vessels do not, however, respond to the increased demand during exercise, and recent work suggests that they may respond to vasodilator drugs differently from other coronary vessels. By dilating collateral vessels, drugs such as the organic nitrates (see later section) may be able to redistribute the coronary flow towards ischaemic areas, even though they do not appreciably increase the total flow.

Angina

Anginal pain occurs when the oxygen supply to the myocardium is insufficient for its needs. The pain has a characteristic distribution in the chest, arm and neck, and is brought on by exertion or excitement. It is a very common clinical syndrome, and an important target for therapeutic intervention (see later section on anti-anginal drugs). A similar type of pain can be produced in skeletal muscle when it is made to contract while its blood supply is interrupted, and the work of Lewis clearly showed that a chemical factor released by the ischaemic muscle is responsible for activating pain afferents in the muscle. Possible candidates for this pain-producing substance include **potassium ion**, **hydrogen ion**, peptides such as **bradykinin** (see Chapter 9), **adenosine**, **ADP**, and **prostaglandins**, all of which have been shown to stimulate pain endings. Since angina can occur in patients suffering from severe anaemia who have no reduction in coronary blood flow, it seems that the substance responsible must be produced in larger quantities when muscle contracts anaerobically, and it is possible that the same substance is responsible both for the regulation of the coronary vessels and the stimulation of pain afferents.

Two kinds of angina are recognized clinically. **Angina of effort** is always produced by an increased demand on the heart (e.g. by exercise) and is usually due to atherosclerosis of the coronary vessels. **Variant angina** occurs at rest and is associated with coronary artery spasm, causing reduced coronary flow.

Myocardial infarction

Death of an area of myocardium occurs usually when a coronary vessel is suddenly blocked by thrombosis. This is the commonest single cause of death in many parts of the world, and death usually results either from mechanical failure of the ventricle or from ventricular fibrillation. The sequence of events leading from vascular occlusion to irreversible cellular damage has been much investigated (Van der Vusse & Reneman, 1985), and it is generally believed that an increase in $[Ca^{++}]_i$ is the trigger for the secondary cellular damage. $[Ca^{++}]_i$ probably rises because the mechanisms responsible for removing calcium from the cytosol (namely uptake by the sarcoplasmic reticulum, and uptake by mitochondria) are affected, so that calcium leaks from these stores into the cytosol. The effect that this may have on the electrical activity of the myocardial cells has already been mentioned (p. 229) and this could account for the tendency to dysrhythmias. Death of the cells may also be secondary to a rise in $[Ca^{++}]_i$ through the activity of a **calcium-dependent protease** which is present in myocardial cells. The possible use of calcium antagonists (see later section) in preventing ischaemic damage follows from the involvement of calcium in its causation.

DRUGS THAT AFFECT CARDIAC FUNCTION

Drugs that have a major action on the heart can be divided into the following groups:

1. Autonomic neurotransmitters and related drugs.
2. Cardiac glycosides.
3. Antidysrhythmic drugs, including calcium antagonists, which also affect other aspects of cardiac function.
4. Antianginal drugs.
5. Various other hormones and endogenous substances, together with related synthetic agents. Most of these are discussed in more detail elsewhere. The most important are:
   a. Methylxanthines (see Chapter 26)
   b. Adenosine derivatives (see Chapter 11)
   c. Histamine (see Chapter 8)
   d. Glucagon (see Chapter 16).

AUTONOMIC TRANSMITTERS AND RELATED DRUGS

Many aspects of autonomic pharmacology have been discussed in Chapters 5, 6 & 7, so here we shall mention only aspects that particularly concern the heart.

Autonomic control of the heart

Both sympathetic and parasympathetic systems normally exert a tonic effect on the heart at rest.

Sympathetic system

The main effects that **sympathetic activity** produces are:

1. Increased heart rate (**positive chronotropic effect**)
2. Increased force of contraction (**positive inotropic effect**), affecting all parts of the heart
3. Increased **automaticity**
4. **Facilitation of conduction** in the AV node
5. **Reduced cardiac efficiency** (i.e. O_2 consumption is increased more than cardiac work).

These effects all result from activation of β_1-receptors. There is also evidence for the existence of α-receptors, activation of which causes an increased refractory period, but this is a small effect that is normally outweighed by the β-effects. Coronary vessels are constricted by α-receptor activation and dilated by β-receptor activation. Sympathetic activity produces a strong coronary vasodilation, and an increase in blood flow that matches the increased oxygen consumption, but this is mediated by the metabolic response of the myocardium rather than by a direct action on the coronary vessels.

The β-effects of catecholamines on the heart, though complex, are probably all due to an increase in the intracellular concentration of cAMP (see Chapter 1). The increase in heart rate results from an increase in the slope of the pacemaker potential (see Fig. 10.7). This slow diastolic depolarization results from a voltage-sensitive inward current which is slowly switched on when the membrane potential is in the diastolic range (about $-70\,\text{mV}$). The effect of β-receptor activation is to shift the voltage-dependence of this process to a less depolarized potential, so that the pacemaker current is switched on earlier and faster, and the firing threshold is reached earlier.

The *shape* of the action potential is also changed

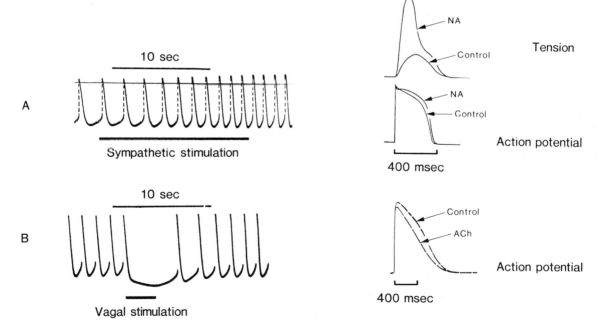

Fig. 10.7 Autonomic regulation of the heart beat.
 A. The effects of sympathetic stimulation and noradrenaline.
 B. The effects of parasympathetic stimulation and acetylcholine.
 Left hand records: spontaneously beating frog sinus venosus (intracellular recording). Sympathetic stimulation increases the slope of the pacemaker potential and increases heart rate. Parasympathetic stimulation abolishes the pacemaker potential, hyperpolarizes the membrane, and temporarily stops the heart.
 Right hand records—Above: calf ventricular muscle showing the effect of noradrenaline (NA) on action potential and tension. Prolongation of the action potential and increased tension result from an increased entry of Ca^{++}. *Below*: frog atrium. Shortening of the action potential produced by acetylcholine (ACh), and reduced tension (not shown) result from inhibition of Ca^{++} entry.
 (From: (Left) Hutter & Trautwein, 1956; (Right-top) Reuter, 1974; (Right-bottom) Giles & Noble, 1976)

by β-receptor activation, the plateau phase becoming more pronounced. At the same time the contraction also becomes larger but briefer (Fig. 10.7). The accentuation of the plateau is due to an increase of the slow inward current. Analysis by the patch clamp method (see Chapter 1) has shown that β-receptor activation, or an increased intracellular cAMP concentration, causes more calcium channels to open in response to a given depolarization and the marked increase in the magnitude of the rise in $[Ca^{++}]_i$ that accompanies the action potential has been measured in atrial cells injected with a light-emitting Ca-indicator protein (Fig. 10.8). It is

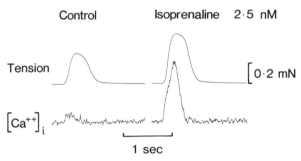

Fig. 10.8 The calcium transient in frog cardiac muscle.

A group of cells was injected with the phosphorescent Ca^{++} indicator, aequorin, which allows $[Ca^{++}]_i$ to be monitored optically. Isoprenaline causes a large increase in the Ca^{++} transient and in the tension produced. (From: Allen & Blinks, 1978)

likely that cAMP-dependent phosphorylation of the membrane protein associated with the calcium channel is required for the channel to function, and that the number of available channels at any moment reflects the relative rates of dephosphorylation and cAMP-dependent rephosphorylation of this protein. The same mechanism probably accounts for the facilitation of AV conduction, where the sodium transient is absent, so that propagation depends on the Ca^{++} current. The increased Ca^{++} entry may also account for the increased automaticity because of the effect of intracellular Ca^{++} on the transient inward current, which can result in after-discharge following a single evoked action potential (see Fig. 10.2). The increased force of contraction is partly due to increased Ca^{++} entry, but β-receptor activation also increases the Ca^{++} sensitivity of the contractile machinery, possibly by phosphorylating troponin C; furthermore it facilitates Ca^{++} capture by the

sarcoplasmic reticulum, thereby increasing the amount of Ca^{++} stored intracellularly which can be released by action potential. The result of catecholamine action is to elevate and steepen the ventricular function curve (see Fig. 10.5).

β-receptor activation causes **hyperpolarization** of some parts of the heart, which is particularly noticeable if the myocardium is damaged or hypoxic. It is due to stimulation of the Na–K pump, which generates a net outward sodium current. This repolarization may suffice to restore conduction, for example in the AV bundle, when heart block has occurred following a myocardial infarction.

The reduction of **cardiac efficiency** by catecholamines is important because it means that the oxygen requirement of the myocardium increases even if the work of the heart is unchanged. Myocardial infarction causes an increase in the concentration of circulating noradrenaline, probably by a reflex mechanism, which has the undesirable effect of increasing the oxygen needs of the damaged myocardium. The mechanism of the reduction of efficiency is not certain, but one explanation is that β-receptor activation stimulates fatty acid production, by promoting lipolysis (see Chapter 7), causing the heart to shift from glucose to fatty acid utilization, which requires more oxygen per ATP molecule generated.

Parasympathetic system

The actions and uses of drugs that act on β-receptors are described in Chapter 7.

The main effects that **parasympathetic activity** produces are, in general, opposite to the effects of the sympathetic, namely:

1. Cardiac slowing and reduced automaticity
2. Decreased force of contraction (mainly in atria)
3. Inhibition of AV conduction.

These effects result from activation of muscarinic acetylcholine receptors, which are abundant in nodal and atrial tissue but sparse in the ventricle. The question of whether an intracellular mediator, corresponding to cAMP in the β-receptor responses just discussed, is involved in muscarinic responses has not been definitely answered, though there is some evidence that cGMP may serve this function (see Chapter 1).

The negative chronotropic effect and reduced automaticity are caused by an increased permeability to potassium ions, resulting in a steady hyperpolarizing current which effectively opposes the inward pacemaker current (see Fig. 10.7). The cardiac slowing caused by vagal stimulation or by administration of muscarinic agonists can amount to complete cardiac standstill for many seconds, though if stimulation is maintained a slow beat, generated by the ventricular conducting tissue normally reappears. The negative inotropic effect in the atria results from an inhibition of the slow inward current, and is associated with a marked shortening of the action potential (see Fig. 10.7). It is very likely that both phenomena—increased K^+ permeability and reduced Ca^{++} current—contribute to the conduction block at the AV node, where propagation is dependent on the Ca^{++} current. The shortening of the atrial action potential causes a reduction of the refractory period which can, paradoxically, increase the probability of re-entrant dysrhythmias in the atria. The coronary vessels have no cholinergic innervation.

As well as producing opposite effects on myocardial cells, the sympathetic and parasympathetic systems interact more directly at the pre-synaptic level. The terminals of sympathetic and parasympathetic nerves are often found close together, and there is evidence for mutual inhibition of transmitter release by the two systems. The parasympathetic system appears to be more effective in opposing sympathetic effects than *vice versa*.

The actions and uses of drugs that act on muscarinic receptors are described in Chapter 6.

CARDIAC GLYCOSIDES

Cardiac glycosides are the active principles of leaves of plants of the foxglove family (*Digitalis*), which have been in clinical use for many centuries, for a whole variety of therapeutic purposes. Their effectiveness in the treatment of cardiac failure was first discovered by Withering in 1775, who wrote on the use of the foxglove: 'it has a power over the motion of the heart to a degree yet unobserved in any other medicine'. He had shown it to be effective in relieving the oedema associated with cardiac failure, though before this it had been used to treat tuberculosis, epilepsy, syphilis and many other diseases. Cardiac glycosides are still the most useful drugs for the treatment of cardiac failure.

Chemistry

The leaves of the foxglove contain several cardiac glycosides with similar actions. Similar substances occur in other plants, such as squill and lily of the valley. The compounds that are therapeutically important are **digoxin**, **digitoxin**, **strophanthin** and **ouabain**. All have the same pharmacological actions, but they differ in their pharmacokinetic behaviour.

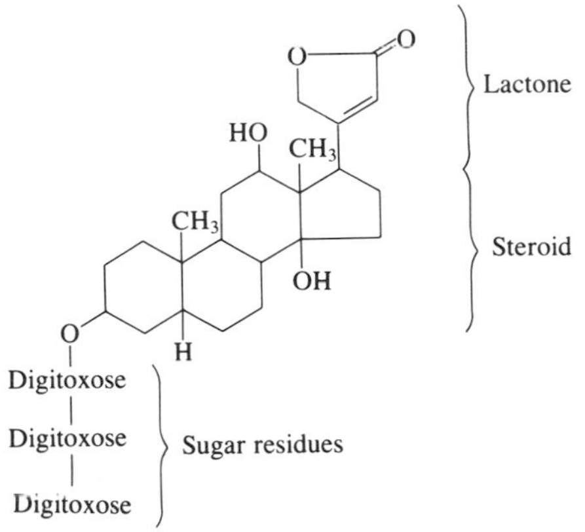

Fig. 10.9 Chemical structure of cardiac glycosides. Individual compounds vary in respect of (1) methyl and hydroxyl groups on steroid nucleus; (2) sugar residues.

Their basic chemical structure is shown in Figure 10.9. They consist of three components, a **sugar moiety**, a **steroid** and a **lactone**. The sugar moiety consists of 1–4 linked monosaccharides, some of which are not found elsewhere in nature. Derivatives in which the sugar has been removed are called **aglycones** or **genins**; these retain the same pharmacological effects as glycosides, but are relatively insoluble and act for only a short time, so they are not clinically useful. The lactone ring is essential for activity, and substituted lactones can retain biological activity even when the steroid moiety is removed.

Pharmacological actions

The main effects of glycosides are on the heart, but

some of their extra-cardiac actions are also clinically important.

The cardiac effects are:

1. Increased force of contraction
2. Disturbances of rhythm
   a. Block of AV conduction
   b. Increased ectopic pacemaker activity
3. Cardiac slowing, associated with increased vagal activity.

The main extra-cardiac effects are:

1. Anorexia, nausea and vomiting
2. Arteriolar constriction and venous dilatation
3. Visual disturbances, particularly the appearance of a yellow-green tinge.

The useful effects are the increased force of contraction and sometimes partial AV block (see below). The other effects constitute side effects which are unpleasant or hazardous.

Mechanism of action

In isolated preparations of cardiac muscle, glycosides cause a large increase in twitch tension. Unlike catecholamines they do not speed up the relaxation phase (compare Figs. 10.8 & 10.10). The increased tension development is due to an increase in the size of the intracellular calcium transient, which has been observed directly by measurements of $[Ca^{++}]_i$ in cells injected with a calcium-sensitive phosphorescent protein (Fig. 10.10). The action potential is, however, only slightly affected; in particular, the inward calcium current during the plateau (the slow inward current) is not changed, so

it appears that the increase in the calcium transient must reflect a greater release of calcium from intracellular stores. The most likely mechanism for this effect is as follows (Fig. 10.11).

1. The primary site on which glycosides act is the Na^+/K^+–ATPase of the cell membrane, which constitutes the Na^+/K^+ pump. Glycosides bind to K^+-binding site of the enzyme, and thus inhibit the pump.

2. Pump inhibition causes a rise in $[Na^+]_i$. Because Na^+/K^+ exchange is normally **electrogenic** (that is, it pumps more Na^+ ions out than K^+ ions in, and thus generates a net hyperpolarizing current) inhibition also causes a partial depolarization, which is important in producing effects on cardiac rhythm.

3. The rise in $[Na]_i$ slows down the rate of extrusion of intracellular Ca^{++} across the membrane. This is because the extrusion of intracellular Ca^{++} is by a Na^+/Ca^{++} **exchange mechanism**. Increasing $[Na^+]_i$ reduces the inwardly-directed gradient for Na^+; the smaller this gradient becomes the slower becomes the extrusion of Ca^{++} by the Na^+/Ca^{++} exchange mechanism, and the more Ca^{++} is retained within the cell.

4. The increase in $[Ca^{++}]_i$, though too small to activate the contractile protein directly, causes an increase in the Ca^{++} content of the sarcoplasmic reticulum, and thus increases the amount released by the action potential.

There is some controversy about whether this mechanism fully accounts for the inotropic effect. Thus at the low concentrations needed to produce the effect, glycosides may actually stimulate the Na^+/K^+ pump, and even with larger concentrations the effect on contraction seems to precede any change in $[Na^+]_i$. There may therefore be an additional mechanism, yet to be discovered.

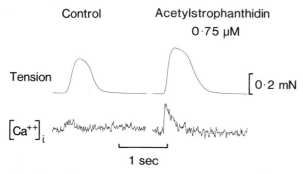

Fig. 10.10 Effect of a cardiac glycoside (acetylstrophanthidin) on the Ca^{++} transient and tension produced by frog cardiac muscle, recorded as in Fig. 10.8. (From: Allen & Blinks, 1978)

Effects on the heart in normal and pathological states

Effects on mechanical performance

In normal individuals, glycosides decrease cardiac output without affecting blood pressure.

The reduction of cardiac output seems paradoxical, because it can be shown that the ventricular function curve (see Fig. 10.5) is elevated, as one would expect. The explanation is that central ven-

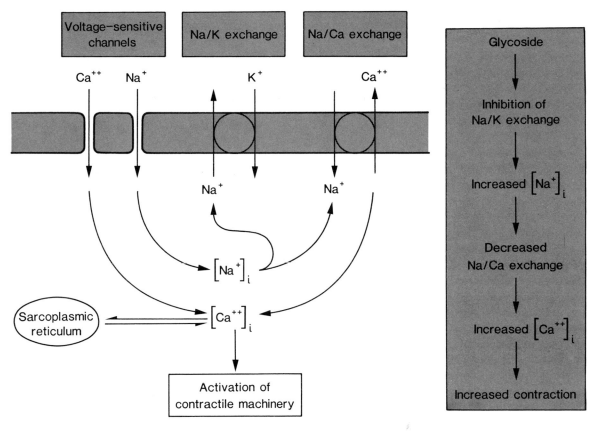

Fig. 10.11 Proposed mechanism of action of cardiac glycosides. Inhibition of Na/K exchange indirectly inhibits Ca^{++} extrusion from the cell, by raising $[Na^+]_i$ (see Fig. 10.4). Thus, the total Ca^{++} increases, so that more Ca^{++} is stored in SR, and more is available for release in response to the action potential.

ous pressure decreases, because of a dilator effect on systemic veins, and this overrides the effect on contractility. At the same time arteriolar vasoconstriction keeps the arterial pressure constant.

In cardiac failure, the effect of elevating the ventricular function curve is all-important (Fig. 10.12) in increasing cardiac output (and thus perfusion of peripheral tissues) and in reducing central venous pressure (thereby relieving pulmonary and systemic oedema). An overall vasodilation occurs, which is a reflex response to the rise in arterial pressure, resulting from the increased cardiac output. This overrides the direct vasoconstrictor action seen in normal subjects. When glycosides are given to patients with heart failure, marked diuresis occurs (as Withering noted in 1775). This is partly the result of increased renal blood flow, but also reflects the inhibition of renal sodium transport (see Chapter

14) by an action on the Na^+/K^+–ATPase of the tubules.

In contrast to catecholamines, glycosides *increase* the efficiency of the failing heart with regard to oxygen consumption, though they do not have this effect on the normal heart. The mechanism is not well understood, but it appears that the efficiency is reduced by the excessive diastolic stretching of the myocardium, so will tend to be improved by any agent that improves contractility.

Effects on rate and rhythm

In a normal subject glycosides cause cardiac slowing. This results from an **increase in vagal activity**, which is due to an action on the central nervous system. Also detectable, particularly at higher dosage is an **increase in AV conduction time**, dis-

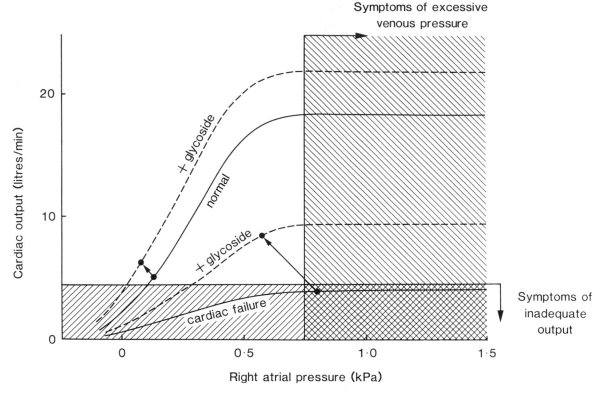

Fig. 10.12 Effect of glycoside in cardiac failure.

The symbols show approximate operating points for a normal subject at rest, and a patient with cardiac failure who has insufficient reserve to maintain an adequate output even at rest. The primary effect of the glycoside is to increase contractility. In the absence of any direct effects on the blood vessels this has the effect of increasing cardiac output and secondarily reducing central venous pressure. In a normal subject the overall haemodynamic effect is insignificant, but in a patient with cardiac failure the effect on both output and central venous pressure is substantial and beneficial. (1 kPa ≡ 7.5 mmHg)

cernible on the ECG as an increased P-R interval, which is due to a slowing of conduction in the AV node. The cells in this region are depolarized (see above) which causes inactivation of the channels responsible for the inward Ca^{++} current by which the action potential propagates in nodal tissue.

Larger doses of glycosides cause overt disturbances of rhythm, which are clinically important because they may occur with doses in, or only slightly above, the therapeutic range. Thus, slowing of AV conduction can progress to an actual **AV block**, with the ventricles either responding intermittently to atrial impulses, or beating quite independently at a low rate.

In addition to depressing AV conduction, glycosides cause ectopic beats to occur, which are associated with the increase in the transient inward current (see previous section) following the action

potential. This tends first to cause **coupled beats** (**bigeminy**), in which a normal ventricular beat is followed by an extra ectopic beat. It can progress to a continuous **ventricular tachycardia**, where there is a continuous succession of such triggered ectopic beats, and eventually to **ventricular fibrillation**, in which the ventricle stops beating because of continuous re-entrant excitation. Some typical ECG patterns associated with glycoside toxicity are shown in Figure 10.13.

Through their effects on AV conduction, glycosides may have a beneficial effect in certain types of dysrhythmia, though they cannot correct the underlying abnormality. Thus, in **atrial tachycardia**, or **atrial fibrillation**, where ectopic beats or re-entrant rhythms occur in the atria, the ventricular rate is excessively high, leading to inefficient ventricular beats because the time for diastolic filling is

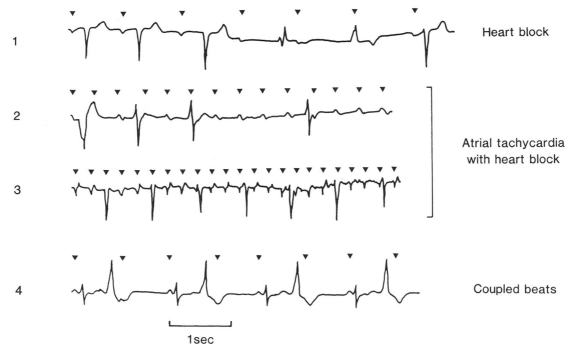

1   Heart block

2   Atrial tachycardia
     with heart block

3

4   Coupled beats

1sec

Fig. 10.13 Example of glycoside-induced cardiac dysrhythmias. The triangles show the position of P waves (atrial beats) on the ECG records.

too short. Increasing the refractory period of the AV node is beneficial under these conditions, because it increases the minimum interval between impulses, and reduces the ventricular rate. The atrial dysrhythmia is unaffected, or even made worse, but the pumping efficiency of the heart improves.

Interaction with extracellular potassium concentration

The effects of glycosides, particularly those on the cardiac rhythm, are increased if the plasma $[K^+]$ decreases. This is probably because of competition between the glycoside and K^+ for the Na–K–ATPase. Increased $[K^+]$ inhibits the binding of glycosides to the enzyme, and reduces their effect on sodium transport. This effect is clinically important, since **diuretic drugs** (see Chapter 14) are often used together with glycosides in the treatment of heart failure, and most of them cause a decrease in plasma $[K^+]$, thereby enhancing the tendency of the glycoside to cause unwanted dysrhythmias.

Pharmacokinetic aspects

The only important differences between the various available glycosides concern their absorption and duration of action (Table 10.1). **Ouabain** is a relatively short-acting compound, and it acts more quickly than the others when given intravenously, so it is useful where a rapid response is important. **Digoxin** and **digitoxin** have much longer-lasting effects, and are used orally for long-term glycoside treatment. Digitoxin is about 90% bound to plasma protein, whereas digoxin only binds weakly. Digoxin is metabolized to only a limited extent, most of it being excreted unchanged in the urine, which means that its duration of action is highly dependent on renal function. It is also incompletely absorbed, so disturbances of gastrointestinal function will affect it. The bioavailability of different digoxin preparations has been found to vary (see Chapter 3), giving rise to problems in clinical use.

The long plasma half-lives of digoxin and digitoxin mean that the time taken for a steady-state to be reached when treatment is first started, or when the dose is changed, is also long (roughly three

Table 10.1 Pharmacokinetic properties of cardiac glycosides

Drug	Oral absorption	Time to peak effect	Approximate duration of action	Plasma half-life	% bound to albumin	Main route of elimination
Ouabain	Poor Given by injection	~ 1 hour (i.v.)	1–3 days	~ 20 hours	—	Hepatic metabolism
Digoxin	About 75%, but varies with pharmaceutical formulation	4–6 hours (oral)	6 days	~ 40 hours	25	Renal
Digitoxin	Good	6–12 hours (oral)	3 weeks	~ 7 days	90	Hepatic metabolism, partly to digoxin

times the half-life; see Chapter 3). An initial loading dose is sometimes given to avoid the slow build-up when a course of treatment is begun.

The glycosides are notable for the small margin between the plasma concentration needed for a therapeutic effect, and the concentration that causes symptoms of toxicity, which means that more care is needed than with most drugs to regulate the dosage in order to keep the plasma concentration in the right range. Radio-immunoassay is used clinically to monitor plasma glycoside concentration when problems arise.

Adverse effects

The main unwanted effects of glycosides are:

1. Nausea and vomiting. This is one of the first signs of impending glycoside toxicity. It is important because it gives warning of cardiac side effects which can be dangerous.
2. Cardiac effects. Many types of dysrhythmia can occur, the commonest being heart block and coupled ventricular extrasystoles. Continued administration can then cause progression to ventricular tachycardia and death from ventricular fibrillation.

These unwanted effects occur at quite clearly-defined plasma glycoside concentrations (Table 10.1), the measurement of which is often important in monitoring glycoside treatment.

Uses

Glycosides are only used for their cardiac effects,

the main clinical applications being: (1) cardiac failure; (2) atrial dysrhythmias. In the latter indication, the object is to induce a degree of heart block, and thus reduce the ventricular rate.

ANTIDYSRHYTHMIC DRUGS

A classification of antidysrhythmic drugs was proposed by Vaughan Williams in 1970. Though not universally accepted, this provides a useful basis for discussing their mechanism of action (see Vaughan Williams, 1980, for a recent account).

The main groups are:

Class I   Drugs that block voltage-sensitive sodium channels, thus reducing the excitability of the non-nodal regions of the heart where the inward sodium current is important for propagation of the action potential

Class II   Drugs that reduce the action of the sympathetic nervous system

Class III Drugs that prolong the refractory period of the myocardium, thus tending to suppress re-entrant rhythms

Class IV   Drugs that block voltage-sensitive calcium channels, thus impairing impulse propagation in nodal areas, and in damaged areas of the myocardium.

The classification is not entirely clear-cut and there are some drugs that do not fit neatly into it. Some authors add two or more extra categories for this reason. One of the weaknesses of the classi-

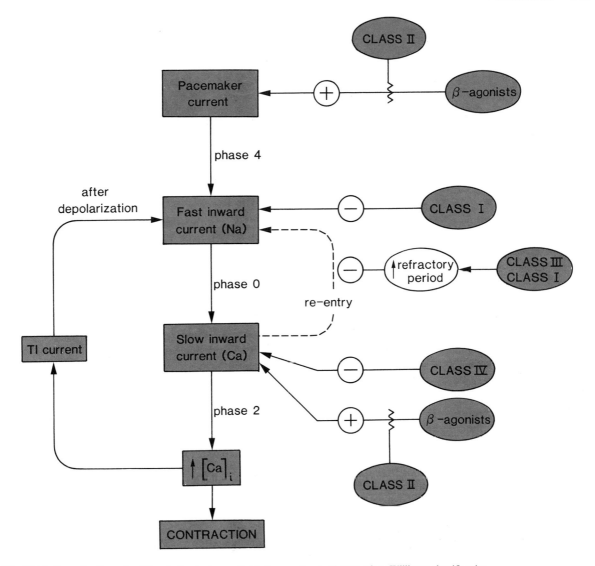

Fig. 10.14 Sites of action of antidysrhythmic drugs, divided according to the Vaughan Williams classification.
TI current = transient inward current.

fication is that Class I covers a wide range of drugs with quite diverse clinical characteristics.

The sites of action of these classes of drug are shown diagrammatically in Figure 10.14.

Class I antidysrhythmic drugs

These drugs act by blocking sodium channels, exactly as local anaesthetics do (see Chapter 27). Because this inhibits action potential propagation in many excitable cells, it has been referred to as 'membrane stabilizing' activity, a phrase best

avoided now that the ionic mechanism is well understood. The characteristic effect of these drugs on the action potential is a **reduction in the rate of depolarization** during phase 0.

The most important examples of drugs in this group are:

1. **Quinidine**
2. **Procainamide**
3. **Lignocaine**
4. **Phenytoin**.

Of these drugs, quinidine and procainamide are

pharmacologically very similar, and they are used mainly to treat dysrhythmias of atrial origin. Lignocaine and phenytoin, on the other hand, are used in ventricular dysrhythmias, and have little effect on atrial dysrhythmias. These differences may be partly explained in terms of the mechanism by which Class I drugs affect the sodium conductance (see below).

Mechanism of action

The work of Hille and others on the action of local anaesthetics on excitable membranes (see Chapter 27) has shown that they bind to a site within the sodium channel and prevent it from conducting Na^+ ions. The channel can exist in three distinct functional states: **resting**, **open** and **refractory**. Channel opening occurs when the channel switches, in response to depolarization, rapidly from resting to open; this is known as **activation**. Maintained depolarization causes it to change more slowly from open to refractory (**inactivation**) and the membrane must then be repolarized for a time to restore the channel to the resting state. Class I drugs can bind to the channel in any of these states, but at different rates. In general they bind most rapidly when the channel is open. Their action therefore shows the property of **use-dependence** (i.e. the more frequently the channels are activated, the greater the degree of block produced). It is this characteristic that enables these drugs to block the high frequency excitation of the myocardium that occurs in dysrhythmias without preventing the heart from beating at normal frequencies.

Though the action of Class I drugs is believed to depend mainly on this kind of interaction with sodium channels, it is not yet clear what distinguishes the effect of drugs such as quinidine and procainamide from those of lignocaine and phenytoin, whose clinical effects are quite different. The main differences in their cellular mechanisms are:

1. Quinidine and procainamide inhibit the pacemaker depolarization, whereas lignocaine and phenytoin do not.
2. Lignocaine inhibits the **transient inward current** (p. 229) that is thought to account for the repetitive ectopic beats that occur in various types of ventricular dysrhythmias.

3. The rate of dissociation from the sodium channels is much lower for quinidine than for lignocaine. This means that each action potential, in the presence of quinidine, causes a small increase in the degree of block, which recovers only slowly after the action potential (resulting in an increase in the **relative refractory period**). In the presence of lignocaine, each action potential causes a more profound, but short-lived, block of the channels (equivalent to a lengthening of the **absolute refractory period**). The latter may be particularly effective in blocking the initiation of a second action potential by the transient inward current in the ventricular myocardium.

Actions of individual drugs

Quinidine and **procainamide**. These will be considered together, as they are pharmacologically very similar. Quinidine is the D-isomer of quinine, an antimalarial drug (see Chapter 33). In addition to its antidysrhythmic action (see above) it causes, in normal individuals, a tachycardia because of its atropine-like effect. In larger doses it reduces the force of contraction of the ventricles, tending to reduce cardiac output, and at the same time dilates arterioles, so causing a fall in blood pressure. It also prolongs AV conduction time, and can produce AV block.

Procainamide, and a newer drug **disopyramide**, are very similar, except that neither has appreciable atropine-like effects.

Adverse effects. Quinidine and, to a lesser extent, procainamide often cause nausea and vomiting. Both drugs also produce hypersensitivity reactions, usually in the form of fever or skin rashes. More seriously, thrombocytopenia or agranulocytosis have been reported. These reactions, though rare, can be fatal, and procainamide is now seldom used because of this risk. Quinidine in overdose can actually *precipitate* dysrhythmias, and even cause death from ventricular fibrillation. The mechanism is not understood. Because of all these side effects, **calcium antagonists** (see below) are increasingly replacing these drugs in clinical use.

Uses. These drugs are used mainly, as oral preparations, in the treatment of atrial tachycardias and atrial fibrillation. A common procedure is to use electrical stimulation to restore normal rhythm, followed by quinidine treatment to prevent recurrence of the dysrhythmia. In atrial dysrhythmias of long standing, the atria often contain thrombi, which may get dislodged when the normal rhythm is restored. To prevent this, anticoagulant drugs (see Chapter 12) are often given for some time before conversion of the rhythm.

Lignocaine. This drug is widely used as a local anaesthetic (see Chapter 27). Its plasma half-life is short (about 2 hours) and it is largely removed from the portal circulation by first-pass metabolism (see Chapter 4) so cannot be used orally.

Its antidysrhythmic action (see above) is confined to the ventricular muscle and conducting system, and it is used, by intravenous infusion to suppress ventricular dysrhythmias.

It has no effect on atrial dysrhythmias, and few other cardiovascular effects.

Adverse effects. These are mainly manifestations of actions on the central nervous system, and include drowsiness, disorientation and, more seriously, convulsions. In practice, the plasma concentration can be adjusted rapidly by varying the infusion rate, because of the short plasma half-life.

Uses. The use of lignocaine is largely confined to intensive care units, where it is used to prevent ventricular fibrillation from developing in patients who have recently suffered a heart attack.

Phenytoin. Phenytoin is widely used as an antiepileptic drug (see Chapter 24) but has antidysrhythmic actions very similar to those of lignocaine. It is likely that the same mechanisms underlie its anticonvulsant and antidysrhythmic effects. It is particularly effective, for reasons that are not clear, in counteracting glycoside-induced dysrhythmias and is mainly used for this purpose.

Class II antidysrhythmic drugs

These drugs act by reducing, in one way or another, the effect of the sympathetic nervous system on the heart, the most important examples being the β-adrenoceptor blocking drugs (see Chapter 7 and earlier section of this chapter).

It is known that adrenaline can cause ventricular extrasystoles, and even fibrillation, by its effects on the pacemaker potential and the slow inward current, carried by calcium ions, in myocardial cells (see

earlier section). There is also evidence that the occurrence of ventricular dysrhythmias following myocardial infarction is partly the result of increased sympathetic activity, and this provides the rationale for using β-adrenoceptor blocking drugs to reduce their occurrence.

AV conduction also depends critically on sympathetic activity, and the refractory period of the AV node is increased by β-adrenoceptor blocking drugs, which can be used, in much the same way as glycosides, to interfere with AV conduction in atrial tachycardias, and slow the ventricular rate.

The most important β-receptor blocking drugs are described in Chapter 7, and several of these, especially **propranolol**, are used for their antidysrhythmic actions.

Propranolol, like several other drugs of this type, has some Class I action in addition to blocking β-receptors, and this may contribute to its antidysrhythmic effects, though probably not very much.

Adverse effects. These are described in Chapter 7, the most important ones being **bronchospasm** and **reduced cardiac output** which can precipitate cardiac failure. Propranolol is most widely used, but the use of β_1-selective drugs (e.g. **metoprolol, acebutolol**) reduces the risk of bronchospasm, while the use of drugs with partial agonist activity (e.g. **alprenolol, pindolol**) may reduce the tendency to cause cardiac failure.

Uses. The main use of β-receptor antagonists as antidysrhythmic drugs is in patients recovering from myocardial infarction. They have been shown to reduce significantly the mortality rate in the first year after a heart attack, and this is partly because of their ability to prevent ventricular dysrhythmias. They may also be effective in treating atrial dysrhythmias when these are provoked by increased sympathetic activity.

Class III antidysrhythmic drugs

This is a small, and poorly understood, group of drugs, whose action is to prolong the action potential and refractory period of cardiac muscle, thus tending to diminish the likelihood of re-entrant rhythms. It includes **amiodarone**, a recently introduced drug that has anti-anginal as well as antidysrhythmic activity (see later section) and some β-receptor antagonists have this effect also. The mechanism cannot at present be explained in electrophysiological terms.

Class IV antidysrhythmic drugs

The mechanism of action common to this group of drugs is that they block calcium channels in cell membranes. In the context of heart muscle, this means that they reduce the slow inward current, thereby shortening the plateau phase of the action potential, and also reducing the force of contraction. This effect impairs conduction in those areas of the heart (including damaged areas of myocardium) where propagation depends on the 'slow response' (p. 230), and also inhibits the transient inward current (p. 229) which produces disturbances of rhythm associated with after-depolarizations.

Calcium antagonists

Calcium antagonists are a chemically and pharmacologically diverse group of drugs. They include **verapamil**, several compounds of the **dihydropyridine** type, such as **nifedipine**, and miscellaneous other drugs including **diltiazem**, **cinnarizine** and **prenylamine** (Fig. 10.15). They affect the entry of calcium rather than its intracellular actions, and are referred to by some authors as '**calcium entry blockers**' to make this distinction clear.

As one might expect, in view of the widespread involvement of intracellular calcium as a regulator of cell function, calcium antagonists have been shown to affect many different physiological processes, including secretion, muscle contraction, platelet function and neurotransmitter release. However, for reasons that are not well understood,

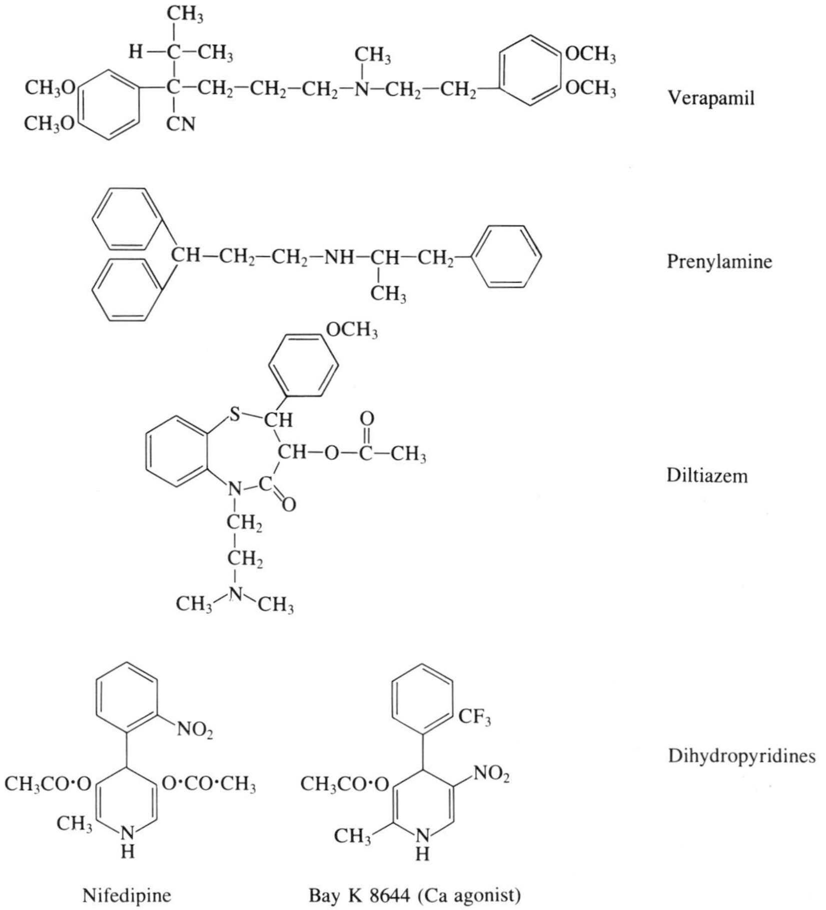

Fig. 10.15 Structures of calcium antagonists, with Bay K 8644 (calcium agonist) included for comparison.

their major effects are produced on (a) the heart and (b) vascular smooth muscle, and when given to man or experimental animals their only important actions are on the cardiovascular system.

Mechanism of action

The calcium channels by which Ca^{++} entry into cells is regulated are of two general kinds:

1. **Voltage-sensitive channels**, which open in response to depolarization of the cell membrane. Such channels occur in the heart, where they are responsible for the slow inward current (see above), and in smooth muscle, where they are responsible for the contracture produced when the cells are depolarized by potassium. They are also responsible for smooth muscle contraction associated with propagated action potentials.
2. **Receptor-operated channels**, which are controlled by the binding of substances such as catecholamines to membrane receptors (see Chapter 1).

The relative importance of these two kinds of Ca^{++} channel evidently varies between different tissues, and between the smooth muscle found in different organs. Calcium antagonists affect both kinds of channel, but most are considerably more effective against voltage-sensitive than against receptor-operated channels. This specificity, which is more marked for some Ca^{++} antagonists than others, is one factor that determines their selectivity of action.

There is some evidence to suggest that calcium antagonists act by competition with Ca^{++} ions, and there is also evidence (Lee & Tsien, 1983) that their effect shows 'use-dependence' of the kind already discussed in relation to Class I antidysrhythmic drugs. In other words, the blocking effect becomes more pronounced if the channels are opened frequently. This is probably important in relation to their actions as antidysrhythmic agents, just as with Class I drugs, for they will tend to act most effectively on cells which are depolarized, or are discharging at an abnormally high frequency. The degree of use-dependence shown by different drugs may be another factor which determines their relative potency on cardiac and smooth muscle, but this is yet to be clarified.

Some reassessment of the mechanism by which calcium antagonists block calcium channels may be required in the light of a newly-discovered type of dihydropyridine, exemplified by **Bay K 8644** (Fig. 10.15). This drug is very similar in structure to nifedipine, but produces the opposite effects (Schramm et al, 1983), namely an *increase* in the force of the cardiac contraction, and *constriction* of blood vessels, and it is competitively antagonized by nifedipine. It appears to work by increasing calcium entry, and it is suggested that voltage-dependent calcium channels are controlled by a regulatory site, to which dihydropyridines bind; depending on the structure of the dihydropyridine, binding to this site either facilitates or inhibits channel opening (Hess et al, 1984). This is clearly a less direct mechanism of action for calcium antagonists than a simple plugging of the channel, and it invites speculation about a possible endogenous dihydropyridine-like mediator with a regulatory effect on calcium entry.

Pharmacological effects

Though voltage-sensitive calcium channels occur in many different types of cell, including neurons, the important pharmacological effects of calcium antagonists are confined to cardiac and smooth muscle. Verapamil and prenylamine mainly affect the heart, whereas most of the dihydropyridines (e.g. nifedipine) exert a greater effect on smooth muscle than on the heart. Diltiazem is intermediate in its actions.

Cardiac actions

Antidysrhythmic effects. Verapamil, prenylamine and diltiazem have useful antidysrhythmic effects. They are much more effective against atrial than against ventricular dysrhythmias, though they appear to inhibit calcium currents in all kinds of cardiac muscle. This may reflect the particular characteristics of the use-dependence of their actions (see Chapter 27), since atrial dysrhythmias generally involve a higher discharge frequency. All calcium antagonists, even those lacking antidysrhythmic activity, can cause AV block and cardiac slowing. They also have a negative inotropic effect, which results from the inhibition of the slow inward current during the action potential plateau. In spite of this the cardiac output usually stays constant or

Table 10.2 Comparison of the haemodynamic effects of nitrates, β-adrenoceptor antagonists and a calcium antagonist

	Nitrate	β-blocker	Nifedipine
Blood pressure	↓	0 or ↓	↓↓
Heart rate	↑	↓↓	0 or ↑
Cardiac output	0 or ↑	↓	↑
R. atrial pressure	↓↓	↑	0 or ↓
Total vascular resistance	↓	↑	↓↓
Coronary flow	0	↓	↓

increases, because of the reduction in peripheral resistance. Verapamil does not affect cardiac output appreciably, whereas dihydropyridines normally increase it (Table 10.2).

Vasodilator effect. Calcium antagonists cause generalized arteriolar dilatation, but do not much affect the veins. They affect all vascular beds, though recent work suggests that the regional effects vary between different drugs to a considerable degree. Vasodilatation causes a fall in arterial pressure.

Nifedipine produces marked vasodilatation without much direct effect on the heart, whereas other calcium antagonists are less selective.

All of these drugs cause coronary vasodilatation in normal individuals and in patients with coronary artery spasm (variant angina), but it is not certain that this happens when coronary atherosclerosis is present (see later section).

Other types of smooth muscle (e.g. biliary tract, urinary tract, uterus) are also relaxed by calcium antagonists (especially dihydropyridines), which may be useful in treating conditions such as biliary colic.

Protection of ischaemic myocardium. Verapamil, in experimental animals, reduces the size of the myocardial necrosis caused by coronary ligation. This may be partly due to inhibition of Ca^{++} entry into the ischaemic cells (since increased $[Ca^{++}]_i$ is partly responsible for cell damage) and partly to the reduced O_2 demand of the myocardium. It is not yet clear whether this effect may be useful in reducing the size of cardiac infarcts in man.

Adverse effects

The main unwanted effects of the calcium antagonists are a direct consequence of their actions on the heart and smooth muscle. They include **constipation, postural hypotension** and **headache**. They can precipitate cardiac failure, and this risk is increased when they are used in combination with β-receptor antagonists, with which there are many overlapping indications.

Uses

Calcium antagonists are used mainly for the following purposes:

1. As antidysrhythmic drugs (verapamil, diltiazem, prenylamine). Their applications are similar to those of quinidine and procainamide, but their side effects are fewer.

2. To treat hypertension (dihydropyridines). Most calcium antagonists combine arteriolar vasodilatation with a negative inotropic effect, and very effectively lower arterial pressure. Their clinical use for this purpose is increasing rapidly (see Chapter 11).

3. To treat angina (diltiazem, dihydropyridines). Reduced cardiac oxygen consumption and coronary vasodilatation are potentially useful effects in angina (see later section), and calcium antagonists are widely used for this purpose.

ANTI-ANGINAL DRUGS

Anginal pain occurs when the coronary blood flow is insufficient to meet the heart's metabolic requirements, and can be counteracted by drugs that either improve myocardial perfusion, or reduce the metabolic demand, or both.

Two of the main groups of drugs that are used in angina, **organic nitrates** and **calcium antagonists**, act as vasodilators, and produce both of these physiological effects. The third group are the **β-receptor antagonists**, which affect only the metabolic demand.

Calcium antagonists are described in the preceding section, and β-receptor antagonists in Chapter 7.

Organic nitrates

The ability of organic nitrates to relieve anginal pain was discovered by Lauder Brunton, a distinguished British physician, in 1867. He had found that angina could be partly relieved by bleeding, and also knew that **amyl nitrite**, which had been synthesized 10 years earlier, caused very marked flushing and tachycardia, with a fall in blood pressure, when its vapour was inhaled. He thought that the effect of bleeding resulted from hypotension, and found that amyl nitrite inhalation worked much better. It was also tried enthusiastically in many other conditions, such as cholera, without effect.

Amyl nitrite, given as a vapour, was used for many years, but has now been replaced by **glyceryl trinitrate (nitroglycerine)**. This substance was discovered by Nobel to be an excellent explosive, and is the major ingredient of dynamite. Organic chemists then were inclined to taste their creations, and nitroglycerine was found early on to cause flushing and a throbbing headache. It was soon realized that its action was the same as that of amyl nitrite, and it was found to be just as effective in angina.

Glyceryl trinitrate is still widely used, but efforts to increase its duration of action have led to many other compounds being tested, of which the two most important are **pentaerythritol tetranitrate**, and **isosorbide dinitrate** (Fig. 10.16). These substances all work in the same way, and differ only in their duration of action.

Mechanism of action

Organic nitrates act solely by relaxing smooth muscle. Considering that their effects were described more than 120 years ago, we are remarkably ignorant about the cellular mechanism underlying this action, though there are a few clues (Bennett & Marks, 1984). The action seems to depend on the production, within the cell, of nitrite ions. Sodium nitrite itself is only a weak vasodilator, presumably because the nitrite ion crosses the membrane much less readily than the lipid soluble organic derivatives. The formation of nitrite from nitrate requires the presence of sulphydryl groups, and if these are blocked (e.g. with **ethacrynic acid**; see Chapter 14) nitroglycerine loses its effect. The relaxant effect is preceded by an increase in cGMP (but not cAMP) content of the tissue, which distinguishes nitrates from many other smooth muscle relaxants (e.g. β-agonists, papaverine). Whether the effect on cGMP production is essential for smooth muscle relaxation is not certain.

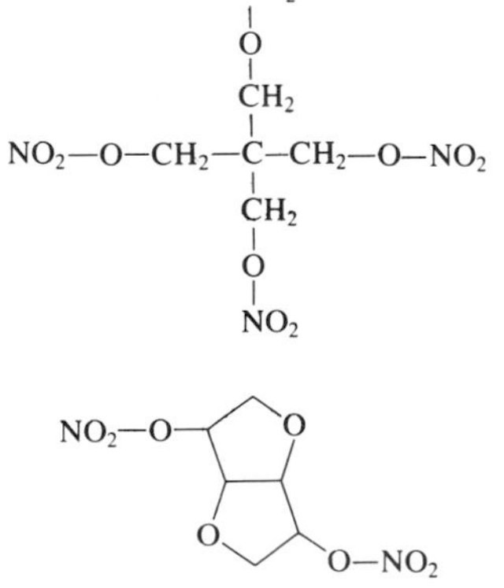

Amyl nitrite

Glyceryl trinitrate

Pentaerythritol tetranitrate

Isosorbide dinitrate

Fig. 10.16 Structures of organic nitrates.

Pharmacological effects

Though organic nitrates can be shown to relax all kinds of smooth muscle, the main effect seen when they are given to normal subjects is on the cardiovascular system. There is marked dilatation of large veins, with a consequent reduction in central venous pressure, which causes reduction of cardiac output. With small doses, there is little effect on the arterioles, and the reduced stroke output is largely compensated by a reflex tachycardia, so arterial pressure does not change. With larger doses, arterioles dilate, and arterial pressure falls, particularly if the subject stands up, causing dizziness. At the same time flushing, and a throbbing headache are produced, by dilatation of cutaneous and cerebral vessels.

Effects on the coronary circulation

Under normal conditions glyceryl trinitrate increases coronary flow, in spite of a decrease in mean arterial pressure, implying a considerable reduction of coronary vascular resistance. Because both arterial pressure and cardiac output are decreased, the myocardial oxygen consumption is reduced. This, and the increased blood flow, cause a large increase in the oxygen content of coronary sinus blood. If the coronary arteries are partially occluded by disease, however, coronary flow is *not* increased by

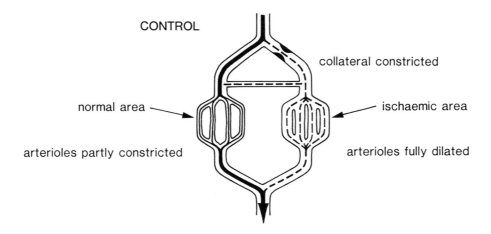

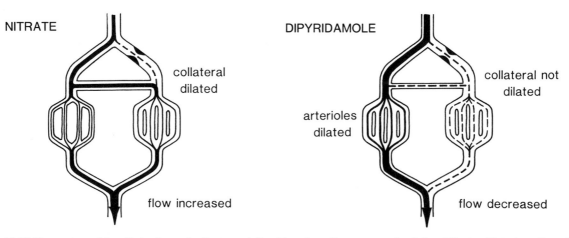

Fig. 10.17 Comparison of the effects of organic nitrates and dipyridamole on the coronary circulation. Nitrates dilate the collateral vessel, thus allowing more blood through to the underperfused region (mostly by diversion from the adequately perfused area). Dipyridamole dilates arterioles, increasing flow through the normal area at the expense of the ischaemic area (in which the arterioles are anyway fully dilated).

nitrates. Several studies in patients who obtain relief from anginal pain with glyceryl trinitrate have shown that during an attack it either has no effect on the total coronary flow, or actually reduces it, because of the fall in the arterial pressure. This might suggest that the benefit results entirely from the reduction of myocardial oxygen consumption secondary to the lowering of arterial and central venous pressure, but this view has been challenged recently by work on the *regional* distribution of coronary flow to different areas of the myocardium in experimental animals, studied by the 'microsphere' technique. Very small radioactive glass beads are injected intravenously and become trapped in capillaries, the number collecting in different tissues providing a good measure of the local blood flow. By this method it has been found that glyceryl trinitrate can divert the blood from normal to ischaemic areas of the myocardium. The mechanism appears to involve collateral vessels, of fairly large calibre, which are dilated by glyceryl trinitrate, enabling a partially blocked vessel to be by-passed (Fig. 10.17).

It is interesting to compare this effect with that of **dipyridamole** (see below) which dilates precapillary arterioles, but not collateral vessels. This drug is as effective as nitrates, or even more so, in increasing coronary flow in normal subjects, but is not effective in angina. This is probably because the arterioles in the ischaemic region are fully dilated anyway, and the drug-induced dilatation of the arterioles in normal areas actually has the effect of diverting blood away from the ischaemic area (Fig. 10.17).

In **variant angina**, where coronary spasm rather than atherosclerotic occlusion is responsible, nitrates act directly to relax the vessel wall.

In summary, the anti-anginal action of nitrates involves: (a) reduction of cardiac oxygen consumption, secondary to reduced arterial pressure and cardiac output; (b) redistribution of coronary flow towards ischaemic areas; (c) in variant angina, relief of coronary spasm. Calcium antagonists also act similarly, whereas β-receptor antagonists work only by mechanism (a).

Tolerance and adverse effects

Repeated administration of nitrates to smooth muscle preparations *in vitro* results in a diminishing relaxant effect, possibly because of a depletion of the free-SH groups that are needed for the production of nitrite ions. Tolerance to the anti-anginal effect of nitrates does not occur clinically to an important extent with short-acting drugs (e.g. glyceryl trinitrate), but may develop with long-acting drugs (e.g. pentaerythritol tetranitrate).

The adverse effects of nitrates consist mainly of the unpleasant sensations of flushing and headache. This was the cause of 'Monday morning sickness' among workers in explosives factories where the content of organic nitrates in the air could be very high. Tolerance to these effects develops quite quickly (which is why the symptoms appeared on Mondays and not later in the week) but the anti-anginal effect remains.

The only toxic effect of any significance with nitrates is the formation of **methaemoglobin**, an oxidation product of haemoglobin that is ineffective as an oxygen carrier. This hardly ever occurs when nitrates are used clinically, but the effect can be induced deliberately in the treatment of cyanide poisoning (see below).

Pharmacokinetic aspects

Glyceryl trinitrate is quickly metabolized by the liver to inorganic nitrite, which has little dilator activity. The drug is quickly absorbed from the oral cavity, and is taken as a tablet which is held under the tongue, producing its effects within a few minutes. If swallowed, the drug is ineffective, because of first-pass metabolism. Given sublingually, glyceryl trinitrate is quickly converted to di- and mono-nitrates, which have some activity and have a half-life of about 2 hours. Its effective duration of action is only about 30 minutes. It is quite well absorbed through the skin, and a more sustained effect can be achieved by applying it as an ointment or skin-patch.

Long-acting organic nitrates

Pentaerythritol tetranitrate and isosorbide dinitrate (see Fig. 10.16) are longer-acting compounds with the same effects as glyceryl trinitrate. Isosorbide dinitrate is rapidly metabolised in the liver to the mononitrate, which is biologically active and has a half-life of about 4 hours. Both drugs are taken orally rather than sublingually, but have the disadvantage that their effect is delayed.

Uses of organic nitrates

By far the most important use is in treating angina, but their smooth muscle relaxant effect can also be used to relax bronchial or biliary tract smooth muscle.

Dipyridamole

Dipyridamole is a pyrimidine, chemically related to **adenosine** (see Chapters 11 and 12). In experimental animals and in normal human subjects it is an effective coronary vasodilator with relatively little effect on smooth muscle elsewhere. Its action is thought to be due to **inhibition of adenosine uptake**, causing tissue accumulation of adenosine, which is an endogenous vasodilator compound. Its vasodilator effect is exerted mainly on precapillary arterioles (see Fig. 10.17). Since these are, in any case, fully dilated in ischaemic areas of the myocardium, it has not proved effective in angina.

β-receptor antagonists (see Chapter 7)

These are important in the treatment of angina. Their action depends entirely on reducing the oxygen consumption of the heart. They probably have no important effects on the coronary vessels, any effect that they do produce being in the direction of constriction rather than dilatation. The effects of nitrates, β-receptor antagonists and calcium antagonists are compared in Table 10.2.

OTHER DRUGS THAT AFFECT THE HEART

The substances considered in this section all have major effects elsewhere in the body, and are described in more detail in other chapters. This discussion is confined to their cardiac effects.

Methylxanthines

Examples include **caffeine** and **theophylline** (see Chapters 13 & 26). These drugs affect many physio-logical systems, including the central nervous system, visceral and vascular smooth muscle, the kidney, heart and skeletal muscle. Their effects in general resemble those of β-receptor agonists, though they do not interact directly with β-adrenoceptors. Thus, their main cardiac effects are **increased contractility** and **increased rate**, together with increased liability to dysrhythmias.

Their mechanism of action has been much debated and may involve one or more of three different processes:

1. *Inhibition of phosphodiesterase*. This intracellular enzyme inactivates cAMP, and the methylxanthines therefore increase the intracellular concentration of cAMP, which explains the similarity of their actions to those of β-receptor agonists.
2. *Antagonism of purines*. Various purines, particularly adenosine (see below) reduce the force and rate of the heart, and this effect is antagonized, probably by a competitive receptor-blocking action, by methylxanthines.
3. *Release of calcium from intracellular stores*. Caffeine, in high concentration, causes contracture of skeletal muscle by releasing calcium from the sarcoplasmic reticulum. It is unlikely that this occurs sufficiently at therapeutic concentrations to contribute to the cardiac effects.

Because of its effect on contractility, theophylline is sometimes used for treating cardiac failure. Its effects on the respiratory system (see Chapter 13) are also therapeutically useful.

Purines

The possible role of ATP and related purines as peripheral neurotransmitters and local hormones is discussed in Chapter 5. Adenosine is particularly active on the heart, where it causes decreased contractility and heart rate, possibly by interacting with a receptor that works to inhibit adenylate cyclase. This may be important in relation to the action of methylxanthines (see above). Adenosine is also a powerful coronary vasodilator, and may act as a local mediator in the physiological regulation of coronary flow (p. 235). This action is clearly not the result of inhibition of adenylate cyclase, and is unaffected by methylxanthines. The coronary dilator action is enhanced by **dipyridamole** (p. 254) which blocks the uptake of adenosine by tissues. Dipyridamole does not, however, reduce myocardial contractility, which suggests that adenosine may not exert a tonic influence on contractility, thus casting doubt on the relevance of the purine antagonistic effect of theophylline to its effect on myocardial contractility.

Other agents

Histamine (see Chapter 8) applied to an isolated heart produces an increase in force and rate similar to that produced by β-adrenoceptor agonists. This is due to an interaction with H_2 receptors, which are linked to activation of adenylate cyclase. It provides a useful means of assaying drugs that affect H_2 receptors, but is probably of no clinical significance.

Glucagon, a peptide hormone produced by the pancreatic islets (see Chapter 16) has the same effect as histamine.

Amrinone is a drug that was recently introduced for the treatment of cardiac failure. It increases myocardial contractility in a manner similar to that of the glycosides, but has less toxicity. Its mechanism of action is uncertain, but is probably related to phosphodiesterase inhibition.

REFERENCES AND FURTHER READING

Bennett B M, Marks G S 1984 How does nitroglycerin induce vascular smooth muscle relaxation? Trends in Pharmacological Sciences 5: 329–332

Braunwald E, Mock M B, Watson J T 1982 Congestive cardiac failure: current research and clinical applications. Grune & Stratton, New York

Canvin C, Loutzenhiser R, van Breeman C 1983 Mechanism of calcium antagonist-induced vasodilatation. Ann Rev Pharmacol 23: 373–396

Cranefield P F 1975 The conduction of the cardiac impulse: the slow response and cardiac arrhythmias. Futura, New York

Flaim S E, Zelis R 1982 Calcium blockers. Mechanisms of action and action and clinical applications. Urban & Schwartzenberg, Munich

Gadsby, D C, Wit A L 1981 Electrophysiological characteristics of cardiac cells and the genesis of cardiac arrhythmias. In: Wilkerson R D (cd) Cardiac pharmacology. Academic Press, New York

Gibbs C L 1978 Cardiac energetics. Physiol Rev 58: 174–254

Hess P, Lansmann J B, Tsien R W 1984 Different modes of Ca-channel gating behaviour favoured by dihydropyridine Ca agonists and antagonists. Nature 311: 538–544

Lee K S, Tsien R W 1983 Mechanism of calcium channel blockade by verapamil, D 600, ditriazem and nitrendipine in single dialysed heart cells. Nature 302: 790–794

Noble D 1975 The initiation of the heart beat. Oxford University Press, Oxford

Noble D 1984 The surprising heart: a review of recent progress in cardiac electrophysiology. J Physiol 353: 1–50

Schramm M, Thomas G. Towart R, Frankowiak G 1983 Novel dihydropyridines with positive inotropic action through activation of Ca^{2+} channels. Nature 303: 535–537

Van der Vusse G, Reneman R S 1985 Pharmacological intervention in acute myocardial ischaemia and reperfusion Trends in Pharmacological Sciences 6: 76–79

Vatner S F, Hintze T H 1982 Effects of a calcium-channel antagonist on large and small coronary arteries in conscious dogs. Circulation 66: 579–588

Vaughan Williams E M 1983 Antiarrhythmic action. Academic Press, London

Zsoter T T, Church J G 1983 Calcium antagonists: Pharmacodynamic effects and mechanism of action. Drugs 25: 93–112 (and other articles in this volume)

The circulation

This chapter is concerned mainly with the pharmacology of peripheral blood vessels. The walls of muscular arteries, arterioles, venules and veins contain smooth muscle, the activity of which is controlled by the sympathetic nervous system, and by various humoral factors. The parasympathetic system has little or no regulatory function on blood vessels except those supplying erectile tissue.

Muscular arteries and arterioles are the main resistance vessels in the circulation, while veins are capacity vessels. In terms of cardiac function, therefore, arteries and arterioles regulate the **after-load**, while veins regulate the **pre-load** of the ventricles. Muscular arteries control not only the **resistance** of the peripheral circulation, but also its **compliance** (i.e. the degree to which the volume of the arterial system increases as the pressure increases), which is an important factor in a circulatory system that is driven by an intermittent, rather than a continuous pump. Much of the blood that is ejected from the ventricle is accommodated, in the first instance, by distension of the arterial system, which absorbs the pulsations in cardiac output and delivers a relatively steady flow to the tissues. The greater the compliance of the system the more effectively will the fluctuations be damped out, and the smaller will be the oscillations of arterial pressure with each heart-beat. This is of some importance, because the **cardiac work**, (see Chapter 10) which is given by $\int P.dV$, can be reduced by introducing additional compliance into the arterial system, even if the cardiac output and mean arterial pressure are unchanged.

In summary, the effects of drugs on the peripheral vascular system can be broken down into:

1. **Effects on total peripheral resistance**, controlled mainly by the arterioles, which is one of the main determinants of **arterial pressure**, and is relevant to the treatment of **hypertension** and **shock**.
2. **Effects on the resistance of individual vascular beds**, which determine the local distribution of blood flow to and within different organs. Such effects are relevant to the drug treatment of **angina** (see Chapter 10), **migraine** and **hypovolaemic shock**.
3. **Effects on arterial compliance**, controlled mainly by muscular arteries, which is relevant in the treatment of **cardiac failure** and **angina**.
4. **Effects on venous capacity**, which determines the central venous pressure, and is relevant to the treatment of **cardiac failure** and **angina**.

In this chapter the effects of various groups of drugs on vascular smooth muscle is first considered, and then the pharmacological approaches to the treatment of hypertension, migraine, shock and cardiac failure are discussed in more detail. The use of drugs in treating angina is discussed in Chapter 10.

VASCULAR SMOOTH MUSCLE

Activation by drugs

Like other muscle cells, vascular smooth muscle cells contract when the intracellular calcium concentration rises, and so pharmacologically-induced contraction is always secondary to a rise in $[Ca^{++}]_i$ (Bolton, 1979; Jones, 1981). Relaxation can occur either by reducing $[Ca^{++}]_i$ or, in some cases, by interfering with the linkage between Ca^{++} and the contractile machinery.

The mechanisms by which stimulant drugs affect $[Ca^{++}]_i$ and initiate contraction are quite complex, as shown by the following facts:

1. In many cases, vasoconstrictor drugs cause a biphasic response, consisting of a **rapid phasic contraction** followed by a **maintained tonic contraction**. Reduction of extracellular calcium concentration, or addition of a calcium antagonist, such as **nifedipine** (see Chapter 10) usually reduces the tonic contraction more than the phasic one.
2. The relative size of the tonic and phasic responses varies in different blood vessels, and also depends on the drug used to elicit contraction.
3. Smooth muscle will still respond tonically to agonists even when it is completely depolarized by immersion in solution containing isotonic KCl.

A generally-accepted scheme to explain the responses of blood vessels (which also applies to other kinds of smooth muscle) is shown in Figure 11.1.

Three separate but interacting mechanisms are postulated:

1. Release of calcium from intracellular stores (mainly the sarcoplasmic reticulum), which can occur without any depolarization of the cell. There is evidence (see Chapter 1) that the calcium permeability of the sarcoplasmic reticulum is controlled by the PI response (see Fig. 1.12) evoked by various agonists.
2. Increase of membrane permeability to Ca^{++} via receptor-operated channels (ROC).
3. Depolarization of the membrane, caused by the increased permeability to Ca^{++} and Na^+ ions, which acts on a separate population of Ca^{++} channels (potential-operated channels, or POC) allowing further entry of Ca^{++}.

The system can act regeneratively in two ways.

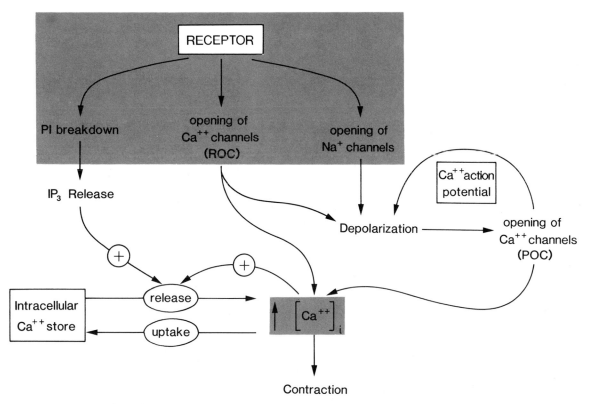

Fig. 11.1 Control of vascular smooth muscle. Receptors for various mediators (e.g. noradrenaline, angiotensin, serotonin) control separate processes which affect the intracellular free calcium concentration, $[Ca^{++}]_i$.
   1. Breakdown of phosphatidylinositols (PI) to yield triphosphoinositol (IP_3), which releases calcium from intracellular stores.
   2. Opening of receptor-operated calcium channels (ROC) which allow calcium to enter the cell, and produce depolarization.
   3. Opening of receptor-operated sodium channels, causing depolarization. Depolarization causes potential-operated calcium channels (POC) to open, which also allows calcium to enter the cell.

Increased $[Ca^{++}]_i$ can cause further release of Ca^{++} from the sarcoplasmic reticulum, and the POCs are activated by depolarization, thus enabling a regenerative Ca^{++} action potential to occur and propagate through the muscle layer.

The tonic phase of the response to agonists probably represents mechanism 2 (see above), whereas the phasic response results from either or both of mechanisms 1 and 3.

Inhibition by drugs

There appear to be two main mechanisms by which drugs can cause smooth muscle relaxation:

1. By interfering with Ca^{++} entry
2. By increasing intracellular cAMP or cGMP concentration (see below).

Drugs that interfere with Ca^{++} entry may do so directly (e.g. Ca antagonists) by blocking ROCs or POCs. Most Ca antagonists appear to be relatively selective for POCs, which partly accounts for the pattern of vasodilation that they produce, affecting arteries and arterioles more than veins. **Papaverine** (see p. 261) owes part of its action to a block of Ca channels. Alternatively, drugs may cause hyperpolarization of the cells, which tends to switch off POCs and secondarily reduce Ca^{++} entry. This occurs in visceral, but not in vascular, smooth muscle.

Drugs that work by increasing intracellular cAMP concentration include **β-adrenoceptor agonists** (see Chapter 7) and **methylxanthines** (see Chapter 10) and probably also vasodilators such as **adenosine** and **dopamine** (see p. 265–6). Exactly how cAMP causes relaxation is not certain. These drugs have little effect on electrical activity, and there is evidence that cAMP affects the linkage between $[Ca^{++}]_i$ and contraction, probably by causing phosphorylation of one of the proteins involved in the contractile machinery. **Organic nitrates** and **nitroprusside** (see p. 260) relax smooth muscle by increasing intracellular cGMP.

An interesting slant on the mechanism of action of vasodilator substances was recently provided by the work of Furchgott (1981), who was puzzled by the fact that the powerful vasodilator effect of acetylcholine-like drugs *in vivo* was hardly ever seen if isolated strips of vascular smooth muscle were examined *in vitro*. In such preparation, acetylcholine usually does nothing or causes a small contraction. Furchgott found that the vascular endothelium needed to be carefully preserved in order to obtain relaxation with acetylcholine, and he showed that acetylcholine acts, not directly on the smooth muscle cells, but on the endothelial cells, causing them to release a vasodilator substance (see Chapter 6). It now appears that several other vasodilators, including **bradykinin** and **purines** such as ADP, work, partly at least, by the same indirect mechanism.

VASOCONSTRICTOR DRUGS

Vasoconstriction is a major effect of three main groups of compounds, namely **sympathomimetic amines**, **angiotensin** and peptides related to it, and **vasopressin-like peptides**. It occurs to a minor extent with other drugs, such as β-receptor antagonists and cardiac glycosides. Mention should also be made of **thromboxane A_2**, an unstable prostaglandin intermediate produced locally in blood vessel walls (see Chapters 7 & 12) which is an extremely potent vasoconstrictor and is probably involved in thrombosis and pathological vasoconstriction.

SYMPATHOMIMETIC AMINES

This group of drugs is discussed fully in Chapter 7. Vasoconstriction is produced by activation of α-adrenoceptors, mainly those of the α_1-subclass, though blood vessels also possess α_2-adrenoceptors. α-adrenoceptors exert a powerful vasoconstrictor effect on the skin and mucous membranes, and on the splanchnic, hepatic and renal vascular beds, with relatively little effect on the cerebral and coronary circulations. Blood flow through skeletal muscle is not very sensitive to α-receptor agonists, but is increased by β-receptor agonists, so drugs such as **adrenaline**, which have a mixed action, effectively divert blood from the skin and splanchnic circulations to skeletal muscle.

α-adrenoceptor agonists constrict arteries, arterioles and veins. They thus increase peripheral resistance and reduce venous capacity, raising the central venous pressure. In the absence of any direct cardiac effect, cardiac output falls, but the reduced arterial compliance and increased arterial pressure tend to increase cardiac work.

Drugs with an almost pure α-receptor action (e.g. **phenylephrine**) cause marked bradycardia, which is a reflex response to the rise in blood pressure that is produced. The same occurs with infusions of noradrenaline (see Fig. 11.8). Drugs with mixed α- and β-actions, which include the indirectly-acting sympathomimetic amines, such as **ephedrine**, cause marked tachycardia because of their β-effects on the heart.

These drugs are used mainly to produce local vasoconstriction. **Adrenaline** is often added to local anaesthetic injections so as to delay removal of the local anaesthetic from the injection site, and thus prolong its action (see Chapter 27).* Adrenaline must not be used with local anaesthetic injections into fingers and toes because the main digital arteries may be so constricted that necrosis occurs.

Other sympathomimetic amines (e.g. **phenylephrine**) may be used to cause shrinkage of congested mucous membranes, e.g. to cause nasal decongestion. Their effects tend to be short-lived, and the congestion returns worse than before. It can also be used to stop superficial bleeding from skin or mucous membranes.

The systemic use of sympathomimetic amines in hypotensive states is a controversial matter (p. 273). It may be useful if the hypotension is due to vasodilatation (e.g. in local anaesthetic toxicity (see Chapter 27) or during spinal anaesthesia) but not in hypovolaemic states.

ANGIOTENSIN

Angiotensin is an endogenous peptide, whose physiological role and possible relevance to hypertension is discussed more fully below. The active substance, **angiotensin II**, is an extremely powerful vasoconstrictor, being roughly 40 times as active as noradrenaline in raising blood pressure. Its peripheral effects resemble those of α_1-receptor agon-

ists, in that it mainly affects cutaneous, splanchnic and renal blood flow, with little effect on the blood flow to brain and skeletal muscle. It does, however, reduce coronary blood flow. It lacks effects on other smooth muscle, and also has less effect on the venous system than α-agonists. Outside the vascular system, its main effects are to increase the force and rate of the heart (which is due to release of noradrenaline from sympathetic nerve terminals) and to increase secretion of aldosterone from the adrenal cortex (see Chapter 14).

Angiotensin has no clinical uses; its pharmacological importance lies in the fact that other drugs (e.g. **saralasin** and **captopril**; see below) may affect the cardiovascular system by altering the production or action of angiotensin.

VASOPRESSIN (ANTIDIURETIC HORMONE)

This posterior pituitary peptide hormone is important mainly for its actions on the kidney and is discussed fully in Chapter 14, but it is also a powerful vasoconstrictor. There is evidence that two distinct types of receptor (V_1 and V_2) are responsible for the effects of vasopressin. The renal effect, mediated through V_1 receptors, occurs at very low concentrations of vasopressin, and involves activation of adenylate cyclase and an increase in intracellular cAMP concentration. The other effects (e.g. on smooth muscle), mediated through V_2 receptors, require much higher concentrations, and involve intracellular calcium mobilization via the inositol phosphate mechanism (see Chapter 1 and Fig. 11.1).

Vasopressin causes a generalized vasoconstriction, affecting all vascular beds about equally, including the coronary vessels. It also affects other smooth muscle (e.g. the gastrointestinal tract and uterus). This is important in relation to its use in treating diabetes insipidus (see Chapter 14) because the large doses needed to produce an antidiuretic effect in patients whose kidneys have become resistant to the hormone, can produce coronary ischaemia and anginal pain, as well as gastrointestinal cramps.

A derivative of vasopressin, **felypressin**, which is more resistant to enzymic degradation, is sometimes used in preference to adrenaline as a vasoconstrictor adjunct to local anaesthetic injections.

---

* The reason for preferring adrenaline to an apparently more suitable agent that acts only on α-receptors seems to be lost in the mists of tradition.

The systemic action of adrenaline is increased, and may be hazardous, in the presence of tricyclic anti-depressant drugs, and the use of felypressin avoids this problem.

VASODILATOR DRUGS

Vasodilators are a heterogenous group of drugs, of which many are clinically important. They may be divided for convenience into those that act directly on vascular smooth muscle and those that act in-directly, by inhibiting the action of a naturally-occurring constrictor. The main groups are listed in Table 11.1. Some of them will be discussed in detail in this chapter; others are discussed elsewhere.

Table 11.1 Vasodilator substances

Substances that act directly on vascular smooth muscle

Drugs

Organic nitrates	Chapter 10
Calcium antagonists	Chapter 10
Methylxanthines	Chapter 10
Hydrallazine	This chapter
Diazoxide	This chapter
Papaverine	This chapter

Endogenous mediators*

Histamine	Chapter 8
Bradykinin	Chapter 8
Prostaglandins	Chapter 8
Serotonin	This chapter
β-adrenoceptor agonists	Chapter 7
Muscarinic agonists	Chapter 6
Dopamine	This chapter
Purines	This chapter

Substances that act indirectly

Drugs that reduce activity or block transmission in the sympathetic nervous system	Chapter 7 & This chapter
Captopril	This chapter
Saralasin	This chapter

* Many of these substances produce mixed vasodilator and vasoconstrictor effects, the predominant effect depending on the location of the vascular bed, the size of the vessel and the species. Furthermore, the vasodilator effect may be indirect, depending on the production of a secondary vasodilator mediator from the vascular endothelium (see Chapter 6).

NITROPRUSSIDE

Sodium nitroprusside (nitroferricyanide) is a very powerful vasodilator with little effect outside the vascular system. It acts equally on arterial and venous smooth muscle, unlike the organic nitrates (see Chapter 10), which act much more on veins than arteries. Both central venous pressure and arterial pressure drop, but cardiac output is not much changed, partly because of a reflex tachycardia. It relieves anginal pain, much as the nitrates do, and has very few side effects.

Although the pharmacological effects of nitroprusside are well-suited to the treatment of hypertension, shock or angina (see below & Chapter 10), its clinical usefulness is limited by the fact that it can only be given intravenously, as a continuous infusion. In solution, particularly when exposed to light, nitroprusside is hydrolysed to **cyanide**, and this means that it would be poisonous if given orally. The intravenous solution has to be made up from dry powder, and must be used within 4 hours. In the body, nitroprusside is rapidly converted to **thiocyanate**, its plasma half-life being only a few minutes, so it must be given as a continuous infusion, with careful monitoring to avoid excessive hypotension. Prolonged use can lead to thiocyanate toxicity (weakness, nausea, and inhibition of thyroid function) because thiocyanate is cleared only slowly from the bloodstream.

Its main uses are as an **anti-hypertensive drug** in emergencies, where a rapid response is essential, or to produce controlled hypotension for certain surgical operations, and in **shock** (see below).

HYDRALLAZINE

This is a vasodilator drug that acts mainly on arteries and arterioles, causing a fall in blood pressure, accompanied by reflex tachycardia and an increased cardiac output; it has little effect on the venous system. Its mechanism of action at the cellular level has not been determined.

Hydrallazine has some pharmacokinetic peculiarities that are important in practice. It is inactivated mainly by acetylation in the liver, and has a plasma half-life of 2–8 hours. One major cause of variation is the **acetylator status** of the individual (see Chapter 4). In slow acetylators, the plasma half-life is longer, and the incidence of side effects much greater, unless the dose is correspondingly reduced. Another complication is that hydrallazine inactivation follows a linear (zero order) rather than an exponential time-course (see Chapter 3), which increases the risk of accumulation of the drug when it is given repeatedly.

Hydrallazine produces a variety of unwanted effects, which occur commonly in clinical use, partly because of the unpredictable variation in metabolism between individuals. The main side effects are headache, nausea and sweating. Drug-induced arthritis and skin rash (lupus syndrome) is also quite common in slow acetylators.

The main use of hydrallazine is as an antihypertensive drug (see below), normally in combination with other drugs.

DIAZOXIDE

This drug belongs chemically to the same group as the **thiazide diuretics** (see Chapter 14) which also have important vasodilator properties as well as their renal actions. Pharmacologically, diazoxide is quite different from the thiazides, however. Its vascular effects are very like those of hydrallazine, though more rapid in onset. It probably acts as a calcium antagonist, and like other such drugs, it acts more on arteries than veins.

Diazoxide has odd pharmacokinetic properties, probably due to its high affinity for plasma albumin. Normally about 90% of the drug is bound in the plasma, and its affinity is such that these sites are saturated before the free concentration reaches an effective level. Relatively small changes in the total dose will then cause disproportionate changes in the free plasma concentration and biological effect. This probably explains why the duration of action of diazoxide is short (1–4 hours) though its plasma half-life (which reflects by the bound, as well as the free concentration) is long (about 30 hours). The drug is not effective orally, and must be given by intravenous injection.

The side effects of diazoxide are considerable. Interestingly, its renal effect is opposite to that of thiazides, for it causes **retention of sodium**, and worsening of oedema, though its other side effects are similar to those of the thiazides, namely **hyperglycaemia** (due to inhibition of insulin release) and retention of uric acid (see Chapter 14).

Diazoxide is used in the emergency treatment of hypertension.

PAPAVERINE

Papaverine is a drug closely related to **morphine** (see Chapter 25) and is also produced by the opium poppy. Pharmacologically it is quite unlike morphine, however, its main action being to relax smooth muscle in blood vessels and elsewhere. The mechanism of action is poorly understood, but seems to involve a combination of phosphodiesterase inhibition (as with methylxanthines) and block of calcium channels. It is no longer used as a vasodilator, having been superseded by more specific and effective drugs.

ENDOGENOUS MEDIATORS THAT DILATE BLOOD VESSELS

Several of these substances are discussed in other chapters (see Table 11.1). In this section we consider in more detail three mediators, namely **serotonin**, **purines** (particularly **adenosine** and **ATP**) and **dopamine**. Though the emphasis is on their cardiovascular effects, it is convenient to include other aspects as well.

These three mediators have a good deal in common. In each case, their acceptance as neurotransmitters has been hard-won (and there remain sceptics who would deny them membership of that exclusive club); they all have numerous pharmacological effects that have proved difficult to categorise unambiguously in terms of different receptor types, a situation that has sometimes been exacerbated rather than improved by the results of numerous binding studies.

Serotonin (5-hydroxytryptamine)

Serotonin was originally discovered in 1948 when the identity of a vasoconstrictor substance released when blood is allowed to clot was being sought, so its inclusion in a section on vasodilator drugs may seem wayward. Further work has shown that it has complex vascular effects, however, including a mixture of vasodilator and vasoconstrictor actions.

Distribution, biosynthesis and degradation of serotonin

Serotonin occurs in the highest concentrations in

three situations in the body, the total amount in a human adult being roughly 10 mg.

1. **In the wall of the intestine.** About 90% of the total amount in the body is present in **chromaffin cells,** which are neural-crest derived cells, similar to those of the adrenal medulla, that are interspersed with mucosal cells, mainly in the stomach and small intestine. Some serotonin also occurs in nerve cells of the myenteric plexus, and there is good evidence that it functions there as an excitatory neuro-transmitter (see Chapter 5).

2. **In blood.** Serotonin is present in high concentration in **platelets**, which accumulate it from the plasma by an active transport system, and release it when they aggregate at sites of tissue damage (see Chapter 12).

3. **In the central nervous system.** Serotonin is a transmitter in the central nervous system (see Chapter 19) and is present in high concentrations in localized regions of the midbrain.

The biosynthesis of serotonin (Fig. 11.2) follows a pathway similar to that of noradrenaline (see Chapter 7), except that the precursor amino-acid is **tryptophan** instead of tyrosine. Serotonin is present in the diet, but is mostly metabolized before entering the bloodsteam. Tryptophan is converted to 5-hydroxytryptophan, in chromaffin cells and neurons, but not in platelets, by the action of **tryptophan hydroxylase.** The 5-hydroxytryptophan is then carboxylated to give serotonin. The same decarboxylase enzyme acts on many other substrates, and is also involved in the synthesis of catecholamines (see Chapter 7) and histamine (see Chapter 9). Platelets (and neurons) possess a high affinity serotonin uptake mechanism, and platelets become loaded with serotonin as they pass through the intestinal circulation, where the local concentration is relatively high. The mechanisms of synthesis, storage, release and re-uptake of serotonin are very similar to those of noradrenaline, and

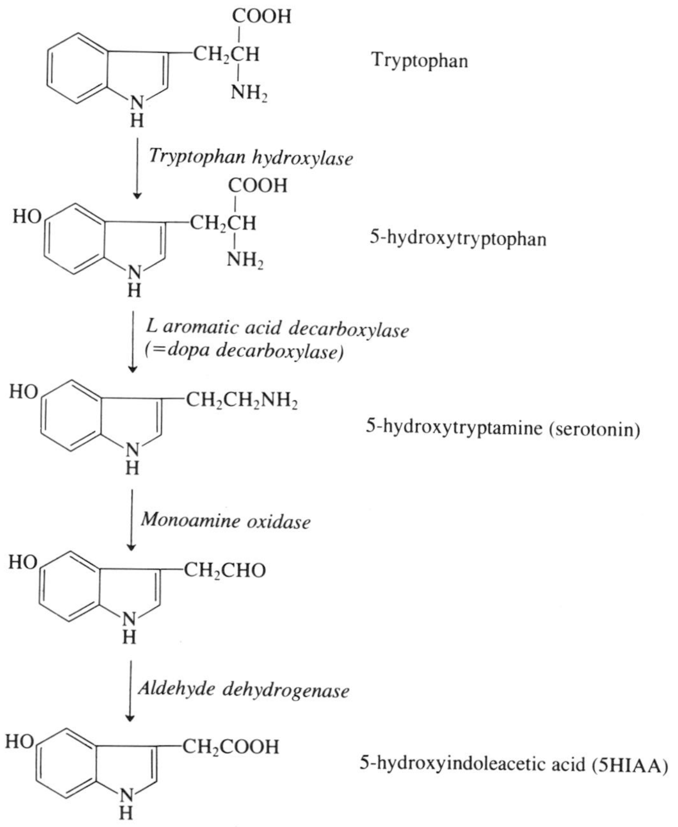

Fig. 11.2 Metabolism and degradation of serotonin.

many drugs affect both processes indiscriminately (see Chapter 7). Recent work has shown that serotonin is often stored, in neurons and chromaffin cells, together with various peptide hormones, such as **somatostatin, substance P** or **vasoactive intestinal polypeptide (VIP)**, and it is suggested that the simultaneous release of more than one active substance—termed **co-transmission** (see Chapter 5) —may be physiologically important.

Degradation of serotonin (Fig. 11.2) occurs mainly through oxidative deamination, catalysed by **monoamine oxidase**, with the formation of an aldehyde; this is followed by oxidation to **5-hydroxy-indoleacetic acid (5HIAA)**, the pathway being exactly analogous to that of noradrenaline catabolism (see Fig. 7.6). 5HIAA is excreted in the urine, and serves as an indicator of serotonin production in the body. It is therefore useful in the diagnosis of **carcinoid syndrome** (see below). Some serotonin is converted by methylation of the ring −OH group to **5-methoxytryptamine**, this reaction being exactly analogous to the formation of normetanephrine from noradrenaline (see Fig. 7.6). 5-methoxytryptamine has actions of its own in the brain, and could be involved in some affective disorders (see Chapter 22).

Pharmacological effects of serotonin

The actions of serotonin are numerous and complex, and show considerable species variation. The main ones are:

Gastrointestinal tract. Serotonin causes increased gastrointestinal motility and contraction of isolated strips of intestine, this being partly due to a direct effect on the smooth muscle cells, and partly due to an indirect effect on enteric neurons. The peristaltic reflex, evoked by increasing the pressure within a segment of intestine, is mediated, partly at least, by the release of serotonin from chromaffin cells in response to the mechanical stimulus. Chromaffin cells also respond to vagal stimulation by releasing serotonin.

Smooth muscle elsewhere in the body (e.g. uterus and bronchial tree) is also contracted by serotonin in many species, but only to a minor extent in man.

Blood vessels. Several effects are produced (Fig. 11.3), the overall effect varying according to the size of the vessel, and the prevailing level of sympathetic

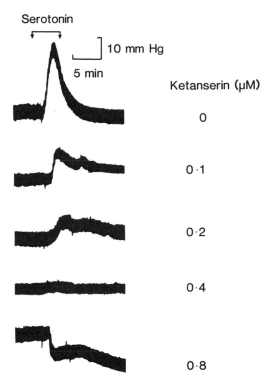

Fig. 11.3 Dual effect of serotonin on blood vessels. The records show changes in the arterial perfusion pressure in a guinea-pig stomach preparation in response to serotonin. The normal response to serotonin is a strong vasoconstriction (upper record). Addition of increasing concentrations of the $5HT_2$ receptor antagonist, ketanserin, reduces the vasoconstriction and reveals a vasodilator effect (lower trace), which is probably mediated by $5HT_1$ receptors. (From: van Nueten et al, 1981)

activity. *Large vessels*, both arteries and veins, are usually constricted by serotonin, though the sensitivity varies greatly. In the *microcirculation*, serotonin causes dilatation of arterioles, together with constriction of venules, with the result that capillary pressure rises and fluid escapes from the capillaries. There is also a direct effect on capillaries, rendering them more permeable to proteins, thus encouraging the formation of tissue fluid (Fig. 11.4).

Serotonin also inhibits the release of noradrenaline from sympathetic nerve terminals, which tends to cause a general vasodilatation.

If serotonin is injected intravenously, the blood pressure usually first rises, due to the constriction of large vessels, and then falls, due to arteriolar dilatation and loss of blood volume.

Nerve endings. Serotonin stimulates sensory nerve endings in various sites. If injected into the

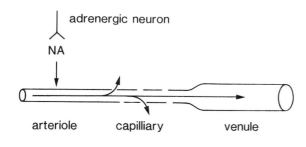

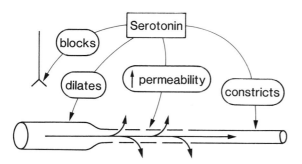

Fig. 11.4 Action of serotonin on microvasculature. Four mechanisms are involved: (1) Inhibition of NA release from sympathetic nerve terminals; (2) Dilatation of pre-capillary vessels; (3) Increase of capillary permeability; (4) Constriction of post-capillary vessel.

skin it causes pain (see Chapter 25), and given systemically it elicits a variety of autonomic reflexes due to stimulation of afferent fibres in the heart and lung, which further complicate the cardiovascular response. Nettle stings contain serotonin, among other things.

Central nervous system. Serotonin excites some neurons, and inhibits others, and also acts, usually in an inhibitory way, on pre-synaptic nerve terminals. The role of serotonin in the central nervous system is discussed in Chapter 19.

Classification of serotonin receptors (*Table* 11.2)

It is clear that the various actions of serotonin are not all mediated by receptors of the same type, but there is still some uncertainty about their classification.

Gaddum originally showed that the excitatory action of serotonin on the gut was produced by two separate actions, which could be independently blocked by different drugs. Part of the effect is due to acetylcholine release from myenteric neurons, and can be blocked by morphine (though this is not

Table 11.2 Classification of serotonin receptors

	M	Receptor type 5HT$_1$	5HT$_2$ (or D)
Effects	Excitation of peripheral neurons, causing: ACh release in periphery → smooth muscle contraction, secretion, etc. NA release → vasoconstriction, tachycardia. Stimulation of C fibres → pain, cardiovascular reflexes.	Pre-synaptic inhibition in CNS and periphery, causing: Inhibition of NA release → vasodilatation. Inhibition of serotonin release in brain	Post-synaptic excitation and inhibition in CNS, causing: Behavioural effects antinociception. Smooth muscle contraction, e.g. blood vessels, uterus, GI tract. Platelet aggregation.
Specific agonists	2-methyl serotonin	5-carboxamide tryptamine Methysergide (partial agonist)	
Specific antagonists	MDL 72222* ICS 205-930*	Quipazine Metergoline	Quipazine Metergoline Methysergide Cyproheptadine Ketanserin LSD
Ligands used in labelling studies	—	Serotonin	Spiperone Ketanserin LSD

* Recently developed compounds (Fozard, 1983; Richardson et al, 1985)
See: Peroutka & Snyder, 1982; Straughan, 1984.

specific for serotonin) and part is a direct action on smooth muscle, blocked in Gaddum's study by dibenamine, so the two receptors were termed M and D respectively.

Subsequent work on the binding of serotonin and of various serotonin antagonists, and on the actions of serotonin peripherally and in the central nervous system has shown that Gaddum's D receptor also occurs in the brain, where it exerts mainly excitatory post-synaptic effects and is responsible for the behavioural arousal caused by serotonin agonists. According to binding studies, this receptor has been classified as the $5HT_2$-receptor, though subsequent pharmacological analysis (Engel et al, 1983) suggests that it is identical with the D receptor (Table 11.2).

The $5HT_1$-site identified originally on the basis of binding studies, exerts a pre-synaptic inhibitory effect on nerve terminals in both the brain and the peripheral noradrenergic nervous system. Various antagonists block $5HT_1$-mediated effects, but none are known which do so selectively (Table 11.2).

Gaddum's M receptors exert an excitatory effect on various peripheral neurons, causing, for example, acetylcholine release (and thus contraction) from the myenteric plexus, noradrenaline release (and thus cardiac stimulation) from sympathetic nerve terminals and stimulation of various sensory nerve terminals.

Serotonin antagonists

There is a group of serotonin antagonists which have been known for many years which act selectively on the D receptor. They include **methysergide**, **cyproheptadine** and **lysergic acid diethylamide** (**LSD**) (Table 11.2). Some compounds also affect $5HT_1$-receptors, but there are no antagonists that act selectively on them. The D receptor antagonists are used clinically to treat carcinoid syndrome and migraine (see later section).

Selective and potent M receptor antagonists have recently been developed, by making modifications to the serotonin molecule (Richardson et al, 1985). These should be useful in elucidating the physiological role of serotonin in the periphery, and may prove clinically useful in the treatment of migraine, but have not yet been fully evaluated.

Antagonism of serotonin responses is also a prop-erty of various other drugs, such as **phenothiazines** and **butyrophenones** (which are anti-psychotic drugs; see Chapter 22) and of some anti-asthmatic drugs (e.g. **pizotifen** and **ketotifen**; see Chapter 13). These drugs are all non-selective in their actions, and it is uncertain whether serotonin antagonism is important to their overall effects.

Purines

Adenosine derivatives produce a wide range of pharmacological effects that are apparently un-related to their role in energy metabolism. It was shown in 1929 that **adenosine** injected into anaes-thetized animals causes cardiac slowing, a fall in blood pressure, vasodilatation and inhibition of intestinal movements, and it has since been sug-gested that adenosine or ATP are implicated in such physiological mechanisms as the regulation of coronary flow, 'antidromic' vasodilatation pro-duced by retrograde stimulation of sensory nerves, and peripheral transmission in the autonomic ner-vous system (see Chapter 5).

Purines as transmitters and local hormones

The evidence for a transmitter role of ATP is con-siderable (Burnstock 1981, 1985). It has long been realized that many actions produced by stimulation of autonomic nerves are not due to acetylcholine or noradrenaline (see Chapter 5). These include effects such as relaxation of intestinal smooth muscle evoked by sympathetic stimulation, and con-traction of the bladder produced by the para-sympathetic. Burnstock's group have shown that ATP is released, in a calcium-dependent fashion, on nerve stimulation, and that exogenous ATP in general mimics the effects of nerve stimulation in various preparations (though not all authors agree on the accuracy of this parallelism). ATP is known to be contained in synaptic vesicles of both adrenergic and cholinergic neurons, and it remains an open question whether it is released simply as a by-product of exocytosis, along with the 'true' transmitter, or has an independent trans-mitter function of its own. Since purines, especially adenosine, are produced by peripheral tissues as well as by neurons, they may also function as local regulatory substances (e.g. in controlling blood flow), whose rate of production varies with the functional state of the tissue.

It has been suggested that ATP is the transmitter responsible for the cutaneous vasodilatation caused by antidromic stimulation of sensory nerves, but recent work has produced more evidence favouring substance P for this role.

Adenosine is actively taken up by many cells, and this uptake is strongly inhibited by **dipyridamole**, a drug which enhances the responses of many test systems to adenosine, and also enhances the neurally-evoked inhibition of intestinal smooth muscle. Dipyridamole is a coronary vasodilator though it is ineffective in the treatment of angina (see Chapter 10). It is postulated that it acts by increasing the local concentration of adenosine, which may be the physiological regulator of the coronary circulation. Dipyridamole is also an inhibitor of platelet aggregation, an effect thought to be due to increased cAMP formation (see Chapter 12).

Pharmacological actions of purines

Four substances have been studied in detail: ATP, ADP, AMP and adenosine, together with various derivatives. All have powerful pharmacological effects that appear to be unrelated to their role in energy metabolism.

The main effects produced are:

1. **Vasodilatation**, affecting most vascular beds. Renal vessels are constricted.
2. **Effects on visceral smooth muscle**. The usual effect is relaxation but some parts of the intestine and genitourinary tracts show mixed stimulant and inhibitory effects. Respiratory smooth muscle is usually contracted.
3. **Cardiac inhibition**, generally producing effects opposite to those of β-adrenoceptor agonists, namely bradycardia, reduced force of contraction and impaired AV conduction.
4. **Inhibition of transmitter release** from cholinergic and adrenergic nerves.
5. **Platelet aggregation** (see Chapter 12). This response is unusual in that adenosine *antagonizes* the effect of ADP.
6. **Inhibition of central neurons**.

Biochemical studies suggest that many of the effects

of purines result from stimulation or inhibition of cAMP production.

Receptor classification

Studies of the relative potencies of different adenosine derivatives in different biological systems suggest strongly that more than one type of purine receptor exists (Satchell, 1984). Burnstock (1978) has postulated two subclasses. One type of receptor (P1) is characterised by higher sensitivity to adenosine than to ATP, and is blocked by **theophylline** whereas the other (P2) is more sensitive to ATP than adenosine, and is unaffected by theophylline. Unfortunately there are problems in using relative agonist potencies as a guide to receptor classification, since ATP is rapidly converted to ADP, AMP and adenosine in tissues, and some tissues have efficient uptake systems which can greatly reduce the concentration reaching the receptors. Measurements of antagonist affinity constants (see Chapter 1) provide, in general, a more secure basis for receptor classification, but this is hampered at present by the absence of selective compounds. Thus, there is no general agreement at present, though the P1/P2 classification provides a reasonable starting point. An alternative classification is based on the effect of adenosine on adenylate cyclase activity in different tissues. According to this scheme, A_1 and A_2-receptor types exist and cause, respectively, stimulation and inhibition of adenylate cyclase. It is now believed that these may represent two sub-types of the P1 receptor.

Compounds related to adenosine have not so far been developed to the point of clinical use, though they have potential use as smooth muscle relaxants and inhibitors of platelet aggregation.

Dopamine

Dopamine as a peripheral transmitter

Dopamine is known to be a precursor of noradrenaline in sympathetic neurons (see Chapter 7) but it also functions as a transmitter in its own right. In the brain (see Chapter 19) there is no doubt that this is so, but the evidence is less clear cut in the periphery (Thorner, 1975; Bell, 1982).

The proposal that dopamine might be a transmitter in the periphery was first made to explain the vasodilatation in the kidney produced by autonomic stimulation, which is not antagonized by blockade of the receptors for any of the well-known transmitters. This, coupled with the fact that dopamine evokes renal vasodilation, and that drugs such as **haloperidol** (which blocks the central actions of dopamine; see Chapter 22) and **ergometrine** block selectively the effect both of nerve stimulation and dopamine infusion, is the main evidence for its transmitter role. Cutaneous vasodilatation in the dog's foot pad has recently been found to have the same characteristics, and there is evidence that dopamine can also dilate coronary and cerebral vessels, so the system may be more widespread than first thought. Dopamine-containing interneurons exist in sympathetic ganglia, where dopamine has an inhibitory effect on transmission. It has been suggested that dopamine is a physiological transmitter in sympathetic ganglia, but this is not proven. Analysis of dopaminergic transmission is complicated by the fact that many agents that affect noradrenergic neurons (e.g. reserpine, 6-hydroxydopamine) also affect dopaminergic neurons, and drugs that affect the receptors may also cross-react.

Actions of dopamine

The main peripheral effects produced by dopamine (Clark, 1981) are:

1. Vasodilatation
2. Increased force of contraction of heart
3. Relaxation of intestinal smooth muscle
4. Inhibition of transmitter release.

In addition, dopamine and some drugs related to it have a weak agonist effect on α-adrenoceptors. The overall effect of dopamine agonists in a normal subject is to cause a fall in arterial pressure, and a decrease in peripheral resistance. This occurs because of the direct vasodilator action, and also because of inhibition of noradrenaline release. In patients suffering from cardiovascular shock, however, dopamine causes a rise in blood pressure rises, because it increases the force of contraction of the heart. Vasodilatation is particularly pronounced in the **renal** and **mesenteric vascular beds**. Other vascular beds may constrict somewhat, possibly because they lack dopamine receptors but are responsive to α-adrenoceptor activation by dopamine.

Veins are not dilated and cardiac output rises. Renal vasodilatation is accompanied by diuresis and an increased rate of sodium excretion. These effects are potentially useful in **hypovolaemic shock** (see below) because blood flow is diverted from other parts of the body to the renal and mesenteric circulations, vascular beds in which the intense vasoconstriction that occurs in response to hypovolaemia can lead to irreversible damage. The effects of dopamine might also be useful in treating hypertension (see below) but at present no drug is available which acts selectively on peripheral dopamine receptors, and yet has satisfactory pharmacokinetic properties.

The inhibitory action of dopamine on transmitter release, in common with that of serotonin and purines, mainly affects peripheral adrenergic neurons. This action probably accounts for the failure of dopamine to cause reflex tachycardia, even though it lowers the arterial pressure.

In many tissues, dopamine activates adenylate cyclase and increases cAMP production, by a mechanism separate from the action of β-receptor agonists. It is likely that the relaxant effects on smooth muscle are produced by this mechanism, as with β-adrenoceptor agonists.

The effects of dopamine in the central nervous system are discussed in Chapters 19 & 22. Dopamine given systemically does not cross the blood-brain barrier and only produces peripheral effects.

Classification of dopamine receptors

Studies of the binding of various dopamine receptor agonists and antagonists in the brain, and their effects on adenylate cyclase, suggest that two kinds of receptor are involved, called D_1 and D_2 (Table 11.3), which show selectivity for both agonists and antagonists.

D_1-receptors, which are coupled to adenylate cyclase and cause an increase in cAMP production, are responsible in the periphery for the vasodilator and positive inotropic effects of dopamine agonists. They are activated, though at relatively high concentration, by **dopamine**, **apomorphine** and **bromocriptine** (a substance derived from ergot; see Chapter 7), though the latter two substances are both partial agonists, or sometimes antagonists, at peripheral D_1-receptors.

Table 11.3 Classification of dopamine receptors

	Receptor type	
	D_1	D_2
Effects	Activation of adenylate cyclase. Vasodilatation. Increased force of contraction of myocardium.	No activation of adenylate cyclase. Inhibition of transmitter release. Central actions (see Chapters 19, 22 & 24).
Agonists:		
Dopamine	+(micromolar)	+(nanomolar)
Apomorphine	± PA* (micromolar)	+(nanomolar)
Bromocriptine	± PA (micromolar)	+(nanomolar)
Antagonists (see Chapter 22)		
Phenothiazines	+(micromolar)	+(nanomolar)
Butyrophenones	+(micromolar)	+(nanomolar)
Sulpiride	Weak	Potent
Domperidone	—	+(nanomolar)

* PA = Partial agonist.
See: Kebabian & Calne, 1979; Goldberg & Kohli, 1983.

These receptors are blocked, though with little selectivity since the same drugs also block serotonin receptors, by neuroleptic drugs of the pheno-thiazine and butyrophenone series (see Chapter 22).

There are at present no highly selective agonists for D_1-receptors, which has made it difficult to ascertain their physiological role.

D_2-receptors are responsible for inhibition of transmitter release, both peripherally and centrally, and also for inhibition of prolactin secretion (see Chapter 16) and other effects in the central nervous system (see Chapter 19). In the periphery, their main effect is to inhibit noradrenaline release, which contributes to the hypotensive action of dopamine. Because, in general, D_2-receptors are affected by much lower agonist concentrations than D_1, and because their effects predominate in the central nervous system, drugs such as bromo-criptine and apomorphine, which enter the brain quite freely, produce mainly central, rather than peripheral actions. Dopamine itself does not enter the brain if given systemically, so is the best drug to use as an agonist for the peripheral receptors.

The classification in Table 11.3, though basically correct, is certainly an oversimplification, and bind-ing studies have revealed some quantitative in-consistencies which have encouraged some authors to propose much more ornate classifications.

Uses of drugs that act on dopamine receptors

Dopamine itself is used for its peripheral cardio-vascular effects, in the treatment of shock (see below). Bromocriptine is used for its central effects (see Chapters 16, 19 & 24) to reduce prolactin secretion and in the treatment of Parkinsonism. Apomorphine has similar central actions, but is a powerful emetic, which limits its usefulness. Dop-amine antagonists form the main group of neuro-leptic drugs, used in the treatment of schizophrenia (see Chapter 22).

Atrial peptides

A new class of peptides which probably play an important role in cardiovascular regulation has recently been characterised (see review by Needle-man et al, 1984). It has been known for many years that distension of the atria (e.g. by an increase in blood volume) evokes a powerful vasodilatation and an increase in renal sodium excretion (natriur-esis). One mechanism by which this occurs appears to involve the secretion of one or more peptides by the atrial muscle cells, which possess struc-tural features characteristic of secretory cells. It was shown in 1981 that extracts of atrial, but not ventricular, muscle cause strong natriuresis, and subsequently a family of closely related peptides containing 21–28 amino acid residues (variously called **atriopeptins**, **atrial natriuretic factors**, or **cardionatrins** by different groups of investigators) has been identified as the mediator of this response. These peptides originate from a common precursor of 151 residues, by proteolytic cleavage at Arg–Arg or Arg–Lys bonds, exactly in the manner of many neuropeptides (see Chapter 19). The atrial peptides have a number of actions, which have the common effect of increasing sodium excretion and increasing the capacity of the vascular system. The natriuresis probably results mainly from renal vasodilatation, but a reduction of aldosterone secretion also occurs, and this would also produce natriuresis (see Chapter 14). Much remains to be discovered about this interesting system, which offers promise for the future development of new types of drug to control extracellular fluid volume.

VASODILATOR DRUGS THAT ACT INDIRECTLY

There are many drugs that cause vasodilatation indirectly by blocking the activity of the sympathetic nervous system; these are discussed in Chapter 7. The other important group of drugs in this category are those that affect the renin-angiotensin system.

The renin-angiotensin system

Renin is a proteolytic enzyme that is secreted into the circulation by cells of the juxta-glomerular apparatus, a specialized island of tissue lying at the point where the afferent arteriole, just before entering the glomerulus, comes into close apposition to a specialized part of the distal tubule (see Chapter 14; Fig. 14.2). The wall of the arteriole contains a cluster of renin-containing **juxta-glomerular cells**, which secrete renin into the bloodstream in response to a rise in the sodium concentration of the fluid in the distal tubule. Renin acts on a plasma globulin, **angiotensinogen**, splitting off a decapeptide, **angiotensin I**, from the N-terminal end of the protein. This happens rapidly, and the renin activity in the plasma disappears within a few minutes. Angiotensin I has no appreciable activity,

but is acted on by a second proteolytic enzyme, **angiotensin converting enzyme** (ACE), which removes two more amino-acids to form the highly active octapeptide, **angiotensin II** (Fig. 11.5). ACE is

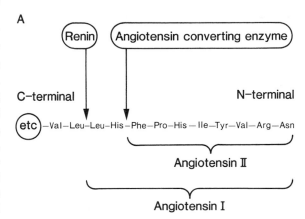

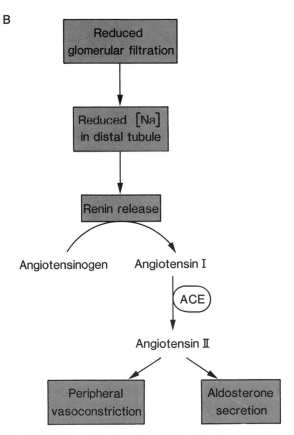

Fig. 11.5 A. Formation of angiotensin I and angiotensin II from the N-terminal of the precursor protein, angiotensinogen. B. The control of angiotensin production and its main physiological effects. (ACE = angiotensin converting enzyme).

a membrane-bound enzyme, and is particularly abundant in the lung, where most of the formation of angiotensin II takes place. The same enzyme is responsible for inactivating bradykinin (see Chapter 8). This pathway, which is important in the pathogenesis of hypertension (see below), can be influenced by drugs at three points: (1) Renin release; (2) ACE; and (3) Interaction of angiotensin II with vascular receptors.

Renin release

This is partly under the control of the sympathetic nervous system. It is known that stimulation of the renal sympathetic nerves causes renin release, and that this is blocked by β-adrenoceptor antagonists. In certain types of hypertension, in which the renin content of the plasma is abnormally high, administration of β-antagonists reduces it. This appears to be one mechanism, but not the only one, to explain the hypotensive action of these drugs.

Angiotensin converting enzyme inhibitors

Several specific ACE inhibitors have been developed, of which **captopril** (Fig. 11.6) is the most important. The enzyme is a carboxypeptidase which splits off pairs of basic amino-acids, and its active site is known to contain a zinc atom. The development of captopril represents one of the first examples of successful drug design based on a chemical knowledge of the target molecule. A variety of small peptides were found to be weak inhibitors of the enzyme, but these were unsuitable as drugs because of their low potency and poor oral absorption. The structure of captopril was designed to combine the steric properties of such peptide antagonists in a non-peptide molecule, which contains a sulfhydryl group appropriately placed to bind to the zinc atom, coupled to a proline residue which binds to the enzyme site normally occupied by the terminal leucine of angiotensin I (Fig. 11.6).

Captopril is a powerful inhibitor of the effects of angiotensin I in the whole animal. It causes a small fall in arterial pressure in normal animals or human subjects, but a much larger fall in subjects in whom renin secretion is enhanced (e.g. in cases of sodium deprivation or renal hypertension). The fall that occurs in normal, sodium replete subjects, in whom

renin secretion is very small, may be related to inhibition of bradykinin inactivation. Captopril has a limited use in the treatment of hypertension (see below).

Angiotensin antagonists

Saralasin, produced in 1970 as a result of determined juggling with the amino-acid composition of angiotensin II, is a competitive inhibitor of the

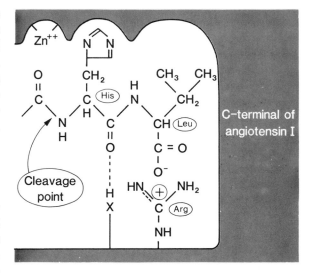

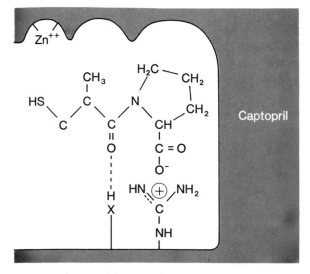

Fig. 11.6 Diagram of the active site of angiotensin converting enzyme showing the binding of angiotensin I (above) and of the inhibitor, captopril (below) which is an analogue of the terminal dipeptide of angiotensin I.

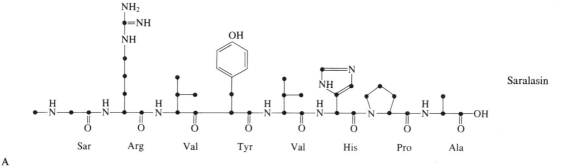

Angiotensin II

Asn   Arg   Val   Tyr   Ile   His   Pro   Phe

Saralasin

Sar   Arg   Val   Tyr   Val   His   Pro   Ala

A

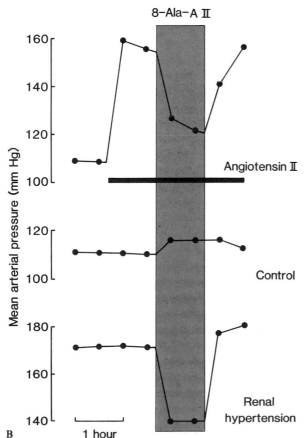

8–Ala–A II

Angiotensin II

Control

Renal
hypertension

1 hour

B

Fig. 11.7 A. The structures of angiotensin II and the competitive antagonist, saralasin.

B. Effects of an angiotensin antagonist, Ala[8]-angiotensin II, on blood pressure of conscious rats. The hypertensive effects of angiotensin II is antagonised (top panel) but the drug causes a small rise in blood pressure when given on its own (middle panel) because it is a partial agonist rather than a pure antagonist. A marked fall in blood pressure occurs in rats with hypertension caused by partial renal artery occlusion (bottom panel).

vasoconstrictor effect of angiotensin. It differs from angiotensin II by two amino-acids (Fig. 11.7A) and is a highly selective antagonist. Like many analogues of peptide hormones, it is not a pure competitive antagonist, but a weak partial agonist, and the agonist/antagonist balance depends on the response that is being measured. Thus saralasin tends to increase aldosterone secretion (an agonist effect), thus causing sodium retention, and to cause slight vasoconstriction in a non-hypertensive subject, while causing vasodilatation in hypertensive subjects (Fig. 11.7B). Because it is a peptide, saralasin can only be given intravenously, and its plasma half-life is only a few minutes, so its clinical use is very limited. It can cause a rise in blood pressure, because of its agonist activity, in patients whose renin secretion is not raised, so must be used with great care.

CLINICAL USES OF VASODILATOR DRUGS

It is beyond the scope of this book to provide a detailed account of the clinical uses of drugs that affect the cardiovascular system, but it is nonetheless useful to consider the various pharmacological approaches that are used in treating certain clinical states. The conditions that will be briefly discussed are: (1) Hypertension; (2) Shock; (3) Cardiac failure; and (4) Migraine.

Hypertension

There are a few recognizable and treatable causes of hypertension, such as phaeochromocytoma, steroid-secreting tumours of the adrenal cortex, renal artery stenosis, etc, but the great majority of cases involve no obvious causative factor, and are grouped as **essential hypertension** (so called because it was originally thought that the raised blood pressure was essential to maintain adequate tissue perfusion). The underlying defect seems to be an

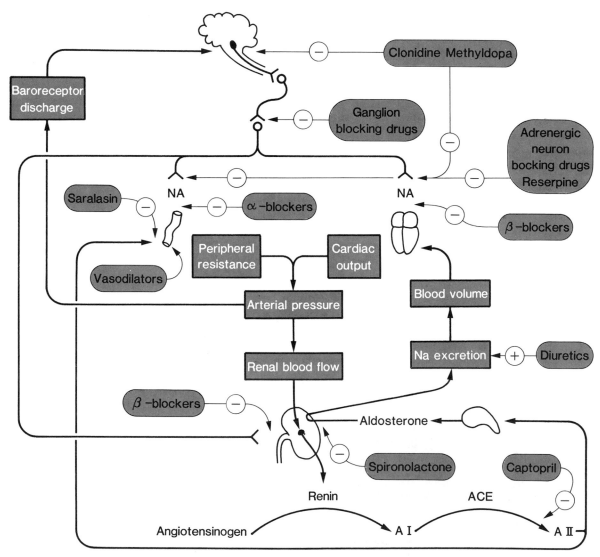

Fig. 11.8 Diagram showing the main mechanisms involved in arterial blood pressure regulation (heavy lines), and the sites of action of antihypertensive drugs (light lines).

excessive tendency for arterioles to constrict, which calls into play a variety of physiological responses involving the cardiovascular system, nervous system and kidney. Certain vicious circles tend to become established, and these provide some of the targets for pharmacological attack.

Figure 11.8 summarizes the major physiological control mechanisms that operate to maintain the arterial blood pressure. The two main systems involved are the sympathetic nervous system and the renin-angiotensin-aldosterone system. One of the ways in which the primary process (which may well be an abnormality of the membrane of smooth muscle cells in blood vessels) tends to lead to progressively worsening hypertension is that renal artery sclerosis occurs in response to the raised pressure, so that the renal blood flow decreases. This results in increased renin secretion and a further increase of the blood pressure. In essence, the control system fails because the normal relationship between renal blood flow and arterial blood pressure is upset by the narrowing of the renal vessels. It is now well established, contrary to the earlier view that hypertension was 'essential' to sustain life, that reducing arterial blood pressure greatly increases the life expectancy of hypertensive patients. The use of drugs to control mild hypertension, which may produce no symptoms, without producing unacceptable side effects, is therefore an important clinical need, and much effort has gone into devising satisfactory therapeutic regimes.

The main points of attack for anti-hypertensive drugs are shown in Figure 11.8. Since these drugs usually have to be continued indefinitely, avoidance of side effects is particularly important, and the protocol usually followed in treating hypertension involves the staged introduction of drugs, starting with those least likely to produce side effects. The main categories of anti-hypertensive drug are summarized in Table 11.4.

Cardiac failure

The underlying abnormality in cardiac failure (see Chapter 10) is inadequate force of contraction of the myocardium, which leads secondarily to an increased central venous pressure (increased preload) and to peripheral vasoconstriction (increased afterload). An increase in body fluid volume occurs

because the increased venous pressure causes increased formation of tissue fluid, and because the reduced renal blood flow leads to sodium retention, partly through activation of the renin-angiotensin system. Hypersecretion of another, so far unidentified, salt-retaining hormone is also postulated. A highly simplified diagram of the sequence of events is shown in Figure 11.9. It can be seen that there are three main points at which drug treatment can act:

1. *Increased force of contraction.* The most important drugs are the **cardiac glycosides** (see Chapter 10) though **dopamine** (see above) and **dobutamine** (a β_1-selective adrenoceptor agonist; see Chapter 7) are also used when a rapid response is needed.

2. *Increased fluid excretion.* **Diuretics** (see Chapter 14) are routinely used to treat cardiac failure. A diuretic may suffice on its own, but is often combined with digoxin treatment.

3. *Vasodilatation.* The use of rapidly-acting vasodilators such as **nitroprusside** or **glyceryl trinitrate** is well established for treating acute episodes of cardiac failure. The venodilator effect of these drugs is helpful in reducing venous pressure, and their effect of increasing the compliance of the arterial system is useful in reducing cardiac work. The use of arteriolar vasodilators, such as calcium antagonists, captopril or hydrallazine for longer term treatment may also be effective.

Shock and hypotensive states

Shock is a condition in which the patient is pale, sweating and anxious, and has a weak, rapid pulse and very low arterial pressure. It can be caused by various kinds of physiological insult, including haemorrhage, burns, bacterial infections and acute myocardial damage (Fig. 11.10). The common feature in each case is a reduction in the circulating blood volume (**hypovolaemia**), caused either directly by a loss of blood or by a movement of fluid from the plasma to the tissues. The dividing line between the normal physiological response to blood loss, and clinical shock is that, in the latter, tissue hypoxia produces secondary effects that tend to magnify, rather than correct, the primary disturbance. Thus, the release of mediators (e.g. histamine, serotonin, bradykinin, prostaglandins and undoubtedly a variety of yet unidentified substances), which cause

Table 11.4 Antihypertensive drugs

Mode of action	Drugs	Adverse effects			
		Postural hypotension	Impotence	Drowsiness	Na-retention
Reduction of sympathetic discharge	Clonidine	—	—	+	—
	Methyldopa	+ +	+	+ +	+
Ganglion	Trimetaphan	+ +	+ +	—	—
Sympathetic neuron	Guanethidine Bethanidine Debrisoquin Methyldopa (see above)	+ +	+ +	—	+
	Reserpine	+	+	+ +	+
Block of adrenoceptors α-receptors	Prazosin	+ +	+	+	—
β-receptors	Propranolol Atenolol Oxprenolol, etc.	—	—	+	—
α- and β-receptors	Labetalol	+	+	+	—
Vasodilatation	Hydrallazine	+	—	—	—
	Diazoxide	+ +	—	—	+ +
	Nitroprusside	+ +	—	—	—
	Thiazide diuretics	—	+	—	—
	Calcium antagonists	+	—	—	—
Block of renin-angiotensin system	Captopril	—	—	—	—
	Saralasin	—	—	—	—
Reduction of blood volume	Diuretics (see Thiazides above)	—	—	—	—

vessels in the microcirculation to become dilated and leaky, is physiologically the opposite of what is required. One of these factors is a small peptide (**myocardial depressant factor**) which comes mainly from the pancreas, where many proteolytic enzymes are likely to be unleashed by tissue damage, and which acts to decrease cardiac output still further. Reduced renal blood flow has two important and harmful consequences, namely renin secretion which, via the angiotensin mechanism, causes further vasoconstriction, and cessation of urine flow, which occurs when the arterial pressure drops below about 50 mmHg. Irreversible renal damage can occur if this goes unchecked.

Therapeutically, the overriding priority in shock is to restore the circulating volume by transfusion, and drug treatment is of limited usefulness. Every imaginable drug has been tried, with a variety of rationalizations, including α-receptor agonists (to increase arterial pressure), α-receptor antagonists and other vasodilators (to increase tissue blood flow), β-receptor agonists (to increase

Other	Special features	Uses
Dry mouth.	Initial pressor effect. Rebound hypertension.	Also in migraine, and treatment of opiate withdrawal.
Disturbance of movement, endocrine disturbance.	Can cause haemolysis, and abnormal haemagglutinin test.	Used if first-line drugs are inadequate.
Constipation, visual disturbance.	Used i.v.	Occasional use in anaesthesia. Not used in hypertension.
Diarrhoea, nasal congestion.	Erratic absorption from gut.	Used if first-time drugs are inadequate.
Severe depression		Little used, because of risk of depression.
Tachycardia		
Bronchoconstriction, cardiac failure, peripheral vasoconstriction.		First treatment of mild hypertension.
		Effective in phaeochromocytoma.
Tachycardia, systemic lupus.	Tolerance. Toxic risk in slow acetylators.	Used in conjunction with β-blockers.
Hyperglycaemia.	Short-acting, must be given i.v.	Emergency treatment of hypertension. Also used in anaesthesia.
Hyperglycaemia, hyperuricaemia, K^+ loss.		First-line treatment of mild hypertension.
Headache, reflex tachycardia, cardiac failure.		Recently introduced, probably similar to hydrallazine, but less toxic.
Rashes, fever, severe hypotension.		Mainly in cases where plasma renin is raised.
Hypertension in some subjects.	Must be given i.v.	Experimental use only.
Hypotension, K^+ loss, deafness.		See thiazides above.

cardiac output and produce vasodilatation), mostly with very limited benefit. The main drugs that are of proven benefit (Fig. 11.10) are **dopamine** and **adrenocortical steroids**.

Dopamine selectively dilates the renal and mesenteric vascular beds, both of which are important in the pathogenesis of shock, and also increases the force of the myocardial contraction.

Adrenocortical steroids (see Chapter 16) have been widely used in treating shock, mainly on the basis of evidence that they protect tissues against the damaging effects of hypoxia. Only in the case of septicaemic shock, however, is there clear evidence that they are effective, and their use in other kinds of shock is controversial.

Migraine

Migraine is a common and unpleasant condition, whose causation is not well understood (Amery et al, 1984). The most generally accepted view is that vascular changes are responsible, and that these are

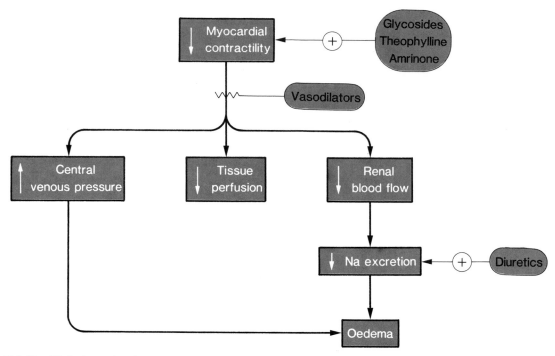

Fig. 11.9 Simplified scheme showing the pathogenesis of heart failure, and the sites of action of some of the drugs, which are used to treat it. The symptoms of heart failure are produced by reduced tissue perfusion, oedema and increased central venous pressure.

triggered by serotonin release. The most common pattern of events in a migraine attack consists of an initial visual disturbance, in which the central area of the visual field is lost, and the surrounding area displays a jagged, flickering pattern. This visual disturbance is followed, about 30 minutes later, by a severe headache, often with nausea and vomiting, which lasts for several hours. These symptoms are accompanied by (and most probably caused by) pronounced vascular changes, the premonitory visual signs being associated with vasoconstriction of intracranial vessels, and the headache with dilatation of extracranial vessels, together with inflammation in their vicinity (Fig. 11.11).

The evidence implicating serotonin in these events is rather strong.

1. There is a sharp increase in the urinary excretion of the main serotonin metabolite, 5HIAA, during the attack. The plasma concentration of serotonin falls, however.
2. Agents that release serotonin (e.g. reserpine) when injected locally, cause a migraine-like headache.

3. Many of the drugs that are effective in treating migraine are serotonin antagonists (Fozard, 1982).

The source of the serotonin, the nature of the stimulus that causes its release, and the mechanism by which this sequence of vascular changes occurs, remain mysterious; there is evidence to suggest that other mediators, such as prostaglandins and substance P, play a part, but no convincing hypothesis. These mediators, including serotonin, can all stimulate pain afferents in tissues, and this may be important in producing the headache.

A possible pattern of events in a migraine attack (Fig. 11.12) is that the prodromal visual disturbance results from cerebral ischaemia caused by excessive release of serotonin (from nerve terminals, platelets or both) which produces cerebral vasoconstriction, while the headache phase is caused by dilatation resulting from too little serotonin release, and also from the action of secondary mediators (e.g. prostaglandins) that are released by the initial excess of serotonin. This, doubtless oversimplified, hypo-

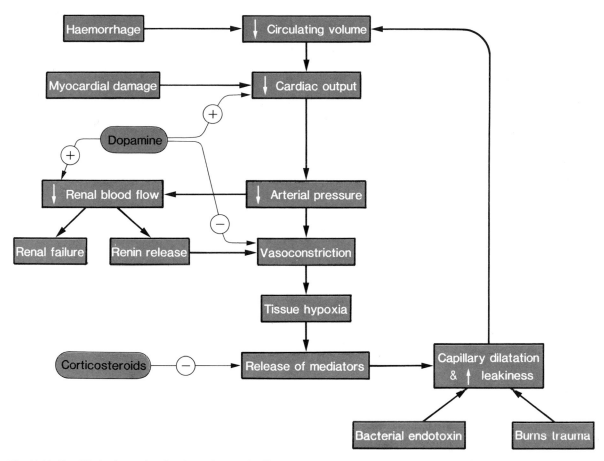

Fig. 11.10 Simplified scheme showing the pathogenesis of hypovolaemic shock, and the sites of action of two types of drug (dopamine and corticosteroids) that may be used to treat it. The most important treatment is to restore circulating volume, normally by intravenous infusion.

thesis would account for the puzzling observation that intravenous serotonin, given during the headache phase when the plasma serotonin concentration is low, alleviates the attack. It also provides a basis for understanding the mode of action of drugs that are used to treat migraine (Fig. 11.12). The main drugs used for this purpose are:

1. Ergotamine
2. Other serotonin antagonists (e.g. methysergide, cyproheptadine, pizotifen)
3. Aspirin-like drugs (see Chapter 9)
4. Clonidine (see Chapter 7)
5. Propranolol (see Chapter 7).

Ergotamine is probably the most effective, though its side effects (see Chapter 7) are trouble-some. It is a partial agonist at both serotonin D-receptors and α-adrenoceptors, and it is likely that the combination of serotonin antagonism with vasoconstrictor activity (Fig. 11.12) is what makes it effective. Its action in a migraine attack is shown in Figure 11.11.

Methysergide is a more selective D-receptor antagonist than ergotamine and has little vaso-constrictor activity. This may explain why it is effective in the prevention of migraine attacks, but (unlike ergotamine) has no effect once the attack has started, for, according to the scheme in Figure 11.12, excessive serotonin activity is involved only at the start of the attack. The clinical usefulness of methysergide is limited by its tendency to cause inflammatory fibrosis of the pleural and peritoneal

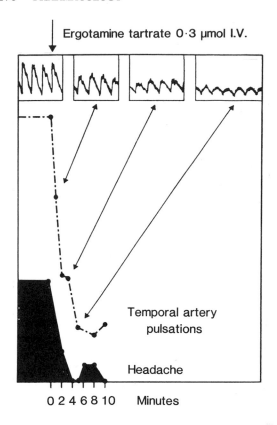

Ergotamine tartrate 0·3 μmol I.V.

Temporal artery pulsations

Headache

0 2 4 6 8 10   Minutes

cavities, an uncommon, but serious side effect. Other serotonin antagonists (cyproheptadine, pizotifen) probably act similarly to methysergide.

The proven effectiveness of **clonidine** and **propranolol** in migraine is rather mysterious. Clonidine is an agonist at α_2-adrenoceptors, used mainly for its hypotensive effect (see Chapter 7). It causes some peripheral vasoconstriction, probably by acting on α_2-receptors in vascular smooth muscle, which could underlie its effectiveness in migraine. Propranolol, a β-adrenoceptor antagonist, also causes peripheral vasoconstriction, and has, in addition, a weak serotonin-blocking effect, but whether these effects are really important, or whether an explanation based on them represents a mere clutching at pharmacological straws, remains to be seen.

Fig. 11.11 Effect of ergotamine in a patient suffering from migraine. The strong extracranial vasoconstrictor effect is seen to occur simultaneously with the relief of the headache. (From: Wolff, 1948; cited in Clark et al, 1978)

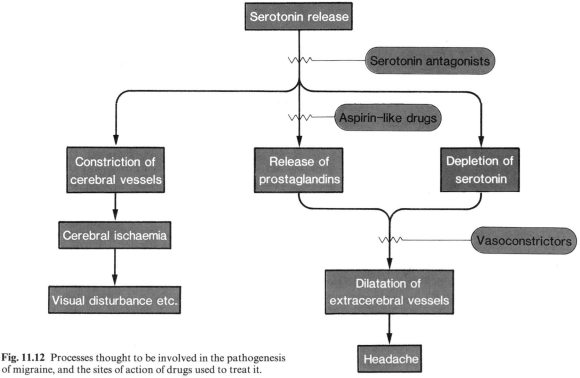

Fig. 11.12 Processes thought to be involved in the pathogenesis of migraine, and the sites of action of drugs used to treat it.

REFERENCES AND FURTHER READING

Amery W K, van Neuten J M, Wauquier A (eds) 1984 The pharmacological basis of migraine therapy. Pitman, London

Bell C 1982 Dopamine as a postganglionic autonomic neurotransmitter. Neuroscience 7: 1–8

Bolton T B 1979 Mechanisms of action of neurotransmitters and other substances on smooth muscle. Physiol Rev 59: 606–718

Burnstock G 1978 A basis for distinguishing two types of purinergic receptor. In: Straub R W, Bolis L (eds) Cell membrane receptors for drugs and hormones. Raven Press, New York

Burnstock G 1981 Purinergic receptors. Chapman & Hall, London

Burnstock G 1985 Purinergic mechanisms broaden their sphere of influence. Trends in Neurosciences 8: 5–6

Clark B 1981 Dopamine receptors and the cardiovascular system. Postgrad Med J 57 (suppl 1): 45–54

Clark B J, Chu D, Aellig W H 1978 In: Berde B, Schild H O (eds) Ergot alkaloids and related compounds. Springer, Berlin

Engel G, Gothert M, Muller-Schweinitzer E et al 1983 Evidence for common pharmacological properties of [^{3}H]5-hydroxytryptamine binding sites, presynaptic 5-hydroxytryptamine autoreceptors in CNS and inhibitory presynaptic 5-hydroxytryptamine receptors on sympathetic nerves. Naunyn Schmiedeberg's Arch Pharmacol 324: 116

Furchgott R F 1981 The requirement for endothelial cells in the relaxation of arteries by acetylcholine and some other vasodilators. Trends in Pharmacological Sciences 2: 173–176

Fozard J R 1982 Basic mechanisms of antimigraine drugs. Adv Neurol 33: 295–307

Fozard J R, Gittos M W 1983 Selective blockade of 5-hydroxytryptamine neuronal receptors by benzoic esters of tropine. Br J Pharmacol 80: 511P

Goldberg L I, Kohli J D 1983 Peripheral dopamine receptors: a classification based on potency series and specific antagonism. Trends in Pharmacological Sciences 4: 64–66

Jones A W 1981 In: Bulbring et al (eds) Smooth muscle. Edward Arnold, London

Kebabian J W, Calne D B 1979 Multiple receptors for dopamine. Nature 277: 93–96

Needleman P, Currie M G, Geller D M, Cole B R, Adams S P 1984 Atriopeptins: potential mediators of an endocrine relationship between heart and kidney. Trends in Pharmacological Sciences 5: 506–509

Peroutka S J, Snyder S H 1982 Recognition of multiple serotonin receptor binding sites. Adv Biochem Psychopharmacol 34: 155–172

Richardson B P, Engel G, Donatsch P, Stadler P A 1985 Identification of serotonin M-receptor subtypes and their specific blockade by a new class of drugs. Nature 316: 126–131

Satchell D 1984 Purine receptors: classification and properties. Trends in Pharmacological Sciences 5: 340–343

Straughan D W 1984 5HT; peripheral and central receptors and function. Trends in Pharmacological Sciences 5: 410–411

Thorner M O 1975 Dopamine is an important neurotransmitter in the autonomic nervous system. Lancet 1: 662

Vanhoutte P M (ed) 1983 Symposium on 5-hydroxytryptamine and the vascular system. Fed Proc 42: 211–237

Van Zweiten P A (ed) 1984 Pharmacology of antihypertensive drugs. Elsevier, Amsterdam

12

Haemostasis and thrombosis

Haemostasis is the arrest of blood loss from damaged blood vessels and is essential to life. It involves three main phenomena: (1) vascular contraction; (2) adhesion and activation of platelets; and (3) fibrin formation. The latter two processes result in the formation of a haemostatic plug which blocks the breach in the vessel and stops the bleeding and, as is explained below, the endothelium of blood vessels also participates. The role of each of the phenomena will depend on the size and the type of vessel (arterial, venous, capillary) which has been injured, but a general outline of their interactions is given in Figure 12.1.

Thrombosis is the unwanted formation of a haemostatic plug or thrombus within the blood vessels or heart. It is a pathological condition usually associated with arterial disease or stasis of blood in the veins or atria of the heart. A **thrombus**, which forms *in vivo*, should be distinguished from a **blood clot**, which can form in static blood *in vitro*. A clot is amorphous in character, consisting of a diffuse fibrin meshwork in which all the cells of the blood are trapped. By contrast, a thrombus has a distinct structure: (1) a white 'head', firm but friable, consisting mainly of platelets and leucocytes in a fibrin mesh; and (2) a jelly-like red 'tail' which is similar in composition to a blood clot.

An arterial thrombus, which is usually associated with **atherosclerosis**, consists largely of the platelet-leucocyte-fibrin head and the main result of its formation is the retardation or interruption of the blood flow, with ischaemia or actual death of the tissue beyond ('infarction'). A venous thrombus, which usually occurs in normal veins in which the blood flow is slowed, consists of a small head and a large tail which streams away in the direction of the flow. A portion of a thrombus may break away

forming an **embolus** which, if it comes from the peripheral veins, may lodge in the lungs, or, if it comes from the heart, may lodge in the brain. In either case, this blocks the blood vessels, causing damage of the tissues supplied. Drug therapy to alter haemostasis is rarely necessary, being required only when this essential phenomenon is defective, which is infrequent. Drug therapy to modify thrombo-embolic diseases, on the other hand, is extensively used because these diseases are very common, being the major cause of death in the developed countries. Drugs may affect haemostasis and thrombosis in three distinct ways: (1) by modifying blood coagulation (fibrin formation); (2) by modifying platelet adhesion and activation; and (3) by affecting the processes involved in fibrin removal (fibrinolysis).

BLOOD COAGULATION

Blood coagulation means the conversion of fluid blood to a solid gel or clot. The main event is the conversion of soluble fibrinogen to insoluble strands of fibrin, although fibrin itself forms only 0.15% of the total blood clot. This conversion is the last step in a complex enzyme cascade. The components (**factors**) are present as **zymogens**, inactive precursors of proteolytic enzymes, which are converted into active enzymes by proteolytic cleavage at specific sites. Activation of a small amount of one factor catalyses the formation of larger amounts of the next factor which catalyses the formation of still larger amounts of the next, and so on, giving an amplication which results in an extremely rapid formation of fibrin.

There are two main pathways to fibrin formation, termed *intrinsic* (because all the components are

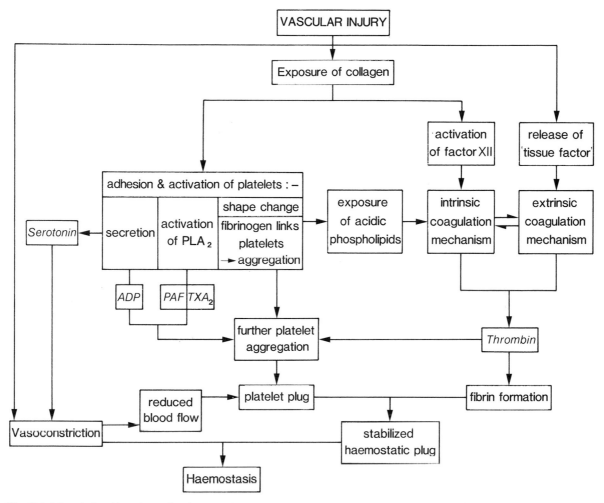

Fig. 12.1 Interrelationships of vascular changes, platelet activities and the coagulation mechanisms in haemostasis after vascular injury. (Modified from: Ogston, 1983)

present in the blood) and *extrinsic* (because some components come from outside the blood), though there are extensive interactions between the factors in each pathway. The cascade is outlined in Figure 12.2.

The **intrinsic pathway** commences when the first zymogen, factor XII or 'Hageman Factor', adheres to a negatively charged surface and in the presence of high molecular weight kininogen and prekallikrein (see Chapter 8), becomes an active enzyme, designated XIIa. The activating surface may be collagen which is exposed by tissue injury. Factor XIIa activates factor XI to give XIa, factor XIa activates factor IX to IXa and this, in the presence

of calcium ions, a negatively charged phospholipid surface and factor VIIIa, activates factor X. The negatively charged phospholipid surface is provided by platelets and *in vivo* this serves to localize the process of coagulation to sites of platelet deposition (see below). Factor Xa, in the presence of calcium ions, a platelet-derived negatively charged phospholipid surface and a binding protein, factor V, activates prothrombin to give thrombin (IIa)—the main enzyme of the cascade. Thrombin, acting on gly–arg bonds, removes small fibrinopeptides from the N-terminal regions of the large dimeric fibrinogen molecules, enabling them to polymerize to form strands of fibrin. Thrombin also activates the *fibrin*

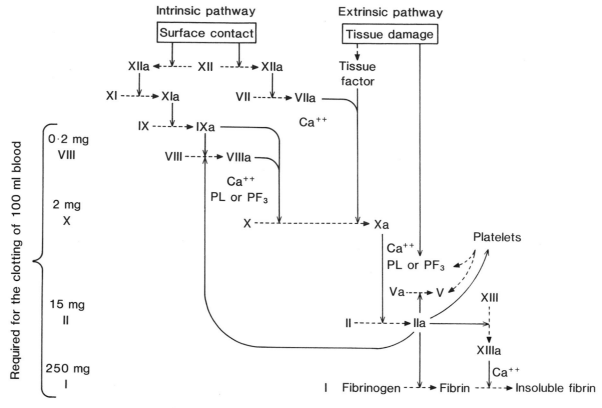

Fig. 12.2 The blood coagulation cascade: PL = a negatively charged phospholipid; PF$_3$ = platelet factor; ⟶ = 'acts on'; ------→ = 'transforms to' or 'gives rise to'.

stabilizing factor, factor XIII, to give XIIIa, a fibrinoligase, which, in the presence of calcium ions strengthens the fibrin-to-fibrin links with intermolecular γ-glutamyl-ξ-lysine bridges. In addition, thrombin acts directly on platelets to cause aggregation and release of subcellular constituents and arachidonic acid (see below). A further function of thrombin is to activate the coagulation inhibitor, protein C (see below). Factors XIIa, XIa, IXa, Xa, and thrombin are all serine proteases.

The **extrinsic pathway** is initiated by a substance generated by tissue damage and termed 'tissue factor', interacting with Factor VII in the presence of calcium ions and phospholipid to activate factor X, after which the sequence proceeds as already described. The precise nature of 'tissue factor' is not known but it is believed to consist of a lipoprotein complex in which the protein portion has peptidase activity when associated with phospholipid. There is evidence that tissue factor occurs in the plasma

membranes of the endothelial cells of blood vessels and also in atheromatous plaques.

The two pathways described are not entirely separate, because both factor IXa and factor XIIa in the intrinsic pathway may activate factor VII in the extrinsic pathway. There are, in addition, various feedback loops between other factors, which enhance reaction rates. For example, thrombin (IIa) enhances the activation of both factor V and factor VIII.

The acidic phospholipids mentioned above are important as **surface catalysts** and are provided by platelets and by damaged tissue. Circulating platelets do not have this procoagulant activity (which is termed 'platelet factor 3'). However, when they are aggregated and activated, the acidic phospholipids (phosphatidyl inositol, phosphatidic acid and, more importantly, phosphatidylserine) which are normally on the cytoplasmic side of the plasma membrane are transposed to the outer surface and provide this procoagulant activity, i.e. a surface which facilitates the localized activation and interaction of the clotting factors. (A possible biochemical basis for a similar transposition is described in Chapter 1.) Platelets also provide some of the factor V which is important in binding, localizing and accelerating the action of factor Xa (see below).

Fibrinogen is not only a principal component in the coagulation pathway—it is a key component in platelet aggregation and some fibrinogen is actually derived from platelets (see below).

As might be expected, this accelerating enzyme cascade has to be controlled and balanced by a series of inhibitors in the plasma. If it were not, all the blood in the body would solidify within minutes of the initiation of clotting. One of the most important inhibitors is an α_2 globulin, **antithrombin III**, which neutralizes not only thrombin, but all the serine proteases in the cascade—X, IX, XI, XII. The endothelium of blood vessels releases **heparan sulphate** and possibly also **heparin**, both co-factors for antithrombin III, (see below). Other inhibitors which play a part are α_2 **macroglobulin** and α_1 **antitrypsin**. One of the inhibitors of the complement cascade (see Chapter 8), **C1 inactivator**, also inhibits some of the coagulation factors, and there are, in addition, inhibitors of XIa and Xa.

An additional system which prevents unwanted coagulation involves '**protein C**', a vitamin K dependent zymogen in the plasma, which is transformed to a serine protease by thrombin acting with a co-factor on the surface of endothelial cells (**thrombomodulin**). Activated protein C inhibits coagulation and stimulates fibrinolysis and plays a pivotal role in the co-ordination of the two phenomena. This protein, which like other vitamin K-dependent factors requires γ-carboxy-glutamic acid and calcium for its activity (see below), inactivates factors Va and VIIIa.

Drugs are used to modify the cascade either when there is a *defect in coagulation* or when there is *unwanted coagulation*.

COAGULATION DEFECTS

Genetically determined deficiencies of clotting factors are relatively rare. Examples are **classical** **haemophilia** which is due to a lack of factor VIII, and an even rarer form of haemophilia which is due to a lack of factor IX (also called Christmas factor). Missing factors can be supplied by giving fresh blood or plasma. Factor VIII is also available as a cryoprecipitate or as a freeze-dried protein concentrate made from plasma. It is possible that factor VIII might eventually be produced in bulk by genetic engineering techniques, which would eliminate the risk of transmitting hepatitis or the acquired immune deficiency syndrome (AIDS) by transfusing blood or plasma.

Acquired clotting defects are more common than the hereditary ones and those most frequently seen are due to **liver disease**, **vitamin K deficiency** or the ingestion of **oral anticoagulant drugs**. Most require treatment with vitamin K—so termed because it is the 'Koagulation' vitamin in German.

Vitamin K

This is a fat-soluble vitamin occurring in nature in two forms—as vitamin K_1 (**phytomenadione**, Fig. 12.3) in plants, and as vitamin K_2 which is synthesized by bacteria in the mammalian gastrointestinal tract. Vitamin K_2 is not a single compound but a series of substance with varying lengths of side chains at C_3 on the napthoquinone ring ('R' in Fig. 12.3A).

Vitamin K is critically important in the synthesis of clotting factors II, VII, IX and X. These factors are all glycoproteins with a number of γ-**carboxyglutamic acid** (Gla) residues clustered at the N-terminal end of the peptide chain. The γ-carboxylation occurs after the synthesis of the chain and is dependent on vitamin K. The role of the vitamin can be made clear by considering the interaction of two of the clotting factors—Xa and prothrombin (factor II). *In vitro* studies show that factor Xa, on its own, is able to convert prothrombin to thrombin, but it does so exceedingly slowly. In the presence of a negatively charged phospholipid surface, calcium ions, and the regulatory protein, factor V, the reaction is localized to the phospholipid surface and its rate is increased about 19 000-fold. The complex of factor Va and the phospholipid surface can be regarded as acting as a receptor of high affinity for factor Xa. Both components of the complex may be supplied *in vivo* by platelets, though

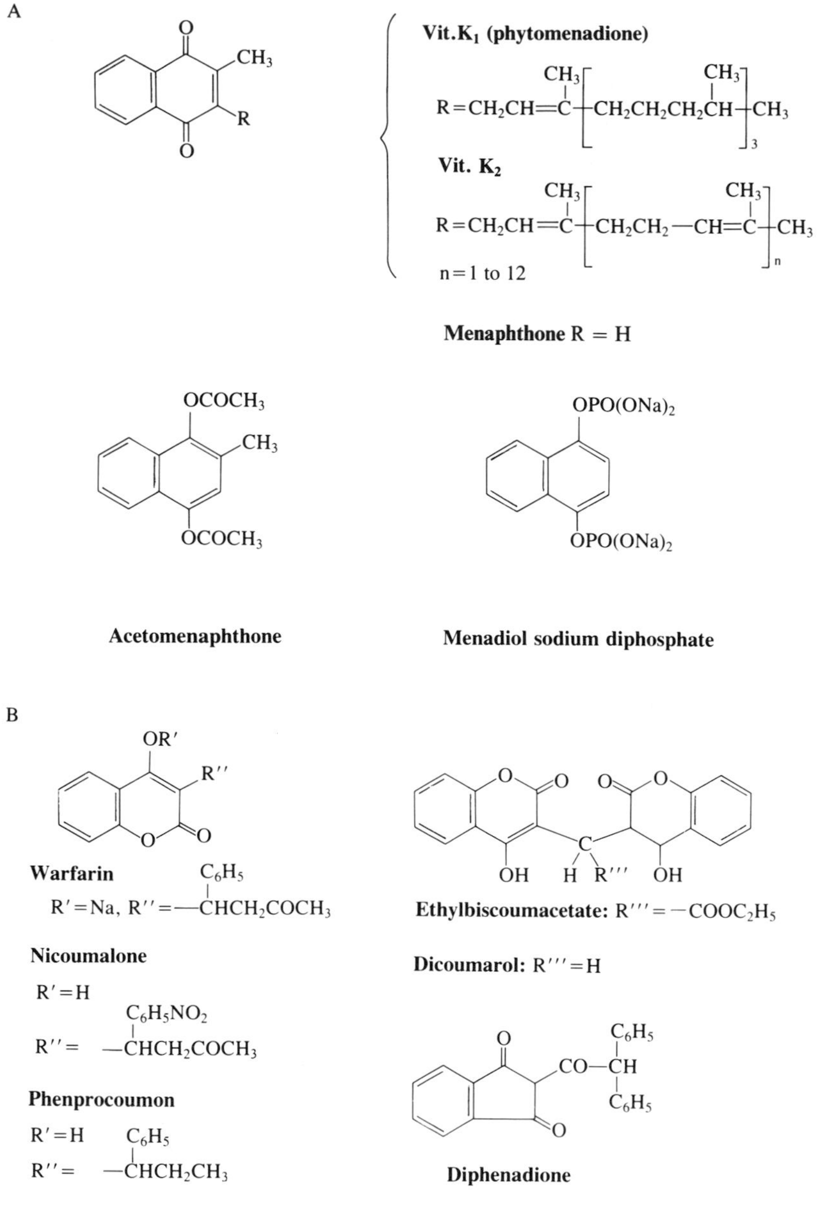

A

Vit.K₁ (phytomenadione)

$R = CH_2CH = C \left[-CH_2CH_2CH_2CH \right]_3 CH_3$

Vit. K₂

$R = CH_2CH = C \left[-CH_2CH_2 -CH = C \right]_n CH_3$

n = 1 to 12

Menaphthone R = H

Acetomenaphthone

Menadiol sodium diphosphate

B

Warfarin
R' = Na, R'' = —CHCH₂COCH₃ C₆H₅

Nicoumalone
R' = H
R'' = —CHCH₂COCH₃ C₆H₅NO₂

Phenprocoumon
R' = H
R'' = —CHCH₂CH₃ C₆H₅

Ethylbiscoumacetate: R''' = —COOC₂H₅

Dicoumarol: R''' = H

Diphenadione

Fig. 12.3 A. Vitamin K and its congeners. B. Vitamin K antagonists: the oral anticoagulant drugs.

some factor V is present in the plasma. Calcium is necessary for the binding of factors Xa and II to the phospholipid, probably acting mainly by bridging, and this binding does not occur unless the 10 or 11 glutamic acid residues clustered at the N-terminal ends of both factors II and Xa have been carboxylated (Fig. 12.4). Vitamin K in the reduced form is

an essential co-factor in the carboxylation of these residues (Fig. 12.5).

Administration and pharmacokinetic aspects

Natural vitamin K, (phytomenadione) may be given orally or by intramuscular or intravenous injection.

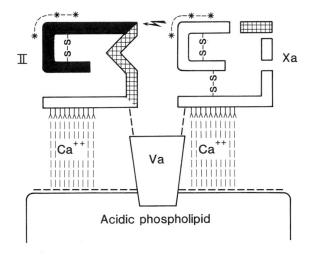

Fig. 12.4 The activation of prothrombin (factor II). The peptide chains of both factors are very similar and are indicated schematically. The complex of factor Va with a negatively charged phospholipid surface (both supplied by aggregated platelets) forms a binding site for factor X and prothrombin. Calcium ions are essential for the binding of these factors. When X is activated, with the removal of an activation peptide, it activates prothrombin, again with the removal of an activation peptide, liberating enzymic thrombin (shown in black). Factor Xa is held at the surface by intrachain sulfhydryl bonds, but thrombin is released. Factor V has to be converted from a non-functional to a functional binding protein (Va)—possibly by thrombin, which is thus autocatalytic.

The enzymic sites are indicated by asterisks, activation peptides by cross-hatching, γ-carboxy glutamic acid residues by inverted Ys and site of cleavage of II by Xa with an arrow. (Modified from: Jackson, 1978)

If given by mouth it requires bile salts for absorption, and this occurs by a saturable energy-requiring process in the top part of the small intestine. Synthetic preparations (see Fig. 12.3A) are also available; some are fat-soluble (**acetomenaphthone**, **menaphthone**); some are water-soluble (**menadiol sodium diphosphate**) and thus do not require bile salts for their absorption. These synthetic compounds take longer to act than phytomenadione.

There is very little storage of vitamin K in the body. It is metabolized to more polar substances which are excreted in the urine and the bile.

Uses

The most important use of vitamin K and its analogues is in the treatment of **bleeding caused by the oral anticoagulants** (see below). It is also used in the syndrome termed '**hypoprothrombinaemia**' seen

frequently in the newborn, in whom the intestinal flora are not established, and in whom consequently there may be inadequate synthesis of vitamin K_2 and thus inadequate clotting capacity. Other reasons for vitamin K deficiency are malabsorption (e.g. associated with sprue, coeliac disease, steatorrhoea, extensive resection of small intestine etc) or a lack of bile (associated with obstructive jaundice, biliary fistulae).

UNWANTED COAGULATION

This occurs mainly in thrombo-embolic diseases, which are very common. The drugs used to modify unwanted coagulation are oral anticoagulants (**warfarin** and related compounds) and injectable anticoagulants (**heparin**, **ancrod**).

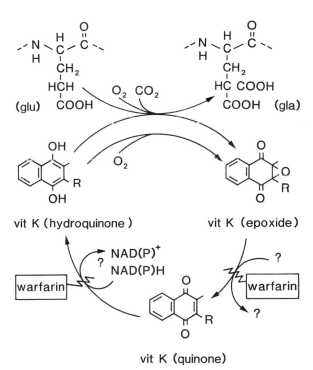

Fig. 12.5 The probable mechanism of action of vitamin K. After the peptide chains have been synthesized, reduced vitamin K, the hydroquinone, acts as a co-factor in the conversion of glutamic acid (glu) to γ-carboxyglutamic acid (gla). During this reaction the reduced form of vitamin K is converted to the epoxide, which in turn is reduced to the quinone and then the hydroquinone. These latter reactions are inhibited by oral anticoagulants. (The physiological reductants for these reactions are not known.)

ORAL ANTICOAGULANTS

This group of drugs became available as an indirect result of a change in agricultural policy in Canada in the 1920s. Sweet clover was substituted for corn in cattle-feed, and soon afterwards an excessive tendency to bleed after minor injury was noticed in animals so fed. This turned out to be due to the presence of **bishydroxycoumarin** in spoiled sweet clover. Congeners of this and related compounds are now used in clinical medicine. **Warfarin** is the most important of these; others are given in Table 12.1. They all act in essentially the same way, differing only in their pharmacokinetic properties and their side effects.

tially), then IX, X and II with half-lives of 24, 40 and 60 hours respectively.

Administration and pharmacokinetic aspects

Warfarin is given orally and is absorbed quickly and totally from the gastrointestinal tract. It has a very small distribution volume, being strongly bound to plasma albumin (see Chapter 3). The peak concentration in the blood occurs within an hour of ingestion, but because of the mechanism of action this does not coincide with the peak pharmacological effect, which occurs 36–48 hours later. The effect does not begin to appear for 12–16 hours, and lasts 4–5 days. The drugs are metabolized by the mixed

Table 12.1 Comparison of some oral anticoagulant drugs

Drug	Duration of action	Half-life	Comment
Warfarin	2–6 days	40 hours	Complete absorption from GIT. The most widely used oral anticoagulant.
Ethylbiscoumacetate	2 days	3 hours	Completely absorbed from the GIT.
Nicoumalone	22 hours	8 hours for drug. Metabolites also active	Some GIT irritation. Dermatitis and urticaria have been reported.
Dicoumarol	Approx. 35 hours	Varies with dose	Slowly and incompletely absorbed from GIT. Mild GIT side effects frequent.
Phenprocoumon	6–10 days	6 days	GIT side effects and dermatitis reported.
Diphenadione	6–21 days	2–3 weeks	Mild gastrointestinal side effects.

Mechanism of action

These drugs interfere with the post-translational γ-carboxylation of glutamic acid residues in clotting factors II, VII, IX, and X (see Fig. 12.5). They do this by **preventing the reduction of vitamin K** which is necessary for its action as a co-factor of the carboxylase. They will therefore act only *in vivo* and will not, of course, have any effect on the clotting of shed blood. Their structural similarity to vitamin K and its analogues is illustrated in Figure 12.3B.

The effect of these drugs on fibrin formation takes several hours to develop because it depends on the balance between the decreased rate of carboxylation and the unaltered rate of degradation of factors already carboxylated. The onset of action of these drugs will thus depend primarily on the half-lives of the relevant factors. Factor VII, with half-life of 6 hours, is affected first (though this does not necessarily influence coagulation very substan-

function oxidases in the liver and the half-life of warfarin is 40 hours.

Oral anticoagulants cross the placenta and they also appear in the milk during lactation. This could be important because the newborn infant is already at risk as a result of inadequate synthesis of vitamin K in the bowel.

The therapeutic use of the oral anticoagulants, particularly if long-continued, requires a careful balance between giving too little, which could leave unwanted coagulation unmodified, and too much, which could lead to haemorrhage. Therapy is complicated not only by the circumstance that the effect of a particular dose is only seen 2 days after giving it, but by the fact that there are numerous conditions which modify the drug's activity (see below), including a number of interactions with other drugs (see Chapter 4).

The action of an oral anticoagulant should be

monitored by its effect on the **prothrombin time**, which is the time taken for the clotting of oxalated plasma to which has been added calcium and standardized reference thromboplastin. The results are reported as a ratio of the patient's prothrombin time to that of a control, and dosage is normally adjusted to give a ratio of between 2 and 4 to 1.

Factors increasing the pharmacological effect of the oral anticoagulants

A decreased availability of vitamin K will obviously exacerbate the action of these drugs. Thus a diet with too little vitamin K as well as various pathological conditions resulting in vitamin K deficiency (previously outlined), will have this effect. Broad spectrum antibiotics such as tetracyclines (p. 636) depress the intestinal flora which normally synthesize vitamin K_2, but this does not have much effect unless there is a concurrent dietary deficiency of the vitamin.

Some pathological conditions, such as liver disease, affect anticoagulant therapy by interfering with the synthesis of the clotting factors. Others increase the effect of the drugs by increasing the rate of degradation of the clotting factors; these include conditions in which there is a high metabolic rate such as fever and thyrotoxicosis.

Many drugs interact with the oral anticoagulants and increase their effect.

1. *Agents which impair platelet aggregation and platelet function* (such as **aspirin** and other non-steroid anti-inflammatory drugs) may cause serious bleeding if given during anticoagulant therapy. They not only prevent the contribution of the platelets to fibrin formation but also inhibit the formation of the crucial plug of aggregated platelets which is the primary event in haemostasis.
2. *Agents which displace the oral anticoagulants from their binding sites* on albumin result in an increase in their concentration in the plasma and an enhanced antiprothrombinaemic effect. Such agents include non-steroidal anti-inflammatory drugs (e.g. **phenylbutazone**), **chloral hydrate** and **ethacrynic acid**.
3. *Agents which inhibit the microsomal enzymes in the liver*, retard the metabolism of the oral anti-

coagulants and result in their attaining higher plasma concentrations and having a longer half-life. Examples include **disulfiram**, **salicylates**, **chloramphenicol**, **imipramine**, **metronidazole**, **cimetidine**.

In addition, various agents may potentiate the action of the anticoagulants by as yet unknown means.

Factors decreasing the pharmacological effect of the oral anticoagulants

There is a decreased response to these drugs during pregnancy (possibly due to the increased concentration of factors VII, VIII and X) and also in some pathological conditions such as the nephrotic syndrome and anaemia.

Drugs which cause induction of the microsomal enzymes in the liver (e.g. **barbiturates**, **glutethimide**) result in increased metabolic degradation of the oral anticoagulants. Some agents, such as **oral contraceptives** decrease the hypoprothrombinaemic effect by mechanisms not yet fully elucidated. (Oral contraceptives with a high oestrogen content may alter the balance of the blood towards hypercoagulability even in the absence of oral anticoagulants. This effect is ascribed to either an increase in the concentration of clotting factors or a reduction in the level of antithrombin III.)

Unwanted effects. Haemorrhage (especially into the bowel), is the only hazard of any importance, and the treatment is administration of vitamin K.

INJECTABLE ANTICOAGULANTS

Heparin

This drug was discovered in 1916 by a second year medical student at Johns Hopkins University. During a vacation project in which he was attempting to extract thromboplastic substances from various tissues, he found powerful anticoagulant activity. Further work made it clear that this was due to the presence of a mucopolysaccharide which was named **heparin** because it was believed to be most abundant in liver.

Strictly speaking 'heparin' is not a single substance but a family of sulphated glycosaminoglycans (mucopolysaccharides) with a range of molecular

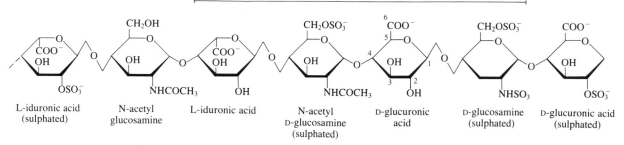

Fig. 12.6 One of the many possible arrangements of the hexosamine and uronic acid residues in the heparin polymer. The tetrasaccharide sequence which is believed to form the binding site for anti-thrombin III is indicated by a bar. The numbering of the carbon atoms is given for D-glucuronic acid.

weights from 4000 to 30 000. The molecules are attached to a protein backbone which, unusually, consists entirely of serine and glycine residues.

The glycosaminoglycan is synthesized as an alternating copolymer of N-acetylglucosamine and glucuronic acid. After synthesis, some of the glucosamine residues are deacylated and N-sulphated, and some are ester-sulphated at C_6. Most glucuronic acid residues are converted to iduronic acid and some of these are ester-sulphated at position 2. A representative portion of a heparin molecule is shown in Figure 12.6. It is important to realize that there is great variability amongst heparin molecules.

In the tissues, heparin is found in **mast cells** (in the form of large polymers of MW 750 000). It is also present in the plasma at about 1.5 mg per litre and in the endothelial cell layer of blood vessels (see below). For clinical use it is extracted from beef lung or hog intestinal mucosa and, since different preparations may differ in potency, it has to be biologically assayed against an agreed international standard.

A related glycosaminoglycan, **heparan sulphate**, occurs extracellularly in many tissues. It differs from heparin in the amino acid composition of its protein backbone and in the relative proportions of iduronic and glucuronic acid. This substance is, like heparin, a co-factor for antithrombin III (see below) and is physiologically important as an anticoagulant, particularly on the endothelium of the microcirculation. It is not used clinically.

Mechanism of action

Heparin inhibits blood clotting both *in vivo* and *in vitro*, its main action being on **fibrin formation**. It also decreases platelet aggregation, but this may be secondary to its effect on thrombin which is a powerful platelet aggregating agent. In addition it has an action which is unrelated to blood coagulation in that it releases lipoprotein lipases from various tissues into the plasma.

Heparin is strongly acidic and its anticoagulant activity is related to its electro-negative charge. Its main mechanism of action is through an effect on **antithrombin III**, which is the naturally occurring inhibitor of thrombin and the other serine proteases in the coagulation cascade, namely XIIa, XIa, IXa and Xa. Antithrombin III forms a 1:1 stoichiometric complex with thrombin in which there is an interaction between the active serine site on the enzyme and the reactive arginine site on the inhibitor. Heparin modifies this interaction by binding to the positively charged lysine in antithrombin III and accelerating the rate of action of this inhibitor so that its effect is virtually instantaneous. The basis of this action is probably that heparin produces a change in the conformation of antithrombin III which renders its active site arginine more accessible. (Some experimental results suggest that in the case of thrombin it may be necessary for heparin to bind to the enzyme as well as to antithrombin III.) After the interaction the serine enzyme and antithrombin III are rendered inactive, but heparin is released from the complex to act on other antithrombin III molecules.

The antithrombin III binding sites in heparin form only a small proportion of the heparin polymer. A particular tetrasaccharide sequence (L-iduronic acid—N-acetylated D-glucosamine 6 sulphate—

D-glucuronic acid—N-sulphated-D-glucosamine 6 sulphate) is critical, though there is also evidence that a longer sequence, an octasaccharide containing the above tetrasaccharide, may be necessary for binding. The critical tetrasaccharide is shown as part of the heparin molecule in Figure 12.6. In terms of the overall anticoagulant action, heparin molecules with a high molecular weight are more effective than those with lower molecular weights, possibly because the probability of the occurrence of the critical sequence is increased. There are also suggestions that within the population of heparin molecules there may be sub-populations which function at different levels of the blood coagulation cascade.

With long-continued heparin therapy there is a depletion of antithrombin III and this decreases the effect of subsequent heparin therapy.

Administration and pharmacokinetic aspects

Heparin is not absorbed from the gastrointestinal tract because of its charge and its large size, and therefore it is given intravenously or subcutaneously. Intramuscular injections are avoided because they result in haematoma formation. A technique still in the experimental stage is the administration of heparin by aerosol inhalation, which is said to give a constant low blood concentration for 14 days after a single application.

The onset of action of heparin is immediate and its half-life is 40–90 minutes. Some may be taken up by endothelial cells in the vessels and this fraction forms a pool from which it may later be released. It is mainly destroyed by heparinase in the liver; though it is possible that a protein released from activated platelets, *platelet factor IV*, which has the capacity to neutralize heparin, may play a part in the inactivation. The amount of this platelet factor is increased in patients with arteriosclerosis.

The effects of heparin can be monitored by testing the whole blood clotting time or the thrombin time,* which should be increased by a factor of 2 to 3.

---

* The 'thrombin time' is the time taken for plasma to clot after the addition of a solution of thrombin. The normal value is about 15 seconds.

Unwanted effects

The main hazard is **haemorrhage** which is treated by stopping therapy and, if necessary, giving a heparin antagonist, **protamine sulphate**. This substance, a strongly basic protein which forms an inactive complex with heparin, is given intravenously as a 1% solution.

A toxic effect reported with long-term treatment, of 6 months or more, is osteoporosis with resultant spontaneous fractures. The reason for this is not known.

As with many drugs, hypersensitivity reactions to heparin may occur in some patients and have also been reported to occur with protamine. A heparin-associated decrease in platelet numbers occurs within 24–36 hours in about 30% of patients. This thrombocytopoenia, which is caused by heparin-induced platelet aggregation, is usually transitory and is not clinically important. In a few cases, however, a profound decrease in platelet numbers occurs 2–14 days after the start of therapy and this may be associated with serious complications, thrombo-embolic as well as haemorrhagic. It is suggested that in these cases, antibodies against a heparin-platelet complex are formed and that these promote aggregation of platelets and the platelet release reaction (see below).

Ancrod

This is a proteolytic enzyme prepared from snake venom. Given intravenously it acts directly on fibrinogen to produce an unstable form of fibrin. This fibrin forms microemboli which are cleared from the blood—possible by the mononuclear phagocyte system—resulting in a depletion of fibrinogen. Ancrod may be used for the same conditions as heparin (see below).

PLATELET ADHESION AND ACTIVATION

Platelets, though non-nucleated and thus, strictly speaking, not entitled to be classified as cells, are capable of a complex variety of reactions. They are essential for haemostasis, important for the healing of damaged blood vessels and play an as yet ill-understood part in inflammation. A low platelet count results in **thrombocytopenic purpura** in which there may be spontaneous bleeding into the skin and other tissues. In this condition the bleeding time is increased but the blood clotting time *in vitro* is normal.*

Platelets have a principal role in the arterial thrombo-embolic diseases which are responsible for a high proportion of deaths from disease in the developed nations. The aetiology and pathogenesis of these conditions is not fully understood and there are as yet no satisfactory anti-platelet agents for their treatment. However, because the development of suitable anti-platelet drugs will depend on further understanding of platelet function and because of the potential future importance of this area, the complex reactions in which the platelets are involved are considered here in some detail.

Platelets or thrombocytes are small non-nucleated disc-shaped bodies derived from megakaryocytes in the bone marrow and present in the blood at a concentration of 150 000 to 400 000 per μl. They are about 0.8 microns in depth and 2.3 microns in diameter and they contain mitochondria, a complex system of tubules, and three sorts of granules— dense granules, alpha granules and lysosomes (see Table 12.2). The plasma membrane has an external coat consisting of protein and glycosaminoglycans (mucopolysaccharides).

Table 12.2 Contents of platelet granules

Alpha granules	Dense granules
Fibrinogen	Serotonin
Factor V	ADP
Platelet factor 4	ATP
Fibronectin†	Calcium pyrophosphate
Thrombospondin	
Factor VIII: vWF	
Albumin	
β-thromboglobulin*	
Platelet-derived-growth factors	

* Biological function unknown
† Glycoprotein of high molecular weight, present on the surface of many cells, is present on platelet surface after activation; may be involved in platelet aggregation
vWF   von Willebrand's factor

* The 'bleeding time', which is normally about 4 minutes, is measured by timing the duration of bleeding from a standard small puncture wound in the skin—the blood being blotted up every 15 seconds.

There is a close inter-relationship between the platelets and the clotting factors, several of which are adsorbed on to the platelet's surface. Factor V in particular is very closely associated with the platelet, and some of this substance may actually be sequestered within it. The platelet plasma membrane contains high affinity sites for factor Va, each site forming part of the 'receptor' for factor X, as described above. Platelets are also reported to contain intrinsic factor XI activity, thus rendering the initiation of clotting possible in the absence of factor XII. Some fibrinogen is stored in the alpha granules.

In a normal undamaged vessel the endothelium plays an active part in the prevention of thrombus formation. It generates and releases not only prostacyclin (see below), plasminogen activator (see below), heparin and heparan sulphate (see above), but also thrombomodulin, a co-factor involved in the activation of the coagulation inhibitor, protein C (p. 283).

When a vessel is cut or injured the endothelium is damaged and the subendothelial tissue is exposed. The damaged endothelium develops tissue factor activity and can bind and activate factors IX, X and V. It thus contributes to haemostasis by promoting blood coagulation and will also play a part in thrombosis. Platelets, which have a strong affinity for collagen, **adhere** within seconds to the subendothelial tissue in the damaged area and become '**activated**'. Activation of platelets involves firstly **shape change**, and then **aggregation**, **secretion** of agents stored in granules and **release of mediators** such as thromboxane A_2. Platelet adhesion to the subendothelial tissue is enhanced by, and may in fact require the presence of, a complex of factor VIII with a component called **von Willebrands factor**—a large glycoprotein of 10^6 daltons (which is missing in von Willebrands disease, a hereditary haemorrhagic disorder). Von Willebrands factor is synthesized by vascular endothelial cells and is also present in platelets. As the platelet adheres, it changes in shape from a disc to a sphere with long pseudopods, and other platelets aggregate to it. The aggregation is accompanied by the secretion of a variety of biologically active substances, some from storage granules, some synthesized *de novo*. This process is referred to as the 'the platelet release reaction' and calcium is a second messenger in

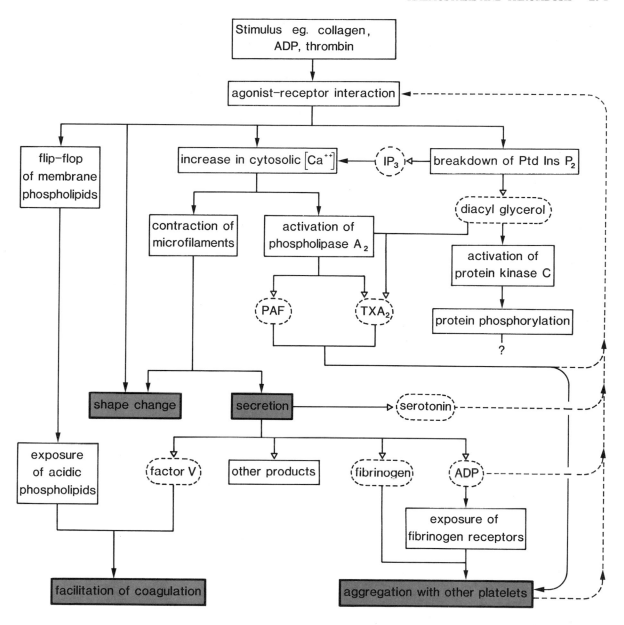

Fig. 12.7 Schematic diagram of events involved in platelet activation. The important events are shape change, the release reaction (secretion of granule constituents and the release of newly formed substances) and aggregation with other platelets. In haemostasis *in vivo*, platelet activation follows adhesion of the platelet to collagen, but platelets can be activated *in vitro* by many agents: thrombin, ADP, thromboxane A_2 (TXA$_2$), platelet-activating factor (PAF) and serotonin, some of which may *in vivo* be involved in autocatalytic feedback events (shown in dashed lines).

The initial loose aggregation of platelets involves cell-to-cell links by fibrinogen, some receptors for which may possibly be exposed as a direct result of agonist-receptor interaction at the membrane. The links formed are subsequently reinforced by thrombospondin, which is also released (not shown).

The role of protein kinase C is not yet understood, although it is known that it can phosphorylate myosin light chain and may thus be involved in the control of microfilaments. Breakdown of phosphotidyl inositol biphosphate (Ptd Ins P_2) may cause influx of calcium (see Chapter 1). IP$_3$ = inositol trisphosphate. Arrow with open head = 'gives rise to'; arrow with solid head = 'causes' or 'acts on'. (This figure is included because of the importance of platelets in arterial thrombosis and the potential future importance of antiplatelet drugs.) (Modified from: Ogston 1983)

this response. *In vitro* studies show that the first event in the transduction mechanism is activation of phospholipase C and stimulation of the turnover of the inositol phospholipids with generation of diacylglycerol which activates protein kinase C (p. 23). This follows very mild stimuli which result only in shape change. A stronger stimulus leads to aggregation which is associated with phospholipase A_2 activation and the production of arachidonate and its metabolites. Calcium is released initially from intracellular sources (probably the endoplasmic reticulum) by inositol trisphosphate, and may also enter the platelet from the plasma. In platelets, in contrast to many other cell types, an increase in cAMP is inhibitory (see Chapter 2). Two of the substances produced during the release reaction, ADP, (which is derived from the dense granules) and thromboxane A_2 (a product of arachidonate metabolism synthesized *de novo* as a result of phospholipase A_2 activation) are powerful promoters of platelet aggregation. Some ADP may be released from damaged cells in the vessel and be instrumental in initiating adhesion, and there is evidence that ADP released from red cells may be important in platelet activation. An outline of some of the events involved in platelet activation is given in Figure 12.7.

Other substances released from the platelets are serotonin, ATP, platelet-activating factor (see Chapter 8), factors which increase vascular permeability, factors chemotactic for white blood cells, and platelet-derived growth factors which can cause proliferation of fibroblasts, of vascular endothelial cells and of vascular smooth muscle cells. Platelets also release the heparin inhibitor (platelet factor 4) mentioned above, as well as lysosomal enzymes, fibronectin, fibrinogen and thrombospondin (a high molecular weight heparin-binding glucoprotein).

Fibrinogen is essential for platelet aggregation and it has been shown that on stimulation with ADP, fibrinogen receptors are exposed on the platelet surface. The primary, loose, reversible aggregation is due to fibrinogen-mediated platelet-to-platelet links. The secondary, irreversible aggregation probably involves reinforcement of these links by thrombospondin. Platelet-activating factors and serotonin stimulate further aggregation.

The mass of aggregated platelets forms a plug which, together with vessel constriction, maintains haemostasis in small vessels until the platelet plug is reinforced by fibrin (see Fig. 12.1). The fibrin formation is associated with the negatively-charged phospholipids which become available on the surface of activated platelets by the 'flip-flop' mechanism previously described. These act as part of the binding site for interacting coagulation factors, facilitating the localized formation of thrombin and thus fibrin (see Fig. 12.4). Thrombin, like ADP and thromboxane A_2, has a powerful action in activating and aggregating platelets. It increases the release reaction and consolidates the platelet plug, rendering the aggregation irreversible. It can be seen that many of the responses of the platelet are autocatalytic.

PLATELETS AND ARACHIDONATE METABOLITES

The arachidonate metabolites seem to have a special role in the regulation of platelet interactions with blood vessels. In the *platelets*, arachidonic acid, which is derived from phospholipid by the action of phospholipases, is metabolized by cyclo-oxygenase to give two cyclic endoperoxides—prostaglandins G_2 and H_2 (see Fig. 8.9). PGG_2 and PGH_2 are in turn acted on by platelet thromboxane synthetase to give **thromboxane A_2**, which, in addition to being a potent platelet aggregating agent, is a vasoconstrictor. TXA_2 has a half-life of 2 minutes. In *blood vessels* on the other hand, the main product of arachidonate metabolism is **prostacyclin (PGI_2)** which is generated enzymatically from PGH_2. Prostacyclin *inhibits* platelet adhesion and aggregation; it can also disaggregate platelet clumps. It has a half-life of 2–3 minutes and is a powerful vasodilator. Thus the cyclic endoperoxides derived from arachidonic acid are precursors for two substances with completely opposite actions—thromboxane A_2 and prostacyclin. The enzymes which generate these two substances may be inhibited in experimental situations—prostacyclin synthetase by lipid peroxides such as **15-hydroperoxyarachidonic acid** and thromboxane synthetase by **imidazole** compounds.

Prostacyclin produces its inhibitory effect on platelet aggregation by stimulating adenylate cyclase and increasing cyclic AMP production. Thromboxane A_2 has the opposite effect and may act mainly by releasing ADP.

The generation of prostacyclin by normal vascular endothelium could serve to limit the platelet plug to areas where the endothelium has been lost. There is evidence that prostacyclin synthetase is abundant in the intima of blood vessels and the concentration decreases progressively from intima to adventitia. Vascular endothelial cells can synthesize prostacyclin not only from their own endogenous precursors but also from the PGH_2 released by platelets, which may be in close association with the vascular endothelium. The concentrations of prostacyclin needed to prevent aggregation are lower than those required to prevent adhesion, so monolayers of adherent platelets may form on the endothelium without clumping of aggregated platelets.

It is possible that, *in vivo*, platelet aggregability is regulated, at least in part, by a balance between thromboxane A_2 and prostacyclin, and that the alteration of this balance is a factor in the aetiology of atherosclerosis and thus of arterial thrombus formation. It is thought, for example, that atheromatous plaques produce lipid peroxides which inhibit prostacyclin synthetase.

ANTIPLATELET AGENTS

Several drugs are able to modify platelet reactions but their effectiveness in the therapy of thrombo-embolic diseases is not very clear.

Acetylsalicylic acid (aspirin; see Chapter 9) alters the balance between those prostanoids which promote and those which inhibit platelet aggregation. It inactivates cyclo-oxygenase by irreversibly acetylating its active enzymic site. This reduces both thromboxane A_2 synthesis in platelets and prostacyclin synthesis in vessel walls. Vascular endothelial cells, however, can synthesize new enzyme whereas platelets cannot. After administration of aspirin, thromboxane A_2 synthesis will not recover until the affected cohort of platelets is replaced, a process which is likely to take 7–10 days. Furthermore, inhibition of the cyclo-oxygenase of the vascular endothelium requires higher concentrations of aspirin than does platelet cyclo-oxygenase. Thus low doses of aspirin given intermittently should decrease the synthesis of thromboxane A_2 without drastically reducing prostacyclin synthesis; and indeed this has been shown to be the case with 3.5 mg/kg of aspirin given every 3 days to healthy volunteers. However, some studies have indicated that high-dose aspirin (over 1 g per day) may also have anti-thrombotic effects. Clinical trials with aspirin in coronary thrombosis are under way but have so far given equivocal results. Aspirin has been reported to be of benefit in reducing the incidence of postoperative venous thrombosis in men and of fatal pulmonary embolism in both sexes. Its antithrombotic action is said to be enhanced by concomitant administration of **dipyridamole** (see below). Specific inhibitors of thromboxane synthesis could possibly be more useful as antiplatelet drugs than cyclo-oxygenase inhibitors, although the fact that thromboxane A_2 is not the only platelet aggregating agent could limit the efficacy of such drugs.*

Epoprostenol (prostacyclin) is a potent inhibitor of platelet aggregation and is also able to disaggregate platelet clumps. It is now available for clinical use but, because of its very short half-life, its place in therapy may be limited to such applications as cardiac by-pass surgery and similar procedures. Stable analogues of prostacyclin could possibly be of great value in thrombo-embolic disease.

Dipyridamole is a vasodilator drug (see Chapter 11) which has been shown experimentally to inhibit platelet-induced thrombo-embolism in rabbits, to decrease adherence of ^{51}Cr-labelled platelets to exposed subendothelium and to decrease platelet aggregation *in vitro*. It acts by inhibiting platelet phosphodiesterase and increasing cAMP and will thus synergise with prostacyclin. Dipyridamole may require the presence of endogeneous prostacyclin for its activity.

A combination of acetylsalicylic acid and dipyridamole seems to offer an effective pharmacological means of modifying platelet aggregation and has proved beneficial in the maintenance of vein-graft patency after coronary by-pass operations.

Sulphinpyrazone is a pyrazole compound related

---

* Thromboxane synthetase inhibitors (eg **dazoxiben**) are now available.

to phenylbutazone (see Chapter 9), but it does not have anti-inflammatory activity. Though it does not inhibit platelet aggregation *in vitro* it inhibits adhesion and the release reactions. It has been shown to reduce the incidence of sudden death in patients who had had an episode of cardiac infarction, but it did not decrease the incidence of stroke. Further evidence of its efficacy is required. It is also uricosuric (p. 328).

FIBRINOLYSIS

When the intrinsic coagulation system is activated the fibrinolytic or clot-dissolving system is also set in motion by two separate mechanisms. The main one involves Factor XIIa which catalyses the formation of **plasminogen activators** from precursor zymogens, though some plasminogen activators may be derived from the endothelium of small vessels and from phagocytic cells. **Plasminogen**, a serum β-globulin of molecular weight 143 000, is a zymogen which is deposited on the fibrin strands within a thrombus. Plasminogen activators, which have a very short half-life in the circulation, are serine proteases which diffuse into the thrombus and cleave a particular arg–val bond in plasminogen to release the enzyme **plasmin** (fibrinolysin) (Fig. 12.8). Plasmin is trypsin-like, acting on arg–lys bonds, and thus can digest not only fibrin but fibrinogen and other blood proteins such as factors II, V, and VIII. It is formed locally and acts on the fibrin meshwork in the clot, generating fibrin degradation products and lysing the clot. In the circulation there is a large excess of various plasmin inhibitors which prevent its action on the other coagulation factors.

A second mechanism for stimulating fibrinolysis involves the activation of protein C by thrombin, as described above.

Drugs may affect the fibrinolytic system by increasing the normal fibrinolytic mechanism (**streptokinase**, **urokinase**) or by inhibiting it (**aminocaproic acid**).

FIBRINOLYTIC DRUGS

Streptokinase is a non-enzymic protein with a molecular weight of 47 000 daltons. It is extracted from cultures of group C β-haemolytic streptococci and has to be biologically assayed and standardized. It acts indirectly, forming a stable complex with plasminogen which gains enzymic activity due to a conformation change. It is antigenic and its action may be reduced by anti-streptococcal antibodies already present.

Urokinase is prepared from human urine or from

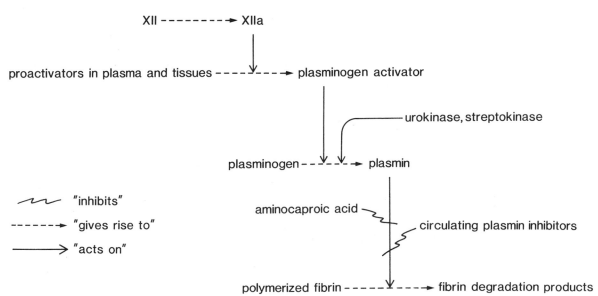

Fig. 12.8 The fibrinolytic system.

cultures of human embryonic kidney cells and has to be biologically assayed and standardized. It is enzymic and acts directly as a plasminogen activator. It is not antigenic.

Administration and pharmacokinetic aspects

Both agents may be given intravenously for systemic effect or through an intravascular catheter for local effect. A large initial loading dose is given to overcome plasma plasmin inhibitors, followed by smaller maintenance doses. The half-life of both agents is about 15 minutes. Their use requires skill and experience.

Toxic effects and contraindications

The main hazard is bleeding which may be treated by giving **aminocaproic acid** (see below) and, if necessary, fresh whole blood. Streptokinase may cause allergic reactions and is reported to produce low grade fever in about 25% of patients treated.

Absolute contraindications to the use of these agents are active internal bleeding and cerebrovascular disease. Relative contraindications include any procedures in which clot formation is important such as surgery, invasive procedures of various kinds and recent serious trauma. Anticoagulants and antiplatelet agents should not be given concurrently with fibrinolytic drugs.

ANTIFIBRINOLYTIC DRUGS

Aminocaproic acid, an analogue of lysine, inhibits streptokinase and urokinase and also prevents the formation of plasmin by plasminogen activator. It is rapidly absorbed from the gastrointestinal tract and thus can be given orally as well as by injection. It may also be used in conditions in which there is bleeding not associated with the use of fibrinolytic drugs.

THERAPEUTIC USES OF ANTICOAGULANTS, ANTIPLATELET AGENTS AND FIBRINOLYTIC DRUGS

Venous thrombo-embolism

The underlying process in a venous thrombus is predominantly coagulation of the blood (fibrin formation) with only a small component of platelet aggregation. As might be expected from the fact that fibrin formation involves an amplifying cascade, anticoagulant agents which interfere with the cascade can be used to *prevent* thrombus formation and as well to prevent extension of a thrombus already formed. In general, heparin is used for short-term effects and the oral anticoagulants for prolonged therapy.

Deep vein thrombosis, which brings the serious hazard of pulmonary embolism, may occur in postoperative patients and in patients immobilized for other reasons, such as stroke, heart failure or myocardial infarction. It may also occur spontaneously in non-immobilized individuals. Subcutaneous injections of heparin in low dosage, repeated 6-hourly, are effective in the prevention of venous thrombosis in moderate- to high-risk patients (e.g. middle-aged patients undergoing major surgery, in whom the risk of venous thrombosis is 10–40% and of fatal pulmonary embolus is 0.1–0.4%).

When thrombosis in the veins has already occurred, larger doses of heparin are required and should be continued for a week or more. Oral anticoagulants are then given—for 3 months if the thrombus has remained localized, for 6 months if there has been embolism to the lungs. In some cases fibrinolytic therapy, with streptokinase, may be used, followed by anticoagulant therapy to prevent recurrence.

Long-term, possibly life-long, therapy with the oral anticoagulants may be necessary in patients who have clinically significant *mitral stenosis, atrial fibrillation* (with the risk of mural thrombi), *prosthetic valves* or *recurrent deep vein thrombosis*.

Arterial thrombo-embolism

Arterial thrombi have a large component of aggregated platelets as well as a component of fibrin-based blood clot and they are usually associated with underlying pathological changes in the vessels. Arterial thrombo-embolism is less easily treated than venous thrombo-embolism and very difficult to prevent. Oral anticoagulants have given poor results in the management of *coronary thrombosis* though it is thought that this might well have been due to inadequate dosage resulting from poor methods of assessment of effect. Results with the current antiplatelet drugs in this condition have been equivocal, both in prevention and treatment, and a definitive assessment of their value awaits further controlled trials. The use of fibrinolysis though essentially still in the experimental stage, has given good results in expert hands when used soon after onset of the condition. In *peripheral arterial thrombo-embolism*, therapy with fibrinolytic drugs can be effective in acute but not chronic disease. Infusions of epoprostenol may also be useful.

In *cerebral vascular disease* with repeated episodes of transient ischaemia and in conditions in which recurrent episodes of thrombo-embolism are expected (e.g. in *atrial fibrillation*) oral anticoagulants with an antiplatelet drug may be used; but continuous monitoring of the anticoagulant drug effect is essential.

Miscellaneous conditions

Both heparin and epoprostenol are useful in preventing thrombi when *extracorporeal circulation of the blood* is used. Some cases of *disseminated intravascular coagulation* may also benefit from treatment with heparin.

REFERENCES AND FURTHER READING

Biggs R (ed) 1976 Human blood coagulation, haemostasis and thrombosis. Blackwell Scientific, Oxford
Brozovic M 1978 Oral anticoagulants in clinical practice. Seminars in Hematology XV: 27–34
Longenecker G L (ed) 1985 The platelets: physiology and pharmacology. Academic Press, London
Lundblad R L, Brown J, Mann K G, Roberts H R (eds) 1981 Chemistry and biology of heparin. Elsevier, North-Holland
Mann K G, Taylor F B 1980 The regulation of coagulation. Elsevier, North-Holland
Moncada S 1982 Biological importance of prostacyclin. Brit J Pharmacol 76: 3–31
Moncada S, Jane J 1984 Prostacyclin and its clinical application. Ann Clin Res 16: 241–252
Ogston D 1983 The physiology of haemostasis. Croom Helm, London

Packham M A, Mustard J F 1980 Pharmacology of platelet-affecting drugs. Circulat 62: V26–V41
Rosenberg R D, Rosenberg J S 1984 Natural anticoagulant mechanisms. J Clin Invest 74: 1–6
Salzman E W 1982 Aspirin to prevent arterial thrombosis. New Engl J Med 307: 113–115
Salzman E W 1983 Progress in preventing venous thromboembolism. New Engl J Med 309: 980–982
Sharma G V R K, Cella G, Parisi A F, Sasahara A A 1982 Thrombolytic therapy. New Engl J Med 306: 1268–1276
Suttie J W 1980 Vitamin K-dependent carboxylation. Trends in Biochemical Sciences 5: 302–304
Wessla S, Gitel S N (1979) Heparin: New concepts relevant to clinical use. Blood 53: 525–544

13

The respiratory system

The chief functions of respiration are to supply oxygen to the body and to remove carbon dioxide. The evaporation of water in the respiratory passages also assists in regulating the temperature of the body.

THE REGULATION OF RESPIRATION

Spontaneous, automatic respiration is controlled by the respiratory centre in the medulla. This centre consists of two groups of neurons, a dorsal and a ventral group. Efferent fibres from this centre pass in the lateral and ventral portions of the spinal cord to the motor neurons controlling the respiratory muscles, and also in the vagus to the accessory muscles of respiration, e.g. those in the larynx. Rhythmic discharge of impulses from the respiratory centre occurs spontaneously but is modulated by vagal afferents from receptors in the lungs and by neurons originating in the pons.

The main pulmonary receptors are sensitive to stretch and are stimulated by inflation. They are situated in the smooth muscle. (Receptors sensitive to deflation are thought to occur, but these are probably more sensitive to congestion of the vessels in the lung. They have been termed J receptors because of their juxtacapillary position.) The respiratory reflex resulting from stimulation of pulmonary receptors is called the 'Hering-Breuer' reflex.

The pontine centres are thought to impose smoothness and regularity on the spontaneous rhythmic discharge of the respiratory centre. They consist of an 'apneustic centre' and a 'pneumotaxic centre'.

The apneustic centre is thought to generate a tonic discharge affecting the medullary neurons which stimulate inspiration. If not interrupted, this tonic discharge would result in maintained contraction of the muscles of inspiration. However, the effect of this discharge is inhibited intermittently by impulses to the medulla from the pontine pneumotaxic centre and from vagal afferents.

There is reciprocal innervation of the inspiratory and expiratory muscles, but this does not involve spinal reflexes, as is the case with reciprocal innervation of the flexor and extensor muscles of the limbs. In the case of respiration, it is the activity in the descending pathways to the inspiratory muscles which results in inhibition of the expiratory muscles through inhibitory interneurons in the brain stem. Similarly, during expiration, the inspiratory muscles are inhibited.

FACTORS AFFECTING THE REGULATION OF RESPIRATION

Apart from the main neurogenic drive outlined above, chemical factors and other neural factors affect the control of respiration.

Chemical factors

The respiratory centre is affected by changes in the arterial blood, being stimulated by a rise in the P_{CO_2} or $[H^+]$ or a fall in P_{O_2}. These effects are mediated through *chemoreceptors* in the carotid and aortic bodies and in the medulla itself.

In each carotid or aortic body (or 'glomus') there are unmyelinated sensory endings among the dopamine containing glomus cells, and both lie in close association with capillaries. The glomus cells and the neurons have unusual reciprocal synaptic connections with each other. There is evidence that it is the nerve endings which are the chemoreceptors since, when the carotid body is removed, the neuroma which develops on the stump of the nerve responds to increases in CO_2 and decreases in O_2 tension. The function of the glomus cells seems to be to modulate the response of the nerve endings, in that, while the Po_2 in the blood is within normal limits, dopamine is released, hyperpolarizing the nerve endings and inhibiting their discharge. When the O_2 in the inspired air falls below 14% (from the normal 21%), the resultant hypoxia reduces this synthesis and release of dopamine, and the sensory nerve endings then generate impulses which stimulate the respiratory centre. The neurons also release acetylcholine on to the glomus cells and this reinforces the inhibition of dopamine release in a positive feedback effect.

The chemoreceptors in the medulla are thought to lie on its ventral surface. It is now known that these receptors are sensitive to the hydrogen ion concentration, not to CO_2 as such. When the Pco_2 in the blood rises, CO_2 diffuses readily through the blood/brain and blood/cerebrospinal fluid barriers as through most membranes; the diffusion of H^+ and HCO_3^- is considerably slower. Having penetrated into the cerebrospinal fluid and the interstitial fluid of the brain, the CO_2 is rapidly hydrated to H_2CO_3 which dissociates to give H^+ and HCO_3^-, and it is this change in H^+ concentration which is sensed by the medullary chemoreceptors.

Metabolic acidosis stimulates respiration and the resultant hyperventilation causes a fall in Pco_2 and thus a decrease in plasma H^+ concentration. Metabolic alkalosis, (which can occur, for example, if persistent vomiting causes loss of HCl), depresses the respiration, which leads to a rise in Pco_2.

Conversely if the increase in respiration is primary, the fall in Pco_2 and thus in plasma H^+ concentration can produce a *respiratory alkalosis*, while a primary decrease in breathing which leads to an increase in Pco_2 and a raised plasma H^+ concentration can produce a *respiratory acidosis*.

Along with the neurogenic factors outlined above, the chemical stimuli specified here—a rise in Pco_2 and a fall in Po_2—are the principal forces driving respiration and drugs which depress respiration may affect these factors differently, as is explained below.

Other neural factors

The processes of swallowing and of vomiting (p. 339) necessitate inhibition of respiration along with closure of the glottis and it is clear that the centres controlling these functions affect the respiratory centre. There is also experimental evidence that movements of joints increases respiration, which implies that proprioceptive impulses in ascending pathways influence the respiratory centre. This carries the connotation that exercise might have a direct effect on respiration.

Pain affects respiration as do emotional factors, which indicates that higher centres also have an input into the medullary centres controlling respiration.

A moderate degree of voluntary control can be superimposed on the automatic regulation of breathing and this implies connections between the neocortex and the motor neurons innervating the muscles of respiration. Bulbar poliomyelitis and certain lesions in the brain stem result in loss of the automatic regulation of respiration without loss of voluntary regulation. This has been referred to as 'Ondine's curse'. Ondine was a water nymph who fell in love with a mortal. When he was unfaithful to her, the king of the water nymphs put a curse on him, eliminating certain automatic functions including that of respiration. Thereafter he had to stay awake and breathe by consciously exerting voluntary control. When exhaustion finally supervened and he fell asleep, he ceased breathing.

DRUGS WHICH AFFECT RESPIRATION

Drugs may produce an effect on respiration because they are intended to (e.g. respiratory stimulants) or inadvertently (e.g. the unwanted effects of some CNS depressants).

RESPIRATORY STIMULANTS

Under some circumstances it may be necessary to stimulate respiration, as for example in acute respiratory failure. Drugs used for this purpose are called **analeptics** (see Chapter 26), the term being derived from the Greek for a restorative because, in the past, these drugs were used in attempts to restore life to dying patients. Most act centrally, stimulating not only the respiratory centre but the vasomotor centre, and in larger doses, the motor cortex as well, causing convulsions. Some analeptic drugs, such as **leptazol**, are used in the laboratory in convulsant doses, in the investigation and screening of potential anticonvulsant drugs.

The use of these drugs in clinical medicine has declined in recent years and they are now employed only in certain specific conditions (e.g. in ventilatory failure due to chronic obstructive disease of the airways) and then only under expert supervision. The main drugs used (see Chapter 26) are **doxapram** which stimulates both carotid chemoreceptors and the respiratory centre, and **nikethamide** and **ethamivan** which stimulate only the respiratory centre (see p. 571). These drugs should not be used in severe acute asthma (*status asthmaticus*) or in respiratory depression which is caused by drug overdose (see below) or by diseases of the nervous system.

Unwanted effects

These are due mainly to the stimulant action on the central nervous system and include tremor, dizziness and convulsions. The stimulation of the vasomotor centre is likely to result in vasoconstriction, and cardiac dysrhythmias may also occur.

DRUGS CAUSING RESPIRATORY DEPRESSION

Many drugs which have a depressant action on the central nervous system, cause a greater or lesser degree of respiratory depression. These include the **narcotic analgesics**, **anaesthetics**, **barbiturates**, many **H$_1$ antihistamines**, some **antidepressants**, **benzodiazepines**, and alcohols such as **ethanol** and **chloral hydrate**. It should be noted, however, that while most of these agents generally depress respiration only in excessive dosage, the opiates cause some degree of respiratory depression in the therapeutic dose range. An additional point is that though the respiratory depression for most of the above agents can prove fatal, this is less likely to be the case with the benzodiazepines. These hazards are discussed in more detail in the chapters devoted to each of these agents.

Opiate analgesics and barbiturates (and possibly other CNS depressant drugs) first affect the sensitivity of respiration to increased P_{CO_2} and only later, in larger doses, do they affect the hypoxic drive.

FUNCTIONS OF THE LUNG UNRELATED TO RESPIRATION

The lung has various functions which have pharmacological and/or physiological relevance but which have nothing to do with breathing.

Angiotensin I is converted to angiotensin II (see Chapter 11) by the angiotensin-converting enzyme, which also inactivates bradykinin (p. 199). The enzyme is present on the luminal surface of the capillary endothelial cells and occurs mainly in the lungs.

Prostaglandins are extracted from the circulation and metabolized in the lung (p. 197) as are noradrenaline and serotonin.

The lung functions as a reservoir for neutrophil polymorphs. Normally, at rest, only about 50% of these cells, which have been released into the circulation from the bone marrow, are present in the circulating blood. The remaining 50% form the 'marginated pool' which can be added to the circulation when needed, virtually doubling neutrophil numbers within seconds. The marginated neutrophils are held mainly in the blood vessels of the lungs and they can be mobilized by a variety of stimuli including exercise and infection. Pharmacological agents such as adrenaline can also mobilize these marginated neutrophils.

THE REGULATION OF THE MUSCULATURE, BLOOD VESSELS AND GLANDS OF THE AIRWAYS

The tone of the bronchial muscle affects the 'airways resistance'. This can be measured indirectly by instruments which record the volume or flow on forced expiration. FEV_1 is the 'forced expiratory volume in 1 sec'. The 'peak expiratory flow rate' (PEFR) can also be quantitated. In the normal individual the state of the mucosa and the activity of the glands play little or no part in determining airways resistance, though these factors may be of prime importance in pathological conditions such as bronchitis and asthma.

Dilatation of the bronchi in a normal individual results in:

1. A fall in airways resistance to three quarters of its normal value.
2. Minor changes in FEV_1 and PEFR.
3. No measurable increase in the anatomical dead space in the lungs.

Constriction of the bronchi results in:

1. An increase in airways resistance.
2. A reduction in FEV_1 and PEFR.
3. Uneven ventilation.

Under physiological conditions, local regulation of bronchial tone contributes to the maintenance of a uniform ventilation:perfusion ratio in different parts of the lung.

In the neuro-humoral control of the airways three different types of sensory receptor are important in the afferent pathways. The efferent pathways to the muscular, vascular and glandular elements include parasympathetic nerves, sympathetic nerves, circulating adrenaline and the 'noradrenergic, non-cholinergic' (NANC) nerves (see Chapter 5).

Afferent receptors

The three types of receptors are: stretch receptors, J-receptors and irritant receptors.

Stretch receptors are located in the bronchial musculature and are stimulated by distension of the airways. Nerve impulses are conducted over myelinated fibres from these receptors at 5–68 m/s. The response to distension is inhibition of inspiration by an effect on the respiratory centre (the Hering-Breuer reflex described above) and relaxation of bronchial muscles. These reflexes operate mainly, if not only, when there is marked pulmonary inflation.

J-receptors are found between the pulmonary capillaries and alveolar walls; the related nerve fibres are unmyelinated and have a conduction velocity of 0.8–2.4 m/s. As explained above these receptors are thought by some to be 'deflation receptors' and by others to respond to congestion of the blood vessels. Stimulation results in cessation of breathing ('apnoea') followed by rapid respiration ('tachypnoea').

Irritant receptors occur in the bronchial epithelium, and the related afferent nerve fibres are thin, unmyelinated fibres with a conduction velocity of < 1 m/s. The receptors respond to a variety of stimuli: ammonia, dust, inhalation of histamine, pulmonary microembolism and marked inflation. Type I hypersensitivity reactions (p. 186) are also thought to cause stimulation of irritant receptors. The responsiveness of these receptors is exacerbated if the epithelium is damaged, e.g. by infection. Stimulation of these receptors is believed to result in bronchospasm.

Efferent pathways

Parasympathetic innervation

Bronchial tone is regulated principally by vagal pathways, and there are also vagal efferents to the glands. Muscarinic receptors can be demonstrated on the smooth muscle and the submucous glands, stimulation causing contraction of the former and secretion from the latter. Muscarinic receptors in the vessels mediate vasodilatation while similar receptors on the epithelial cells mediate ion transport. The vagus influences the smooth muscle from the trachea down to bronchioles of 0.5 mm diameter, but binding studies show that there are few muscarinic receptors in the small as compared to the large airways, and stimulation of the vagus or the use of agonists at muscarinic receptors causes, predominantly, narrowing of the larger airways.

Sympathetic innervation and catecholamines

It is currently held that there is no sympathetic innervation of the bronchial smooth muscle and that 'sympathetic' effects are due to circulating catecholamines. This is based on the following evidence:

1. Histochemical studies (in which the presence of dopamine β-hydroxylase, an enzyme necessary for the synthesis of noradrenaline, is detected by a fluorescent antibody technique), show sympathetic nerves around blood vessels and submucosal glands in the bronchi but none in the smooth muscle.

2. Studies of *in vitro* preparations show that though muscle contraction following nerve stimulation can be inhibited by atropine, muscle relaxation following nerve stimulation is not affected by either β- or α-blockers; in addition, dose-response curves of relaxation with exogenous noradrenaline are not altered by cocaine. For explanation of these effects see Chapter 7. The relaxation is thought to be mediated by the NANC system; see below.

3. *In vivo* studies with tyramine, which releases noradrenaline from sympathetic nerve terminals (scc Chapter 7), indicate that though there is a dose-related increase in blood-pressure and a decrease in heart rate, there is no change in FEV_1 or in peak flow in the airways. Salbutamol, on the other hand, a β-adrenoceptor agonist, *does* increase FEV, and peak flow.

As regards adrenoceptors in the lungs, studies with labelled atenolol indicate a very high density of β-receptors in the lung. Autoradiography shows that these occur in the smooth muscle, the epithelium and glands and also, in very large numbers, in the alveoli. In man virtually all the β-receptors in the airways are β_2; those in the alveoli are both β_1 and β_2. (The function of the alveolar receptors is not known). In contrast with the muscarinic receptors, the number of β-receptors increases as one goes from trachea to bronchioles.

Stimulation of the airway β-receptors with drugs results in relaxation of smooth muscle, inhibition of mediator release from mast cells, and increased muco-ciliary clearance. A decrease in cholinergic transmission is also reported, possibly by an effect on receptors on local parasympathetic ganglia.

α-adrenoceptor agonists have no effect on normal airways but cause contraction if the airways are diseased. Histamine increases the response to α-agonists.

Non-adrenergic, non-cholinergic (NANC) innervation

There is experimental evidence that some aspects of airway function are influenced by nerves which are neither cholinergic nor adrenergic, and there are grounds for believing that, in some respects, the intrinsic nerve plexuses of the airways may resemble those in the gastrointestinal tract (see Chapter 15). The principal NANC pathways mediate mainly **smooth muscle relaxation** and the identify of the transmitter is, at present, a matter of debate. Evidence is against these nerves being purinergic. Most evidence points to a peptide—vasointestinal peptide ('VIP')—being the transmitter causing relaxation of smooth muscle, the effect being more marked in large than in small airways.

A separate system of non-cholinergic peptidergic excitatory nerves is also thought to exist. Here again the neurotransmitter is not known for certain and candidates include substance P as well as other peptides. This system when stimulated, results in bronchospasm. There is evidence that substance P can release histamine from mast cells, and axon reflexes involving this non-cholinergic system may be important in non-allergic asthma (see below).

DISORDERS OF RESPIRATORY FUNCTION

Two of the main disturbances of respiratory function which require pharmacological intervention are bronchial asthma and cough.

BRONCHIAL ASTHMA

Asthma may be defined as a syndrome in which there is recurrent reversible obstruction of the airways in response to stimuli which are not in themselves noxious and which do not affect non-asthmatic subjects. The asthmatic subject has intermittent attacks of dyspnoea and wheezing which are usually debilitating as well as unpleasant; the dyspnoea (disorder of breathing) consisting of difficulty in breathing out. Acute severe asthma ('*status asthmaticus*') can be fatal. Because of its prolonged course and recurrent nature, asthma ranks high in economic importance in terms of demands on medical services. The pathogenesis of the condition is still a matter of debate and the drugs available for treatment are still far from ideal; consequently there is active research into the pathogenesis of asthma and many drug firms are attempting to find better anti-asthma drugs. The eliciting stimuli, the type of airway obstruction, the contribution of inflammation and the response to treatment may vary widely between different individuals, but virtually all patients show a greater or lesser degree of **bronchial hyper-reactivity** (i.e. increased tendency to bronchoconstriction and secretion in response to a variety of physical and chemical stimuli).

According to the classical concept of asthma, the condition is a simple Type I hypersensitivity reaction (see page 186) and occurs as a result of the following sequence of events: (1) a sensitization phase, consisting of exposure to an allergen (such as pollen or animal danders), production of IgE antibodies, followed by binding of IgE molecules to the IgE receptors on mast cells; (2) The actual asthma attack on second exposure to allergen, the attack being due to the interaction of allergen with cell-fixed IgE, leading to the release of mast cell histamine and other mediators, which constrict bronchial smooth muscle, dilate blood vessels and stimulate mucous glands. It is now recognized that this concept is an oversimplification. Only 30% of asthma is due to allergy and, even in these cases, elements other than interaction of allergen with mast cell-fixed IgE are almost certainly involved.

Underlying the tendency to develop attacks of asthma is bronchial hyper-reactivity, as specified above. This is mainly hyper-reactivity of the smooth muscle, in that rapid reversible bronchoconstriction occurs when the subject is given histamine or muscarinic agonists by inhalation in doses that do not affect normal individuals. Mechanisms thought to be important in this increased sensitivity include changes in airway smooth muscle contractility and changes in autonomic regulation. There is evidence for a variety of autonomic changes including an increase in parasympathetic activity, an increase in α-adrenoceptor activity, a decrease in β-adrenoceptor activity or in non-adrenergic, non-cholinergic (NANC) inhibitory activity, and an in-

crease in NANC excitatory activity (see above). However, the precise role of these changes is not yet clear.

Local **inflammatory changes** in the bronchial mucosa are probably important in bronchial hyper-reactivity and there may well be an interaction between neuronal and inflammatory factors. **Platelets** are now believed to play a part in the hyper-reactivity by producing substances which increase the sensitivity of the smooth muscle to stimuli and which cause its proliferation.

Asthma in the past has been classified as either 'extrinsic', when attacks are provoked by external agents, or 'intrinsic', in which no external causative factors can be identified. Stimuli which cause asthmatic attacks are many and various and include allergens (in atopic subjects), exercise (in which the stimulus may be cold air), respiratory infections, cigarette smoke, atmospheric pollutants such as sulphur dioxide, and emotional states.

In many subjects the asthmatic attack consists of two main phases as can be demonstrated by tests of FEV_1 (Fig. 13.1).

The initial phase or *immediate response* occurs abruptly and is due mainly to **spasm of the bronchial smooth muscle**. This phase can be reversed by giving bronchodilator drugs such as **β-adrenoceptor agonists** or **theophylline**. The cells involved in this

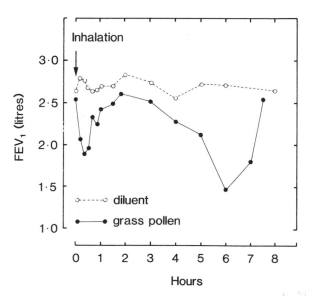

Fig. 13.1 The two phases of asthma as demonstrated by the changes in the forced expiratory volume in 1 sec (FEV_1) after inhalation of grass pollen. (From: Cockcroft, 1983)

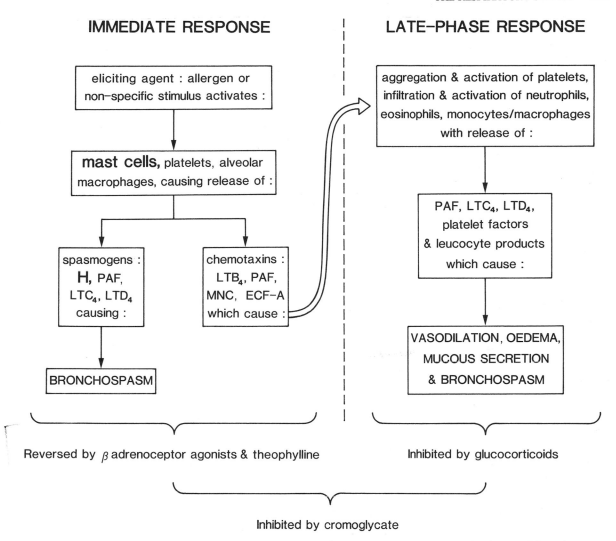

IMMEDIATE RESPONSE

eliciting agent : allergen or non–specific stimulus activates :

mast cells, platelets, alveolar macrophages, causing release of :

spasmogens :
H, PAF,
LTC_4, LTD_4
causing :

chemotaxins :
LTB_4, PAF,
MNC, ECF-A
which cause :

BRONCHOSPASM

Reversed by β adrenoceptor agonists & theophylline

LATE–PHASE RESPONSE

aggregation & activation of platelets, infiltration & activation of neutrophils, eosinophils, monocytes/macrophages with release of :

PAF, LTC_4, LTD_4,
platelet factors
& leucocyte products
which cause :

VASODILATION, OEDEMA,
MUCOUS SECRETION
& BRONCHOSPASM

Inhibited by glucocorticoids

Inhibited by cromoglycate

Fig. 13.2 Outline of the reactions thought to occur in asthma. H = histamine; PAF = platelet activating factor; LTC_4 and D_4 = leukotrienes C_4 and D_4; MNC = mast cell derived chemotactic factor for neutrophils; ECF-A = eosinophil chemotactic factor of anaphylaxis. (Based on: Kay, 1986)

phase are thought to be primarily mast cells, but platelets, and possibly alveolar macrophages, are also believed to play a part and the spasmogenic mediators include histamine, platelet activating factor (PAF) and possibly leukotrienes C_4 and D_4 (Fig. 13.2). Both platelets and macrophages have receptors for IgE, albeit of low affinity, and there is clinical evidence of platelet activation *in vivo* during allergic bronchospasm. It is possible that in non-allergic asthma, irritants may stimulate the irritant receptors and cause release of peptide mediators by antidromic impulses in sensory nerve fibres and

that these mediators then activate mast cells and other cells.

The second, *late-phase response* (see Fig. 13.1) occurs at a variable time after exposure to the eliciting stimulus and may be nocturnal. This phase is in essence, an **acute inflammatory reaction** and is associated with infiltration and activation of neutrophils, eosinophils, platelets and monocyte/macrophages (and possibly lymphocytes) which occurs in response to chemotactic agents released during the first phase (Fig. 13.2). The chemotactic agents include platelet activating factor, leukotriene B_4, and chemotactic factors for neutrophils and eosinophils derived from mast cells. This phase is characterized by vasodilatation, oedema of the mucosa, and mucus secretion as well as bronchospasm. There is evidence that platelet aggregation and activation have a role in the bronchospasm. The mediators causing these phenomena are believed to be those usually associated with acute inflammatory responses (see Chapter 8), in particular platelet activating factor and the spasmogenic leukotrienes. Peptide mediators, released from sensory nerve endings as a result of antidromic impulses may also play a part and some investigators suggest that complement components are involved. Membrane and granule-derived products (such as the eosinophil 'major basic protein') are thought to be responsible for cell damage, particularly to the bronchial mucosa.

This late-phase response cannot be reversed by bronchodilators but can be blocked by the **anti-inflammatory steroids**.

Cromoglycate inhibits both phases in many patients, but is not effective if given *after* the initial phase.

In patients who die from acute severe asthma (*status asthmaticus*) there is evidence of marked inflammation of the bronchi with narrowing of the airways due to oedema of the mucosa, associated with extensive secretion of thick mucus which plugs the bronchi and in which inflammatory cells are embedded, particularly eosinophils.

DRUGS USED TO TREAT ASTHMA

β-adrenoceptor agonists

This group of drugs is dealt with in Chapter 7. Their mechanism of action in the asthmatic attack is two-fold. The main effect is a bronchodilator action directly on the β_2-adrenoceptors on smooth muscle. As indicated above, recent studies have shown that there is little or no sympathetic innervation of airway smooth muscle as opposed to blood vessels and submucosal glands, but β-receptors are abundant both on smooth muscle and in the alveoli. Stimulation of the β-adrenoreceptors on smooth muscle produces relaxation by activation of cAMP-dependent kinase which is thought to

enhance calcium efflux, to prevent PIP_2 breakdown or to inactivate myosin light chain kinase thus inhibiting the formation of the contractile actin-myosin complex (see Chapter 1). Another action of the β-adrenoceptor agonists which may contribute to the reversal of bronchoconstriction is inhibition of mediator release from mast cells. The endogenous agent which acts on the pulmonary β-receptors is circulating **adrenaline** and in the past this was the main drug used in the therapy of acute asthmatic attacks. However, since it acts on the β_1-receptors in the heart as well as the β_2-receptors in the lungs, it is likely to cause tachycardia and even dysrhythmias. These unwanted effects occur to an even greater extent with isoprenaline, which is now no longer recommended for asthma.

The main drugs in this group used clinically are β_2-agonists such as **salbutamol**, **terbutaline** and **rimiterol**. These are usually given by inhalation of aerosol, powder or nebulized solution, but may be given orally in some subjects, or by the parenteral route in severe attacks. Given by inhalation, salbutamol and terbutaline start to act within a few minutes and the effects last for 3–5 hours. Rimiterol has a shorter duration of action. Some degree of tolerance to the effects of these broncho-dilators can develop if they are used for 2–3 weeks, but thereafter the response does not alter much. The decreased responsiveness can be reversed by parenteral steroids, and this can be important in treating a severe acute attack.

These agents may also be used prophylactically, as may oral **ephedrine** preparations, though this latter drug has the disadvantage of not having a selective effect on β_2-receptors.

It should be mentioned that β-adrenoceptor antagonists, such as propranolol, though having no effect on airway function in normal individuals, cause wheezing in asthmatics and can precipitate an acute asthmatic attack.

Methylxanthine drugs

There are three pharmacologically active methyl-xanthines—theophylline, theobromine and caffeine (Fig. 13.3; see also Chapters 10 & 26). The xanthine used in clinical medicine is **theophylline** (1,3-dimethylxanthine), used usually as theo-phylline–ethylenediamine, known as **amino-**

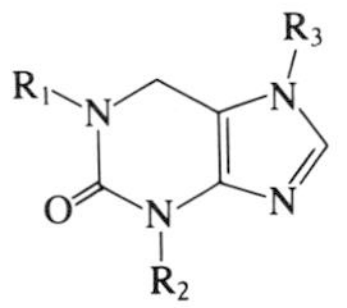

Drug	R_1	R_2	R_3
Caffeine	CH_3	CH_3	CH_3
Theophylline	CH_3	CH_3	H
Theobromine	H	CH_3	CH_3

Fig. 13.3 Methylxanthine drugs.

phylline. Theophylline was used at one time as a diuretic, but its main therapeutic use at present is as a bronchodilator. Caffeine and theophylline are constituents of coffee and tea, and theobromine is a constituent of cocoa.

Actions and mechanism of action

1. *Bronchial smooth muscle.* Theophylline has a relaxant effect on this tissue but the mechanism of this action is not entirely clear. It has been thought to be due to an inhibitory effect on phosphodiesterase, leading to an increase in cAMP, with the results outlined above, and possibly part of the action of this drug may be due to this effect. However, the concentration of theophylline necessary for inhibition of the enzyme is 20 times higher than the concentration which relaxes the smooth muscle of the airways (20 μM). Furthermore, other drugs which are more potent inhibitors of phosphodiesterase, such as papavarine and dipyridamole, do not effect the tone of bronchial smooth muscle.

Part of the action of theophylline on smooth muscle may be due to antagonism of endogenously produced adenosine (see Chapter 11). This latter agent has been shown to potentiate the IgE-dependent release of mediators from mast cells, to stimulate afferent nerve endings, and to have an inhibitory effect on sympathetic neurotransmission. Theophylline may also act, at least in part, by releasing endogenous catecholamines from the adrenal medulla.

2. *Central nervous system.* The methylxanthines (and in particular caffeine), have a stimulant effect on the CNS causing increased alertness (see Chapter 26). They may cause tremor and nervousness and may interfere with sleep.

3. *Cardiovascular system.* This group of drugs stimulates the heart (see Chapter 11), having positive chronotropic and inotropic actions. They cause vasodilation in most blood vessels, though the effect on the cerebral blood vessels may be constrictor.

4. *Kidney.* Methylxanthines have a weak diuretic effect involving both an increased glomerular filtration rate (which may be related to the vasodilator effect and consequent increased blood flow) and reduced reabsorption in the tubules (see Chapter 14).

Unwanted effects

When theophylline is used in asthma, most of its other effects, such as those on the CNS, cardiovascular system and gastrointestinal tract, are unwanted side effects. Furthermore theophylline has a relatively low therapeutic index; clinical improvement in asthma occurs with concentrations of 27–80 μM, and adverse effects are likely to occur with concentrations greater than 110 μM. There are various immunoassay techniques for measuring the theophylline concentration in the plasma. (See Chapter 2) Gastrointestinal symptoms (anorexia, nausea and vomiting) and nervousness and tremor may be seen with concentrations slightly higher than the clinically effective levels. Serious cardiovascular and CNS effects can occur when the plasma concentration exceeds 200 μM.

Pharmacokinetic aspects

Aminophylline and theophylline can be given orally and preparations for rectal administration are also available. Rapid-release oral preparations are rarely used now because of the possibility of side effects. Sustained-release preparations have a lower incidence of side effects and furthermore result in effective plasma concentrations for as long as 12 hours. Aminophylline may also be given by slow intravenous injection.

Theophylline is well absorbed from the gastrointestinal tract, and is metabolized in the liver. 10% is excreted unchanged in the urine. The plasma half-life is 8–9 hours in adults but is less than half this in children. Liver disease results in a prolongation of the half-life.

Muscarinic receptor antagonists

These drugs are only of use in asthmatic attacks in which there is a marked component of reflex bronchospasm mediated by parasympathetic nerves. This applies mainly to asthma produced by irritant stimuli. They are, however, useful as bronchodilators in some cases of chronic bronchitis.

This group of agents is dealt with in detail in Chapter 6. The compound used specifically as an anti-asthmatic is **ipratropium bromide**. This is a quaternary derivative of N-isopropylatropine and it is given by aerosol inhalation. It is not well absorbed into the circulation and thus does not have much action at muscarinic receptors other than those in the bronchi. It does not cross the blood-brain barrier to any great extent and, unlike many other muscarinic antagonists, it does not decrease the mucociliary clearance of bronchial secretions, nor does it produce an increase in the viscosity of these secretions. The maximum effect is not seen until after 30 minutes or so, but then lasts for 3–5 hours. It can be used with β_2-agonists.

Cromoglycate

This drug was the result of research aimed at finding congeners of the naturally occurring drug, khellin. It is unique in that it was firsted tested, and its efficacy demonstrated, in allergic asthma in man, without prior testing in animals. Its structure is shown in Figure 13.4.

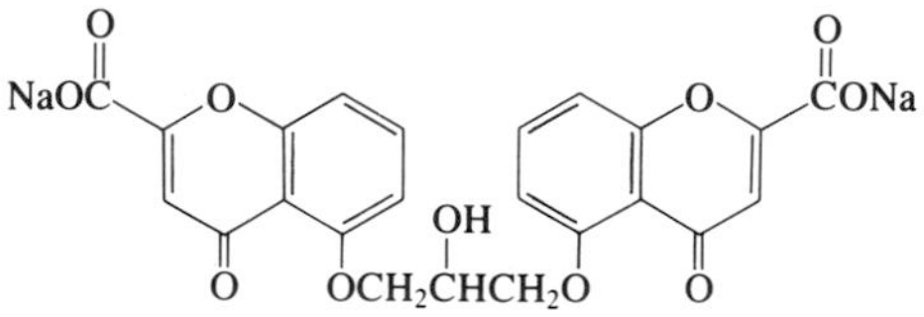

Fig. 13.4 Cromoglycate.

Action and mechanism of action

Cromoglycate is not a bronchodilator and does not have any direct effects on smooth muscle, nor does it inhibit the actions of any of the known smooth muscle stimulants. If given *prophylactically* it inhibits both the immediate and the late-phase asthmatic responses. It is effective in antigen-induced, exercise-induced and irritant-induced asthma, though not all asthmatic subjects respond. Pre-treatment before exposure to an eliciting stimulus may be dramatically effective in preventing an asthmatic attack in many patients. Continuous treatment with cromoglycate is thought to result in a decrease in bronchial hyper-reactivity.

Its mechansim of action is a matter of debate. It was originally thought to act by preventing mediator release from mast cells and indeed it can be shown to have this effect in animal models of Type 1 or immediate hypersensitivity (p. 186). It is also active against human mast cells of the lung, the nose and the conjunctivae but inactive against human skin mast cells and basophils. However, even in those human tissues in which it is active cromoglycate is not very effective as a 'mast cell stabilizing agent', being in fact 1000 times less effective than salbutamol in this respect. Furthermore, at least 20 other compounds have been produced, by various pharmaceutical companies, which are equally potent or, in some cases, considerably more potent than cromoglycate as 'mast cell stabilizers' in the animal models specified, but none has so far proved to have any anti-asthmatic effect in man.

There is evidence that cromoglycate depresses exaggerated neuronal reflexes generated by stimulation of the 'irritant receptors', which are thought to be important in bronchial hyper-reactivity and which might indirectly cause release of mast cell mediators. It has been claimed to suppress the response of sensory C fibres to the irritant, capsaicin.

An effect on the interaction of platelets and platelet-activating factor may be of significance for the action of cromoglycate in asthma in man. Platelet activating factor can produce both early and late-phase responses in experimental animals. This mediator produces a biphasic broncho-constriction if given into the trachea in rabbits, and a biphasic change in the vascular responses (similar to that seen in antigen-induced reactions) if injected intradermally in both animals and man. Cromoglycate inhibits these reactions, in particular the late-phase responses, although it is known not to affect mast cells in the skin and so cannot be acting as a mast-cell stabilizer in this situation.

A full understanding of its mechanism of action awaits the results of further study.

Pharmacokinetic aspects

Cromoglycate is extremely poorly absorbed from the gastrointestinal tract. It is given by inhalation as an aerosol, as a nebulized solution, or in powder form; about 10% is absorbed into the circulation when it is given in this way. It is excreted unchanged—50% in the bile and 50% in the urine. Its half-life in the plasma is 90 mins.

Unwanted effects

These are few and consist mostly of the effects of irritation in the upper respiratory tract. Hypersensitivity reactions have been reported (urticaria, anaphylaxis), but are rare. Eosinophil infiltration in the lungs has also occurred.

Ketotifen

This drug has some actions resembling those of cromoglycate. It is a serotonin antagonist, and also has some degree of antihistamine activity, including sedation which constitutes the commonest unwanted effect. It is given orally and its full action is not expressed for 3–4 weeks. It has been shown to be effective for prophylaxis of bronchial asthma; in a recent trial involving over 8000 patients, 70% reported that it was efficacious.

Glucocorticoids

These drugs are dealt with in detail in Chapter 16 (p. 394). They are not bronchodilators and are not effective in the treatment of the immediate response to the eliciting agent. Given prophylactically they inhibit the late-phase response and given continuously they may reduce bronchial hyperreactivity. Their effect is believed to be largely due to their anti-inflammatory actions.

The main compounds used are **beclomethasone** and **betamethasone** which are given by inhalation with a metered-dose inhaler. The full effect is attained only after several days of therapy. Oral prednisolone, or corticotrophin or tetracosactrin may be required in some cases (p. 393).

Calcium antagonists

These drugs may have a role in asthma therapy, but more research on this topic is required. This group of drugs is dealt with in Chapter 11.

SEVERE ACUTE ASTHMA (STATUS ASTHMATICUS)

This condition is a medical emergency requiring hospitalization. Treatment includes oxygen, systemic glucocorticoids and bronchodilator drugs such as aminophylline given intravenously, or salbutamol given either intravenously or by inhalation.

DRUGS USED FOR COUGH

Cough is a protective reflex mechanism, the purpose of which is to remove foreign material and secretions from the bronchi and bronchioles. It may be inappropriately stimulated by conditions not associated with either excess secretion or foreign material—conditions such as inflammation or neoplasia. In these cases **antitussive** or (**cough suppressant**) drugs may be used. It should be understood that these drugs merely suppress the symptom without influencing the underlying condition.

Antitussive drugs act by an ill-defined central action in the nervous system. They may depress a 'cough centre' in the brain stem. The **narcotic analgesics** have effective antitussive action in doses below those required for pain relief, and various isomers of these agents, which are neither analgesic nor addictive, are also effective against cough.

Codeine

Codeine, or methylmorphine, is one of the opium alkaloids (see Chapter 25). It has considerably less addiction liability than the main opioid analgesics and is an effective cough suppressant. Its antitussive action is accompanied by an inhibitory action on both secretion and the muco-ciliary clearance of sputum. Constipation also occurs because of the well known action of opiates on the gastrointestinal tract (see Chapters 15 & 25).

Dextromethorphan

This drug is related to levorphanol, a synthetic narcotic analgesic, but it itself is non-narcotic, non-analgesic and non-addictive. Its antitussive potency is equivalent to that of codeine but it does not produce constipation or an inhibition of ciliary activity in the bronchioles.

REFERENCES AND FURTHER READING

Barnes P J 1986 Asthma as an axon reflex. Lancet i: 242–244
Buckle D R, Smith H (eds) 1984 Development of anti-asthma drugs. Butterworths, London
Flenley D C 1983 New drugs in respiratory disorders. Brit Med J 286 (i): 871–875
Goetzl E J 1984 Asthma: new mediators and old problems. N Engl J Med 311: 252–253
Kay A B, Austen K. Lichtenstein L M (eds) 1984 Asthma: physiology, immunopharmacology and treatment. Third International Symposium. Academic Press, London
Kay A B 1986 Mediators and inflammatory cells in asthma. In: Kay A B (ed) Asthma: clinical pharmacology and therapeutic progress 1–10. Blackwell Scientific Publications, Oxford
Morley J (ed) 1982 Bronchial hyperreactivity. Academic Press, London
Morley J, Sanjar S, Page C P 1984 The platelet in asthma. Lancet ii: 1142–1144
Nadel J A, Barnes P J 1984 Autonomic regulation of the airways. Ann Rev Med 35: 451–467

14

The kidney

One of the main functions of the kidney is the excretion of waste products such as urea, uric acid and creatinine. In the course of this activity it fulfils another function, crucially important in homeostasis—the regulation of the salt and electrolyte content and the volume of the extracellular fluid. It also plays a part in acid-base balance.

The kidneys receive about a quarter of the cardiac output. From the huge volume of plasma which flows through them each day, they filter an amount equivalent to about 15 times the extracellular fluid volume. This filtrate is identical in composition to plasma, except that it has very little protein. As it passes through the renal tubule, about 99% of it is reabsorbed while some substances are secreted, and eventually about 1.5 litres of the filtered fluid is voided as urine (Table 14.1).

Table 14.1 Reabsorption of fluid and solute in the kidney

	Filtered/day	Excreted/day	% reabsorbed
NaCl	20 000 mEquiv	100 mEquiv	99 +
NaHCO$_3$	5000 mEquiv	2 mEquiv	99 +
K$^+$	700 mEquiv	50 mEquiv	93 +
H$_2$O	170 litres	1.5 litre	99 +

Renal blood flow = 1200 ml/mm (20–25% of cardiac output)
Renal plasma flow 660 ml/min
Glomerular filtration rate 125 ml/min

The most important group of drugs employed for their effect on the kidney are the **diuretics**. These are used mainly in the therapy of oedema (a defect in salt and water balance in which there is an accumulation of extracellular fluid), but in addition they have an important role in the treatment of hypertension. Drugs may also be used to alter the pH of the urine and to modify the excretion of some organic compounds such as uric acid.

In structure each kidney consists of an outer cortex, an inner medulla and a hollow pelvis which empties into the ureter. The functional unit is the nephron, of which there are about 1.3×10^6 in each kidney.

THE STRUCTURE AND FUNCTION OF THE NEPHRON

The nephron consists of a glomerulus, proximal convoluted tubule, loop of Henle, distal tubule and collecting duct (Fig. 14.1). The glomerulus comprises a tuft of capillaries projecting into the blind dilated end of the renal tubular system. Most nephrons lie largely or entirely in the cortex. The remaining 12%, called the juxtamedullary nephrons, have their renal glomeruli and convoluted tubules next to the junction of the medulla and cortex and their loops of Henle pass deep into the medulla.

The blood supply to the nephron

This possesses the special characteristic of having two capillary beds in series with each other (see Fig. 14.1). The main arteries to the kidney give rise to the arcuate arteries which run between the cortex and medulla. The vessels to the glomeruli come from branches of the arcuate arteries which radiate outwards through the cortex.

The details of the blood supply to nephrons at various levels of the cortex are complex, but there are two main patterns of vascular supply. For those nephrons which lie entirely in the cortex the afferent arterioles branch to form the capillaries of the glomerulus. These empty into the efferent arterioles which in turn branch to form a second capillary

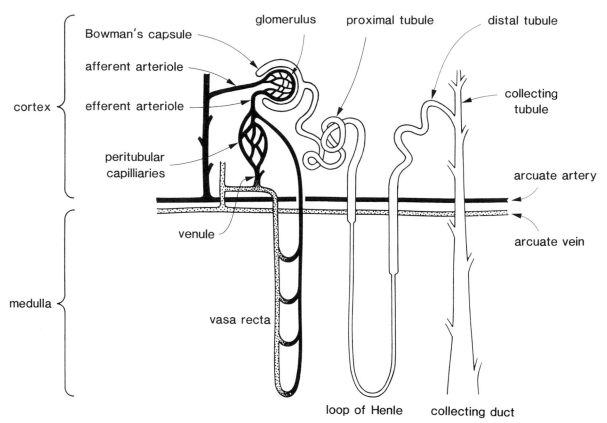

Fig. 14.1 Simplified diagram of the nephron and its blood supply. The tubules and the blood vessels are shown separately for clarity. In the kidney the peritubular capillary network surrounds the convoluted tubules, and the distal convoluted tubule passes close to the glomerulus, between the afferent and efferent arterioles.

network in the cortex, around the convoluted tubules and loops of Henle of other nephrons, before emptying into the veins. In the case of the juxtamedullary nephrons the pattern of blood vessels is slightly different in that some of the branches of the afferent arterioles do not supply the convoluted tubules, but instead form bundles of vessels which pass deep into the medulla with the thin loops of Henle. These loops of vessels are called *vasa recta.* Some of the blood from these juxtamedullary glomeruli therefore bypasses the proximal convoluted tubules. (The usual methods of measuring renal blood flow involving substances which are secreted into the urine from the proximal convoluted tubules will thus miss this part of the blood flow through the kidney.)

The juxtaglomerular apparatus

A conjunction of afferent arteriole, efferent arteriole

and distal convoluted tubule near the glomerulus comprises the juxtaglomerular apparatus (Fig. 14.2). At this site there are specialized cells in both the afferent arteriole and in the tubule. The latter, termed *macula densa* cells, are able to respond to changes in the rate of flow and the composition of tubule fluid, and are thought to control renin release from the specialized granular renin-containing cells in the afferent arteriole. The juxtaglomerular apparatus is important in controlling the blood flow to the nephron and the glomerular filtration rate. Factors extrinsic to a kidney can influence these processes through circulating hormones and through noradrenergic sympathetic fibres which supply the afferent and efferent arterioles and the specialized cells. The role of the juxtaglomerular apparatus in the control of sodium metabolism is dealt with below and in Chapter 16. Its role in cardiovascular dynamics is considered in Chapter 11.

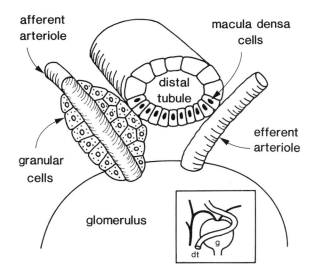

Fig. 14.2 The juxtaglomerular apparatus with cutaway sections to show the granular renin-containing cells round the afferent arteriole and the *macula densa* in the distal convoluted tubule. The inset shows the general relationships between the structures. (g = glomerulus, dt = distal tubule) (Modified from: Sullivan & Grantham, 1982)

Glomerular filtration

Fluid is driven from the capillaries into the tubular capsule (Bowman's capsule) by hydrodynamic force. It crosses three layers — the capillary endothelium, basement membrane and the epithelial cell layer of the capsule. These form a complex filter which excludes large molecules. The passage of substances above a molecular weight of 5000 will depend largely on their size and shape and partly on their ionic charge. About 50% of the glomerular basement membrane is Type IV collagen, with which negatively charged components are associated—glycoproteins containing carboxyl groups and proteoglycans carrying sulphate groups. This forms a physical and electrostatic barrier to the passage of large anionic molecules such as albumin. Normally all constituents in the plasma, except the plasma proteins, appear in the filtrate, and the blood which passes on through the efferent arteriole to the peritubular capillaries has a higher concentration of plasma proteins and thus a higher oncotic pressure than normal. (The term 'oncotic pressure' refers to osmotic pressure created by large molecules such as the plasma proteins.)

Tubular function

In the epithelium of the tubules, as in all epithelia, the apex or luminal surface of each cell is surrounded by a *zonula occludens*, a specialized region of membrane which forms a tight junction between it and neighbouring cells and which separates the intercellular space from the lumen (see Fig. 14.7). The movement of ions and water across the epithelium can occur both through the cells (the transcellular pathway) and between the cells through the *zonulae occludentes* (the paracellular pathway). The *zonulae* in different parts of the nephron vary in their degree of functional tightness, i.e. their relative permeability to ions. The tightness or leakiness of the epithelium of various portions of the nephron is an important factor in their function. The tight epithelium is the site of action of the major hormones involved in the control of salt and water excretion, and is found in the distal portions of the nephron.

Normally 70–75% of the volume of the ultrafiltrate is absorbed back into the blood in the proximal convoluted tubule, with virtually no change in the sodium concentration or the osmotic pressure of the remaining tubular fluid. In the rest of the renal tubule the electrolyte concentrations and osmotic pressure of the ultrafiltrate vary a great deal under the influence of the antidiuretic hormone, mineralocorticoids and the counter current exchange system in the medulla.

The proximal convoluted tubule

The cells of this part of the tubule are tall and the apical or luminal surface of each is extensively increased by numerous microvilli, forming a brush

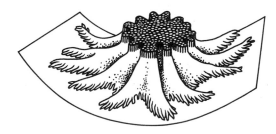

Fig. 14.3 Simplified three-dimensional reconstruction of a cell in the proximal convoluted tubule. (Modified from: Sullivan & Grantham, 1982)

border. The surface area at the sides of the cells is moderately increased and that against the basement membrane is markedly increased by numerous ridges and folds (Fig. 14.3). The epithelium is 'leaky', i.e. the 'zonula occludens' is permeable to ions and water and permits passive flows in either direction. This prevents the build-up of ionic gradients and also means that separate regulation of the movement of ions of water is not possible.

Reabsorption of the filtrate in the proximal convoluted tubule is due to the Na^+/K^+ ATPase which transports sodium out of the tubule. *Water* is reabsorbed as a result of the osmotic force generated by this solute reabsorption, the increased colloid osmotic pressure in the peritubular capillaries contributing to this effect.

The *sodium* reabsorption is related to *potassium* exchange. The tubule cell, like most cells, is freely permeable to potassium, but while being virtually impermeable to sodium at the basolateral surface, is permeable to sodium at the luminal surface. The crucial Na^+/K^+ ATPase is in the basolateral membrane. It transports sodium out of the cell and potassium in, sodium entering the cell at the permeable luminal surface down its electrochemical gradient.

In the first part of the proximal tubule the movement of sodium into the cell is facilitated by *symport* systems for other molecules.* *Glucose* enters the cell with sodium by such a symport process, the co-transport being driven by the electrochemical gradient for sodium across the apical membrane. There are similar symport processes for various *amino-acids* with sodium. It is assumed that in these symport systems there is a two-site carrier in the membrane with one site for sodium and one for glucose or an amino-acid. On the luminal side, where the concentration of sodium is high, sodium combines with its specific site and this increases the affinity of the other site for the other solute. Re-orientation of the binding sites to the inner side of the membrane, where the sodium concentration

is low, favours dissociation of the sodium and consequently of the other solute.

Chloride absorption is largely passive. Some may diffuse through the *zonula occludens*.

Mercurial diuretics exert part of their effect in this part of the nephron. They cause an increase in urine output by preventing the reabsorption of sodium chloride and thus retaining both salt and water in the tubules (Fig. 14.4).

Bicarbonate is returned to the plasma by an indirect method (see Fig. 14.5a). In the cell, carbonic anhydrase catalyses the formation of carbonic acid from CO_2 and water: the acid dissociates to form hydrogen and bicarbonate ions. The bicarbonate ion passes into the plasma and the hydrogen ion is secreted into the lumen, the secretion being balanced electrically by the opposite transport of sodium and involving an antiport system driven by the electrochemical gradient for sodium. In the lumen the hydrogen ions combine with filtered bicarbonate ions to form carbonic acid which breaks down to form water and carbon dioxide. This latter reaction is catalysed by carbonic anhydrase associated with the cell surface. The carbon dioxide diffuses back into the cell. The net effect of these processes is that virtually all the filtered bicarbonate is reabsorbed by the proximal tubule. Drugs, such as **acetazolamide**, which inhibit carbonic anhydrase, increase the volume of urine flow (i.e. are diuretic) by preventing bicarbonate reabsorption (Fig. 14.4). They also result in a depletion of extracellular bicarbonate.

The cells of the proximal convoluted tubule secrete various organic substances into the tubular fluid, including exogenous materials. *Uric acid* excretion (see p. 328) is also regulated by this part of the nephron.

After passage through the proximal tubule the remaining 25–30% of the filtrate, which is still isosmotic with plasma but almost free of potassium and bicarbonate, passes on to the loop of Henle.

The loop of Henle

The loop of Henle plays an important part in regulating the osmolarity of the urine, and hence in regulating the osmotic balance of the body as a whole. Its function is summarized in Figure 14.5.

The loop consists of a descending and an ascend-

---

* In a *symport* or co-transport system, the transport of one substance is coupled to that of another, both being transported across a membrane in the same direction, as opposed to an *antiport* system in which two substances are exchanged across a membrane.

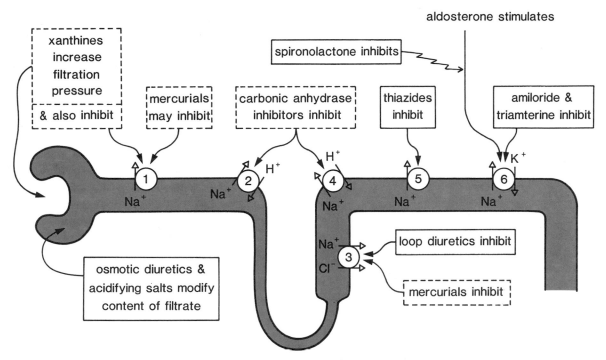

Fig. 14.4 Sodium absorption in the nephron and the main sites of action of diuretic drugs.

Sites of sodium absorption: (1) Na^+ (passive Cl^- absorption); (2) Na^+/H^+ exchange; (3) Na^+Cl^- co-transport; (4) Na^+/H^+ exchange; (5) Na^+ transport (passive Cl^- absorption); (6) Na^+/K^+ exchange.

Currently used diuretics are boxed in with solid lines, obsolete or near obsolete diuretics in dashed lines.

ing portion, each with both thick and thin segments, the thin segments having flattened epithelium and the thick segments having cuboidal epithelium fairly similar to that of the proximal convoluted tubule.

The *descending* limb is highly permeable to water which moves out passively under the influence of osmotic forces. These forces arise because the interstitial fluid of the medulla is hypertonic (see below), and possibly also because the capillaries surrounding the loop may be derived from the efferent arteriole and the plasma within them has a relatively high oncotic pressure. In juxtamedullary nephrons with long loops there is extensive movement of water out of the tubule (and also movement of urea in) so that the fluid eventually reaching the tip of the loop has a high osmolarity—up to 1500 mosm/litre under conditions of dehydration.

The *ascending* limb has very low permeability to water. In the thick segment of this limb there is **active reabsorption of sodium chloride, not accompanied by water**, which reduces the osmolarity of the tubular fluid and causes the interstitial fluid of the medulla to be hypertonic.

The mechanism of sodium chloride absorption in this portion of the nephron has been a matter of controversy. In *in vitro* experiments the transepithelial potential difference was found to be 4–10 mV, lumen positive, indicating that chloride absorption was occurring against an opposing electrochemical gradient. This led to the view that chloride absorption was an active process, that it generated the electrical gradient and that sodium reabsorption was secondary. However, it was difficult to reconcile this hypothesis with the fact that there is a high concentration of Na^+/K^+ ATPase in the basolateral surface of the cells in this segment of the nephron and the fact that ouabain (an inhibitor of this enzyme) blocks chloride absorption. It is now considered that sodium and chloride move into the cell by a co-transport system, this process being driven by the electrochemical gradient for sodium produced by the Na^+/K^+ ATPase in the baso-lateral membrane; chloride then passes into the circulation while some sodium diffuses back into the lumen via the *zonula occludens* which in this part of the nephron forms a cation-selective tight junction. This partial back-flux of sodium contributes to the generation of the transepithelial lumen-positive potential difference.

The **'loop' diuretics** (which are described in detail below) act by inhibiting the co-transport of sodium and chloride into the cells of the thick segment of the ascending limb of the loop of Henle. The absorption of sodium and chloride and the site of action of these drugs are illustrated in Figures 14.4 & 14.11.

Mercurial diuretics also have some degree of inhibitory action on the co-transport system for sodium and chloride (see Fig. 14.4).

The tubular fluid, after passage through the loop of Henle, has been reduced in volume by a further 5% and rendered hypotonic by absorption of salt. As it enters the distal convoluted tubule, its osmolarity is about 150 mosm/l. The thick ascending limb of the loop of Henle is sometimes referred to as the 'diluting segment' because the absorption of salt with very little water results in this marked dilution of the filtrate.

As the ascending part of the loop of Henle is virtually impermeable to *urea* the concentration of this substance will be fairly high in the fluid which reaches the distal nephron.

The distal tubule

This is a zone of transition between the 'diluting segment' and the cortical collecting tubule rather than a distinct functional unit. This portion of the nephron has 'tight' epithelia, i.e. the *zona occludens* has low permeability to both ions and water. Because of this property, ion and water movement can be dissociated and individual regulation of each can be influenced by hormones.

In this section of the nephron, **active salt transport** continues to dilute the tubular fluid until its osmolarity is below that of plasma. The transport is driven by the sodium-potassium pump in the basolateral membrane, sodium diffusing into the cell from the lumen, accompanied by chloride. The mineralocorticoid hormone, **aldosterone**, enhances sodium reabsorption and potassium excretion in this region. As explained in Chapter 17 (page 404), it acts by binding to high affinity, low capacity receptors in the nucleus and directing the synthesis of specific messenger RNA and subsequently of a

mediator protein or proteins. The ultimate effect is an increase in the number of apical membrane sodium channels. In addition aldosterone may exert long-term effects on the number and/or activity of the basolateral sodium pumps.

Aldosterone secretion is controlled indirectly by the juxtaglomerular apparatus (see Fig. 14.2) which is sensitive to the composition of the fluid in the distal tubule. A decrease in the sodium chloride concentration of the filtrate is sensed by the *macula densa* cells of the distal tubule, which stimulate renin release. This leads to the formation of angiotensin I and subsequently angiotensin II (see Chapter 11), which in turn stimulates the synthesis and release of aldosterone. The sympathetic nervous system has a role in renin secretion through β-receptors, and β-adrenoreceptor antagonists such as propranolol reduce renin release (see Chapter 11). The renin-angiotensin-aldosterone system and the mechanism of action of aldosterone are considered in more detail in Chapters 11 (p. 269) & 16. **Spironolactone** exerts a diuretic effect by antagonizing the action of aldosterone in this part of the nephron (see Fig. 14.4).

Bicarbonate is exchanged for hydrogen ions as in the proximal tubule and carbonic anhydrase inhibitors act by preventing this exchange (see Fig. 14.4).

Ammonia may be produced and pass into the tubular fluid (see below).

In the distal convoluted tubule and in the collecting tubules (see below) the absorption of water is under the control of the **antidiuretic hormone** (ADH), also termed **vasopressin** (see Chapter 11), which produces a sustained increase in the permeability to water, allowing its passive reabsorption. This hormone is secreted by the posterior pituitary gland (p. 366) and binds to receptors in the basolateral membrane. These receptors, which are different from those involved in vascular responses (p. 260), are termed V_2-receptors and the ligand/receptor binding results in stimulation of adenylate cyclase and the activation of a cyclic AMP-dependent kinase. (This contrasts with the effect of stimulation of the V_1-receptors on smooth muscle and other cells such as hepatocytes in which the transduction mechanism involves calcium influx and polyphosphoinositide turnover; see p. 23 & 260.) The eventual result of stimulation of the V_2-receptors is an increase in the number of water channels in the apical membrane, thought to be derived from pre-existing vesicles in the sub-apical cytoplasm. Microfilaments and microtubules are important in this effect, possibly in the translocation of the vesicles. Changes in the cytosolic calcium are thought to be involved in this process. The passive movement of water is dependent on the osmotic gradient which in turn is dependent on the counter-current system (see below).

Thiazide diuretics act in this part of the nephron, as do the potassium-sparing diuretics, **triamterene** and **amiloride**.

The collecting tubules and ducts

Several distal tubules empty into each collecting tubule which carries the tubular fluid straight down from the cortex to the medulla. Collecting tubules join to form collecting ducts (see Fig. 14.1). This part of the nephron has 'tight' epithelium, i.e. **low permeability to water and ions in the absence of ADH or aldosterone**. Permeability to *water* is controlled by ADH throughout the length of this portion of the nephron. Water reabsorption occurs particularly in the medulla where the interstitial tissue has a high osmolarity. *Sodium* and *chloride* are absorbed as in the distal convoluted tubule (though at lower rates) and absorption is stimulated by aldosterone. In addition to increasing water permeability, ADH also causes a transient increase in active transport of sodium ions mainly by increasing sodium permeability in the apical membrane. *Hydrogen* ions and *ammonia* may be added to the tubular fluid. *Urea* is reabsorbed from the medullary section of the tubule and passes into the interstitial tissue where it plays a part in increasing the osmolarity of this area.

The potassium-sparing diuretics may exert some of their diuretic action in the early parts of the collecting duct system.

THE CONTROL OF EXTRACELLULAR FLUID OSMOLARITY

The *volume* and *osmolarity* of the extracellular fluid are determined by the amount of sodium in this fluid compartment and are maintained within narrow limits despite continuous variation in the intake of salt and water in the diet. The renal processes for regulating the reabsorption of salt and water constitute the primary means of controlling the volume and osmolarity of the extracellular fluid. The interaction of the various renal and vascular elements to provide the concentrating and diluting mechanisms of the kidney are outlined below.

Receptors sensitive to *osmotic* changes occur in the hypothalamus and affect the kidney through the secretion of the posterior pituitary antidiuretic hormone, which controls water excretion. This is the most powerful of the mechanisms which control the osmolarity of the extracellular fluid.

A detailed treatment of *volume* regulation is beyond the scope of this textbook. In summary, receptors sensitive to changes in extracellular fluid volume occur in the heart and arteries, and possibly also in the liver and the central nervous system. They act on the kidney through both nervous pathways and hormonal influences. These latter include not only the renin-angiotensin-aldosterone system, but also prostaglandins, kinins and the recently-discovered atrial natriuretic peptides* (see Chapter 11).

CONCENTRATING MECHANISMS: THE COUNTER-CURRENT MULTIPLIER SYSTEM IN THE MEDULLA

The structures involved in this system are the long loops of Henle, the *vasa recta* and the collecting tubules, which by virtue of their anatomical arrangements allow for counter-current flow. The tubular fluid and plasma flowing down into the medulla run in close proximity to tubular fluid and plasma flowing up out of the medulla. The main principle of the counter-current exchange is that a small horizontal osmotic gradient is multiplied vertically, establishing and maintaining a hyperosmotic environment in the medulla. **The primary generating force is the active reabsorption of salt in the ascend-**

---

* Atrial natriuretic peptides (atriopeptius) are a family of peptides released from the heart in response to atrial stretch, volume expansion and increased body sodium. The peptides act primarily on the kidney, producing marked vasodilatation, natriuresis and diuresis. They also reduce aldosterone release.

ing limb of the loop of Henle. This, with the differences in epithelial permeability of the structures in the medulla, outlined above, particularly the low permeability to water in the ascending limb of the loop of Henle, results in an osmotic gradient in the medulla which ranges from isotonicity (300 mosm/litre) at the cortical boundary to 1200–1500 mosm or more in the innermost area (see Fig. 14.5). It is postulated that urea contributes to this gradient because it is more slowly reabsorbed than water throughout most of the nephron (it may be *added* to the descending limb; Fig. 14.5) and so its concentration rises until it reaches the collecting tubules in the medulla where it diffuses out into the interstitia. It is thus 'trapped' in the inner medulla.

The main site at which the urine is concentrated is in the collecting tubule as it passes into the medulla where there is passive reabsorption of water due to the increasing osmolarity of the interstitium. This absorption depends on the **antidiuretic hormone** which controls the permeability to water of this part of the nephron. When there is adequate hydration, secretion of ADH is very low and water is not reabsorbed in the latter part of the distal convoluted tubule and the collecting ducts; then hypotonic urine is formed corresponding to the low osmolarity of the fluid entering the distal tubule.

An inhibition of the action of antidiuretic hormone is seen as a side effect of some drugs—lithium carbonate (used in psychiatric disorders; see Chapter 23), demeclocycline (an antibiotic) and agents which affect the microtubules such as colchicine and the vinca alkaloids.

ACID-BASE BALANCE

The kidneys participate in the regulation of the hydrogen ion concentration of the body fluids. Though either an acid or alkaline urine can be excreted according to need, the basic requirement is the formation of an acid urine to compensate for the tendency to a decrease in body pH consequent on the metabolic production of CO_2. The main renal mechanism is the secretion of hydrogen ions into the tubular fluid and the conservation of bicarbonate. This depends on the carbonic anhydrase-catalysed reactions outlined above and illustrated in Figure 14.6a. In the *proximal* convuluted tubule

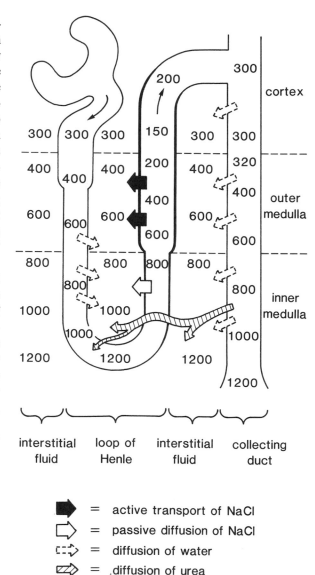

= active transport of NaCl

= passive diffusion of NaCl

= diffusion of water

= .diffusion of urea

Fig. 14.5 The counter-current mechanisms for concentrating the urine. The figures are in milliosmoles per litre. The three main requirements for a counter-current multiplier are shown:
1. counter-current flow
2. differences in permeability between tubules carrying fluid in opposite directions. The thickened outline of the ascending limb of Henle's loop indicates decreased permeability to water in contrast to the water-permeable descending loop
3. a source of energy, which is supplied by the active transport of sodium chloride. (Loop diuretics act by inhibiting this active transport, thus interfering with the counter-current concentrating mechanism).

The absorption of water in the collecting ducts is controlled by the antidiuretic hormone. Additional active reabsorption of sodium chloride, which is not part of the counter-current mechanism, occurs in the distal tubule and is controlled by aldosterone.

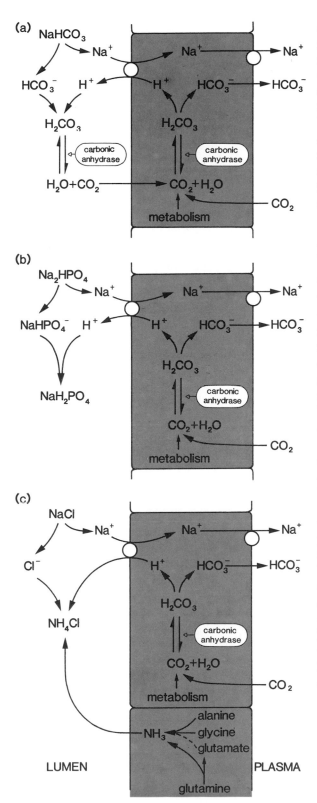

about 80–99% of the bicarbonate in the filtrate, is reabsorbed by this process. The process of conserving bicarbonate and excreting hydrogen ions also occurs in the *distal* and *collecting* tubules. Here the sodium ions in the tubular fluid are accompanied mainly by chloride and phosphate ions, since the bicarbonate has been largely reabsorbed (Fig. 14.6b & c). One of the buffering systems in this part of the nephron depends on the fact that ammonia is generated in the distal tubules and collecting tubules, mostly from glutamine, but also from other amino acids such as glycine and alanine (Fig. 14.6c).

POTASSIUM BALANCE

The extracellular potassium concentration is controlled rapidly and within narrow limits by regulation of potassium excretion by the kidney. This regulation is very important because small changes in extracellular $[K^+]$ affect the function of many excitable tissues, particularly the heart, brain and skeletal muscle. Urinary potassium excretion is normally about 50–100 mEq in 24 hours, but can be as low as 5 mEq or as high as 1000 mEq. The amount which normally appears in the urine represents potassium secreted into the filtrate in the *distal* parts of the nephron, as virtually all of the filtered potassium is reabsorbed in the proximal tubule and loop of Henle.

The mechanisms whereby potassium is added to the filtrate in the distal nephron are not completely clear. Potassium is transported into the cell from the blood and the interstitial fluid by the Na^+/K^+-ATPase in the basolateral membrane. It can then enter the lumen passively, the electrochemical gradient being favourable because of the small potential difference (~ 30 mV) across the luminal membrane. However, it is thought that there is also an active transport mechanism in the luminal membrane which may transport potassium either into or out of the cell. A high flow rate of

Fig. 14.6 Renal mechanisms for conserving base. Sodium is absorbed and hydrogen ions secreted at the luminal surface; an antiport mechanism may be involved. Most bicarbonate in the filtrate is 'reabsorbed' in the proximal tubule (shown in a). In the distal tubule (b & c) bicarbonate is added to the plasma and monobasic phosphate or ammonium chloride is added to the urine.

filtrate through the distal tubules favours potassium excretion by continually flushing it away, decreasing its concentration in the tubules and increasing the gradient from cell to lumen. Increased delivery of sodium to the distal nephron also augments the rate of potassium excretion because the increased sodium concentration decreases the luminal membrane potential and increases the electrochemical gradient for potassium from cell to lumen. It also stimulates Na^+/K^+ exchange by the Na^+/K^+-ATPase. This consequence of increased sodium delivery to the distal nephron is an important side effect of many diuretics.

Mineralocorticoids facilitate potassium excretion by an increase in transport of potassium into the cell at the basolateral membrane, or an increase in potassium conductance at the lumenal membrane, or both.

EXCRETION OF ORGANIC MOLECULES

There are different mechanisms for the excretion of organic anions and organic cations (see Chapter 3).

Organic anions may be bound to plasma albumin and consequently will not appear in the glomerular filtrate, but when the blood from the glomerulus passes into the peritubular capillary plexus some of these substances, such as *urate* and *p-aminohippuric acid* are secreted into the proximal convoluted tubules. The secretion involves a transport process in the relatively impermeable basolateral membrane followed by diffusion down a concentration gradient into the lumen through the more permeable luminal membrane. Amongst the drugs excreted in this way are the **thiazides**, **ethacrynic acid**, **frusemide**, **salicylates** and **penicillin G**.

Organic cations are secreted by transport processes in both the basolateral and luminal membranes. Many drugs are eliminated by this route: **atropine**, **morphine**, **quinine**, etc.

This topic is dealt with in more detail in Chapter 3.

ARACHIDONIC ACID METABOLITES AND RENAL FUNCTION

The metabolites of arachidonic acid, the eicosanoids, which are generated in the kidney, are now recognized as important modulators of its haemodynamics and excretory functions. Details of the eicosanoids are given in Chapter 8 (p. 192).

Prostanoids, the products of the cyclo-oxygenase pathway, are synthesized in all parts of the kidney, the predominant products being PGE_2 and $PGF_{2\alpha}$. Factors which stimulate their synthesis include ischaemia, mechanical trauma, circulating angiotensin II, catecholamines, antidiuretic hormone and bradykinin.

Influence on haemodynamics. Under basal conditions prostaglandins derived from endogenous synthesis probably do not have a significant part to play in the control of renal blood flow and the glomerular filtration rate, although the fact that angiotensin II stimulates the release of vasodilator prostaglandins implies that they may provide a local braking mechanism on its vasoconstrictor action. Prostaglandins play a part in the control of renin release under basal conditions and also in conditions of intravascular volume depletion.

Influence on the renal handling of salt and water. Medullary prostaglandins may influence three aspects of this process. It is believed that they can reduce ADH-dependent water permeability in the distal nephron, that they can reduce NaCl reabsorption in the thick segment of the ascending limb of Henle's loop and that they can enhance medullary blood flow. An increase in the production of medullary prostaglandins thus results in a decrease in the solute content in the medullary interstitium and an increase in water excretion. Their overall action, therefore, is to cause a reduction in the effect of antidiuretic hormone, and it is believed that their function is the 'fine tuning' of water excretion. Whether this is an important consideration when NSAIDs are used in therapy is still a matter of controversy.

DRUGS ACTING ON THE KIDNEY

DIURETICS

Diuretics are drugs which cause a net loss of sodium and water from the body by an action on the kidney. Their primary effect is to decrease the reabsorption from the filtrate of sodium and chloride, increased water loss being secondary to the increased excretion of salt. This can be achieved by (1) a direct action on the cells of the nephron, or (2) indirectly modifying the content of the filtrate. Since a very large proportion of the salt and water which passes into the tubule in the glomerulosa is reabsorbed (Table 14.1) a small decrease in reabsorption can result in a marked increase in excretion. A summary diagram of the mechanisms and sites of action of various diuretics is given in Figure 14.4.

THE DEVELOPMENT OF DIURETIC DRUGS

The diuretics used prior to 1920 were **xanthines** (e.g. theophylline, caffeine) and **osmotic diuretics** (e.g. urea). These were subsequently supplemented by the organic **mercurial diuretics**, the action of these drugs on the kidney having been discovered inadvertently in 1919 when they were used to treat syphilis. Large numbers of organic mercurial compounds were synthesized and tested for diuretic action during the next 30 years, and although this group of diuretics is now no longer used, this period was important in that it became clear that potent and effective diuretics could be generated in the laboratory and that clinicians need no longer rely on natural products. The next group of compounds introduced were the **carbonic anhydrase inhibitors**. These were developed from the sulphonamides, following on the observation that sulphanilamide (p. 628) caused, as a side effect, a metabolic acidosis, with alkaline urine and a mild diuresis. This effect was found to be due to inhibition of renal carbonic anhydrase. The programmes of molecular modification and research which followed have led to the introduction of some very important and useful compounds into clinical medicine. Since this gives an indication of how modern drugs are developed, a brief outline of the sequence of events will be given.

Sulphanilamide was soon superseded, as an anti-

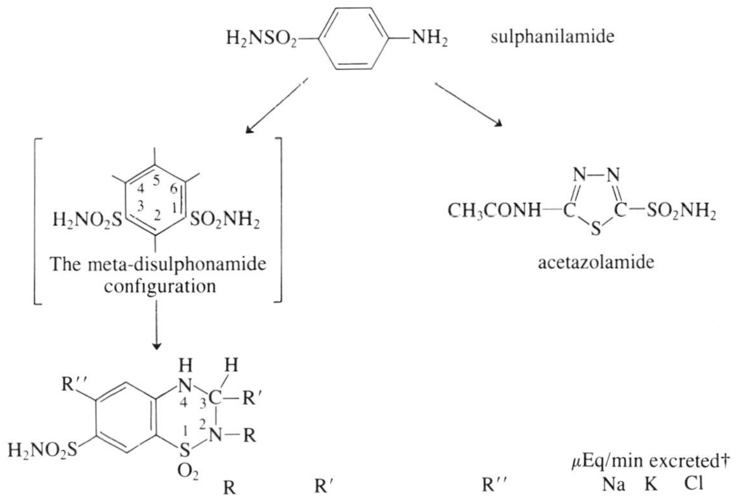

	R	R′	R″	μEq/min excreted† Na	K	Cl
chlorothiazide*	H	H	Cl	20	24	7
hydrochlorothiazide	H	H	Cl	265	33	291
bendrofluazide	H	CH_2—	CF_3	493	61	455
cyclopenthiazide	H	CH_2—	Cl	—	—	—

Fig. 14.7 Development of diuretics from sulphanilamide by molecular modification.
* This compound has a double bond between N-4 and C-3
† the effect on excretion of ions with an intravenous dose of 0.5 mg/kg per hour

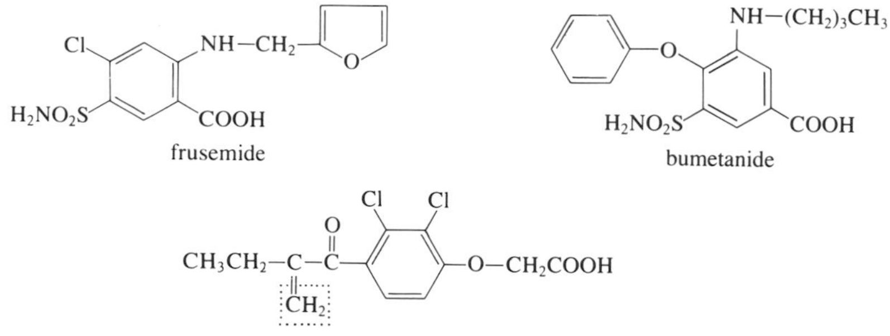

frusemide bumetanide ethacrynic acid

Fig. 14.8 Loop diuretics. The boxed methylene group of ethacrynic acid forms an adduct with cysteine *in vivo* and this adduct is thought to be the pharmacologically active form of the drug.

bacterial agent, by safer compounds all of which had substituents on the sulphonamide nitrogen (p. 629). None of these new compounds, however, had carbonic anhydrase inhibitory activity and it became clear that such activity required the free primary amine of the sulphonamide moiety (Fig. 14.7). As a result of further modifications of the original structure, the heterocyclic compond **acetazolamide** (Fig. 14.7) was introduced in 1950. Acetazolamide, unlike the mercurials, could be given orally and was 300 times more potent than sulphanilamide in inhibiting carbonic anhydrase. Further molecular modifications, in which diuretic activity was sought rather than carbonic anhydrase inhibition, resulted in studies of meta-disulphonamides and gave rise eventually to **chlorothiazide** and **hydrochlorothiazide**, then **bendrofluazide**, the series showing increasing potency in promoting sodium excretion, not accompanied by equivalent potency on potassium excretion. Numerous other similar compounds have been produced.* (A by-product of the research on thiazides was the development of **diazoxide**, an antihypertensive agent (see Chapter 11).

Further molecular modifications led in the early 1960s to the compounds **frusemide** and **bumetanide** which, though also sulphonamides, have very few chemical features in common with the thiazides (Fig. 14.8). Their mechanism of action is also different from that of the thiazides. They are **loop diuretics** with a 'ceiling' of diuresis much higher than that of the thiazides; their action is similar to that of **ethacrynic acid**, a compound which was developed in a quite different research programme in which attempts were being made to find drugs that acted, like mercurials, by combining with sulphydryl groups.

Although all these compounds proved to be very effective in promoting sodium excretion, all resulted in potassium loss and this prompted the search for potassium-sparing diuretics. Aldosterone antagonists such as **spironolactone** (Fig. 14.9), introduced in 1962, partially satisfied this requirement, but they had several drawbacks. Numerous compounds were screened and eventually **amiloride** and **triamterene** emerged (Fig. 14.9). These drugs were

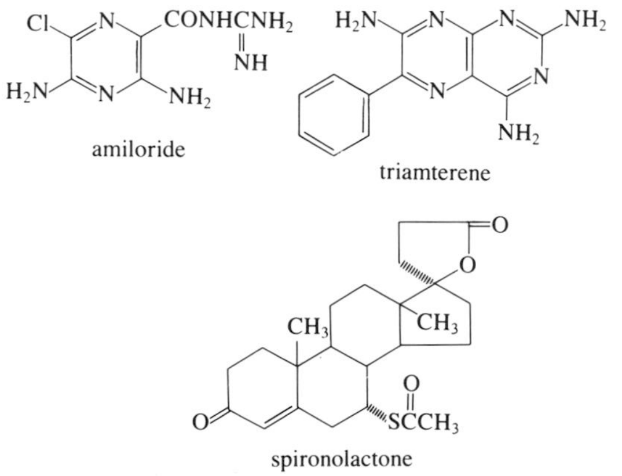

amiloride triamterene spironolactone

Fig. 14.9 Potassium-sparing diuretics.

* It would be apposite to mention, in this context, that molecular modification of an isopropylthiadiazole derivative of sulphanilamide gave rise to the oral antidiabetic agents, the sulphonylureas and that investigation of the goitrogenic action of sulphaguanidine led to the development of the antithyroid drugs thiouracil, prophylthiouracil and methimazole (see Chapter 16).

developed from two different research programmes but they have rather similar sites of action.

The most recent development in this area is the attempt to develop uricosuric diuretics to overcome the problem that most currently used diuretics tend to result in an increase in the plasma uric acid concentration.

DIURETICS ACTING DIRECTLY ON THE CELLS OF THE NEPHRON

Drugs which cause a net salt loss by an action on cells must obviously affect those parts of the nephron where most of *active* and selective solute reabsorption occurs—(a) the ascending loop of Henle, and (b) the distal nephron.

LOOP DIURETICS

These are the most powerful of all diuretics, capable of causing 15–25% of the sodium in the filtrate to be

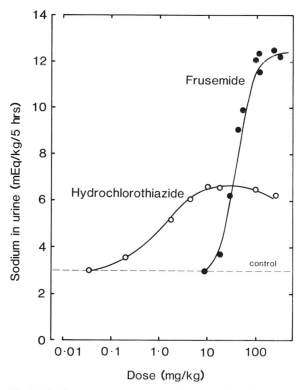

Fig. 14.10 The dose-response curves for frusemide and hydrochlorothiazide. (Adopted from: Timmerman et al, 1964)

excreted and are termed 'high ceiling' diuretics (see Fig. 14.10). The main examples are **frusemide**, **ethacrynic acid** and **bumetanide**. They are drugs which act primarily on the thick segment of the ascending loop of Henle inhibiting the transport of sodium chloride out of the tubule into the interstitium (see Fig. 14.4). As has been explained above, the reabsorption of solute at this site is the basis for the ability of the kidney to concentrate the urine by creating a hypertonic interstitium in the medulla, which provides the osmotic force by which water is reabsorbed from the collecting tubules under the influence of the antidiuretic hormone. This action of the drugs on the loop has the additional effect that more solute is delivered to the distal portions of the nephron where its osmotic pressure further reduces water reabsorption. Essentially some of the solute which normally passes into the medullary interstitium and draws water out of the collecting ducts, now remains in the tubular fluid and holds water with it. As much as 25% of the glomerular filtrate may pass out of the nephron resulting in an intense diuresis.

The molecular basis of the action of these drugs is not clear, but it has been shown that if frusemide is placed in the lumen of the thick ascending limb it very rapidly abolishes the transepithelial potential difference and inhibits absorption of sodium chloride. It acts only on the apical, luminal side of the cell, and has no effect on the contraluminal side, which implies that it inhibits the cotransport of sodium of chloride into the cell (Fig. 14.11). The action of bumetanide is very similar, the principal difference being that it is 40–50 times more potent. Ethacrynic acid forms a complex with cysteine which may be the active form of the drug. This compound may act in a similar manner to frusemide, but there is also evidence that it inhibits the supply of energy for ion transport.

The loop diuretics are thought to have a subsidiary action in that they are all capable of increasing renal blood flow (RBF) without affecting glomerular filtration rate (GFR), more particularly when they are given intravenously. The result of this is that the filtration fraction, which is given by GFR/RBF, is decreased, i.e. a smaller proportion of the blood passing through the kidney is filtered into the nephrons. The protein in the peritubular capillaries is therefore less concentrated, there is de-

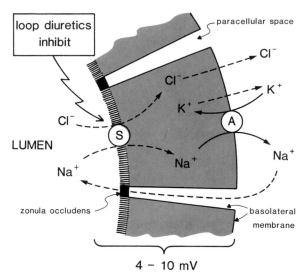

Fig. 14.11 Electrolyte transport in the cells of the thick ascending segment of the loop of Henle. Solid lines indicate active transport, dashed lines, passive transport; S = symport (co-transport); A = anti-port. (The *zonula occludens* in this portion of the nephron is thought to function as a cation-selective tight junction, allowing partial backflux of sodium ions; this contributes to the generation of the lumen-positive potential difference.) Potassium is also absorbed from the lumen (not shown). The transepithelial potential difference (4–10 mV) is lumen positive.

creased oncotic pressure, less reabsorption from the proximal convoluted tubule and thus increased solute and therefore water in the tubular filtrate. In addition, frusemide increases blood flow through the medulla, dissipating somewhat the hypertonicity of the medulla, and thus decreasing the efficiency of the counter-current exchange system.

Some of the effects of frusemide, in particular the vascular effects, may be mediated by prostaglandins, PGE_2 and PGI_2, because indomethacin produces a slight reduction in its diuretic action. Both frusemide and ethacrynic acid have been shown to inhibit prostaglandin degradation.

The action of these drugs is independent of acid/base balance in that they are effective in alkalosis and acidosis. But they themselves cause a pronounced electrolyte imbalance, not only loss of sodium and chloride, but also potassium. This last effect is the result of both the increased sodium load and the increased volume of filtrate delivered to the distal tubule enhancing potassium excretion. Loop diuretics may produce a metabolic alkalosis because volume depletion (either absolute or relative), and potassium depletion both stimulate hydrogen ion

secretion and bicarbonate generation. A decrease in $[K^+]_0$ also causes loss of K^+ from cells in exchange for H^+, causing alkalosis.

An increase in magnesium and calcium excretion is associated with the increased excretion of sodium chloride.

Pharmacokinetic aspects

The loop diuretics are readily absorbed from the gastrointestinal tract and may also be given by injection. They are strongly bound to plasma protein and so do not pass into the glomerular filtrate to any marked degree. They reach their site of action by being secreted in the proximal convoluted tubule by the organic acid transport mechanism and the fraction thus secreted will be excreted in the urine. Given orally, they act within the hour and their duration of action is 4–6 hours. Given intravenously the peak effect occurs within 30 minutes. In the case of all three compounds a proportion of the dose is excreted in the faeces. The rates of elimination are high and cumulation does not occur.

Unwanted effects

Some unwanted effects are common with loop diuretics, and are directly related to their renal actions. The **loss of potassium** and of **hydrogen ions** causes a **hypokalaemic metabolic alkalosis** as described above. Hypokalaemia can be averted or treated by concomitant use of potassium-sparing diuretics (see below) or by potassium supplements. **Depletion of magnesium and calcium** is common, and **hypovolaemia** and **hypotension** may follow the torrential diuresis produced by these agents.

Unwanted effects which are not related to the renal actions of the drugs are infrequent. A potentially serious toxic effect is ototoxicity; concomitant use of an aminoglycoside antibiotic will compound the problem. Allergic reactions (skin rashes, blood dyscrasias) may be seen, rarely, but with frusemide and bumetanide are more likely to occur in patients who have developed hypersensitivity to other sulphonamide derivatives. An allergic interstitial nephritis has been described with frusemide and the kidney damage produced by cephalosporin antibiotics is exacerbated by this drug.

Bumetanide can cause myalgia. Ethacrynic acid is more likely than the other loop diuretics to cause gastrointestinal upsets.

Clinical use

Loop diuretics are used in:

1. Acute pulmonary oedema, where a rapid decrease of extracellular fluid volume is required
2. Oedema due to heart failure and liver disease, and some cases of renal oedema, particularly if refractory to less powerful diuretics
3. Hypercalcaemia, where their action in increasing calcium excretion may be of benefit
4. Electrolyte disturbances. Hyperkalaemia and the toxic effect of halides (which are absorbed in the thick ascending limb of the loop) may be countered by loop diuretics, though the use of these drugs should be accompanied by saline infusion.

DIURETICS ACTING ON THE DISTAL NEPHRON

The term 'distal nephron' refers to the distal convoluted tubules, collecting tubules and collecting ducts. Drugs active at this site include **thiazides**, **spironolactone**, **triamterene** and **amiloride**.

Thiazides and related drugs

The development of this group of drugs is outlined above. The main thiazides are **hydrochlorothiazide**, **bendrofluazide** and **cyclopenthiazide**, but many similar drugs are available. Of the drugs related to the thiazides and having similar actions the main one is **chlorthalidone**, and newer ones are **indapamide** and **xipamide** (Fig. 14.12).

This group of drugs has a moderately powerful diuretic action. They inhibit active reabsorption of sodium and accompanying chloride in the distal tubule resulting in 5–10% of sodium in the filtrate being excreted (see Fig. 14.4). They do not have any action on the thick ascending loop of Henle. The precise mode of action on the cells is not known, but experimental evidence suggests a luminal site of action involving a decreased membrane permeability to both sodium and chloride. They may also have some action on the proximal convoluted tubule. Some have a slight inhibitory effect on carbonic anhydrase, but this is not a significant aspect of their diuretic action, though, as described above, this group of drugs was developed from studies with carbonic anhydrase inhibitors.

Potassium excretion with these drugs is significant and can be serious. The loss of potassium is consequent on the increased delivery of sodium to the distal tubules and resultant increased potassium secretion, as explained previously.

Subsidiary effects are decreases in both uric acid excretion and calcium excretion and an increase in magnesium excretion. Thiazide diuretics have a paradoxical effect in diabetes insipidus (p. 367), where they *reduce* the volume of urine.

The action of this group of drugs is unaffected by changes in the acid-base balance (i.e. they are effective in alkalosis and acidosis) but they may themselves give rise to a hypochloraemic alkalosis.

They have some extra-renal actions. Thus they

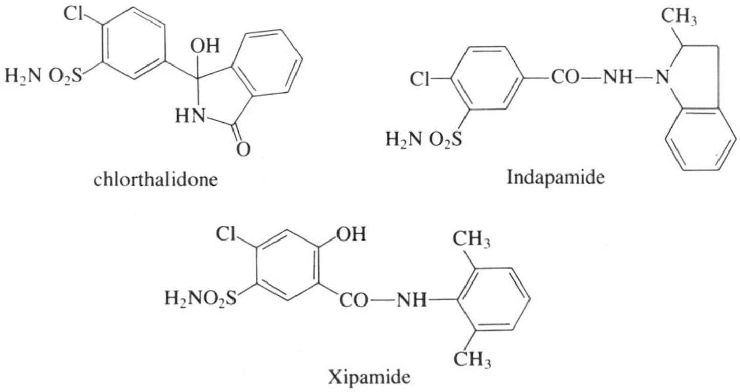

Fig. 14.12 Some diuretics related to the thiazide compounds.

are thought to have some *vasodilator* effects. When used in the treatment of hypertension the initial fall in blood pressure is due to decreased blood volume resulting from diuresis, but the later phase seems to be due to a direct and ill-understood action on the blood vessels. Diazoxide, a non-diuretic thiazide, has powerful vasodilator effects (see Chapter 11). This action may be related to another extra-renal effect which is sometimes seen, that of increasing the blood sugar. Diazoxide also has this latter effect, though whether by the same mechanism is not clear. Indapamide is said to lower blood pressure with less metabolic disturbance.

Pharmacokinetic aspects

The thiazides and related drugs are all effective orally, being well absorbed from the gastrointestinal tract. All are excreted both by glomerular filtration and tubular secretion. Their tendency to increase plasma uric acid is due to competition with uric acid for tubular secretion. With the shorter-acting drugs such as hydrochlororothiazide, chlorothiazide and cyclopenthiazide, onset of action is within 1–2 hours, maximum effect at about 4–6 hours and duration between 8 and 12 hours. The longer-acting drugs, such as bendrofluazide, have a similar onset but a duration of 24 hours. Chlorthalidone's action may last for 2–3 days.

Unwanted effects

The main unwanted effects are repercussions of the renal actions—**hypokalaemia** and **metabolic alkalosis**. An increased plasma uric acid is likely to occur but usually does not cause any problems except in individuals susceptible to gout. Hyperglycaemia has been reported and will exacerbate diabetes mellitus.

These agents have a fairly large therapeutic index and toxic effects are relatively rare, but hypersensitivity reactions may occur and include dermatitis, blood dyscrasias, acute pancreatitis, and acute pulmonary oedema. In cases of hepatic failure, thiazides may precipitate encephalopathy.

Clinical use

Thiazides are the diuretics of choice in cardiac failure and are also used to treat hypertension. Their paradoxical anti-diuretic effect in patients with diabetes insipidus may be made use of to treat this condition, and the capacity to increase calcium excretion may be of value in hypercalcaemia.

Spironolactone

This drug has a limited diuretic action, causing only about 5% of the sodium in the filtrate to be excreted. It is an antagonist of aldosterone, the main endogenous mineralocorticoid, competing with aldosterone for intracellular receptors in the cells of the distal tubule (see Chapter 16). The spironolactone-receptor complex does not apparently attach to the DNA and the subsequent processes of transcription, translation and production of mediator proteins do not occur. The result is an inhibition of the sodium-retaining action of aldosterone (see Fig. 14.4), and a concomitant decrease in its potassium-secreting effect.

Spironolactone has subsidiary actions in decreasing hydrogen ion secretion and also uric acid excretion.

Pharmacokinetic aspects

Spironolactone is well absorbed from the gastrointestinal tract. Its plasma half-life is only 10 minutes but its active metabolite, **canrenone**, has a plasma $t_{\frac{1}{2}}$ of 16 hours. The action of spironolactone is believed to be largely due to canrenone. The onset of action is very slow, taking several days to develop.

Unwanted effects

Gastrointestinal upsets occur fairly frequently. If spironolactone is used on its own it will cause hyperkalaemia and this may also occur if it is given with thiazides in patients with poor kidney function. Actions on steroid receptors in tissues other than the kidney may result in gynaecomastia, menstrual disorders and testicular atrophy. Peptic ulceration has been reported.

Clinical use

Spironolactone is commonly given with the potassium-losing diuretics to **prevent excessive po-**

tassium loss. It is also used to treat patients suffering from hyperaldosteronism, either primary (e.g. due to ectopic ACTH production) or secondary (due to cardiac failure, nephrotic syndrome, hepatic cirrhosis).

Triamterene and amiloride

These drugs, (see Fig. 14.9) like spironolactone, have a limited diuretic efficacy, causing excretion of about 5% of the sodium in the filtrate. They act on the distal convoluted tubule and also the collecting tubules, inhibiting both sodium reabsorption and potassium excretion (see Fig. 14.4). Amiloride decreases the sodium permeability of the luminal membrane (blocking the sodium channels by which aldosterone produces its main effect) making less sodium available for transport across the baso-lateral membrane. Triamterene probably has a similar action. Their effect on potassium secretion may be secondary to this or they may have an effect on potassium secretion by a mechanism which is independent of their action on sodium. By preventing Na^+ entry into the tubular cells, they also reduce Na^+/H^+ exchange, and thus inhibit H^+ excretion resulting in some degree of alkalinization of the urine. This action is less marked in the case of amiloride. Their action is not impaired by alkalosis or acidosis. Both are mildly uricosuric, i.e. they promote the excretion of uric acid.

The main importance of these diuretics lies in their **potassium-sparing ability**. They can be given with potassium-losing diuretics like the thiazides in order to maintain potassium balance.

Pharmacokinetic aspects

Triamterene is well absorbed in the gastrointestinal tract. Its onset of action is within 2 hours and its duration of action 12–16 hours. Amiloride is poorly absorbed and has a slower onset, with a peak action at 6 hours and a duration of action of about 24 hours. Most of the drug is excreted unchanged in the urine.

Unwanted effects

The main unwanted effect is related to the phar-macological actions—hyperkalaemia. Gastrointestinal disturbances may also occur but are infrequent.

DIURETICS WHICH ACT INDIRECTLY BY MODIFYING THE CONTENT OF THE FILTRATE

These are agents which increase either the osmolarity or the sodium load of the filtrate.

Osmotic diuretics

Osmotic diuretics are pharmacologically inert substances (e.g. **mannitol**, **urea**, **isosorbide**) which are filtered in the glomerulus but not (or incompletely) reabsorbed by the nephron (see Fig. 14.4). They can be given in amounts sufficiently large for them to constitute an appreciable fraction of the plasma osmolarity. Within the nephron, their main effect is exerted on the proximal tubule, where passive water reabsorption is reduced by the presence of the non-reabsorbable solute within the tubule. Thus a larger volume of fluid remains within the proximal tubule. This has the secondary effect of reducing sodium reabsorption, since the sodium concentration within the proximal tubule is lower, because of the greater volume, than it otherwise would be, and this alters the electrochemical gradient for sodium reabsorption. Further down the nephron, where the fluid is no longer isotonic, the extra solute is no longer balanced exactly by an osmotically equivalent volume of water, but it still results in a substantial increase in urine volume.

Thus the main effect of osmotic diuretics is to increase the amount of water excreted, with a relatively smaller increase in sodium excretion. They are therefore not useful in treating conditions associated with sodium retention, for which conventional diuretics are widely used, but have much more limited therapeutic applications. These include **acute renal failure** and **acutely raised intra-cranial or intraocular pressure**.

In acute renal failure, which may occur after haemorrhage or in other kinds of hypovolaemic shock, the glomerular filtration rate is reduced, and absorption of salt and water in the proximal tubule becomes almost complete, so that more distal parts of the nephron virtually dry up, and urine flow ceases. This can result in irreversible renal damage, as well as the metabolic consequences of anuria. Retention of fluid within the proximal tubule by administration of an osmotic diuretic prevents these effects. Where there is hypovolaemia, it is of course essential to increase the blood volume, which would otherwise be further reduced by the restoration of urine flow.

The treatment of acute cerebral oedema and glaucoma relies on the increase in plasma osmolarity by solutes which do not enter the brain or eye, which results in extraction of water from these compartments. It has nothing to do with the kidney; indeed the effect is lost as soon as the osmotic diuretic appears in the urine.

Osmotic diuretics can also be used to accelerate the renal excretion of drugs taken in overdose (e.g. salicylates, barbiturates; see Chapter 3), but it is not clear that they are better than conventional diuretics for this purpose.

Osmotic diuretics are usually given intravenously, though isosorbide is given orally to reduce intra-ocular pressure.

Acidifying salts

Acidifying salts, of which the only important one is **ammonium chloride**, produce a weak and transient diuresis. The diuresis occurs because ammonium chloride has the effect of replacing bicarbonate in the plasma and glomerular filtrate by chloride. Ammonium chloride gives rise to ammonia (which is metabolized, mainly to urea), hydrogen ion and chloride ion. The hydrogen ion combines with bicarbonate to produce carbonic acid, so the net result is replacement of bicarbonate by chloride. Since bicarbonate is completely reabsorbed by the proximal tubule, but chloride is not, the result is a diuresis.

At one time acidifying salts were used in conjunction with mercurial diuretics, whose action is limited by the alkalosis that they cause, but this form of diuretic therapy has been superseded.

OBSOLETE OR NEAR-OBSOLETE DIURETICS

Some drugs which were originally used as diuretics have found clinical applications in other fields.

Carbonic anhydrase inhibitors cause increased excretion of bicarbonate with accompanying sodium, potassium and water, resulting in an increased flow of an alkaline urine and a mild metabolic acidosis. The effect is self-limiting as the blood bicarbonate falls. These agents, though not now used as diuretics, may be used in the treatment of glaucoma to reduce the formation of aqueous humor and also in some types of epilepsy. Examples of carbonic anhydrase inhibitors are **acetazolamide** (see Fig. 14.8), **ethoxzolamide**, **methazolamide** and **dichlorphenamide**.

Methylxanthines are compounds with a variety of pharmacological actions—increasing cardiac output (see Chapter 10), relaxing some smooth muscle (see Chapters 11 and 13) and causing stimulation of the central nervous system (see Chapter 26). They have a weak diuretic action attributed partly to inhibition of salt and water reabsorption and partly to an increased glomerular filtration rate by virtue of their action on the heart and the glomerular arteries (see Fig. 14.4). Their use as diuretics has become very rare, **aminophylline** being the only one retained for occasional use.

Organic mercurial compounds such as **mersalyl**, are powerful diuretics, but they have to be given by intra-muscular injection and they may have significant nephrotoxicity. They have been superseded by the thiazides and the loop diuretics.

GENERAL ASPECTS OF THE ACTION OF DIURETIC DRUGS

The 'braking phenomenon' and volume depletion

Though diuretics cause an increase in the excretion of sodium, a negative sodium balance and weight loss, this does not continue indefinitely. In a subject given diuretics, together with a constant sodium intake, the sodium loss decreases gradually over several days until the weight stabilizes and a new steady state occurs in which urinary sodium loss is equal to dietary sodium intake. This reflects adaptation of those parts of the nephron not affected by the diuretic and is a response to the depletion of the volume of the extracellular fluid. However, some degree of depletion of the extracellular fluid volume may occur with loop diuretics.

Alterations in potassium balance

An effect on potassium homeostasis is a clinically important side effect of some diuretics which needs to be emphasized. The **thiazides**, **loop diuretics** and **carbonic anhydrase inhibitors** can cause potassium depletion. Loop diuretics do this by increasing the flow rate, the volume and the sodium content of the filtrate reaching the distal nephron. Thiazides also increase the sodium load to distal parts of the nephron. The higher the sodium content in the filtrate at this point, the greater the Na^+/K^+ exchange and the greater the potassium loss. With a high flow rate, potassium is continually swept away, and a low tubular concentration, and thus a high electrochemical gradient is maintained, favouring secretion. Carbonic anhydrase inhibitors decrease the absorption of bicarbonate in the proximal tubule and the higher concentration of this anion in the distal tubule results in an increase in the secretion of potassium.

Prolonged use of diuretics may cause some depletion of the volume of the extracellular fluid below normal values. This may activate the renin-angiotensin system and result in increased secretion of aldosterone which causes potassium excretion and can thus exacerbate potassium loss.

The metabolic alkalosis which may occur with some diuretics (see below) may also be a factor in increasing potassium excretion. In acute alkalosis there is an increase in cellular potassium in the tubule cells and this apparently stimulates its excretion.

Some diuretics (amiloride, triamterene and spironolactone) *inhibit* potassium excretion as explained above, and may be used in conjunction with potassium-losing diuretics.

Potassium supplements may be required with the potassium-losing diuretics.* **Potassium chloride** is available as preparations for both oral and parenteral use and combinations of diuretics with potassium chloride are also marketed. However, some authorities have put forward the view that potassium supplements are not generally necessary when diuretics are used in the treatment of non-oedematous states and should only be used if there is evidence of hypokalaemia. They recommend that potassium should only be used on a routine basis for digitalized patients and patients susceptible to complications of potassium depletion (e.g. hepatic encephalpathy).

Hyperkalaemia can be a hazard when potassium is given, especially in aged patients. Gastrointestinal disturbances may occur with oral potassium chloride.

Diuretic-induced alterations in acid-base balance

Prolonged use of diuretics causes increased delivery of solute to the distal nephron with enhanced exchange of sodium for hydrogen and therefore an alkalosis which is maintained. Depletion of potassium can exacerbate this alkalosis since it reduces Na^+/K^+ exchange in the distal tubule and thus favours Na^+/H^+ exchange.

Uric acid retention

The loop diuretics and the thiazides can cause hyperuricaemia (an increased blood uric acid). This may be due to a direct inhibition of uric acid excretion in the proximal tubule. The condition is usually symptomless, but may be important in patients who have gout. The handling of uric acid by the kidney is considered in more detail below.

Alterations in calcium balance

Thiazides may decrease calcium excretion in some individuals, particularly if there is increased parathyroid activity. Loop diuretics increase calcium excretion. This effect is usually not a problem with therapy of short duration, but could be a disadvantage in the elderly patient who may already be in negative calcium balance.

DRUGS WHICH ALTER THE pH OF THE URINE

In various conditions it is of advantage to alter the

---

* In addition to its use with the potassium-losing diuretics, potassium administration may be necessary in patients being treated with corticosteroids, (see Chapter 16) and with carbenoxelone (see Chapter 15).

pH of the urine and it is possible to produce urinary pH values ranging from 5 to 8.5.

Agents which increase the urinary pH

Sodium or potassium citrate or others salts (acetate, lactate) are metabolized and the cations are excreted with bicarbonate to give an alkaline urine. This increases the action of some antibacterial drugs (sulphonamides, streptomycin) and may by itself have some antibacterial effect, as well as decreasing irritation or inflammation in the urinary tract. Alkalinization is important in preventing some drugs, such as the sulphonamides, from crystallizing out in the urine. It also decreases the formation of uric acid and cystine stones.

Agents which decrease urinary pH

This can be accomplished with **ammonium chloride**. The ammonia is metabolized to urea leaving chloride and hydrogen ion so that a hyperchloraemic acidosis results. The chloride, with accompanying sodium, appears in the glomerular filtrate and passes out in the urine with an osmotic equivalent of water causing a mild diuresis. After several days the tubules secrete hydrogen ions in exchange for sodium, the ammonium-generating mechanism comes into play and an acid urine is excreted.

Acidification of the urine may enhance the activity of some antibacterial agents such as tetracycline and penicillin, and increase the excretion of basic drugs such as pethidine and amphetamine (see Chapter 3).

DRUGS WHICH ALTER THE EXCRETION OF ORGANIC MOLECULES

The main organic molecules to be considered are *uric acid* and *penicillin*.

Uric acid is derived from the catabolism of the purine bases and is present in plasma mainly as ionized urate. In man it passes freely into the glomerular filtrate and most is then reabsorbed in the proximal convoluted tubule while a small amount is simultaneously secreted into the tubule. The net result is excretion of approximately 8–12% of the filtered urate. Under physiological conditions a rise in the level of urate in the plasma results in increased secretion into the proximal tubule. This process keeps the plasma urate concentration within the normal range, but in some conditions (e.g. gout) blood levels remain high. Urate crystals are then deposited in joints resulting in the arthritis of gout. Drugs which *increase* the elimination of urate (uricosuric agents) may be useful in such cases. (Drugs used to treat gout are dealt with in more detail in Chapter 9 (p. 216). Some uricosuric agents *decrease* the secretion of penicillin and may also be used for this purpose. The two main uricosuric agents are probenecid and sulphinpyrazone.

Probenecid is a lipid soluble derivative of benzoic acid which inhibits the reabsorption of urate in the proximal convoluted tubule. It has the opposite effect on penicillin, inhibiting its *secretion* into the tubules and raising its plasma concentration. Given orally probenecid is well absorbed in the gastrointestinal tract, maximal concentrations in the plasma occurring in about 3 hours. The greater proportion of the drug (90%) is bound to plasma albumin. The free drug passes into the glomerular filtrate, but more is actively secreted into the proximal tubule from whence it may diffuse back due to its high lipid solubility.

Sulphinpyrazone is a congener of phenylbutazone (see Chapter 9) with powerful inhibitory effects on uric acid reabsorption in the proximal convoluted tubule. It is absorbed from the gastrointestinal tract, highly protein-bound in the plasma and secreted into the proximal convoluted tubule. This drug also has effects on platelet aggregation (see Chapter 12).

Both these agents if given in sub-therapeutic doses actually inhibit *secretion* of urate. Salicylates on the other hand have this action in doses within their therapeutic range, and produce an increase in urate levels in the blood. They may thus exacerbate gouty arthritis and will antagonize the effects of uricosuric agents.

REFERENCES AND FURTHER READING

Barter D C 1983 Pharmacodynamic considerations in the use of diuretics. Ann Rev Pharmacol 23: 45–62

Burg M, Good D 1983 Sodium chloride coupled transport in mammalian nephrons. Ann Rev Physiol 45: 533–547

Cragoe E J (ed) 1983 Diuretics: chemistry, pharmacology and medicine. John Wiley, New York

Jamison R, Maffly R H 1976 The urinary concentrating mechanism. N Eng J Med 295: 1059–1067

Karnovsky M J 1979 The ultrastructure of glomerular filtration. Ann Rev Med 30: 213–224

Levenson D J, Simmons C E, Brenner B M 1982 Arachidonic acid metabolism, prostaglandins and the kidney. Am J Med 72: 354–374

Maclean D, Tudhope G R 1983 Modern diuretic treatment. Brit Med J 286 (i): 1419–1422

Needleman P, Greenwald J E 1986 Atriopeptin: a cardiac hormone intimately involved in fluid, electrolyte, and blood pressure homeostasis. N Eng J Med 314: 828–834

Reineck H J, Stein J H 1981 Mechanism of action and clinical use of diuretics. In: Brenner B M, Rector F C (eds) The kidney, 2nd ed. W B Saunders, Philadelphia, Ch 22, p1097–1131

Skorechi K L, Brenner H M 1981 Body fluid homeostasis in man. Am J Med 70: 77–88

Sullivan L P, Grantham J J 1982 The physiology of the kidney, 2nd ed. Lea and Febiger, Philadelphia

Taylor A, Palmer L G 1982 Hormonal regulation of sodium chloride and water transport in epithelia. In: Goldberger R F, Yamamoto K R (eds) Biological regulation and development, Vol 3A. Plenum Press, New York 253–298

15

The gastrointestinal tract

An understanding of the innervation of the gastro-intestinal tract and of its hormonal secretions is relevant to the understanding both of its physiological functions and of the various pathological states which can affect it (peptic ulcer, diarrhoea, constipation, etc) and is also necessary for an appreciation of the action of drugs which are used in the treatment of these conditions. Furthermore the gastrointestinal tract is one of the major endocrine systems of the body and information derived from a study of its hormones has enlarged our awareness of the role of peptides in the control of physiological processes and of their potential pharmacological significance. A brief overview of these aspects of the function of the tract will therefore be given.

THE INNERVATION AND THE HORMONES OF THE GASTROINTESTINAL TRACT

The elements under neuronal and hormonal control are the smooth muscle, the blood vessels and the glands (exocrine, endocrine and paracrine).

Neuronal control

There are two principal intramural plexuses in the tract—the **myenteric plexus (Auerbach's plexus)** between the outer, longitudinal and the middle, circular muscle layers and **Meissner's plexus** or **submucous plexus**, on the luminal side of the circular muscle layer, The plexuses are interconnected and their ganglion cells receive preganglionic **parasympathetic fibres** from the vagus which are mostly cholinergic and mostly excitatory. However, some vagal fibres are inhibitory and there is strong evidence that they release transmitters other than

acetylcholine (see Chapter 5). Some have been shown to contain peptides—substance P, vasoactive intestinal peptide, enkephalin-like substances and gastrin (see below). Incoming **sympathetic fibres** are largely postganglionic and these, in addition to innervating blood vessels, smooth muscle and some glandular cells directly, may have endings in the plexuses where they inhibit acetylcholine secretion (see Chapter 5).

The neurons within the plexuses are regarded by some investigators as constituting an additional part of the autonomic nervous system—an enteric nervous system—which should be classified separately from the sympathetic and parasympathetic nervous systems, i.e. a nonadrenergic, noncholinergic (NANC) system. This is partly because these intrinsic plexus neurons secrete not only acetylcholine and noradrenaline but serotonin, and a variety of pharmacologically active peptides—substance P, vasoactive intestinal peptide (VIP), somatostatin, the enkephalins, bombesin, cholecystokinin and neurotensin. Angiotensin II may also be released. There appears to be a close embryological relationship between the neurons and the cells of the mucosal glands since these latter cells also contain many of the peptides (see below). The enteric plexus also contains sensory neurons which respond to mechanical and chemical stimuli. These afferents are involved in local reflexes within the intrinsic networks of the gastrointestinal tract, as well as in reflexes mediated through the coeliac plexus and the central nervous system.

In whatever manner the neurons within the gastrointestinal tract are classified it is clear that the control of the functions of the tract is very complex, and it has long been known that the plexuses can regulate and co-ordinate motor activity (peristalsis, and pendular and other movements) in the complete absence of extrinsic nerves, a fact known to all pharmacology students who have carried out experiments with lengths of intestine *in vitro*.

Hormonal control

The hormones of the gastrointestinal tract include both **endocrine** secretions and **paracrine** secretions. The endocrine secretions (i.e. substances released into the blood stream) are mainly peptides synthesized by endocrine cells in the mucosa and the most important is **gastrin**. Others of this group, especially gastric inhibitory peptide (GIP), are important in giving an 'anticipatory' signal to the pancreatic islets as explained in Chapter 16.

Table 15.1 Gastrointestinal hormones

Hormone	No of amino-acid residues	Site of occurrence	Main stimulus for secretion	Action
Cholecysto-kinin (pancreo-zymin)	33	Mucosal cells of the duodenum and jejunum (also in brain and pancreatic islets)	Proteins, peptides amino-acids and triglycerides in the lumen	Stimulates secretion of pancreatic enzymes, contracts gallbladder. May induce satiety. Stimulates peristalsis.
Secretin*	27	Mucosal cells of duodenum	Low pH: < pH 4.5	Stimulates pancreatic secretion and the flow of bile. Inhibits gastric acid secretion and motility. Increases pepsin secretion.
Vasoactive intestinal polypeptide (VIP)	28	Release from nerve endings and endocrine cells throughout GIT (in high concentration in CNS; also found in pancreatic islets, GUS and lung	Vagal stimulation	Vasodilator actions. Relaxes smooth muscle of GIT and GUS. Increases GIT secretions.
Motilin	22	Duodenum (also pineal and pituitary)	Not fully understood	Stimulates intestinal peristalsis. (Action occurs 2 hours *after* food ingestion.)
Gastric inhibitory polypeptide (GIP)	43	Mucosa of duodenum and jejunum (also in brain)	Glucose, triglyce-ride, mixtures of amino-acids (after absorption into intestinal mucosa)	Stimulates insulin release. Inhibits gastric acid and pepsin secretion and gastric motility
Bombesin	14	In nerves and endo-crine cells throughout GIT (mainly in stomach), in wall and mucosa (? in CNS)	Not clearly known	Releases gastrin; increases gastric acid secretion. Contracts sphincters and relaxes muscle in GIT. Increases both endocrine and exocrine secretions of pancreas.
Somato-statin	2 forms: 14a.a. and 28a.a. residues	Gastric mucosa, pan-creatic islets. Present in nerves in GIT, in posterior pituitary and in CNS	Vagal stimulation. Intragastric fat, glucose	Inhibits gastric secretion and motility. (In pancreas it inhibits both glucagon and secretion. In hypothalamus/pituitary axis it inhibits growth hormone release).
Substance P	11	In special endocrine cells. In GIT and in nerve cells throughout body		Contracts ileal smooth muscle. (Vasodilator, lowers b.p., is a sensory neurotransmitter in spinal cord and has transmitter actions in brain. Causes natriuses and diuresis.)
Neurotensin	13	Mucosa of ileum (also in brain)	(not clearly known)	Contracts fundus of stomach; relaxes duodenum. (Has general vascular and neuroendocrine actions.)
Pancreatic polypeptide	36	Special endocrine in islets	Protein in GIT	Stimulates basal acid secretion. Increases gastric emptying and motility in GIT.

GIT = gastrointestinal tract; GUS = genitourinary system.
* There is considerable degree of homology between secretin, GIP, VIP, and the pancreatic hormone, glucagon.

The paracrine secretions, or local hormones, are released from paracrine cells, particularly in the mucosa, but also throughout the wall of the tract. These hormones act on nearby cells, and the most important of these in the stomach, is **histamine**. It is of interest that, as mentioned above, many of the hormones which are released by endocrine cells are also released by neurons in the tract and function as neurotransmitters. Histamine, gastrin and acetylcholine are considered below in the context of the local control of acid secretion. The other hormones have no immediate relevance to the understanding of therapy for gastrointestinal disorders but are of great potential interest as pharmacological tools, particularly as many of them have been found elsewhere in the body, e.g. in nervous tissue. Since these peptides, and others derived from them or related to them, are likely to be of considerable pharmacological significance in the future, a brief consideration of them is given in Table 15.1.

The main functions of the gastrointestinal tract which are important from a pharmacological point of view are: gastric secretion, vomiting (emesis), the formation and excretion of bile, the motility of the bowel and the expulsion of the faeces. These are considered below.

GASTRIC SECRETION

The stomach secretes about 2.5 litres of gastric juice daily. The principal exocrine secretions are pepsinogens, from the **chief** or **peptic cells**, and hydrochloric acid and intrinsic factor (see Chapter 18) from the **parietal** or **oxyntic cells**. These substances are secreted by glands in the body of the stomach. In addition, mucus is secreted by mucus-secreting cells found throughout the gastric mucosa and, according to recent evidence, bicarbonate is also secreted though the cell type involved is not known. Disturbances in all these secretory functions are thought to be involved in the pathogenesis of peptic ulcer and the therapy of this condition may involve drugs which modify each of these factors.

The control of gastric secretion involves both neuronal and humoral mechanisms and is generally classified under the headings 'cephalic', 'gastric' and 'intestinal' according to the location of the afferent stimuli initiating the response.

The cephalic phase

Afferent impulses initiated by the taste and smell of food or the thought of an appetizing meal are relayed through vagal efferent fibres to the stomach. Emotional factors can influence gastric secretion through these pathways. Cutting the vagus blocks the cephalic phase; stimulation of specific areas in the frontal cortex and the anterior hypothalamus results in gastric secretion.

The gastric phase

The gastric phase is brought about partly by *distension* of the stomach with food and partly by a *chemical mechanism* operating through amino-acids and other products of digestion. These stimuli act on receptors in the mucosa and the stomach wall, initiating local neuronal reflexes which involve the same post-ganglionic cholinergic neurons that are stimulated by vagal pre-ganglionic fibres. One of the effects of activity of these neurons is the release of **gastrin** (see below). Protein digestion products also act on gastrin-secreting 'G' cells in the pyloric mucosa causing gastrin release; these products may, in addition, have a direct stimulant effect on the acid-secreting parietal cells. As acid secretion proceeds and the pH falls, gastrin secretion is inhibited.

The intestinal phase

Protein digestion products, on entering the duodenum may still influence the secretory activity of the stomach. This is evident from the fact that addition of chyme or 10% peptone to this area results in gastric acid secretion. The mechanism of this effect is uncertain but may involve either a **bombesin-like** hormone released from the duodenum into the blood, or another peptide termed **entero-oxyntin** which has been isolated from the mucosa in this area and which is said to have the requisite action.

Fats and carbohydrates, on entering the duodenum, tend to inhibit gastric secretion and it is thought that this action is mediated by the hormone **gastric inhibitory peptide** (GIP).

Other factors which stimulate gastric secretion are hypoglycaemia and the intake of alcohol or caffeine-containing drinks.

THE REGULATION OF ACID SECRETION BY PARIETAL CELLS

This is especially important in peptic ulcer and constitutes a particular target for drug action. It will therefore be considered here in some detail. The secretion of the parietal cells appears to be an isotonic solution with a pH of less than 1, and contains 150 mEq/litre each of H^+ and Cl^-, which is in contrast to the 4×10^{-8} mEq of H^+ and 100 mEq of Cl^- per litre of plasma.

The Cl^- is actively transported into canaliculi in the cells which communicate with the lumen of the gastric glands and thus with the lumen of the stomach. K^+ accompanies the Cl^- and is then exchanged for H^+ from within the cell by a K^+/H^+ ATPase (Fig. 15.1). H_2CO_3 formed from CO_2 and H_2O in a carbonic anhydrase-catalysed reaction dissociates to form H^+ and HCO_3^-. The HCO_3^- exchanges across the basal membrane for Cl^-. Consequently during gastric secretion, the venous blood from the stomach has a higher pH than arterial blood and this is reflected in an increased pH in the urine   the 'alkaline tide'.

ATP is the main source of energy for gastric acid

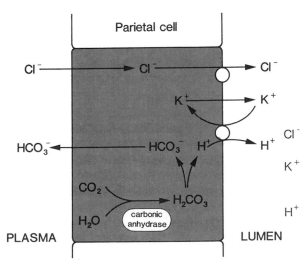

Fig. 15.1 A schematic illustration of the secretion of hydrocholoric acid by the gastric parietal cell. See text for details.

secretion and three main stimuli act on the parietal cells: **gastrin**, **acetylcholine** and **histamine**. These substances represent a hormone, a neuro-transmitter and a paracine secretion (or local hormone) respectively and will be considered below.

There has been a long-running controversy as to the relative roles of histamine and gastrin as gastric acid secretagogues. The development of the hist-amine H_2-receptor antagonists has made it clear that histamine is important as a physiological regulator of secretion and further clarification of the problem is likely to result from techniques for studying isolated gastric glands and parietal cells *in vitro* which are currently being developed and exploited.

Other substances influencing acid secretion are amino-acids (phenylalanine, histidine) and alcohol, which stimulate secretion by a direct action on the parietal cell, and some peptide hormones which inhibit it. These include gastric inhibitory peptide (GIP) and enterogastrone—which are endocrine secretions of the intestinal mucosa—and somato-statin, a paracrine secretion of the gastric mucosa. When injected, urogastrone, a peptide found in normal male human urine, which may be identical with epidermal growth factor, inhibits acid secretion stimulated by histamine or by penta-gastrin (see below).

Gastrin

That gastrin is a true hormone was demonstrated in experiments in which the gastric antrum (the endo-crine organ) and the stomach (the receptor organ) were transplanted in such a way that there was a vascular connection but no neuronal connection between them. Addition of liver extract to the antral mucosa caused the release of a chemical messenger into the blood which stimulated acid secretion from the transplanted stomach. This turned out to be gastrin, which is synthesized in, and released into the portal blood and the lumen of the stomach from, the G cells in the glands in the mucosa of the gastric antrum and the upper portion of the duodenum. These cells are thought to be derived, embryo-logically, from the neural crest and they contain in addition to gastrin, amines related to noradrenaline and serotonin. Similar cells, termed TG cells, which secrete a modified form of gastrin, are found throughout the gastrointestinal tract. Gastrin itself is also found in the CNS and in the vagus and sciatic nerves.

Gastrin is, strictly speaking, not a single substance but a family of straight-chain peptides. In man there are three main forms, containing 34, 17 and 14 amino-acids and termed respectively G34 or big gastrin, G17 or little gastrin, and G14 or minigastrin. G17 appears to be the main form of gastrin involved in the control of gastric secretion. The four amino-acids (trp-met-asp-phe) at the C terminal end, which are common to all three forms of gastrin exhibit all the physiological activity, though this fragment has only 10% of the potency of G17. G17 and G14 have half-lives in the plasma of 2–7 min and G34 a half-life of 40 mins. The plasma concentrations are measured by radio-immunoassay, the normal fasting concentration being 50–100 pg/ml.

Physiological actions of gastrin

The main action of gastrin is stimulation of the secretion of acid by the parietal cells. This action is thought by some investigators to be a direct action on the parietal cell, by some to be entirely through the release of histamine and by some to be partly direct and partly histamine-mediated. It is reported that gastrin receptors on the parietal cells have been demonstrated using radioactively labelled gastrin. However, there are no specific competitive gastrin antagonists, which makes a definitive assessment of its role difficult. It may be pertinent to this assessment that, in many species, H_2-antagonists inhibit the action of gastrin which suggests that if it does have a direct action it requires histamine for full effect. The results of recent studies imply that, like cholecystokinin on the pancreatic acinar cell, gastrin may stimulate polyphosphoinositide breakdown with generation of inositol trisphosphate which mobilizes intracellular calcium (Fig. 15.2).

Pepsinogen secretion is also increased indirectly by gastrin and there are stimulant effects on blood flow and gastric motility, and a long-term trophic action on the mucosa of the intestine and the pancreas.

Control of gastrin release

This involves both neuronal mediators, blood-borne mediators and the direct effects of the stomach contents. As regards this last factor the principal stimuli are the products of protein digestion, more particularly amino-acids but also small peptides, which act directly on the G cells. Milk and solutions of calcium salts are also effective, and it is inappropriate, therefore to use calcium-containing salts as antacids (see below).

Neuronal factors are important, impulses reaching the cells from the vagus and from the intramural plexuses. The neurotransmitter causing gastrin release is believed to be a peptide, said by some to be bombesin, by others, vasoactive intestinal peptide (VIP). Acetylcholine inhibits gastrin release and low doses of atropine enhance the effect of positive stimuli on the G cells—an effect which should be borne in mind when muscarinic receptor antagonists are used in the treatment of peptic ulcer (see below). Somatostatin, produced locally, is a potent inhibitor of gastrin secretion. Adrenaline releases gastrin, an action which is blocked by β-adrenoceptor antagonists. Gastrin secretion is inhibited when the pH of the gastric contents falls to 2.5 or lower. This effect is mediated through cholinergic nerves and is inhibited by atropine.

An excessive secretion of gastrin resulting in excessive secretion of acid is seen with tumours of gastrin-secreting cells—gastrinomas—the complex of signs and symptoms being called the Zollinger–Ellison syndrome.

Acetylcholine

Acetylcholine is released from neurons and stimulates specific muscarinic receptors on the surface of the parietal cells and on the surface of histamine-containing cells, as determined by studies with competitive antagonists (see Chapter 6). The signal-transduction mechanism in the parietal cell involves a rise in cytosolic calcium and is dependent on an adequate extracellular calcium concentration. In pancreatic acinars cells a similar increase in calcium caused by acetylcholine is dependent on the turnover of polyphosphoinositides and the generation of inositol trisphosphate (see Chapter 1), and it is believed that a similar mechanism of raising cytosolic Ca^{++} operates in the parietal cell (Fig. 15.2).

Histamine

Histamine is discussed fully in Chapter 8. Only those aspects of its pharmacology relevant to gastric secretion will be dealt with here.

Considerable clarification of the role of histamine has followed from the development of the histamine H_2-antagonists by Black and his colleagues. It is now known that the parietal cell has H_2-receptors and is sensitive to histamine, responding to amounts which are below the threshold concentration which acts on H_2-receptors on blood vessels.

In man and in the dog the histamine is derived from mast cells or histamine-containing cells similar to mast cells, which lie close to the parietal cell; in the rat it is derived from enterochromaffin cells. Rabbit gastric glands which have no mast cells nevertheless contain 50–100 nmol histamine per gram of wet weight. There is a steady basal release of histamine which can be increased by gastrin and acetylcholine.

The action of histamine on H_2-receptors in the parietal cell and elsewhere involves stimulation of adenylate cyclase and an increase in cyclic AMP.

The role of acetylcholine, histamine and gastrin in acid secretion

The exact mechanism of action of the three secretagogues on the parietal cell is not yet entirely clear. One problem is that there are considerable species differences in the responses of the experimental animals used to investigate this problem. A general scheme is given in Figure 15.2 which summarizes the two main theories—the *single cell* hypothesis and the *two cell* hypothesis. According to the former, the parietal cell has specific H_2-receptors for histamine and specific muscarinic receptors for acetylcholine; stimulation of the former increases cAMP and of the latter increases cytosolic calcium and these intracellular messengers synergize to produce acid secretion. (There is evidence that synergism of this sort, between cAMP and cytosolic calcium, is implicated in the mechanism of action of secretagogues acting on a related cell—the pancreatic acinar cell). Gastrin, in this scheme, acts directly on the parietal cell. According to the *two cell* hypothesis on the other hand, gastrin acts either only by

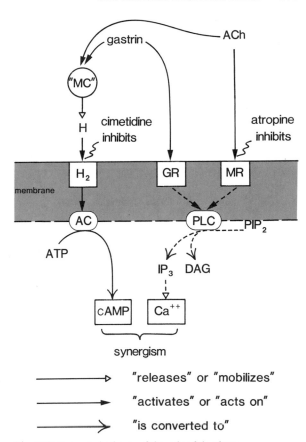

Fig. 15.2 Suggested scheme of the role of the three secretagogues: histamine (H), acetylcholine (ACh), and gastrin on the acid-secreting gastric parietal cell. MR = muscarinic receptor; H_2 = histamine H_2-receptor; GR = gastrin receptor; 'MC' = histaminocyte, (mast-cell like); PLC = phospholipase C; PIP_2 = phosphotidylinositol biphosphate; DAG = diacylglycerol; IP_3 = inositol trisphosphate; cAMP = cyclic AMP. Dashed lines indicate reactions for which definitive evidence has yet to be obtained in gastric parietal cells. (Synergism of the sort depicted occurs in pancreatic acinar cells.)

releasing histamine, or partly by releasing histamine and partly by a direct action on a gastrin receptor on the parietal cell. Similarly, acetylcholine released from the vagus is believed to act either only by releasing histamine or partly by releasing histamine and partly directly on the parietal cell.

DRUGS USED IN THE DIAGNOSIS AND TREATMENT OF GASTRIC AND DUODENAL DISORDERS

One of the principal pathological conditions in this

area is **peptic ulceration**. The reason why ulcers develop in the stomach and duodenum is not really understood though it is assumed that one factor is a defect in the mechanisms which normally prevent the gastric secretions from damaging and digesting the mucosa. Another factor, particularly in duodenal ulcers, is excessive secretion of acid. Measurements in subjects with duodenal ulcer have shown that their acid output, 1 hour after a steak meal is very considerably higher than that of normal subjects (approximately 65 mEq/h as compared to 15 mEq/h). Gastrin secretion is also higher in ulcer patients and, in addition, parietal cells appear to have increased sensitivity to the action of gastrin.

Drug treatment of peptic ulcer is aimed at decreasing the secretion of acid with **H_2-receptor antagonists** and neutralizing secreted acid with **antacids**. **Anticholinergic drugs** may be used as adjuncts to other therapy. **Drugs which promote healing** are also used. These four categories of drugs are dealt with below.

Another disorder of gastric function is **achlorhydria**, in which there is total inability to secrete acid. This is seen in pernicious anaemia (see Chapter 18) and is thought to be an autoimmune disorder in which the parietal cells are damaged by an inappropriate cell-mediated immune reaction (see Chapter 8) and are unable to secrete either acid or the intrinsic factor necessary for absorption of vitamin B_{12}. Gastric acid stimulants used diagnostically to test acid secretion are **pentagastrin**, **histamine** and **betazole**; these are dealt with below.

STIMULANTS OF GASTRIC ACID SECRETION

Pentagastrin consists of the 'working end' of the gastrin molecule (trp-met-asp-phe) to which a substituted β-alanine has been added. It is stable and water soluble and has all the physiological actions of endogenous gastrin in that it stimulates gastric acid secretion, pepsinogen secretion, gastric blood flow and contraction of the circular muscle of the stomach. It also has other, probably non-physiological, effects in that it stimulates pancreatic secretion, and contracts the smooth muscle of the lower oesophageal sphincter, the gallbladder, the intestine and the colon. It inhibits gastric emptying and the absorption of glucose and electrolytes in the small intestine.

It is used diagnostically to test gastric acid secretion, given in a single dose of 6 μg/kg by subcutaneous or intramuscular injection. Secretion begins within 10 minutes and the maximum response occurs within half an hour. The plasma half-life of pentagastrin is about 10 minutes. Unwanted effects are few, minor and transient and are mostly related to the action of the drug on the gastrointestinal tract. Thus patients may feel nausea, and be aware of increased intestinal noises (borborygmi) and an urge to pass faeces. Flushing of the skin, increased heart rate and dizziness may also occur. Hypersensitivity reactions are rarely seen.

Histamine injected subcutaneously causes an increase in gastric acid secretion with 5–10 minutes with a peak response in approximately 45 minutes and a duration of 90 minutes. An H_1-receptor antagonist (see Chapter 9) may need to be given to abrogate the other, systemic effects of histamine—particularly those on blood vessels which cause headache and other symptoms.

Betazole is pyrazolethylamine—an isomer of histamine which is a relatively specific stimulant of H_2-receptors (see Chapter 8) and as such has been used as a gastric acid stimulant, being more effective than histamine in producing acid gastric secretion without evoking H_1 side effects. Its action is slower in onset than that of histamine but more prolonged.

Histamine and betazole are rarely used nowadays having been superseded by pentagastrin for tests of gastric secretory capacity.

H_2-RECEPTOR ANTAGONISTS

Studies in man have shown that effective pharmacological control of gastric acid secretion has now become practicable. H_2-receptor antagonists are capable not only of decreasing both basal and food-stimulated acid secretion by 90% or more, but have a very significant effect in promoting healing of duodenal ulcers, as shown by the results of ten endoscopically-controlled double-blind trials, involving nearly one thousand patients. The drugs can also produce full clinical remission of symptoms in the Zollinger–Ellison syndrome.

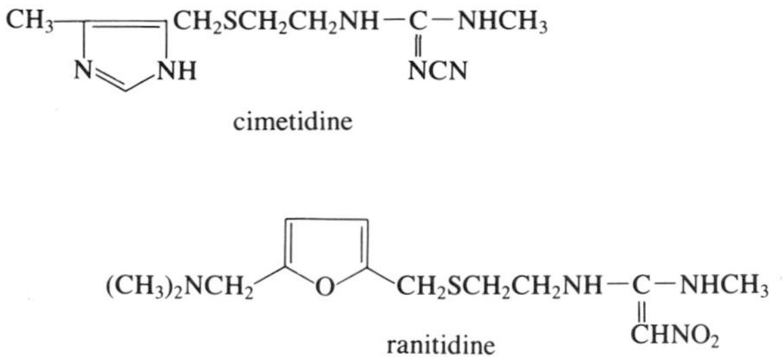

$$CH_3-\text{[imidazole]}-CH_2SCH_2CH_2NH-\underset{NCN}{\overset{\parallel}{C}}-NHCH_3$$

cimetidine

$$(CH_3)_2NCH_2-\text{[furan, O]}-CH_2SCH_2CH_2NH-\underset{\overset{\parallel}{CHNO_2}}{C}-NHCH_3$$

ranitidine

Fig. 15.3 Histamine H_2-receptor antagonists.

The pharmacology of histamine and the H_1 and H_2-antagonists is discussed in Chapter 9 and mentioned in Chapter 1. The drugs used are **cimetidine** and **ranitidine** (Fig. 15.3). The results of an early experiment with cimetidine on gastric secretion in a dog are given in Figure 15.4.

Pharmacokinetic aspects

The drugs are given orally, and are well absorbed. Preparations for intramuscular and intravenous use are also available. The half-life of cimetidine is

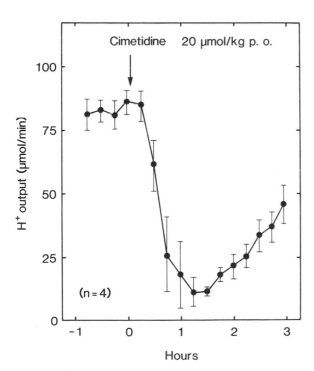

Fig. 15.4 The inhibitory effect of a single oral dose of cimetidine on maximal histamine-stimulated gastric secretion in the Heidenhain pouch dog. (After: Parsons, 1977)

shorter than that of ranitidine, oral doses of the former being given four times daily and of the latter, twice daily.

Unwanted effects

These are rare. Diarrhoea, dizziness, muscle pains and transient rashes have been reported. Cimetidine has a propensity to bind to androgen receptors and in some cases this may result in gynaecomastia and, rarely, in decrease in sexual function. Cimetidine also inhibits cytochrome P450 and may retard the metabolism of drugs such as the oral anticoagulants, phenytoin and theophylline and thus potentiate their effects. It may cause confusion in the elderly. Ranitidine appears to have less effect on androgen receptors and the P450 system.

Relapses are likely to follow when treatment with H_2-antagonists is stopped.

ANTICHOLINERGIC AGENTS

These drugs are discussed in detail in Chapter 6. The main effects of parasympathetic stimulation on the gastrointestinal tract are an increase in motility and an increase in secretory activity. However, the effects may be complicated by the fact that acetylcholine also inhibits gastrin release (see above). Anticholinergic drugs such as **atropine** can be shown experimentally to abolish completely the gastric secretion provoked by parasympathomimetic agents, but to have only a partial effect on histamine-induced secretion. In patients with peptic ulcer these agents reduce basal acid secretion by 50% but food-induced secretion by only 30%. Their anti-spasmodic effect may be of some value in peptic ulcer since this condition may be accompanied by a greater or lesser degree of smooth muscle spasm. Other conditions in which the reduction of spasm by these drugs may be useful are *irritable bowel syndrome* and *diverticular disease*. But in general this group of compounds is used mainly as adjuncts to other treatment in all these conditions. The main agents used are **propantheline**, **dicyclomine**, and **pirenzepine** (Table 6.2 and Fig. 15.5) though many other similar drugs are available. They are all given orally. Effective therapeutic doses necessarily have inhibitory effects

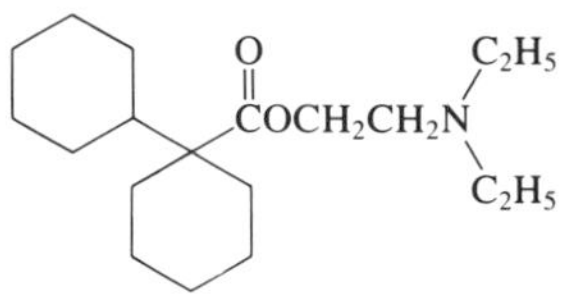

Fig. 15.5 Dicyclomine. The structures of other muscarinic receptor antagonists used in treating gastrointestinal disorders (eg propantheline and pirenzepine) are given in Table 6.2

at other muscarinic cholinoceptors. These are unwanted effects in this context, and thus a high incidence of side effects is to be expected. These include dry mouth, blurred vision, constipation, sedation, urinary retention and tachycardia. Muscarinic receptor block in the eye may precipitate glaucoma in elderly patients. Pirenzepine is said to have fairly specific effects on gastric secretion and may have fewer side effects than other anticholinergic agents.

ANTACIDS

Antacids are drugs used to produce relief of the gastric pain associated with hyperchlorhydria. They act by neutralizing gastric acid and thus raising the gastric pH, which has the effect of inhibiting peptic activity, which practically ceases at pH 5.

The following properties are required in an antacid:

1. it should be neutral in aqueous suspension but be capable of neutralizing acid
2. it should produce its effect rapidly and maintain its action for several hours
3. it should not cause irritation of the stomach and intestine
4. it should not cause gastrointestinal disturbances such as diarrhoea or constipation
5. it should not produce acid-rebound
6. it should not disturb the acid-base balance, cause alkalosis or alkalinize the urine, (which would carry the risk of the precipitation of calculi in the urinary tract).

Magnesium hydroxide is an insoluble powder which, when ingested, neutralizes the hydrochloric acid of the stomach, forming magnesium chloride. Its action is more delayed than that of sodium bicarbonate (see below) but it lasts longer since, as the drug is insoluble, some of it remains in the

stomach forming a reservoir of antacid. Some of the magnesium chloride formed in the stomach passes unchanged into the intestine and acts as a mild saline purgative, but most is converted to magnesium carbonate and excreted as such. Magnesium hydroxide, unlike sodium bicarbonate, does not produce systemic alkalosis since magnesium ion is only partially absorbed from the gut.

Magnesium trisilicate is an insoluble powder which reacts slowly with the gastric juice forming magnesium chloride and colloidal silica. During the first 60 minutes about 75% of the available magnesium is neutralized and the remaining drug is neutralized slowly over the succeeding three hours; thus this agent has a prolonged antacid effect. An excess of magnesium trisilicate results in a pH of 6.5–7 and even large doses do not result in an alkaline gastric juice. This drug also has adsorptive properties.

Alumimium hydroxide gel consists of a 4% suspension of aluminium hydroxide, which neutralizes hydrochloric acid in the stomach, forming aluminium chloride and water. Aluminium hydroxide acts rather gradually and raises the pH of the gastric juice to about 4. Its effect continues for several hours. When the aluminium chloride reaches the intestine it forms insoluble aluminium compounds, releasing chloride which is reabsorbed. Aluminium hydroxide is not absorbed and there is no loss of chloride and alkalosis does not occur. Long-continued use can cause constipation.

Colloidal aluminium hydroxide combines with phosphates in the gastrointestinal tract and this may lead to a phosphorus deficiency. The increased excretion of phosphate in the faeces which occurs results in decreased excretion of phosphate via the kidney. This effect may be clinically useful for the prevention and treatment of phosphatic renal stones, the compound used being basic aluminium carbonate.

Sodium bicarbonate acts rapidly and raises the pH of gastric juice to about 7.4. Carbon dioxide is liberated leading to the eructation of gas. This evolution of CO_2 stimulates gastrin secretion and results in a secondary rise in acid secretion. Some sodium bicarbonate is absorbed in the intestine, thus, frequent administration of this antacid can cause alkalosis, the onset of which may be insidious. The main effects vary from increased irritability to drowsiness and coma. Headache, gastrointestinal disturbances and tetany may also be seen. Because of its propensity to cause systemic alkalosis, sodium bicarbonate should not be prescribed for the long-term treatment of peptic ulcer. It should not be given to patients who are on a sodium-restricted diet.

Calcium carbonate is an effective antacid which may have other actions on the gastrointestinal tract in that it may cause constipation, an effect which may be ameliorated by giving it with magnesium oxide. The calcium may be partly absorbed, raising the concentration of calcium in the serum and this may have systemic effects—headache, nausea and, in some cases, damage to the kidneys. An additional drawback is that calcium stimulates gastrin release (see above).

DRUGS WHICH PROMOTE THE HEALING OF ULCERS

With the drugs cited below, as with the H_2-antagonists, relapses may follow when treatment is stopped.

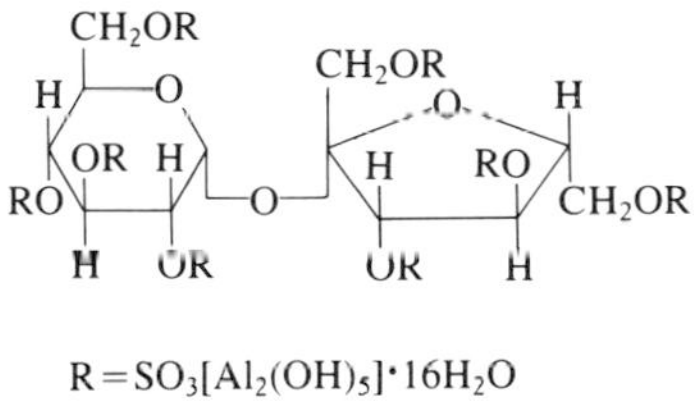

$$R = SO_3[Al_2(OH)_5] \cdot 16H_2O$$

Fig. 15.6 Sucralfate.

Sucralfate (Fig. 15.6) is a complex of aluminium hydroxide and sulphated sucrose, which has been shown in double-blind trials to promote healing of ulcers as assessed by endoscopic examination. It is thought to act by coating the ulcer surface, the anion of sucralfate binding to the positively charged protein molecules exposed in the ulcer base. It does not adhere as well to normal mucosa. *In vitro* studies indicate that it may inhibit the action of pepsin and prevent the diffusion of hydrogen ions. It is given orally, 4 times daily before meals and forms a viscous paste in the acid environment of the stomach. 30% is still present in the stomach 3 hours after administration. A small amount is absorbed into the systemic circulation and 1–2% of the drug

given appears in the urine. The unwanted effects are few, the most common being constipation which in a recent study occurred in 1.4% of patients treated. Other gastrointestinal disorders occurred even more rarely.

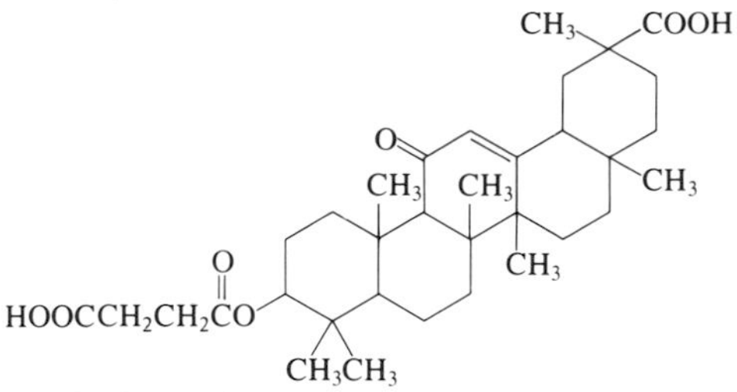

Fig. 15.7 Carbenoxolone

Carbenoxolone is a synthetic derivative of glycyrrhizic acid (a constituent of liquorice) which has been shown to be of value in promoting healing of peptic ulcers. The mechanism of action is not really understood but it is believed to involve an effect on intestinal mucus, increasing its secretion and its viscosity and thus protecting the mucosa from attack by acid and pepsin. It has an aldosterone-like action and results in sodium retention and hypokalaemia and may exacerbate oedema and hypertension. (Interestingly, spironolactone, which abrogates the renal effects of carbenoxolone also abolishes its ulcer-healing effects; whereas, diuretics with a different mechanism of action—the thiazides—abrogate the renal effects without abolishing the ulcer-healing action.)

Tripotassium dicitratobismuthate is a bismuth chelate which promotes the healing of peptic ulcers. It may act by coating the ulcer and protecting it.

Prostaglandin E_2 (PGE_2) an arachidonate metabolite, which is generated by gastric mucosal cells, is believed to play a part in protecting the gastric mucosa. It has been demonstrated experimentally that methyl derivatives of PGE_2, when given by mouth, can assist the healing of peptic ulcer and of aspirin-induced gastric erosions. However, the prostaglandins given in this way also induce diarrhoea which limits their clinical usefulness. Prostaglandins are discussed in Chapter 8.

VOMITING

Vomiting, usually preceded by a sensation of

nausea, is accomplished by a complex series of movements which are controlled by a centre situated in the reticular formation of the lower medulla. When vomiting occurs there is contraction of the pyloric portion of the stomach and relaxation of the cardiac portion. The cardiac sphincter opens and the gastric contents are expelled by a simultaneous contraction of the diaphragm and the stomach wall, the fundus of the stomach having merely a passive role. Thus the act of vomiting is a complicated one necessitating co-ordinated activity of the somatic respiratory and abdominal muscles and the involuntary muscles of the gastrointestinal tract. Furthermore, the preceding nausea is often accompanied by secretion of saliva, pallor, sweating, fall of blood pressure, tachycardia and irregular respiration. Vomiting is often associated with anti-peristaltic movements of the small bowel and after repeated episodes, the ejected fluid may contain bile.

The reflex mechanism of vomiting

Borison & Wang (1953) showed that the central neural regulation of vomiting is vested in two separate units in the medulla: the *vomiting centre*, mentioned above, which controls the interrelated movements of the smooth muscle and striated muscle involved, and the *chemoreceptor trigger zone*. This latter is contained in the *area postrema* on the floor of the fourth ventricle, close to the vagal nuclei.

The chemoreceptor trigger zone (CTZ) is sensitive to chemical stimuli and is analogous to the chemoreceptive element of the carotid body. It is the site of action of drugs such as **apomorphine**, **morphine** and the **cardiac glycosides**, which reach the CTZ through the blood stream and it lies, functionally, *outside* the blood-brain barrier. An action on the CTZ is also probably the mechanism by which endogenous substances produced in uraemia, radiation sickness and various clinical disorders, stimulate vomiting. The CTZ is also concerned in the mediation of motion sickness, since it is not possible to induce motion sickness in dogs in which the *area postrema* has been destroyed. The cerebellum also appears to be implicated in the vomiting of motion sickness.

Motion sickness is caused by certain kinds of motion and the origin of the stimuli is primarily the vestibular apparatus, although movement of the visual field when the body is stationary may also induce a degree of nausea. The manner in which impulses arising in the vestibular apparatus reach the CTZ is not yet understood. It seems clear that there is at least one primary afferent relay, in the vestibular nucleus, and the cerebellum may function as a secondary relay. However, it is not clear how stimuli impinge on the CTZ. The CTZ has no ganglionic or synaptic functions. It appears to act purely as a chemosensor of substances in the blood and cerebrospinal fluid; no *throughput* reflex connections have been found for axons entering it from surrounding structures, although it is possible that nerves to the CTZ could modulate chemosensory activity, as appears to happen in the carotid body. Accordingly, it has been postulated that a chemical substance mediates the connection between the vestibular nuclei and the CTZ. There is recent preliminary experimental evidence that a neuro-humoral factor in the cerebrospinal fluid may be implicated in motion sickness.

Impulses from the CTZ in the *area postrema* pass to the vomiting centre. The nuclei which constitute part of this neuroanatomical region, in which vomiting is controlled, include the *nucleus tractus solitarius*, the dorsal motor nucleus of the vagus and the *nucleus ambiguus*. The latter two nuclei comprise the main vomiting centre where the motor components of vomiting are initiated. Borison et al (1981) have stressed the role of the *nucleus tractus solitarius* in nausea and vomiting. 80% of vagal fibres terminate in this nucleus, as do many of the sensory fibres of the VIIIth and IXth cranial nerves. Thus much information as to visceral status reaches this nucleus, including data on the state of the blood pressure, pH and gas composition of the blood, content of the gastrointestinal tract, lung volume, etc. It has been suggested that the vomiting centre co-ordinates the action of both visceral and somatic effectors in response to the sensory information it receives from both the *nucleus tractus solitarius* and the *area postrema*. An outline of the suggested interrelationship is given in Figure 15.8.

Vomiting can be triggered by a variety of stimuli:

1. Stimulation of the sensory nerve endings in the stomach and duodenum. Some drugs act locally

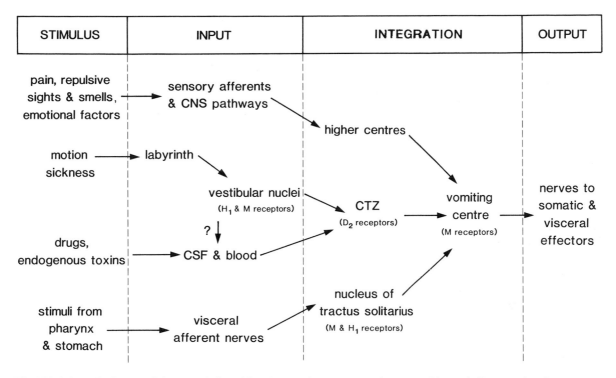

Fig. 15.8 Schematic diagram of the control of vomiting. CTZ = chemoreceptor trigger zone. The cerebellum may function as a second relay or as a gating mechanism in the link between labyrinth and CTZ. H_1 = histamine H_1; M = muscarinic; D_2 = dopamine D_2-receptors. (Based partly on a diagram from: Borison et al, 1981)

in the gastrointestinal tract and can produce vomiting even when the CTZ is destroyed. Examples are copper sulphate, and hypertonic solutions of sodium chloride.

2. Stimulation of the vagal sensory endings in the pharynx, e.g. by tickling.
3. Drugs or endogenous emetic substances produced as a result of radiation damage or disease, acting on the CTZ.
4. Disturbance of the vestibular apparatus, e.g. motion sickness.
5. Various stimuli to the sensory nerves of the heart and viscera, e.g. distension or damage to the uterus, renal pelvis or bladder, injury to the testicles. These stimuli probably act through higher centres in the CNS, but may have a direct action in the medulla.
6. A rise in intracranial pressure.
7. Nauseating smells, repulsive sights, emotional and psychic factors, acting through higher centres in the CNS.
8. Endocrine factors, as for example in the

'morning sickness' of pregnancy. The increased concentration of oestrogen is thought to be the cause, acting on the CTZ.

The receptors and neurotransmitters involved in the vomiting reflex

A variety of different substances are thought to be transmitters in the areas of the brain which control vomiting. These include acetylcholine, noradrenaline, dopamine, serotonin, histamine, glutamate, GABA, ATP, substance P, endorphins and various neurophysins. However, their precise roles and interrelationships have yet to be established.

The *area postrema* contains dopamine receptors as evidenced by the fact that exogenous dopamine causes vomiting and that labelled spiroperidol (a dopamine antagonist) binds to *area postrema* membranes with high affinity. The radioactive drug is displaced by various agents, the order of potency being apomorphine (a dopamine receptor agonist) > dopamine > serotonin > clonidine. The receptor is thought to be a D_2-type dopamine receptor (see Chapter 11) since dopamine does not activate adenylate cyclase in cell membranes from this area and domperidone, a selective D_2-antagonist inhibits the binding of labelled spiroperidol.

Whether endogenous dopamine acts on these receptors and if so whether it is implicated in motion sickness is not clear. Dopamine receptor blocking drugs are not useful in motion sickness though they have a value in other types of vomiting as explained below.

Apart from dopamine, the main neurotransmitters believed to be involved in the reflex pathways controlling vomiting are *acetylcholine* and *histamine*. Muscarinic receptors have been demonstrated in the *nucleus tractus solitarius* and the *nucleus ambiguous*, and histamine H_1-receptors in the *nucleus tractus solitarius* and the dorsal motor nucleus of the vagus (see Fig. 15.8). Both muscarinic and histamine H_1-receptors are found in the lateral vestibular nuclei.*

Antagonists of acetylcholine at muscarinic receptors and of histamine at H_1-receptors are useful anti-emetic drugs (see below).

EMETIC DRUGS

In some circumstances, such as when a toxic substance has been swallowed, it may be necessary to stimulate vomiting. This should never be attempted unless the patient is fully conscious or if the substance is corrosive.

In the past the centrally acting emetic, apomorphine which acts on the CTZ (see Fig. 15.8 and above), has been used to produce vomiting, subcutaneous injections resulting in ejection of stomach content within a minute or so. However, this procedure is regarded as dangerous and is no longer employed. For similar reasons the use of the

---

* It has been hypothesized that enkephalins are implicated in the mediation of vomiting, acting, possibly, at δ-receptors in the CTZ and at μ receptors in the vomiting centre, and that cytotoxic drugs which cause emesis may act by inhibiting the metabolizing enzymes which break down the enkephalins in the CTZ.

salts of heavy metals, zinc sulphate and copper sulphate, which act locally in the stomach (Fig. 15.8), has been discontinued.

The drug now used to produce vomiting is **ipeca-chuanha**, which acts locally in the stomach (Fig. 15.8), its irritant action being due to the presence of two alkaloids *emetine* and *cephaeline*. Emetine has also been used in the treatment of amoebiasis (see Chapter 33).

ANTI-EMETIC DRUGS

It is probable that the ability to sense and eject potentially toxic substances was developed during evolution because it had survival value. However, it does not always have a protective function, and in clinical practice drugs which stop vomiting (anti-emetic drugs) may be required in various circumstances, such as the following:

1. For the prevention of motion sickness
2. For the prevention and treatment of the nausea and vomiting associated with vestibular disorders such as Meniere's disease, labyrinthitis and positional vertigo
3. As an adjunct to cancer chemotherapy to combat the nausea and vomiting produced by many cytotoxic drugs (see Chapter 29). (It is reported that a young medically-qualified patient being treated by combination chemotherapy for sarcoma stated that 'the severity of the nausea and vomiting at times made the thought of death seem like a welcome relief'.)
4. As a result of the production of endogenous toxins in uraemia and other clinical disorders, and after radiation treatment
5. For the prevention and treatment of postoperative vomiting
6. For the prevention and treatment of morning sickness. Drug treatment is to be avoided for the normal degree of morning sickness of pregnancy but may be necessary in *hyperemesis gravidarum*—a condition in which severe vomiting occurs, which may endanger life
7. For the treatment of vomiting associated with gastrointestinal disorders.

Different anti-emetic agents are used for different conditions though there may be some overlap. The

Table 15.2 Anti-emetic drugs

| Drug | Potency at receptors (Ki nM)* | | | Main clinical use in vomiting due to: |
	Dopamine D$_2$	Muscarinic	Histamine H$_1$	
Antimuscarinics				
hyoscine	10 000	0.8	> 10 000	motion sickness
H$_1$-antihistamines				
diphenhydramine	10 000	120	17 ⎫	motion sickness
			⎬	*hyperemesis gravidarum*; post-operative;
promethazine	240	21	2.9 ⎭	labyrinthine disorders
Dopamine antagonists				
chloropromazine	25	130	28 ⎫	cancer chemotherapy; radiation sickness
fluphenazine	3.7	340	60 ⎬	uraemia; post-operative; labyrinthine disorders;
prochlorperazine	15	2100	100 ⎭	
metochlopromide	270	>10 000	1100	⎰ motion sickness; GIT disorders;
				⎱ cancer chemotherapy
haloperidol	4.2	>10 000	1600	cancer chemotherapy
domperidone	+	—	—	cancer chemotherapy
Tricyclic antidepressants				
nortriptyline	800	57	27 ⎫	cancer chemotherapy
amitryptyline	290	10	3.2 ⎭	
Miscellaneous				
cannabinoids	—	—	—	cancer chemotherapy
high dose steroids	—	—	—	cancer chemotherapy

Data from: Peroutka & Snyder, 1982; Seigel & Longo, 1981.
* The smaller the Ki, the more potent the anti-emetic drug.

main drugs and their potencies at neurotransmitter receptor sites are given in Table 15.2 along with a general indication of their clinical use. Details of the main categories of agents are given below.

H$_1$-antihistamines

This group of drugs is dealt with in Chapter 9. H$_1$-antihistamine drugs have little or no activity against apomorphine-induced vomiting but are effective against copper sulphate-induced emesis and the nausea and vomiting of labyrinthine origin, such as motion sickness. There are histamine H$_1$-receptors in the lateral vestibular nucleus and in the nucleus of the *tractus solitarius* (see Fig. 15.8) and also in the dorsal motor nucleus of the vagus and it follows that the drugs could block impulses from the labyrinths and from afferent visceral pathways to the vomiting centre. However, there is no correlation between the potency of the drugs at H$_1$-receptors and their ability to protect against motion sickness and thus their precise mechanism of action remains to be determined. It is possible that the component of antimuscarinic activity in

some H$_1$-antihistamines plays a part in their effects.

Several large well-controlled trials on the effect of various agents on motion sickness have been carried out, using as subjects, soldiers and airmen on transatlantic sea voyages. The most effective drugs were the H$_1$-antihistamines, in particular the piperazine derivatives, **meclozine** and **cyclizine**, and the phenothiazine, **promethazine**. This last agent produced rather more drowsiness than the other two. **Diphenhydramine** and **dimenhydrinate** have also been used for motion sickness but have fairly marked sedative effects.

Promethazine and **diphenhydramine** have proved of value in the nausea associated with Meniere's disease and other disorders of the labyrinth. In using drugs to treat the morning sickness of pregnancy, the problem of potential damage to the fetus has to be borne in mind. **Piperazine** antihistamines are effective and there is no evidence of teratogenicity in man.

In general H$_1$-antihistamines are most effective if given before the onset of nausea and vomiting but may have some action in controlling it when established.

Antimuscarinic agents

Drugs which antagonize acetylcholine at muscarinic receptors are dealt with in Chapter 6. **Hyoscine** is active against nausea and vomiting of labyrinthine origin and against copper sulphate-induced vomiting, but is ineffective in apomorphine-induced emesis. **Atropine** and other related drugs are less active. As explained above, there are muscarinic receptors in the lateral vestibular nucleus, the nucleus of the *tractus solitarius* and in the *nucleus ambiguus* of the vomiting centre. It seems probable that the anti-emetic action of hyoscine is due to blockade of impulses from the labyrinth and from visceral afferents which normally act via these receptors, but the precise mechanism of action is not yet clear.

Hyoscine is the drug of choice for the prevention of motion sickness, though it is less useful once it occurs. The usual unwanted actions of this drug (drowsiness, dry mouth, blurring of vision, retention of urine) are not necessarily very marked with the doses employed for anti-emetic effect. The sedative action may be of value in some cases.

Phenothiazines

Phenothiazines are dealt with in Chapter 22; only those aspects relevant to the control of vomiting will be considered here.

Neuroleptic phenothiazines, such as **chlorpromazine**, **prochlorperazine** and **trifluoperazine** are effective anti-emetics, while some phenothiazines, such as **thiethylperazine** (Fig. 15.9) are employed only for this purpose. They are active against apomorphine-induced vomiting, but most are not active against copper sulphate-induced vomiting and, as they are known to be dopamine receptor antagonists, they are thought to act at the chemoreceptor trigger zone (see Fig. 15.8). However, they also have some degree of antihistaminic and antimuscarinic activity and may have other sites of action. Their action at the chemoreceptor trigger zone is not equivalent to surgical ablation since they are ineffective in digitalis-induced vomiting. Apart from chlorpromazine, the phenothiazines specified above as being potent anti-emetics have a piperazine side chain (see Figs. 15.9 & 22.3) as do the non-sedative antihistamines with anti-emetic activity (see Fig. 9.12).

The main *unwanted effects* are sedation, orthostatic hypotension and extrapyramidal symptoms, this last being particularly likely to occur in children.

Halogenation of the R_1 side chain, as in trifluoperazine and prochlorperazine, increases anti-emetic activity and extrapyramidal effects and decreases the occurrence of sedation and hypotension. Chlorpromazine has less prominent extrapyramidal action. Other, less frequent unwanted effects are liver dysfunction, gynaecomastia, blood dyscrasias and photosensitivity.

Phenothiazines are the drugs of choice for the prevention and control of the nausea and vomiting associated with uraemia, radiation sickness and acute viral gastroenteritis. They are valuable against the vomiting caused by cancer chemotherapy agents, oestrogens, and narcotic analgesics. Thiethylperazine may be used in hyperemesis gravidarum.

Phenothiazines can be given orally, rectally or parenterally, which means that unlike some anti-emetics they can be given after a patient starts to vomit.

Butyrophenones

Butyrophenones are dealt with in detail in Chapter 22. They are dopamine receptor antagonists and are powerful inhibitors of the chemoreceptor trigger zone, as evidenced by their prevention of vomiting after apomorphine challenge in human subjects.

Unwanted effects include agitation and restlessness in some subjects and sedation in others. Extrapyramidal reactions are common, as with phenothiazines. **Haloperidol** and **droperidol** have given good results as anti-emetics against strongly emetic cytotoxic drugs such as cisplatin, mechlorethamine and doxorubicin.

Metoclopramide

Metoclopramide (Fig. 15.9) is a dopamine receptor antagonist and acts at the chemoreceptor trigger zone, being considerably more potent against apomorphine-induced vomiting than chlorpromazine, in experiments in dogs.

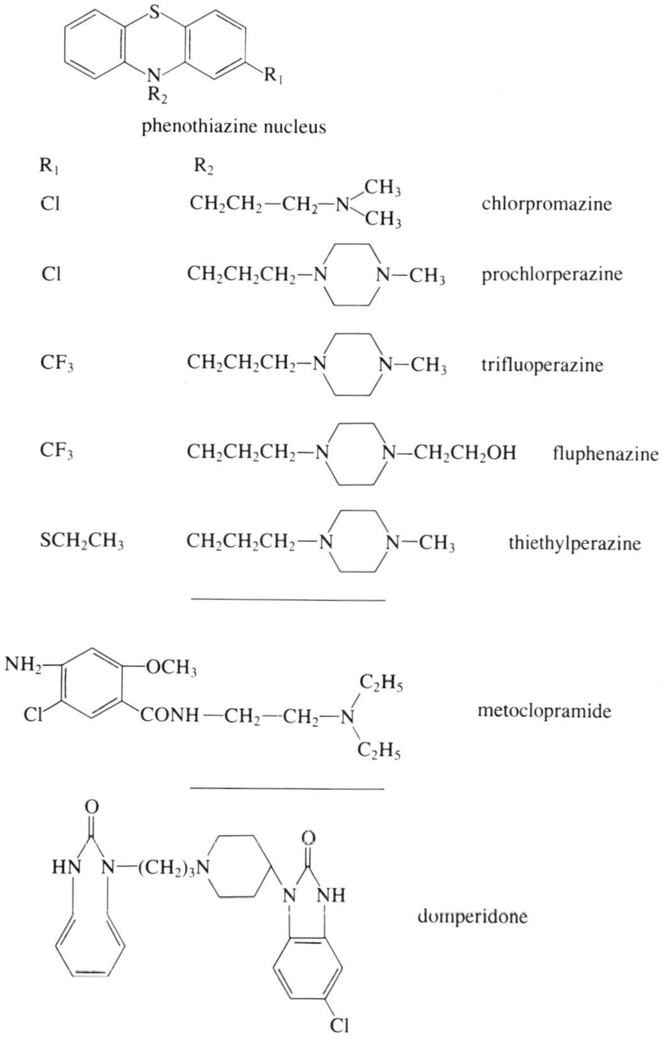

Fig. 15.9 The structures of some anti-emetic drugs. (The structure of promethazine is given in Fig. 9.12)

Like the phenothiazines its unwanted effects are related to its blockade of other CNS dopamine receptors. Extrapyramidal reactions are more common in children and young adults, but most patients experience mild sedation, and about 20% restlessness. It stimulates prolactin release (see Chapter 16) and may cause galactorrhea and disorders of menstruation. It is given orally, has a plasma $t_{\frac{1}{2}}$ of 4 hours and is excreted in the urine.

Metoclopramide is of value in the treatment of the nausea and vomiting associated with uraemia, radiation sickness and gastrointestinal disorders. It is ineffective in motion sickness and the vomiting which occurs in disorders of the labyrinth. High

doses of metoclopramide have proved effective in preventing the normally intractable vomiting which occurs during therapy with cisplatin, and may well be of value in other cancer treatment regimes.

Metoclopramide also has peripheral actions, increasing the motility of the stomach and intestine, which add to its anti-emetic effect and which may be used in therapy of gastrointestinal disorders (see below).

Domperidone

Domperidone (Fig. 15.9) is a dopamine-receptor antagonist and, like metoclopramide, is anti-emetic by actions at two sites. Its primary focus of anti-emetic action is on the chemoreceptor trigger zone but it also has a peripheral effect, increasing the motility of the gut. This latter action is discussed later in this chapter.

It can be given both parenterally and orally, though after oral administration, bioavailability is only 17%. Its plasma half-life is approximately 7 hours and it is excreted in the urine. It is said not to cross the blood-brain barrier. (Note that, as explained above, the chemoreceptor trigger zone is functionally outside this barrier.)

Unwanted effects referrable to actions on the basal ganglia are less frequent with domperidone than with metoclopramide since its penetration of the brain is limited. Cardiac dysrhythmia has been reported following intravenous bolus injections and infusion of the drug is advised.

Its main use as an anti-emetic is in the prevention of vomiting after treatment with moderately emetogenic cytotoxic drugs. Given intravenously, it has also proved effective against postoperative vomiting.

Cannabinoids

Following the observation that smoking marijuana decreased the nausea and vomiting produced by cytotoxic drugs, studies have been conducted on the anti-emetic properties of cannabinoids (see Chapter 35). Tetrahydrocannabinol (THC) was reported to be effective and **nabilone**, a synthetic derivative, is now available for clinical use. It appears to act at the chemoreceptor trigger zone since, given intravenously in a cat, it blocks apomorphine-induced vomiting. Its anti-emetic effect is antagonized by naloxone which implies that opioid receptors may be important in the reduction of vomiting produced by this drug.

Nabilone is given orally, is well absorbed from the gastrointestinal tract and is metabolized in many tissues. Its plasma half-life is approximately 120 minutes and its metabolites are excreted in the urine and in the faeces.

In well-controlled clinical trials it has proved superior to prochlorperazine in the treatment of patients on most cytotoxic drug regimes and equal to prochlorperazine in patients being given high-dose cisplatin.

Unwanted effects are common, especially drowsiness, dizziness and dry mouth. Mood changes and postural hypotension are also fairly frequent. Some patients experience hallucinations and psychotic reactions. Earlier reports of neurotoxicity in experimental animals have proved to be due to a metabolite which is not formed to any significant extent in man.

Tricyclic antidepressants

Nortriptyline and **amitriptyline** are antidepressant drugs (see Chapter 23) which have significant potency as antagonists at muscarinic and H_1-receptors (see Table 15.2). Preliminary clinical trials have indicated that these drugs are effective against moderately emetogenic cytotoxic agents when used in combination with fluphenazine.

Steroids

There are now several reports of the anti-emetic effect of high-dose steroids either alone or in combination with a phenothiazine. The steroids used were the glucocorticoids, **dexamethasone** and **methylprednisolone** (see Chapter 16) and given parenterally they proved to be useful in relieving the nausea and vomiting of the strongly emetogenic cytotoxic agents cisplatin, doxorubicin and mechlorethamine. Their mechanism of action as anti-emetics is not known.

THE MOTILITY OF THE GASTRO-INTESTINAL TRACT

The normal motility of the gastrointestinal tract is designed both to produce a thorough mixing of the contents and to propel them in a caudal direction. It is essentially under local neurohumoral control, although evacuation of the contents (defaecation) is under voluntary control. The relevant neurohumoral factors are outlined at the beginning of this chapter. Apart from the effects on vomiting, described above, drugs can be used to increase or to decrease gastrointestinal movements.

Drugs which increase movements include the *purgatives*, which accelerate the passage of food through the intestine, and *agents which increase the motility* of the gastrointestinal smooth muscle without causing purgation. The main agents decreasing movements are the *anti-diarrhoeal* drugs. These three groups of agents are dealt with below.

PURGATIVES

For love of God do take some laxative;
Upon my soul that's the advice to give
For melancholy choler; let me urge
You free yourself from vapours with a purge.

(Pertelote to Chanticleer, on hearing that he had had bad dreams; in the Nun's Priest's Tale, *Canterbury Tales*, Chaucer, Coghill's translation. See page 349 for the reply.)

The transit of food through the intestine may be hastened by several different methods:

1. by increasing the volume of non-absorbable solid residue with bulk laxatives
2. by increasing the water content with osmotic laxatives
3. by altering the consistency of the faeces with faecel softeners
4. by using drugs which stimulate the mucosa and reflexly increase peristalsis (stimulant purgatives).

Some agents are given rectally.

Bulk laxatives

This group of substances includes **methylcellulose** and certain plant gums, e.g. **sterculia**, **agar**, **bran** and **ispaghula**. These agents are polysaccharide polymers which are not broken down by the normal processes of digestion in the upper part of the gastrointestinal tract. It is thought that they act by virtue of their capacity to retain water in the gut lumen and so promote peristalsis, since their ability to hold water *in vitro* parallels *in vivo* ability to increase faecal bulk.

Their use is favoured by many because they are considered to increase faecal bulk by 'natural' means.

Faecal softeners

Dioctyl sodium sulphosuccinate is a surface active compound which acts in the gastrointestinal tract in a manner similar to a detergent, and produces softer faeces.

Liquid paraffin is a mixture of the higher paraffins of the methane series. It is rarely used now because of the disadvantages associated with its use. The main practical objection is that the oil may leak through the anal sphincter. Other disadvantages are more serious in that it may interfere with the digestion and absorption of food. Furthermore, it dissolves α- and β-carotenes, the chief precursors of vitamin A, preventing their absorption. Liquid paraffin may be absorbed and form 'paraffinomas' in the mesenteric lymph ducts.

Osmotic laxatives

Osmotic laxatives consist of poorly absorbed solutes which maintain an increased volume of fluid in the lumen of the bowel by osmosis. They include **saline purgatives** and **lactulose**. Their principal effect is to accelerate the transfer of the gut contents through the small intestine, resulting in an abnormally large volume entering the colon. This causes distension which leads to purgation about an hour later.

The entrance of hypertonic salt solutions into the duodenum leads to closure of the pylorus, and vomiting may ensue. An amount of a saline purgative dissolved in sufficient water to produce an isotonic or hypotonic solution causes more rapid purgation than the same amount used as a hypertonic solution.

Saline purgatives should be given on an empty stomach, since this allows the solution to pass directly through the stomach into the duodenum and intestine. Given on a full stomach, a saline purgative will only pass in driblets into the intestine, and its action will be much reduced.

A large number of non-toxic salts act as saline purgatives. These include all soluble salts of magnesium and some salts of sodium, particularly the sulphate, phosphate and tartrate.

Magnesium sulphate is a saline purgative widely used in spite of its bitter taste. It is not irritant and it is very slowly absorbed. The osmotic pressure which is created by the presence of the salt in solution in the intestine results in sufficient fluid being retained within the lumen to maintain a solution of the salt isotonic with the body fluids. 8 g of magnesium sulphate retain about 120 ml of water in the lumen of the gut. This doubles the volume of the faeces.

If given intravenously, magnesium salts do not cause purgation, but produce depression of the central nervous system, neuromuscular block and relaxation of smooth muscle. The amount of magnesium absorbed after an oral dose is usually too small to have these actions although there have been reports that, in small children, oral administration resulted in sufficient absorption to produce unconsciousness. The central effects can be treated by giving calcium salts intravenously.

Magnesium carbonate and **magnesium hydroxide** (an antacid, see above) act as mild purgatives by virtue of their magnesium content.

Sodium sulphate is a saline purgative which is as effective as magnesium sulphate. It has a rather more unpleasant taste than magnesium sulphate but it lacks the potential toxicity of the magnesium ion.

Lactulose is a semisynthetic dissacharide of fructose and galactose. In the bowel, bacteria convert it to its two component sugars and when these are fermented, the lactic and acetic acid formed function as osmotic laxatives. It takes much longer to act than a saline purgative. After lactulose administration the gut contents have a lower pH than normal and this decreases the activity of ammonia-producing organisms. Because of this effect, lactulose is used in the treatment of hepatic encephalopathy. (This condition is associated with chronic liver failure; its pathogenesis is not understood but it is known that there is an imbalance between different types of amino-acids along with a retention of nitrogenous metabolites such as ammonia.)

Stimulant purgatives

Many agents increase peristalsis by stimulating the mucosa of the gut, probably by irritating local reflexes, the impulses arising in the mucosa and being transmitted through the intramural plexuses to the smooth muscle of the intestine. The following are the more important purgatives in this group: castor oil, cascara, bisacodyl, dantron, sodium picosulphate and preparations of senna and fig.

Castor oil is obtained from the seeds of *Ricinus comunis*. It, itself, is non-irritant but in the small intestine it is hydrolysed by lipase with the liberation of ricinoleic acid which has a strong irritant effect on the gut mucosa. It probably acts in both the small and large intestine and results in the evacuation of the bowel in 3–6 hours. Its action is self-limiting as the expulsion of the gut contents eliminates the unhydrolysed oil. The hydrolysis of the castor oil necessitates the presence of bile and pancreatic juice and thus this agent is without effect in patients with obstructive jaundice.

Senna and **cascara** have laxative activity because they contain derivatives of anthracene — emodin (tri-hydroxyl-methyl-anthraquinone) and chryso-phanic acid (di-hydroxy-methyl-anthraquinone). These substances are combined with sugars to form glycosides which must be hydrolysed before the active principles are free to act.

The drugs pass unchanged into the colon where bacteria hydrolyse the glycoside bond releasing the free anthracene derivatives; these are then absorbed and have a direct stimulant effect on the myenteric plexus, resulting in smooth muscle activity and thus defaecation. Some emodin is excreted in the urine and some may appear in the milk. Cascara sagrada is the mildest of the anthracene purgatives when given in ordinary doses.

Senna is a relatively mild purgative. A single dose usually produces a laxative action within 8 hours, which may be accompanied by griping. Senokot is a biologically standardized dry extract of senna, the biological standardization being based on the measurement of the number of wet faeces produced after administration of the preparation to mice.

Danthron is an effective anthraquinone purgative which produces evacuation of the bowel in 6–12 hours. It may colour the urine red. **Bisacodyl** has similar actions; it can be given orally, but is usually administered as a suppository, when it causes stimulation of the rectal mucosa resulting in peristaltic action and defaecation in 15–30 minutes. Other rectally administered laxatives include, **dioctyl sodium sulphosuccinate** given as enema or suppository, **glycerol** given as suppository and **arachis oil** given as enema. Magnesium sulphate may also be given as an enema.

Misuse of purgatives

It is commonly believed that if the bowels are not

evacuated each day, the retained contents constitute a source of toxins which will be absorbed and cause ill health, the belief being based partly on the fact that constipation produces a sense of discomfort. Consequently purgatives are very widely used, often quite unnecessarily. The belief that daily defaecation is an absolute prerequisite for good health is embedded in folklore and tradition but there is little to support it in modern medicine.

Upon your laxatives I set no store,
For they are venomous. I've suffered by them
Often enough before and I defy them.

(Chanticleer's reply to Pertelote; in the Nun's Priest's Tale, *Canterbury Tales*, Chaucer, Coghill's translation.)

DRUGS WHICH INCREASE GASTRO-INTESTINAL MOTILITY

Agents which increase the motility of the gastrointestinal tract without causing purgation are used mostly for disorders of motility in the gastrointestinal tract, though some may also be employed as anti-emetics, for diagnostic radiography or duodenal intubation. The main groups of drugs used are : (1) muscarinic agonists and anti-cholinesterases; (2) domperidone; and (3) metoclopramide.

Muscarinic agonists and anticholinesterases

This group of drugs is dealt with in detail in Chapter 6. For action in the gastrointestinal tract **bethanechol**, a muscarinic agonist, is the drug of choice since it has no action on nicotinic receptors and is not hydrolyzed by cholinesterases. Given subcutaneously, the peak response is seen within 30 minutes. It increases the lower oesophageal sphincter pressure, stimulates motor activity in the stomach and increases gastric acid secretion but does not affect blood gastrin concentrations. It is an effective therapy for gastro-oesophageal reflux. It can be used to treat postoperative paralytic ileus, as can cholinesterase inhibitors such as **neostigmine**. The muscarinic effects of neostigmine are manifested by a powerful stimulant action on the intestine and the bladder. It can be administered in the early postoperative period when parenteral medication for intestinal atony is necessary.

Stimulation of gastrointestinal activity can be brought about by upsetting the normal balance of parasympathetic and sympathetic innervation of the intestine. Thus the adrenergic neurone blocking drug guanethidine frequently causes diarrhoea.

Domperidone

Domperidone (see Fig. 15.9) is a dopamine antagonist acting at D_2-receptors and is used as an anti-emetic as described above. It is also effective in increasing gastrointestinal motility. However, although it is thought that in some vagal fibres the neurotransmitter is dopamine, there is no real evidence that dopamine receptors per se occur in the gastrointestinal tract. Dopamine can be shown to produce relaxation of guinea-pig gastro-oesophageal smooth muscle but the order of potency of antagonists of this action (prazosin > phentolamine > domperidone > haloperidol) suggests that it is acting on α-adrenoreceptors. Domperidone is thought to enhance motility by blocking α_1-adrenoceptors and thus decreasing the relaxant effect mediated through these receptors. Clinically, it increases lower oesophageal sphincter pressure (thus inhibiting gastro-oesophageal reflux), increases gastric emptying and enhances duodenal peristalsis. It does not stimulate gastric acid secretion. It is useful in disorders of gastric emptying and in chronic gastric reflux.

Metoclopramide

In addition to its central effects as an anti-emetic, metoclopramide (see Fig. 15.9) exerts a significant local stimulant effect on gastric motility causing a marked acceleration of gastric emptying with no concomitant stimulation of gastric acid secretion. In comparison with muscarinic agonists it appears to have less effect on the motility of the lower bowel. Since its effects can be blocked by tetrodotoxin or muscarinic receptor antagonists it is believed to act by activation of cholinergic neurons.

Clinically, the lower oesophageal sphincter pressure is increased as is the amplitude of oesophageal contractions. Gastric emptying is facilitated with no concomitant increase in gastric acid secretion. Metoclopramide is useful in gastro-oesophageal reflux and in disorders of gastric emptying, but is ineffective in paralytic ileus.

ANTIDIARRHOEAL AGENTS

Diarrhoea is the too frequent passage of faeces which are too liquid. It can be caused by infectious agents, toxins, food, anxiety or drugs. The repercussions will depend not only on the cause but on the state of nutrition and health of the patient. They can range from discomfort and inconvenience in a healthy well-nourished adult, to a medical emergency requiring hospitalization and parenteral fluid and electrolyte therapy. On a worldwide basis acute diarrhoeal disease is one of the principal causes of death in infants, particularly if malnourished.

Diarrhoea involves both an increase in the motility of the gastrointestinal tract and a decrease in the absorption of fluid and thus a loss of electrolytes (particularly sodium) and water. In man about 8000 ml of fluid enters the intestine daily but normally only 100 ml are voided. In severe diarrhoea due to infective agents, fluid loss is due not only to decreased absorption but increased secretion. The principal intracellular messengers for stimulus-secretion coupling in the gastrointestinal tract are cyclic nucleotides and calcium. Cholera toxins and some other bacterial toxins produce a profound increase in secretion through their effect on the guanine nucleotide regulatory proteins which couple the surface receptors of the mucosal cells to adenylate cyclase (see Chapter 1). Some bacterial toxins release serotonin from enterochromaffin cells, and this can itself directly stimulate secretion or may do so indirectly by releasing acetylcholine or vasoactive intestinal peptide from neurons. Inflammatory responses to invasive micro-organisms can result in generation of kinins (see Chapter 8) for which there are receptors on the basolateral membrane of the mucosal cell. Kinins can initiate the arachidonate cascade (see Chapter 8) and arachidonate metabolites are believed to have a significant role in the stimulation of intestinal secretion. PGE_2, for example, is a potent stimulant of adenylate cyclase.

There are three approaches to the treatment of severe acute diarrhoea.

1. *The maintenance of fluid and electrolyte balance.* This is the first priority and many cases may require no other treatment. An increase in the understanding of the absorptive and secretory processes in the gastrointestinal tract during the past decade has led to the use of glucose-containing salt solutions for *oral* rehydration. This approach makes use of the knowledge that in the ileum, as in parts of the nephron, there is co-transport of sodium and glucose across the epithelial cell and that therefore glucose enhances sodium absorption and thus water uptake. Amino-acids have a similar effect. Preparations of sodium chloride and glucose for oral use are available in powder form. When reconstituted these may be particularly valuable not only in small children with acute diarrhoea but in other salt-losing conditions such as the diuretic phase of acute renal failure.

2. *The use of anti-infective agents.* These are usually not necessary in simple gastroenteritis. In developed countries the majority of these are viral in origin and those that are bacterial generally resolve without antibacterial therapy. *Campylobacter* is the commonest bacterial organism causing gastroenteritis in the UK and severe cases may require erythromycin. Chemotherapy may be necessary in some types of enteritis (e.g. typhoid, amoebic dysentery, cholera). Anti-infective agents are dealt with in Chapter 30).

3. *The use of non-antimicrobial antidiarrhoeal agents.* These are dealt with below and include antimotility agents, adsorbents and agents which modify fluid and electrolyte transport.

Antimotility agents

The main pharmacological agents which decrease motility are **opiates** (see Chapter 25) and **anticholinergic drugs** (Chapter 6). Agents in this latter group are seldom used nowadays because of their actions on other systems, when they are used in doses likely to reduce diarrhoea.

The mechanism of action of **morphine** on the alimentary tract is complex and furthermore varies in different species. Studies of this action initiated the understanding of the different receptors on which opiates act. This subject is dealt with in detail in Chapter 25.

In man, morphine increases the tone and rhythmic contractions of the intestine but diminishes propulsive activity. Its overall effect is constipating. The pyloric, ileocolic and anal sphincters are contracted and the tone of the large intestine is markedly increased. Morphine also reduces awareness of the normal stimuli for defaecation and patients with diarrhoea who are treated with morphine or opium may notice the call for defaecation only after the intestinal contents have left the body.

Morphine increases the tone of the intestine, but **papaverine** diminishes it. Opium, which contains papaverine as well as morphine, may be slightly more effective than morphine in reducing the motor activity of the gut, but the difference is very small.

The main opiates used in diarrhoea are **codeine**, **diphenoxylate** and **loperamide** (see Figs. 25.5 & 15.10). All have unwanted effects which include nausea, vomiting, abdominal cramps, drowsiness and dizziness. Paralytic ileus may also occur. They should not be used in young children.

Adsorbents

This type of agent is used extensively in the treatment of diarrhoea although properly controlled trials proving adequacy have not been carried out.

The main preparations used are **kaolin**, **pectin**, **chalk**, **charcoal**, **methyl cellulose** and **activated attapulgite** (magnesium aluminium silicate).

It has been suggested that these agents may act by adsorbing micro-organisms or toxins, by altering the intestinal flora or by coating and protecting the intestinal mucosa.

Agents which modify fluid and electrolyte transport

Drugs which reduce secretion and/or stimulate absorption may well be of value in acute diarrhoea. Preparations with the potential for producing these effects have been tested in the laboratory and are being investigated in man. **Non-steroidal anti-inflammatory agents** such as **aspirin** and **indomethacin** have been shown to have significant anti-diarrhoeal actions both in experimental animals

Fig. 15.10 Structures of two antimotility drugs used as antidiarrhoeal agents.

Loperamide has a relatively selective action on the gastrointestinal tract which is related to its distribution in the body. In rats, after oral dosing, 85% is found in the gastrointestinal tract, and 5% in the liver. There is evidence that there is efficient entero-hepatic cycling of the drug.

Codeine and loperamide have anti-secretory actions in addition to their effects on intestinal motility.

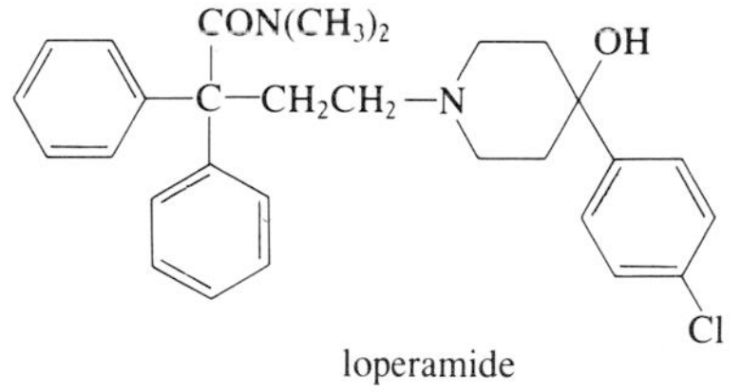

and in man. The effect is probably largely due to inhibition of prostaglandin synthesis (see Chapter 9) though other, as yet unknown, mechanisms may play a part, since both drugs reduce the effect of cholera toxin, which is independent of prostaglandin synthesis. **Bismuth subsalicylate** has been shown to be effective in travellers' diarrhoea and may work largely by virtue of its salicylate component.

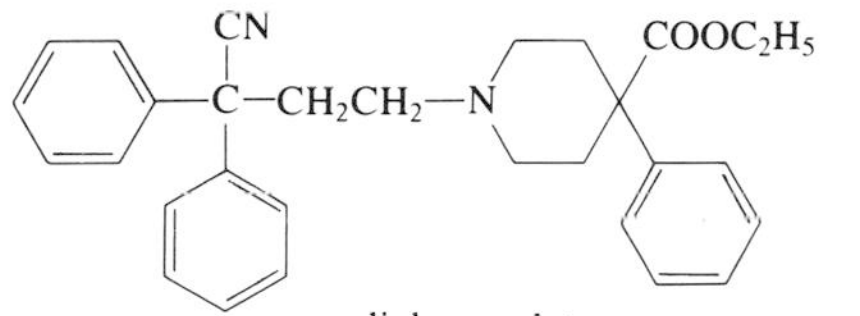

Phenothiazines, e.g. chlorpromazine, have been shown to have antisecretory activity in the intestine in experimental animals and have proved of value in the treatment of diarrhoea in preliminary controlled clinical trials. Their mechanism of action is probably due to modification of a step distal to cyclic nucleotide production in stimulus-secretion coupling and may involve inhibition of calmodulin or of protein kinase C since both these effects can be shown with phenothiazines in isolated cells *in vitro*. These drugs are dealt with in Chapter 22.

PHARMACOLOGY OF BILE

Bile is excreted by the liver as a dilute salt solution containing about 0.4% of organic solids. Since the presence of bile in the gut is required only during the digestion of food, the dilute bile is stored in the gall bladder where about 90% of the water content is absorbed and mucin is added. The concentrated bile is passed periodically into the small intestine. The process involves relaxation of the sphincter of Oddi at the termination of the common bile duct and contraction of the gall bladder. The wall of the gall bladder contains smooth muscle, and when the organ contracts it can produce a pressure of about 30 cm of water.

Drugs affecting bile flow

A 'cholagogue' is a substance which increases bile secretion by the liver; but since the bile in the gall bladder is normally concentrated tenfold it is al-

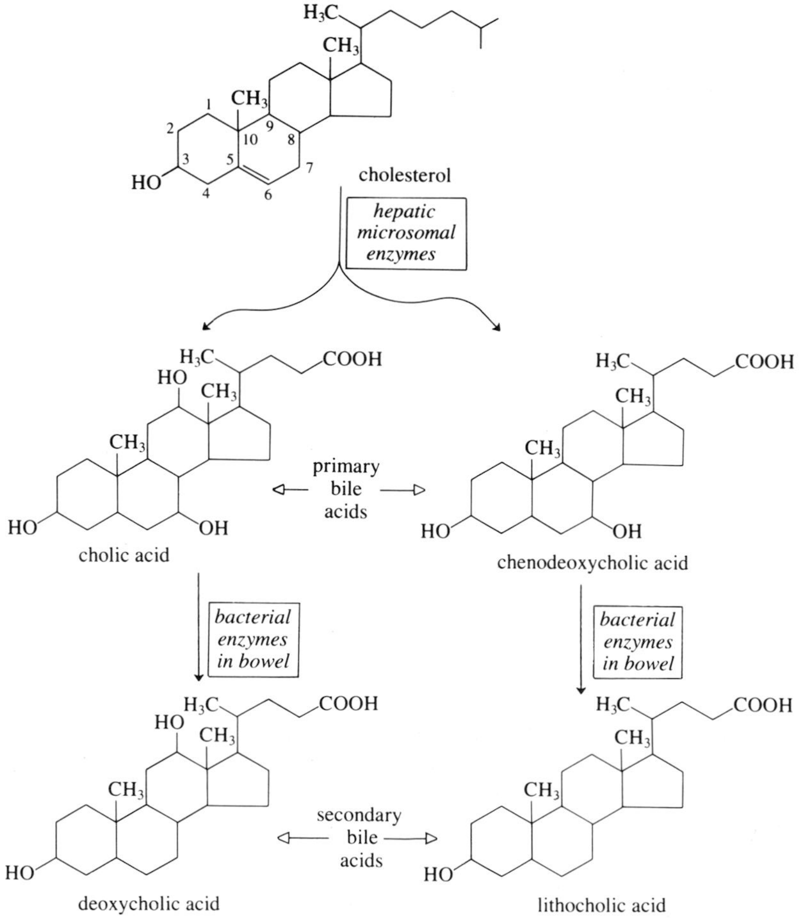

Fig. 15.11 Formation of bile acids from cholesterol. The hydroxyl groups on carbons 3, 7 and 10 are in the α-position. Chenodeoxycholic acid and its 7-β-hydroxy epimer, ursodeoxycholic acid, are used in the medical treatment of cholesterol gallstones.

most impossible to assess whether a drug increases the quantity of bile *entering* the gall bladder.

The presence in the duodenum of lipids causes contractions of the gall bladder. A variety of other stimuli are effective, e.g. a hypertonic solution of magnesium chloride introduced into the duodenum by intubation produces immediate contraction of the gall bladder. Numerous drugs are reputed to increase the flow of bile but the evidence is not very convincing since it depends on the fact that they hasten the transit of the intestinal contents and partially check putrefactive processes, resulting in more bile pigment being present in the faeces.

The organic constituents of bile

The most abundant group of organic compounds in bile, (constituting about 50% of organic constituents in human bile) are the bile acids: cholic acid, chenodeoxycholic acid, deoxycholic acid and lithocholic acid. These acids differ from each other mainly in the number of hydroxyl groups and their position. Cholic acid and chenodeoxycholic acids are made in the liver by oxidation of cholesterol and they are known as *primary bile acids*. Deoxycholic acid and lithocholic acid are formed in the intestine by dehydroxylation of the primary bile acids and they are termed *secondary bile acids* (Fig. 15.11). Another major group of organic compounds in bile are the phospholipids, the main ones being the phosphatidylcholines. A third organic component, cholesterol, is present in only small amounts, about 4% of the total solids of bile, while the bile pigments constitute about 2% of total organic solids.

When secreted, bile acids undergo entero-hepatic cycling. They are stored in the gallbladder, and discharged into the intestine during the digestion of a meal and they take part in the digestion and absorption of lipids. In the terminal ileum they are reabsorbed and pass in the portal blood to the liver where they are taken up by the liver cells and eventually resecreted. Much of the work on elucidating the biology of bile acids has been done by Hofman and his co-workers.

Bile has striking dispersant properties having the capacity to disperse polar lipids in micellar form. This property is the basis of absorption of fats and fat-soluble vitamins in the form of mixed micelles consisting of bile acids, fatty acids and mono-glycerides and fat soluble vitamins. The biliary route is also the only significant route for the excretion of cholesterol from the body.

Bile is a concentrated micellar solution. According to the model proposed by Small et al (Hofman, 1979), the core of the micelle is made up of phosphatidylcholine and cholesterol in a bilayer in which the rigid cholesterol molecules fit in between the flexible hydrocarbon chains of the phosphatidylcholine. The outside of the micelle has a layer of bile acid molecules which are bifacial detergents and have their hydrophobic sides against the fatty acid chains of the phosphatidylcholine molecule. (Other bifacial molecules, e.g. some drug metabolites, may also adsorb to the phosphatidylcholine and be excreted in the bile.) According to this model, cholesterol molecules are dissolved by the phosphatidylcholine, which is dispersed by the bile acids.

The bile acids adsorbed onto the micelle are in dynamic equilibrium with the surrounding bile acids which are in true molecular solution. The molar ratios of the constituents are as follows: bile acids to phosphatidylcholine 3:1, bile acids to cholesterol 10–20:1.

The formation of gall-stones

The commonest pathological condition of the biliary tract is cholesterol cholelithiasis, i.e. the formation of cholesterol gall-stones. Cholesterol cholelithiasis is very common in Western Europe and the USA, its incidence being nearly 30% in the members of some European population groups by the time they have reached middle age. It should be stressed that though gall-stones may cause gall bladder disease, the two conditions are not synonymous and gall-stones can occur without gall bladder disease.

Cholelithiasis is caused by an excess of cholesterol in the bile relative to the amounts of phosphatidylcholine and bile acids. This may result from a reduced secretion of bile acids or an increase in cholesterol.

Drugs used in cholelithiasis

Patients with cholelithiasis may require surgical treatment and indeed surgery is in general the preferred method of dealing with gall-stones. However, pharmacological agents may have a place in therapy.

Drugs used to dissolve non-calcified cholesterol gall-stones are **chenodeoxycholic acid (CDCA)** (Fig. 15.11) and **ursodeoxycholic acid (UDCA)**. CDCA is one of the two primary bile acids (Fig. 15.11). UDCA, the 7 β-hydroxy epimer of CDCA, occurs in small amounts in human bile and is the main bile acid in the bear (hence 'urso'). UDCA and CDCA are interconvertible during entero-hepatic cycling in man.

The original rationale for using bile acids in cholelithiasis was to increase its secretion by the liver and hence correct the disproportion between bile acids and cholesterol. However, it appears that the proportion is changed not by an increased secretion of bile acids but mainly by reduced secretion of cholesterol into the bile. Both CDCA and UDCA decrease cholesterol synthesis by inhibition of an enzyme which catalyses an early rate-limiting reaction in cholesterol formation. UDCA may also have an action on the surface characteristics of cholesterol crystals.

When the cholesterol saturation of the bile is lowered sufficiently, cholesterol passes slowly from the stone to the bile. The rate of dissolution depends partly on the size of the stone. Stones with a diameter greater than 15 mm are unlikely to dissolve. Stones with a diameter less than 5 mm have been shown to dissolve in 66–76% of patients treated with UDCA or CDCA for 6–12 months.

Given orally, UDCA and CDCA are handled by the body in the same way as endogenous bile acids.

Unwanted effects

One-third of patients taking CDCA have diarrhoea. This occurs only rarely with UDCA. Calcification of stones may occur, and this is less frequent with CDCA than with UDCA.

Drugs such as oestrogens, which cause an increase in the secretion of cholesterol in the bile will reduce the effect of UDCA and CDCA as will lipid-lowering agents (see below).

Clinical use

The clinical use of these agents is appropriate only in selected patients with gall-stones since, as has been pointed out, surgery is the preferred treatment in most cases.

Drugs affecting biliary spasm

The pain produced by the passage of gall-stones down the bile duct (biliary colic) can be very intense and immediate relief may be required. **Morphine** relieves the pain owing to its central narcotic analgesic action, but locally it may have an unfavourable effect since it constricts the sphincter of Oddi and raises the pressure in the bile duct. **Pethidine** has similar actions although it relaxes other smooth muscle, e.g. that of the ureter. **Atropine** is commonly employed to relieve biliary spasm since it has antispasmodic action. It may be used in conjunction with morphine.

The **nitrites** (see Chapter 10) produce a marked fall of intrabiliary pressure and if biliary colic is due primarily to spasm, a tablet of **glyceryl trinitrate** taken sublingually may relieve the attack.

Drugs altering the metabolism and excretion of cholesterol and other lipids

An increase in plasma lipid is a common feature of **atherosclerosis**, a condition which may lead to ischaemic heart disease, myocardial infarction and cerebral vascular accidents. Some types of hyperlipidaemia are associated with an increased risk of **pancreatitis** and in many types, deposits of lipid (**xanthomas**) occur in skin and tendons. Since the high lipid content of plasma is believed to underlie these conditions, attempts have been made to develop pharmacological agents which reduce the concentration of plasma lipids.

Lipids are insoluble in water and they are transported in the plasma as lipoproteins. Hyperlipidaemia (more correctly termed hyperlipoproteinaemia) reflects changes in the plasma concentration of these substances.

Lipoprotein transport in the blood

Lipoproteins consist of a central core of hydrophobic lipid (triglycerides or cholesteryl esters) encased in a more hydrophilic coat of polar substances—phospholipids, free cholesterol and associated proteins (apoproteins). There are four main classes of lipoprotein, differing in the relative proportion of the core lipids and in the type of apoprotein. They also differ in size and density and it is this latter property, as measured by centrifugation, which is the main basis of their classification. Thus, they are classified as: (1) High density lipoproteins (HDL); (2) Low density lipoproteins (LDL); (3) Very low density lipoproteins (VLDL); and (4) Chylomicrons. Each of these lipoprotein classes has a specific role in lipid transport in the circulation and there are different 'pathways' for exogenous and for endogenous lipids (Goldstein et al., 1983).

In the *exogenous pathway*, cholesterol and triglycerides derived from the gastrointestinal tract are transported as **chylomicrons** (diameter 100–1000 nm) to muscle and adipose tissue. Here, on the vascular endothelial cells, the core triglycerides are hydrolysed by a surface-bound lipoprotein lipase (which requires one of the apoproteins as a co-factor) and the free fatty acids are taken up by the tissues. The chylomicrons, smaller now (diameter 30–50 nm)*, but still containing their full complement of cholesteryl esters, pass to the liver, are bound to receptors on the liver cells which recognize two apoproteins on the chylomicrons, and undergo receptor-mediated endocytosis. Cholesterol is liberated within the cell and may be stored, or oxidized to bile acids, or secreted in the bile unaltered, or it may enter the endogenous pathway of lipid transport in VLDL.

In the *endogenous pathway*, triglycerides and cholesterol, derived from liver cells, are transported as VLDL (diameter 30–80 nm) to muscle and adipose tissue where the triglycerides are hydrolysed and fatty acids enter the tissues as described above. The lipotrotein particles become smaller (diameter 20–30 nm), but still have a full complement of cholesteryl esters and are now termed low density lipoproteins (LDL). These esters constitute a major reservoir of cholesterol for synthesis of steroids (see Chapters 16 and 17), new plasma membrane and bile acids. Cells requiring cholesterol for any of these purposes synthesize receptors for the requisite

apoproteins of LDL and take up these lipoproteins by receptor-mediated endocytosis. Some drugs may reduce the LDL concentration in the blood by stimulating the synthesis of these receptors. When cells die and their plasma membranes are degraded, cholesterol molecules are returned to the plasma and are adsorbed onto HDL particles (diameter 7–20 nm) where they are esterified with long-chain fatty acids. The resulting cholesteryl esters are subsequently transferred to VLDL or LDL particles by a transfer protein present in the plasma. HDL may contribute cholesterol for steroid synthesis in the adrenal cortex (see Chapter 16).

Types of hyperlipoproteinaemia

Hyperlipoproteinaemia may be primary or secondary. The **primary** forms are genetically determined and are classified into five types (Table 15.3) which vary in the extent to which (1) the plasma triglyceride and cholesterol concentrations are raised, and (2) particular lipoprotein classes are increased. The **secondary** forms may occur as a consequence of other conditions such as diabetes, alcoholism, chronic renal failure, hypothyroidism, liver disease, administration of oestrogen.

An essential component of the treatment of hyperlipoproteinaemia is the reduction of caloric intake and the restriction of saturated fats in the diet, but several **lipid-lowering drugs** have been introduced. These act either by reducing the production of lipoproteins or increasing their removal

Table 15.3 Frederickson classification of the primary hyperproteinaemias

	I	IIa	IIb	III	IV	V
Cholesterol	.	+	+	+		
Triglycerides	+ +		+	+	+	+
HDL						
LDL		+	+			
VLDL			+	abn	+	+
Chylomicrons	+					+

+ = increased concentration; abn = abnormal; HDL = high density lipoproteins; LDL = low density lipoproteins; VLDL = very low density lipoproteins.

Types IIa and IIb carry a markedly increased risk, and types III and IV a moderately increased risk of coronary artery disease. Types IV and V are associated with an increased incidence of pancreatitis. Type I is rare.

---

* At this stage the particle is referred to as a chylomicron remnant.

from the blood. The drugs used include cholestyramine, clofibrate, benzafibrate, nicotinic acid and probucol.

Whether treating hyperlipoproteinaemia is of value in decreasing the complications of atherosclerosis has been a controversial issue, although epidemiological studies have indicated that high blood concentrations of LDL-cholesterol and of total cholesterol are a principal risk factor in the development of these conditions. However, recently, evidence from a major multicentre, randomized double-blind trial carried out in the USA (Lipid Research Program, 1984) has shown that decreasing the blood concentration of LDL-cholesterol in patients with *primary* hypercholesterolaemia can lower the risk of coronary arterial disease. The drug used in the trial was cholestyramine.

In *secondary* hyperlipoproteinaemia the main therapeutic approach should be to treat the primary condition and to adjust the diet.

The main lipid-lowering drugs are described below. Current opinion is that combinations of these drugs are more effective than single drug therapy.

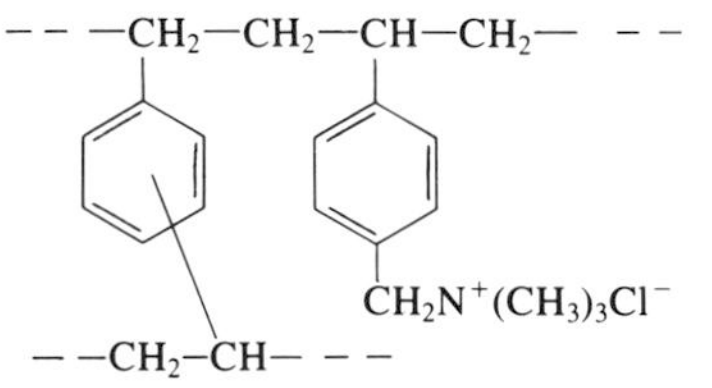

skin. Since cholestyramine is not absorbed, its systemic toxicity is low, but it may cause nausea, heartburn and constipation. Hyperchloraemic acidosis can occur. Cholestyramine may interfere with the absorption of fat-soluble vitamins, and of drugs such as chorothiazide, phenobarbitol, digitalis preparations and anticoagulants, if these are given concurrently.

Clofibrate (Fig. 15.12) reduces elevated plasma concentrations of triglycerides and, to a lesser extent, of cholesterol. It particularly reduces elevated concentrations of VLDL. Its main action appears to be stimulation of lipoprotein lipase. It is effective in type III hyperlipoproteinaemia, but is also used in types IV and V. The results of several recent clinical trials indicate that it does not necessarily reduce the mortality of coronary artery disease.

Bezafibrate is more potent than clofibrate and reduces high density lipoprotein and low density lipoprotein to a greater extent.

Nicotinic acid is a vitamin which has been used as a lipid-lowering agent. It has antilipidaemic activity and is used in type II, III, IV and V. Unwanted effects are common and include flushing, palpitations and gastrointestinal disturbances. High

part of cholestyramine polymer

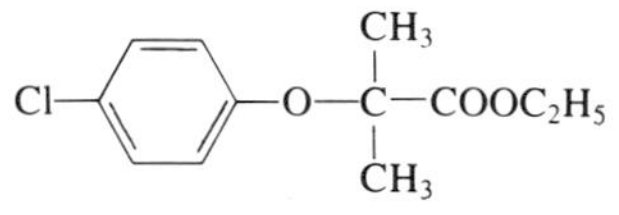

clofibrate

Fig. 15.12 Structures of two 'lipid-lowering' agents.

Cholestyramine (Fig. 15.12) is the insoluble chloride salt of a basic anion exchange resin which sequesters bile acids in the intestine and prevents their reabsorption and their enterohepatic recirculation. This results in a decreased absorption of exogenous cholesterol and an increase in the metabolism of endogenous cholesterol into bile acids in the liver. The consequence is a **reduction in the cholesterol** concentration in the plasma.

Cholestyramine is used in the therapy of types II and III hyperlipoproteinaemia. The drug is also effective in relieving pruritis in biliary obstruction which is due to the accumulation of bile acids in the

doses can cause disorders of liver function. It may impair glucose tolerance and may increase the risk of gout.

Probucol is a recently introduced agent which lowers the concentration in the plasma of both LDL-cholesterol and HDL-cholesterol. It acts in part by increasing the catabolism of cholesterol to bile acids. It is markedly hydrophobic and sequestrates in fat, remaining in the body for several months. Its peak effect on plasma cholesterol occurs only after 1–3 months administration. Gastrointestinal disturbances occur in 1 in 10 patients.

REFERENCES AND FURTHER READING

Angus J A, Black J W 1982 The interaction of choline esters, vagal stimulation and H_2 receptor blockade on acid secretion in vitro. Eur J Pharmac 80: 217–224

Awouters F, Niemegeers C J E, Jansen P A J 1983 Pharmacology of antidiarrhoeal drugs. Ann Rev Pharmacol Toxicol 23: 279–301

Berglindh T 1984 The mammalian gastric parietal cell in vitro. Ann Rev Physiol 46: 377–392

Black J W 1979 The riddle of gastric histamine. In: Yellin T O (ed) Histamine receptors. SP Medical and Scientific Books, New York 23–33

Borison H L, Wang S C 1953 Physiology and pharmacology of vomiting. Pharmacol Rev 5: 193–230

Borison H L, Borison R, McCarthy L E 1981 Phylogenic and neurologic aspects of the vomiting process. J Clin Pharmacol 21: 235–295

Code C F 1965 Histamine and gastric secretion: a later look. 1955–1965 Fed Proc 24: 1311–1321

Davenport H W 1982 Physiology of the digestive tract, 5th Ed. Year Book Publishers Inc, Chicago

Frytak S, Moertel C G 1981 Management of nausea and vomiting in the cancer patient. J Am Med Assoc 245: 393–396

Goldstein J L, Kita T, Brown M S 1983 Defective lipoprotein receptors and atherosclerosis; lessons from an animal counterpart of familial hypercholesterolemia. N Engl J Med 309: 288–295

Grossman M I, Konturek S J 1974 Inhibition of acid secretion in the dog by metiamide, a histamine antagonist acting on H_2 receptors. Gastroent 66: 517–521

Havel R, Goldstein J L, Brown M S 1980 Lipoproteins and lipid transport. In: Bondy P K, Rosenberg L E (eds) Metabolic Control and Disease. W B Saunders, Philadelphia, 393–494

Hofman A F 1979 The medical treatment of gallstones: a clinical application of the new biology of bile acids. Harvey Lecture Series No 74, 23–48

Kilbinger H, Weihrauch T R 1982 Drugs increasing gastrointestinal motility. Pharmacol 25: 61–72

Lipid Research Clinics Program 1984 The lipid research clinics coronary primary prevention trial results. I Reduction in incidence of coronary heart disease. II The relationship of reduction in incidence of coronary heart disease to cholesterol lowering. JAMA 251: I: 351–364, II: 365–374

Machen T E, Rutten M J, Ekblad E B M 1982 Histamine, cAMP and activation of piglet gastric mucosa. Amer J Physiol 242: G79–84

Mutt V 1982 Chemistry of the gastrointestinal hormones and hormone-like peptides and sketch of their physiology and pharmacology in vitamins and hormones volume. Academic Press 39: 231–431

Peroutka S J, Snyder S H 1982 Anti-emetics: neurotransmitter receptor binding predicts therapeutic actions. Lancet (i): 658–659

Recent Advances in the Development of Non-microbial Antidiarrhoeal Agents. Report of the scientific working group on drug development and management of acute diarrhoeas. WHO Document CDD/DDM/81.2

Seigel L J, Longo D L 1981 The control of chemotherapy-induced emesis. Ann Intern Med 95: 352–359

Soll A H, Grossman M K 1981/82 The interaction of stimulants on the function of isolated canine parietal cells. Phil Trans Roy Soc Lond 296B: 5–15

Soll A H, Walsh J H 1979 Regulation of gastric acid secretion. Ann Rev Physiol 41: 35–53

Stoudemire A, Cotanch P, Laszlo J 1984 Recent advances in the pharmacologic and behavioural management of chemotherapy-induced emesis. Arch Intern Med 144: 1029–1033

Williams R H 1981 Gastrointestinal hormones. In: Williams R H (ed) Endocrinology. W B Saunders, Philadelphia, 685–715

Wood C D, Graybiel A 1970 A theory of motion sickness based on pharmacological reactions. Clin Pharmacol and Ther 11: 621–629

16

The endocrine system

THE PITUITARY

The pituitary gland is composed of two sections, each of separate embryological origin. The anterior pituitary or **adenohypophysis** is derived from the ectoderm of the buccal cavity while the posterior pituitary **neurophypophysis** is derived from neural tissue. Both parts have an intimate functional relationship with the hypothalamus, the neurones of which can be shown to consist of two quite distinct systems influencing the anterior and posterior pituitary respectively.

THE ANTERIOR PITUITARY (ADENOHYPOPHYSIS)

The anterior pituitary secretes a number of different hormones vital to normal physiological function, some of which are involved in the regulation of other endocrine glands (corticotrophin, thyrotrophin and the gonadotrophins) while others have direct effects on peripheral target tissues (growth hormone, prolactin) (Table 16.1).

The cells of the anterior pituitary, originally classified purely on the basis of the staining properties of the cytoplasm into chromophobe, acidophil and basophil cells are now, using more complex criteria, classified into somatotrophs, mammotrophs (lactotrophs), corticotrophs, gonadotrophs and thyrotrophs, according to the substances secreted (see below).

Secretion from the anterior pituitary is largely regulated by factors (hormones) derived from the hypothalamus, which reach the pituitary through the blood stream. Blood vessels to the hypo-

thalamus divide in its tissue to form a meshwork of capillaries—the primary plexus (Fig. 16.1). This drains into the hypophyseal portal vessels, which pass through the pituitary stalk to feed a second plexus of sinusoidal capillaries in the anterior pituitary. (Some portal veins which drain into these sinusoid capillaries originate from a different primary plexus in the posterior pituitary.) Peptidergic neurones in the hypothalamus secrete a variety of releasing or release-inhibiting factors or hormones directly into the capillaries of the primary plexus. (Table 16.1 & Fig. 16.1). These substances regulate the secretion of hormones from the various cells of the anterior pituitary—**corticotrophin** (ACTH) from corticotrophs, **prolactin** from lactotrophs, **growth hormone** from somatotrophs, **thyroid-stimulating hormone** from thyrotrophs, and **gonadotrophins** from gonadotrophs. There is a delicate balance between the hypothalamic factors, the trophic hormones whose release they regulate, and the secretions of the peripheral endocrine glands. This balance may in each case involve one or more negative feedback pathways. The long negative feedback pathways affect both the hypothalamus and the anterior pituitary and are mediated by the hormones which are secreted from the peripheral glands. The short negative feedback pathways are mediated by anterior pituitary hormones acting on the hypothalamus. There is some evidence that the anterior pituitary hormones reach the hypothalamus by retrograde blood flow in the pituitary stalk.

The peptidergic neurons in the hypothalamus which secrete the factors which regulate the anterior pituitary are themselves influenced by higher centres in the CNS. This action is mediated through dopamine, noradrenaline and serotonin. The opi-

Table 16.1 Hormones secreted by the hypothalamus and the anterior pituitary

Hypothalamic factor (or hormone)	Hormone affected in anterior pituitary	Main effects of anterior pituitary hormone
Corticotrophin-releasing factor (CRF)	Corticotrophin	Stimulates secretion of adrenal cortical hormones (mainly glucocorticoids). Maintains integrity of adrenal cortex.
Thyrotrophin-releasing hormone (TRH; Protirelin)	Thyrotrophin	Stimulates synthesis and secretion of thyroid hormones, T_3 and T_4. Maintains integrity of thyroid gland.
Growth hormone-releasing factor (GHRF) Growth hormone-release inhibiting factor (GHRIF; Somatostatin)	Growth hormone	Regulates growth, partly directly, partly through evoking the release of somatomedins from the liver and elsewhere. Increases protein synthesis, increases blood glucose, stimulates lipolysis.
Gonadotrophin-releasing-factor (GRF)	Follicle-stimulating hormone (FSH)	Stimulates the growth of the ovum and the Graffian follicle in the female and gametogenesis in the male. With LH, stimulates the secretion of oestrogen throughout the menstrual cycle and progesterone in the second half.
	Luteinizing hormone (LH) or Interstitial cell-stimulating hormone (ICSH)	Stimulates ovulation and the development of the corpus luteum. With FSH, stimulates secretion of oestrogen throughout the menstrual cycle, and progesterone in the second half. In male, regulates testosterone secretion.
Prolactin release-inhibiting factor (PRIF). Probably dopamine. Prolactin-releasing factor (PRF)	Prolactin	Together with other hormones, prolactin promotes development of mammary tissue during pregnancy. Stimulates milk production in the post-partum period.
Melanocyte-stimulating hormone releasing factor (MSH-RF) MSH release inhibiting factor (MSH-RIF)	Melanocyte-stimulating hormone (MSH)	Darkens the skin in amphibia and fish. Function in man not known.

oid pentapeptides, which are found in highest concentration in the hypothalamus, also affect the peptidergic neurons which control the anterior pituitary.

Another means of hypothalamic control of the anterior pituitary is exerted through the tubero-infundibular dopaminergic pathway, the neurones of which lie in close apposition to the primary capillary plexus (see Chapter 19). Dopamine can be secreted directly into the hypophyseal portal circulation and thus reach the anterior pituitary.

It is now considered that the anterior pituitary, in addition to being a complex endocrine gland, has some similarity to neural tissue and paracrine tissue in that some of its cells communicate with and influence each other through paracrine association (local hormone effects) and possibly also through gap junctions and electrical coupling.

HYPOTHALAMIC HORMONES

There are at least six hormones or factors which originate in the hypothalamus and which regulate the secretion of anterior pituitary hormones. These are listed in Table 16.1 and are described in more detail below. Those which are available for use constitute valuable research tools as well as being of actual or potential clinical use in treatment and in diagnosis.

GROWTH HORMONE-RELEASING FACTOR (GHRF)

GHRF* is a peptide with 40–44 amino-acid re-

* There is a proposal that the acronym GHRF be replaced by the name 'somatocrinin'.

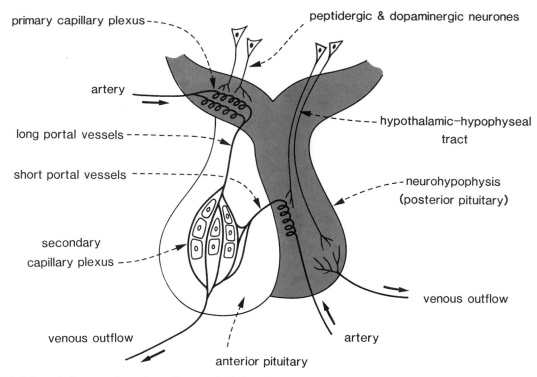

Fig. 16.1 Schematic diagram of vascular and neuronal relationships between the hypothalamus, the posterior pituitary and the anterior pituitary. The main portal vessels to the anterior pituitary lie in the pituitary stalk and arise from the primary plexus in the hypothalamus, but some arise from the vascular bed in the posterior pituitary. The neurons secreting into the primary plexus may be peptidergic or dopaminergic.

sidues, the sequence of which was worked out on material from patients with acromegaly-producing pancreatic tumours. It has strong homology with glucagon and with various gastrointestinal hormones such as vasoactive intestinal polypeptide (VIP), secretin, and gastric inhibitory peptide (GIP). However, although these latter peptides have some stimulatory effect on growth hormone secretion from cultured pituitary cells, none is as potent as GHRF, which is active in a concentration of 10^{-15} M. A preparation of the first 29 amino-acids has been shown to have full intrinsic activity and potency *in vitro*. The actions of GHRF are calcium dependent, are accompanied by a rise in cAMP (see Chapter 1) and are potentiated by prior exposure of these cells to glucocorticoids or thyroid hormone.

Actions

The main action of GHRF is summarized in Figure 16.2. Synthetic preparations of GHRF containing

the first 40 and the first 29 amino-acids of the peptide derived from human pancreatic tumours have been tested in man. These two peptides are termed respectively hpGHRF(1–40) and hpGHRF(1–29), the 'hp' referring to their derivation from 'human pancreas'. Both have been shown to stimulate the release of growth hormone in normal subjects and in growth hormone-deficient subjects. Given i.v. in a dose of 0.5 µg/kg body weight they caused secretion of growth hormone within minutes and peak concentrations were reached in 60 minutes. A similar response has been reported after intranasal administration of GHRF. The action appears to be selective for the somatotrophs in the anterior pituitary, no other pituitary hormones being released.

Clinical use

Preliminary trials have indicated that GHRF is effective in restoring the secretion of growth hor-

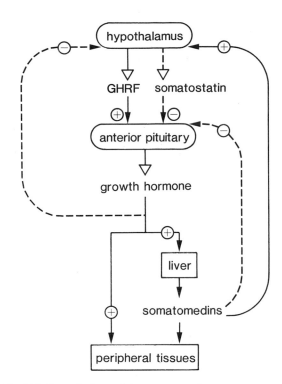

Fig. 16.2 Control of growth hormone secretion.
Arrow with open head = releases
Arrow with closed head = acts on
----⊖---- = inhibits; ———⊕——— = stimulates

(Fig. 16.2) and also that of thyrotrophin from the anterior pituitary as well as the release of secretions from other endocrine glands—insulin, glucagon (p. 379) and most gastrointestinal hormones. It also appears to reduce gastric acid and pancreatic secretion (p. 331).

A long-acting analogue of somatostatin is undergoing clinical trial. This is an octapeptide protected from breakdown by a D-phenylalanyl residue at the N terminus and an amino-alcohol at the C terminus and it is more potent than somatostatin itself. It is given by subcutaneous injection twice daily and has been used in preliminary trials to treat acromegally. It is expected to be of value in a variety of hyperfunctioning endocrine tumours including insulinomas, glucagonomas and growth-hormone-secreting adenomas. Further applications are likely to be in pancreatitis and in gastric bleeding due to ulcer or stress gastritis, since results in preliminary trials with somatostatin itself for these conditions have been very promising.

mone, with its resultant physiological effects, in growth hormone-deficient children. An increase in linear growth was reported during the 6 month period of administration, 1–3 μg/kg of the peptide being given subcutaneously every 3 hours through an indwelling catheter. It has also stimulated growth hormone release in individuals in whom growth hormone deficiency has resulted from radiotherapy.

SOMATOSTATIN

Somatostatin is a cyclic peptide of 14 amino-acid residues. It is derived from a larger precursor protein (MW 15 000) and in addition to being found in the hypothalamus is present elsewhere in the CNS as well as in the pancreas (p. 378) and gastrointestinal tract. Its action is mediated partly by an effect on calcium permeability.

When injected it has a half-life of less than 4 minutes. It inhibits the release of growth hor-

THYROTROPHIC-RELEASING HORMONE (PROTIRELIN; TRH)

Protirelin (called 'thyroliberin' in the USA) is a tripeptide (pyroglutamyl-histidyl-proline amide), which releases thyrotrophin from the anterior pituitary. Its action involves stimulation of adenylate cyclase. It is found not only in the hypothalamus, but in other parts of the CNS and also in the pancreas and the gastrointestinal tract. It may have neurotransmitter and paracrine functions as well as endocrine functions.

Its action in releasing thyrotrophin involves binding to a specific receptor on the membrane of pituitary cells with activation of adenylate cyclase, but does not involve protein synthesis.

The main clinical use of TRH is in diagnosis of mild thyroid disorders. It is given intravenously and in normal subjects it elicits an increase in plasma thyrotrophin concentration which reaches a peak in 20–30 minutes. In cases of hyperthyroidism, the blood thyroxine concentration is raised, which has a negative feedback effect on the anterior pituitary resulting in a blunted response to protirelin. The opposite occurs with hypothyroidism, in which the defect is in the thyroid itself.

CORTICOTROPHIN-RELEASING FACTOR (CRF)

CRF is a peptide containing 41 amino-acid residues. Synthetic preparations are available and can be shown to release corticotrophin from corticotrophs in cultures of pituitary cells. It acts synergistically with arginine vasopressin. In the body both its action and its release are inhibited by glucocorticoids (see Fig. 16.20).

Its main use is likely to be in diagnostic tests—to assess the ability of the pituitary to secrete corticotrophin, to assess whether a deficiency of corticotrophin is due to a pituitary or a hypothalamic defect, or to evaluate hypothalamic-pituitary function after therapy for Cushing's syndrome. It may be of value in detecting an early Cushing's syndrome (see Fig. 16.19).

GONADOTROPHIN-RELEASING FACTOR

This is a decapeptide which releases both follicle-stimulating hormone and luteinizing hormone. It has been called luteinizing hormone releasing hormone (LHRH) and is available as a preparation called *gonadorelin*. Its structure, actions and uses are described in Chapter 17 (p. 413).

ANTERIOR PITUITARY HORMONES

GROWTH HORMONE

Growth hormone is found in the anterior pituitary in larger quantities, (5–15 mg/g), than any other pituitary hormone. It is a single polypeptide (21 500 MW) of 191 amino-acids, with two intrachain disulphide bonds, derived by proteolysis from a precursor protein and secreted by the somatotroph cells. It is somewhat similar in structure to prolactin and to the chorionic somatomammotrophin secreted by the placenta, and there is some overlap in the activities of these hormones. Fragments prepared from the whole molecule also have moderate metabolic activity on injection, but their physiological significance is a matter of conjecture.

The secretion of growth hormone is high in the newborn, decreasing at 4 years to a steady level, which is then maintained until after puberty when there is a further decline.

Regulation of growth hormone secretion

This occurs by the action of hypothalamic **growth hormone-releasing factor (GHRF)** modulated by **somatostatin** or growth hormone release-inhibiting factor (GHRIF), as described above and is outlined in Figure 16.2.

One of the mediators of growth hormone action, **somatomedin C**, which is released from the liver (see below) has an inhibitory effect on growth hormone secretion by stimulating somatostatin release from the hypothalamus (Fig. 16.2).

Hypothalamic neurotransmitters which are implicated in the release of growth hormone include noradrenaline, dopamine and serotonin and opioid peptides (which increase the release). α-adrenoceptor antagonists prevent the repetitive surges of secretion. There are also dopamine receptors on the somatotrophs of the anterior pituitary and the stimulant action of **levodopa** may be used in normal subjects as a test for growth hormone reserve.

Growth hormone release, like that of other anterior pituitary secretions, is pulsatile, and its plasma concentration, which can be measured by radioimmunoassay, may fluctuate 10–100 fold. These surges occur repeatedly during the day and night and reflect changes in hypothalamic control. They can be abolished by measures which interrupt α-adrenergic pathways in the CNS. The concentration of growth hormone rises after fasting and falls after a meal and is increased by stress, exercise and emotional factors. Deep sleep is another potent stimulus to secretion, more particularly in children.

Actions

The main effect of this hormone is, as its name implies, on normal growth. In childhood the lack of it causes **pituitary dwarfism** and an excess, **gigantism**. In both these conditions the normal proportions of the body may be maintained. Increased secretion in adults results in **acromegaly**, a condition in which there is enlargement of facial structure and of hands and feet. (Acral means distal.) In exercising control of normal growth, this endocrine secretion affects many tissues, acting in conjunction with other hormones secreted from the thyroid, the gonads and the adrenal cortex.

Growth hormone stimulates the production, mainly from the liver, of several polypeptides termed **somatomedins** which are responsible for many if not most of its anabolic actions (see Fig. 16.2). These polypeptides have a certain degree of structural homology with insulin and they cross react with it. Receptors for somatomedins exist on liver cells, fat cells and cartilage cells. (Other growth hormone-dependent factors, with specific effects on particular tissues, such as nerve growth factor and epidermal growth factor, are considered by some to be 'somatomedins'.)

Protein synthesis is stimulated by growth hormone and the uptake of amino-acids into cells is increased, especially in skeletal muscle. This action involves an effect on DNA and the production of specific messenger RNA and protein. Increased DNA synthesis with subsequent mitosis is also stimulated, resulting in proliferation of various tissues. Somatomedins mediate many of these anabolic effects, influencing skeletal muscle and also the synthesis of cartilage at the epiphyses of long bones, and thus bone growth, by a direct action on the cartilage cells.

The effects on *carbohydrate metabolism* are complex. The early 'insulin-like' effect (e.g. a decrease in blood glucose; see below) which is seen soon after administration both *in vivo* and *in vitro* is only produced by unphysiologically high concentrations. With lower, physiological concentrations insulin-like reactions do not occur. The long-term effects of growth hormone, a decrease of glucose uptake and an enhancement of potassium uptake, are the opposite of those produced by insulin, and in fact growth hormone inhibits the action of insulin if both are given together. It is, however, insulinotrophic in that it enhances the secretion of insulin in response to a rise in blood glucose.

The main action on *fat metabolism* is to cause lipolysis, an effect which, *in vitro*, necessitates the presence of a glucocorticoid and appears to require the synthesis of RNA and proteins.

Growth hormone also has prolactin-like effects (see below).

Disturbances in growth hormone production and clinical treatment

Pituitary dwarfism, in which growth hormone production is deficient, can result from a lack of GHRF, or a failure of somatomedin generation, or defects in the somatomedin receptors in target tissues. In patients with GHRF deficiency, satisfactory linear growth can be achieved by giving human growth hormone. At present this is extracted from the pituitaries of cadavers and is expensive and difficult to obtain. It is given intramuscularly three times a week. It may provoke antibody formation and there is a potential risk of hepatitis transmission. Material produced from microorganisms by genetic engineering techniques should soon be available.

An excessive production of growth hormone in children results in increased growth before the epiphyses are closed and therefore gigantism. The pathogenesis of this condition is not clearly known; it is possible that it is hypothalamic in origin.

An excessive secretion of growth hormone in adults, resulting in acromegaly, is usually the result of a benign pituitary tumour. Treatment consists of removal or irradiation of the tumour. Pharmacological agents which may ameliorate the condition include **levodopa** (p. 541) and **bromocriptine**. Levodopa, which stimulates growth hormone secretion in normal subjects, paradoxically suppresses it in acromegalic patients. Bromocriptine, which is a dopamine agonist (see Chapter 19) suppresses prolactin secretion, and may also suppress growth hormone production. The long-lasting analogue of **somatostatin** is reported to be of value in acromegaly.

PROLACTIN

Prolactin, a pituitary hormone which is also known as mammotrophin, lactogenic hormone, or luteogenic hormone, is, in structure, a single peptide chain (23 000 MW) consisting of 198 amino-acid residues with three loops formed by three intrachain disulphide bonds. Prolactin is secreted by mammotroph (lactotroph) cells which are abundant in the anterior pituitary and which increase in number during pregnancy, probably under the influence of oestrogen. The hormone is present in only very small amounts in the gland, the total quantity being 100–200 µg. In plasma its average concentration is normally about 8 ng/ml in women and 5 ng/ml in men. There is an increase at night which does not reflect a circadian periodicity but the effect of sleep itself, because it does not occur if subjects are kept awake and does occur during daytime if subjects are allowed to sleep.

It is structurally related to growth hormone (see above) but its main known function in humans is the control of lactation in females. Its function in males is not known.

Regulation of prolactin secretion

Prolactin is unusual in that its secretion is under tonic *inhibitory* control by the hypothalamus (Fig. 16.3 & see Table 16.1). This is shown by the fact that

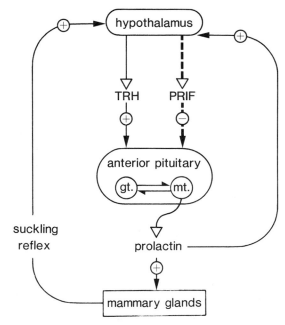

Fig. 16.3 Control of prolactin secretion. The dominant inhibitory effect of dopamine (or PRIF) may be modulated post-natally by the stimulatory effect of TRH whose release is indirectly triggered by the suckling reflex. Both PRIF and TRH act directly on the mammotrophs. Prolactin is thought to have an inhibitory influence on its own secretion by stimulating the inhibitory, hypothalamic, dopaminergic pathways which affect the anterior pituitary. Paracrine secretion from gonadotrophs modulates the response of the mammotrophs.
gt = gonadotroph; mt = mammotroph
----⊖---- = stimulates
———⊕——— = stimulates
Arrow with open head = releases
Arrow with closed head = acts on

section of the pituitary stalk results in an increase of prolactin secretion but a decrease in all other anterior pituitary hormones. The inhibitory influence is exerted through the dopaminergic tubero-infundibular pathway (see Chapter 19); the **prolactin release-inhibiting factor** (**PRIF**) secreted by the hypothalamus is generally thought to be dopamine itself. That there are dopamine receptors in the anterior pituitary has been demonstrated by pharmacological experiments (see below). However, the full suppressive action of the hypothalamus probably requires a second inhibitor which may be gamma-aminobutyric acid (for which there are receptors in the pituitary) or the metabolites of TRH and/or oestrogen.*

Two other hypothalamic factors, **prolactin-releasing factor** (PRF) and **thyrotrophin-releasing hormone** (TRH) *stimulate* prolactin secretion but their full physiological significance *in vivo* is uncertain. There are receptors for TRH on the mammotrophs.

Gonadotrophs are thought to be involved, modulating the response of the mammotrophs to hypothalamic hormones, possibly by a paracrine mode of communication (see Fig. 16.3).

There is no long negative feedback pathway influencing prolactin secretion, but there is experimental evidence in animals that prolactin can regulate its own secretion through a short feedback loop, *stimulating* dopaminergic neurons in the hypothalamus.

Neural reflexes arising in breast tissue are also important in the control of prolactin secretion (see below).

Oestrogens are known to increase prolactin secretion but the physiological role of this action is not known.

Several drugs affect prolactin secretion and provide evidence for the presence of dopamine receptors in the anterior pituitary. Dopamine antagonists such as the **phenothiazines** and **butyrophenones** (see Chapter 22) and also dopamine-depleting agents such as **reserpine** (see Chapter 7) are potent stimulants of prolactin release. **Domperidone**, a po-

---

* A peptide associated with the gonadotrophin releasing hormone (the **GnRH-a**ssociated **p**eptide, GAP) is also thought to have a role in inhibiting prolactin secretion.

tent dopamine receptor-blocking agent which does not cross the blood-brain barrier, causes a prompt, marked rise in prolactin concentration by its action on the pituitary.

Dopamine agonists suppress prolactin release but vary in the extent and duration of their action. **Levodopa** which is decarboxylated *in vivo* to give dopamine (see Chapter 24) has a transient suppressant effect when given orally. **Apomorphine** has a similar effect. The ergot derivative **bromocriptine** is a potent agonist having a prolonged suppressive effect on both basal and stimulated release (see below).

Actions of prolactin

A wide range and diversity of effects of prolactin can be shown in animals, but there are marked species differences, and limited supplies of the compound for studies in humans have meant that its role in man is still not fully delineated.

Prolactin clearly has mammotrophic activity in rats and indeed one of the main mammotrophic hormones, oestrogen, is ineffective in experimental animals in the absence of prolactin. It is possible that this holds true in humans as well. Development and proliferation of the secretory alveoli of the mammary glands during pregnancy requires the coordinated action of many hormones—of the ovary, placenta, thyroid and adrenal cortex as well as the anterior pituitary. If the requisite hormonal environment is provided *in vitro*, prolactin can be shown to bind to specific receptors and to stimulate proliferation and differentiation of mammary tissue. It has been demonstrated that this mammotrophic action contributes to the development of mammary tumours in rodents, but there is no evidence that prolactin plays a direct part in the production of breast tumours in humans, though an indirect, permissive role cannot be ruled out.

The main specific function of prolactin is the control of milk production. In experimental animals, the synthesis of milk protein requires the presence of insulin and glucocorticoids but is critically dependent on prolactin. At parturition, when the placenta is expelled and the blood level of oestrogen falls the prolactin concentration rises and lactation is initiated. Maintenance of lactation depends on suckling, which stimulates a reflex se-

cretion of prolactin by neural pathways, causing a 10–100-fold increase within 30 minutes. There is mounting evidence that the increased prolactin release in these circumstances involves a stimulation by TRH and the development of a substantial increase in responsiveness of the mammotrophs to this hormone.

Prolactin's effect on gonadal function varies in different species but in man it may inhibit gonadotrophin release and/or the response of the ovaries to these trophic hormones. This may be one of the reasons why ovulation does not usually occur during breast feeding, constituting a natural contraceptive mechanism.

According to one rather attractive hypothesis the high post-natal concentration of prolactin reflects its biological function of 'parental' hormone. Certainly broodiness and nest-building activity can be induced in birds by prolactin injections, and equivalent 'parental' behaviour can be induced in mice and rabbits. However, its relevance for primates is still conjectural.

Disorders of prolactin secretion

Hyperprolactinemia (increased concentration of prolactin in the blood) is relatively rare. It may occur with pituitary tumours, conditions in which TRH is increased, disorders of the hypothalamus and as a side effect of neuroleptic drugs (see Chapter 22) or oral contraceptives.

In females an excessive prolactin secretion frequently but not invariably results in galactorrhea, i.e. nonpuerperal lactation, (though not all cases of galactorrhea have hyperprolactinemia). Increased prolactin concentration is usually associated with amenorrhea, and in males it causes gynaecomastia and impotence.

Bromocriptine, a dopamine agonist, has a powerful inhibitory action on prolactin release. It may be used after parturition to prevent lactation without causing pain or engorgement of the breast, as well as to suppress established lactation, being more effective than oestrogens in this latter action.

In hyperprolactinaemia due to pituitary adenoma, bromocriptine rapidly reduces prolactin levels to normal. In females this results in the restoration of ovulatory menstruation and the suppression of galactorrhea. In males this may relieve the gynaecomastia and restore potency. It is also used in Parkinsonism (see Chapter 24).

Bromocriptine is well absorbed orally and peak concentrations occur after 2 hours. It is metabolized in the liver and excreted in the bile. Unwanted reactions include nausea and vomiting, which may be ameliorated by taking the drug with meals. Dizziness, constipation and postural hypotension may also occur.

CORTICOTROPHIN

Corticotrophin, (also termed adrenocorticotrophic hormone or ACTH) is the adenohypophyseal endocrine secretion which controls the synthesis and release of most of the hormones of the adrenal cortex. It is derived from a larger precursor molecule, pro-opiomelanocortin, which is also the precursor for β-lipotrophin (and thus for β-endorphin) as well as α, β and γ-melanocyte-stimulating hormone (α, β and γ-MSH). The relationship of these peptides is outlined in Figure 19.10 and is discussed in more detail in Chapters 19 & 25.

The precursor is found in the hypothalamus and the intermediate lobe of the pituitary as well as in the anterior pituitary. In the anterior pituitary, endopeptidases cleave pro-opiomelanocortin to give mainly ACTH and β-lipotrophin, whereas in the hypothalamus and intermediate lobe the molecules are further processed to give γ-MSH and β-endorphin respectively.

Corticotrophin secretion from the anterior pituitary is under the control of corticotrophin-releasing factor from the hypothalamus (see Table 16.1 & Fig. 16.20) and the system is modulated by negative feedback by the glucocorticoids released from the adrenal cortex. This topic is dealt with in more detail later in this chapter.

MELANOCYTE-STIMULATING HORMONES (MSH)

These are derived from the same precursor as corticotrophin namely pro-opiomelanocortin (see Fig. 19.10) and are released mainly from the cells of the intermediate lobe under the influence of two hypothalamic hormones—a releasing-factor (MSHRF) and a release-inhibiting factor (MSH-RIF)—see Table 16.1. In fish and amphibians MSH has a skin-darkening effect by virtue of its action in dispersing the pigment granules of melanocytes. Its action in man is a matter of conjecture.

GONADOTROPHIC HORMONES

These endocrine secretions are involved in the control of gonadal function and are dealt with in Chapter 17.

POSTERIOR PITUITARY (NEUROHYPOPHYSIS)

The posterior pituitary is a downward extension of the hypothalamic area of the brain (see Fig. 16.1) and consists largely of the axons of nerve cells which lie in the supraoptic and paraventricular nuclei of the hypothalamus. These axons form the hypothalamic-hypophyseal tract and the fibres terminate in dilated nerve endings in close association with capillaries in the posterior pituitary. A few also terminate near the primary capillary plexus of the portal vascular system which passes to the anterior pituitary.

The two main hormones of the posterior pituitary are **oxytocin** and the **antidiuretic hormone**

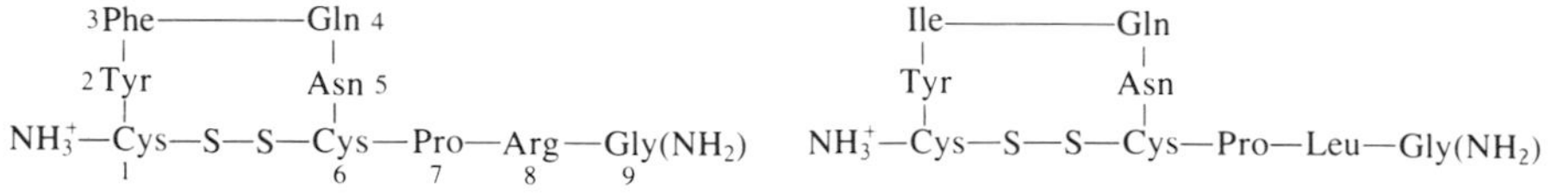

ADH (Arginine-vasopressin)

Oxytocin

Fig. 16.4 The structures of the two posterior pituitary peptides.

(**ADH**) (Fig. 16.4). The latter hormone is also called vasopressin (see Chapters 14 & 11). The hormones are synthesized, initially as part of larger precursor proteins, in the cell bodies of the neurons of the supraoptic and paraventricular nuclei in the hypothalamus. Separate neurones are involved in the synthesis of ADH and oxytocin. The peptides, in neurosecretory granules, pass down the axons of the neurons to the posterior pituitary where they are stored. Within the granules the hormones are bound to carrier proteins, termed 'neurophysins' (10 000 MW), the neurophysins for oxytocin and vasopressin being quite specific and separate. The stimulus for secretion is a nerve impulse which depolarizes the axon terminal and results in the discharge of the granules by a calcium dependent exocytosis. Both the hormone and its binding protein pass into the bloodstream. Some ADH-secreting neurones release their granules into the hypophyseal portal system and are involved in the control of ACTH secretion (see later in this chapter) and some may release ADH into the CSF.

The structure of the posterior pituitary hormones was determined by du Vigneaud and his co-workers in the 1950s. This same group synthesized the peptides and worked out the main structure/activity relationships. Natural ADH is a nonapeptide with a sulphydryl bridge connecting residues 1 and 6 which is necessary for physiological activity. Residue 8 is arginine in all mammalian species except swine in which it is lysine. Oxytocin differs from ADH in having leucine at position 8 and isoleucine at position 3 (Fig. 16.4).

Several peptides have been synthesized which vary in their antidiuretic, vasopressor and oxytocic (uterine stimulant) properties.

Desmopressin, 1-deamino-8-D-arginine vasopressin has 12 times the antidiuretic potency of ADH, less than 1% of its pressor activity and a much longer duration of action.

Felypressin (2-phenylalanine-8-lysine vasopressin) has predominantly pressor activity and is used as a local vasoconstrictor with local anaesthetics. The synthetic peptide **1-deamino-oxytocin** is several times more potent as a uterine stimulant than natural oxytocin. **Arginine vasotocin**, a naturally occurring peptide found in the pituitaries of many non-mammalian vertebrates, has the same structure as oxytocin except that it has arginine in

position 3. It has both oxytocic and antidiuretic properties.

ANTIDIURETIC HORMONE (ADH)

The control of secretion of ADH and its physiological role

ADH has a crucial role in the control of the water content of the body through its action on the cells of the distal part of the nephron and the collecting tubules in the kidney (see Chapter 14). Specific nuclei in the hypothalamus which control water metabolism lie close to the nuclei which synthesize and secrete ADH.

One of the main stimuli to ADH release is an *increase in plasma osmolality*. The mean set point of plasma osmolality is 282 mosm/kg, ADH release being stimulated in response to stimulation of 'osmoreceptors' if this rises to 287 mosm/kg or above. A *decrease in circulating blood* volume is the other major factor causing secretion of ADH. The sensation of thirst is produced by both these factors.

The main disorder of ADH secretion is **diabetes insipidus**, a condition in which, usually, there is decreased circulating ADH and thus continuous production of copious amounts of hypotonic urine. Any pathological lesion which interferes with the hypothalamic hypophyseal tract is likely to result in diabetes insipidus, the threshold level of secretion of ADH below which the syndrome occurs being 7% of normal. Causes of damage in this area include surgery, neoplasia and trauma. Diabetes insipidus can also occur with normal ADH secretion if the kidney does not respond to the hormone. This is termed 'nephrogenic diabetes insipidus'.

Actions of ADH

Renal actions

ADH binds to receptors in the basolateral membrane of the cells of the distal tubule and collecting ducts of the nephron (see Chapter 14). Its main effect is to increase the permeability of the luminal membrane to water. The interaction with the receptor results in activation of adenylate cyclase, an increase in cAMP and activation of protein kinase A. The current theory is that the actual increase in water permeability involves an increase in the number of water channels which are derived by aggregation of pre-existing vesicles in the subapical cytoplasm. These channels are thought to have diameter close to that of the water molecule ($\sim 2A°$). Microtubules and microfilaments are important in the action of ADH, possibly being necessary for the translocation of the vesicles from cytoplasm to membrane, and an increase in cytosolic calcium also appears to be involved in this process. Water moves passively from the tubule lumen to interstitia under the influence of the osmotic gradient created by the counter-current mechanism.

In addition to this action (the promotion of a sustained increase in passive movement of water across the cell), ADH transiently stimulates the active transport of sodium ions. This involves an increase in the apical membrane permeability to sodium ions through sodium-specific entry sites and is independent of the effect on water permeability.

The receptors on the tubule cells have a high affinity for ADH, are different from the ADH receptors on smooth muscle cells and are termed V_2-receptors.

Numerous pharmacological agents interact with ADH in its action on the kidney: ADH stimulates phospholipase A_2 and the generation of prostaglandins, predominantly PGE_2 (see Chapter 8) which inhibits ADH actions, functioning as a 'braking' mechanism; drugs which inhibit prostaglandin formation (**indomethacin**, **paracetamol**) thus enhance ADH activity; **chlorpropamide** which enhances sensitivity to ADH is believed to have the same mechanism of action. ADH action is counteracted by the general anaesthetic **methoxyflurane** (see Chapter 20), by **lithium carbonate** (see Chapter 23) and by the antibiotic **demeclocycline**. These last two agents are used to treat patients with excessive water retention due to excessive secretion of ADH.

Agents which modify microtubules, such as colchicine (see Chapter 9) and the vinca alkaloids (see Chapter 29) will also reduce ADH effects.

Non-renal actions

ADH has effects on *smooth muscle* particularly in the cardiovascular system in which it has a vaso-constrictor action (see Chapter 11). ADH binds to V_1-receptors on smooth muscle cells causing stimulation. The transduction mechanism for these receptors involves the turnover of polyphosphoinositides and an increase in cytosolic calcium (see Chapter 1). The affinity of these V_1-receptors for ADH is lower than that of the V_2-receptors and the responses are only seen with doses somewhat larger than those affecting the kidney. The main effects occur in the blood vessels of the skin and gastrointestinal tract; higher doses affect the coronary and pulmonary vessels as well. The effects on the heart and the blood pressure will depend on the baroreceptor reflexes. The smooth muscle of the uterus and gastrointestinal tract is also stimulated.

In addition to its actions on the kidney and on smooth muscle, ADH has actions on a variety of other tissues. It accelerates glycogen breakdown in liver cells, stimulates aggregation and degranulation of platelets and increases the concentration of factor VIII of the blood coagulation cascade. Released into the pituitary 'portal' circulation, it promotes the release of corticotrophin from the anterior pituitary (see Fig. 16.20) and within the central nervous system it probably acts as a neurotransmitter.

Preparations used and pharmacokinetic aspects

The preparations of antidiuretic peptides available for clinical use are **vasopressin**, (which is ADH itself) **lypressin**, (8-lysine vasopressin), and **desmopressin** (1-deamino-8-D-arginine vasopressin). These have 80% and 120% of the antidiuretic potency of vasopressin and 60% and 0.4% of its vasopressor potency respectively. Vasopressin is given by subcutaneous or intramuscular injection or by intravenous infusion and can also be given intranasally. The other two are usually given intranasally as snuff or spray, though preparations of desmopressin for injection are available.

Vasopressin and lypressin are rapidly eliminated having a plasma half-life of 10 minutes and a short duration of action. Metabolism is by tissue peptidases and 33% of vasopressin is removed by the kidney. Desmopressin is less subject to degradation by peptidases and its plasma half-life is 75 minutes.

Clinical use

The main use of antidiuretic peptides is in the treatment of diabetes insipidus of pituitary origin, intranasal desmopressin being the treatment of choice; they are valueless in nephrogenic diabetes insipidus.

Chlorpropamide (a sulphonylurea used in diabetes; see p. 390) and **carbamazepine** (an antiepileptic drug; see Chapter 24) potentiate the action of endogenous and exogenous ADH and may also be used in the therapy of diabetes insipidus. Other drugs which may be effective not only in diabetes insipidus of pituitary origin but in the nephrogenic type, are, paradoxically, the thiazide diuretics and the related compound chlorthalidone.

Vasopressin, given intravenously, has a use as an adjunct in the treatment of bleeding oesophageal varices, since it has a particularly marked vasoconstrictor action on splanchnic blood vessels.

Both vasopressin and desmopressin may be useful as prophylactics in haemophilia because of an unexplained effect in increasing the plasma concentration of factor VIII (see Chapter 12).

Unwanted effects

These are few if the antidiuretic peptides are used intranasally in therapeutic doses. Nausea and abdominal cramps, and hypersensitivity reactions have been reported. Intravenous vasopressin may result in spasm of the coronary arteries and frequently causes abdominal and uterine cramps.

OXYTOCIN

The control of the secretion of oxytocin and its physiological significance

Oxytocin is important in milk 'let-down', i.e. the secretion of milk in response to suckling. A neurogenic reflex from the nipple to the hypothalamus *via* the spinal cord and the midbrain results in the release of oxytocin which causes contraction of the myoepithelial cells in the mammary acini. Whether oxytocin is also important in the initiation and maintenance of labour is still uncertain, though it seems probable that it has a role in the postpartum contraction of the uterus.

Oxytocin is discussed in more detail in Chapter 17.

THYROID

In 1883 it was first suggested by Semon that *cretinism* and *myxoedema* might both result from the loss of thyroid function. In the following year, Schiff showed that the adverse effects of total thyroidectomy in dogs could be reversed by transplantation of normal thyroid; this suggested to him that the thyroid gland was the source of an internal secretion which passed into the circulation. In the following 10–15 years numerous workers showed that thyroidectomy or loss of thyroid function in humans could be successfully treated with grafts, injections and oral administration of thyroid tissue. It was not until Christmas Day, 1914, that Kendall isolated crystalline **thyroxine** (T_4); this was subsequently synthesized by Harrington & Barger in 1927. The presence in the thyroid of **triiodothyronine**, (T_3), a substance 3–5-fold more active than thyroxine, was shown by Gross & Pitt-Rivers in 1952.

The T_4 and T_3 secreted by the thyroid are critically important for normal growth and development and for energy metabolism. A third hormone secreted, **calcitonin**, is involved in the control of plasma calcium, and is dealt with later in this chapter (p. 410). The term 'thyroid hormone' will be used here to refer to T_4 and T_3.

Synthesis, storage and secretion of thyroid hormone

The functional unit of the thyroid is the follicle or acinus. Each follicle consists of a single layer of epithelial cells around a cavity, the follicle lumen, which is filled with a thick colloid containing principally **thyroglobulin**. Thyroglobulin is a large glycoprotein (660 000 MW) each molecule of which contains about 115 tyrosine residues. It is synthesized by the ribosomes, undergoes glycosylation in the smooth reticulum and Golgi apparatus and is then secreted into the lumen of the follicle where iodination of the tyrosine residues occurs. Surrounding the follicles is a rich capillary network, and the rate of blood flow through the gland (about 6 ml/g per minute) is very high in comparison with other tissues. There is a complex interrelationship between plasma, follicle cells and the thyroglobulin

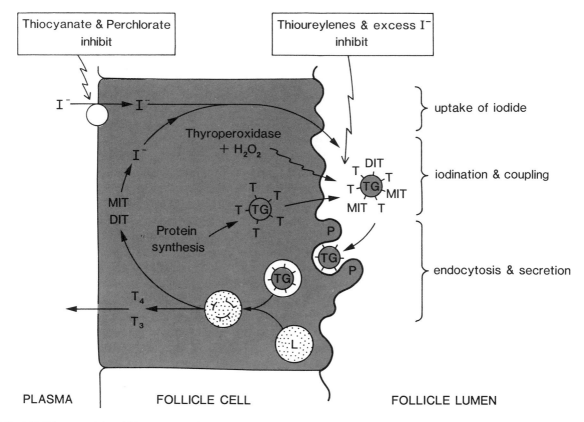

Fig. 16.5 Diagram of thyroid hormone synthesis secretion. TG = thyroglobulin; T = tyrosine; MIT = monoiodotyrosine; DIT = diiodotyrosine; T_4 = thyroxine; T_3 = tri-iodothyronine; L = lysosome; P = pseudopod. (See text for details)

of the colloid in the synthesis, storage and secretion of thyroid hormone. The steps in this process, (Fig. 16.5) are as follows:

1. *Uptake of plasma iodide by the follicle cells.* This is an energy-dependent transport process occurring against a gradient, which is normally about 25:1. It is clear that Na^+/K^+ ATPase activity is required for this transport because uptake is inhibited by ouabain. Thiocyanate and perchlorate also inhibit the uptake of iodide.

2. *Oxidation of iodide and iodination of tyrosine residues in the thyroglobulin of the colloid.* This process is brought about by an enzyme, thyroperoxidase, at the inner, apical surface of the cell at the interface with the colloid. It is very rapid—labelled iodide (^{125}I) can be found in the lumen within 40 seconds of intravenous injection—and requires H_2O_2 as an oxidising agent. This latter is probably produced by an NAPH-dependent cytochrome c reductase. Iodin-

ation (referred to as 'organification' of iodine) occurs *after* the tyrosine has been incorporated into thyroglobulin, but the nature of the process is not clearly known. It seems not to involve molecular iodine and probably not enzyme-bound iodinium (I^+), as has been proposed. (Iodide ions can be oxidized sequentially, the removal of the first electron giving the free radical, I°, and the removal of a second electron, the iodinium ion, I^+.) It is probable that iodination involves two active sites on the enzyme, one of which preferentially oxidizes I^- to the iodine atom or free radical, I°, and the other tyrosine to tyrosine free radical. Iodotyrosine formation is then thought to occur by a reaction between the two radicals while both are attached to the enzyme (Fig. 16.6). Tyrosine is iodinated first at position 3 on the ring and then, in some molecules, on position 5 as well, forming **monoiodotyrosine (MIT)** in the first case, and **diiodotyrosine (DIT)** in the second. Two of these molecules are then

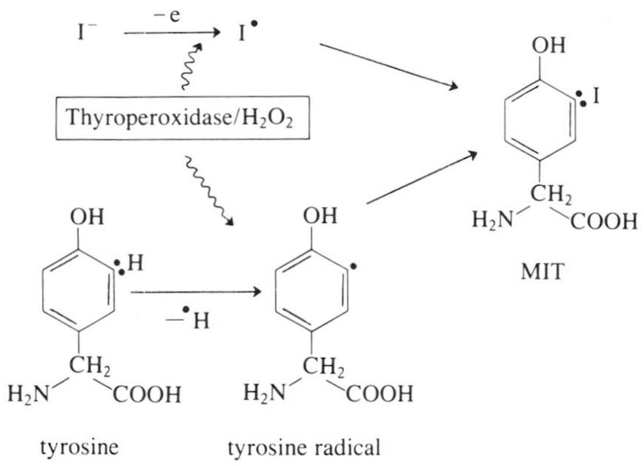

Fig. 16.6 Iodination of tyrosyl by the thyroperoxidase-H_2O complex probably involves two sites on the enzyme, one of which removes an electron from iodide to give the free radical, $I^\bullet$, and another removes a monohydrogen (monoelectron) from tyrosine to give the tyrosine radical. Formation of moniodotryosine (MIT) results from addition of the two radicals.

creted by the anterior pituitary or the hormones of the adrenal cortex, which are synthesized on demand.

3. *Secretion of thyroid hormone*. Although T_4 and T_3 comprise only a small proportion of the thyroglobulin, the whole molecule is broken down when the hormones are secreted. The process involves the endocytosis of thyroglobulin by the follicle cells (see Fig. 16.5). This starts with the formation of pseudopods which engulf some of the colloid in the lumen. The endocytic vesicles then fuse with lysosomes, proteolytic enzymes act on thyroglobulin, and T_4 and T_3 are released and secreted into the plasma by a process which involves microtubules and microfilaments. The MIT and DIT which are released at the same time are normally metabolized within the cell, the iodide being removed enzymically and reused.

Regulation of thyroid function

The main controlling mechanism (see Fig. 16.8) is through **thyrotrophin (thyroid stimulating hormone, TSH)**, a large glycoprotein (28 000 MW) released from the thyrotroph cells of the anterior pituitary under the influence of the hypothalamic hormone, TRH (see p. 361). Another pituitary secretion which affects thyrotrophin release is somatostatin (p. 361) which reduces basal thyrotrophin release.

The production of thyrotrophin is also influenced by a negative feedback effect of T_3 and T_4 (Fig. 16.8). This action on the pituitary cells, unlike that of TSH, *does* require protein synthesis. Thyroid hormone may also stimulate secretion of somatostatin, though the importance of this action

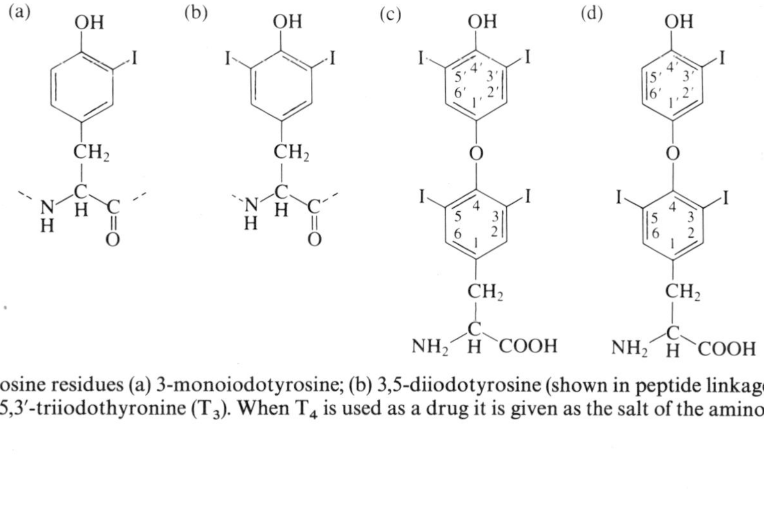

coupled—either MIT with a DIT to form T_3 or two DIT molecules to form T_4 (Fig. 16.7). The mechanism for coupling is not fully known but is believed to involve a peroxidase system similar to that involved in iodination. About one-fifth of the tyrosine residues in thyroglobulin are iodinated and the distribution of the four different iodo-amino-acids per molecule of thyroglobulin is as follows:

MIT: 6.5%, DIT: 4.8%, T_4: 2.3%, T_3: 0.29%.

The iodinated thyroglobulin of the thyroid forms a large store of thyroid hormone and, as is explained below, there is a relatively slow turnover of hormone in the tissues. This is in contrast to other endocrine secretions such as growth hormone se-

Fig. 16.7 Iodinated tyrosine residues (a) 3-monoiodotyrosine; (b) 3,5-diiodotyrosine (shown in peptide linkage, as in thyroglobulin) (c) thyroxine (T_4); (d) 3,5,3'-triiodothyronine (T_3). When T_4 is used as a drug it is given as the salt of the amino-acid.

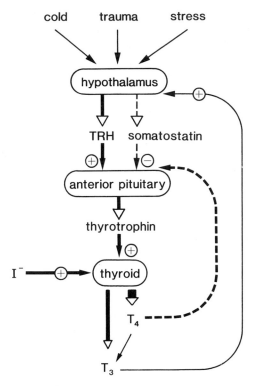

Fig. 16.8 Regulation of thyroid hormone secretion; TRH = thyrotrophin releasing hormone. The thickness of the lines indicates the relative importance of each factor. An excess of iodide (30 × the daily requirements) inhibits the increased thyroid hormone production which occurs in thyrotoxicosis. Arrow with open head = releases Arrow with closed head = acts on
----⊖---- = inhibits; ——⊕—— = stimulates

in the control of thyrotrophin is not yet clear. The extent of conversion of T_4 to T_3 and its degradation in the tissues (see below) will affect the plasma concentration and thus influence the negative feedback effect on thyrotrophin release.*

The control of the secretion of thyrotrophin thus depends on a balance between the actions of T_4 and TRH and probably also somatostatin on the pituitary, but even high concentrations of thyroid hormone do not *completely* inhibit thyrotrophin secretion.

---

* A preparation of TRH, *protirelin*, is used in a diagnostic test of thyroid function. Injected intravenously, it produces a rapid increase in thyrotrophin in the blood in normal patients, but not in patients with hyperthyroidism (see below) in whom there is an excess of circulating thyroid hormones and thus marked feedback inhibition.

Thyrotrophin secretion has a circadian rhythm with a peak at 3 a.m. and a nadir in the afternoon. It acts on receptors on the membrane of thyroid follicle cells and, like TRH, its main second messenger is cAMP. However, it also stimulates phosphatidylinositol turnover, the phosphorylation of one or more proteins and the redistribution of intracellular calcium (see Chapter 1). It has a half-life of about 50 minutes in the circulation.

Thyrotrophin influences all aspects of thyroid hormone synthesis, stimulating the following processes:

1. The uptake of iodide by follicle cells, an effect which is blocked by puromycin, implying an action on the synthesis of the transport proteins. This is the main mechanism by which it regulates thyroid function
2. The synthesis and secretion of thyroglobulin
3. The generation of hydrogen peroxide and the iodination of tyrosine (effects which probably depend on a rise in cytosolic calcium ions)
4. Endocytosis and proteolysis of thyroglobulin
5. Secretion of T_3 and T_4. This is the first effect seen when thyrotrophin is administered experimentally—pseudopod formation occurring within 2 minutes in thyroid tissue studied *in vitro*
6. The blood flow through the gland
7. Hypertrophy and hyperplasia of the thyroid. This is a long-term effect seen if there is prolonged administration of thyrotrophin, and it implies that the hormone has trophic action on the cells themselves. This effect involves protein synthesis and the hormone may act on transcription.

The other main factor influencing thyroid function is the **plasma iodide concentration**. About 100 nmol of T_4 is synthesized daily, necessitating the gland taking up approximately 500 nmol iodide each day (equivalent to about 70 µg of iodine). A reduced iodine intake with reduced plasma iodide concentration will result in a decrease of hormone production and an increase in thyrotrophin secretion. An increased plasma iodide has the opposite effect, though this may be modified by other factors (see below). The overall feedback mechanism does not respond immediately to changes of iodide but apparently senses the average of iodide intake over fairly long periods—days or weeks. There is a large reserve capacity for the binding and uptake of iodide in the thyroid which can thus be increased five-fold. The size and vascularity of the thyroid are reduced by an increase in plasma iodide. A prolonged decrease of iodine in the diet results in a continuous excessive secretion of thyrotrophin and eventually in an increase in vascularity and hypertrophy of the gland.

The iodide transport system in the thyroid cells appears to be regulated by a dual control mechanism. It can be modified not only by thyrotrophin but also by an intracellular autoregulatory system, not clearly understood, which adapts to iodide excess or deficiency independently of the pituitary. With prolonged iodide excess there is a decrease in uptake and/or augmentation of the 'leak' of unbounded iodide from the gland.

Actions of the thyroid hormones

The physiological actions of the thyroid hormones fall into two categories—those affecting metabolism and those affecting growth and development.

Metabolism

The hormones are regulators of metabolism in most tissues, T_3 being 3–5 times more active than T_4 (Fig. 16.9). They produce a general increase in the metabolism of carbohydrates, fats and proteins.

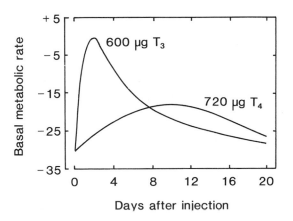

Fig. 16.9 Schematic diagram of the effect of single equimolar doses of T_3 and T_4 on basal metabolic rate in a hypothyroid subject. (From: Blackburn et al, 1954)

Most of these effects involve modulation of the actions of other hormones such as insulin, glucagon, the glucocorticoids and the catecholamines, although the thyroid hormones also control, directly, the activity of some of the enzymes of carbohydrate metabolism. There is an increase in O_2 consumption and heat production which is manifested as an increase in basal metabolic rate. This reflects action on some tissues, such as heart, kidney, liver and muscle, but not others, such as the gonads, brain and spleen. The calorigenic action is important as part of the response to a cold environment. Administration of thyroid hormone results in augmented cardiac rate and output and increased tendency to dysrhythmias such as atrial fibrillation.

Growth and development

The thyroid hormones have a critical effect on growth, partly by a direct action on cells and partly indirectly by influencing growth hormone production and potentiating its effects. They are important for a normal response to parathormone and calcitonin and for skeletal development and are particularly necessary for normal growth and maturation of the CNS.

Mechanism of action

Although this is not clearly known, it is probable that, as the thyroid hormones act relatively slowly, with a lag time of 12–48 hours, their primary action involves protein synthesis. Certainly T_3 causes a rise in nuclear RNA polymerase activity and protein synthesis and the T_3-induced rise in basal metabolic rate can be inhibited by actinomycin D. The hormones seem to act by a mechanism rather similar to that of the steroids. After they enter the cell, T_4 is converted to T_3 which binds with high affinity to a specific, acidic (non-histone) receptor protein (51 000 MW approx.) which is associated with DNA in the nucleus. More than 85% of the bound hormone is in fact T_3. The binding of T_3 induces a conformational change in the receptor protein and this leads to the synthesis of specific messenger RNA and protein. The effects produced depend on the cell type. Expression of activity is related to the degree of occupancy of the receptor and in liver and kidney cells about 50% of the sites are saturated at normal plasma T_3 concentrations. The affinity of the receptors for T_4 is less by a factor of four to ten, and only small amounts of T_4 are bound. Thus T_4 can be regarded mainly as a *pro-hormone*.

It has been suggested that thyroid hormone may produce some of its effects, particularly those on calorigenesis and oxygen consumption, by a direct action on mitochondria. High affinity binding sites for T_3 in mitochondrial membranes in liver, kidney and muscle, but not in thyroid-unresponsive tissues, have been described. The significance of these sites, however, is at present a matter of conjecture.

Transport and metabolism of thyroid hormones

The normal plasma concentrations of the hormones, which can be measured by radio-immunoassay (see Chapter 3) are 10^{-7} M for T_4 and 2×10^{-9} M for T_3. Virtually all of the T_4 and T_3 in the circulation is bound to plasma protein and only 0.3% of the T_3 and about 0.05% of the T_4 is free. The main proteins involved are thyroxine-binding globulin (TBG), thyroxine-binding prealbumin (TBPA) and albumin. TBG is a glycoprotein (50 000 MW) each molecule of which binds one molecule of thyroid hormone, the affinity for T_3 being greater than for T_4. Most of the T_4 (about 75%) is bound to this protein, 15% to TBPA and 10% to albumin. TBG also binds most of the T_3, the rest being bound to albumin.

The concentration of total thyroid hormone-binding proteins (TBP) is slightly reduced in hyperthyroid states but more of the T_4-binding sites are occupied. In hypothyroid states the converse is true. An overall increase of TBP is seen in pregnancy, during administration of oestrogens and during prolonged phenothiazine treatment, and in these conditions more T_4 is bound both in relative and in absolute terms. Phenytoin and salicylates block the binding sites on TBP and displace thyroid hormone.

In the tissues T_4 is monodeiodinated; one-third is converted to T_3 which is the main hormone regulating energy metabolism, while about 40% is converted to the inactive 3,3',5'-triiodothyronine (also termed reverse T_3, rT_3), which may inhibit the calorigenic actions of T_3. The conversion rate of T_4 to T_3 depends on the body concentration of T_4—an increase resulting, rather unexpectedly, in reduced conversion. The generation of T_3 thus remains fairly constant over a wide range of T_4 concentrations. In starvation, the activity of the enzymes which catalyze monodeiodination at position 5' is reduced. There is therefore less production of T_3 from T_4 and also decreased degradation of rT_3, resulting in a possibly protective reduction in the overall metabolic effect of the thyroid hormones.

The thyroid hormones are eventually degraded by deiodination, deamination and conjugation with glucuronic and sulphuric acids. This occurs mainly in the liver, and the free and conjugated forms are excreted partly in the bile and partly in the urine. The metabolic clearance of T_3 is 20 times faster than that of T_4.

In summary, there is a large 'pool' of T_4 in the body, it has a low turnover rate and is found mainly in the circulation, while T_3 has a small 'pool' in the body, a fast turnover rate and is found mainly intracellularly.

ABNORMALITIES OF THYROID FUNCTION

Hyperthyroidism (thyrotoxicosis)

In thyrotoxicosis there is excessive activity of the thyroid hormones with a high metabolic rate, an increase in temperature and sweating and a marked sensitivity to heat. Nervousness, tremor, tachycardia, fatiguability and increased appetite associated with loss of weight also occur. There are several types of hyperthyroidism but only two are commonly seen: **diffuse toxic goitre** (also called Graves' disease or exophthalmic goitre) and **toxic nodular goitre**.

Diffuse toxic goitre is an organ-specific autoimmune disease caused by thyroid-stimulating immunoglobulins directed at a component of the follicle cell membrane which may be the receptor for thyrotrophin. Several different types of thyroid-stimulating immunoglobulins have been reported, the commonest being the **long-acting thyroid stimulator (LATS)**, the effect of which is similar to thyrotrophin although its action is slower in onset and longer lasting. As is indicated by the name, patients with exophthalmic goitre have protrusion of the eyeballs. The pathogenesis of this condition is not understood but there is some evidence that it, also, may have an immunological basis, being possibly due to the effect of an antibody or antigen-antibody complex on the retro-orbital tissues and eye muscles.

Toxic nodular goitre is due to a benign neoplasm or adenoma and may develop in patients with long-continued simple goitre (see below). This condition does not usually have concomitant exophthalmos.

Hypothyroidism

A decreased activity of the thyroid results in hypo-thyroidism, one form of which is termed **myxoedema**. It is immunological in origin and the manifestations are low metabolic rate, slow speech, deep hoarse voice, lethargy, bradycardia, sensitivity to cold and mental impairment. Patients also develop a characteristic thickening of the skin which gives the condition its name. Another form of hypothyroidism termed **Hashimoto's disease** is due to a chronic autoimmune thyroiditis in which there is an immune reaction against thyroglobulin or some other component of thyroid tissue, which results eventually in fibrosis of the gland. Therapy of thyroid tumours with radio-iodine (see below) is another cause of hypothyroidism.

When there is congenital absence or incomplete development of the thyroid the result is **cretinism** which is characterized by gross retardation of growth and mental deficiency.

Several drugs may depress thyroid function by interfering with the synthesis, secretion or transport of thyroid hormone. Examples are non-steroidal anti-inflammatory agents, glucocorticoids, X-ray contrast agents, α- and β-blockers, sulphonylureas and tranquillizers. The antidepressant lithium also has antithyroid activity, inhibiting thyroid hormone release, and it is used in some countries for the treatment of hyperthyroidism.

A dietary deficiency of iodine, if prolonged, causes a rise in plasma thyrotrophic hormone (see above) and eventually an increase in the size of the gland. This condition is known as **simple** or **non-toxic goitre** and is endemic in some areas. The enlarged thyroid usually manages to produce normal amounts of thyroid hormone though if the iodine deficiency is very severe, hypothyroidism may supervene.

DRUGS THAT AFFECT THYROID FUNCTION

Thyroid function may be modified by the following agents:

1. *Inhibitors of thyroid hormone synthesis or release (see Fig. 16.5):*

a. Drugs that block organification of iodine e.g. thioureylenes (see below)
b. Iodide. In large doses iodide paradoxically inhibits thyroid secretion (see below)
c. Drugs that block iodine uptake e.g. thiocyanate, perchlorate (see below)
d. Radioactive iodine (^{131}I) which kills thyroid follicle cells by selective irradiation.
e. Other drugs which may inhibit thyroid function as an unwanted side effect, e.g. glucocorticoids, sulphonylureas, lithium (see above).

2. *Drugs that affect the peripheral effects of thyroid hormones*

There are no drugs that reduce the peripheral actions directly, but sympathetic blocking drugs (especially β-adrenoceptor antagonists, such as propranolol) are effective in controlling the tachycardia, dysrhythmias, tremor and agitation associated with hyperthyroidism. Guanethidine, used as eye drops, is also effective in relieving exophthalmos (which is not relieved by antithyroid drugs) by relaxing the sympathetically innervated muscle which causes eyelid retraction. There are no drugs that specifically augment the synthesis or release of thyroid hormones, and no clinically useful analogues that mimic their peripheral effects. The only effective treatment of hypothyroidism, unless it is due to iodine deficiency, is to administer T_4 or, in special circumstances, T_3 (see below).

DRUGS USED IN HYPERTHYROIDISM

Hyperthyroidism may be treated surgically or pharmacologically. In general, the treatment of choice for toxic nodular goitre is surgical whereas for diffuse toxic goitre it is pharmacological, the agents employed being thioureylene drugs or radioiodine.

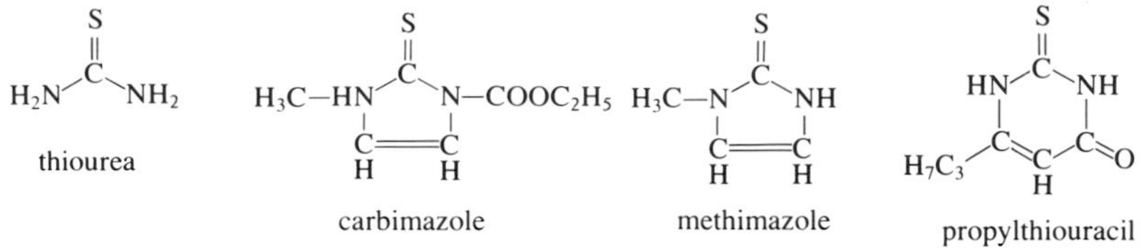

Fig. 16.10 Formulae of antithyroid drugs.

Thioureylenes

These are the most important antithyroid agents and the main compounds are **carbimazole**, **methimazole** and **propylthiouracil** (Fig. 16.10). They are related to thiourea—the thiocarbamide group (S=C—N) being essential for antithyroid activity.

Pharmacological actions

The compounds decrease the output of thyroid hormones from the gland and cause a gradual reduction in the signs and symptoms of thyrotoxicosis, the basal metabolic rate and pulse rate returning to normal over a period of 3–4 weeks. Their mode of action is not completely understood but there is evidence that they are general inhibitors of thyroperoxidase-catalysed oxidation reactions. They have been shown *in vitro* to inhibit the iodination of tyrosyl residues in thyroglobulin (see Fig. 16.5 & 16.11). It was originally proposed that they interefered with iodination by acting as substrates for the postulated peroxidase-iodinium complex thus competitively inhibiting the interaction with tyrosine. However, this hypothesis for the mechanism of iodination is now thought to be incorrect and more recent evidence indicates that the drugs act by inhibiting the formation of the enzyme-iodide complex. They may, in addition, inhibit the coupling reactions which occur subsequent to iodination and which are believed to be thyroperoxidase-catalyzed reactions. Propylthiouracil has the additional effect of reducing the deiodination of T_4 to T_3 in peripheral tissues. It has been suggested that these drugs may also suppress the synthesis of the antibodies which are implicated in the pathogenesis of Graves' disease and that their use increases the possibility of spontaneous remission. There is certainly some evidence that they cause a fall in the production of autoantibodies both *in vivo* and *in vitro* and it seems that this is not due to an action on the lymphocytes, but on the antigen-presenting accessory cells.

Pharmacokinetic aspects

All three drugs are given orally. Carbimazole is rapidly converted to methimazole and it is this which has the pharmacological activity. Methimazole is distributed throughout the body water and has a plasma half-life of 6–15 hours. An average dose of carbimazole produces more than 90% inhibition of thyroid organification of iodine within 12 hours. The clinical response however may take many weeks or even months (Fig. 16.12). This is because the thyroid may have large stores of hormone which need to be depleted before the drug's action can be manifest.

Propylthiouracil is distributed throughout the extracellular water. It has a plasma half-life of about $2\frac{1}{2}$ hours. An average dose results in 60–70% inhibition or organification of iodine within 7 hours, but as with carbimazole, the clinical response is delayed. Both methimazole and propyl-

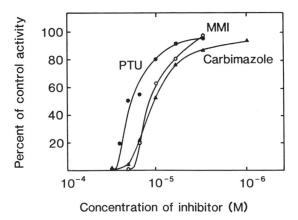

Fig. 16.11 Dose-response curves for inhibition of thyroperoxidase-catalysed iodination of thyroglobulin. The IC_{50} for carbimazole: 10.5 μM, for methimazole (MMI): 11.5 μM and for propylthiouracil (PTU): 18.5 μM. (Modified from: Taurog, 1976)

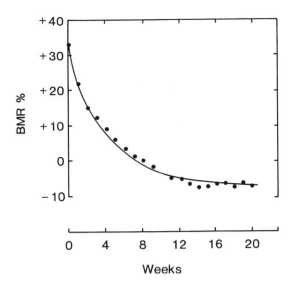

Fig. 16.12 Average time course of fall of BMR during treatment with an antithyroid drug, carbimazole. Curve is plotted on linear scales. When the data are replotted with a logarithmic ordinate and fit a straight line, it is clear that there is a daily fall in BMR of 3.4% of the previous day's BMR. (From: Furth et al, 1963)

thiouracil cross the placenta and also appear in the milk. After degradation, their metabolites are excreted in the urine, propylthiouracil being excreted more rapidly than methimazole. The thioureylenes are not concentrated in the thyroid.

Unwanted reactions

The most important of these is agranulocytosis, which, fortunately, is relatively rare, having an incidence of 0.2%, and is reversible if the drug is stopped. Rashes are more common and other symptoms such as headaches, nausea and pain in the joints may occasionally occur.

Clinical use

The drugs may be used as the main treatment of diffuse toxic goitre or as a preliminary treatment in preparation for subsequent surgery. They are sometimes given to decrease symptoms while waiting for radioactive iodine to take effect.

Iodide

This is the original agent used to treat thyro-

toxicosis but its effect is unreliable when it is used as a sole agent in therapy.

Pharmacological action

When high doses of iodide—30 times the average daily requirement or more—are given to thyrotoxic patients, the symptoms subside within 1–2 days. There is inhibition of the secretion of thyroid hormones and over a period of 10–14 days a marked reduction in vascularity of the gland, which becomes smaller and firmer. The mechanism of action is not entirely clear but may be related to the fact that, as seen in experiments in rats, excess iodide inhibits organification of iodide.

In *in vitro* experiments with purified thyroperoxidase, excess iodide inhibited iodination of thyroglobulin, but this did not happen when thyroid particles were used as a source of thyroperoxidase. It may be that, *in vivo*, excess iodide inhibits another process necessary for iodination of thyroglobulin, such as H_2O_2 generation.

Pharmacokinetic aspects

Potassium iodide is given orally. With continuous administration its effect reaches maximum within 10–15 days and then decreases.

Clinical uses

Its main use is in the preparation of hyperthyroid subjects for surgery and in the treatment of severe thyrotoxic crises (thyroid storm). In preparation for surgery a common regime is to use propranolol (see below) for about 2 weeks or antithyroid drugs such as carbimazole or propylthiouracil for about 6 weeks and then give iodide as well in the 10 days immediately before operation.

Iodide added to food (bread or salt) may be used prophylactically to prevent simple goitre in areas where this is endemic due to iodine deficiency.

Unwanted effects

Allergic reactions such as angio-oedema may occur; these include rashes, drug fever, lacrimation, conjunctivitis, pain in the salivary glands and a coryza-like syndrome.

Radioiodine

The isotope used is ^{131}I. It is taken up and processed by the thyroid in the same way as the stable form of iodide, eventually becoming incorporated into thyroglobulin. It emits both β-particles and X-rays. The X-rays pass through the tissue, but the β-radiation has a very short range and exerts a cytotoxic action virtually restricted to the cells of the thyroid follicles. ^{131}I has a half-life of 8 days and by 2 months its radioactivity has effectively disappeared. It is used in one single dose, but its effect on the gland is delayed for 1–2 months and does not reach its maximum for a further 2 months.

The uptake of ^{131}I and other isotopes of iodine may be used as a test of thyroid function. A tracer dose of the isotope is given orally or intravenously and the amount accumulated by the thyroid is measured by a gamma scintillation counter placed over the gland.

Unwanted effects

Hypothyroidism will eventually occur after treatment with radioiodine, particularly in patients with Graves' disease. The risk of development of carcinoma of the thyroid, once considered to be a hazard, is now known to be negligible. However, radioiodine is best avoided in children and also in pregnant patients because of the potential damage to the foetus.

Perchlorate and other anions

A number of inorganic anions compete with iodide for the iodide transport system in the membrane of the follicle cell, the main ones being perchlorate and thiocyanate (see Fig. 16.5). They also cause loss of inorganic iodide which has already been taken up. Their effects can be overcome by increasing the concentration of iodide.

Perchlorate, though effective in hyperthyroidism, carries the risk of aplastic anaemia and is no longer used in treatment.

Lithium

This inhibits thyroid hormone release; its mechanism of action is not known but it may inhibit a membrane bound adenylate cyclase.

Propranolol

This β-blocking drug (see Chapter 7), although not an anti-thyroid agent, is useful for decreasing many of the signs and symptoms of hyperthyroidism, particularly the tremor and tachycardia. In addition to its employment in preparation for surgery it is used for the initial treatment of most hyperthyroid patients while the thioureylenes or radioiodine are taking effect.

DRUGS USED IN HYPOTHYROIDISM

The thyroid hormones themselves are used for replacement therapy. **Thyroxine** and **triiodthyronine (liothyronine)** are available and are given orally. Thyroxine has a plasma half-life of 6 days. The time taken to reach peak effect with this drug is 9 days and the half-life of decline of response is 11–15 days (see Fig. 16.9). Liothyronine has a shorter plasma half-life (2–5 days), and reaches its peak effect in 1–2 days. Its half-life for decline of response is 8 days. Both accumulate if given daily.

The drug of choice for general use is thyroxine. Liothyronine is virtually never used except in the rare condition of myxoedema coma when its more rapid action is required for emergency treatment.

Unwanted effects

These may occur with overdose and in addition to the signs and symptoms of hyperthyroidism there is a risk of precipitating angina pectoris, cardiac dysrhythmias or cardiac failure.

THE ENDOCRINE PANCREAS AND THE CONTROL OF BLOOD GLUCOSE

The endocrine portion of the pancreas, the islets of Langerhans, contains cells which secrete **insulin, glucagon** and **somatostatin**. The glucagon-secreting cells (α_2 or A cells) and the somatostatin-secreting cells (the α_1 or D cells) are found peripherally in the islet and the predominant, insulin-secreting cells (β or B cells) in the centre (see Fig. 16.14). Insulin and glucagon have crucial roles in the control of blood

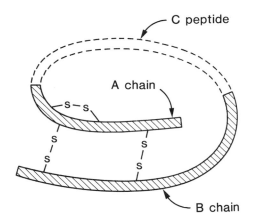

Fig. 16.13 Schematic diagram of proinsulin structure. Hatched areas indicate the 2-chain insulin peptide.

glucose, and somatostatin has an indirect paracrine role in that it has inhibitory actions on both insulin and glucagon secretion. Somatostatin is also released from the hypothalamus and inhibits the release of growth hormone from the pituitary (p. 361).

INSULIN

In structure insulin is a small polypeptide (6000 MW approx) consisting of two polypeptide chains connected by two disulphide bridges. Its amino-acid sequence was determined by Sanger and his co-workers in 1955. It is derived by proteolytic cleavage from a larger single-chain protein precursor (9000 MW approx.) termed proinsulin. Proteolysis removes a connecting peptide, the C peptide (Fig. 16.13) and the molecules of insulin so produced, together with the associated C peptide, are stored in the β-cells, in granules, until a stimulus for secretion occurs, when they are released in equimolar amounts.

Synthesis and secretion of insulin

The main factor controlling the synthesis and secretion of insulin is the *blood glucose* concentration (Fig. 16.14). The β-cell responds to both the *actual glucose concentration* and also to the *rate of change* of blood glucose. There is thus a steady basal release of insulin and also a response to a rise in blood glucose. In both *in vitro* and *in vivo* experiments it can be shown that this response has two phases—an initial rapid phase which reflects the release of stored hormone and a slower second, delayed phase which reflects both release of stored hormone and new synthesis (Fig. 16.15). The response is often abnormal in diabetes, as discussed later.

A product of glucose metabolism may provide the signal for insulin synthesis and/or secretion, though a putative glucoreceptor in the cell membrane may also participate. One possibility is that stimulation of a glucoreceptor initiates secretion

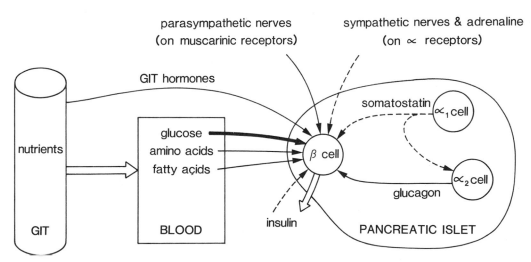

Fig. 16.14 Endogenous factors regulating the secretion of insulin by the β-cells of the islets of Langerhans in the pancreas.
————— = stimulation; ------- = inhibition
The blood glucose is the most important factor.

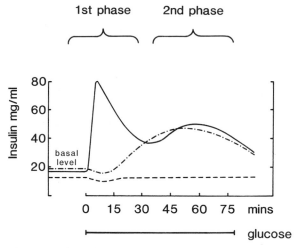

Fig. 16.15 Schematic diagram of the two-phase release of insulin which occurs with constant glucose infusion (indicated by bar) in normal subjects (———), in non-insulin-dependent diabetes (—·—·—), and in insulin-dependent diabetes (-----). The first phase can also be produced by amino-acids, sulphonylureas, glucagon and GIT hormones. (Data from: Pfeifer et al, 1981)

and that a metabolic product of glucose within the cell is responsible for the potentiation of the effect of other secretogogues (see below).

Stimulus/secretion coupling in the β-cell involves a rise in cytosolic calcium and also increased phosphatidylinositol turnover with generation of diacylglycerol and activation of protein kinase C (see Chapter 1). There is evidence that calcium is involved primarily in the first phase of the response to glucose and that the second phase, the sustained response, requires protein kinase C activity. On stimulation with glucose there is an initial depolarization which leads to Ca^{++} entry through voltage-dependent channels. cAMP, though not the main second messenger, has a potentiating effect, possibly by virtue of its ability to promote release of Ca^{++} from internal stores.

Secretion occurs by exocytosis, a process which depends on microtubules and microfilaments. The granules, which are surrounded by a membrane, move towards the plasma membrane, the two membranes fuse and the granule contents are discharged.

Other factors, besides glucose, which stimulate insulin release are glucagon, amino-acids (particularly arginine and leucine), fatty acids, various hormones from the gastrointestinal tract (GIT), and the sulphonyl urea drugs (see below). Insulin release is inhibited by somatostatin (see Fig. 16.14).

The action of the GIT hormones (gastrin, secretin, cholecystokinin, gastric inhibitory polypeptide (GIP) and enteroglucagon) which are released after the absorption of food (p. 331) may explain the observation that oral glucose causes a greater insulin release than intravenous glucose, although only GIP has been shown to have a significant effect in physiological concentrations. GIT hormones, (in particular GIP), may be said to provide, after ingestion of food, an anticipatory signal from the GIT to the islets. It has been pointed out that, if one considers the digestive and hormonal functions of the GIT and the exocrine and endocrine functions of the pancreas, there is clearly a complex interrelationship between the two organs not only in digestion and absorption of food but also in the regulation of its utilization.

Of the secretogogues cited above, only glucose causes both phases of insulin release; all the others stimulate only the first phase.

The *autonomic nervous system* has a significant modulating effect on insulin secretion (see Fig. 16.14). The islets of Langerhans have both parasympathetic and sympathetic innervation and though the network of nerve terminals is not very extensive, the presence of gap junctions and electrical coupling between islet cells means that neural signals can be amplified, and islet cells are known to be electrically active during insulin secretion. Acetylcholine is a glucose-dependent stimulant of insulin release by an action on muscarinic receptors, and β-agonists also stimulate insulin secretion while α-agonists inhibit it. Adrenaline's effect on the β-cell is predominantly on α-receptors; thus when it is released into the circulation in stress, this action, together with its general glycogenolytic effect (see Chapter 7), will increase blood glucose.

The integration of parasympathetic and sympathetic control of the islets occurs in the hypothalamus. Stimulation of the ventrolateral areas causes an increase of insulin secretion, and stimulation of the ventromedial area, a decrease.

About one-fifth of the insulin store in the pancreas of the human adult is secreted daily (this is equivalent to about 5 mg) and the mean plasma concentration after an overnight fast is 0.6 ng/ml. The concentration in the portal vein is usually three-fold higher than in the rest of the circulation, reflecting the removal of a large amount (approximately 50%) of insulin by the liver, but this differential may rise to a ratio of 10:1 after the islets have been stimulated by glucose.

Circulating insulin is measured by radioimmunoassay. In insulin-treated diabetic patients, in whom there may be circulating antibodies to the exogenous hormone which could interfere with this measurement, determination of the C peptide concentration may provide an estimate of the patient's insulin secretion.

Actions of insulin

Insulin is the main factor controlling the storage and metabolism of ingested metabolic fuels. In doing so it affects directly or indirectly the function of every tissue in the body and its overall effect is the conservation of body fuel supplies. Its most obvious action when secreted or injected is to cause a *reduction in blood sugar* and this reflects its general physiological function of *facilitating the uptake, utilization and storage of glucose, amino acids and fats after a meal.* Conversely a fall in plasma insulin leads to reduced uptake of these substances into cells and a mobilization of endogenous fuel sources.

Insulin affects all three main sources of metabolic energy—carbohydrate, fat and protein—and its actions involve the three principal tissues—liver, muscle and adipose tissue (Table 16.2), as detailed below.

regulation of carbohydrate homeostasis. This is partly because ingested glucose goes first to the liver, partly because the blood reaching the liver in the portal vein has a higher insulin concentration than the rest of the circulation, and partly because the membrane of the liver cell is highly permeable to glucose. After oral ingestion of 100 g of glucose, about 60 g are taken up and metabolized by the liver, 25 g are retained in and used by the CNS, and only about 15 g are taken up by muscle and adipose tissue. (A high concentration of blood glucose (hyperglycemia) produced by *intravenous* injection does *not* cause hepatic uptake of glucose and this has given rise to the hypothesis that a GIT hormone regulates the action of insulin on the liver.) The action of insulin on the liver is to decrease both glycogenolysis (glycogen breakdown) and gluconeogenesis (synthesis of glucose from noncarbohydrate sources). It also increases glucose utilization (glycolysis) but the overall effect is to increase glycogen stores. It produces its effects, partly directly on the relevant enzymes (see below), and partly through an indirect action by inducing the synthesis of specific enzymes involved in glucose breakdown and repressing specific gluconeogenic enzymes. (Glucocorticoids, adrenaline and glucagon induce these same gluconeogenic enzymes.) Insulin has a further action on gluconeogenesis in that it decreases the release and breakdown of fatty acids (see below) which results in lessened availability of acetyl coenzyme A, a necessary co-factor for one of the key enzymes in gluconeogenesis. It

Table 16.2 Summary of the effects of insulin on carbohydrate, fat and protein metabolism in liver, muscle and adipose tissue

	Liver cells	Fat cell	Muscle
Carbohydrate metabolism	↓ gluconeogenesis ↓ glycogenolysis ↑ glycolysis ↑ glycogenesis	↑ glucose uptake ↑ glycerol synthesis	↑ glucose uptake ↑ glycolysis ↑ glycogenesis
Fat metabolism	↑ lipogenesis	↑ synthesis of triglycerides ↑ fatty acid synthesis	—
Protein metabolism	↓ protein breakdown	—	↑ amino-acid uptake ↑ protein synthesis

Carbohydrate metabolism

Insulin influences glucose metabolism in all tissues, but the *liver* is the main organ involved in its

has a particularly important effect on glucose metabolism by affecting the state of phosphorylation of some of the enzymes involved. As many enzymes are phosphoenzymes, which may be very rapidly activated or inactivated by phosphorylation or dephosphorylation, this effect has significant metabolic repercussions (see p. 20). For example, dephosphorylation enhances the activity of key enzymes involved in glycogen synthesis. These effects may be controlled by one or more mediators (see below) which may act at the level of protein kinases or protein phosphatases.

In *muscle*, unlike liver, uptake of glucose is slow and is the rate-limiting step in carbohydrate metabolism. The main effect of insulin is to increase the active transport of glucose, but it also increases glycogen synthesis and the metabolism of glucose.

A similar effect on glucose uptake and metabolism is seen in *adipose tissue*. One of the main end products of glucose metabolism in adipose tissue is glycerol which esterfies with fatty acids to form triglycerides—thus a product of the action of insulin on glucose,—glycerol—facilitates its action on fat metabolism (see below and Table 16.2).

Fat metabolism

Insulin causes lipogenesis in the *liver*. Indeed, when adequate amounts of insulin and carbohydrate are available there is more de novo synthesis of fatty acids in the liver than in adipose tissue. However, insulin does increase fatty acid synthesis in *adipose tissue*, and also triglyceride formation (Table 16.2), and it decreases lipolysis, partly by promoting dephosphorylation of the lipases and thus inactivating them. Insulin also depresses the lipolytic action of adrenaline and growth hormone (and possibly glucagon) by opposing their stimulant action on adenylate cyclase.

Protein metabolism

Insulin stimulates the uptake of amino-acids into *muscle* and increases protein synthesis. It also decreases protein catabolism, and the oxidation of amino-acids, particularly in the *liver* (see above).

Other metabolic effects

Other metabolic effects of insulin are increased transport into cells of K^+, Ca^{++}, nucleosides and inorganic phosphate, and increased synthesis of nucleic acids.

Mechanism of action

Insulin binds to a specific receptor on the surface of its target cells. The receptor is a glycoprotein complex (350 000 MW) consisting of two α and two β subunits linked by disulphide bridges (Fig. 16.16). Insulin receptors are synthesized continuously, the subunits being derived from larger precursor molecules. The α subunits are associated with the outer surface of the membrane and are of particular importance in insulin binding. The β subunits are transmembrane proteins, and when insulin binds to the receptor these β subunits manifest kinase activity (see Fig. 16.17), acting upon themselves (autophosphorylation) and also possibly on other target proteins, phosphorylating tyrosine and probably serine. Phosphorylation does not influence insulin binding, and there is evidence that the kinase remains active so long as the β subunit is phosphorylated, irrespective of whether insulin remains bound.

The binding of insulin to its receptor is not a simple reversible interaction with a single equilibrium constant as discussed in Chapter 1, but appears to show negative co-operativity. By this is meant that the initial binding of insulin to some sites reduces the affinity of unoccupied sites. Purified α subunits have a lower affinity for insulin than receptors in situ, and do not show negative co-operativity, which appears to be a function of the complex of α and β subunits. To complicate matters

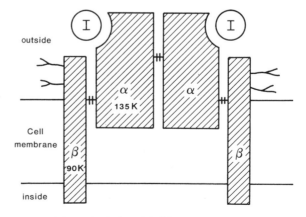

Fig. 16.16 Hypothetical model of the insulin receptor. The α and β subunits are linked by disulphide bridges. I = insulin

still further there may be, particularly in fat cells, two classes of receptor—a high affinity, low capacity class and a low affinity, high capacity class.

On interaction with insulin, the receptors aggregate into clusters and the insulin-receptor complexes are subsequently internalized in vesicles by an energy-dependent procedure (see Fig. 16.17). This process seems to be important for the increased glucose transport by insulin as well as for other insulin actions. (Similar clustering and internalization can be triggered by antibodies against the insulin receptor and these antibodies can mimic virtually all the biological activities of insulin.) The internalized insulin is degraded but the receptor is recycled back to the plasma membrane.

At concentrations of insulin which produce maximum effects, only a small proportion (less than 10%) of the receptors are occupied. It has been suggested that the affinity of the receptors may be subject to control and that this could enable the cell to regulate its sensitivity to insulin. A high molecular weight protein which affects insulin binding affinity has been found associated with the receptor so it seems possible that the cells can regulate the affinity of the receptors and thus insulin binding.

In some circumstances the number rather than the affinity of the receptors is altered. When there is a high concentration of circulating insulin such as occurs in obesity or with a high carbohydrate diet, there is 'down-regulation' of receptors (i.e. reduction in the number). When there is a low concentration of plasma insulin (e.g. in starvation) the converse occurs. The process of internalization and recycling of receptors cited above is clearly of great importance in determining the number of receptors expressed at the surface in these conditions.

The transduction mechanisms in the insulin response (i.e. the events which link receptor-binding to the biological response) are still a matter of debate, but it seems likely that several pathways are involved.

One important question concerns the mechanism by which the rapid increase in glucose transport is produced. It appears that the basis of this is an increase in the number of carriers in the membrane by recruitment from intracellular sites, as well as specific activation of these carriers. Another significant question concerns the mechanism by which

metabolic pathways are regulated. It appears that this regulation is mediated largely through alteration of the state of phosphorylation of key enzymes and thus activation of the relevant kinases, phosphates and phosphodiesterases must be one of the principal transduction events. However, the mechanisms involved in transporter recruitment and activation and in the control and activation of kinases and phosphatases are not known with any clarity.

One hypothesis is that the insulin-receptor interaction activates a protease which generates one or more peptide mediators and that it is these mediators which are responsible for many of the actions of insulin (see Fig. 16.17). Such mediators have been shown to exist and there is evidence that they stimulate not only various phosphatases and kinases relevant to the effects of insulin on metabolism, but also Ca^{++} transport in mitochondrial and cell membranes and mRNA synthesis. It is postulated that these mediators may also be responsible for insulin's action on the glucose transporters.

Another hypothesis, for which some evidence is forthcoming, is that the endocytosis of insulin-receptor complexes with subsequent recycling of the receptors triggers the transfer of inactive glucose carriers from an internal vesicle pool to the plasma membrane.

A different hypothesis concerns the role of a putative guanine nucleotide regulatory protein (see Fig. 16.17). There is some evidence that the insulin-receptor interaction affects membrane bound kinases (cAMP-dependent and cAMP-independent) through a regulatory protein of this nature. It is further suggested that this protein may be responsible for activating the glucose carriers.

A rise in cytosolic Ca^{++} appears to be implicated in the increase in glucose transport, but not in any of the other actions of insulin.

A summary diagram of the current hypotheses on the mechanism of action of insulin is given in Figure 16.17, but it is clear that the ideas and information on this topic are still in a state of flux.

GLUCAGON

Glucagon is a single chain polypeptide of 21 amino-acid residues with a molecular weight of about

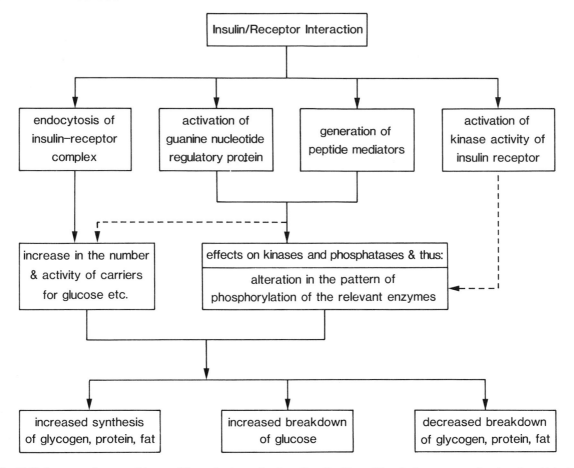

Fig. 16.17 Summary diagram of the possible mechanisms of action of insulin. (Dotted lines indicate proposed actions for which the evidence is, at present, limited.)

3000. Unlike insulin, it is identical in all mammalian species. Its primary site of synthesis is the α_2-cell of the islet but an immunologically identical peptide of similar molecular weight is synthesized by cells in the stomach, which are very similar to α_2 cells. Glucagon itself has considerable structural homology with other GIT hormones such as secretin, vasoactive intestinal peptide and gastric inhibitory peptide. Glucagon is also found in the CNS and may function as a neuromodulator (see Chapter 19). In the pancreas it is derived from a large precursor molecule (9000 MW) which can on occasion be found in the circulation.

One of the main physiological stimuli to glucagon secretion is the concentration of aminoacids, in particular arginine, in the plasma. Thus an increase in secretion follows ingestion of a high protein meal. Secretion is stimulated by low, and inhibited by high plasma glucose. The latter inhibitory response is sensitive to quite small increases in glucose and may require the presence of insulin, which itself has an inhibitory effect on glucagon release. The response to fatty acids parallels the response to glucose in that low concentrations increase and high concentrations decrease glucagon secretion.

Sympathetic nerve activity and circulating adrenaline stimulate release by an action on β-receptors. Parasympathetic nerve activity and acetylcholine also increase secretion, the relevant receptors being muscarinic.

GIT hormones appear to give an anticipatory signal to the α-cells, augmenting glucagon release, the principal hormone being cholecystokinin, which is secreted during absorption of protein. Gastrin and GIP may also participate in this communication between the GIT and the pancreas.

Somatostatin, from the adjacent α_1-cells in the islets, has an inhibitory action on glucagon release.

The concentration of glucagon in the plasma is measured by radioimmunoassay, but only 40–50% of the total measured in this way represents biologically active hormone. However, changes in the levels of immunoreactive substance generally reflect changes in the biologically active component.

In contrast to insulin, which fluctuates with ingestion of meals, there is no very marked change in plasma glucagon concentration throughout the day, although prolonged exercise may cause a rise.

Actions

Glucagon increases glycogen breakdown and gluconeogenesis and inhibits glycogen synthesis and glucose oxidation. The main initial action is a stimulation of adenylate cyclase in liver cell membranes, an enzyme which is particularly sensitive to glucagon. The consequent rise in cAMP activates a protein kinase which starts a cascade of phosphorylations and dephosphorylations of enzymes which result in the above changes in carbohydrate metabolism. In both liver and adipose tissue, the kinase activated by increased cAMP activates the hormone sensitive lipase and increases breakdown of fats. The fatty acids so produced further increase gluconeogenesis. Glucagon may also increase ketogenesis. A prolonged rise in plasma glucagon results in *induction* of the enzymes involved in the above effects as well as their stimulation through elevated cAMP.

Glucagon's actions on target tissues are thus the opposite of those of insulin. In general, its actions of glycogenolysis and lipolysis are similar to those of adrenaline, but glucagon is proportionally more active on liver and adrenaline on muscle and fat.

It increases the rate and force of contraction of the heart in a manner similar to adrenaline, and has occasionally been used clinically to treat acute cardiac failure (see Chapter 10).

SOMATOSTATIN

Somatostatin is secreted by the α_1 (or D) cells of the pancreas. It is also the growth hormone release-inhibiting factor generated in the hypothalamus. Its main function is probably the local, paracrine, inhibitory regulation of insulin and glucagon release within the islet. However, it is also secreted into the potential circulation in response to stimulation by glucose or amino-acids. It can affect several gastrointestinal activities, inhibiting both emptying of the stomach and gut motility, and may thus be another factor in the regulatory interrelationship between the pancreas and the gastrointestinal tract in the absorption and metabolism of food.

CONTROL OF BLOOD GLUCOSE

The control of blood glucose must be seen in the context of the necessity of maintaining adequate fuel supplies in the face of intermittent food intake along with variable exercise and thus variable demand. After food intake more fuel is available than is immediately required. Glucose is the main fuel utilized, and the excess calories are stored as glycogen or fat. After fasting, the energy stores need to be mobilized in a regulated manner.

The blood glucose concentration is controlled by a feedback system between liver, muscle and fat and the pancreatic islets, the main regulatory hormone being insulin.

As the overall pattern of control of blood glucose is different in the basal state (i.e. with no influx of nutrients) and in the fed state, after a meal, these two conditions will be considered separately.

The basal state

In the absence of food intake, as for example after fasting overnight, homeostatic processes come into play which maintain the blood glucose concentration. This is important for those tissues (e.g. brain, kidney) that cannot use free fatty acids as a source of energy. The homeostatic processes function as follows: as glucose is utilized, its plasma concentration falls, resulting in a decrease of insulin output and an increase of glucagon output by the islets. The effect on the liver is to produce a slow efflux of glucose which restores the blood glucose concentration. Thus the liver is the main source of blood glucose in these circumstances, and glucose utilization is non-insulin dependent and occurs mainly

Table 16.3 The effect of hormones on the control of blood glucose

		Main actions	Main stimulus for secretion	Main effect
Main regulatory hormone	Insulin	↑ glucose uptake ↑ glycogen synthesis ↓ glycogenolysis ↓ gluconeogenesis	Moment-to-moment fluctuations in blood glucose	↓ blood glucose
Main counter-regulatory hormones	Glucagon	↑ glycogenolysis ↑ gluconeogenesis		
	Catecholamines	↑ glycogenolysis ↓ glucose uptake	Hypoglycaemia, i.e. blood glucose less than 50 mg/100 ml (e.g. with exercise, stress, high proteins meals, etc)	↑ blood glucose
	Glucocorti-coids	↑ gluconeogenesis ↓ glucose uptake and utilization		
	Growth hormone	↓ glucose uptake		

Adapted from: Felig, 1981

in the brain. Basal insulin secretion continues however and prevents the rate of glucose and ketone production from exceeding their rate of utilization. (This control is disrupted in juvenile diabetes as is explained below.) This basic feedback loop, (the effect of plasma glucose on the pancreas) may be modulated by the 'counter regulatory hormones' all of which counteract the actions of insulin and tend to raise the blood sugar (Table 16.3). The glucocorticoids decrease the uptake and utilization of glucose and promote gluconeogenesis. This latter function is facilitated by their protein-catabolic action which provides amino-acids, and is further increased by their induction of the enzymes involved. Adrenaline increases glycogen breakdown particularly in muscle, and growth hormone decreases glucose uptake.

The fed state

After a meal there is an influx of the breakdown products of food into the circulation. The glucose, and to a lesser extent the amino-acids and fatty acids, stimulate an increased output of insulin, which constitutes the primary regulatory factor controlling the level of blood glucose. Insulin lowers the concentration of glucose in the blood by a combination of the factors outlined above and summarized in Tables 16.2 & 16.3. The principal organ involved in the response to a meal is the liver,

which takes up to 30–60% of the glucose load in the portal vein. However, as explained above, although insulin controls the disposal of glucose within the liver cell, it does not regulate glucose uptake into this organ. Glucose passes freely into the cells of the liver and is phosphorylated to glucose-6-phosphate by glucokinase. This enzyme, unlike the equivalent hexokinase in extrahepatic tissues, is not subject to inhibitory negative feedback control by its product. Its activity increases with the increase in glucose delivered to the liver after a meal.

'Counter-regulatory' hormones such as adrenaline and the glucocorticoids play little or no part in the control of blood glucose in the fed state (Table 16.4). The type of food ingested determines the participation of other 'counter-regulatory' hormones such as glucagon and growth hormone (Table 16.4).

DIABETES MELLITUS

Diabetes mellitus is a chronic metabolic disorder characterized by a **high blood glucose concentration (hyperglycaemia)** which is due to insulin deficiency or insulin resistance. The hyperglycaemia is due to the fact that the liver and skeletal muscle cannot store glycogen and the tissues are unable to utilize glucose. When the kidney threshold for glucose is exceeded, glucose spills over into the urine (**gly-**

Table 16.4 Hormonal response to altered fuel availability

Condition	Insulin	Glucagon	Growth hormone	Adrenaline	Glucocorticoids
Fuel availability					
Glucose ingestion	↑	↓	↓	—	—
Protein ingestion	↑	↑	↑	—	—
Mixed meal	↑	—	—	—	—
Fuel need					
Starvation	↓	↑	↑ or —	↑ or —	↓
Acute hypoglycaemia	↓	↑	↑	↑	↑
Exercise	↓	↑	↑	↑	↑

↑ = increased secretion; ↓ = decreased secretion; — = unchanged
Adapted from: Felig, 1981

cosuria) and causes an osmotic diuresis (**polyuria**) which in turn results in dehydration and increased fluid intake (**polydipsia**). The decreased insulin action allows increased catabolism of nutrients. In florid diabetes **ketosis** and **protein wasting** are seen. Protein wasting occurs when protein metabolism in the liver is deranged and an excessive amount of protein is converted to carbohydrate. Ketosis occurs because there is less synthesis of lipids along with increased fat breakdown. As a result of the effects of the liberated fatty acids on various metabolic pathways, some acetyl-CoA is shunted to the synthesis of cholesterol or ketone or both since not all of it enters the citric acid or fatty acid synthesis pathways. The result is an increase in ketone bodies in the plasma and tissue fluids.

Apart from the metabolic derangements in diabetes, various vascular and neurological complications develop often over many years.

Most diabetics show **reduced glucose tolerance**, which is determined by monitoring blood glucose concentration for 2 hours following a dose of oral glucose after an overnight fast. In diabetic subjects, the rise in blood glucose is abnormally large and prolonged.

There are two main forms of diabetes.

1. **Juvenile-onset diabetes**, in which there is a profound decrease in the number of β-cells in the islets and thus an absolute deficiency of insulin. This is also referred to as 'insulin-dependent' or Type I diabetes and the main treatment is insulin. A viral aetiology is proposed for some severe forms of this condition. Impaired counter-regulation by catecholamines, glucocorticoids and growth hor-

mone may also be a feature of this type of diabetes, especially in long-standing cases.

2. **Maturity-onset** diabetes, in which there may be varying degrees of insulin deficiency and insulin resistance in individual patients. This is also referred to as 'insulin-independent' or Type II diabetes. The patients are usually obese and the treatment is usually dietary, though supplementary oral hypoglycaemic drugs or insulin may be necessary. There is evidence that the resistance to insulin is, in some cases, associated with a decrease in the number of insulin receptors in peripheral tissues. However, as only 10% of receptors need to be occupied for an adequate response this may be unimportant and a post-receptor defect may be implicated. An increased sensitivity to insulin occurs with weight loss.

The alterations in insulin secretion in the two forms of diabetes are shown schematically in Figure 16.15 and are contrasted with the normal response.

In a *normal* individual there is a basal level of insulin secretion and the response to an intravenous infusion of glucose (equivalent to what might happen after a meal) has two phases. The first phase is rapid and short-lived and the second is prolonged. In *non-insulin-dependent diabetes* there is hyperglycaemia and a normal or slightly raised basal insulin concentration. The first phase of the insulin-secretory response to i.v. glucose is virtually absent but the delayed response to glucose is present. The response to the non-glucose secretagogues (e.g. amino-acids, sulphonylureas, glucagon, GIT hormones) is nearly normal (not shown). In *insulin-dependent diabetes* there is a severe β-cell dysfunction. Basal insulin secretion is extremely low and there is virtually no response to glucose, or any other stimuli. The minimal insulin secretion is insufficient to maintain metabolic homeostasis with the result that there is hyperglycaemia, proteolysis, lipolysis and ketosis.

DRUGS USED IN TREATMENT OF DIABETES MELLITUS

The aim of treatment is to keep the glucose concentration in the plasma within normal levels as far as possible. The drugs used are insulin and the oral hypoglycaemic agents, which have to be combined with dietary control. Overdosage with insulin may necessitate the use of oral or intravenous glucose or, in some circumstance, intramuscular glucagon.

Insulin

The effects of insulin and its mechanism of action have been described above. Being a peptide, it is destroyed in the gastrointestinal tract, and must always be given parenterally, usually subcutaneously, but occasionally intravenously. One of the main problems in using it is to avoid wide fluctuations in plasma concentration and thus in the blood glucose, for there is evidence that precise control of blood glucose, with avoidance of sharp peaks and troughs, is important for preventing the long-term complications which are responsible for the morbidity and mortality associated with diabetes.

Insulin for clinical use is extracted from bovine or porcine pancreatic tissue and is not identical with the human hormone. Beef insulin differs in three

Table 16.5 Insulin preparations*

Category	Preparations	Source	With subcutaneous injection		Comments
			Peak action (hours)	Duration of action (hours)	
Fast-action	Neutral insulins	Human (emp, & crb)	2–4		Important in emergencies e.g. ketoacidosis. Can be given i.v. when peak effect in 30–60 min and duration 3–4 hours. If used on their own, two or more injections are necessary daily. Can be mixed in the syringe with any intermediate or long-acting insulin except protamine zinc insulin.
		Porcine		6–8	
Intermediate action	Isophane insulins	Human (emp & crb); bovine; porcine	6–12	12–24	Can be used for starting twice daily injection regimes. Can be mixed with neutral insulin. Ready-mixed preparations are available.
	Insulin zinc suspensions (amorphous; semilente)	Porcine	5–10	12–16	
	Biphasic insulins	Human (emp & crb); porcine; bovine	3–8	16–22	Mixtures of neutral insulin with either crystalline insulin or isophane insulin
Long-action	Insulin zinc suspension (crystalline; ultralente)	Bovine; porcine	10–24	24–36	(Human crb insulin zinc suspension crystalline is intermediate, not long-acting)
	Insulin zinc suspension, (mixed; lente)	Bovine; porcine	6–14	18–30	30% amorphous + 70% crystalline
	Protamine zinc insulin	Bovine	10–20	20–36	Given once daily, in conjunction with a short-acting insulin, (but not in same syringe). Use is declining.

* See: MacPherson & Feely, 1983

amino-acid residues and pork insulin in one. Two recent developments have meant that 'human' insulin is now also available—the use of techniques involving chain recombinant DNA is bacteria (crb insulin) and enzymic techniques to modify pork insulin (emp insulin).

Insulin has to be biologically assayed against an international standard and its dosage is therefore expressed in 'units'.

There is a confusing variety of insulins available. They may be classified according to their peak effect and duration of action. Details of some preparations are given in Table 16.5.

Early preparations of insulin were made with amorphous (i.e. non-crystalline) insulin and the solutions were of low pH. The possibility of precipitation in the tissues or when mixed with other insulin formulations led to the introduction of acetate-buffered neutral solutions. This type of insulin is freely soluble and produces a rapid and short-lived effect. **Soluble insulins** are the only ones which can be given intravenously. Longer-acting insulin preparations are made by precipitating the insulin in the presence of zinc, thus forming relatively insoluble crystals, which are injected as a suspension and are only slowly absorbed. The crystal size can be adjusted to provide preparations of varying rates of absorption (**semilente**, **lente** and **ultralente** preparations). **Protamine-zinc insulin** is a protamine-insulin complex crystallized in the presence of zinc; this results in a preparation with a long action but a very slow onset. **Isophane insulin** is a modified preparation of protamine zinc insulin with more rapid onset.

It needs to be remembered that the objective is to maintain a steady concentration of blood glucose, not of insulin, and none of these long-lasting preparations can substitute effectively for an endogenous source of insulin which responds rapidly to changes in blood glucose. One problem is that endogenous insulin secretion is stimulated mainly by glucose and other nutrients after a meal; the insulin is released into the hepatic portal vein and goes directly to the liver whose sensitivity to insulin is much greater than that of the peripheral tissues. Attempts are now being made to supply insulin from a small infusion pack, and to regulate the dose by means of a sensor that continuously monitors blood glucose. If technically feasible, this should greatly improve the control that can be achieved. Administration by the intraperitoneal route has been investigated in an attempt to provide direct hepatic utilization. Intranasal delivery has also been described.

There has recently been a strong emphasis on improving the purity of insulin preparations, to reduce the incidence of immune responses leading to anti-insulin antibodies (see below). 'Monocomponent' insulins are purified by anion exchange chromatography and most types of insulin (soluble, lente, semilente and ultralente) are also obtainable in the purer monocomponent form.

Combinations of different forms of insulin with different speeds of action (**biphasic insulins**) extend the range of preparations available. The preparations in common use are the short-acting soluble insulins and the medium acting isophane and zinc suspensions. They are often used singly or in combination in treatment regimes involving 1–4 injections per day.

Patients may vary widely in their responses to particular preparations. Insulin regimes must be tailored to each individual patient's need and must be constantly monitored and adjusted since a variety of factors (exercise, infection, etc) alters the requirement. Home testing by the patient of urine or of blood glucose capillary samples using reflectance meters or enzyme-impregnated strips has improved the control which can be achieved.

In terms of the cost of treatment the cheapest insulins are the bovine insulins. Human crb insulin and the purified porcine insulins are more expensive and comparable in price, whereas the semisynthetic human emp insulin is the most expensive.

Uses

Insulin is essential in the treatment of insulin-dependent (juvenile-onset) diabetes and may be required in maturity-onset diabetes if dieting fails. The type of insulin used and the regime of administration is adjusted according to urinary and blood glucose measurement and treatment has to be tailored to each individual's requirement by the clinician. If conditions such as pregnancy, infection or endocrine disorders supervene, the regime may need to be adjusted. Insulin resistance is very rare but may complicate treatment. In practical terms a patient may be considered to have insulin resistance if his or her daily requirement is 200 units or more, in the absence of ketoacidosis, intercurrent infection or endocrine disorders. The main cause is a high titre of circulating anti-insulin antibodies, which is more likely to occur with bovine insulin than with porcine insulin. Note, however, that virtually all patients treated with animal insulin have antibodies against the hormone, albeit usually of low titre. 'Human' insulin is less immunogenic than animal insulin but may still evoke an antibody response, since the source of the hormone is not the only determinant of immunogenicity; insulins undergo physical changes before and after injection which can increase their potential for provoking antibodies.

Unwanted effects

The main undesirable effect is *hypoglycaemia*, for which the treatment is to administer carbohydrate orally or, in an emergency, intravenously. Glucagon injected intramuscularly may be used if intravenous administration of glucose is not feasible.

Allergy to insulin may occur and may take the form of local or systemic reactions.

Lipodystrophy involves the proliferation of adipose tissue or, less commonly, its loss at the site of injection. It is cosmetically undesirable but harmless, and may be related to an antibody response to less purified insulin preparations. A *rebound hyperglycaemia* may follow excessive insulin administration. This results from the release of the insulin-opposing or counter-regulatory hormones (catecholamines, hydrocortisone, growth hormone and glucagon) in response to an insulin-induced hypoglycaemia.

Oral hypoglycaemic agents

There are two groups of oral agents which are able to lower the blood sugar effectively, the sulphonylureas and related compounds, and the biguanides.

Sulphonylureas

This group of drugs was developed as a result of the finding that a substituted sulphonamide, p-amino benzene sulfonamido-isopropylthiadazole, used to treat typhoid, resulted in a marked lowering of blood glucose.

There are now numerous sulphonylureas available for therapy, the main ones being **tolbutamide** and **chlorpropamide** (Fig. 16.18). Others are **glibenclamide**, **glipizide**, **acetohexamide**, **glibornuride** and **tolazamide**. They all contain the sulphonylurea moiety, but different substitutions result in differ-

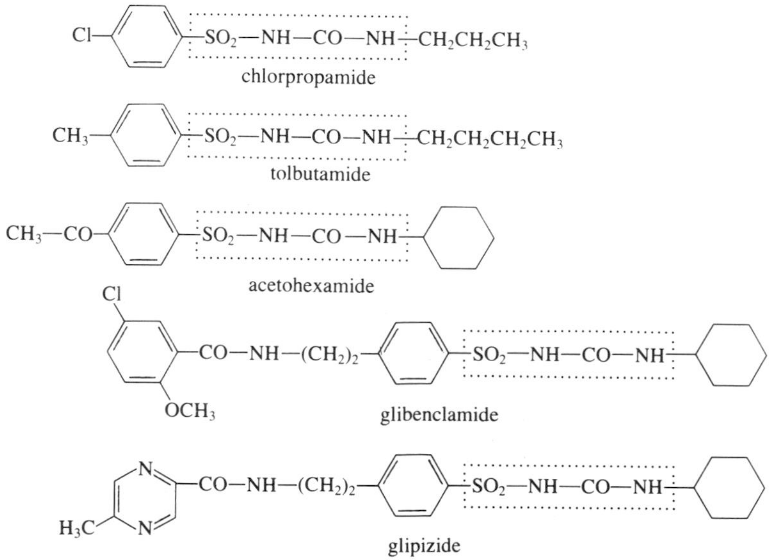

Fig. 16.18 The structure of some oral hypoglycaemic drugs, and with the sulphonylurea moiety within the dotted box.

ences in potency, pharmacokinetics and duration of action (see Table 16.6). **Glyuridine**, though not chemically a sulfonylurea, is closely related and pharmacologically very similar to tolbutamide.

Mechanism of action

The principal action is on the β-cells of the islets, stimulating the secretion of insulin (the equivalent of phase 1 in Fig. 16.15) and thus causing a fall in the plasma glucose concentration.

The mechanism of stimulation of the β-cells is unknown. *In vitro* studies imply that the sulphonylureas do not act in the same way as glucose, in that they do not enter the cell or stimulate the synthesis of insulin, as glucose does.

In the first few days of treatment with these drugs the basal insulin levels and the insulin secretory response to various stimuli are enhanced. With longer treatment both the basal insulin concentration and the insulin response to various non-glucose signals return to pre-treatment values, whereas the decrease in blood glucose is maintained. It has therefore been suggested that the effects on the β-cell are transient and that the long-term effects are due to other actions, such as an increase in insulin sensitivity of the liver and peripheral tissues, or an increase in the number of insulin receptors. Other effects of the drugs on the liver have also been postulated, such as a reduction in hepatic uptake of insulin or a direct inhibition of hepatic glucose production. However, it may well be that the stimulatory effects on the β-cells do, in fact, persist after the first few days of therapy but

Table 16.6 Oral hypoglycaemic sulphonylurea drugs

Drug	Duration of action and half-life	Pharmacokinetic factors	Specific toxic effects and general comments
Chlorpropamide	24–72 h (36 h)	Poorly metabolized. Tightly bound to plasma protein. Excreted virtually unchanged over 10–14 days.	Contraindicated in renal impairment. Has ADH-like effect on renal tubules and may cause hyponatraemia and water intoxication. May cause hypoglycaemia. May cause flushing and headache after alcohol. May interact with other protein-bound drugs.
Tolbutamide	6–12 h (4–8 h)	Bound to plasma protein. Carboxylated in liver to inactive compound which is excreted in the urine.	Least likely to cause hypoglycaemia or toxicity. May decrease iodide uptake by thyroid. Contraindicated in liver failure.
Acetohexamide	10–16 h (1 h for parent, 45 h for active metabolite)	Rapidly metabolized to more active compound:-hydroxyhexamide. Weakly bound to plasma protein. 75% excreted unchanged in urine.	Contraindicated in impaired renal function.
Tolazamide	10–16 h (7 h)	Rapidly metabolized to at least six metabolic products, many having hypoglycaemic activity. Renal excretion.	More potent than acetohexamide.
Glibenclamide	12 h (6–12 h)	About 25% is oxidized in the liver and is excreted in urine; the rest is excreted unchanged in the faeces. Not protein bound.	20–100 times more potent than above drugs. May actually increase the number of β-cells in the islets. Contraindicated in liver failure. Interactions due to displacement from plasma proteins less likely.
Glipizide	8 h (3–5 h)	Metabolized in the liver.	
Glicazide	12–18 h (12 h)	Metabolized in liver.	

that these effects are masked by the decrease in plasma glucose which has occurred.

There is no evidence that the effect of the sulphonylureas on impaired islets exhausts the β-cells or decreases their number. In fact some 'second-generation' sulphonylureas, such as glibenclamide and glipizide, may actually increase the number of β-cells in the islets.

Pharmacokinetic aspects

These drugs are well absorbed after oral administration. The duration of action varies (Table 16.6) and this determines the number of doses required per day, e.g. a single dose of chlorpropamide, two to three of tolbutamide. They bind strongly to plasma albumin, and are therefore involved in interactions with other drugs (e.g. salicylates, sulphonamides) which compete for these binding sites (see below and Chapter 4). Most rely largely on renal excretion for their elimination from the body, so their action is enhanced in elderly patients or in those with renal disease. It is also affected by diuretics (see below). Further details of pharmacokinetic factors are given in Table 16.6.

Uses

These drugs are only effective if there is adequate β-cell function and are therefore not useful in juvenile-onset insulin-dependent diabetes. They are used mainly in maturity-onset diabetes and then only if dietary therapy aimed at weight reduction is not effective. However, even in this type of diabetes only 60–75% of patients respond and many of these cease to respond eventually. A satisfactory continued response is achieved in only 20–30%.

Unwanted effects

Side effects and toxic effects which occur more frequently with some agents than others are specified in Table 16.6. Hypoglycaemia may occur with any of the agents but is more common with chlorpropamide because of its long duration of action; this particular toxic effect can be serious especially in elderly patients and in patients with impaired renal function. An effect which can be troublesome is the occurrence of flushing, nausea and headache after consuming alcohol, similar to the reaction produced by disulfiram (see Chapter 35). This occurs only in certain individuals, and appears to have a genetic origin, though the mechanism is not known. Hepatic effects (canalicular bile stasis) occur infrequently, the incidence being related to the hypoglycaemic potency of the drug. Allergic skin rashes have been observed and bone marrow damage, though very rare, has been reported.

A vexed question is whether prolonged therapy with oral hypoglycaemic drugs has effects on the cardiovascular system. A study on the treatment of Type II diabetes sponsored by the National Institutes of Health in the USA in 1970 found that after 4–5 years of treatment there was an increase in cardiovascular-related deaths in the sulphonylurea-treated group as compared with the groups treated with insulin or placebo. However, there was no statistically significant increase in total mortality in the sulphonylurea group as compared with the others. The significance of these findings for therapy with the sulphonylureas is still a matter of controversy.

Drug interactions

Several compounds *augment* the hypoglycaemic effect of the sulphonylureas. Phenylbutazone, salicylates, bishydroxycoumarin, alcohol, monoamine oxidase inhibitors, sulphaphenazole and sulphisoxazole have all been reported to produce severe hypoglycaemia when given with the sulphonylureas. The probable basis of the interaction is competition for the metabolizing enzymes, but interference with plasma protein binding or with excretion may play a part. Aspirin has been shown to interfere with the protein binding of tolbutamide and the urinary excretion of chlorpropamide, and phenylbutazine with the binding of acetohexamide.

Agents which *decrease* the action of the sulphonylureas include thiazides, corticosteroids, chloramphenicol, frusemide, and the oral contraceptives.

Biguanides

These are orally active hypoglycaemic agents whose mode of action is quite different from that of the sulphonylureas in that they do not requite functioning β-cells. They appear to affect the peripheral tissues directly by increasing glucose uptake, and they may also increase glycolysis and decrease gluconeogenesis. The main compound is **metformin** which has a half-life of about 3 hours. In addition to the fact that they produce minor gastrointestinal toxic effects more frequently than the sulphonylureas, the biguanides have a propensity to cause a severe lactic acidosis. This has resulted in their withdrawal from the market in the USA and a decline in their use in the UK.

ACTH AND ADRENAL STEROIDS

The steroids secreted by the adrenal cortex are crucial for survival in that they are necessary for the response to a threatening environment, an animal deprived of its adrenal cortex being able to survive only in rigorously controlled conditions. The main adrenal steroids are those with **mineralocorticoid** and **glucocorticoid** activity, but some **sex steroids**—mainly androgens—are also secreted. The mineralocorticoids affect water and electrolyte balance and the main endogenous hormone is **aldosterone**. The glucocorticoids affect carbohydrate and protein metabolism and the main endogenous hormones are **hydrocortisone** and **corticosterone**. The two actions are not completely separated in naturally occurring steroids, some glucocorticoids having quite substantial effects on water and electrolyte balance. Synthetic steroids have

Table 16.7 Comparison of the main corticosteroid agents (using hydrocortisone as a standard)

Compound	Relative affinity for glucocorticoid receptors*	Approx relative potency in clinical use:		Duration of action after oral dose	Comments
		Anti-inflam.	Sodium-retaining		
Hydrocortisone (cortisol)	1	1	1	S	Drug of choice for replacement and emergencies.
Cortisone	0.01	0.8	0.8	S	Cheap. Inactive until converted to hydrocortisone. Not used as anti-inflammatory because of mineralocorticoid effects.
Corticosterone	0.85	0.3	15	S	—
Prednisolone	2.2	4	0.8	I	Drug of choice for anti-inflammatory and immunosuppressive effects.
Prednisone	0.05	4	0.8	I	Inactive until converted to prednisolone. Anti-inflammatory and immunosuppressive.
Methyl-prednisolone	11.9	5	minimal	I	Anti-inflammatory and immunosuppressive.
Triamcinolone	1.9	5	none	I	Relatively more toxic than others. Anti-inflammatory and immunosuppressive.
Dexamethasone	7.1	30	minimal	L	Anti-inflammatory and immunosuppressive, used especially where water retention is undesirable, e.g. cerebral oedema. Drug of choice for suppression of ACTH production.
Betamethasone	5.4	30	negligible	L	Anti-inflammatory and immunosuppressive, used especially where water retention is undesirable. Used for suppression of ACTH production.
Beclomethasone		+	—	—	Anti-inflammatory and immunosuppressive. Used topically and as an aerosol.
Deoxycortone	0.19	neg.	50	—	
Fludrocortisone	3.5	15	150	S	Drug of choice for mineralocorticoid effects.
Aldosterone	0.38	none	500	—	Endogenous mineralocorticoid.

* Human foetal lung cells
Duration of action: S: $t_\frac{1}{2}$ = 8–12 h; I: $t_\frac{1}{2}$ = 12–36 h; L: $t_\frac{1}{2}$ = 36–72 h
Data for relative affinity obtained from: Baxter & Rousseau, 1979

been developed which show a much clearer separation of these two actions (Table 16.7). In addition to their metabolic effects, glucocorticoids also have anti-inflammatory and immunosuppressive activity and it is for these actions that they are most commonly used therapeutically.

A deficiency in corticosteroid production, **Addison's disease**, is characterized by muscular weakness, low blood pressure, depression, anorexia, loss of weight and hypoglycaemia. Addison's disease may have an auto-immune aetiology or be due to destruction of the gland by chronic inflammatory conditions such as tuberculosis. A decreased production of endogenous corticoids also occurs when glucocorticoids are given therapeutically; this can result in deficiency after a period of prolonged therapy.

When corticosteroids are produced in excess, the clinical picture depends on which of the steroids predominate. An excess of glucocorticoid activity results in **Cushing's syndrome**, the manifestations of which are outlined in Figure 16.19. This is usually due to hyperplasia of the adrenal glands but a somewhat similar picture can be produced by long continued administration of glucocorticoids. An excess production of mineralocorticoids results in disturbances of sodium and potassium balance. This may occur with hyperactivity of the adrenals or tumours of the glands (**primary hyperaldosteronism**, or with excess renin/angiotensin action such as occurs in nephrosis, cirrhosis of the liver or congestive cardiac failure (**secondary hyperaldosteronism**). Hypersecretion of aldosterone may also occur in hypertension (see Chapter 11). Excess production of adrenal androgens results in '**adrenal virilism**'. These three syndromes may overlap.

GLUCOCORTICOIDS

Synthesis and release

Adrenal steroids are not stored preformed—they are synthesized and released as needed, and the main physiological stimulus for synthesis and release of the glucocorticoids is **corticotrophin** (adrenocorticotrophic hormone; **ACTH**) secreted from the anterior pituitary gland. Corticotrophin secretion is regulated partly by **cortico-**

trophin-releasing factor (**CRF**) derived from the hypothalamus and partly by the level of glucocorticoids in the blood. The release of CRF in turn is controlled by the level of glucocorticoids and, to a lesser extent, of corticotrophin in the blood and it is influenced by input from higher central nervous system centres. Opioid peptides normally exercise a tonic inhibitory control on the secretion of CRF,

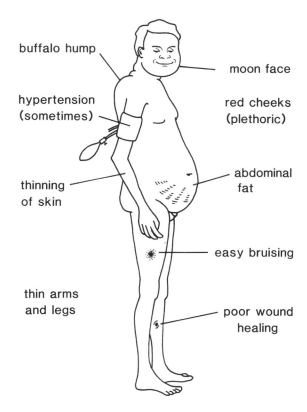

Euphoria

(though sometimes depression or psycotic symptoms, and emotional lability)

also:

Osteoporosis

Tendency to hyperglycemia

Negative nitrogen balance

Increased appetite

Increased susceptibility to infection

Increased weight

Fig. 16.19 Effects of prolonged glucocorticoid excess: Cushing's syndrome. Italicized effects are particularly common. (Adapted from: Baxter & Rousseau, 1979)

but in conditions of stress they may be instrumental in stimulating its release. Emotional changes may affect release of CRF, as may stimuli such as excessive heat or cold, injury or infections; this release is the mechanism, in fact, by which the pituitary-adrenal system is activated in response to a threatening environment. The inter-relationship of these factors is outlined in Figure 16.20.*

There is a diurnal variation in the concentration of endogenous corticosteroids in the blood, between approximately 450 nM at 8 a.m. and 110 nM at 4 p.m.

The starting substance for synthesis of glucocorticoids is **cholesterol** which is obtained mostly from the plasma and is present in the lipid granules of the cells of the fascicular zone—the middle layer of cells in the adrenal cortex. The steps involved in synthesis are outlined in Figure 16.21. The first step, the conversion of cholesterol to **pregnenolone** is the rate-limiting step and is regulated by ACTH. Some of the reactions in the synthesis can be inhibited by drugs:

Metyrapone prevents the β-hydroxylation at C_{11} and thus the formation of hydrocortisone and corticosterone. Synthesis is stopped at the 11-desoxy corticosteroid stage and as these substances have no negative feedback effects on the hypothalamus and pituitary, there is a marked increase in ACTH in the blood. Metyrapone can therefore be used to test ACTH production and may also be used in some cases of Cushing's syndrome.

Aminoglutethimide, an experimental tool rather than a therapeutic agent, inhibits an earlier stage in the synthetic pathway and has the same effect as metyrapone.

Mitotane, a derivative of DDT, decreases corticosteroid synthesis mainly by a cytotoxic action on the cells and is used only in inoperable tumours of the adrenal cortex. It has a selective action on the adrenal cortex, but its precise mechanism of action is not known.

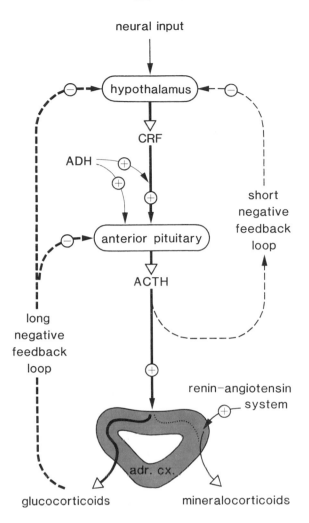

Fig. 16.20 Regulation of synthesis and secretion of adrenal corticosteroids ACTH = adrenocorticotrophic hormone (corticotrophin); adr.cx = adrenal cortex; ADH = anti-diuretic hormone; CRF = corticotrophin-releasing factor. Arrow with open head = releases. Arrow with closed head = acts on;
———⊕———→ = stimulates; ----⊖---→ = inhibits.
ACTH has only a minimal effect on mineralocorticoid production, indicated by dotted line.

PHARMACOLOGICAL ACTIONS

The pharmacological actions of the glucocorticoids may be considered under three main headings: (1) general effects on metabolism, water and electrolyte balance and organ systems; (2) negative feedback effects on the anterior pituitary and hypothalamus;

---

* When released, the corticosteroids pass first through the adrenal medulla because both the medulla and cortex of the adrenal gland have a common blood supply. Glucocorticoids play a part in controlling the conversion of noradrenaline to adrenaline, through a stimulant action on the relevant methyl-transferase (see Chapter 7).

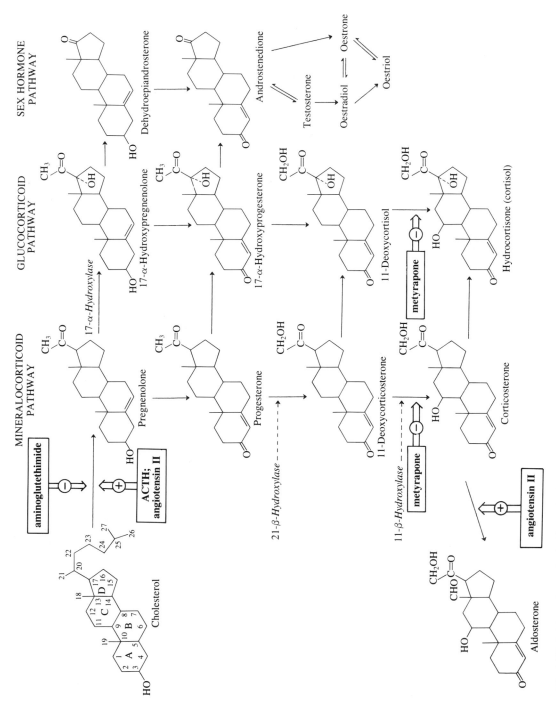

Fig. 16.21 Main pathways in the biosynthesis of corticosteroids and adrenal androgens with sites of action of drugs indicated.

and (3) anti-inflammatory and immunosuppressive effects.

General metabolic and systemic effects

The main metabolic effects are on carbohydrate and protein metabolism. The hormones cause both a decrease in the uptake and utilization of glucose and an increase in gluconeogenesis, resulting in a tendency to hyperglycaemia, as explained in the section on blood glucose earlier in this chapter (see Table 16.3). There is a concomitant increase in glycogen storage which may be due to insulin secretion in response to the increase in blood sugar. There is decreased protein synthesis and increased protein breakdown, particularly in muscle. Glucocorticoids have a 'permissive' effect on the lipolytic response to catecholamines and other hormones, which act by increasing intracellular cAMP concentration (see Chapter 1). Such hormones work through a cAMP-dependent protein kinase, the synthesis of which requires the presence of glucocorticoids (see below). The protein kinase converts an inactive lipase to an active one. Large doses of glucocorticoids given over a long period result in the redistribution of fat characteristic of Cushing's syndrome (see Fig. 16.19).

The glucocorticoids have some mineralocorticoid actions (see below), causing a degree of sodium retention and potassium loss. This may be due to the fact that glucocorticoids, when present in concentrations above those found physiologically, can occupy mineralocorticoid receptors and induce mineralocorticoid activity. They may also in some circumstances have a different action—increasing the glomerular filtration rate and promoting diuresis. The mechanism of this action is not understood, but can be seen if they are administered in adrenal insufficiency in which there is impaired diuresis after water loading.

Glucocorticoids tend to produce a negative calcium balance by decreasing calcium absorption in the gastrointestinal tract and increasing its excretion by the kidney. This may result in osteoporosis (see below).

Negative feedback effects on the anterior pituitary and hypothalamus

As mentioned above, endogenous glucocorticoids have a negative feedback effect on the secretion of CRF and ACTH (see Fig. 16.20). Thus, one of the pharmacological effects of exogenous glucocorticoids is to depress the secretion of these hormones, with a resultant decrease in secretion of endogenous glucocorticoids and atrophy of the adrenal cortex. If therapy is prolonged it may take many months for the pituitary-adrenal system to return to normal function when the drugs are stopped.

Anti-inflammatory and immunosuppressive effects

When given therapeutically glucocorticoids have powerful anti-inflammatory and immunosuppressive effects. They inhibit both the early and the late manifestations of inflammation, i.e. not only the initial redness, heat, pain and swelling, but also the later stages of wound healing and repair and the proliferative reactions seen in chronic inflammation. They affect *all* types of inflammatory reactions whether caused by invading pathogens, by chemical or physical stimuli or by inappropriately deployed immune responses such as are seen in hypersensitivity or autoimmune disease (p. 186).

They reduce the degree of dilatation of *blood vessels* and there is less fluid exudation. This may be, in part, due to a direct vasoconstrictor action on small blood vessels. One of their main anti-inflammatory actions is to decrease accumulation of *blood leucocytes* at the site of inflammation. With *neutrophil leucocytes* glucocorticoid action is associated with increased release from the bone marrow and a neutrophil leucocytosis; whereas with *monocytes* the action of the drug results in a decreased release of monocytes from the bone marrow and thus fewer monocytes in the blood. In the tissues *mononuclear phagocytes* are less effective in dealing with those bacteria, (such as the organism which causes tuberculosis) whose destruction requires 'activated' macrophages*. There is less secretion of neutral proteases from macrophages and

---

* 'Activated', in this context, refers to an increased microbicidal activity brought about by lymphokines (factors released from lymphocytes) or by endotoxin. Activated macrophages are also capable of generating more toxic oxygen products and secreting more enzymes than non-activated macrophages.

thus a decrease in those sorts of tissue damage (e.g. in arthritis) associated with extracellular release of these enzymes.

Fibroblasts are less active in the presence of glucocorticoids, producing less collagen and glyco-saminoglycans, and in consequence chronic inflammation may be reduced, but so also is healing and repair. The activity of *osteoblasts* (which lay down the bone matrix) is inhibited. The activity *osteoclasts* (which digest bone matrix) is indirectly increased because a decrease in intestinal calcium absorption results in increased secretion of para-thyroid hormone which stimulates these cells (see parathyroid section: p. 405). Thus there is a tendency to develop osteoporosis.

The concentration of various *complement components* is decreased by the glucocorticoids. In experiments on guinea-pigs, all components except C1 and C9 were affected, C4 and C8 being most markedly depressed. During the first 2 weeks of administration there was a progressive fall in complement components followed by stabilization at lower levels.

The effect of glucocorticoids on *lymphocytes* varies in different species. In steroid-susceptible animals (rabbit, rat, mouse) they cause lympholysis, with a decrease in both T and B cells and their products. In 'steroid-resistant' species (man, monkey, guinea-pig) there is little or no lympholysis. Much of the previous confusion about the effect of these agents on lymphocytes arose not only because most *in vivo* studies had been carried out on mice, but also because much of the *in vitro* work had employed very high concentrations of steroid. These studies have dubious applicability to the action of the drugs in man. *In vitro* tests on human cells with more therapeutically relevant concentrations (about $3\,\mu M$) have shown that corticosteroids result in a decreased proliferative response to mitogens and antigens. The main reason for this is probably a decreased production of the T cell growth factor (interleukin 2), the hormone produced by a clone of lymphocytes when it 'recognizes' an antigen. This hormone is necessary for the proliferation of activated T cell clones and has been shown to be important in the provision of T cell 'help' in a number of immune responses (see Fig. 8.4). This effect of the steroids may be the basis for the fact that, certainly as far as graft rejection is

concerned, glucocorticoids suppress more efficiently the initiation and generation of a 'new' immune response than one which is already established, and in which clonal expansion has already occurred. *In vivo* studies in man show that after a single intravenous dose, glucocorticoids cause a marked, though transient, lymphocytopenia which is maximal at 4–6 hours with a return to normal counts by 24 hours. The depletion is due to redistribution of the cells, the T lymphocytes being affected to a greater degree than the B lymphocytes. Steroids also result in decreased entry of lymphocytes into areas of cell-mediated immune reactions and decreased production of the lymphokines which are required for mobilizing and activating other cells such as macrophages (see Chapter 8). This is probably one of the reasons why there is a decrease in 'activated' macrophages, though the drugs also reduce the sensitivity of macrophages to activation by lymphokines.

The consequence of these powerful actions of the glucocorticoids is that they can be of immense value in certain conditions in which there is hypersensitivity and unwanted inflammation, but they carry the hazard that they can suppress the necessary protective responses to infection and can decrease essential healing processes.

Mechanism of action

Most steroid effects involve interactions with intracellular receptors (see Chapter 1), possible exceptions being some of the actions on the hypothalamic-pituitary axis and on adipose tissue. In most tissues the glucocorticoids, after entering cells, bind to specific receptors in the nucleus (Fig. 16.22), the binding involving hydrophobic interactions. The receptors are found in virtually all tissues and have a high affinity for glucocorticoids, the equilibrium dissociation constant for dexamethasone, for example, being 10^{-9}–10^{-8} M. The receptors, which number about 3000 to 10000 per cell, are large proteins of about 1000000 daltons with one or more sub-units. After interaction with the steroid the receptor becomes activated—a temperature and calcium dependent process. This involves a change of conformation of the receptor which results in the exposure of nuclear binding sites, possibly involving basic amino-acid residues. It is thought that

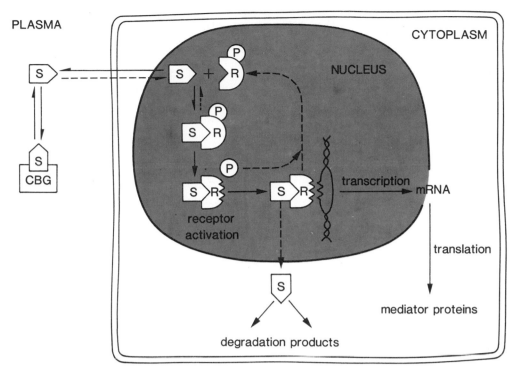

Fig. 16.22 Diagram of mechanism of action of the glucocorticoids at the cellular level. Steroid (S) interacts with the phosphorylated receptor protein. (Receptor: R; Phosphate: P). The complex becomes activated, which involves dephosphorylation and an alteration of conformation. This latter step exposes basic amino-acid residues which interact with DNA at specific acceptor sites resulting in the production of specific messenger RNA, and subsequent mediator proteins. After interaction the complex dissociates, the steroid is degraded and the receptor is phosphorylated and recycled. (The receptor is shown as being in the nucleus, but it may be present in the cytoplasm and translocate to the nucleus after interaction with steroid.) CBG = corticosteroid binding globulin.

the unoccupied receptor is phosphorylated and that activation involves dephosphorylation. Activation may also involve the dissociation of a low molecular weight factor that inhibits activation while associated with the receptor. The steroid-receptor complex is thought to bind to both the DNA and chromatin protein, the binding with chromatin protein increasing the affinity of the interaction with the DNA. The receptor determines the specificity for a particular DNA sequence and hence regulates the formation of specific messenger RNAs, which direct the synthesis of specific proteins. It is these proteins which are believed to mediate the effects of the glucocorticoids. The receptor binding in the nucleus is reversible, as is the binding of steroid to receptor.

As far as the metabolic effects are concerned, several enzymes can be shown, *in vitro*, to be induced by glucocorticoids, but these do not explain all of the metabolic actions seen *in vivo*. A full understanding of the protein mediators of the

effects of glucocorticoids on metabolism and on organ systems awaits further investigation. There has however been progress in elucidating some of the mediators of the anti-inflammatory actions of these drugs. There is evidence that glucocorticoids induce the formation of various polypeptides which have anti-inflammatory effects. One such polypeptide, of approximately 15 000 daltons which was described by Flower & Blackwell in 1979 has been called 'macrocortin' (Flower, 1984). This appears to be formed from a larger glycoprotein of 40 000 daltons, which is the equivalent of an anti-inflammatory mediator protein found by Hirata & Axelrod and their co-workers in 1980 and termed 'lipomodulin'.* In studies carried out so far the

---

* Added in proof: It has recently been agreed that the term **'lipocortin'** be used collectively for the anti-inflammatory protein mediators of glucocorticoid action. The gene for lipocortin has been cloned.

source of lipomodulin has been the neutrophil and the source of macrocortin the macrophage. Macrocortin when injected *in vivo* has anti-inflammatory actions in some but not all experimental models of inflammation. *In vitro* both macrocortin and lipomodulin, and also larger glucocorticoid-induced proteins (170 000 daltons and more), have an inhibitory effect on phospholipase A_2 and therefore on the production from phospholipid of platelet activating factor and of arachidonate and the eicosanoids (see Chapter 8). Lipomodulin also has a lesser inhibitory effect on phospholipase C which, in some cells, also liberates arachidonate from phospholipid (see Chapter 9). Furthermore, because certain arachidonate metabolites are believed to participate in the stimulus-activation coupling mechanism in some inflammatory cells, the activity of these cells may be reduced.

In vitro studies with isolated phospholipase have indicated that lipomodulin is inactivated through phosphorylation by a calcium-dependent protein kinase, and it has been shown that inactivation by phosphorylation occurs in intact neutrophils as well. There is further evidence that macrocortin requires dephosphorylation for optimum activity. Lipomodulin/macrocortin thus constitutes a 'brake' on phospholipase A_2 in inflammatory cells, holding them quiescent and preventing the generation of the powerful inflammatory mediator systems derived from phospholipid (see Fig. 8.7). When the cell is activated during an inflammatory response, lipomodulin is phosphorylated and the brake is removed (see Fig. 16.23).

Neither the transduction mechanisms in inflammatory cells nor the effect of glucocorticoids on them are as yet fully understood, but a simplified outline of the possible relationships is as follows: In neutrophils and other inflammatory cells, phospholipase C initiates the turnover of phosphatidyl inositol bi-phosphate (PIP_2) which is believed to be important in stimulus-activation coupling (see Chapter 1). The action of phospholipase C on PIP_2

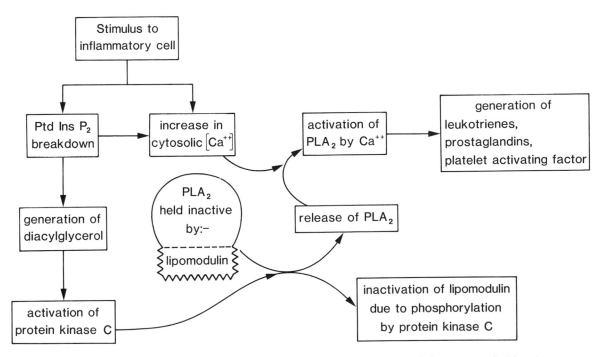

Fig. 16.23 Schematic diagram of effect of lipomodulin on stimulus-activation coupling in an inflammatory cell. (Phosphatases probably subsequently dephosphorylate lipomodulin which then interacts with phospholipase A_2 (PLA_2) inactivating it.) Ptd. Ins P_2 = phosphatidylinositol biphosphate. (It is known that lipomodulin is inactivated through phosphorylation by a calcium-dependent protein kinase. In this diagram, protein kinase C, which is known to be activated in stimulated inflammatory cells, is shown as carrying out the necessary phosphorylation, but the phosphorylation process may be more complex than indicated here, and may involve other kinases.)

results in the production of diacylglycerol which is involved in the activation of a calcium-dependent protein kinase, which phosphorylates several proteins, one of which is lipomodulin (see Figure 16.23).

It is probable that a phosphorylation-dephosphorylation process such as is outlined in Figure 16.23 is a mechanism for regulating the inflammatory response. The full role of the anti-phospholipase A_2 mediator proteins under *physiological* conditions remains to be clarified, but it is thought that they serve to modulate, and thus prevent 'overshoot' of, the body's immensely powerful and potentially damaging defence reaction—the inflammatory response (see Chapter 8)—which comes into play when a pathogen causes infection (see Munck et al, 1984).

It has been shown that many patients with severe inflammatory disease, such as rheumatoid arthritis, systemic lupus erythematosus and dermatomyositis, have plasma antibodies to lipomodulin, and that these antibodies decrease the activity of lipomodulin.

Though the production of lipomodulin/macrocortin explains many of the anti-inflammatory effects of the glucocorticoids, it is not the whole story. Preliminary evidence indicates that some of the anti-inflammatory effects of the glucocorticoids, such as those on blood vessel permeability, may involve mediator proteins other than the two cited above and may, possibly, not involve inhibition of phospholipase A_2.

The actions of glucocorticoids on the hypothalamus and pituitary may occur by mechanisms different from those outlined above. The evidence for this is two-fold: firstly, the structure/activity relationships for the effects of various glucocorticoids on the hypothalamus and pituitary differ from those in other tissues; secondly, the *immediate* response to a sudden change in glucocorticoid concentration (the 'rate-sensitive negative-feedback response') occurs too quickly for transcription and translation to be involved—a decrease in plasma ACTH being detectable within 5 minutes. Receptors in the plasma membrane of the cells may be involved in this response. The *delayed* negative-feedback response however appears to depend on synthesis of protein.

Another exception may be the inhibitory effect of glucocorticoids on glucose uptake into adipose tissue, which can be produced by hydrocortisone linked to agarose beads, and which cannot therefore be due to intracellular action.

Therapeutic uses

These fall into two main categories:

Replacement therapy. This is necessary when the adrenal cortex is not functioning adequately. All the actions of the corticoids are required and a mineralocorticoid may need to be given along with a glucocorticoid. The drugs should be given twice daily to mimic the normal diurnal rhythm of corticoid secretion.

Anti-inflammatory therapy or immunosuppression. This is the commonest use of the glucocorticoids and is largely empirical. Conditions in which they are used include severe asthma and various other hypersensitivity states, collagen diseases such as systemic lupus erythematosis and rheumatoid arthritis, and a wide range of eye and skin disorders.

When they are used as anti-inflammatory and immunosuppressive agents all of their other actions are unwanted side effects. Synthetic steroids have been developed in which it has been possible to separate the glucocorticoid from the mineralocorticoid actions (see Table 16.7) but it has not been possible to separate the anti-inflammatory actions from the other actions of the glucocorticoids.

Unwanted effects

These effects are inherent in the three categories of pharmacological action of the drugs. They are more likely to occur with large doses or prolonged administration and should not occur with replacement therapy.

1. *Suppression of the response to infection or injury.* An intercurrent infection can be potentially very serious unless recognized and treated with antimicrobial agents along with an increase in the dose of steroid. Wound healing may be impaired, but peptic ulceration is probably not the problem it has been considered to be in the past, the incidence being only slightly higher in patients treated with steroids than in controls. However, patients on concurrent high doses of aspirin (e.g. in rheumatoid arthritis) may be more at hazard from peptic ulceration.

2. *The suppression of the patients' own capacity*

to synthesize corticosteroids. Sudden withdrawal of the drugs after prolonged therapy may result in acute adrenal insufficiency. Careful procedures for phased withdrawal should be followed, the rate of withdrawal depending mainly on duration of therapy. Recovery of full adrenal function usually takes about 2 months though in some cases it may take 18 months or more.

3. *Metabolic effects*: when the drugs are used in anti-inflammatory and immunosuppressive therapy, the metabolic actions and the effects on water and electrolyte balance and organ systems are unwanted side effects and iatrogenic Cushing's syndrome may occur (see Fig. 16.19). The osteoporosis previously mentioned, with the attendant hazard of fractures, is probably one of the main limitations to long-term glucocorticoid therapy. Another is muscle wasting and weakness.

In children the metabolic effects, particularly those on protein metabolism, may result in inhibition of growth even with fairly low doses, though this is not likely to occur unless treatment is continued for more than 6 months. A depressant effect on DNA synthesis and cell division in some tissues may also be implicated in this effect, though this anti-proliferative action is not as general as that produced by antimitotic drugs.

There is often euphoria, but some patients may become depressed or develop psychotic symptoms.

The incidence of cataracts is higher after prolonged administration of the glucocorticoids in patients with rheumatoid arthritis, and cataracts have occurred in children as well.

Other toxic effects which have been reported are glaucoma, raised intracranial pressure, hypercoagulability of the blood, fever and disorders of menstruation.

Pharmacokinetic aspects

Glucocorticoids may be given by a variety of routes. Most are active when given orally. All can be given systemically, either intramuscularly or intravenously. They may also be given topically—injected intra-articularly, given by aerosol into the respiratory tract, administered as drops into the eye, or the nose, or applied in creams or ointments to the skin. There is much less likelihood of systemic toxic effects after topical administration, though such effects can occur if large quantities are used.

The drugs are carried in the plasma bound to corticosteroid binding globulin (CBG) and to albumin. The distribution of steroid between free and bound forms depends both on the type of steroid and on the level of CBG and albumin in the plasma. CBG has one hydrocortisone binding site per molecule and has a high affinity for naturally occurring glucocorticoids $(3 \times 10^7 \, \text{l/mol}$ for both hydrocortisone and corticosterone). It is present in plasma in very low concentration—about $0.037 \, \text{g/l}$—and accounts for about 77% of hydrocortisone bound. At hydrocortisone concentrations above $25 \, \mu\text{g}/100 \, \text{ml}$, CBG-binding sites are saturated and more hydrocortisone exists unbound or bound to albumin. CBG does not bind synthetic steroids. Albumin has 1–20 binding-sites per molecule with a lower affinity for hydrocortisone $(0.5 \times 10^4 \, \text{l/mol})$, but its concentration is very much higher, being approximately $4 \, \text{g/l}$. It accounts for 15% of bound hydrocortisone but it binds both natural and synthetic steroids, including conjugated steroids, the affinity being inversely related to the number of polar groups in the steroid. Both CBG-bound and albumin-bound steroids are biologically inactive.

It is generally assumed that steroids, being small lipophilic molecules, enter their target cells by simple diffusion, and experimental studies on hepatoma cells and thymocytes bear this out.

Hydrocortisone has a plasma half-life of 90 mins, though its main biological effects occur only after 2–8 hours. The main step in inactivation is the reduction of the double bond between C_4 and C_5. This occurs in liver cells and elsewhere. The ketone at C_3 is reduced in the liver and most compounds are then linked enzymically to sulphate or glucuronic acid at the C_3 hydroxyl, and finally excreted in the urine. Hydrocortisone may undergo an oxidation at C_{17} to give a 17-ketosteroid along with a 2 carbon fragment. Virtually all of the metabolites are excreted within 72 hours. Metabolism is slowed if there is a double bond between carbon atoms 1 and 2 (methylprednisolone, prednisolone, dexamethasone, betamethasone, beclomethasone) and if there is a fluorine atom at C_9 (dexamethasone, betamethasone). Cortisone and predisone are inactive until converted *in vivo* to hydrocortisone and prednisolone respectively.

CORTICOTROPHIN

Corticotrophin (ACTH) is a polypeptide hormone with 39 amino-acid residues. A peptide consisting of the first 20 residues from the N-terminal end retains the full biological activity of the whole molecule, but removal of even one residue from the N-terminal end inactivates the hormone completely. The polypeptide precursor of corticotrophin is also the precursor for several other peptides, such as the endorphins, and there is complete sequence homology between corticotrophin and the first 39 amino-acid residues of the lipotrophins (see Fig. 19.10). Residues 1 to 13 are identical with α-melanocyte-stimulating hormone. The first 24 amino-acids of corticotrophin are the same in all species investigated, the remainder of the chain varying in different species. Corticotrophin extracted from animal tissues is available for clinical use, but may provoke the formation of antibodies. A synthetic polypeptide consisting of the first 24 amino-acids—**tetracosactrin**—is also available and is less immunogenic than corticotrophin because the immunogenicity resides mainly in the 15 amino-acids at the C-terminal end.

Actions of corticotrophin

This hormone has two separate actions on the adrenal cortex.

1. It stimulates the synthesis and release of glucocorticoids from the two inner layers of cells of the adrenal cortex. (It has a slight effect on the release of aldosterone from the outer layer of cells and it also releases small amounts of steroids with a weak androgenic action.) It is believed to act on a receptor in the cells and to increase cAMP formation by stimulating adenylate cyclase. The principal locus at which cAMP regulates steroid synthesis is the formation of pregnenolone from cholesterol, which is the rate limiting step in the sequence (Fig. 16.21). The main effect is to increase the concentration of the starting substrate for steroid synthesis, cholesterol, which it does both by activating cholesterolesterase and by stimulating the up-

take of cholesterol from plasma lipoproteins. It acts very rapidly, producing a release of glucocorticoids within minutes of injection, and at low dosage the amount released is linearly related to the log of the dose. The main biological actions of corticotrophin are those of the steroids it releases.

2. It has a trophic action on adrenal cortical cells, and also regulates the levels of key mitochondrial steroidogenic enzymes.

Control of corticotrophin secretion

The physiological release of corticotrophin is controlled by a balance between stimulatory and inhibitory factors (see Fig. 16.20). Its release is *stimulated* by corticotrophin-releasing factor (CRF; see Table 16.1). CRF-release from the hypothalamus is under control of higher centres in the CNS, particularly the limbic system. Stimuli which cause CRF to be released are, as explained above, various stressful physical and emotional conditions and factors which interfere with the body's ability to maintain homeostasis—heat, cold, infections, toxins, injury, etc. Opioid receptors may be physiologically important in CRF release. Other hormones which can stimulate corticotrophin release are the catecholamines and the posterior pituitary hormone, ADH (vasopressin: p. 367). This last also potentiates the action of CRF.

Corticotrophin release is *inhibited* by corticosteroids, acting partly directly on the anterior pituitary and partly on the secretion of CRF. The effect of the steroids on the hypothalamus is referred to as the 'long negative-feedback loop'. Corticotrophin concentration in the blood also influences CRF release (the 'short negative-feedback loop'), but this is less important.

A peptide of 41 amino-acids with CRF activity has been isolated from hypothalamic tissue. This peptide has been synthesized and is under investigation.

Pharmacokinetic aspects

As might be expected, corticotrophin and tetracosactrin are broken down in the gastrointestinal tract and therefore cannot be given parenterally. They have to be injected, the usual route being intramuscular, though it is possible to give the drugs intravenously. The plasma half-life after intravenous injection is 15 minutes and the peak effect on the adrenal cortex occurs within 30 minutes. A slow-release preparation of corticotrophin is available, which requires only twice-weekly injection. The naturally occurring hormone which is extracted from pituitary glands may be measured by radio-immunoassay (p. 49).

Clinical use

The main use of both agents is in the diagnosis of adrenal cortical insufficiency. The drugs are given intramuscularly and then the concentration of hydrocortisone in the plasma is measured, using a radio-immunoassay (see Chapter 1). They may sometimes be used in treatment—to stimulate an adrenal cortex which is not functioning adequately, or very occasionally as an alternative to the use of the glucocorticoids in the treatment of inflammatory disorders. The advantages of using these drugs rather than the glucocorticoids themselves are that there is no depression of the production of endogenous corticosteroids and also that there is release of some androgens which may partially counter-balance the predominantly catabolic effect of the glucocorticoids. This latter effect may be of importance for long-term administration in children. A disadvantage is that it is not possible to achieve selective anti-inflammatory and immunosuppressive effects with the peptide hormones, as corticosteroids with mineralocorticoid actions are also released from the adrenal. A further disadvantage is that they have to be given by injection.

MINERALOCORTICOIDS

The main endogenous mineralocorticoid is **aldosterone**, which is produced in the outermost of the three zones of the adrenal medulla, the *zona glomerulosa*. Its main action is to increase sodium reabsorption by an action on the distal tubules in the kidney, with concomitant increased excretion of potassium and hydrogen ions (see Chapter 14). An excessive secretion of mineralocorticoids, as in Cushing's syndrome, causes marked sodium and water retention with resultant increase in the volume of extra-cellular fluid, hypokalaemia and some degree of alkalosis. There is also, commonly, hypertension. A decreased secretion, as in Addison's disease, causes increased sodium loss which is relatively more pronounced than water loss. The osmotic pressure of the extracellular fluid is thus reduced, resulting in a shift of fluid into the intracellular compartment and a marked decrease in extracellular fluid volume. There is a concomitant decrease in the excretion of potassium ions resulting in hyperkalaemia and there is also a moderate decrease in plasma bicarbonate.

Regulation of aldosterone release

The control of the synthesis and release of aldosterone is complex. Though corticotrophin plays some part, the control depends mainly on the electrolyte composition of the plasma and on the angiotensin II system (Fig. 16.20 & Chapters 11 & 14). Low plasma sodium or high plasma potassium concentration affects the zona glomerulosa cells of the adrenal directly, stimulating aldosterone release. A depletion in body sodium also activates the **renin-angiotensin system.** One of the effects of angiotensin II is to increase the synthesis and release of aldosterone. It has been shown that the action of angiotensin II on the glomerulosa cells involves synergism between an increase in cytosolic calcium and the generation of diacylglycerol which results in protein kinase C activation (see Chapter 1).

Mechanism of action of aldosterone

Aldosterone, like other steroids, binds to specific intracellular receptors. Unlike the glucocorticoid-binding receptors which occur in most tissues, aldosterone receptors occur in only a few target tissues such as the kidney, and in the transporting epithelia of the colon and bladder.

As with the glucocorticoids, the interaction of ligand with receptor initiates a change in conformation of the receptor. The complex binds to nuclear material, and regulation of specific messenger RNAs occurs, resulting in the production of specific protein mediators.

The mechanism whereby these actions of aldosterone produce an effect on sodium excretion in the kidney is not clearly understood. One hypothesis is that the protein or peptide mediator(s) induced by aldosterone increases the activity of the specific Na^+/K^+-ATPase which pumps sodium from the cells of the distal convoluted tubule out into the peritubular space from where it passes into the blood; and that active transport of K^+ into these cells from the peritubular space is facilitated. Another hypothesis, based on work on the toad bladder, is that aldosterone induces a permease which increases the permeability of the apical membrane to sodium (p. 314).

Spironolactone is a competitive antagonist of aldosterone and also prevents the mineralocorticoid effects of other adrenal steroids (p. 324).

Administration and therapeutic use

The main clinical use of mineralocorticoids is in replacement therapy (Table 16.7). Aldosterone has to be given intramuscularly and, having a short duration of action, needs to be given several times a day. **Deoxycortone**, which is a precursor of aldosterone in the biosynthetic pathway, is available in slow release preparations for intramuscular injection which need to be given every 2–4 weeks. The drug of choice is **fludrocortisone** which can be taken orally.

PARATHYROID HORMONE, VITAMIN D, AND BONE MINERAL HOMEOSTASIS

Calcium and phosphate both have intracellular and extracellular roles in the body. Intracellularly, calcium is a second messenger, regulating the activity of a variety of enzymes. Phosphate is an integral component of nucleic acids, nucleotides, phospholipids and many proteins. It is important in the 'energy-currency' of the cell, and phosphorylation-dephosphorylation reactions control the state of activity of many, if not most, enzymes. Extracellularly, calcium and phosphate are critically important constituents of bone.

Calcium and phosphate homeostasis is controlled by parathyroid hormone and a family of hormones derived from vitamin D (Fig. 16.24).

THE STRUCTURE OF BONE

The cells involved in bone formation are osteoblasts, which synthesize and secrete the organic matrix of bone (the osteoid) and osteoclasts, which resorb it. The principal component of bone matrix is collagen, but there are also other components such as osteocalcin, (a vitamin K-dependent protein which binds calcium by virtue of γ-carboxyglutamic acid residues; p. 284) and various phosphoproteins, one of which, osteonectin, binds to both calcium and collagen and thus links these two major constituents of bone matrix. Calcium phosphate crystals, in the form of hydroxyapatite $[Ca_{10}(PO_4)_6(OH)_2]$ are deposited in the osteoid converting it into hard bone matrix. Bone is continuously being remodelled, a process whereby the synthesis of bone matrix and the deposition of mineral salts is balanced by bone resorption. This latter process is stimulated mainly by parathyroid hormone and calcitriol, a hormone derived from vitamin D (see below), but other agents such as prostaglandin E_2 (see Chapter 8), the lymphokine termed osteoclast-activating factor (see Chapter 8 and below) also play a part.

Calcium

Virtually all the calcium in the body (more than 95%) is in the skeleton, most as crystalline hydroxyapatite (see above) but some as noncrystalline phosphates and carbonates. Together these make up half the bone mass. The daily turnover of the minerals in bone involves about 700 mg of calcium, as the bone is continuously remodelled.

Intracellular calcium constitutes only about 1% of body calcium but it has a major role in cellular function. An increase in calcium permeability with an increase in cytosolic calcium is part of the transduction mechanism of many cells and thus the concentration of calcium in the extracellular fluid and the plasma needs to be controlled with great precision. The plasma concentration of calcium is approximately 2.5 mM. About 40% is bound to plasma proteins and 10% is in the form of complexes with various anions. The remaining 50% is present as diffusible ionized calcium.

The normal plasma calcium concentration is regulated by complex interactions between para-

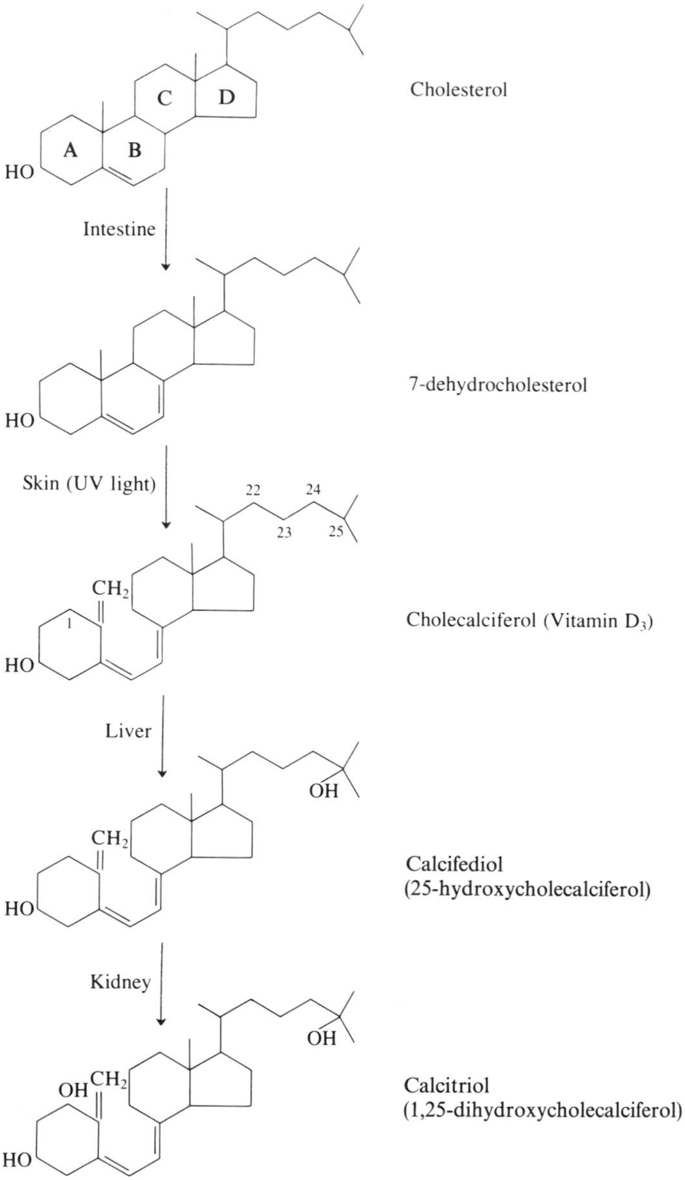

Fig. 16.24 The basic structure of vitamin D_3, cholecalciferol. The B ring of the precursor 7-dehydrocholesterol is cleaved by u.v. irradiation. Vitamin D_2 (calciferol) and its precursor, ergosterol, both have a double bond between C22 and C23 and a methyl group at C24. Hydroxylation at various sites results in the active human D metabolites.

thormone and various forms of vitamin D (Fig. 16.25). Calcitonin and a variety of other hormones also play a part.

Calcium absorption in the intestine involves a calcium-binding protein whose synthesis is regulated by calcitriol (see Fig. 16.25 and below). It is probable that the overall calcium content of the body is regulated largely by this absorption mechanism, since urinary calcium excretion remains more or less constant, the amount of calcium in the faeces varying considerably with the changing calcium content of the diet. However, with high blood calcium concentrations, urinary excretion increases somewhat and with low blood concentrations uri-

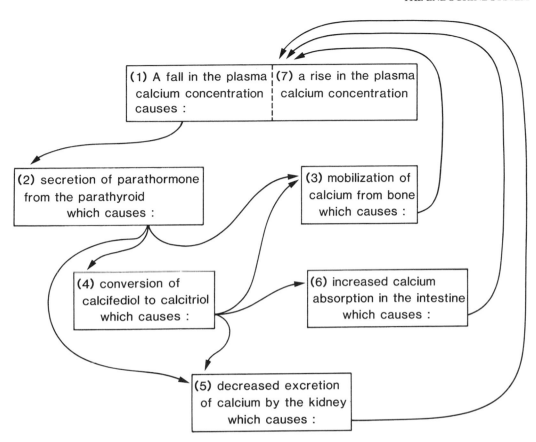

Fig. 16.25 The main factors involved in maintaining the concentration of calcium in the plasma. Calcifediol and calcitriol are metabolites of vitamin D_3 being the 'hormones' 25-hydroxy vitamin D_3 and 1,25-dihydroxy vitamin D_3 respectively.

nary excretion can be modulated by parathormone, and calcitriol, both of which enhance calcium reabsorption in the renal tubules.

Calcium salts are used in therapy as oral supplements when dietary calcium is deficient, and by injection for the treatment of hypocalcaemic tetany. Oral preparations include **calcium gluconate** and **calcium lactate** preparations. Calcium gluconate is used for injection. An oral preparation of **hydroxyapatite** is also available. It is prepared from bovine bone and contains traces of fluoride, and has been used in the prevention of osteoporosis.

Phosphate

Phosphates are critically important in the structure and function of the cells of the body. They play a significant part in enzymic reactions in the cell; they have roles as intracellular buffers and in the excretion of hydrogen ions in the kidney (see Fig. 14.5). They comprise a major component of bone and constitute one of the factors which modify the calcium concentration in tissues.

Phosphate absorption is an energy-requiring process regulated by calcitriol (see below). Its deposition in bone, as hydroxyapatite, depends on the plasma concentration of parathormone, which, with calcitriol, tends to mobilize both calcium and phosphate from the bone matrix. Phosphate excretion occurs in the kidney. 90% is filtered in the glomerulus and most of this is reabsorbed in the proximal tubule. Parathormone inhibits reabsorption and thus increases excretion, while vitamin D metabolites promote reabsorption. This latter effect is usually masked by the former.

Parathyroid hormone (parathormone)

Parathormone is a single chain polypeptide of 84 amino-acids, the essential activity of which is contained in residues 1–34 of the N terminal part of the molecule. It is the most important regulator of the extracellular calcium concentration. When the blood calcium is lowered, parathormone increases it by mobilizing calcium from bone, promoting its retention in the kidney and, in particular, stimulating the synthesis of calcitriol which in turn increases calcium absorption from the intestine and synergizes with parathormone in mobilizing bone calcium (Fig. 16.25). Parathormone promotes phosphate excretion and thus its net effect is to increase the concentration of calcium in the plasma and lower that of phosphate. However, under some circumstance parathormone can stimulate bone formation and patients treated intermittently with this hormone may have an increase in trabecular mass.

The mobilization of calcium from bone by parathormone is mediated, at least in part, by stimulation of osteoclast activity, and the effect on these cells and on the cells of the kidney tubules involves activation of adenylate cyclase (see Chapter 1). Osteoblast activity is also inhibited, thus decreasing calcium deposition by decreasing the amount of matrix available for mineralization.

Parathormone is not stored in the cells of the parathyroid glands. It is synthesized and secreted continuously, the principal factor controlling this being the concentration of ionized calcium in the plasma. The phosphate concentration has no effect on the secretion of the hormone.

There is little or no clinical use for parathormone as such (though preparations of bovine hormone have been available in the past). Hypoparathyroidism is best treated by vitamin D. Therapy of acute hypoparathyroidism necessitates the use of intravenous calcium and injectable vitamin D preparations.

VITAMIN D

Vitamin D is a prohormone which is converted in the body into a number of biologically active metabolites. These function as true hormones, circulating in the blood and regulating the activities of various cell types. The main action is the maintenance of plasma calcium by increasing calcium absorption in the intestine, mobilizing calcium from bone and decreasing its renal excretion (see Fig. 16.25). Vitamin D itself is really a family of sterol derivatives. In man there are two sources of vitamin D. Dietary **ergocalciferol**, (D_2) derived from ergos-

Table 16.8 Vitamin D and its main derivatives

Compound	Alternative name	Notes
Vitamin D_3	Cholecalciferol	Formed in skin from dehydrocholesterol by u.v. irradiation. Available for clinical use of calciferol.
Vitamin D_2	Ergocalciferol	Formed in plants by u.v. irradiation of ergosterol. Available for clinical use as calciferol.
25-hydroxy-vitamin D_3	Calcifediol	Formed in liver from cholecalciferol or ergocalciferol. Main 'storage' form of vitamin D. Thought to be important in reabsorption of calcium in the renal tubules and the regulation calcium flux in muscle.
1,25-dihydroxy vitamin D_3	Calcitriol	Formed from calcifediol in kidney. Most potent metabolite in regulating plasma $[Ca^{++}]$. Available for clinical use.
Dihydro-tachysterol	—	A crystalline compound prepared by reduction of vitamin D_2. Available for clinical use.
1α-hydroxy-cholecalciferol	Alfacalcidiol	A synthetic derivative of vitamin D_3 by hydroxylation.

terol in plants, and **cholecalciferol** (D_3) generated in the skin from 7-dehydrocholesterol by ultraviolet irradiation, the 7-dehydrocholesterol having been formed from cholesterol in the wall of the intestine (Table 16.8). The basic structure is outlined in Figure 16.24. Vitamin D_3 is converted to 25,hydroxyvitamin D_3 (**calcifediol**) in the liver, and this is converted to a series of other metabolites of varying activity in the kidney, the most potent of which is 1,25,dihydroxyvitamin D_4 (**calcitriol**) (see Fig. 16.24).

Calcifediol is the main metabolite found in the circulation and constitutes a storage form of the hormone. The synthesis of calcitriol from calcifediol is regulated by parathyroid hormone and is also influenced by the phosphate concentration in the plasma and by the calcitriol concentration itself through a negative feedback mechanism. The importance of this substance is evidenced by the fact that in experimental animals calcitriol, in physiological amounts, is able to regulate the plasma calcium concentration in the absence of the parathyroids and the kidneys, and the fact that receptors for it have been identified in almost every tissue examined except liver and skeletal muscle.

The main action of calcitriol is to stimulate the absorption of calcium and phosphate in the intestine and the mobilization of calcium from bone (Fig. 16.25). The effect on the intestine involves the binding of calcitriol to an intracellular receptor. The complex then interacts with the nucleus and results in the synthesis of carrier proteins which bind calcium and transport it across the membrane. Calcitriol also affects calcium absorption through another mechanism by which calcium flux is increased without increased protein synthesis. The absorption of phosphate appears to involve a separate transport system, and this is also increased by calcitriol, but the mechanism has not been clarified. Calcitriol can stimulate bone resorption on its own, as shown by *in vitro* studies, but *in vivo* it probably synergizes with parathormone. It decreases collagen synthesis by osteoblasts, and its effect on these cells is believed to be by the classical steroid pathway, involving intracellular receptors and an effect on the DNA. However, the effect on bone is a complex one; the action of vitamin D is clearly not confined only to mobilizing calcium, since in clinical vitamin D deficiency (see below) in which the

mineralization of bone is impaired, administration of vitamin D restores bone formation. Whether this is primarily an indirect effect of calcitriol due to increased calcium and phosphate absorption or a direct effect brought about by a vitamin D metabolite other than calcitriol is not clear. An explanation may lie in the fact that calcitriol has been shown to stimulate synthesis of osteocalcin, the vitamin K-dependent calcium-binding protein of bone matrix.

Calcitriol increases calcium reabsorption in the kidney tubules (see Fig. 16.25), though 25,hydroxyvitamin D_3 (calcifediol) may be more important for this action and may also be of more significance in the regulation of calcium flux, and thus contractility, in muscle.

Calcitriol stimulates phosphate reabsorption in the kidney but as mentioned above this effect is usually overriden by the contrary action of parathormone.

The vitamin D preparations available for clinical use are **calciferol**, **dihydrotachysterol**, **alfacalcidol** and **calcitriol** (Table 16.8). The latter three preparations are more expensive than calciferol and for most purposes offer little advantage over it. All can be given orally and are well absorbed from the intestine. Vitamin D is fat soluble and bile salts are necessary for absorption. Injectable forms of calciferol are available.

Pharmacokinetic aspects

Vitamin D is bound to a specific α-globulin in the blood and the plasma half-life is about 22 hours but it can be found in the tissues, particularly the fat depots, for many months. Enterohepatic recirculation of the vitamin occurs and the main route of elimination from the body is in the faeces.

Unwanted effects

Excessive intake of vitamin D causes hypercalcaemia, the manifestations of which are gastrointestinal disturbances, physical weakness and fatigue. Osteoporosis is likely to occur as a result of the mobilization of calcium from bone. Renal effects are also seen—proteinuria, and a reduced ability to concentrate the urine, resulting in polyuria and polydipsia. If the hypercalcaemia continues for a long period calcium salts may be deposited in the kidney and, in some cases, also in the skin, the vascular system, the heart and the lungs.

Some anticonvulsant drugs can interact with vitamin D, in that they decrease the sensitivity of the target organs (bone, intestine) to the hormones. Thus prolonged administration of phenytoin or phenobarbitone may cause rickets or osteomalacia.

Clinical use

Vitamin D is used to prevent and to treat various forms of rickets and osteomalacia, and also the hypocalcaemia associated with hypo-parathyroidism.

CALCITONIN

Calcitonin is a hormone secreted by the 'C' cells found in the thyroid gland. It is a single chain polypeptide of 3600 MW, containing 32 amino-acid residues and the entire peptide is necessary for its biological activity. It is derived from a precursor of 15 000 MW and there is considerable heterogeneity in the forms found in the plasma, which may represent linked oligomers.

The main action of calcitonin is to decrease the plasma calcium concentration by effects on kidney and on bone. Its action on the kidney is to decrease the reabsorption of both calcium and phosphate in the proximal tubules; the reabsorption of sodium potassium and magnesium is also reduced. Its principal action, however, is on bone where it in-hibits resorption by inhibiting the action of the osteoclasts and possibly enhancing that of the osteoblasts.

The main factor determining the secretion of calcitonin is the concentration of calcium in the plasma, but other factors may also play a part. Pentagastrin stimulates its secretion suggesting an inter-relationship between gastrin and calcitonin. Its plasma half-life is 4–12 minutes and its duration of action is short.

Calcitonin is available for clinical use, the prepar-ations being porcine (natural) **calcitonin** and **salca-tonin** (synthetic 'salmon' calcitonin). Synthetic human calcitonin is now also available. Porcine calcitonin may contain traces of thyroid and can

lead to the production of antibodies. It is given by subcutaneous or intramuscular injection, and there may be a local inflammatory action at the injection site. Nausea and vomiting may occur, as may facial flushing, an unpleasant taste in the mouth and a tingling sensation in the hands.

Clinical use

This drug is used to lower the plasma calcium in hypercalcaemia, for example that associated with neoplasia. It is also of value in Paget's disease of bone (a condition associated with excessive thick-ening and calcification), in which it not only relieves the pain but may reduce some of the neurological complications.

OTHER AGENTS USED IN DISORDERS OF CALCIUM AND PHOSPHATE METABOLISM

Several other substances may be of value in conditions of disturbed calcium and phosphate homeostasis. These include diphosphonates, mith-ramycin, glucocorticoids, oestrogens and cellulose phosphate.

Diphosphonates

Diphosphonates are related to pyrophosphate, the P-O-P structure of pyrophosphate being replaced by P-C-P. They are adsorbed on to the surface of hydroxyapatite crystals, slowing both further growth of these crystals and also their dissolution. They therefore reduce the turnover of bone.

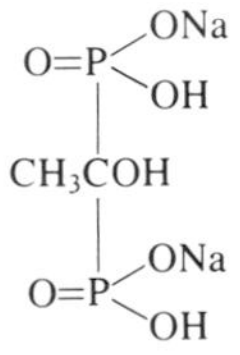

$$O=P \begin{array}{l} ONa \\ OH \end{array}$$
$$| $$
$$CH_3COH$$
$$| $$
$$O=P \begin{array}{l} ONa \\ OH \end{array}$$

Fig. 16.26 Disodium etidronate.

The main diphosphonate at present available for clinical use is **disodium etidronate** (Fig. 16.26). It is given orally, about 10% is absorbed and 50% of the absorbed drug accumulates in bone, the rest being excreted unchanged by the kidney. That portion of the drug which is taken up by bone remains for several weeks. Its effect in reducing bone turnover is of value in Paget's disease of bone, in which there are foci of increased bone turnover with alterations in its structure. Disodium etidronate also inhibits calcitriol production and has other effects on bone metabolism such as causing alterations in alkaline and acid phosphatase activities. A high dose may cause demineralization of bone and result in iatrogenic osteomalacia.

Mithramycin

Mithramycin is an antibiotic used in cancer chemotherapy which also inhibits resorption of bone. Its cytotoxic action is attributed to its binding to DNA and interrupting DNA-directed RNA and protein synthesis. It is believed to have a relatively specific action on osteoclasts and thus to block calcium mobilization from bone.

It is used in Paget's disease and hypocalcaemia and for these conditions can be used in doses one-tenth those required for cancer chemotherapy.

Glucocorticoids

It has been pointed out earlier in this chapter that

one of the unwanted effects of glucocorticoid therapy is osteoporosis. This is due partly to decreased intestinal absorption of calcium and phosphate associated with increased renal excretion, and partly to an inhibition of bone formation. This latter action is thought to be due to an inhibition of osteoblast precursors. These effects can be made use of in the therapy of some types of hypercalcaemia, particularly if associated with sarcoidosis.

Oestrogens

Oestrogens may have a place in the prevention of postmenopausal osteoporosis. They are thought to act by opposing the calcium-mobilizing, bone-resorbing effect of parathormone.

Sodium cellulose phosphate

This agent, given orally, binds calcium and reduces its absorption in the intestine, and can be used as an adjunct in the treatment of hypercalcaemia. An unwanted effect which may be associated with its use is an increase in plasma phosphate.

REFERENCES AND FURTHER READING

The pituitary
De Groot et al (eds) 1979 The pituitary gland and its hormones. In: Endocrinology, Vol 1, (8 Chapters by many authors). Grune & Stratton, New York
Jackson I M D 1982 Thyrotropin-releasing hormone. N Engl J Med 306: 145–155
Leong D A, Frawley S, Neill J D 1983 Neuroendocrine control of prolactin secretion. Ann Rev Physiol 45: 109–127
Ontjes D A, Walton J, New R L 1980 The anterior pituitary gland. In: Bondy P K, Rosenberg L E (eds) Metabolic control and disease. W B Saunders, Philadelphia 1165–1239
Page R B 1982 Pituitary blood flow. Am J Physiol 243: E427–442
Reichlin S 1983 Somatostatin. N Engl J Med 309: 1495–1501 & 1556–1563
Taylor A, Palmer L G 1982 Hormonal regulation of sodium chloride and water transport in epithelia. Biological Regulation and Development 3A: 253–298

The thyroid
De Groot L J 1979 Thyroid hormone action. In: De Groot et al (eds) Endocrinology, Vol 1. Grune & Stratton, New York, p 357–363
Dumont J E, Vassart G 1979 Thyroid gland metabolism and the action of TSH. In: De Groot et al (eds) Endocrinology, Vol 1. Grune & Stratton, New York, p 311–329
Marchant B, Lees J F H, Alexander W D 1978 Antithyroid drugs. Pharmac Ther 3: 305

Nunez J, Pommier J 1982 Formation of thyroid hormones. In: Munson P L et al (eds) Vitamins and hormones, Vol 39. Academic Press, New York, p 175–229
Ramsden D B, Hoffenberg R 1983 The actions of thyroid hormones mediated via the cell nucleus and their clinical significance. Clin Endocrinol Metab 12: 101–115

Pancreas and the control of blood glucose
Ensinck J W, Williams R H 1981 Disorders causing hypoglycaemia. In: Williams R H (ed) Endocrinology. W B Saunders, Philadelphia, Ch 16, p 844–875
Felig P 1981 The endocrine pancreas: diabetes mellitus. In: Felig P, Baxter J D, Broadus A E, Frohman L A (eds) Endocrinology & metabolism. McGraw Hill, New York, p 761–868
Harvey R F 1983 Choice of insulin. Brit Med J 287: 1571–1574
Houslay M D, Heyworth C M 1983 Insulin in search of a mechanism. Trends in Biochemical Science: 449–452
Jacobs S, Cuatrecasas P 1983 Insulin receptors. Ann Rev Pharmacol Toxicol 26: 461–479
Larner J 1983 Mediators of postreceptor action of insulin. Amer J Med 74: 38–51
Levine R 1982 Insulin: the effects and mode of action of the hormone. In: Munson P L, Diczfalusy E, Glover J, Olson R (eds) Vitamins & hormones. Academic Press, New York, 39, 145–173
MacPherson J N, Feely J 1983 Diabetes I: Insulins. Brit Med J 286: 1502–1504

Peden N, Newton R W, Feely J 1983 Oral hypoglycaemic
agents. Brit Med J 286: 1564–1567

Pfeifer M A, Halter J B, Porte D 1981 Insulin secretion in
diabetes mellitus. Am J Med 70: 579–588

Porte D, Halter J 1981 The endocrine pancreas and diabetes
mellitus. In: Williams R H (ed) Endocrinology. W B Saunders
& Co, Philadelphia, Ch 16, p 716–843

ACTH & adrenal corticosteroids

Baxter J D, Rousseau G G (eds) 1979 Glucocorticoid hormone
action. Monographs on Endocrinology 12

Fink G 1981 Has corticotropin-releasing factor finally been
found. Nature 294: 511–512

Flower R J, Dale M M 1987 The glucocorticoid steroids and
lipocortin. In: Dale M M, Foreman J C (eds) Textbook of immunopharmacology, 2nd ed. Blackwell Scientific Publications, London

Hirata F, Notsu Y, Iwata M, Parente L, di Rosa M, Flower R J
1982 Identification of several species of phospholipase inhibitory proteins by radioimmunoassay for lipomodulin. Biochem Biophys Res Comm 109: 223–230

Kelso A, Munch A 1984 Glucocorticoid inhibition of lymphokine secretion by alloreactive T lymphocyte clones. J Immunol 133: 784–791

Munck A, Guyre P M, Holbrook N J 1984 Physiological functions of glucocorticoids in stress and their relation to pharmacological actions. Endocr Rev 5: 25–44

Schleimier R P, Jacques A, Shin H S, Lichtenstein L M, Plaut M
1984 Inhibition of T cell-mediated cytotoxicity by anti-
inflammatory steroids. J Immunol 132: 266–271

Parathyroid hormone, vitamin D, and bone mineral homeostasis

Avioli L V, Haddad J G 1984 The vitamin D family revisited. N
Engl J Med 311: 47–49

Bikle D D 1981 The vitamin D endocrine system. Adv Intern
Med 27: 45–71

Fraser D R 1981 Biochemical and clinical aspects of vitamin D
function. Br Med Bull 37: 37–42

Habener J F 1981 Regulation of parathyroid hormone secretion
and biosynthesis. Ann Rev Physiol 43: 211–223

Norman A W, Roth J, Orci L 1982 The vitamin D endocrine
system: steroid metabolism, hormone receptors and biological response (calcium binding proteins). Endocr Rev 3:
331–366

Raisz L G, Kream B E 1983 Regulation of bone formation. N
Engl J Med 309: 29–35, 83–89

General reading

Greep R O 1984 Recent progress in hormones research: 40

Litwack G (ed) Biochemical actions of hormones, 1984 Vol 11,
1983 Vol 10, 1982 Vol 9

17

The reproductive system

ENDOCRINE ASPECTS

Hormonal control of the reproductive system in both male and female involves the sex steroids, the hypothalamic peptides and the glycoprotein gonadotrophins from the anterior pituitary.

HORMONAL CONTROL OF THE FEMALE REPRODUCTIVE SYSTEM

At puberty an increased output of the hormones of the hypothalamus and anterior pituitary stimulates secretion of oestrogenic sex steroids which are responsible for the maturation of the reproductive organs and the development of the secondary sexual characteristics, and also for a phase of accelerated growth followed by closure of the epiphyses of the long bones. These hormones are thereafter involved in the regulation of the cyclic changes expressed in the menstrual cycle and are important in pregnancy. A simplified outline of the complex inter-relationship of these substances in the physiological control of the menstrual cycle is given in Figures 17.1 and 17.2.

The **menstrual cycle** is taken as beginning with the start of menstruation. This lasts for 3–6 days during which the superficial layer of the endometrium of the uterus is shed. When the menstrual flow stops, the endometrium is regenerated. In the first phase of the cycle a **releasing factor, LH/FSH-RF**, secreted by the hypothalamus (see Chapter 16) stimulates the anterior pituitary to release gonadotrophic hormones, mainly **follicle stimulating hormone (FSH)**. This acts on the ovaries promoting the development of small groups of follicles each of which contains an ovum. One of these develops faster than the others and forms the **'Graafian follicle'** and the rest degenerate. Cells of

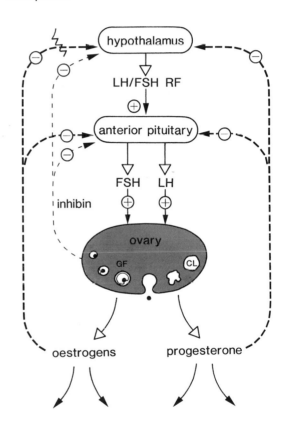

clomiphene

Fig. 17.1 Hormonal inter-relationship in the control of the female reproductive system.
————⊕———— indicates a positive effect; ---⊖--- indicates a negative effect
An open-headed arrow = releases
Arrow with closed head = acts on
GF = Graafian follicle; CL = corpus luteum;
LH = luteinizing hormone;
FSH = follicle stimulating hormone;
RF = releasing factor.

act on reproductive tract & other tissues

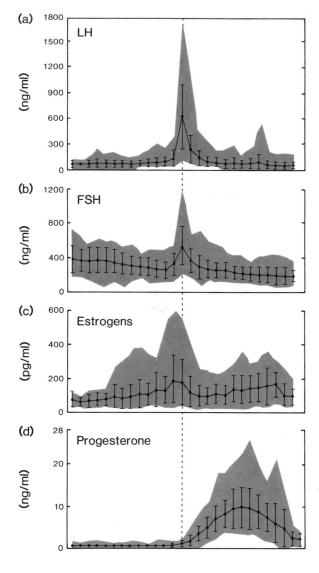

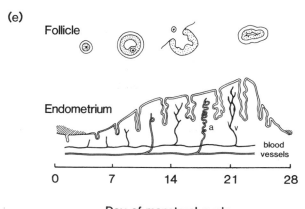

Day of menstrual cycle

the ripening Graafian follicle secrete **oestrogens** which are responsible for the early, *proliferative* phase of endometrial regeneration which occurs from day 5 or 6 until midcycle (see Fig. 17.2e). During this phase the endometrium increases in thickness and vascularity and at the peak of oestrogen secretion there is a prolific cervical secretion of mucous of pH 8–9, rich in protein and carbohydrate, which is thought to make the passage of sperm easier. The secreted oestrogens have a negative feedback effect on the anterior pituitary, decreasing FSH release. It is thought that, in addition, they sensitize LH-releasing cells of the pituitary to the action of the releasing factor and thus are instrumental in determining the midcycle surge of secretion of **luteinizing hormone (LH)** which causes rapid swelling and rupture of the main follicle, resulting in ovulation. If fertilization of the ovum by a spermatozoon occurs, the fertilized ovum passes down the Fallopian tubes to the uterus, starting to divide as it goes.

An important action of the oestrogens is to promote the formation of **progesterone** receptors in target tissues. They also have mild anabolic effects and tend to increase retention of salt and water.

There is some evidence that, in addition to its effect on oestrogen secretion, FSH stimulates the Graafian follicle to secrete **inhibin**, a peptide of molecular weight 20 000, which also has a negative feedback effect on FSH production.

Under the influence of luteinizing hormone (LH), the cells of the ruptured follicle proliferate and the follicle develops into the **'corpus luteum'** which secretes progesterone. During the second part of the menstrual cycle, this hormone acts on the oestrogen-primed endometrium stimulating the *secretory* phase of its regeneration which renders the endometrium suitable for the implantation of a fertilized ovum. At this stage the cervical mucus becomes more viscid, less alkaline, less copious and in general less welcoming for the sperm. Pro-

Fig. 17.2 Plasma concentrations of ovarian hormones and gonadotropins in women during normal menstrual cycles are given in (a)–(d). Values are the mean ± standard deviation of 40 women. The shaded areas indicate the entire range of observations. Day 1 is the onset of menstruation. Ovulation on day 14 of the menstrual cycle occurs with the midcycle peak of LH, represented by the dashed line. (e) shows diagrammatically the changes in the ovarian follicle and the endometrium during the cycle. (After: Van de Wiele & Dyrenfurth, 1974)

gesterone has a negative feedback effect on the hypothalamus and pituitary, decreasing the release of LH. It also has a **thermogenic** effect causing a slight rise in body temperature of about 0.5°C which commences at ovulation and is maintained until the end of the cycle. If implantation of the ovum does not occur, progesterone secretion stops and its sudden cessation is the main cause of the onset of menstruation. If implantation does occur and pregnancy results, the corpus luteum continues to secrete progesterone, which, by its effect on hypothalamus and anterior pituitary, prevents further ovulation. As pregnancy proceeds the placenta develops hormonal functions and secretes gonadotrophins, progesterone and oestrogens. Progesterone secreted during pregnancy controls the development of the secretory alveoli in the mammary gland while oestrogen stimulates the lactiferous ducts. After parturition, oestrogens, along with prolactin (see Chapter 16), are responsible for stimulating and maintaining lactation, though high doses of exogenous oestrogen will inhibit it.

THE BEHAVIOURAL EFFECTS OF SEX HORMONES

As well as exerting a cyclical control over the menstrual cycle, sex steroids affect sexual behaviour. Two types of control are recognized, namely *organizational* and *activational*. The former refers to the fact the sexual differentiation of the brain can be permanently altered by the presence or absence of sex steroids at a key stage in development. In rats, administration of androgens to females within a few days of birth modifies their development, resulting in virilization of behaviour. Conversely, neonatal castration of male rats causes them to develop behaviourally as females. It is believed (Larsson & Beyer, 1981) that brain development in the absence of sex steroids follows female lines, but that it can be switched to the male pattern by exposure of the hypothalamic cells to androgen at a key stage of development (Harris, 1964). In rats this sensitive phase extends for a few days either side of birth, but in guinea pigs it occurs earlier in foetal development. In primates, similar but less complete behavioural virilization of female offspring has been demonstrated following administration of testosterone to the pregnant mothers. This probably happens in humans also, if pregnant women secrete, or are treated with, androgens. One cause of concern has been the fact that certain types of oral contraceptive pill (see below) contained progestogens which are metabolized to androgens; it was felt that if a woman became pregnant during a gap in pill-taking, and then resumed taking the pill, this could affect foetal sex development. Progestogens that are metabolized in this way are no longer included in oral contraceptives.

The *activational* effect of sex steroids refers to their ability to modify sexual behaviour after brain development is complete. In general, oestrogens and androgens increase sexual activity in the appropriate sex. If given to animals of the inappropriate sex, they do not affect sexual behaviour markedly.

OESTROGENS

These hormones are synthesized mainly by the ovary, the stimulus being FSH, for which cAMP is a second messenger. Oestrogens are also synthesized in large amounts by the placenta, and in small amounts by the testis in males and by the adrenal cortex in both sexes. Some other tissues, such as liver, muscle, fat and hair follicles, can also convert steroid precursors into oestrogens.

The starting substance for oestrogen synthesis is cholesterol (see Fig. 16.21). The immediate precursors to the oestrogens are androgenic substances—androstenedione or testosterone—and the significant reaction is aromatization of ring A of the steroid molecule.

There are three main endogenous oestrogens in humans—**oestradiol**, **oestrone** and **oestriol** (Fig. 17.3). Oestradiol is the most potent and is the principal oestrogen secreted by the ovary. At the beginning of the menstrual cycle, the plasma concentration is 50 pg/ml (0.2 nM) rising to 350–850 pg/ml (1.3–3.1 nM) in midcycle (see Fig. 17.2c). In the liver, oestradiol is converted to oestrone which may be converted to oestriol (Fig. 17.3). Oestradiol and oestrone are the two main endogenous oestrogens and exist in equilibrium with each other in a ratio of 1:2–1:4. Oestrone may be sulphated in the liver and the **oestrone sulphate** so formed can be converted back to oestrone by sulphatases. Oestrone sulphate is in equilibrium with

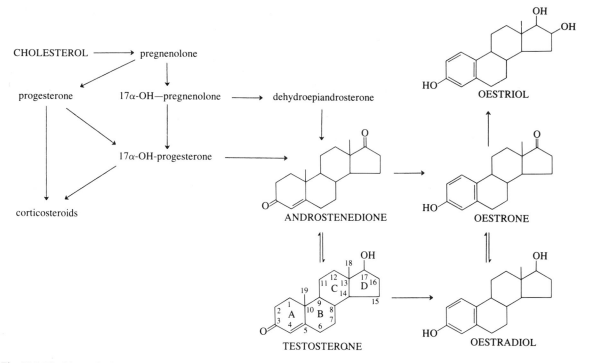

Fig. 17.3 The biosynthetic pathway for the oestrogens. (See also Fig. 16.21)

oestrone and thus with oestradiol, and it has been suggested that it constitutes a storage form of the hormones.

Oestriol is sometimes referred to as an 'impeded' oestrogen. It is regarded as a partial agonist, i.e. an oestrogen of low potency which competes with oestradiol and reduces its effect. However, the true situation is probably that it is short-acting (see below) and if its concentration in the plasma is maintained (as under physiological conditions) it is as potent as oestradiol.

Pharmacological actions

The pharmacological actions of exogenous oestrogens are in essence the same as the physiological actions of endogenous hormones, especially if they are given as replacement therapy in hypo-ovarian conditions. Their effects as drugs will depend on the age at which they are administered. Given at age 11–13 (with progestogens) for primary hypogonadism, oestrogens stimulate the development of the secondary sexual characteristics and the phase of accelerated growth. In the adult with primary amenorrhea, oestrogens, given cyclically with a progestogen, will induce an artificial cycle. Their main use in adult women however is for oral contraception and their pharmacological actions when thus used are described below. They may also be used in the post-menopausal period and here again their actions are in general similar to their physiological effects. They reduce menopausal symptoms associated with the decline in oestrogen production—hot flushes, inappropriate sweating, paraesthesias, palpitations, atrophic vaginitis, etc. They are also believed to decrease post-menopausal osteoporosis, by decreasing the loss from bone of calcium phosphate complexes and protein matrix. The osteoporosis may be partly due to the loss of the physiological effect of oestrogen in antagonizing parathormone and thus decreasing bone resorption (see Chapter 16).

These agents have several metabolic actions which may become manifest when they are used as drugs. They cause some degree of retention of salt and water, as occurs with endogenous oestrogens in the latter half of the menstrual cycle. However, when used as drugs they rarely cause oedema as such unless given in large doses, although they may accentuate oedema due to other causes such as cardiac failure or kidney disease. They have mild anabolic actions.

Oestrogens increase the coagulability of the blood. The exact reason for this action is not clear. Increases in the plasma concentration of various clotting factors (II, VII, IX & X) occur (p. 281) as does an increase in platelet aggregation. The antithrombin III concentration is decreased and there are changes in the fibrinolytic system. This increase in coagulability is the basis for the increased risk of thrombo-embolism which occurs with contraceptive pills containing a high oestrogen content. This is discussed below.

Although plasma glucose concentrations under fasting conditions are normal, an impairment in glucose tolerance may occur in some individuals. The concentration of serum triglycerides and of low density lipoproteins is raised; that of high density lipoproteins is decreased.

Mechanism of action

As with other steroids, the action of oestrogen involves its binding to intracellular receptors, the interaction of the resultant complexes with nuclear sites and subsequent DNA-directed RNA and protein synthesis (see Chapters 1 & 16). Most of the information on how oestrogen acts derives from experimental work with mouse or rat uterus or chick oviduct.

Oestrogen receptors occur mainly in cells of its principal target tissues: the reproductive system (uterus, vagina, mammary glands) and the anterior pituitary and hypothalamus. These tissues contain about 15 000–20 000 high affinity oestrogen binding sites per cell (Kd ~ 0.6 nM), but smaller numbers of sites also occur in the liver, kidney, adrenal and ovary.

In the absence of hormone, the oestrogen receptor, which is a 4S protein (M_r 75 000), is associated with an inhibitory macromolecule. Activation by the hormone involves dissociation of the receptor from this molecule and the conversion of the 4S protein to a 5S protein (M_r 140 000) by dimerization or by association with another protein. This 5S protein has a high affinity for nuclear sites and it is

probable that one portion of the dimer contains a site for interaction with DNA while the other interacts with chromatin protein.

In considering the relationship between the binding of the steroid/receptor complexes in the nucleus and the magnitude of the subsequent response, a distinction has to be made between *short-term* and *long-term* effects. Short-term responses are taken as those which occur within the first 6 hours, such as an increase in uterine fluid and early RNA and protein synthesis. Long-term responses include the late increases in RNA synthesis, DNA synthesis, an increase in uterine weight and, in the case of immature animals, actual growth of the uterus. The early responses are a necessary but not sufficient preliminary for the late effects. For many responses, particularly short-term ones, there is a linear relationship between the nuclear binding of the complexes and the magnitude of the effect. In the case of some long-term effects the situation is more complex in that it is not only the degree of binding which is important but the maintenance of the complexes in the nucleus for critical periods of time. Full uterine growth can be produced by the binding of the hormone-receptor complex to only 20% of the nuclear sites, if maintained for a sufficient length of time, although this degree of binding does not stimulate maximally the early responses. The significance of the duration of nuclear binding is exemplified by experimental data obtained with oestriol. This oestrogen, which was found experimentally to be of very low potency on long-term responses when compared to oestradiol, was as effective as oestradiol in producing early responses. The explanation for its lack of effect on long-term responses is that, under the experimental conditions used, oestriol complexes are not retained in the nucleus. Oestriol can, however, be made as effective as oestradiol on the late responses if its concentration in the plasma is maintained at high levels for long periods, or if it is injected repeatedly. Similar temporal factors are of importance in the effects of oestrogens on the hypothalamus and pituitary.

The fate of the receptors after interaction in the nucleus is not yet clear. In the presence of inhibitors of RNA and protein synthesis, 60% of the receptors seem to disappear after their interaction with oestrogens, which indicates a requirement for de novo synthesis. The remaining 40% appear to be recycled.

Table 17.1 Oestrogens

Drug	Formula	Comment
Oestradiol		A natural oestrogen. Usually given i.m. Long-acting preparations are available. Oestradiol valerate is active by mouth.
Oestriol		A natural oestrogen. Can be given orally.
Oestrone		Given orally as piperazine oestrone sulphate. Oestrone sulphate is the main ingredient of an oral preparation of equine oestrogens.
Ethinyloestradiol		Semi-synthetic. Given orally. Effective and cheap. The drug of choice.
Mestranol		Synthetic. Used in many oral contraceptive preparations. Converted to ethinyloestradiol in the body.
Chlorotrianisene		Given orally. Taken up in fat depots from which it is slowly released. Converted into a more active compound in the body.
Stilboestrol		Orally active. Depot preparations are available. Its use during pregnancy has been associated with an increase in genital tract cancer in female offspring of the pregnancy when they reach maturity. Not much used now except in therapy of cancer. (R = C_2H_5)

The number of oestrogen receptors in the cells of target tissues is affected by other hormones. Progesterone decreases oestrogen receptor levels in the reproductive tract even in the presence of continuously high plasma oestrogen concentrations, the effect being produced by interference with the de novo synthesis of the receptors. Prolactin, on the other hand, increases the numbers of oestrogen receptors in the mammary gland and liver but has no effect on those in the uterus.

One of the principal effects of the oestrogens on DNA is the induction of synthesis of progesterone receptors in target tissues such as uterus, vagina, anterior pituitary and hypothalamus.

Preparations

Many preparations of oestrogens are available. Some of the more commonly used ones are listed in Table 17.1. Others are **quinestradol** (which has low potency), **hexoestrol**, **dienoestrol**, **quinestrol** and **methallenoestril**.

Pharmacokinetic aspects

Both the natural and synthetic oestrogens used in therapy, are well absorbed in the gastrointestinal tract, but after absorption the natural oestrogens are rapidly metabolized in the liver. The synthetic oestrogens and non-steroidal oestrogen-like compounds are less rapidly degraded. Most oestrogens are readily absorbed from skin and mucous membranes. They may be given topically in the vagina as creams or pessaries for local effect, but will also be absorbed into the circulation from these sites. In the plasma, natural oestrogens are bound to albumin and to a sex steroid-binding globulin. Natural oestrogens are excreted in the urine as glucuronides and sulphates.

Uses

Oestrogens may be used for:

1. Replacement therapy, as in hypo-ovarian conditions, or to treat post-menopausal symptoms
2. Contraception (see below)
3. Therapy of prostatic and breast cancer (see Chapter 29)
4. Menstrual disorders
5. Acne.

Unwanted effects

These include tenderness in the breasts, nausea, vomiting, anorexia, thrombo-embolism, alteration of carbohydrate metabolism (see below) and retention of salt and water with resultant oedema.

Long-term administration in post-menopausal women also increases the risk of gall bladder disease and endometrial carcinoma. When administered to males, oestrogens result in feminization.

Oestrogens should not be given to pregnant women especially during the first few months of pregnancy when development of the reproductive organs of the foetus is occurring. There is clear evidence that carcinoma of the vagina and the cervix may occur in young women whose mothers were given the synthetic oestrogen preparation, stilboestrol, in early pregnancy. Whether this particular effect occurs with other oestrogen preparations is not known, but an increased incidence of genital abnormalities in both male and female progeny has been reported.

ANTI-OESTROGENS

These are substances which are inactive or weakly active themselves, but which compete with natural oestrogens for binding sites in target organs (Fig. 17.4).

Tamoxifen is an anti-oestrogen which is used mainly in the treatment of oestrogen-dependent breast cancer (see Chapter 29). It produces the same side effects as the oestrogens themselves but they are less marked. This drug binds to the oestrogen receptor in the nucleus but there is little or no stimulation of transcription, possibly because the complex binds to a different nuclear acceptor site. Moreover, the complex does not readily dissociate, so there is interference with the recycling of receptors. **Clomiphene** (see Fig. 17.1) and **cyclofenil** inhibit oestrogen binding in the hypothalamus and anterior pituitary, so preventing the normal feedback inhibition and causing increased secretion of the releasing-hormone and of gonadotrophins. This results in a marked stimulation and enlargement of the ovaries and increased oestrogen secretion. The main effect of their anti-oestrogen action is that they *induce ovulation*. These compounds are used in treating infertility due to lack of ovulation. Multiple pregnancies may occur.

PROGESTOGENS

The natural progestational hormone or progestogen is **progesterone** (see Fig. 17.1) which is secreted mainly by the *corpus luteum* in the second part of the menstrual cycle. Small amounts are also secreted by the testis in the male and the adrenal cortex in both sexes and large amounts are secreted by the placenta.

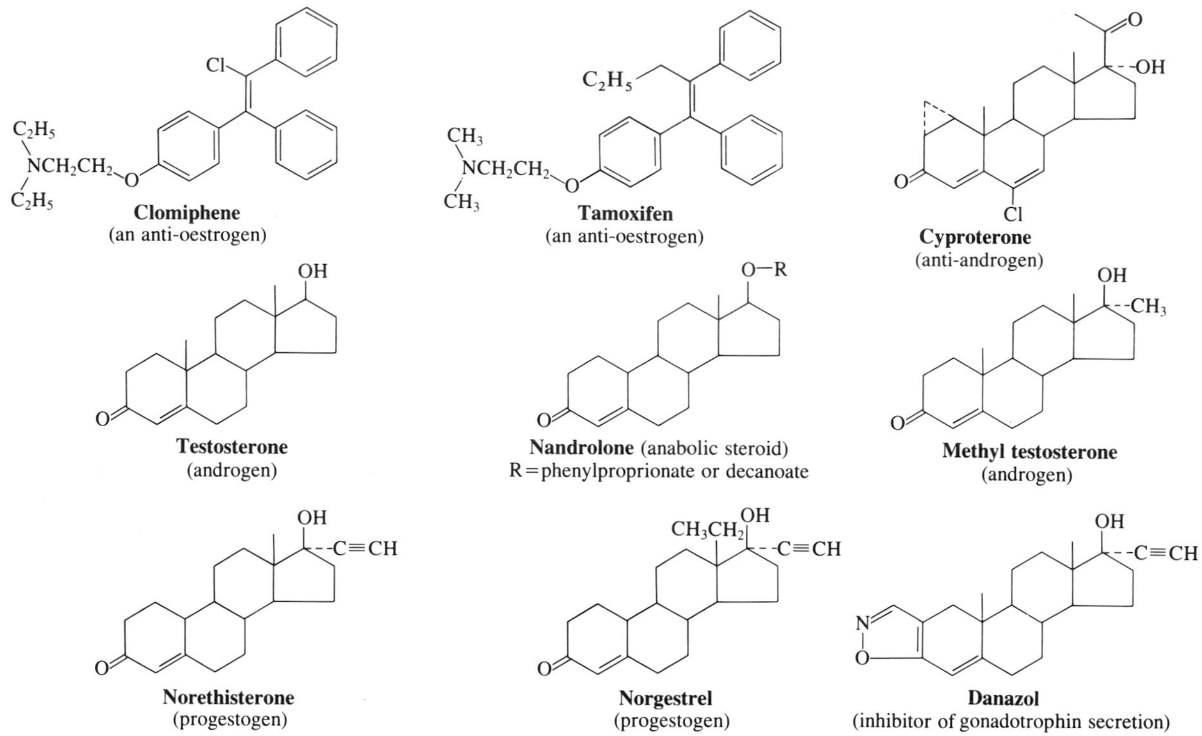

Fig. 17.4 Structures of various sex steroids and related compounds.

Mechanism of action

This is similar to that of other steroids, involving binding to specific receptors with subsequent DNA-directed RNA and protein synthesis (see above). The presence of adequate numbers of progesterone receptors depends on the prior action of oestrogens (see above). Progesterone administration results in a decrease of both oestrogen and progesterone receptors in the reproductive tract.

Preparations

There are two main groups of progestogens:

1. The naturally occurring hormone and its derivatives (see Figs. 16.21 & 17.4). **Progesterone** itself is virtually inactive orally because after absorption it is metabolized in the liver. Preparations are available for intramuscular injection and for topical use in the vagina and rectum. Hydroxyprogesterone is an intermediate in the pathway of synthesis of hydrocortisone and testosterone (see Fig. 16.21) and has progesterone-like activity. It is given as **hydroxyprogesterone hexanoate**—the esterification

at C_{17} inhibiting its further enzymic conversion—and is administered by intramuscular injection. **Medroxyprogesterone** can be given orally or by injection. **Dydrogesterone**, which is given orally, has only the peripheral actions of progesterone and does not have an inhibitory action on gonadotrophin release.

2. Testosterone derivatives. **Ethisterone, norethisterone, lynoestrol, norgestrel, ethynodiol, allyloestrenol** and **dimethisterone** are all derivatives of testosterone with progesterone-like activity and all can be given orally. The first three all have some androgenic activity and are metabolized to give oestrogenic products.

Pharmacological actions

These are in essence the same as the physiological actions. Specific effects relevant to contraception are detailed below.

Pharmacokinetic aspects

Injected progesterone has a very short half-life of

about 15 minutes. In the plasma it is bound to albumin, not to the sex steroid-binding globulin. Some is stored in adipose tissue. It is metabolized in the liver, and the products, **pregnanolone** and **pregnanediol**, are conjugated with glucuronic acid and excreted in the urine.

Unwanted effects

Some of the progestogens which are derived from testosterone have weak androgenic actions.

Uses

The main use of progestogens is in contraception (see below). They have an ill-defined place in the therapy of various gynaecological conditions such as menstrual disorders, endometriosis and dysmenorrhea. They are also used in the treatment of endometrial carcinoma, and, in conjunction with oestrogen, for hormone replacement therapy.

ANTI-PROGESTOGENS

A recent development has been the synthesis of compounds which bind avidly to progesterone receptors but which do not have progestogen-like activity. They have been tested as abortifacients, but used on their own have not proved to have any specific advantage over vacuum aspiration or the use of prostaglandin analogues (p. 431) in termination of early pregnancy. However, combination of an anti-progestogen agent with the prostaglandin, sulprostone, has proved to be very effective in early trials.

The anti-progestogens presently available for trial also have a significant antagonist action at the glucocorticoid receptor, though in higher concentration. Attempts are being made to develop agents with more selectivity.

HORMONAL CONTROL OF THE MALE REPRODUCTIVE SYSTEM

As in the female, endocrine secretions from the hypothalamus, anterior pituitary and gonads control the male reproductive system. A simplified outline of the interrelationships of these factors is given

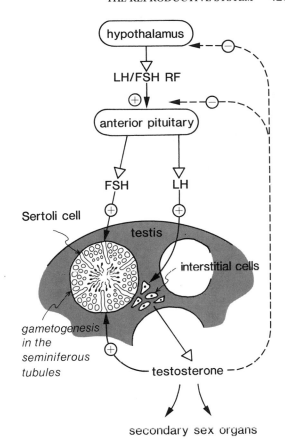

Fig. 17.5 Hormonal inter-relationships in the control of the male reproductive system.
———⊕——— indicates a positive, stimulant effect
– – –⊖– – – indicates an inhibitory effect
An open-headed arrow = releases
Arrow with closed head = acts on

in Figure 17.5. LH/FSH-releasing hormone controls the secretion of gonadotrophins by the anterior pituitary. This secretion is not cyclical as in the female but constant, though in both sexes it is pulsatile (see below). FSH is responsible for the integrity of the seminiferous tubules and, after puberty, is important in gametogenesis through an action on the Sertoli cells which nourish and support the developing spermatozoa. LH, which in the male is also called '**interstitial cell stimulating hormone**' (**ICSH**) stimulates the interstitial cells (Leydig cells) to secrete androgens—in particular **testosterone**. The secretion of LH begins at puberty and the testosterone secreted is responsible for the maturation of the reproductive organs and the development of the secondary sexual characteristics.

Thereafter the primary function of testosterone is the maintenance of spermatogenesis and hence fertility—an action mediated by the Sertoli cells. This steroid is also important in the maturation of the spermatozoa as they pass through the epididymis and vas deferens. A further action is a feedback effect on the anterior pituitary, modulating its sensitivity to LH/FSH releasing hormone and thus influencing the concentration of LH in the circulation. In addition it has marked anabolic effects causing development of the musculature and increased bone growth resulting in a rapid increase in height. This is followed by closure of the epiphyses of the long bones.

Though the secretion of testosterone is controlled largely by LH, FSH may play a part, possibly by inducing the release from the Sertoli cells (which are its primary target) of a factor similar to LH/FSH-releasing hormone. The interstitial cells which synthesize testosterone also have receptors for **prolactin** and this substance may influence testosterone production by increasing the number of receptors for LH.

ANDROGENS

Testosterone is the main natural androgen and it is synthesized not only by the interstitial cells of the testis in males, but in small amounts by the ovary in females and the adrenal cortex in both sexes. Adrenal production of androgens is under the control of corticotrophin. Cholesterol is the starting substance (see Fig. 16.21) and an increase in cAMP is involved. Precursor substances are dehydroepiandrosterone and androstenedione, which may be released from the gonads and the adrenal cortex in both sexes and subsequently converted to testosterone in the liver. (see Fig. 17.3).

Pharmacological actions

In general the effect of exogenous androgens are the same as those of the endogenous hormones and will depend on the age of the patient to whom they are given.

If administered to males at the age of puberty, there is rapid development of the secondary sexual characteristics, and maturation of the reproductive organs. A marked increase in muscular strength occurs fairly soon (within days). Height increases more gradually. The anabolic effects may be accompanied by retention of salt and water. The skin becomes thickened and may darken and the sebaceous glands become more active (which may result in acne). There is growth of hair on the pubic and axillary regions and on the face. The vocal cords hypertrophy resulting in a lower pitch to the voice. Androgens cause a feeling of well-being and an increase in physical vigour and may increase libido. Whether they are responsible for sexual behaviour as such is controversial as is their contribution to aggressive behaviour.

If given to prepubertal males, the individuals concerned may not reach their full height because of premature closure of the epiphyses of the long bones.

Administration to women results in masculinization changes similar to those seen in the pubertal male. The initial effects will be on the skin (acne and growth of facial hair) and the voice. These are reversible. If treatment is continued there is development of the musculature and of the male pattern of baldness, hypertrophy of the clitoris and further deepening of the pitch of the voice. With long continued administration many of the effects are irreversible.

Mechanism of action

Testosterone is converted to dihydrotestosterone in most target cells, though in skeletal muscle, bone marrow and some other tissues, other metabolites are probably involved in the ultimate action of the steroid. In the hypothalamus it may be converted to an oestrogen. Its action requires DNA-directed synthesis of RNA and protein (see Chapters 1 & 16 and the discussion of oestrogens above).

Preparations

Testosterone is rapidly metabolized in the liver if given orally, though this does not happen if it is absorbed from the buccal mucosa or from rectal suppositories. It can be given by subcutaneous implantation. Testosterone propionate and testosterone enanthate are given by intramuscular depot injection.

Methyltestosterone (Fig. 17.4) may be given

sublingually. It is more resistant to metabolism than testosterone. **Fluoxymesterone** is active by mouth and is fairly potent.

Other androgens which are active when given orally are **mesterolone** and **stanolone**.

Pharmacokinetic aspects

Virtually all testosterone in the circulation is bound to plasma protein—mainly to the sex steroid-binding globulin though small amounts are bound to albumin and to the sex steroid-binding globulin. The half-life of free testosterone is 10–20 minutes. It is inactivated in the liver by conversion to androstenedione which has weak androgenic activity (see Fig. 17.3) and 90% of its metabolites are excreted in the urine. Synthetic androgens are less rapidly metabolized and some are excreted in the urine unchanged.

Uses

1. For replacement therapy in testicular failure. This condition may occur in hypogonadism and in hypopituitarism. In the latter condition growth hormone therapy is used until puberty, when androgens may be added to the treatment regime.
2. In the treatment of refractory anaemias of various aetiologies. Androgens are reported to be fairly efficient, non-specific stimulants of erythropoiesis.
3. As anabolic agents: see below.
4. In the treatment of mammary carcinoma in women. When receptors for oestrogens or progestogens are present in the cancer cells the modification of the hormonal environment by the use of androgens may result in regression of the tumour (see Chapter 29).

Unwanted effects

These include liver damage (which is more likely to occur with methyltestosterone and fluoxymesterone than with testosterone), eventual decrease of gonadotrophin release with resultant infertility, and salt and water retention leading to oedema. In children the androgens cause disturbances in growth and in females, acne and masculinization.

ANABOLIC STEROIDS

It is possible to modify the structure of androgens so as to enhance the anabolic effects and decrease the other effects. Many have been produced and one example, **nandrolone**, is given in Figure 17.4. Others are **ethyloestrenol, oxymetholone and stanozolol**. They are believed to increase protein synthesis and enhance muscle development, resulting in weight gain. They have a place in the treatment of debilitating and wasting conditions and in terminal disease, in which they may improve appetite and promote a welcome feeling of well-being. They increase healing of fractures and wounds and can be employed in the treatment of osteoporosis. They are used in some cases of hormone-dependent metastatic mammary cancer. The rationale for this use is explained above.

Side effects may occur, in particular cholestatic jaundice.

These agents are used, illegally, by some athletes to increase muscle bulk.

ANTI-ANDROGENS

Both oestrogens and progestogens have anti-androgen activity, oestrogens mainly by inhibiting gonadotrophin secretion and progestogens by competing with androgen receptors in target organs. This latter effect has been the basis for the development of more specific and more potent anti-androgen agents:

Cyproterone. This is a derivative of progesterone (see Fig. 17.4) and has weak progestational activity. It is a partial agonist on androgen receptors, competing with dihydrotestosterone for receptors in androgen-sensitive target tissues. Through its effect in the hypothalamus it depresses the synthesis of gonadotrophins. It seems also to have an effect in the central nervous system, decreasing libido.

It has been effective in treating precocious puberty, masculinization in females and prostatic carcinoma. It has been proposed for use in the treatment of male sexual offenders.

Anti-androgens are under investigation for their possible usefulness as oral contraceptives for males.

GONADOTROPHIN-RELEASING HORMONE

It was originally thought that there were two hypothalamic releasing hormones—one for FSH and one for LH—but a decapeptide which has both activities has been isolated and has since been synthesized. It is referred to as the **LH/FSH-releasing hormone (LH/FSH, RH)** or as **gonadorelin** and its amino-acid sequence is pyroglu-his-trp-ser-tyr-gly-leu-arg-pro-gly-NH_2. Physiologically, its secretion is controlled by neural input from higher centres and, in the female particularly, through negative feedback by the sex steroids.

Binding sites for the sex steroids occur in the relevant cells in the hypothalamus. Exogenous androgens, oestrogens and progestogens all inhibit the secretion of the peptide but only the progestogens when given on their own seem to have this effect without having marked hormonal actions on peripheral tissues. This is presumably because in the absence of oestrogen there is less induction of progesterone receptors in the reproductive tract.

Clinical use

Gonadorelin may be used in the female to induce ovulation. It is very potent, a dose of 10–100 µg producing a very marked increase of gonadotrophin concentration in the plasma. Administration needs to be *pulsatile* to be effective in stimulating ovulation. Continuous infusion has the opposite effect, of desensitizing the pituitary, and has been used in the treatment of precocious puberty. Long-acting analogues of gonadotrophin-releasing hormone similarly cause desensitization and are being tested in the management of sex hormone-dependent cancers and some analogues, given by intranasal spray, are being tested for contraceptive activity in both males and females.

GONADOTROPHINS

These hormones are produced in moderate amounts by the anterior pituitary (see Chapter 16 & Table 16.1) in both males and females and in large amounts by the placenta during pregnancy in the female. They are glycoproteins with two different subunits, designated α and β. Biological specificity depends on the β subunit, the α subunit being virtually identical in all the gonadotrophins and also nearly identical with the α subunit of thyrotrophin (see Chapter 16). There are similarities between the β subunits, the first 115 residues being about 80% homologous. The glycoproteins differ, however, in their carbohydrate content.

Preparations

These hormones have to be extracted from biological tissues and standardized by bioassay. **Human chorionic gonadotrophin (HCG)**, a glycoprotein with a molecular weight of 30 000 is prepared from the urine of pregnant women. It has mainly LH activity. **Menotrophin** is a preparation of gonadotrophins extracted from the urine of post-menopausal women. It consists largely of a degraded product of FSH with a molecular weight of 17 000 (FSH itself has a MW of 32 000), but it has some LH activity as well.

Pharmacokinetic aspects

These agents have to be given by injection. Their degradation occurs in two phases with distinct half-lives which are, for example, 11 hours and 23 hours for chorionic gonadotrophin.

Clinical use

In females the gonadotrophins are used primarily to treat infertility due to lack of ovulation. In males they are used for some types of failure of spermatogenesis and for some cases of failure of development of the testis.

MISCELLANEOUS DRUGS AFFECTING THE REPRODUCTIVE SYSTEM

Danazol

Most of the sex steroids inhibit gonadotrophin secretion, but a fairly selective action has been produced by modifying the structure of the progestogen, ethisterone, to produce **danazol** (see Fig. 17.4). This is effective in inhibiting the output of gonadotrophins, affecting particularly the midcycle surge in the female. It is also active in males, reducing spermatogenesis. It inhibits the synthesis of sex steroids and binds competitively to sex steroid receptors, manifesting anti-oestrogen, anabolic and weak androgenic activity.

It is useful in various conditions in which decreased sex hormone production would be beneficial: gynaecomastia in men and endometriosis, menorrhagia and cystic disease of the breast in women. Unexpectedly, recent studies report efficacy in idiopathic thrombocytopoenic purpura, in which glucocorticoids and other therapies had proved ineffective, as well as in classic haemophilia and hereditary angioneurotic oedema. The mechanism of action of danazol in these conditions is not obvious.

Bromocriptine

This is an ergot alkaloid which acts as a dopamine agonist (p. 365 & Chapter 19). It inhibits both basal and stimulated prolactin secretion from the pituitary and is the most effective agent available for inhibiting lactation being able, unlike oestrogens, to suppress established lactation.

DRUGS USED FOR CONTRACEPTION

Oral contraceptives

There are two main types of preparations taken orally on a regular basis to prevent conception.

Combinations of an oestrogen with a progestogen. The oestrogen in most combined preparations is **ethinyloestradiol** though a few preparations contain **mestranol** instead. The progestogen may be **norethisterone**, **levonorgestrel** or **norgestrel**. This combined pill is taken for 21 consecutive days followed by 7 pill-free days. The mode of action is thought to be as follows: the oestrogen inhibits the release of FSH and thus suppresses the development of the ovarian follicle; the progestogen inhibits the release of LH and thus prevents ovulation and it also makes the cervical mucus less suitable for the passage of sperm; together they alter the endometrium in such a way as to discourage implantation. They may also interfere with the coordinated contractions of cervix, uterus and Fallopian tubes which are thought to be necessary for successful fertilization and implantation.

When administration ceases after 21 days it is the withdrawal of the progestogen which precipitates menstruation.

This form of oral contraception is the most effective available, but there are drawbacks (see below).

Progestogen alone. The drugs used are **norethisterone**, **norgestrel**, **megestrol** or **ethynodiol**. They are taken daily without interruption. Their mode of action is primarily on the cervical mucus which is made inhospitable to sperm. They probably also hinder implantation through their effect on the endometrium and on the motility and secretions in the Fallopian tubes. Inhibition of ovulation is variable and inconsistent. Their contraceptive effect is less reliable than that of the combination pill and missing a dose may result in conception. There is liable to be break-through bleeding.

An advantage is that they can be taken after parturition as, unlike oestrogen-containing pills, they do not interfere with lactation.

Unwanted effects

These are more pronounced with the combined pill.

1. The possibility of increased risk of thromboembolism. This is related to the increased coagulability of the blood described above and the main manifestation is deep vein thrombosis which may result in pulmonary embolism. The incidence is said to be 3 per 1000 woman years (as compared to 1 per 1000 woman years in individuals *not* taking oral contraceptives). There is also reported to be a slightly increased risk of cerebrovascular disease and myocardial infarction. The alteration in the concentrations of low density and high density lipoproteins described above are thought to contribute to the increased risk of these latter two conditions. The risk of thrombo-embolism is due to the oestrogen content in the combined pill and is only significant if the dosage is high (e.g. above 50 µg for ethinyloestradiol or 100 µg for mestranol). With low oestrogen dosage the risk is small and is confined to specific subgroups in whom other factors contribute, such as smoking and long-continued use of the pill, especially in women over 35 years.

2. An impairment of glucose tolerance which may precipitate diabetes in a small number of individuals. Such individuals may have had preclinical diabetes.

3. A slight increase in the risk of cervical cancer from 1 in 1000 woman years to 2 in 1000 woman years.

4. Gain in weight due to fluid retention or an anabolic effect or both. The anabolic effect is seen particularly with progestogens derived from testosterone.

5. Impairment of liver function, sometimes with mild jaundice in some individuals who may have a genetic predisposition for this effect. It appears to be related mainly to the progestogen component and is associated with bile thrombi in the bile canaliculi. There is said to be an increased risk of benign liver tumours.

6. The occurrence, in some individuals, of general symptoms such as nausea, flushing, dizziness, depression or irritability.

7. Skin changes: an increase in pigmentation may occur and may be troublesome in dark skinned individuals. Acne and hirsutism is reported and are more likely to occur with preparations containing progestogens derived from testosterone.

8. Infections in the vagina. These have a higher incidence in individuals taking oral contraceptives.

9. An increase in blood pressure may occur. This is normally minimal, but may be fairly marked in some individuals.

Beneficial effects

These include less risk of rheumatoid arthritis, thyroid disease, cancer of the ovaries, and iron deficiency anaemia. In general oral contraceptives with low oestrogen content appear to be an effective form of contraception and are reasonably safe in young women who do not smoke.

Post-coital oral contraceptives

Various regimes have been tried. One which has been reported to be safe and effective is the use of an oestrogen-progestogen combination in 2 doses, 90 mins apart, with the total oestrogen content being equivalent to 6 low-dose combined pills. Nausea occurs in 50–60% of those treated and vomiting in 30%. To be effective, treatment must be instituted within 72 hours of unprotected intercourse.

Contraception with depot progestogen

Medroxyprogesterone can be given intramuscularly as a contraceptive—50 mg a month, or 150 mg every 3 months. This is effective, and medical opinion is that it has no significant dangers. However, menstrual irregularities are very common, and infertility may persist for many months after cessation of treatment.

Oral contraceptives for males are still in the experimental stage.

THE UTERUS

The physiological and pharmacological responses of the uterus vary in different species. In animals, the physiological activity shows cyclical changes which are different in dioestrus and oestrus. Profound changes occur during pregnancy in that both the weight and the volume of the uterus are increased. Thus the human uterus enlarges so that its capacity increases from about 5 ml to 5000 ml and its weight from 50 g to 1 kg, while the individual muscle fibres increase about ten-fold in length. Along with these changes are alterations in the response to pharmacological agents. After parturition the uterus undergoes rapid involution, but it does not return to its initial size and weight.

The motility of the uterus

Several methods have been employed for assessing the movements of the human uterus:

1. by measuring intrauterine pressure with a balloon inserted into the cavity of the uterus
2. by using an external recording instrument (tocograph) which records changes in shape of the pregnant uterus
3. by observing the movements with X-rays after filling the cavity with a radio opaque material
4. by measuring *in vitro* the contractions of strips of myometrium removed at operation.

Uterine muscle contracts rhythmically both *in vitro* and *in vivo*. These contractions originate in the muscle itself and are not abolished by interference with the nerve supply. There is no evidence for the existence of an intrinsic nerve plexus which controls the muscle, such as occurs in the gastrointestinal tract.

Both the force and the frequency of contractions of uterine muscle vary greatly during the menstrual cycle, the variation being due to the effect of the complex hormonal changes which occur during the cycle.

The non-pregnant human uterus shows weak spontaneous contractions during the first part of the cycle. At about the 14th day, larger and more prolonged contractions can be recorded and during menstruation strong co-ordinated contractions occur, rather similar to those observed in the pregnant uterus during parturition (Fig. 17.6). The condition of the endometrium also changes as explained in the first section of this chapter.

In early pregnancy uterine movements are depressed but towards the end of the nine month period the movements increase in force and the contractions become fully co-ordinated during parturition. The fundus is the origin of these co-ordinated contractions; myometrial cells in this area function as pacemakers and give rise to conducted action potentials. The waves of contraction which result take about 10–20 seconds to pass from the fundus to the cervix. The electrophysiological activity of the myometrial pacemaker cells is regulated by the sex hormones.

Administration of oestrogen increases the membrane potential and subsequent administration of progesterone can increase it still further. The electrical activity of the uterus is inhibited if the membrane potential is very high and there is evidence that during pregnancy a condition of electrical and mechanical quiescence and relative inexcitability is produced by endogenous progesterone acting locally at the site of implantation of the foetus.

Innervation of the uterus and the action of sympathomimetic amines

The nerve supply to the uterus includes both excitatory and inhibitory sympathetic fibres. The uterus also receives some parasympathetic fibres from the sacral outflow but there is no definite evidence that cholinergic fibres have any role in the control of uterine motility.

Sympathetic stimulation causes mixed stimula-

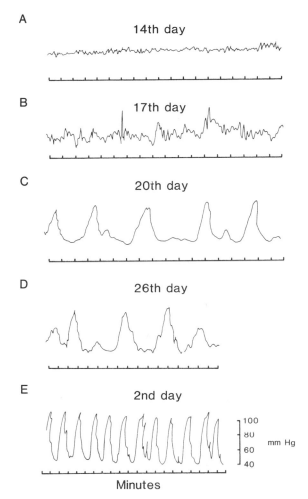

Fig. 17.6 Uterine tracings obtained at various stages of the menstrual cycle (different women). Time marked in minutes. (From Moir, 1944)

tory and inhibitory actions on the uterus, the predominant effect depending on the species. Within a species the result of sympathetic stimulation will depend on the hormonal condition of the uterus. Thus electrical stimulation of the hypogastric nerve results in relaxation of uterine muscle in the virgin cat but contraction of the muscle in the pregnant cat. The importance of endocrine factors is shown by the fact that if an ovariectomized cat is pretreated with oestrogen, adrenaline causes uterine relaxation, while pre-treatment with a combination of oestrogen and progesterone results in an adrenaline-induced contraction.

Noradrenaline stimulates the uterus in both pregnant and non-pregnant women, by an action on α-adrenoceptors. With an intravenous infusion of 2–10 µg/min of noradrenaline there is an immediate increase in the tone, the force and the frequency of uterine contractions. These contractions are not co-ordinated and thus noradrenaline is not useful for stimulating the uterus during parturition.

Adrenaline, given systematically, inhibits the uterus in both pregnant and non-pregnant women by an action on β-adrenoceptors. This effect cannot be made use of clinically since after the end of an adrenaline infusion there is a rebound increase of uterine activity and tone. However, selective β₂-adrenoceptor agonists have a limited place in obstetric practice. **Isoxsuprine**, **salbutamol**, **terbutaline** and **orciprenaline** (see Chapter 7) inhibit both the spontaneous and oxytocin-induced contractions of the pregnant uterus, and are of value in selected patients to prevent premature labour. They are also used to prevent fetal asphyxia when myometrial stimulants have resulted in hypertonus and excessive uterine contractions.

Adrenoceptor antagonists, are without effect on the motility of the human uterus.

The role of posterior pituitary hormones in uterine function

As explained in Chapter 16, the neurohypophyseal hormones are important in the regulation of myometrial activity. Oxytocin release can be stimulated by certain peripheral stimuli such as suckling

Day 5

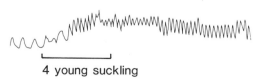

4 young suckling

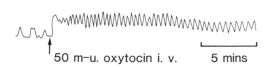

50 m–u. oxytocin i. v.   5 mins

Fig. 17.7 Uterine contractions in rabbits 5 days after parturition. The effect of suckling compared to that of an intravenous injection of oxytocin. The effect of suckling is believed to be due to oxytocin release. (After: Fuchs, 1966)

(Fig. 17.7). Cervical dilatation can also cause its release.

Whether oxytocin has a physiological role in the *initiation* of parturition is not clear, but there is evidence that an oestrogen-mediated increase in oxytocin receptors in the myometrium plays a part in the regulation of the contractility of uterine muscle during pregnancy and during the oestrus cycle in animals. Certainly the uterus develops a high degree of sensitivity to oxytocin at parturition and the myometrial contractions induced by infusion of exogenous oxytocin at term are very similar to the normal uterine movements which occur during labour.

The non-pregnant human uterus and the uterus in early pregnancy have greater sensitivity to vasopressin than to oxytocin. The uterus becomes more sensitive to oxytocin as pregnancy progresses and at term it is more sensitive to oxytocin than to vasopressin.

OXYTOCIC DRUGS

Three types of oxytocic agent stimulate the pregnant uterus and are of clinical importance: **oxytocin**, **ergometrine** and the **E & F type prostaglandins**.

Oxytocin

Oxytocin for clinical use is prepared synthetically. Its chemical structure is given in Figure 16.4. The S–S bond of cystine is crucial for its activity, the biological action being completely lost if it is reduced. Oxytocinase, an enzyme which destroys the peptide, is present in the serum of pregnant women.

Pharmacological activity

1. *On the uterus.* Oxytocin contracts the mammalian uterus. Figure 17.8 illustrates the effect of oxytocin and other spasmogens on the uterus of the stilboestrol-primed rat. On the human uterus at term, oxytocin, given by slow intravenous infusion causes regular coordinated contractions which travel from fundus to cervix, and both the amplitude and the frequency of the contractions are related to dose, the uterus relaxing completely

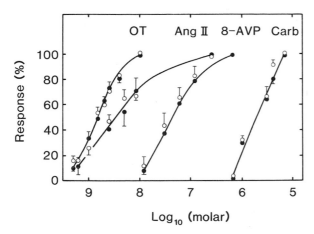

Fig. 17.8 Dose-response curves for uterine contraction. Uterine tissue was obtained from rats pre-treated (24 h) with stilboestrol. Two different strains of rats were used as indicated by the two types of symbol. OT = oxytocin; Ang II = angiotensin II; 8-AVP = vasopressin; carb = carbachol. (Adapted from: Hollenberg et al., 1983)

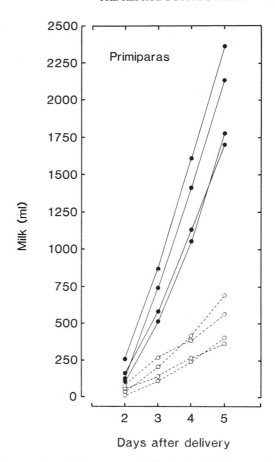

Fig. 17.9 Cumulative amount of milk obtained during second to fifth days after delivery by using breast pump on four occasions each day in primiparous women. The subjects were given either oxytocin or a placebo by nasal spray. Solid lines = oxytocin; dotted lines = placebo. (Data from: Ruis et al, 1981)

between contractions. There may be a slight transient increase in tone when the infusion is started.

Large doses cause an increase in the frequency of the contractions such that there is incomplete relaxations between them. Very high doses cause tetanic contractions which interfere with blood flow through the placenta and lead to foetal distress or death.

2. On the mammary gland. Oxytocin causes contraction of the myoepithelial cells of the mammary gland, which leads to 'milk let-down'—the expression of milk from the alveoli and ducts. This process is essential for the total evacuation of the gland—this cannot be effected solely by suckling. This action of oxytocin has been reported to be of value in enhancing lactation in the mothers of premature infants. Establishing adequate lactation by manual expression or breast pump is frequently unsatisfactory, especially in women who have had a first child. Increasing plasma prolactin concentrations with dopamine antagonists such as **metoclopramide** or **phenothiazines** (see Chapter 16) has the drawback that these agents are excreted in the milk and could harm the infant. Oxytocin given by intranasal spray facilitates milk let-down and results in significantly enhanced milk collection when a breast-pump is used (Fig. 17.9). There is no interference with the normal milk let-down reflex since there is no negative feedback effect of oxytocin.

3. On the vasculature. Oxytocin has a vasodilator action especially in birds and this effect can be made use of in bioassays of the peptide. A similar vasodilator effect, with a transient fall in blood pressure, is seen in man when oxytocin is given by intravenous injection.

4. On the kidney. Oxytocin has a weak vasopressin-like anti-diuretic action, which can result in water intoxication if large doses are infused.

Ergometrine

Ergot (*Claviceps purpurea*) is a fungus which grows on rye and on certain grasses (see also Chapter 7). Extracts of ergot contain an extraordinary variety of pharmacologically active substances, including histamine, acetylcholine, tyramine and ergosterol. Outbreaks of ergot poisoning due to the eating of bread made from ergot-infected rye have occurred frequently in Europe in the past, the manifestations being of two types: (a) gangrene of the extremities and (b) convulsions. In both types, abortions were frequent and it was clear that ergot contained an active principle which had powerful effects on the uterus.

In 1906 Barger & Carr, and independently, Kraft, isolated an alkaloid from ergot which was named **ergotoxine**. Ergotoxine was subsequently found to be, not a single substance, but a mixture of three alkaloids—**ergocristine**, **ergokryptine** and **ergocornine**. Later, in 1920, another alkaloid was isolated, by Stoll, and was named **ergotamine**. None of these alkaloids, however, produced on the uterus the powerful effect of the crude extracts of ergot. In 1935 **ergometrine** was isolated and was recognized as the oxytocic principle in ergot.

The central chemical moiety in the ergot alkaloids is lysergic acid and the chemical structure of this substance and of ergometrine is given in Figure 7.11. Of the ergot alkaloids only ergometrine is present in aqueous extracts of ergot since it is soluble in water whereas ergotoxine and ergotamine are relatively insoluble in water but soluble in alcohol.

Pharmacological activity

Ergometrine has a selective action on the myometrium though this effect is not marked when the muscle is tested *in vitro*. On the post-partum human uterus *in vivo*, ergometrine has a rapid stimulant effect. Its action depends partly on the state of the organ; thus on a normally contracting uterus, ergometrine has little effect, but if the uterus is quiescent, it initiates a prolonged series of strong contractions (Fig. 17.10).

Mechanism of action

The mechanism of action is not understood. It is possible that it acts on α-adrenoceptors, like the related alkaloid ergotamine, which is a partial agonist on these receptors (see Chapter 7), though it may produce effects through stimulation of 5-HT receptors in the myometrium.

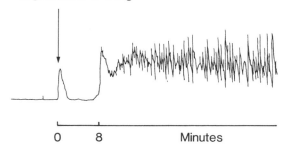

Ergometrine 0·5 mg

0   8   Minutes

Fig. 17.10 Contractions of the human uterus at the end of the first week of puerperium recorded by intrauterine balloon. Ergometrine 0.5 mg by mouth gave a series of rapid uterine contractions after 8 min. (After: Moir, 1935)

Given intravenously, its action starts within 30 seconds to 1 minute; given intramuscularly, effects are seen after 2–4 minutes. It can be administered by mouth, when it is rapidly absorbed and produces a response of the uterus in 4–8 minutes. Its action lasts for 3–6 hours.

Unwanted effects

Ergometrine may produce vomiting. A rather more serious unwanted effect is an increase in blood pressure, which may continue for several hours, but fortunately this is rare.

Prostaglandins

Endogenous prostaglandins

The endometrium and the myometrium of the uterus have significant prostaglandin-synthesizing capacity, particularly in the second, proliferative phase of the menstrual cycle. The vasoconstrictor prostaglandin, $PGF_{2\alpha}$, is generated in particularly large amounts and is thought to be implicated in the ischaemic necrosis of the endometrium which precedes menstruation. The vasodilator prostaglandins, PGE_2 and prostacyclin, are also generated by the uterus. (Prostaglandins are discussed in detail in Chapter 8).

In addition to their vasoactive properties the E and F type prostaglandins cause contractions of both the non-pregnant and the pregnant uterus.

In two of the main disorders of menstruation, dysmenorrhea (painful menstruation) and menorrhagia (excessive blood loss via menstruation), prostaglandins play a significant role.

Menorrhagia, in the absence of uterine pathology, appears to be due to a combination of increased vasodilatation and reduced haemostasis. There is evidence that the increased vasodilatation is associated with an increased production of PGE_2 and PGI_2 as compared to $PGF_{2\alpha}$. Haemostasis depends on both platelet aggregation and fibrin formation, the former being important in providing a surface for the latter (p. 292). There are fewer platelets in menstrual blood than in normal blood and they have a reduced capacity to aggregate and to synthesis thromboxane A_2. Increased generation by the uterus of prostacyclin (which inhibits platelet aggregation) will clearly impair haemostasis as well as causing vasodilatation.

It is possible to reduce the excessive blood loss of menorrhagia with a combined oestrogen-progestogen preparation or with danazol (p. 424) but the first is likely to have side effects and the second is very expensive. Non-steroidal anti-inflammatory drugs such as mefenamic acid (see Chapter 9) have proved to be of value in double-blind randomized placebo-controlled cross-over trials, though 20% of patients do not respond at all. The drugs are taken only for a few days immediately before and during the marked blood loss.

Dysmenorrhea of the spasmodic type is now known to be associated with increased production of the spasmogenic prostaglandins, PGE_2 and $PGF_{2\alpha}$ and can be successfully treated with non-steroidal anti-inflammatory drugs.

Exogenous prostaglandins

On the pregnant uterus prostaglandins of the E and F series promote a series of co-ordinated contractions of the body of the organ, along with relaxation of the cervix. It is possible that this latter action is due to a direct relaxant effect of prostaglandins on cervical smooth muscle. The action of the prostaglandins on the uterus differs from that of oxytocin in that, although both types of drug produce co-ordinated contractions of the myometrium, the prostaglandins have a greater propensity to increase uterine tone. In early and middle pregnancy oxytocin generally cannot cause expulsion of the uterine contents (since, at this time, the myometrial cells are not very sensitive to its action), whereas the prostaglandins can, and are therefore abortifacient.

The prostaglandins used in obstetrics are **dinoprostone** (PGE_2), **dinoprost** ($PGF_{2\alpha}$) and **sulprostone** (15-methyl prostaglandin $E_{2\alpha}$ methyl ester). They are administered intravenously or, preferably, by the extra-amniotic or intra-amniotic route. This latter route is only feasible after 14–16 weeks gestation.

Since they are able to activate co-ordinated contractions and cause the uterus to expel its contents even in the early stages of pregnancy, the prostaglandins specified above are sometimes used in the second trimester of pregnancy for therapeutic abortion. They may also be used for evacuation of the contents of the uterus in cases of missed abortion or hydatidiform mole. However, they may fail to produce complete expulsion of uterine contents and subsequent surgical evacuation may be necessary. During the first trimester surgical methods are altogether more effective. However, because of their relaxant action on the cervix, the prostaglandins may be of value in the pre-treatment of patients who have not had children, prior to termination of pregnancy by suction techniques.

Prostaglandins, given by slow intravenous infusion, have also been employed for the induction of labour at term, but they are not the drugs of choice since they may produce prolonged uterine contractions which cause foetal distress. Furthermore, they can cause nausea and vomiting or diarrhoea and may also produce phlebitis at the site of infusion. Systemic side effects are also likely to occur when prostaglandins are given, as abortifacients, by intravaginal pessary.

REFERENCES AND FURTHER READING

Endocrine aspects

Brotherton J 1976 Sex hormone pharmacology. Academic Press, New York

Buckingham J 1984 LHRH: fertility and anti-fertility drugs. Trends in Pharmacological Sciences 5: 136–137

Chaudhury R R 1981 Pharmacology of estrogens. International Encyclopaedia of Pharmacology & Therapeutics Section 106 Pergamon Press

Harris G W 1964 Endocrinology 75: 627–648

Jänne O A, Bardin C W 1984 Androgen and antiandrogen receptor binding. Ann Rev Physiol 46: 107–118

Larsson K, Beyer C 1981 In: Hrdina P D, Singhal R L (eds) Neuroendocrine regulation and altered behaviour. Croom Helm, London 95–118

Liao S 1977 Molecular actions of androgens. In: Litwack G (ed) Biochemical actions of hormones. Academic Press, New York, 351–406

O'Malley B W, Birnbaum L (eds) Receptors and hormone action 1978 Vol II and Vol III. Academic Press, New York

Segal S J, Koide S S 1979 Molecular pharmacology of oestrogens. Pharmac Ther 4: 183–220

Uterus

Berde B (ed) 1968 Neurohypophysial hormones. Handbook of Experimental Pharmacology, vol 32

Berde B, Schild H O (eds) 1978 Ergot alkaloids. Handbook of Experimental Pharmacology, vol 49

Dingfelder J R 1981 Primary dysmenorrhea treatment with prostaglandin inhibitors: a review. Am J Obstet Gynecol 140: 874–879

Elder M G 1983 Prostaglandins and menstrual disorders. Brit Med J 287: 703–704

Fuchs A-R 1966 The physiological role of oxytocin in the regulation of myometrial activity in the rabbit. In: Pickles V R, Fitzpatrick R J (eds) Endogenous substances affecting the myometrium. Cambridge University Press, London 229–248

Moir J C 1964 The obstetrician bids, the uterus contracts. Brit Med J (ii): 1025–1029

Moir D D 1974 Drugs used during labour; analgesics, anaesthetics and sedatives. In: Hawkins D F (ed) Obstetric therapeutics. Baillere Tindall, London 380–441

Saameli K 1979 Effects on the uterus. In: Berde, Schild (eds) Ergot alkaloids and related compounds. Handbook of Experimental Pharmacology, vol 49, Springer, Berlin 233–319

The haemopoietic system

The main components of the haemopoietic system are the bone marrow and the blood, but the spleen and the liver are important accessory organs. The spleen constitutes a blood store and also acts as a graveyard for effete red blood cells. The liver synthesizes many of the principal constituents of the plasma and is involved in the process of breakdown of the haemoglobin liberated when the red blood cells are destroyed. In addition, the kidney manufactures a factor termed 'erythropoietin' which stimulates red cell synthesis.

The term 'erythron' is used to describe the circulating red blood cells and their precursors. In a healthy adult the erythron is in a steady-state, cell loss being precisely balanced by new production of cells.

Red blood corpuscles (erythrocytes) are formed and developed in the bone marrow and, after entering the circulation, have an average life of about 120 days. The bone marrow is one of the few tissues in the body in which very rapid cell multiplication continues throughout life. It has been estimated that a normal man needs to replace daily the number of red cells contained in about 50 ml blood. To do this he requires only about a quarter of the capacity of his bone marrow.

The main function of the red cells is to carry oxygen and their oxygen-carrying power depends on their haemoglobin content. 1 g of haemoglobin contains about 3.3 mg of iron and the production of haemoglobin depends on the supply of iron. Anaemia results when the red cells are too few in number, or do not contain the normal amount of haemoglobin, or are abnormal in other respects.

Types of anaemia

Severe acute haemorrhage will produce anaemia, but a normal healthy person has remarkable powers of regenerating erythrocytes, and the haemoglobin content of the blood may be restored to normal within a relatively short time. Chronic anaemia results from chronic minor blood loss, from dietary deficiency, or from the disorder of an organ concerned in the manufacture of the factors essential for the formation of red blood cells. The symptoms are mainly a result of anoxia and are usually more severe if the anaemia develops rapidly.

The following is a convenient classification of anaemias according to their aetiology:

1. *Anaemias caused by deficiency of factors necessary for erythropoiesis* such as:
   a. Iron (microcytic hypochromic anaemia)
   b. Folic acid and vitamin B_{12} (megaloblastic anaemia)
   c. Vitamin C, thyroxine.
2. *Anaemias caused by depression of the bone marrow.* Aplastic or hypoplastic conditions of the bone marrow may affect the formation and development of the red cells, leucocytes or platelets. In complete aplastic anaemia the formation of all these blood cells is deficient. Aplastic anaemia affecting only red cells or only platelets is rare, but agranulocytosis, a condition in which leukocytes and other cells of the myeloid series are absent, occurs relatively frequently as a result of the administration of certain drugs, exposure to radio-active substances or to severe infection.
3. *Anaemias caused by excessive destruction of red blood cells.* These are termed 'haemolytic' anaemias and are due either to the breakdown of red corpuscles which are defective or to the effects of poisons or infection.

The principal agents used in the treatment of

anaemia are **iron**, **vitamin B$_{12}$** and **folic acid**, and this chapter will deal mainly with these agents. **Vitamin C** will only be mentioned briefly.

IRON

Iron is a transition metal with two important properties relevant to its biological role, the ability to exist in several oxidation states and the tendency to form stable co-ordination complexes.

The body of a 70 kg man contains about 4 g of iron, 65% of which circulates in the blood as the oxygen-transporting molecule, haemoglobin. About one-half of the remainder is stored in the liver, spleen and bone marrow chiefly as ferritin and haemosiderin. The iron of these molecules is available for fresh haemoglobin synthesis. The rest, which is not available for haemoglobin synthesis, is present in myoglobin, cytochromes and various other enzymes. The distribution of iron in an average normal adult male is shown in Table 18.1. The figures for an average 55 kg female would be about 55% of these. Since most of the iron in the body is either part of, or destined to be part of, the haemoglobin in red cells, the most obvious clinical result of iron deficiency is anaemia, and the only *pharmacological* action of iron used therapeutically is to provide material for haemoglobin synthesis.

Haemoglobin is made up of four protein chain subunits (globins), each of which contains one *haem* moiety. Haem consists of a tetrapyrrole porphyrin

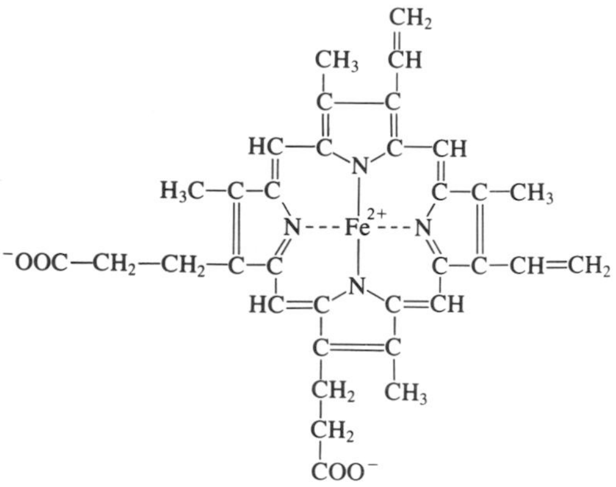

Fig. 18.1 The structure of haem.

ring containing ferrous (Fe^{2+}) iron (Fig. 18.1). Each haem group can carry one O$_2$ molecule, which is bound reversibly to the Fe^{2+} and to a histidine residue in the particular globin chain to which the haem is linked. This reversible binding is the basis of O$_2$ transport.

Iron turnover and iron balance

Both the normal physiological turnover of iron and *pharmacokinetic factors* affecting iron given therapeutically will be dealt with here.

The normal daily requirement for iron is approximately 5 mg for a man, and 15 mg for a woman during the reproductive period and for a growing child. A pregnant woman needs between two and ten times this amount because of the demands of the fetus and the increased requirements of the mother. The average diet in Western Europe provides 15–20 mg of iron daily, the main sources being green vegetables, peas, beans, oatmeal, eggs, chocolate and dried fruits and, more particularly, meat. Iron in meat is generally present as haem and this form of iron is very readily absorbed intact by the intestinal mucosa. About 20–40% of haem iron is available for absorption and this is not altered by other factors in the diet. The human body appears to be specifically adapted to absorb iron in the form of haem. It is thought that one reason why man has problems in maintaining iron balance (there are an estimated 500 million people with iron deficiency in the world) is that the change from hunting to grain cultivation 10 000 years ago led to cereals constituting a much larger proportion of the diet and

Table 18.1 The distribution of iron in the body of a normal 70 kg male

Protein	Tissue	Iron content (mg)
Haemoglobin	Erythrocytes	2600
Myoglobin	Muscle	400
Enzymes (cytochomes catalase etc)	Liver and other tissues	25
Transferrin	Plasma and extracellular fluid	8
Ferritin and hemosiderin	Liver	410
	Spleen	48
	Bone marrow	300

Data from: Jacobs & Worwood: in Hardisty & Weatherall, (1982)

cereals have relatively small amounts of readily absorbable iron, in comparison with meat.

Non-haem iron in food is mainly in the ferric state and both this iron, as well as ferric iron preparations used therapeutically, need to be converted to ferrous iron for absorption. Ferric iron, and to a lesser extent ferrous iron, has low solubility at the neutral pH of the intestine, but in the stomach iron dissolves and binds to mucoprotein which functions as a carrier, transporting the iron to the intestine. In the presence of ascorbic acid, fructose and various amino-acids, iron is detached from the carrier, forming soluble low molecular weight complexes. This process enables iron to remain in soluble form in the intestine. Ascorbic acid stimulates iron absorption partly by forming soluble iron-ascorbate chelates and partly by reducing ferric iron to the more soluble ferrous form.

Phosphates and phytates inhibit iron absorption by forming insoluble iron complexes. Tetracycline forms an insoluble iron chelate resulting in impaired uptake of both substances; tannates (e.g. in tea) also interfere with iron absorption.

The amount of iron in the diet and the various factors affecting its availability are thus important determinants in absorption, but the *regulation* of iron absorption is a function of the intestinal mucosa, influenced by the body's iron stores. In fact the absorptive mechanism holds a central role in iron balance since it is the sole mechanism by which body iron can be controlled.

The site of iron absorption is the duodenum and upper jejunum and it is a two-stage process involving firstly a rapid uptake across the brush border and then transfer from the interior of the cell into the plasma (Fig. 18.2). The second stage, which is rate-limiting, is known to be energy-dependent. Haem iron, as explained above, is absorbed as intact haem and the iron is released in the mucosal cell by the action of haem oxidase. Non-haem iron is absorbed in the ferrous state. Within the cell, ferrous iron is oxidized to ferric iron which is bound to an intracellular carrier, a transferrin-like protein; the iron is then either held in storage in the mucosal cell as *ferritin* (if body stores of iron are high) or passed on to the plasma (if iron stores are low).

Iron is carried in the plasma bound to *transferrin*—a β-globulin with two binding sites for ferric iron—which is normally only 30% saturated.

(a) normal

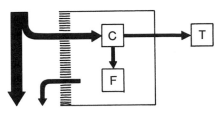

(b) iron deficiency

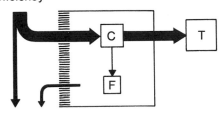

(c) iron overload

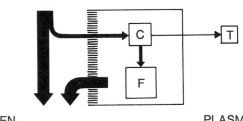

LUMEN   PLASMA

Fig. 18.2 Schematic illustration of one of the main theories of iron absorption (and thus the regulation of iron balance) by intestinal mucosal cells. Iron in the food is absorbed into the mucosal cells and bound to a transferrin-like carrier molecule (C), from where it is transferred to either transferrin (T) in the plasma or ferritin (F) within the cell, the amount transferred being influenced by the degree of iron-saturation of plasma transferrin. The iron in the ferritin is lost when the cell sloughed off. The thickness of the arrows indicates the amount of iron transferred. (Modified from: Ganong, 1983)

Plasma contains 4 mg of iron at any one time but the daily turnover is about 30 mg (Fig. 18.3). Most of the iron which enters the plasma is derived from the mononuclear phagocyte system following the degradation of time-expired erythrocytes. Intestinal absorption and mobilization of iron from storage depots contribute only small amounts. Most of the iron which leaves the plasma daily is used for haemoglobin synthesis by red cell precursors. These cells have receptors which bind transferrin molecules, releasing them after the iron has been taken up. This process may involve internalization of the complex.

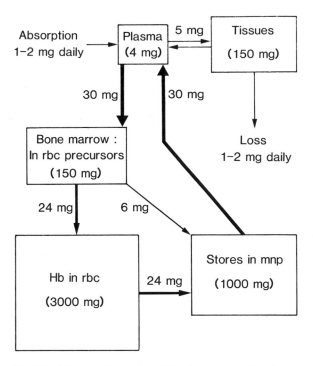

Fig. 18.3 Schematic illustration of the distribution of iron in the body with an indication of the daily intake, movement between compartments and loss. Hb = haemoglobin; rbc = red blood cells; mnp = mononuclear phagocytes. Data from: Jacobs & Worwood: in Hardisty & Weatherall (1982)

The body has no means of actively excreting iron. Small amounts leave the body through the peeling off of mucosal cells containing ferritin and even smaller amounts leave in the bile, the sweat and the urine. A total of about 1 mg is lost daily. The iron balance is therefore critically dependent on the active absorption mechanism in the intestinal mucosa. This absorption is influenced by the iron stores in the body but the precise mechanisms of this control are still a matter of debate. It is suggested that the amount of ferritin in the intestinal mucosa may be important in regulating absorption and possibly also the balance between ferritin and the transferrin-like carrier molecule in these cells. The daily movement of iron in the body is illustrated in Figure 18.3 and one of the main theories of the regulation of iron absorption and iron balance is illustrated schematically in Figure 18.2.

Clinical use of iron

Iron is used only for the treatment or prevention of *iron deficiency anaemia*, which may result from increased loss, increased demand, inadequate dietary intake or malabsorption of iron.

The commonest cause of iron deficiency is *chronic blood loss* and the usual sites from which this loss occurs are the gastrointestinal tract and uterus. In Western Europe and the USA the gastrointestinal lesions most frequently associated with chronic blood loss are haemorrhoids, peptic ulcer and salicylate-induced damage (this last effect is dealt with in Chapter 9). Outside these areas a very common cause is hookworm infestation (see Chapter 34). If iron reserves are normal the body is able to replace relatively easily the iron lost during a single sudden acute haemorrhage even if this involves as much as one-third of the blood volume, but the steady loss of as little as 3–4 ml per day can result, in time, in a negative iron balance and iron deficiency anaemia requiring iron treatment.

Women in the reproductive period of life lose an average of 40 ml of blood during each period of menstruation and since 2 ml of blood contains about 0.5 mg of iron, about 20 mg of iron is lost each month over and above that leaving the body by other routes. A loss of more than 80 ml of blood in each menstrual period is likely to lead eventually

Iron is stored in two forms—soluble ferritin and insoluble haemosiderin. *Ferritin* is found in all cells, the mononuclear phagocytes of liver, spleen and bone marrow containing especially high concentrations. It is also present in plasma. Apoferritin is a large protein of molecular weight, 450 000, composed of 24 identical polypeptide subunits which enclose a cavity in which up to 4500 iron molecules can be stored. Apoferritin takes up ferrous iron, oxidizes it and deposits the ferric iron in its core. In this form it constitutes ferritin—the primary storage form of iron—from which the iron is most readily available. The life span of this iron-laden protein is only a few days. *Haemosiderin* is a degraded form of ferritin in which the iron cores of several ferritin molecules have aggregated, following partial disintegration of the outer protein shells. The ferritin in plasma has virtually no iron associated with it. It is in equilibrium with the storage ferritin in cells and its concentration in the plasma provides an estimate of total body iron stores.

to iron deficiency anaemia and will require treatment with iron.

There is an *increased demand* for iron during pregnancy and in early infancy. Each pregnancy 'costs' the mother 680 mg of iron, equivalent to 1300 ml of blood, due to the demands of the fetus, plus an extra 450 mg to meet the requirements of the expanded blood volume. Adequate pre-natal care necessitates iron supplements if iron deficiency anaemia is to be prevented.

Infants are also likely to require iron supplements during the first 6 months of life since milk is a poor source of iron.

Inadequate iron intake is common in developing countries where dietary iron may be of low availability (see above). This will exacerbate a negative iron balance caused by hookworm infestation.

Malabsorption of iron may occur in patients with partial gastrectomy and in patients with steatorrhea or coeliac disease.

Preparations of iron for clinical use

Iron is usually given orally but may be given parenterally in special circumstances. A number of different preparations of ferrous iron salts are available for oral administration. These include **ferrous sulphate**, **ferrous succinate**, **ferrous gluconate** and **ferrous fumarate** which are all absorbed to a comparable extent. The elemental iron content of ferrous sulphate is 200 µg per mg, of ferrous succinate 350 µg per mg, of ferrous gluconate 120 µg per mg and of ferrous fumarate 330 µg per mg.

An individual who has an established iron deficiency may utilize as much as 50–100 mg of iron for haemoglobin synthesis each day. As only 20–25% of orally administered ferrous iron can be absorbed, 200–400 mg of elemental iron may need to be given daily to provide this amount. The red cell defect can be repaired within 30–60 days. However, treatment will need to be continued for 3–6 months to ensure replenishment of the iron stores since the rate of absorption of iron decreases as the anaemia is reversed. Some individuals cannot tolerate this amount of iron and lower doses are then given for longer periods. The time factor is usually not critical.

Parenteral iron is rarely given but may be necessary in patients who have extensive continuing chronic blood loss, or in individuals who are not able to absorb oral iron as a result of surgical procedures or inflammatory conditions involving the gastrointestinal tract, or malabsorption syndromes. The preparations used are **iron-dextran** or **iron-sorbitol**, both given intramuscularly. Iron-dextran, but not iron-sorbitol can be given by slow intravenous infusion, but this method of administration should only be used if absolutely necessary.

Unwanted effects

The side effects of oral iron administration include nausea, abdominal cramps and diarrhoea. These are dose-related and less likely to occur if doses of 100 mg are used. *Acute toxicity* is usually seen in young children who have swallowed attractively coloured iron tablets in mistake for sweets. The result of the ingestion of large quantities of iron salts is severe necrotizing gastritis with vomiting, haemorrhage and diarrhoea followed by circulatory collapse. **Desferrioxamine** may be used to treat acute toxicity. It is a powerful iron chelating agent which is given both intragastrically and intramuscularly in the treatment of acute iron toxicity. In severe poisoning it can be given by slow intravenous infusion. Adequate supportive therapy for shock and haemorrhage may also be required.

Chronic iron toxicity or iron overload is virtually always due to causes other than ingestion of iron salts, the commonest cause being the giving of repeated blood transfusions to treat haemolytic anaemias.

VITAMIN B$_{12}$ AND FOLIC ACID

Vitamin B$_{12}$ and folic acid are necessary constituents of man's diet, the active forms of these agents being essential for DNA synthesis and cell proliferation. Deficiency of either vitamin B$_{12}$ or folate will have effects principally in those tissues in which there is rapid cell turnover—bone marrow and the gastrointestinal tract—though dividing cells in other tissues are also likely to be affected. The main manifestation of such deficiency is *megaloblastic haemopoiesis* in which there is a marked disorder of erythroblast (pronormoblast) proliferation and defective erythropoiesis. There are increased numbers of large abnormal erythrocyte precursors in the bone marrow due to the fact that during the cell cycle of the proliferating cells (see Fig. 29.1) absence of these substance results in decreased DNA synthesis but little change in RNA and protein synthesis. The nucleated red blood cell precursors consequently have a high RNA:DNA ratio and many do not go on to form erythrocytes. Those erythrocytes which are produced are large cells (macrocytes) with normal cytoplasm and haemoglobin but with an increased susceptibility to destruction. Many, instead of being neat biconcave discs, are distorted in shape. Some degree of leucopenia and thrombocytopenia usually accompanies the anaemia.

The principal cause of vitamin B_{12} deficiency is decreased absorption of the vitamin due either to a lack of **intrinsic factor** (see below) or to conditions which interfere with its absorption in the ileum.

Intrinsic factor is secreted by the stomach and is essential for B_{12} absorption (p. 441). It is lacking in patients with *pernicious anaemia* or individuals who have had gastrectomies. Pernicious anaemia is a condition in which there is atrophic gastritis, thought to be due, in most cases, to a local, genetically-determined cell-mediated autoimmune reaction. There is often a concurrent neurological disorder—*subacute combined degeneration of the spinal cord*. The anaemia was originally termed 'pernicious ' because it seemed to be untreatable, but in 1926 Minot & Murphy showed that there was a remarkable response to the feeding of raw liver. Castle and his associates subsequently established that liver contained an **extrinsic factor** (later defined as **vitamin B_{12}**), that this, together with an 'intrinsic factor' present in normal gastric juice, was necessary for normal maturation of red cells and that pernicious anaemia was due to a deficiency of the intrinsic factor.

Other conditions resulting in B_{12} deficiency include malabsorption syndromes (e.g. sprue), ileal resection, various inflammatory conditions of the bowel and fish tapeworm infestations. (The effect of the last is ascribed to sequestration of the vitamin by the worm and is common in Finland.) Some drugs may cause a degree of B_{12} deficiency. Neomycin and colchicine have a toxic effect on the ileal mucosa. Phenformin, oral contraceptives, anticonvulsants and cimetidine are other, rare, causes of reduced B_{12} absorption.

Part of the reason for the response to liver seen in pernicious anaemia was the presence in this tissue of **folic acid**.

Wills suggested in the 1930s that the vegetable extract 'Marmite' also contained an anti-anaemia factor, and established that it could correct nutritional anaemia in monkeys. This, too was eventually shown to be folic acid—though the Marmite factor was transiently named vitamin M. Mitchell and his colleagues isolated pure folic acid from spinach in 1941 and Spies and his co-workers demonstrated that folic acid itself produced an initial clinical improvement in pernicious anaemia comparable with that obtained with liver extract. However, treatment with folic acid does not stop the development of the neurological lesions and may indeed precipitate their onset. Furthermore, continuous treatment of pernicious anaemia with folic acid fails to maintain a satisfactory response.

Although folic acid is an unsatisfactory treatment in those anaemias which are due to lack of vitamin B_{12}, it is very effective in other megaloblastic anaemias in which the underlying defect is a specific deficiency of folate. Folate deficiency is usually due to poor diet, but also occurs in malabsorption syndromes. Liver disease exacerbates the effect of inadequate diet. Conditions in which there is increased utilization of folate may also result in folate deficiency particularly if associated with a marginally adequate dietary intake. These include pregnancy, haemolytic anaemia, malignancy and various chronic inflammatory conditions. Folate deficiency may follow the use of some drugs—phenytoin, barbiturates and oral contraceptives. It may also occur with folate antagonists such as methotrexate (p. 598 & 614) and, to a smaller extent, trimethoprim and pyrimethamine (p. 630 & 664).

Folic acid

Structure and sources

Folic acid (pteroylglutamic acid) consists of a pteridine ring, para-amino benzoic acid and glutamic acid (Fig. 18.4). It probably does not occur in nature as such but can be regarded as the parent compound of a group of naturally occurring folates. These differ from folic acid in several respects. Different states of reduction of the pteri-

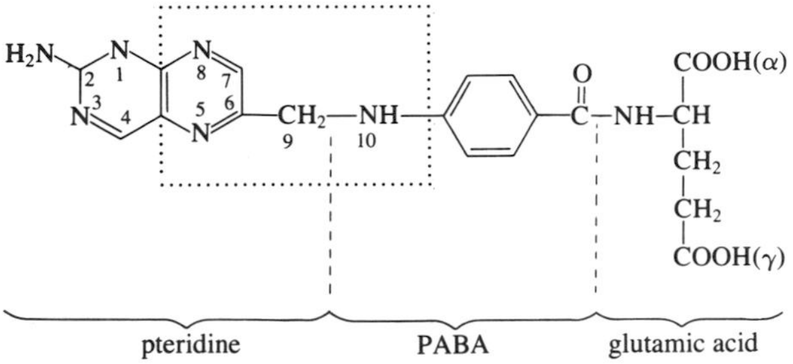

Fig. 18.4 Folic acid (pteroylglutamic acid). Folates may also contain: (a) extra hydrogens at positions 7 and 8 (dihydrofolate) or at 5, 6, 7 and 8 (tetrahydrofolate); (b) one-carbon units such as—a methyl group ($-CH_3$) at N^5, a formyl group ($-CHO$) at N^5 or N^{10}, a methylene ($-CH_2-$) or a methenyl ($=CH-$) group between N^5 and N^{10}; (c) additional glutamic acid residues attached to the γ-carboxyl of the glutamate moiety. The area in the box is the part of the molecule involved in one-carbon transfers in purine and pyrimidine synthesis.

dine ring may occur, several one-carbon units may be attached to N^5 or N^{10} or both, and additional glutamic acid residues may be attached to the glutamate moiety by unusual γ-peptide bonds, giving folate polyglutamates. (Some aspects of folate structure and metabolism are dealt with in Chapter 29).

Folates are found in liver, green vegetables, yeast, nuts, cereals, fruit, etc, and the average daily diet in Western Europe contains about 600 µg, of which about 100 µg is absorbed. The folates in food are in the form of polyglutamates. They are converted to the monoglutamate 5,methyltetrahydrofolate, before absorption and are transported in the blood in this form, most bound loosely to α_2 macroglobulin but some tightly bound to a specific folate-binding protein. The folates in tissues are mostly polyglutamates.

Physiological and pharmacological actions of folates

Folates are essential for DNA synthesis in that they

are cofactors in the synthesis of purines and pyrimidines. They are also necessary for reactions involved in amino-acid metabolism. In all reactions folate polyglutamates are considerably more active than monoglutamates. For activity folate must be in the tetrahydro-form, in which it is maintained by the enzyme dihydrofolate reductase. This enzyme reduces dietary folic acid to tetrahydrofolate (FH_4) in a two step reaction and also reduces the dihydrofolate (FH_2) produced from FH_4 during thymidylate synthesis (see Figs. 18.5 & 29.8). Folate antagonists act by inhibiting dihydrofolate reductase (see also Chapters 28, 29 & 33).

The *de novo* synthesis of purines requires two folate-dependent one-carbon transfer reactions. The insertion of the carbon atom at position 2 of the purine ring requires methenyl ($-CH=$) tetrahydrofolate and the insertion of the carbon at position 8, formyl ($-CHO$) tetrahydrofolate (Fig. 18.6).

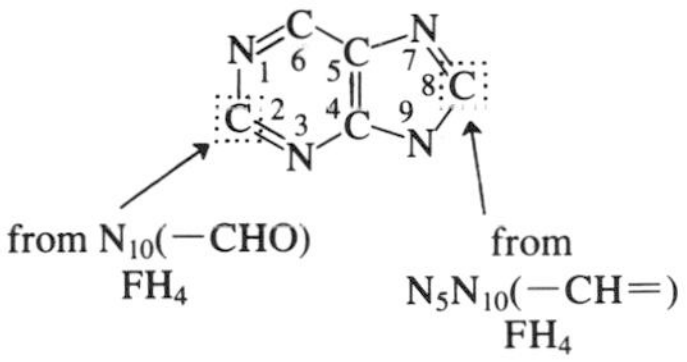

Fig. 18.6 The purine ring. Carbon atoms 2 and 8 are derived from one-carbon transfers from N^{10} formyl-tetrahydrofolate ($N^{10}(-CHO)FH_4$) and N^5N^{10} methenyl-tetrahydrofolate ($N^5N^{10}(-CH=)FH4$) respectively.

Folates are especially important in pyrimidine synthesis, for the methylation of deoxyuridylate monophosphate (DUMP) to thymidylate monophosphate (DTMP) which is catalysed by the enzyme, thymidylate synthetase. During this reaction, in contrast to other folate-dependent reactions, tetrahydrofolate is oxidized to dihydrofolate (see Figs. 18.7 & 29.8) and must therefore be reduced before it can act again.

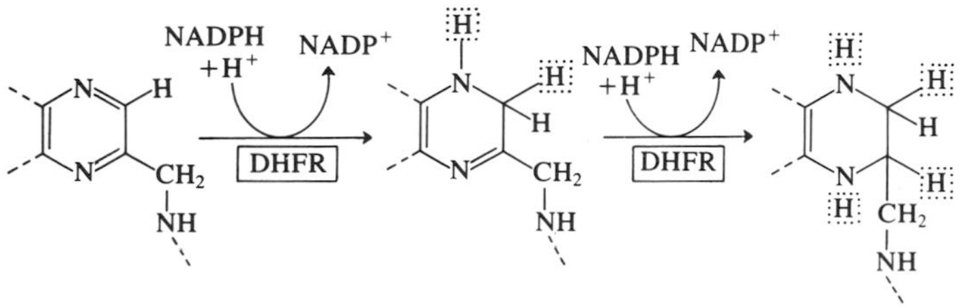

Fig. 18.5 The reduction of folic acid to dihydrofolate then to tetrahydrofolate by the enzyme dihydrofolate reductase (DHFR). Only a portion of the pteridine moiety of the folate molecule is included—that portion shown in a box in Fig. 18.4.

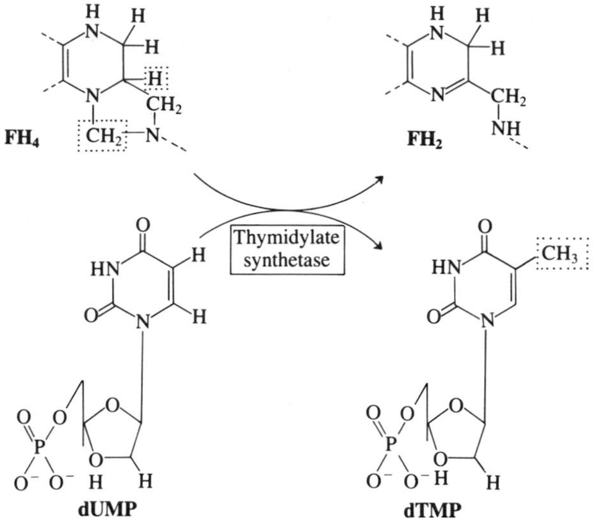

Fig. 18.7 The synthesis of 2-deoxythymidylate (dTMP) by the transfer of a methyl group from N^5N^{10}-methylene tetrahydrofolate (FH_4) to 2-deoxyuridylate (dUMP), the FH_4 being oxidized to dihydrofolate (FH_2) in the process. Only a portion of the pteridine moiety of the folates is included.

The thymidylate synthetase reaction is rate-limiting in mammalian DNA synthesis and since, after the reaction, the tetrahydrofolate coenzyme requires regeneration by sequential action of dihydrofolate reductase and serine transhydroxymethylase (to give the necessary methylene tetrahydrofolate) this step in DNA synthesis is particularly susceptible to the effect of folate antagonists, acting as they do by inhibition of dihydrofolate reductase (see Fig. 29.8).

Folates are also important in amino-acid interconversion—in glycine-serine interconversion, in the methylation of homocysteine to methionine, and in the formation of glutamic acid from formiminoglutamic acid. These reactions are of less relevance for the role of folates in haemopoiesis than those specified above.

Pharmacokinetic aspects

Folic acid is usually given orally but preparations for parenteral use are available. In the intestine, folic acid is transferred across the mucosa unchanged. Whether this is an active or a passive process is still a matter of debate. The results of animal experiments point to a passive process but some studies suggest that a specific permease may

be involved in absorption in man. Folates are taken up into the liver and into bone marrow cells by active transport—there being separate carrier mechanisms for folic acid and for reduced folates and methotrexate (p. 616). The carrier-mediated uptake of reduced folate is considerably more effective than that of folic acid. Within the cells, folic acid is reduced and methylated or formylated before being converted by polyglutamate synthetase to the polyglutamate form, through sequential addition of two to five glutamate moieties. Folinic acid, a synthetic tetrahydrofolic acid, is converted much more rapidly to the polyglutamate form. Recent studies suggest that methyltetrahydrofolate is a poor substrate for polyglutamate formation, unlike dihydrofolate, tetrahydrofolate and formyltetrahydrofolate. (This has relevance for the effect of vitamin B_{12} deficiency on folate metabolism, as is explained below).

Clinical use

Folate is used to treat megaloblastic anaemia which is due to folate deficiency and is also used prophylactically in individuals at hazard from developing such a deficiency—pregnant women, premature infants, patients with severe chronic haemolytic anaemias, those in intensive care and those undergoing regular renal dialysis.

Unwanted effects

These do not occur even with large doses of folic acid.

It is important to determine whether a megaloblastic anaemia is due to a folate or a vitamin B_{12} deficiency, since, if vitamin B_{12} deficiency is treated with folic acid, the blood picture may improve and give the appearance of cure while the neurological lesions get worse. Haematological investigations should be carried out and if necessary, an examination of the bone marrow. Other necessary investigations should include assays of serum folate and B_{12} concentrations and of red cell folate content.

Vitamin B_{12}

Structure and sources

Vitamin B_{12} is a cobalamin compound (Fig. 18.8).

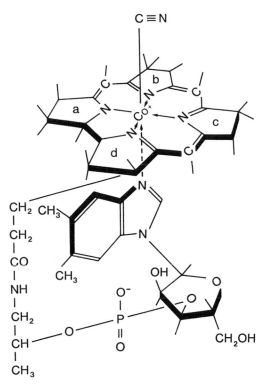

Fig. 18.8 Cyanocobalamin (vitamin B_{12}). The corrin ring containing a cobalt atom is at the top of the illustration. The cobalt atom is attached to the nucleotide structure which lies below and at right angles to the ring, while above is the cyano group. In 5'-deoxyadenosylcobalamin the CN is replaced by a deoxyadenosyl group and in hydroxocobalamin by a hydroxy group. (Adapted from: Thompson & Proctor, 1984).

Cobalamins are complex molecules having two main components:

1. A planar, corrin ring. This is a porphyrin-like ring consisting of four reduced pyrrole rings, with a central cobalt atom. Three of the pyrrole rings are linked by bridged carbon atoms, as in the porphyrin nucleus, but there is a direct bond between the a and d rings.
2. A nucleotide portion—a 5,6-dimethylbenzimidazole attached to ribose phosphate—which is set nearly at right angles to the corrin ring and is linked to it by bonds to the cobalt atom at one end and to the proprionate side-chain of the d ring through an aminopropanol group esterified with the phosphate, at the other.
3. A group, co-ordinated to the cobalt atom, which may be cyanide, methyl, hydroxyl or deoxyadenosyl. The term 'vitamin B_{12}' is sometimes

used specifically for the compound in which this group is cyanide (—CN), i.e. for **cyanocobalamin**, but is often used (and will be used here) to include other pharmacologically active cobalamins.

Vitamin B_{12} is sometimes referred to as 'extrinsic factor' to differentiate it from the 'intrinsic factor' produced by the parietal cells of the gastric mucosa and necessary for the absorption of B_{12}. In nature, B_{12} occurs mainly as **methyl-cobalamin** (methyl-B_{12}) and **5'-deoxyadenosylcobalamin** (ado-B_{12}). These are the active forms of the vitamin but they are unstable and convert spontaneously to **hydroxocobalamin** on exposure to light.

Vitamin B_{12} for medical use consists of cyanocobalamin and hydroxocabalamin and is obtained commercially as a by-product of the manufacture of streptomycin, since the streptomyces organism is one of the many microorganisms which synthesize the vitamin. In the diet the principal source of vitamin B_{12} is meat (particularly liver) eggs and dairy products. Its presence in these is due to microbial synthesis. All cobalamins, dietary and therapeutic, must be converted to the methyl and ado forms for activity in the body.

The average daily diet in Western Europe contains $5–25\,\mu g$ of B_{12} and the daily requirement is $2–3\,\mu g$. Absorption requires intrinsic factor—a glycoprotein of $45\,000\,MW$ which is a secretory product of the parietal cells of the stomach. One molecule of intrinsic factor binds one molecule of B_{12}, with high affinity. A complex is formed in which surface peptide bonds of intrinsic factor that are susceptible to the action of proteolytic enzymes are protected by infolding. The stomach secretes a huge excess of intrinsic factor; what limits absorption is the amount the ileum is capable of absorbing. The complexes attach passively to receptors on the mucosa of the ileum, at neutral pH and in the presence of calcium ions. B_{12} is transferred across the cell in an energy-requiring step, intrinsic factor being removed by lyosomal enzymes on the way.

B_{12} is transported in the plasma by B_{12}-binding proteins called *transcobalamins* (TCs), of which there are three—TCI, TCII and TCIII. TCI, an α_1-globulin of $57\,000\,MW$ secreted mainly by granulocyte precursors carries virtually all the B_{12}

present in serum and is normally about 60% saturated. It takes up B_{12} which is released from the liver and gives it up only very slowly to tissues. The complex of TCI-B_{12} has a plasma half-life of about 10 days and it is thought that it may constitute a storage form of the vitamin. TCIII is very similar. TCII is a β-globulin of 38 000 MW secreted mainly by macrophages but also by liver and ileal cells. It is a more selective carrier for B_{12} since it does not, like TCI and TCIII, bind B_{12} analogues. It normally carries 5–10% of plasma B_{12} but is largely unsaturated and capable of binding considerably more of the vitamin. The TCII-B_{12} complex is thought to attach to receptors on cells and to be taken up by pinocytosis.

The vitamin is stored in the body, 80% in the liver and the rest in the kidney, adrenal, pancreas and other organs, the mean total body store being 4 mg with a range of 2–11 mg.

Since the daily requirement is so low, if B_{12} absorption is stopped suddenly—as after a total gastrectomy—it takes 2–4 years for evidence of deficiency to become manifest.

Physiological and pharmacological actions

Vitamin B_{12} is required for two main biochemical reactions in man—methionine synthesis and isomerization of methylmalonyl CoA to succinyl CoA.

1. *The conversion of homocysteine to methionine.* The enzyme involved is homocysteine-methionine methyl transferase. The reaction requires B_{12} and 5-methyltetrahydrofolate as methyl donor. It is thought that the 5-methyltetrahydrofolate donates the methyl group to B_{12}, the co-factor, which is bound to the apoenzyme. The methyl group is then transferred to homocysteine (Fig. 18.9). Vitamin B_{12}-dependent methionine synthesis thus has a significant role in the generation of tetrahydrofolate from methyltetrahydrofolate.

Methyltetrahydrofolate, (the form in which folates are usually carried in blood and in which they enter cells) is a functionally inactive form of folate. Vitamine B_{12} deficiency results in the 'trapping' of folate in the inactive methyltetrahydrofolate form, and the consequent depletion of all intracellular folate polyglutamates co-enzymes, since methyltetrahydrofolate is a poor substrate for polyglutamate synthetase (see above).

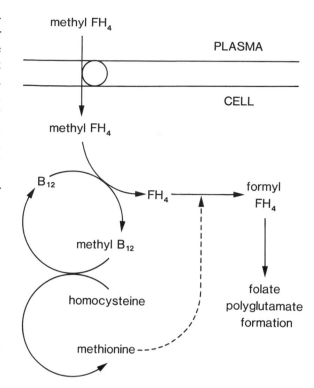

Fig. 18.9 The role of vitamin B_{12} in the synthesis of folate polyglutamate co-enzymes. 5-methyltetrahydrofolate monoglutamate (methyl FH$_4$) enters the cells by active transport. The methyl group is transferred to homocysteine to form methionine via vitamin B_{12}, which is bound to the apoenzyme: homocysteine-methionine methyl-transferase. (Vitamin B_{12} is shown as 'B_{12}' and as 'methyl B_{12}', but the enzyme is not shown). Methionine is important in the donation of formate (shown by dashed line) for the conversion of tetrahydrofolate (FH$_4$) to formyl tetrahydrofolate (formyl FH$_4$) which is the preferred substrate for the formation of folate polyglutamates.

B_{12}-dependent methionine synthesis may also affect the synthesis of folate-polyglutamate co-enzymes by an additional mechanism. There is evidence that the preferred substrate for polyglutamate synthesis is formyltetrahydrofolate and the conversion of tetrahydrofolate to formyltetrahydrofolate requires a formate donor such as methionine. The proposed role of vitamin B_{12} in folate co-enzyme synthesis is indicated in Figure 18.9.

2. *Isomerization of methylmalonyl CoA to succinyl CoA.* This reaction is part of a route by which propionate is converted to succinate. Through this

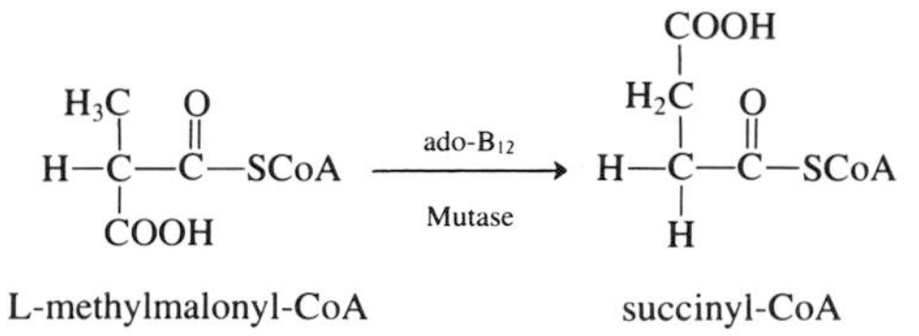

Fig. 18.10 The conversion of L-methyl-malonyl-CoA to succinyl-CoA by methyl-malonyl CoA mutase. 5'-deoxydenosyl B_{12} (ado-B_{12}) acts as a co-enzyme.

pathway cholesterol, odd-chain fatty acids, some amino-acids and thymine may be used for energy production via the Krebs cycle, or for gluconeogenesis. Vitamin B_{12}, in the form of deoxyadenosyl cobalamin (ado-B_{12}) is a co-factor in the reaction (Fig. 18.10). In vitamin B_{12} deficiency states the reaction cannot occur and methylmalonyl-CoA accumulates. It has been postulated that this causes fatty acid synthesis in neural tissue to be distorted and that this is the basis of the neuropathy which occurs in these states. The results of other studies suggest that the neurological lesions may be due to a block of methionine synthesis (see above) and thus of S-adenosylmethionine formation and hence defective methylation reactions in lipid (e.g. phosphatidylcholine) synthesis.

Administration and pharmacokinetic aspects

When vitamin B_{12} is used as a drug it is almost always given by intramuscular injection since B_{12} deficiency is virtually always due to malabsorption of the vitamin. Plasma transport and distribution of therapeutically administered B_{12} are similar to that of vitamin B_{12} absorbed from the diet (see above).

The preparations available are **hydroxocobalamin** and **cyanocobalamin**. Hydroxocobalamin binds tightly to protein and remains in the body three times longer than cyanocobalamin.

At the beginning of treatment of pernicious anaemia, six or more injections are given at 2 or 3 day intervals, to saturate body stores; thereafter maintenance therapy is required. This may consist of one injection every 2 or 3 months or four injections over a period of 2 weeks once each year. Most patients require life-long therapy. Unwanted effects do not occur.

The sole *clinical* use of vitamin B_{12} is for the treatment of deficiency of this substance. As specified under the clinical use of folic acid, above, it is important to determine whether a megaloblastic anaemia is due to a vitamin B_{12} or a folate deficiency.

VITAMIN C

Vitamin C is ascorbic acid. Deficiency of this vitamin leads to *scurvy*, in which there is tenderness and swelling of the joints, tenderness of the gums with loosening of the teeth and, frequently, anaemia. Ascorbic acid is important in the maintenance of the integrity of the intercellular material of skin, cartilage periosteum and bone and for the integrity of the capillary endothelium. It may have a role in the synthesis of collagen. It may also have a role in folate metabolism but its exact role in erythropoiesis is not known. The anaemia of scurvy responds to small doses of vitamin C as do the other manifestations of the scorbutic state.

REFERENCES AND FURTHER READING

Chanarin I et al 1981 How vitamin B_{12} acts. Br J Haematol 47: 487–491
Finch C A, Hueber S H 1982 Perspectives in iron metabolism. N Engl J Med 306: 1520–1528
Hardisty R M, Weatherall D J (eds) 1982 Blood and its disorders. Blackwell Scientific Publications, Oxford Chapter 5

Jacobs A, Worwood M Iron metabolism, deficiency and overload, p 149–197
Chapter 9 Hoffbrand A V Vitamin B_{12} and folate metabolism, p 199–263
Steinberg S E 1984 Mechanisms of folate homeostasis. Amer J Physiol 246: G319–324

The central nervous system

Chemical transmission and drug action in the central nervous system

There are two reasons why understanding the action of drugs on the CNS presents a particularly challenging problem. One is that centrally acting drugs are of special significance to mankind. Not only are they of major clinical and therapeutic importance,* but they include the drugs that human beings most commonly administer to themselves without the intervention of the medical profession (e.g. alcohol, tea and coffee, cannabis, nicotine, opiates, amphetamines, etc). The second reason is that the CNS is functionally far more complex than any other system in the body, and this makes the understanding of drug effects very much more difficult. Thus, the relationship between the behaviour of individual cells, and that of the organ as a whole, is far less direct in the brain than, for example, in the heart or kidney. In these latter organs, a detailed understanding of how a drug affects the cells gives us a fairly clear idea of what effect it will produce on the organ (and on the animal) as a whole. In the brain, this is simply not true. Thus, we may know that a drug mimics the action of serotonin in its effect on nerve cells, and we know empirically that this type of action is often associated with drugs that cause hallucinations, but the link between these two events remains wholly mysterious. In recent years investigation of the cellular and biochemical effects produced by centrally-acting drugs has progressed rapidly, but the gulf between the description of drug action at this level and the description of drug action at the functional and behavioural level remains, for the most part, very wide. Attempts to

bridge it seem, at times, like throwing candy floss into the Grand Canyon. A few bridgeheads have nonetheless been established, some more firmly than others. Thus, the relationship between dopaminergic pathways in the extrapyramidal system and the effects of drugs in alleviating or exacerbating the symptoms of Parkinsonism (see Chapter 24) is clear-cut. Less well established are the postulated connections between hyperactivity in dopaminergic pathways and schizophrenia (see Chapter 22), and between the actions of noradrenaline and serotonin in certain parts of the brain and the symptoms of depression (see Chapter 23). At the other end of the spectrum, attempts to relate the condition of epilepsy to an identifiable cellular disturbance (see Chapter 24) have been very disappointing, even though the abnormal neuronal discharge pattern in epilepsy seems, on the face of it, a much simpler kind of disturbance than, for example, the abnormal perception and behaviour of a schizophrenic patient.

The aim of this chapter is to describe briefly the present state of knowledge about some of the main transmitter systems that are important in the brain, concentrating on those systems which form the basis of reasonably coherent explanations of the effects of centrally-acting drugs. More detailed accounts will be found in textbooks such as Ryall (1979), Palmer (1981), Cooper et al (1982) and Feldman & Quenzer (1984) all of which are recommended. At the end of this chapter a simple classification of the main groups of psychotropic drugs is given.

In the last decade, ideas about transmitter action in the CNS have changed quite radically, particularly in two respects:

1. The number of putative transmitters has

---

* A recent (1977) study of general practitioners prescribing in UK showed that 1 person in 6 was given a prescription for a centrally-acting drug in 1 year. In women aged 45–49 the figure was 1 in 3.

jumped from about ten 'classical' transmitters, mainly monoamines and amino-acids, to 40 or more, with the discovery of a host of neuro-peptides.

2. The concept of what is meant by a neuro-transmitter has broadened considerably. The ori-ginal concept envisaged a substance released by one neuron and acting rapidly, briefly, and at short range on the membrane of an adjacent neuron, producing a change in conductance which either increased or decreased the excitability of the post-synaptic cell. It is now clear that chemical medi-ators within the brain can produce slow and long-lasting effects (over minutes or hours); that they can act rather diffusely, at a considerable distance from their site of release; and that they can produce diverse effects, for example on transmitter synthesis and on the expression of neurotransmitter recep-tors, in addition to affecting the ionic conductance of the post-synaptic cells.

These 'atypical' characteristics have been ascribed mainly to neuropeptides, and the term **'neuromodu-lator'** (**'neuroregulator'** in some texts) has been coined to denote a neuronally-released mediator whose actions do not conform to the conventional (if un-written) view of how a neurotransmitter should act. The term 'neuromodulator' has a nebulous meaning, however, and is in danger of being used indiscriminately to describe any chemical mediator whose actions are ill-understood.

Both of the conceptual developments cited above have come largely through the explosion of new information about neuropeptides, and their impact on the interpretation of how centrally-acting drugs exert their effects is yet to come. The increasing number of putative chemical mediators, and the diversity of the effects ascribed to them (both of which are still in a stage of rapid expansion) have increased enormously the range of potential points of attack for centrally acting drugs, compared with the situation existing during the 'monoamine' period of neuropharmacology. It will take a good many years before this new information can be translated into a better understanding of how drugs produce their effects.

The best that can be done, in this transitional stage, is to present some of the well-established information about monoamines and related trans-mitters in the brain, and to discuss theories of drug action based on these systems, recognizing that a good deal of reappraisal may be needed in the future.

INDIVIDUAL NEUROTRANSMITTERS

The following chemical transmitters will be dis-cussed in this chapter:

1. Noradrenaline
2. Dopamine
3. Serotonin
4. Acetylcholine
5. Amino-acids
   a. γ-aminobutyric acid (GABA)
   b. Glutamate and other excitatory amino acids
6. Neuropeptides
7. Other putative neurotransmitters
   a. Histamine
   b. Purines

NORADRENALINE

Many aspects of noradrenergic transmission have been discussed in Chapter 7. The basic processes responsible for the synthesis, storage, release and reuptake of noradrenaline are the same in the brain as in the periphery, and the same types of adrenergic receptor are found in pre- and post-synaptic locations in the brain. Here we will consider ana-tomical and functional aspects of central noradren-ergic pathways and their possible involvement in different types of mental disorder.

Central noradrenergic pathways

Though the existence of noradrenaline in the brain was demonstrated biochemically in the 1950s, and its transmitter role was suspected, detailed analysis of its neuronal distribution only became possible when the fluorescence technique, based on the formation of a fluorescent derivative of catechol-amines when tissues are exposed to formaldehyde, was devised by Falck & Hillarp. This technique enabled detailed maps of the pathways of noradren-ergic, as well as dopaminergic and serotonergic, neurons to be produced. Very detailed information is available for laboratory animals, such as the rat, and the same basic features have been found in more limited studies of human brains.

The cell bodies of noradrenergic neurons are found exclusively in the pons and medulla, where they form a number of discrete clusters. These rather small clumps of neurons send extensively branching axons to many other parts of the brain (Fig. 19.1) including the cerebral cortex, limbic

on the locus coeruleus button and large areas of the brain are diffusely sprayed with noradrenaline.

Other noradrenergic neurons lie close to the locus coeruleus in the pons and medulla. Axons from these cells run via the **ventral noradrenergic bundle**, and provide a similarly diffuse innervation to the hypothalamus, hippocampus and other parts of the forebrain. The cells also project to the cerebellum

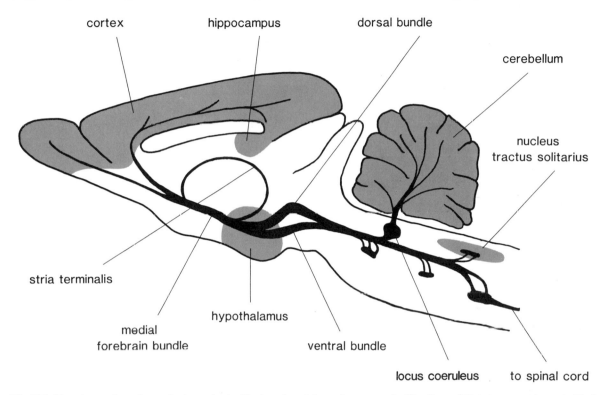

Fig. 19.1 Noradrenergic pathways in the rat brain. The location of the main groups of cell bodies and fibre tracts are shown in black. Grey areas show the location of noradrenergic terminals.

system, hypothalamus, cerebellum and spinal cord. The most prominent cluster of noradrenergic neurons is the **locus coeruleus** which is found in the grey matter of the pons. Although it contains, in the rat, only 1000–2000 neurons, axons from these cells, running in a discrete **dorsal noradrenergic bundle**, give rise to many millions of noradrenergic nerve terminals throughout the cortex, hippocampus and cerebellum. It is an extremely diffuse system, and the nerve terminals do not form close, discrete, synaptic contacts, but appear to release transmitter at some distance from the target cell. These characteristics have caused the noradrenergic system to be likened to a neural aerosol—one press

and spinal cord, and here, too, the terminals form a diffuse network rather than discrete synaptic contacts.

Functional aspects

If noradrenaline is applied by microionophoresis to individual cells in the brain, the effect most often seen is inhibitory, and in most cases it is produced by activation of β-adrenoceptors. Activation of adenylate cyclase with resulting accumulation of cAMP, has been unequivocally demonstrated as the mechanism of action in several types of CNS neuron. In some situations, however, noradrenaline has an excitatory effect, which is mediated by either α- or β-adrenoceptors.

There is still, as mentioned above, a wide gulf between these fairly well-characterized neuronal mechanisms and an understanding of the behavioural and physiological responses in which noradrenergic neurons are believed, on the basis of lesioning studies and drug effects, to participate. The most important of these behavioural and physiological functions are: (a) Reward system and mood; (b) Arousal; and (c) Blood pressure regulation.

Reward system and mood

If electrodes are implanted in the region of the noradrenergic projection from the locus coeruleus to the limbic system and cortex of experimental animals, and the electrodes are connected to a switch which the animal can operate, the animals quickly establish a high rate of self-stimulation. This response is inhibited by drugs that prevent noradrenergic transmission. Studies of this kind have led to the suggestion that the noradrenergic pathways constitute a 'reward' system, though the relationship of this psychological construct to subjective feelings in man is uncertain.

The catecholamine hypothesis of affective disorders, originally formulated by Schildkraut (1965) suggests that **depression** results from a functional deficiency of noradrenaline in certain parts of the brain, while **mania** results from an excess. The evidence is discussed in Chapter 23.

Arousal

Various lines of evidence suggest that activation of noradrenergic pathways can produce behavioural arousal. One is that amphetamine-like drugs, which are known to act by releasing catecholamines in the brain, increase wakefulness, alertness and exploratory activity. Another is that the electrical activity of locus coeruleus neurons in conscious animals is highly responsive to sensory stimuli. Stimuli of an unfamiliar or threatening kind excite these noradrenergic neurons much more effectively than familiar stimuli. Furthermore, there is a close relationship between mood and state of arousal. Depressed patients are usually lethargic and unresponsive to external stimuli; this association of symptons may reflect the dual role of noradrenergic neurons in controlling both mood and arousal.

Blood pressure regulation

The realization that central, as well as peripheral, noradrenergic synapses play a role in blood pressure regulation, comes mainly from investigation of the mechanisms of action of hypotensive drugs such as **clonidine** and **methyldopa** (see Chapter 11), both of which were shown to decrease the discharge of sympathetic nerves emerging from the central nervous system. It was then shown that they cause marked hypotension when injected locally into the vasomotor centres or into the fourth ventricle, in much smaller amounts than are required when the drugs are given systemically. Noradrenaline, injected locally into the region of the vasomotor centres, has a similar effect. Pharmacological studies with agonists and antagonists show that these responses are due to activation of α_2-adrenoceptors, which, on the basis of lesion studies, appear to be located post-synaptically (in contrast to most peripheral α_2-receptors, which are pre-synaptic). Noradrenergic synapses in the medulla probably form part of the baroreceptor reflex pathway (see Fig. 19.2), since stimulation or antagonism of α_2-receptors in this part of the brain has a powerful effect on the activity of baroreceptor reflexes. Thus, clonidine markedly increases the bradycardia and hypotension that occur in response to mechanical distension of the carotid sinus, and α_2-receptor blocking drugs have the opposite effect. Other noradrenergic neurons, apart from those in the baroreceptor reflex arc, are important as well. Ascending fibres run to the hypothalamus, and descending fibres run to the lateral horn region of the spinal cord, acting to increase sympathetic discharge in the periphery. Noradrenergic transmission does not actually form an essential link in the baroreceptor reflex pathway, since the reflex still occurs when noradrenergic transmission is prevented; nevertheless, noradrenergic neurons greatly influence the activity of the reflex, presumably by forming synaptic connections on neurons in the pathway (Fig. 19.2). These noradrenergic regulatory neurons probably originate in one or more of the groups of noradrenergic neurons in the pons and medulla;

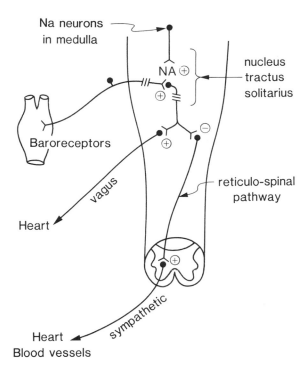

Fig. 19.2 Simplified diagram of pathways in the medulla involved in the central regulation of blood pressure. Interruptions indicate the existence of polyneuronal pathways.

there is evidence that a similar type of regulation also occurs in the spinal cord. It has recently been suggested that these regulatory neurons may release *adrenaline*, rather than noradrenaline. Some catecholamine containing cells in the brainstem contain PNMT (the enzyme that converts noradrenaline to adrenaline; see Chapter 7) and inhibition of this enzyme appears to prevent the normal regulation of the baroreceptor reflex. Attention is currently being given to this mechanism as a possible factor in the aetiology of hypertension.

DOPAMINE

Appreciation of the role of dopamine in the brain, as a transmitter in its own right and not merely as a precursor of noradrenaline, came in the mid-1960s, during a remarkable decade of progress—the 'monoamine years'—when a combination of neurochemistry and neuropharmacology led to many important discoveries about the role of CNS transmitters, and about the ability of drugs to

influence these systems. It was found that the distribution of dopamine in the brain is highly non-uniform, and more restricted than the distribution of noradrenaline. A large proportion of the dopamine content of the brain is found in the **corpus striatum**, a part of the extrapyramidal motor system concerned with the co-ordination of movement (see Chapter 24), and there is also a high concentration in certain parts of the **limbic system**.

The synthesis of dopamine follows the same route as that of noradrenaline (see Chapter 7), namely conversion of tyrosine to dopa (the rate-limited step, catalysed by tyrosine hydroxylase) followed by decarboxylation (catalysed by dopa decarboxylase). Dopaminergic neurons lack dopamine β-hydroxylase, and thus do not produce noradrenaline.

Dopamine is largely recaptured, following its release from nerve terminals, by a mechanism very similar to uptake 1 for noradrenaline (see Chapter 7), and is metabolized by MAO and COMT, the pathways being exactly analogous to those for noradrenaline (Fig. 19.3). The main products are **dihydroxyphenylacetic acid (DOPAC)** which is formed by oxidative deamination (MAO) followed by enzymic oxidation of the resulting aldehyde, and **homovanillic acid (HVA)** the methoxy-derivative of DOPAC, formed by the action of COMT. These substances are present in the brain, and the content of HVA is often used as an index of **dopamine turnover**. Drugs that cause the release of dopamine increase HVA concentration, often without changing the dopamine concentration. DOPAC and HVA, and their sulphate conjugates, are excreted in the urine, which provides another index of dopamine release that can be used in human subjects.

Dopamine pathways in the CNS

The mapping studies of Dahlstrom & Fuxe in 1965, based on fluorescence staining, showed that dopaminergic neurons form three main systems (Fig. 19.4). The main system, accounting for about 75% of the dopamine in the brain, is the **nigrostriatal pathway**, whose cell bodies lie in the **substantia nigra** (forming the A9 cell group) and whose axons terminate in the **corpus striatum**. These fibres run in the medial forebrain bundle along with many nor-

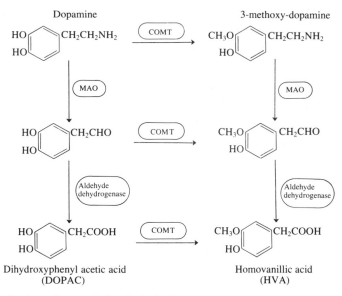

Fig. 19.3 The main pathways for dopamine metabolism in the brain. MAO—monoamine oxidase; COMT—catechol-O-methyl transferase.

adrenergic and serotoninergic fibres. The second important system is the **mesolimbic pathway**, whose cell bodies lie in various groups in the midbrain (mainly the A10 cell group) and whose fibres pro-

ject, also via the medial forebrain bundle, to parts of the limbic system, especially the nucleus accumbens.

Finally, the **tuberoinfundibular system** is a group

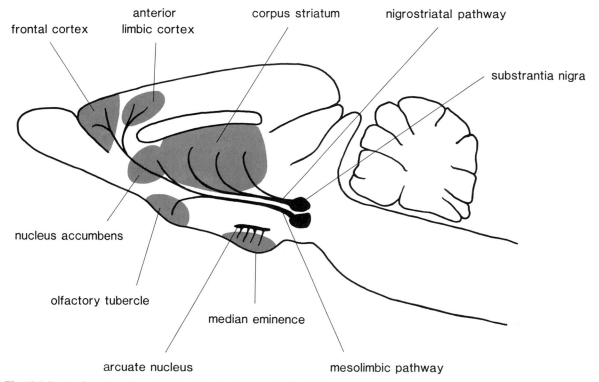

Fig. 19.4 Dopaminergic pathways in the rat brain, drawn as in Fig. 19.1.

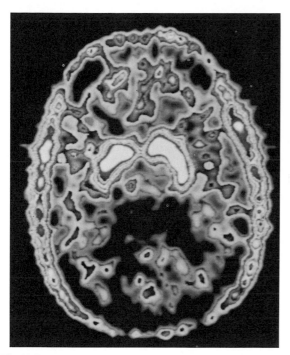

Fig. 19.5 Dopamine in the basal ganglia of a human subject. The subject was injected with 5-fluoro-dopa, labeled with the positron-emitting isotope ^{18}F, which was localized 3 hours later by the technique of positron emission tomography. White areas are regions of maximum radioactivity. The isotope is accumulated by the dopa uptake system of the neurons of the basal ganglia, and to a smaller extent in the frontal cortex. It is also seen in the scalp and temporalis muscles. (From: Garnett et al, 1983)

of short neurons running from the arcuate nucleus of the hypothalamus to the median eminence and pituitary gland, whose secretion they regulate.

The abundance of dopamine-containing neurons in the human striatum can be appreciated from the remarkable image shown in Figure 19.5 which was obtained by injecting a dopa derivative containing radioactive fluorine, and scanning with a computerized detection system to display the distribution of radio-activity in the brain 3 hours later.

Dopamine receptors in the CNS

There is strong evidence for the existence of more than one type of dopamine receptor in the central nervous system, as in the periphery (see Chapter 11), but little agreement on the correct basis on which to make the classification. The scheme proposed by Kebabian & Calne (see Table 11.3) provides a useful basis, but may well be an oversim-

plification. This scheme suggests that two types of receptor, D_1 and D_2, can be distinguished, D_1 being linked to activation of adenylate cyclases, while D_2 is responsible for most of the excitatory post-synaptic effects of dopamine. The antipsychotic effects of drugs that act on dopamine receptors appear to be correlated with their action on D_2-receptors, which can be labelled selectively with dopamine antagonists such as spiroperidol.

Dopamine, like many other transmitters and modulators, acts pre-synaptically, as well as post-synaptically. Pre-synaptic dopamine receptors occur mainly on dopaminergic neurons, for example those in the striatum and limbic system, where they act to inhibit dopamine release. Dopamine antagonists, by blocking these receptors, increase dopamine release, and cause accumulation of dopamine metabolites in these parts of the brain. There are reports of pharmacological differences between pre- and post-synaptic receptors, and the pre-synaptic receptors possibly represent a third category, D_3 (Offermeier & van Rooyen, 1982). The functional role of D_1 receptors in the brain is not clear at present, though recent work on the retina has shown that dopamine, acting through adenylate cyclase, causes an uncoupling of electrically-conducting junctions between adjacent horizontal cells, thus restricting the interaction between them (Watling, 1983). It is too early to say whether similar mechanisms operate elsewhere in the CNS.

Functional aspects

The functions of dopaminergic pathways are rather better understood than those of pathways involving other transmitters. This is partly because selective agonists and antagonists are available for dopamine receptors, and partly because dopaminergic neurons can be selectively destroyed by local injection of 6-hydroxydopamine (see Chapter 7) into small areas of the brain.

Dopamine and motor systems

Ungerstedt showed, in 1968, that bilateral destruction of the substantia nigra in rats, which destroys the nigrostriatal neurons, causes profound catalepsy, the animals becoming so inactive that they die of starvation unless artificially fed. Unilateral lesions produced by 6-hydroxydopamine injection caused the animal to turn in circles *towards* the lesioned side. There is evidence that this abnormal locomotion results from an unequal action of dopamine in the corpus striatum on the two sides of the brain. Thus, unilateral injection of apomorphine (a dopamine-like agonist) into the striatum causes circling *away from* the injected side. If apomorphine is given systemically to normal rats it causes, as one would expect, no asymmetrical pattern of locomotion, but if given systemically to animals with unilateral substantia nigra lesions made days or weeks earlier, apomorphine causes circling away from the lesioned side. This is thought to be due to denervation supersensitivity (see Chapter 5) which arises because the destruction of dopaminergic terminals on one side causes a proliferation of dopamine receptors, and hence supersensitivity to apomorphine, in the cells on that side of the striatum. In these animals, administration of drugs that act by *releasing* dopamine (e.g. amphetamine) cause turning *towards* the lesioned side, since the dopaminergic nerve terminals are only present on the normal side. This 'turning model' has been extremely useful in investigating the action of drugs on dopaminergic neurons and dopamine receptors (Ungerstedt, 1971).

Parkinson's disease (discussed in more detail in Chapter 24) is a progressive motor disturbance that occurs mainly in elderly patients, whose main symptoms are **rigidity** and **tremor**, together with extreme slowness in initiating voluntary movements (**hypokinesia**). It is known to be associated with a deficiency of dopamine in the nigro-striatal pathway. **Huntington's chorea**, an inherited disease that results in severe involuntary movements, may be the pathological opposite of Parkinsonism, in which the symptoms are associated with an excess, rather than a deficit, of dopamine (see Chapter 24).

Behavioural effects

Administration of amphetamine to rats, which releases both dopamine and noradrenaline, causes a cessation of normal 'ratty' behaviour (exploration and grooming) and the appearance of repeated 'stereotyped' behaviour (rearing, gnawing, etc) unrelated to external stimuli. These effects are prevented by dopamine antagonists, and by destruction of dopamine-containing cell bodies in the midbrain, but not by drugs that inhibit the noradrenergic system. These amphetamine-induced motor disturbances in rats probably reflect hyperactivity in the nigro-striatal dopaminergic system (A9 cell group; see Fig. 19.4) since they are abolished by lesions in this area.

Amphetamine also causes a general increase in motor activity, which can be measured, for example, by counting electronically the frequency at which a rat crosses from one part of its enclosure to another. This effect, in contrast to stereotypy, appears to be related to the mesolimbic dopaminergic pathway originating from the A10 cell group (see Fig. 19.4). There is strong evidence (see Chapter 22) that schizophrenia in man is associated with dopaminergic hyperactivity, and many attempts have been made to detect behavioural effects of dopamine in animals that might be related to the symptoms of human schizophrenia. It has been found that chronic administration of amphetamine to a few rats in a large colony produces various types of abnormal social interaction, including withdrawal and aggressive behaviour, but it is extremely difficult to quantify such effects or to establish their relationship to schizophrenia in man.

Dopamine and the anterior pituitary gland

The tuberoinfundibular dopaminergic pathway (see Fig. 19.4) is involved in the control of **prolactin** secretion. The hypothalamus secretes various mediators (mostly small peptides; see Chapter 16) which control the secretion of different hormones from the pituitary gland. One of these, which has an inhibitory effect on prolactin release, is dopamine. This system is of considerable clinical importance. It was observed many years ago that **ergot derivatives** (see Chapter 7) tend to suppress lactation, whereas antipsychotic drugs (see Chapter 22) have the opposite effect, even to the point of causing breast development and lactation in males. These effects were subsequently found to be due to changes in prolactin secretion, and studies on isolated pituitary glands confirmed that dopamine and related agonists strongly inhibit prolactin secretion, an effect that is abolished by many antipsychotic drugs, which block dopamine receptors. One dopamine receptor agonist, **bromocriptine**, derived from ergot, is used clinically to suppress prolactin secretion by tumours of the pituitary gland.

Another hormone whose secretion is regulated

by dopamine is **growth hormone**. In normal subjects dopamine receptor activation increases growth hormone secretion, but it paradoxically inhibits the excessive secretion responsible for acromegaly, a condition in which bromocriptine has a useful therapeutic effect, provided that it is given before the excessive growth has taken place (see Chapter 16).

Vomiting

Pharmacological evidence strongly suggests that dopaminergic neurons have a role in the production of nausea and vomiting (see Chapter 15). Thus, nearly all dopamine receptor agonists (e.g. bromocriptine) and other drugs which increase dopamine release in the brain (e.g. levodopa; see Chapter 24), cause nausea and vomiting as side effects, while many dopamine antagonists (e.g. **phenothiazines**, Chapter 22; **metoclopramide**, Chapter 15) have anti-emetic activity. The neural pathways are not well understood, however, and there are several effective anti-emetic drugs (e.g. hyoscine, Chapter 6; antihistamines, Chapter 8) which are not dopamine antagonists.

SEROTONIN

The occurrence and functions of serotonin in the periphery are described in Chapters 5 & 11. Interest in serotonin as a possible CNS transmitter dates from 1953, when Gaddum found that **lysergic acid diethylamide (LSD)**, a drug known to be a powerful hallucinogen, acted as a serotonin antagonist in peripheral tissues, and suggested that its central effects might also be related to this action. Its presence in the brain was demonstrated a few years later. Even though brain serotonin accounts for only about 1% of the total body content, it occupies a central position in the neurochemical hegemony (Jacobs & Gelperin, 1981; Osborne, 1982).

The formation, storage and release of serotonin (see Fig. 11.2) are very similar to those of noradrenaline. The precursor substance is **tryptophan**, an amino-acid derived from dietary protein, the plasma content of which varies considerably according to food intake and time of day. Tryptophan is taken up into neurons by an active transport process, converted by tryptophan hydroxylase to **5-hydroxytryptophan** and then decarboxylated by a non-specific amino-acid decarboxylase to serotonin. Tryptophan hydroxylase is the rate limiting enzyme, and can be selectively and irreversibly inhibited by **p-chlorophenylalanine (PCPA)**. It is at the tryptophan hydroxylase step that physiological regulation of serotonin synthesis occurs. The decarboxylase is very similar, if not identical, to DOPA decarboxylase, and does not seem to play any role in regulating serotonin synthesis. Following release, serotonin is largely recovered by neuronal uptake, this mechanism being inhibited by many of the same drugs (e.g. tricyclic antidepressants) that inhibit catecholamine uptake. The carrier is not identical, however, and inhibitors show some specificity between the two systems (see Chapter 23). Serotonin is degraded almost entirely by MAO (see Fig. 11.2), which converts it to 5-hydroxyindoleacetaldehyde, most of which is dehydrogenated to form 5-hydroxyindoleacetic acid (5HIAA) which is excreted in the urine.

Central serotonin pathways

Mapping of serotonin-containing neurons has been carried out by techniques similar to those used for noradrenergic neurons, namely fluorescence histochemistry, immunofluorescent labelling of specific enzymes (tryptophan hydroxylase) and the observation of specific markers that are taken up by nerve terminals or cell bodies and transported to other parts of the neuron. The distribution of serotonin-containing neurons (Fig. 19.6) is very similar to that of noradrenergic neurons, and quite different from that of dopamine-containing neurons. The cells occur in several large clusters in the pons and upper medulla, which lie close to the midline (raphe) and are often referred to as **raphe nuclei**. The rostrally-situated nuclei project, via the median forebrain bundle, which also contains many noradrenergic fibres, in a diffuse way to many parts of the cortex, hippocampus, limbic system and hypothalamus, the whole arrangement being very similar to that of the noradrenergic system. The caudally-situated cells project to the medulla and spinal cord.

Functional aspects

Many studies on the effects of serotonin and related

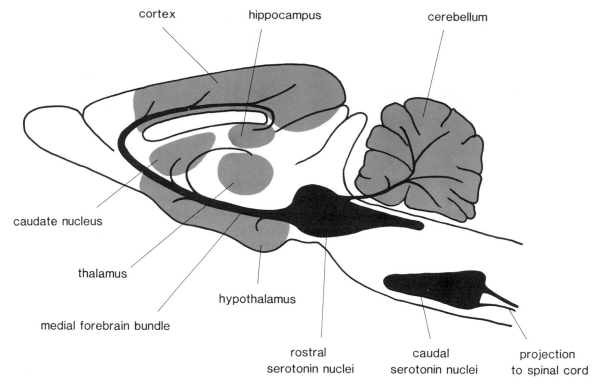

Fig. 19.6 Serotonin pathways in the rat brain, drawn as in Fig. 19.1.

compounds on individual neurons have shown that it can interact with at least two types of receptor (up to six according to some authors) and elicit many different kinds of response. The main types of response reported in vertebrate CNS neurons are:

1. Post-synaptic excitation, which may be fast or slow, and may act either to cause depolarization directly or to facilitate the depolarizing effect of excitatory synaptic inputs
2. Post-synaptic inhibition
3. Pre-synaptic inhibition, affecting both serotoninergic terminals and terminals releasing other transmitters.

The pharmacological classification of the receptors producing these varied effects is not completely clear, though there is reasonable correspondence between the two receptor types (designated $5HT_1$ and $5HT_2$) that have been described in the brain, and two of the three types that have been recognized in peripheral tissues (see Table 11.2). The two receptor types in the brain have been distinguished mainly on the basis of binding studies (Table 11.2),

$5HT_1$ receptors having a high affinity for serotonin itself, but a low affinity for most antagonists, whereas $5HT_2$ receptors bind a variety of antagonists (e.g. **ketanserin**) at much higher affinity than serotonin. It appears that $5HT_1$ receptors are located on pre-synaptic nerve terminals in both the central and peripheral nervous systems, and act to inhibit the release of transmitters, including serotonin itself. $5HT_2$ receptors are located post-synaptically, and may be excitatory or inhibitory. They are equivalent to the D receptors originally described by Gaddum (see Table 11.2), and probably responsible for many of the central effects of serotonin, including its behavioural effects, and its inhibitory effect on transmission through the nociceptive afferent pathways (see Chapter 25). A detailed correlation of the various functional effects of serotonin in the brain with individual receptor types is, however, still not possible.

In vertebrates, the main physiological and behavioural functions that are believed to involve serotonin pathways are: (a) sleep, wakefulness and mood; (b) control of motoneuron excitability; (c)

control of sensory transmission; and (d) autonomic and endocrine function.

Sleep, wakefulness and mood

Lesions of the raphe nuclei, or depletion of serotonin by PCPA administration, abolish sleep in experimental animals, whereas micro-injection of serotonin at specific points in the brainstem induces sleep. Attempts to cure insomnia in man by giving serotonin precursors (tryptophan or 5-hydroxytryptophan) have, however, proved unsuccessful. There is evidence that serotonin, as well as noradrenaline, may be involved in the control of mood (see Chapter 23), and the use of tryptophan to enhance serotonin synthesis has been tried in depression, with equivocal results.

Control of motoneuron excitability

Motoneuron excitability is increased by the influence of descending serotoninergic neurons, which thereby increase monosynaptic reflexes. Conversely, polysynaptic reflexes are inhibited, and the threshold for drug or stimulation-induced convulsions is increased by lesions to these serotoninergic pathways or by drugs that block serotonin synthesis.

Sensory transmission

After lesions of the raphe nuclei, or administration of PCPA, animals show exaggerated responses to many forms of sensory stimulus. They are startled much more easily, and also quickly develop avoidance responses to stimuli that would not normally produce this effect. It appears that the normal ability to disregard irrelevant forms of sensory input requires intact serotonin pathways. The 'sensory enhancement' produced by various hallucinogenic drugs (e.g. LSD; see Chapter 26) may be due to antagonism of serotonin.

Serotonin also exerts an inhibitory effect on transmission in the pain pathway, both in the spinal cord and in the brain, and there is a synergistic effect between serotonin and analgesics such as morphine (see Chapter 25). Thus depletion of serotonin by PCPA, or selective lesions to the descending serotonin-containing neurons that run to the dorsal horn, antagonize the analgesic effect of morphine, while serotonin uptake inhibitors have the opposite effect. Serotonin is also thought to be an inhibitory transmitter in the retina. These effects, on nociception and retinal function, may be an aspect of the more general inhibitory effect of serotonin on sensory input (see above).

Autonomic and endocrine function

There is evidence for a role of serotonin in temperature regulation. The hypothalamus, which coordinates the physiological responses that control body temperature, is rich in serotonin-containing nerve terminals, and local injection of serotonin causes, in cats and monkeys, a sharp rise in temperature. A cold environment increases serotonin release in this region, and PCPA interferes with the heat-conserving response to a cold environment. The secretion of various anterior pituitary hormones is affected by serotonin-containing neurons in the hypothalamus. These neurons appear to inhibit the production of the hypothalamic factors that control secretion from the anterior pituitary gland. They therefore inhibit the secretion of hormones, such as gonadotrophins, whose release is enhanced by hypothalamic factors, and increase the secretion of those (e.g. growth hormone) that are normally held in check by the hypothalamus (see Chapter 16).

It will be realized that serotonin is involved in many very important physiological processes, and there would seem to be scope for producing useful therapeutic effects with drugs that influence serotoninergic transmission in a selective way. Such drugs are beginning to appear, but their range and specificity are still very limited in comparison to the many drugs that affect catecholamine transmission.

ACETYLCHOLINE

There are numerous cholinergic neurons in the central nervous system, and the basic processes by which acetylcholine is synthesized, stored and released are apparently the same as in the periphery (see Chapter 6). Various biochemical markers have been used to locate cholinergic neurons in the brain, including choline acetyltransferase (CAT), acetylcholinesterase, high affinity choline uptake and acetylcholine receptor labelling. Acetylcholine itself cannot be made visible by histochemical techniques. Acetylcholinesterase can readily be stained, but its distribution is widespread and not specific to cholinergic pathways. Recently, monoclonal antibodies to CAT have been used for immunofluorescent staining, and this provides a very useful method for labelling cholinergic neurons. Biochemical studies on acetylcholine precursors and metabolites are also more difficult than corresponding studies on other amine transmitters, because the relevant substances, choline and acetate, are less distinctive biochemically, and involved in many processes other than acetylcholine metabolism. Furthermore, the widespread distribution of cholinergic neurons limits the usefulness of surgical lesioning techniques, and no chemical agents have so far been discovered that are able to damage cholinergic neurons selectively.

Central cholinergic pathways

Acetylcholine is very widely distributed in the brain, occurring in all parts of the forebrain (including the cortex), midbrain and brainstem, though there is rather little in the cerebellum. Some of the main cholinergic pathways in the brain (see Pepeu, 1983) are shown in Figure 19.7. The anterior horns and roots of the spinal cord, and the motor nuclei of the cranial nerves contain about five times as much acetylcholine as other parts of the CNS, reflecting the presence of cholinergic motoneurons supplying skeletal muscle. In the rat, there is a diffuse cholinergic innervation supplying all areas of the forebrain, and the cell bodies of these cholinergic neurons lie in a small area of the basal forebrain, forming the **magnocellular forebrain nuclei** (so-called because the cell bodies are conspicuously large). Other groups of cholinergic neurons occur in the septum, from which the septo-hippocampal projection arises, and in the pons, from which fibres run to the thalamus and cortex (Fig. 19.7).

Short cholinergic interneurons are also found in the striatum and in the nucleus accumbens (two areas where dopaminergic neurons are important). The role of the striatal cholinergic neurons in

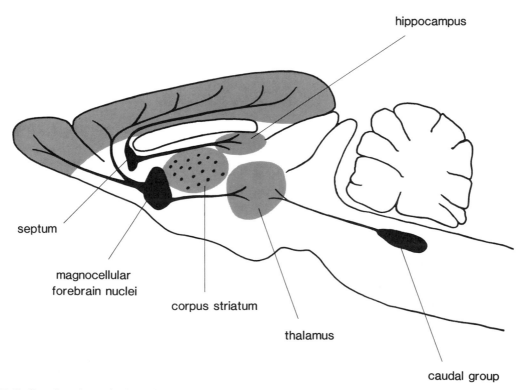

Fig. 19.7 Cholinergic pathways in the rat brain, drawn as in Fig. 19.1.

connection with Parkinsonism and Huntington's chorea is discussed in Chapter 24.

Acetylcholine receptors in the brain

The effect of acetylcholine on individual neurons is usually excitatory, and may be mediated by either nicotinic or muscarinic receptors. Some neurons show an inhibitory response, mediated by muscarinic receptors.

The muscarinic receptors in the brain are very similar in their pharmacological properties to those elsewhere, and it is believed that the central actions of muscarinic antagonists and anticholinesterases depend on block and stimulation of these receptors respectively. Muscarinic receptors act pre-synaptically to inhibit acetylcholine release from cholinergic neurons, and muscarinic antagonists, by blocking this inhibition, markedly increase acetylcholine release. Most of the behavioural effects associated with cholinergic pathways seem to be produced by acetylcholine acting on muscarinic, rather than nicotinic receptors.

Very little is known about nicotinic receptors in the brain, though they are known to exist. They probably mediate the effects of nicotine itself (see Chapter 35). Many of the drugs that block nicotinic receptors (e.g. tubocurarine; see Chapter 6) do not cross the blood-brain barrier, and even those that do (e.g. mecamylamine) produce no major CNS side effects.

Functional aspects

The first cholinergic synapse to be investigated in the CNS was that of the **Renshaw cell** in the ventral horn of the spinal cord. These small interneurons receive an excitatory cholinergic innervation from a branch of the axon of the motoneuron. This synapse works through nicotinic receptors, and its pharmacological properties are very similar to those of the neuromuscular junction (see Chapter 6). The Renshaw cell in turn activates interneurons which form inhibitory synaptic connections with motoneurons.

Other functional characteristics of cholinergic pathways have been deduced mainly from studies of the action of drugs that mimic, accentuate or block the actions of acetylcholine on muscarinic

receptors, so the evidence tends to be indirect and circumstantial.

The main functions ascribed to cholinergic pathways are related to (a) arousal and learning, and (b) motor control.

Electroencephalographic (EEG) recording has often been used to monitor the state of arousal in man or in experimental animals. A drowsy, inattentive state is associated with a large amplitude, low frequency EEG record, which switches to a low amplitude, high frequency pattern on arousal by any sensory stimulus (Fig. 19.8). Administration of **physostigmine** (an anticholinesterase which crosses the blood-brain barrier) produces EEG arousal, whereas **atropine** has the opposite effect. It is presumed that the cholinergic projection from the ventral forebrain to the cortex mediates this response. The relationship of this response to behaviour is confusing, however, for the EEG changes produced by physostigmine are the same as those produced by amphetamine, whereas the behavioural effects are not. Thus physostigmine in man causes a state of lethargy and anxiety, and in rats it depresses exploratory activity, whereas amphetamine has the opposite effects. Furthermore, atropine

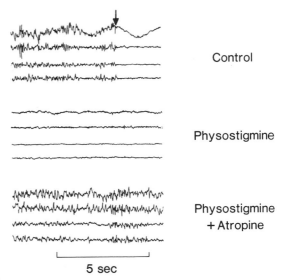

Fig. 19.8 The effect of physostigmine and atropine on EEG activity in a conscious cat. *Top.* Normal resting EEG, with a sudden cessation of slow wave activity (the arousal response) following a sharp sound (↓). *Centre.* After physostigmine, showing the arousal pattern throughout. *Bottom.* After atropine, which antagonizes the effect of neostigmine, re-establishing the resting EEG pattern. (From: Bradley & Elkes, 1957)

causes excitement and agitation, and increases exploratory activity in rats.

The evidence that cholinergic pathways are involved in learning and short-term memory is also mainly pharmacological, though experiments involving lesioning and stimulation of the septo-hippocampal pathway have lent support to the idea that cholinergic neurons in this region play an important role. Several studies have shown that hyoscine impairs memory in human subjects, and amnesia is a well-documented effect of hyoscine used as pre-anaesthetic medication in clinical practice. Hyoscine also impairs the ability of experimental animals to learn to press a bar in response to specific visual stimuli. It is notable that most of these positive results have been obtained with hyoscine, and that atropine in similar studies has often been found to have no effect. Some studies have also shown improvement of learning by anticholinesterase drugs or muscarinic agonists, such as **arecoline**, which enter the brain, but this finding has not been universal, and in several studies in man it has been found that the state of lethargy, nausea and general misery produced by physostigmine adversely affects learning.

Senile dementia and Alzheimer's disease

Senile dementia, a slowly progressive loss of intellectual ability, occurs in about 5% of the population over the age of 65 and 20% over 80. **Alzheimer's disease** or **presenile dementia** (Reisberg, 1983) is a pathologically identical syndrome occurring in younger patients; from a functional point of view there is no reason to distinguish the two conditions.

Dementia is associated with a general shrinkage of brain tissue, but with relatively little loss of cortical neurons. The microscopic features (**plaques of degenerating nerve terminals** mainly in the cortex, and **neurofibrillary tangles** occurring in the cell bodies of the cortex and hippocampus) are characteristic of the disease. Though changes in many transmitter systems have been demonstrated, mainly from measurements on post-mortem brain tissue, a relatively selective loss of cholinergic neurons is characteristic. Thus CAT activity in the cortex and hippocampus is reduced considerably (30–70%) in senile dementia, but not in other psychological disorders, such as depression or

schizophrenia, and acetylcholinesterase activity is also greatly reduced (Reisberg, 1983). The number of muscarinic receptors, determined by binding studies, is not affected.

This relatively selective loss of cholinergic neurons in dementia has led to attempts to treat it by using the strategy that was successful for Parkinsonism (see Chapter 24), namely administration of a precursor of the missing transmitter (Fovall et al, 1983; Pomara et al, 1983). Various clinical trials of the use of **choline** and **lecithin** (a choline-containing phospholipid) in doses of several grams per day, for treating dementia have been reported. Most have been discouraging, though in two studies apparent improvement in about one-third of the patients treated with lecithin was reported. The biochemical basis for expecting this treatment to increase acetylcholine release is far from clear, and a more rational approach, since the muscarinic receptors appear to remain, might be to use centrally-acting muscarinic agonists in conjunction with a peripherally-acting antagonist to avoid parasympathetic side effects.

The intrinsic cholinergic neurons of the corpus striatum (which has the highest content of ACh, CAT and AChE in the brain) are involved in the disease processes that lead to Parkinsonism and Huntington's chorea. ACh release from the striatum is strongly inhibited by dopamine, and it is suggested that hyperactivity of these cholinergic neurons (associated with a lack of dopamine) leads to hypokinesia, rigidity and tremor (characteristic of Parkinsonism) whereas hypoactivity (associated with a surfeit of dopamine, secondary to a deficiency of GABA) results in hyperkinetic movements and hypotonia (characteristic of Huntington's chorea). The use of muscarinic antagonists in the treatment of Parkinsonism, and of anticholinesterase drugs in the treatment of Huntington's chorea fits in with this general scheme. Up to a point, redressing the balance between the dopaminergic and cholinergic neurons appears to be able to compensate for an overall deficit or surfeit of dopaminergic function.

AMINO-ACID TRANSMITTERS

There is now very strong evidence that three amino-acids, **γ-aminobutyric acid (GABA)**, **glycine** and

glutamate, function as neurotransmitters in the central nervous system, and it is quite likely that others do as well. It has been much more difficult to obtain convincing evidence for the transmitter role of these substances than for monoamines, and there are still substantial gaps in the evidence, particularly in the case of glutamate. The difficulty in providing clear evidence stems partly from the fact that amino-acids are biochemically involved in many metabolic pathways, so that it is not easy to distinguish a putative transmitter pool from other metabolic pools. Furthermore, enzymes that synthesize and destroy amino-acids are found in many cells and are not specific to transmitter-synthesizing neurons. One particular difficulty in the central nervous system is that glial cells, as well as neurons, often take up and release amino-acids, and this confuses attempts to measure neuronal release.

There is unequivocal evidence that glutamate and GABA function as excitatory and inhibitory transmitters at the neuromuscular junction of various insects and crustacea, where the release has been measured directly, and the post-synaptic action of these substances has been shown to mimic exactly the action of the endogenous transmitter. This finding obviously lends support to the idea that they might have similar functions in the mammalian brain, but it is only recently, mainly through studies of the action of antagonists of these amino-acids on transmission at certain well defined synapses, that this has received strong experimental support.

The main amino-acids with a claim to neurotransmitter status are shown in Table 19.1.

GABA

GABA occurs in brain tissue, but not in other mammalian tissues, except in trace amounts. In the brain it is particularly abundant (about $10\,\mu\text{mol/g}$ tissue) in the nigro-striatal system, but occurs at lower concentrations ($2-5\,\mu\text{mol/g}$) throughout the grey matter.

GABA is formed from glutamate (Fig. 19.9) by the action of glutamic acid decarboxylase (GAD), an enzyme which has been used, with immunohistochemical labelling, to map the distribution of GABA-synthesizing neurons in the brain. GABA is destroyed by a transamination reaction, in which the

Table 19.1 Amino-acid transmitters

Substance		Action	Transmitter role
GABA		Inhibitory	Definite
Glycine		Inhibitory	Definite
β-alanine		Inhibitory	Possible
Glutamate		Excitatory	Definite
Aspartate		Excitatory	Probable
Cysteine		Excitatory	Possible

amino group is transferred to α-oxoglutaric acid (to yield glutamate), with the production of succinic semialdehyde, and then succinic acid. This reaction is catalysed by GABA-transaminase (GABA-T), a widespread enzyme believed to be located in mitochondria. GABA-ergic neurons have an active GABA uptake system, and it is this, rather than GABA-T, which removes the GABA after it has been released.

GABA is thought to function as an inhibitory transmitter in many different CNS pathways. The most detailed studies have been carried out on the cerebellum, cerebral cortex, hippocampus and striatum (see earlier section). In most situations GABA is found in short interneurons, the only long GABA-ergic tracts being those running to the cerebellum and striatum. The widespread distribution of GABA, and the fact that virtually all neurons are sensitive to its inhibitory effect, suggest that its function is ubiquitous in the brain.

GABA receptors

Two distinct types of GABA receptor are recognized in vertebrates, known as GABA_A and GABA_B respectively (see review: Simmonds, 1983). The GABA_A receptor resembles, but is not identical with, the inhibitory GABA receptor of invertebrates.

Electrophysiological studies of the action of GABA on CNS neurons have shown that its post-synaptic inhibitory effect depends on an increase in chloride permeability of the post-synaptic membrane, which has the effect of reducing the depolarization produced by excitatory transmitter action. GABA also exerts a pre-synaptic inhibitory effect on pre-synaptic nerve terminals at many sites in the brain and peripheral nervous system (e.g. dopamine-releasing terminals of the striatum, peripheral sympathetic terminals, etc). It was thought likely that a GABA-like substance might prove to be effective in controlling epilepsy and other convulsive states, and since GABA itself fails to penetrate the blood-barrier, a search was begun for more lipophilic GABA analogues. One such substance is the p-chlorophenyl derivative of GABA (**baclofen**; see Bowery, 1982) which was introduced in 1972. When detailed comparisons of the actions of GABA and baclofen were made, however, some important differences became evident. Baclofen, like GABA, inhibits the release of transmitter from many types of nerve terminal, but, unlike GABA, has little post-synaptic inhibitory effect. Furthermore, the post-synaptic inhibitory effect of GABA is blocked competitively by the convulsant drug, **bicuculline**, but the actions of baclofen are not antagonized. Other GABA-like substances (e.g. **muscimol**) produce the post-synaptic bicuculline-sensitive effects of GABA, but not the pre-synaptic, bicuculline-resistant effects. The former effects are thus associated with GABA$_A$ receptors, and the latter with GABA$_B$ receptors (Table 19.2). The ionic mechanism underlying the GABA$_B$ effects is still uncertain, though recent studies have shown that these receptors, in some neurons, act to inhibit a voltage-sensitive calcium channel, which may well account for the reduction of transmitter release.

Evidence of a physiological role of GABA$_B$ receptors in the brain is still lacking, and is likely to remain so until selective GABA$_B$ antagonists are developed.

A remarkable relationship exists between GABA$_A$ receptors and the actions of the **benzodiazepine** group of drugs, which have powerful sedative and anxiolytic effects (see Chapter 21). These drugs selectively potentiate the effects of GABA on GABA$_A$ receptors, and there is evidence that they bind with high affinity to an accessory site on the GABA$_A$ receptor, in such a way that the binding of GABA is facilitated and its pharmacological activity is enhanced. It is interesting that GABA$_A$ receptors occur in a variety of peripheral neurons (e.g. autonomic ganglion cells) where GABA has no transmitter role; at these sites, however, there is no potentiating effect of benzodiazepines. Certain **barbiturates** (see Chapter 21) also potentiate GABA$_A$ effects, but they are much less selective than benzodiazepines, and the relevance of this phenomenon to their overall depressant actions on the nervous system is uncertain.

Glycine

This amino-acid is present in particularly high concentration (5 µmol/g) in the grey matter of the

Table 19.2 Classification of GABA receptors

	Receptor type	
	GABA$_A$	GABA$_B$
Effects	Post-synaptic inhibition ↑ chloride conductance	Pre-synaptic inhibition ?.↓ calcium conductance
Agonists		
GABA	+	+
Baclofen	−	+
Muscimol	+	−
Antagonists		
Bicuculline	Competitive	−
Picrotoxin	Non-competitive	−
Potentiators		
Benzodiazepines	+	−
Barbiturates	+	−

spinal cord. Applied ionophoretically to moto-neurons or interneurons it produces an inhibitory hyperpolarization that is indistinguishable from the inhibitory synaptic response. Most significantly, **strychnine** (see Chapter 26), a convulsant drug that acts mainly on the spinal cord, blocks the synaptic inhibitory response and the response to glycine. This, together with direct measurements of glycine release in response to nerve stimulation, provides strong evidence for its physiological transmitter role.

β-alanine has pharmacological effects, and a pattern of distribution, very similar to glycine, but its action is not blocked by strychnine.

EXCITATORY AMINO-ACIDS

L-glutamate and **L-aspartate** (see Table 19.1) are naturally occurring excitatory amino-acids. Synthetic derivatives with similar actions include **N-methyl-D-aspartate (NMDA)** and **quisqualate**.

Glutamate, like GABA, is widely and fairly uni-formly distributed in the CNS, and virtually all neurons seem to respond to it by depolarization and excitation (Nistri, 1983). It has an important metabolic role, being involved in both carbohydrate and nitrogen metabolism, and the transaminase enzymes which catalyse the interconversion of glutamate and α-oxoglutarate (Fig. 19.9) are by no means confined to neurons. Glutamate is released from brain tissue by electrical stimulation or by potassium-evoked depolarization, but it is not clear that this shows the dependence on extracellular calcium that is characteristic of neurotransmitter release; nor is it clear (except in a few well-studied pathways, such as the olfactory tract) that the release originates from nerve terminals. The evidence for a transmitter role of glutamate is most complete for the olfactory tract, the hippocampus and the corticostriate pathway. It is clearly established as the excitatory transmitter at the neuro-muscular junction of insects and crustacea.

The action of glutamate on most nerve cells is to cause depolarization, which is due to an increase

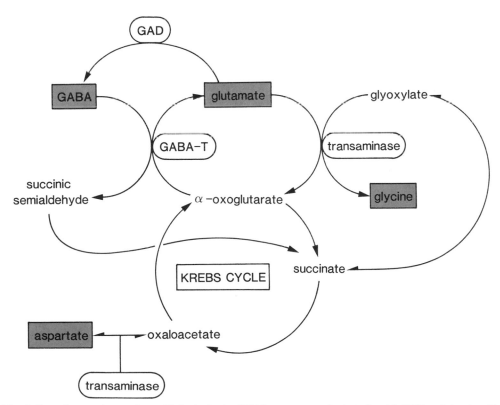

Fig. 19.9 Metabolism of transmitter amino-acids in the brain. GABA—gamma-aminobutyric acid; GAD—glutamic acid decarboxylase; GABA-T—GABA transaminase. Transmitter substances are marked with grey boxes.

in membrane conductance to sodium and other cations (essentially similar to the action of acetylcholine on nicotinic receptors at the neuromuscular junction). Recent studies on different types of glutamate receptor (see below) suggest, however, that different receptors may be coupled to other types of effector mechanism.

Excitatory amino-acid receptors

Recent work on derivatives of L-glutamate and L-aspartate, some of which have antagonistic activity, have suggested that at least two types of receptor exist (Watkins & Evans, 1981; Krogsgaard-Larsen & Honoré, 1983; Watkins, 1984). One type (the NMDA receptor) responds strongly to the glutamate analogue, NMDA, and is specifically blocked by **2-amino phosphonovalerate (APV)** and a series of related compounds. Ketamine, and other 'dissociative' anaesthetics (see Chapter 20) have also been reported to act as antagonists at the NMDA receptor (Lodge et al, 1982). The ion channels controlled by these receptors are highly sensitive to block by magnesium ions. The use of selective NMDA receptor antagonists has shown that some, but not all, CNS synapses where glutamate is the transmitter substance operate through NMDA receptors. In the spinal cord excitatory interneurons appear to act mainly on NMDA receptors, whereas primary afferent neurons do not. There is evidence for two other types of excitatory amino-acid receptor, which are sensitive respectively to **quisqualic acid** (the QUIS receptor) and to **kainic acid** (the KAI receptor). Neither of these is blocked by APV, and there are so far no selective blocking agents known for them, though several compounds are known that block all three receptor types indiscriminately. All three receptors are excitatory, and cause depolarization by similar ionic mechanisms, though they differ in their time-course. The NMDA receptor produces a more rapid response than the other two, and sometimes causes phasic oscillations of the membrane potential (see Fig. 24.2), which may be a consequence of the channel blocking action of magnesium ions mentioned above.

Kainic acid, which is obtained from seaweed, is about 50 times as potent as glutamate, but also has a delayed toxic effect on neurons whose cell bodies are exposed to it. This toxic effect is known to result from an interaction with glutamate receptors, though the detailed mechanism is not understood. Microinjection of kainic acid into the brain provides a useful way of destroying small groups of nerve cells, for it acts only on cell bodies and not on axons or nerve terminals. Its selective neurotoxic action somewhat resembles that of **capsaicin** (see Chapter 25) a substance that stimulates, and in larger doses destroys, unmyelinated primary afferent fibres. It has been suggested that these agents cause an increase in calcium permeability and produce an excessively large rise in $[Ca]_i$, possibly leading to protease activation and cell death, as is postulated in myocardial infarction (see Chapter 10).

Functional aspects

The role of excitatory amino-acids in epilepsy has been much studied, and it has been shown that in experimentally-induced focal epilepsy there is an increased release of glutamate from the cortical areas involved. More recently, a glutamate antagonist closely related to APV has been found to be an anti-convulsant in mice, so there is a possibility that this will lead to new types of anti-epileptic drug.

The neurotoxic action of kainic acid can also occur with other excitatory amino-acids, if their action is prolonged, and it has been suggested that some degenerative brain lesions (e.g. Huntington's chorea) may be due to abnormal glutamate metabolism resulting in a prolonged (and toxic) excitatory effect. At a more down-to-earth level, the copious addition of monosodium glutamate to food, as a 'flavour enhancer' raises the question of possible neurotoxicity. The 'Chinese restaurant syndrome'—an acute attack of neck stiffness and chest pain—is known to result from excessive glutamate, but so far the possibility of more serious neurotoxicity is only hypothetical.

NEUROPEPTIDES

Though the existence in the central nervous system of a number of peptides with powerful biological actions (such as vasopressin, oxytocin and substance P) has been known for many years, the realization that these substances play a major role as chemical mediators is much more recent (see Krieger et al, 1984). In 1975 Hughes & Kosterlitz succeeded in isolating from brain tissues two penta-peptides, which compete strongly with morphine-like drugs for binding to receptors in the brain, and whose pharmacological actions closely resemble those of morphine itself. This outstanding work showed that the hitherto mysterious actions of morphine (see Chapter 25) reflected its ability to mimic the actions of a family of endogenous mediators, the opioid peptides. These studies stimulated a great deal of interest in the role of peptides as neurotransmitters, and since 1975 the number of neuropeptides (defined as peptides that show activity on pharmacological test systems and are found within individual neurons) described in the literature has increased to more than 30. Iversen

(1983) lists 33 neuropeptides (Table 19.3) and several are being added to the list each year. As he points out 'almost overnight, the number of puta-tive transmitters in the mammalian nervous system has jumped from the ten or so monoamine and amino-acid candidates to more than 40'.

So far it cannot be claimed that this cataract of new information has produced more than a frag-mentary understanding of the functional role of neuropeptides; nonetheless, work on this subject at present dominates, and seems likely to continue to dominate, the study of chemical mediators in the CNS.

The original work on enkephalins and the opioid peptides, which did much to clarify the mode of action of morphine-like analgesics, fuelled the ex-pectation that the discovery of other neuropeptides might similarly illuminate the actions of other types

Table 19.3 Neuropeptides

Pituitary peptides	Corticotrophin (ACTH)
	Growth hormone
	Lipotropin
	α-melanocyte stimulating hormone (α-MSH)
	Oxytocin
	Vasopressin
Circulating hormones	Angiotensin
	Calcitonin
	Glucagon
	Insulin
Gut hormones	Cholecystokinin (CCK)
	Gastrin
	Motilin
	Pancreatic polypeptide
	Secretin
	Substance P
	Vasoactive intestinal polypeptide (VIP)
Opioid peptides	Dynorphin
	β-endorphin
	Met-enkephalin
	Leu-enkephalin
	Kytorphin
Hypothalamic releasing hormones	Corticotropin releasing factor (CRF)
	Luteinizing hormone releasing factor (LHRH)
	Somatostatin
	Thyrotropin releasing hormone (TRH)
Miscellaneous peptides	Bombesin
	Bradykinin
	Calcitonin gene related peptide (CGRP)
	Carnosine
	Neurokinin
	Neuromedin
	Neuropeptide Y
	Neurotensin
	Proctolin

of drug that affect the CNS, and also point the way to the development of new and potentially useful drugs. In the event, neither expectation has, so far, been realized. The satisfying realization that morphine owes its effects to its ability to mimic, at the receptor level, the actions of endogenous peptides, has not yet been repeated for any other class of drug; nor has the discovery of new endogenous peptides with highly selective actions on the brain and peripheral nervous system so far enabled synthetic analogues with clinically useful patterns of pharmacological activity to be developed. From a pharmacological point of view, the opioid peptides are the most important and thoroughly studied group at present, and will be discussed further in this section. Substance P is discussed in Chapter 25. Useful sources of information on other neuropeptides are given at the end of this chapter.

One striking feature of the neuropeptide scene is the frequent discovery that peptides, such as somatostatin, insulin, glucagon, thyrotrophin releasing hormone (TRH) and many others, which were originally recognized as circulating hormones with actions on peripheral target tissues (see Chapter 16), have also been shown by immunocytochemical labelling to be located in individual neurons, both in the CNS and in the peripheral autonomic nervous system. Though we cannot say from evidence of localization alone that a peptide functions as a chemical messenger, such a role is, for many peptides, now well supported by other evidence.

It has, in general, been difficult to obtain evidence that the key criteria needed to demonstrate neurotransmitter function for a putative mediator (see Chapter 8)—namely cellular localization, release by physiological stimuli, post-synaptic action corresponding to that produced by synaptic activity, including susceptibility to blocking agents, and a mechanism for rapid removal following release—are satisfied by the neuropeptides. In particular, the identification of a well-defined post-synaptic action has often been difficult, and selective antagonists of neuropeptides have proved extremely difficult to find. In the absence of good evidence for a clear-cut neurotransmitter role (i.e. involvement in passing signals at high frequency from one neuron to another, along precisely defined anatomical pathways) alternative roles as *neuro-modulators* or *neuroregulators* are frequently discussed (see Chapter 5).

One of the major disappointments of the neuropeptide field has been the failure to discover or synthesize compounds (apart from very closely-related peptides) that mimic or antagonize the effects of endogenous peptides. The sole exception is in the opioid field, where the opium alkaloids and their synthetic derivatives produce their effects by binding specifically to receptors for opioid peptides. For the other thirty or so neuropeptides, we still (with a few exceptions) lack either selective antagonist or non-peptide agonists. The former are badly needed if we are to gain a better understanding of the physiological function of the various neuropeptides, while the latter are needed if all of this new information is to be translated into clinically useful drugs. Peptides themselves generally make poor drugs, as they are usually not well absorbed, fail to penetrate the blood-brain barrier, and are chemically unstable and short-acting owing to rapid metabolic degradation.

Opioid peptides

The numerous actions of morphine, and particularly the discovery of specific antagonists (e.g. naloxone) made it clear at least 20 years ago that opiate analgesics must be acting on specific receptors, and raised the possibility of an endogenous chemical mediator. The development of binding techniques for measuring the binding of these drugs to receptors in the brain led Hughes & Kosterlitz to show that brain extracts contain substances that can inhibit the binding of naloxone. They identified two pentapeptides, **leu-enkephalin** and **met-enkephalin**, and also noted that the sequence of met-enkephalin is contained in the structure of a pituitary hormone, β-lipotropin. At the same time, in other laboratories, three other peptides with powerful morphine-like actions were discovered, α-, β- and γ-endorphin, which also consisted of stretches of the β-lipotropin molecule (Fig. 19.10). At first there was much speculation that the enkephalins might be preparative artefacts resulting from proteolysis of the larger peptides, but further work has shown that the cellular location of the enkephalins is quite distinct from that of β-endorphin. β-endorphin is concentrated in the pituitary; it is also found in particular cell groups of the hypothalamus but is absent from the spinal cord. Met-enkephalin, on the other hand, is widely distributed in the central and peripheral nervous systems, including the spinal cord.

The nesting of active peptide fragments within larger protein molecules is a feature of peptide neurobiology. In the case of opioid peptides, three large precursor proteins are known to be coded for genetically, and the subsequent snipping of these proteins into active neuropeptides occurs by 'post-translational processing', which involves mainly the enzymatic cutting of the chain at points where there are two adjacent basic amino-acids (Arg–Arg or Arg–Lys). The three large precursor proteins and some of their offspring are shown in Figure 19.10. **Pro-opiomelanocortin** (265 residues) was first characterized from the pituitary, and is the source of the pituitary hormones ACTH and MSH as well as β-endorphin. It is not certain whether any of the leu-enkephalin in the nervous system actually derives from this source, though it could do so in principle. **Pro-enkephalin** (267 residues) was isolated from the adrenal medulla. It contains six molecules of met-enkephalin and one of leu-enkephalin embedded within its sequence, and is pro-bably a major source of these peptides in the brain. It does not possess the dynorphin or β-endorphin sequences. **Pro-dynorphin** (256 residues), isolated from the hypothalamus, contains the highly active dynorphin sequences, which themselves incorporate leu-enkephalin. Altogether 18 opioid peptides, derived from these three precursors, have so far been identified and interest in the control of the proteolytic enzymes responsible for the post-translational processing is now intense.

The pharmacological actions of the opioid peptides, and related opiate drugs, together with a discussion of the various types of receptor on which they act, are presented in Chapter 25.

It is not possible here to discuss other neuropeptides individually, and recent reviews and monographs (for example Iversen et al, 1982; Krieger et al, 1984) should be consulted for further information. Certain broad generalizations may, however, be summarized:

1. Peptides are produced by proteolytic cleavage of large precursor molecules. These are relatively few in number and each can give rise to a variety of hormones and neuropeptides. The precursor proteins are synthesized in the cell body, where cleavage occurs to form the active peptides. The

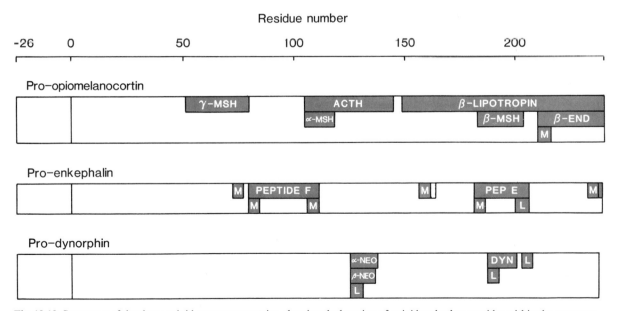

Fig. 19.10 Structures of the three opioid precursor proteins, showing the location of opioid and other peptides within the sequence. These contained peptides are bounded by pairs of basic amino-acids, which form points of attack for enzymic cleavage. MSH—melanocyte stimulating hormone; ACTH—adrenocorticotrophic hormone; β-END—β-endorphin; M—methionine enkephalin; DYN—dynorphin; NED—neoendorphin.

peptides are then conveyed by fast axonal transport to the nerve terminals.

2. Many peptides appear to function both as peripheral hormones and as transmitters (or modulators) in the central and peripheral nervous systems. It is suggested that a single peptide may thus have control, through its central and peripheral actions, of an integrated physiological or behavioural response.

3. Peptide receptors are extremely selective. There are only a few examples of specific competitive antagonists, and very few examples of non-peptide compounds that interact with peptide receptors. The opioid system is an exception in both respects; for other neuropeptide systems the lack of specific antagonists makes it very difficult to assess their biological function. The angiotensin antagonist, saralasin (Chapter 11), is another example of a potent peptide antagonist.

4. There are several examples of peptides being released as co-transmitters with conventional neurotransmitters from the same neuron. So far there is no evidence for the co-release of more than one peptide, or of more than one conventional transmitter from the same neuron. However, there is convincing evidence for the co-localization of more than one peptide in the same neuron, so it would not be surprising if both were released simultaneously.

PURINES

The possibility that purines, particularly the adenine nucleotides, may function as peripheral neurotransmitters has been mentioned in Chapter 11. Their role as CNS transmitters, or 'modulators' remains uncertain (for reviews see Stone, 1981; Phillis & Wu, 1981). Adenine nucleotides of course play a central role in energy metabolism in all cells, and studies of the content, turnover and release of ATP under various conditions are likely to be dominated by the 'metabolic' pool of ATP, making any transmitter pool hard to detect. Furthermore, ATP and ADP are rapidly hydrolysed in tissues, and the product, adenosine, is actively taken up by many cells, so that studies of nucleotide release are often difficult to interpret. Add to that the fact there are few potent purine antagonists at present, and it

is not hard to see why the transmitter role of these substances in the CNS remains undecided.

The effect of purines on CNS neurons is predominantly inhibitory. A pre-synaptic inhibitory effect occurs at many central and peripheral synapses. It is mediated by P_1-receptors (see Chapter 11), which are more sensitive to adenosine than to ATP and are blocked by methylxanthines. Both inhibitory and excitatory post-synaptic effects have been described. The mechanism of action of the methylxanthines (e.g. caffeine, theophylline; see Chapter 26) is interesting in relation to the hypothesis of purinergic transmission. These drugs have a stimulant effect on the central nervous system, and are known to be antagonists at the P_1-receptor. However, they also inhibit the enzyme phosphodiesterase which destroys cAMP (see Chapter 1), and it is not clear which (if either) of these biochemical effects underlies their actions on the CNS.

HISTAMINE

Histamine has been discussed as a possible neurotransmitter for many years, but the evidence for its role in the vertebrate CNS is still equivocal (Schwartz et al, 1980). It is present in the brain in much smaller amounts than in other tissues, such as skin and lung, and much of the brain content of histamine is due to mast cells rather than neurons. If the mast cells are depleted, however, some histamine remains, and this is associated with the nerve-ending fraction of the brain homogenate.

The biosynthetic enzyme, histidine decarboxylase, is present mainly in neurons, and is probably a better marker than histamine itself, since mast cells, whose histamine store turns over much more slowly than that of neurons, have relatively little histidine decarboxylase.

Anatomically, histamine-containing neurons have been found to run from the brainstem to large areas of the cortex, and to the hippocampus, via the medial forebrain bundle, which carries a variety of monoamine-containing neurons. Stimulation of the medial forebrain produces an inhibitory response in cortical and hippocampal neurons which is partly blocked by the H_2-receptor antagonist metiamide (see Chapter 15).

Histamine applied ionophoretically to central

neurons produces either excitatory or inhibitory effects. In most cases the excitatory effects are blocked by H_1 antagonists and the inhibitory effects by H_2 antagonists. A histamine-sensitive adenylate cyclase has been found in the brain; the receptors involved in its activation by histamine are of the H_2 type.

Other pieces of evidence which point towards a transmitter role for histamine in the vertebrate brain are:

1. There is good evidence for the existence of histaminergic neurons in the nervous system of some molluscs.

2. Antagonists at H_1-receptors all have sedative and anti-emetic effects. The anti-emetic effect of drugs such as cyclizine is often used to combat motion sickness (see Chapter 15). The sedative effect of such drugs is well known to those who take them to relieve the symptoms of hay fever (see Chapter 13).

It seems very likely that histamine will gradually emerge as a recognized transmitter, but unlikely, in view of the rather modest central effects produced by the available histamine antagonists, that it will prove to be of major importance.

THE CLASSIFICATION OF PSYCHOTROPIC DRUGS

Psychotropic drugs are defined as those which affect *mood* and *behaviour*. Because these are extremely complex functions, arriving at a satisfactory classification of drug effects is far from straightforward, and no single basis for classification has been found to be satisfactory. Thus classification on a chemical basis, which produces categories such as benzodiazepines, butyrophenones, etc, does not give much guide to pharmacological effects. A pharmacological or biochemical classification, on the other hand, is appealing for those drugs whose mechanism of action is reasonably well understood (e.g. monoamine oxidase inhibitors, catecholamine uptake blockers, etc), but there are still many instances (e.g. hallucinogens) where the mechanism of action is too poorly understood to form the basis of a reliable classification. Another possibility is to adopt an empirical classi-

fication based on clinical use, and divide drugs into categories such as 'antidepressants', 'antipsychotic agents' etc, but this has the weakness that some important psychotropic drugs have no clinical use, or their use may have changed or been superseded according to clinical fashion. Amphetamine, for example, a drug with well-characterized effects on mood and behaviour, has had an extremely chequered clinical career and would have been dismissed, revived and reclassified many times if a purely clinical classification had been adopted.

Because no single basis for classifying psychotropic drugs is feasible, different authorities tend to offer a variety of hybrid, and often incompatible schemes, and the scene is one of some confusion.

The following classification (Tyrer, 1982) is based on that suggested by the World Health Organization in 1967; although not watertight it provides a useful basis for the material represented later (see Chapters 21–23 & 26).

1. **Anxiolytic sedatives**
   Synonyms: Hypnotics, sedatives, minor tranquillizers
   Definition: Drugs that cause sleep and reduce anxiety
   Examples: Barbiturates, benzodiazepines, ethanol
   See Chapters 21 & 35

2. **Neuroleptics***
   Synonyms: antipsychotic drugs, antischizophrenic drugs, major tranquillizers
   Definition: Drugs that are effective in relieving the symptoms of schizophrenic illness
   Examples: Phenothiazines, butyrophenones
   See Chapter 22

3. **Antidepressant drugs**
   Synonym: thymoleptics*
   Definition: Drugs that alleviate the symptoms of depressive illness

---

* These strange terms are the remnants of a classification proposed by Javet in 1903, who distinguished psycholeptics (depressants of mental function) psychoanaleptics (stimulants of mental function) and psychodysleptics (drugs which produce disturbed mental function). The term neuroleptic (literally 'nerve-seizing') was coined 50 years later to describe chlorpromazine-like drugs (see Chapter 22). It gained favour, presumably by virtue of its brevity rather than its literal meaning.

Examples: Monoamine oxidase inhibitors, tricyclic antidepressants
See Chapter 23

4. **Psychomotor stimulants**
Synonym: Psychostimulants
Definition: Drugs that cause wakefulness and euphoria
Examples: Amphetamine, cocaine, caffeine
See Chapter 26

5. **Psychodysleptics***
Synonyms: Hallucinogens, psychotomimetic agents
Definition: Drugs that cause disturbance of perception and behaviour in ways that cannot be

simply characterized as sedative or stimulant effects, but resemble the symptoms of schizophrenia
Examples: Lysergic acid diethylamide (LSD), mescaline, phencyclidine
See Chapter 26

Some drugs defy classification in this scheme; for example, **lithium** (see Chapter 23), which is used in the treatment of manic-depressive psychosis; and **ketamine** (see Chapter 20), which is classed as a dissociative anaesthetic, but produces psychotropic effects rather similar to those produced by phencyclidine.

REFERENCES AND FURTHER READING

Bowery N G 1982 Baclofen: 10 years on. Trends in Pharmacological Sciences 3: 400–403
Cooper J R, Bloom F E, Roth R H 1982 Biochemical basis of neuropharmacology. Oxford University Press, New York
Feldman R S, Quenzer L J 1984 Fundamentals of neuropsychopharmacology. Sinauer, New York
Fink G, Whalley L J (eds) 1982 Neuropeptides: basic and clinical aspects. Churchill Livingstone, Edinburgh
Fovall P, Dysken M W, Davis J M 1983 Treatment of Alzheimer's disease with choline salts. In: Reisberg B (ed) Alzheimer's disease. Free Press, New York
Green A R, Costain D W 1981 Pharmacology and biochemistry of psychiatric disorders. Wiley, Chichester
Iversen L L, Iversen S D, Snyder S H (eds) 1982 Neuropeptides. Handbook of Psychopharmacology, Vol 16. Plenum, New York
Iversen L L 1983 Neuropeptides—What next? Trends in Neurosciences 6: 294–295
Jacobs B L, Gelperin A (eds) 1981 Serotonin transmission and behaviour. MIT Press, Boston
Krieger D T, Brownstein M J, Martin J B (eds) 1984 Brain peptides. Wiley, New York
Krogsgaard-Larsen P, Honoré T 1983 Glutamate receptors and new glutamate agonists. Trends in Pharmacological Sciences 4: 31–33
Lodge D, Anis N A, Buron N R 1982 Effect of optical isomers of ketamine on excitation of cat and rat spinal neurones by amino acids and acetylcholine. Neuroscience Letters 29: 281–286
Nistri A 1983 Glutamate. In: Barker J L, Rogawski M A (eds) Neurotransmitter actions in the vertebrate nervous system. Plenum Press, New York
Offermeier J, van Rooyen J M 1982 Is it possible to integrate dopamine receptor terminology? Trends in Pharmacological Sciences 3: 326–328
Osborne N N (ed) 1982 Biology of serotonergic transmission. Wiley, Chichester
Palmer G (ed) 1981 Neuropharmacology of central nervous system and behavioural disorders. Academic Press, New York
Pepeu G 1983 Brain acetylcholine: an inventory of our

knowledge on the 50th anniversary of its discovery. Trends in Pharmacological Sciences 4: 416–418.
Phillis J W, Wu P H 1981 The role of adenosine and its nucleotides in central synaptic transmission. Prog Neurobiol 16: 187–239
Pomara N, Brinkman S, Gershon S 1983 Pharmacologic treatment of Alzheimer's disease. In: Reisberg B (ed) Alzheimer's disease. Free Press, New York
Reisberg B (ed) 1983 Alzheimer's disease. Free Press, New York.
Ryall R W 1979 Mechanisms of drug action on the nervous system. Cambridge University Press, Cambridge.
Schildkraut J J 1965 The catecholamine hypothesis of affective disorders: a review of supporting evidence. Am J Psychiat 122: 509–522
Schwartz J-C, Pollard H, Quach T T 1980 Histamine as a neurotransmitter in mammalian brain: neurochemical evidence. J Neurochem 35: 26–33
Simmonds M A 1983 Multiple GABA receptors and associated regulatory sites. Trends in Neurosciences 6: 279–281
Stone T W (ed) 1981 Physiological roles for adenosine and adenosine 5'-triphosphate in the nervous system. Neuroscience 6: 523–555
Swanson L W 1983 Neuropeptides—new vistas on synaptic transmission. Trends in Neurosciences 6: 294–295
Tyrer P J 1982 Drugs in psychiatric practice. Butterworth, London
Ungerstedt U 1971 On the anatomy, pharmacology and function of the nigrostriatal dopamine system. Acta Physiol Scand (Supp) 367
Watkins J F 1984 Excitatory amino-acids and central synaptic function. Trends in Pharmacological Sciences 5: 373–376
Watkins J F, Evans R H 1981 Excitatory amino acid transmitters. Ann Rev Pharmacol Toxicol 21: 165–204
Watling K J 1983 A function for dopamine-sensitive adenylate cyclase in the retina? Trends in Pharmacological Sciences 4: 327–328
Weber E, Evans C J, Barchas J D 1983 Multiple endogenous ligands for opioid receptors. Trends in Neurosciences 6: 333–336.

General anaesthetic agents

General anaesthetics are used as an adjunct to surgical procedures in order to render the patient unaware of, and unresponsive to, painful stimulation. They are given systemically, and exert their main effects on the central nervous system, in contrast to local anaesthetics (see Chapter 27) which work by producing a local block of conduction of sensory impulses from the periphery to the central nervous system.

Many drugs, including for example ethanol and morphine, can produce a state of insensibility and obliviousness to pain, but are not used as anaesthetics. For a drug to be useful as an anaesthetic it must be rapidly controllable as well as having appropriate pharmacological actions, so that induction and recovery from anaesthesia occur rapidly, enabling the level of anaesthesia to be adjusted as required during the course of the operation. For this reason it was only when inhalation anaesthetics were first discovered, in 1846, that surgical operations under controlled anaesthesia became a practical possibility. Until that time surgical skill consisted largely of being able to operate at lightning speed, and most operations were amputations. Inhalation is still the most useful route of administration for anaesthetics, though there are also some drugs which are sufficiently rapidly metabolized or redistributed in the body to be given as anaesthetics by the intravenous route.

The usefulness of nitrous oxide in relieving the pain of surgery was first suggested by Humphrey Davy in 1800. He was the first person to make nitrous oxide and he tested its effects on several people, including himself and the Prime Minister, noting that it caused euphoria, analgesia and loss of consciousness. The use of nitrous oxide, billed as 'laughing gas', became a popular fair-ground entertainment, and came to the notice of an American dentist, Horace Wells, who had a tooth extracted under its influence while he himself squeezed the inhalation bag. Ether, too, first gained publicity in a disreputable way, through the spread of 'ether frolics' at which it was used to produce euphoria among the guests (explosions, too, one might have thought). Henry Morton, also a dentist, and a student at Harvard Medical School, used it successfully to extract a tooth in 1846 and then suggested to Warren, the chief surgeon at Massachusetts General Hospital, that he should administer it for one of Warren's operations. Warren grudgingly agreed, and on 16 October 1846 a large audience was gathered in the main operating theatre; after some preliminary fumbling, Morton's demonstration was a spectacular success. 'Gentlemen, this is no humbug' was Warren's comment to the assembled audience. A somewhat more wordy appreciation came later from Oliver Wendell Holmes (1847), the neurologist who first coined the word 'anaesthesia'. 'The knife is searching for disease, the pulleys are dragging back dislocated limbs—Nature herself is working out the primal curse which doomed the tenderest of her creatures to the sharpest of her trials, but the fierce extremity of suffering has been steeped in the waters of forgetfulness, and the deepest furrow in the knotted brow of agony has been smoothed forever'. Morton subsequently sank into an endless and bitter dispute with one of his collaborators over the patent rights, and contributed nothing more to medical science.

In the same year James Simpson, professor of obstetrics in Glasgow, used chloroform to relieve the pain of childbirth, bringing on himself fierce denunciation from the clergy, one of whom wrote: 'Chloroform is a decoy of Satan, apparently offering itself to bless women; but in the end it will harden society and rob God of the deep, earnest cries which arise in time of trouble, for help'. Opposition was effectively silenced in 1853 when Queen Victoria gave birth to her seventh child under the influence of chloroform, and the procedure became known as 'anaesthésie à la reine'.

PHYSICOCHEMICAL THEORIES OF ANAESTHESIA

Unlike most drugs, inhalation anaesthetics, which include a diverse group of substances such as **halothane**, **nitrous oxide** and **xenon**, belong to no recognizable chemical class. The shape and electronic configuration of the molecule is evidently unimportant, and the pharmacological action requires only that the molecule has certain physicochemical properties. The lack of chemical specificity argues against there being any distinctive 'receptor' for anaesthetics (see Chapter 1); instead we need to consider in which 'phase' of the cell the drugs are acting. The three possibilities that have received most attention are:

1. *Lipid.* It is suggested that by dissolving in the membrane lipid, anaesthetic drugs affect its physical state in such a way as to alter the function of the membrane.
2. *Water.* Anaesthetic molecules cause the ordering of water molecules in their vicinity ('iceberg' formation). It is suggested that this, occurring at the surface of a membrane, can disturb the function of membrane proteins, and possibly also interfere with ionic movements.
3. *Protein.* It is established that the interaction of anaesthetic molecules with hydrophobic domains of various protein molecules may affect their function in such a way as to disrupt the normal mechanisms by which the ion permeability of the membrane is controlled.

Lipid theory

The lipid theory derives from the extensive work of Overton & Meyer, published in 1899–1901, who showed a close correlation between **anaesthetic potency** (measured in terms of the concentration needed to produce reversible immobilization of swimming tadpoles) and **lipid solubility** (measured as the olive-oil:water partition coefficient) in a diverse group of simple and unreactive organic compounds. This led to the theory, formulated by Meyer in 1937: 'Narcosis commences when any chemically indifferent substance has attained a certain molar concentration in the lipids of the cell. This concentration depends on the nature of the animal or cell but is independent of the narcotic.'

The relationship between anaesthetic activity and lipid solubility has been repeatedly confirmed. Figure 20.1 shows results obtained in man where the **minimal alveolar concentration** (**MAC**) required to produce a lack of response to painful stimulation is plotted against lipid solubility, for various inhalation anaesthetics whose oil:water partition coefficient varies over a 10 000-fold range. MAC is inversely proportional to the potency of an anaesthetic.

The Meyer-Overton studies did not suggest any particular mechanism, but revealed an impressive correlation, which any theory of anaesthesia needs to take into account. It was later suggested that the introduction of anaesthetic molecules into the lipid phase of the membrane resulted in a **volume expansion** of this phase, leading to disturbance of function. An observation which has been held to support this view is that of **pressure reversal** of anaesthesia. If animals, such as newts, are immobilized by addition of anaesthetic to the water in which they swim, application of hydrostatic pressure to about 100 atmospheres immediately restores their mobility, and anaesthesia returns as soon as the pressure is lowered (Miller et al, 1973). Quantitative analysis of this phenomenon suggests that hydrostatic compression of the lipid phase of the membrane is responsible, and the results are compatible with the suggestion that anaesthesia occurs when the volume of the lipid phase is expanded by about 0.4% as a result of the intrusion of anaesthetic molecules. Pressure is thought to act simply by opposing this volume expansion. There is independent evidence that anaesthetics do indeed cause membranes to expand (e.g. in the red cell) slightly, but there are quantitative discrepancies between these results and those of pressure reversal experiments, so the interpretation is not clear at present. It is interesting that pressure reversal has also been observed when anaesthesia is produced

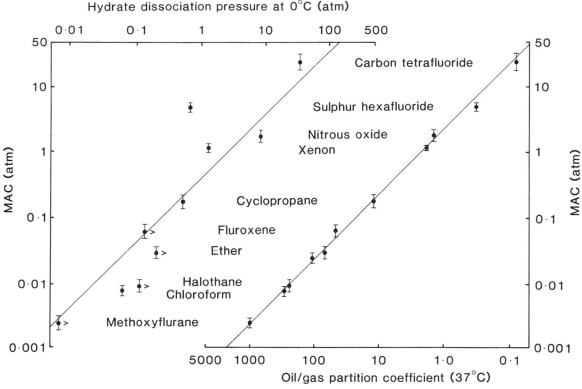

Fig. 20.1 Correlation of anaesthetic potency with hydrate dissociation pressure and oil:gas partition coefficient. Anaesthetic potency in man is expressed as minimum alveolar partial pressure (MAC) required to produce surgical anaesthesia, MAC being inversely proportional to potency. The correlation with oil:gas partition coefficient is much higher than with hydrate dissociation pressure. (From: Eger et al, 1969)

by intravenous agents such as barbiturates, and with local anaesthetics, though there are discrepancies which mean that lipid volume expansion cannot explain all of the actions of these drugs.

By the technique of electron spin resonance (e.s.r.) spectroscopy it is possible to measure the **fluidity** of the lipid encironment of cell membranes and of artificial lipid bilayers. Many studies have shown that anaesthetics increase fluidity. This effect correlates, in general, with anaesthetic activity, though relatively high concentrations are needed. The effect of clinical concentrations would correspond only to a minute increase in fluidity, such as might occur if the temperature was increased by less than 1°C, so the relevance of this phenomenon to the pharmacological actions of anaesthetics is not clear.

Hydrate theory

In 1961 Pauling & Miller independently suggested

that anaesthetics might act by 'freezing' water molecules in the form of an anaesthetic-hydrate complex close to the surface of the cell membrane. They showed that the potency of anaesthetic agents correlates with their ability to form hydrate complexes almost as well as with their lipid solubility. More recent studies have produced evidence against this hypothesis. For example, certain anomalous compounds, such as SF_6, which have high lipid solubility but do not readily form hydrates, have an anaesthetic potency which correlates well with their lipid solubility, and in general it has been found that there is a much poorer correlation of anaesthetic potency with hydrate formation than with lipid solubility (see Fig. 20.1). The hydrate theory has therefore now been abandoned.

Protein theory

Though there is good evidence that anaesthetics can bind to protein molecules, well-documented for haemoglobin and myoglobin as well as for various enzymes, there is little direct evidence to suggest that this can account for anaesthesia. Where functional studies have been carried out, e.g. with *luciferase* which forms part of the light-emitting system of fireflies and is inhibited by anaesthetics, it has usually been found that the concentrations needed are much higher than those that affect the nervous system.

One observation that may support the protein theory is the **cut-off phenomenon**. Within many homologous series, anaesthetic potency increases steadily, along with lipid solubility, as the length of the hydrocarbon chain is increased. Beyond a certain point, however, potency suddenly drops even though lipid solubility continues to increase. This may mean that anaesthetics do, after all, bind to a site of predetermined size, which is more likely to correspond to a particular domain of a protein molecule than to interaction with an essentially fluid lipid phase (Franks & Lieb, 1982).

At present, it seems clear from the correlation of potency with lipid solubility that the interaction of anaesthetic molecules with one or more hydrophobic regions of the cell membrane underlies their effects, and that hydrate function is not important. Whether the effect involves mainly lipid or protein or both cannot be resolved yet.

THE EFFECTS OF ANAESTHETICS ON THE NERVOUS SYSTEM

At the cellular level, anaesthetics inhibit the conduction of action potentials, and also inhibit transmission at synapses. The effect on axonal conduction, however, requires considerably higher concentrations than the effect of synaptic transmission. During surgical anaesthesia there is little or no effect on transmission along peripheral motor or sensory nerves, while experiments on transmission within the central nervous system in experimental animals have revealed that excitatory synaptic transmission is much more susceptible to anaesthetic action than axonal conduction.

The inhibitory effect on synaptic transmission could be due to reduction of transmitter release, inhibition of the post-synaptic action of the transmitter, or reduction of the electrical excitability of the post-synaptic cell. Though all three effects have been described, most studies suggest that reduced transmitter release and reduced post-synaptic sensitivity to the transmitter are the main factors. A reduction of acetylcholine release has been demonstrated directly in studies on peripheral synapses, and reduced sensitivity to excitatory transmitters has been shown at both peripheral and central synapses.

The action of inhibitory synapses may be enhanced or reduced by anaesthetics. Enhancement of inhibitory synaptic action occurs particularly with barbiturates; volatile anaesthetics either reduce it or have no effect.

Much effort has gone into identifying a particular brain region on which anaesthetics act to produce their anaesthetic effect (see Richards, 1980; Angel, 1980). Unconsciousness can be produced by damage to the brainstem reticular formation, the hypothalamus or the thalamus. Cortical damage produces profound sensory and motor disturbances, but not actual loss of consciousness. Activity of the reticular formation is responsible for cortical 'arousal' and also for facilitation of transmission through the thalamic sensory relay nuclei which lie en route from peripheral sensory receptors to the cortex. Inhibition of activity in this part of the reticular formation may thus be important in causing cortical inactivity together with a lack of awareness of sensory input.

Anaesthetics, even in low concentrations, cause short-term **amnesia**, i.e. experiences occurring during the influence of the drug are not recalled later even though the subject was responsive at the time. It is likely that interference with hippocampal function produces this effect, for it is known the hippocampus is involved in short-term memory and that certain hippocampal synapses are highly susceptible to inhibition by anaesthetics.

Thus, the reticular formation and the hippocampus may be the most important sites at which anaesthetics work in the brain. As the concentration is increased, however, many other functions are affected, including motor control and reflex activity, respiration and autonomic regulation. It is clear that the cellular effects produced by anaesthetics can influence the function of the nervous system in many different ways, and it is therefore unrealistic to seek a critical 'target site' in the brain responsible for all the phenomena of anaesthesia.

Stages of anaesthesia

When a slowly-acting anaesthetic, such as ether, is given on its own, certain well-defined stages are passed through as its concentration in the blood increases.

Stage I—analgesia

The subject is conscious but drowsy. Responses to painful stimuli are reduced. The degree of analgesia actually varies greatly with different agents; it is pronounced with ether and nitrous oxide, but not with halothane.

Stage II—excitement

The subject loses consciousness, and no longer responds to non-painful stimuli, but responds reflexly to painful stimuli. He may talk incoherently, hold his breath, choke or vomit. Increased muscle tone and involuntary movement may also occur. It is a dangerous state, and modern anaesthetic procedures are designed to eliminate it as far as possible.

Stage III—surgical anaesthesia

Spontaneous movement ceases and respiration becomes regular. If anaesthesia is light, some reflexes (e.g. responses to pharyngeal and peritoneal stimulation) are still present, and muscles show appreciable tone. With deepening anaesthesia, these reflexes disappear, and the muscles relax fully. Respiration becomes progressively shallower, with the intercostal muscles failing before the diaphragm.

Stage IV—medullary paralysis

Respiration and vasomotor control cease, and death occurs within a few minutes.

The use of a single anaesthetic agent on its own is now uncommon, and the orderly progression through the above-listed stages of anaesthesia is seldom observed in practice. The anaesthetic state, for clinical purposes, consists of three components, namely **loss of consciousness**, **analgesia**, and **loss of reflexes**, and it has proved more satisfactory to produce these effects with a combination of drugs rather than with a single anaesthetic agent. Thus, a common practice would be to produce unconsciousness rapidly with an intravenous induction agent (e.g. **thiopentone**); to maintain unconsciousness and produce analgesia with one or more inhalation agents (e.g. **nitrous oxide**, **halothane**), which might be supplemented with an intravenous analgesic agent (e.g. an **opiate**; see Chapter 25); and to produce muscle paralysis with a neuromuscular blocking drug (e.g. **tubocurarine**; see Chapter 6). Such a procedure results in much faster induction and recovery, avoiding long (and hazardous) periods of semi-consciousness, and it enables surgery to be carried out with relatively little impairment of homeostatic reflexes.

EFFECTS ON THE CARDIOVASCULAR AND RESPIRATORY SYSTEMS

Though all anaesthetics decrease the contractility of isolated heart preparations, their effects on cardiac output and blood pressure in man vary, mainly because of concomitant actions on the sympathetic nervous system. Thus **ether** causes an increased sympathetic discharge and increased plasma noradrenaline concentration, and tends to increase blood pressure, whereas **halothane** and other halogenated anaesthetics have the opposite effect. **Nitrous oxide** has little effect on the cardiovascular system.

Many anaesthetics, particularly halogenated agents, cause **cardiac dysrhythmias**, particularly ventricular extrasystoles. The mechanism is not well understood, but involves an interaction with catecholamines. Thus an injection of noradrenaline which would not normally produce dysrhythmia will do so if given in the presence of halothane. The usual manifestation is the appearance of ventricular ectopic beats, and careful ECG monitoring shows that these occur very commonly in patients under halothane anaesthesia, without producing any harmful effect. If catecholamine secretion is excessive, however, there is a risk of precipitating ventricular fibrillation, which is a particular hazard if stage II of the induction process is unduly prolonged.

With the exception of nitrous oxide and ether, all anaesthetics depress respiration markedly, and increase arterial P_{CO_2}. Nitrous oxide has much less effect, mainly because its low potency prevents very deep anaesthesia from being produced with this drug (see below). Ether, in the concentrations used clinically, has a powerful irritant effect on the respiratory tract, which elicits a reflex stimulation of breathing. This counteracts its direct effect and allows deep surgical anaesthesia to be produced with little respiratory depression.

INHALATION ANAESTHETICS— PHARMACOKINETIC ASPECTS

An important characteristic of an inhalation anaesthetic is the speed at which the arterial blood concentration, on which the pharmacological effect closely depends, follows changes in the concentration of the drug in the inspired air. Ideally, the blood concentration should follow as quickly as possible, so that the depth of anaesthesia can be controlled rapidly. In particular, it is important that the blood concentration should fall to a sub-anaesthetic level rapidly when administration is stopped, so that the patient recovers consciousness without delay. A prolonged semi-comatose state, in which respiratory reflexes are weak or absent, represents a distinct hazard to life.

The only quantitatively important route by which inhalation anaesthetics enter and leave the body is via the lungs. They are all small, lipid soluble molecules, which cross the alveolar membrane with great ease. It is therefore the rate at which the drug enters and leaves the lungs, via the inspired air and the bloodstream, that determines the overall kinetic behaviour of a given anaesthetic. The reason that anaesthetics vary in their kinetic behaviour is that the relative solubilities in blood, and in body fat, vary between one drug and another.

The main factors that determine the speed of induction and recovery (and also the speed with which the level of anaesthesia responds to changes in the concentration added by the anaesthetist to the inspired air) can be summarized as follows:

1. *Properties of the anaesthetic*
   a. Blood:gas partition coefficient
   b. Oil:gas partition coefficient
2. *Physiological factors*
   a. Alveolar ventilation rate
   b. Cardiac output

The solubility of anaesthetics

For practical purposes anaesthetics can be regarded physicochemically as ideal gases: their solubility in different media can thus be expressed as **partition coefficients**, defined as the *ratio* of the concentration of the agent in two phases at equilibrium.

The **blood:gas partition coefficient** is the main factor that determines the **rate of induction** and **recovery** of an inhalation anaesthetic, and the *lower* the blood:gas partition coefficient the *faster* the induction and recovery.

The **oil:gas partition coefficient**, or lipid solubility, is the main determinant of the **potency** of an anaesthetic (as already discussed) and also in-

Table 20.1 Characteristics of inhalation anaesthetics

Drug	Partition coefficient blood:gas	oil:gas	MAC (% v/v)	Induction	Metabolism	Flammability
Ether	12.0	65	1.9	slow	Some oxidation → ethanol, acetaldehhyde, acetic acid	+ +
Halothane	2.4	220	0.8	medium	About 5% → trifluoroacetic acid, bromide	—
Nitrous oxide	0.47	1.4	100*	fast	Not metabolized	—
Enflurane	1.9	98	0.7	medium	About 5% → fluoride	—
Methoxyflurane	13.0	950	0.16	slow	About 50% → fluoride, oxalate	—
Cyclopropane	0.55	11.5	9.2	fast	Not known	+ +

* Theoretical value based on measurements under hyperbaric conditions.

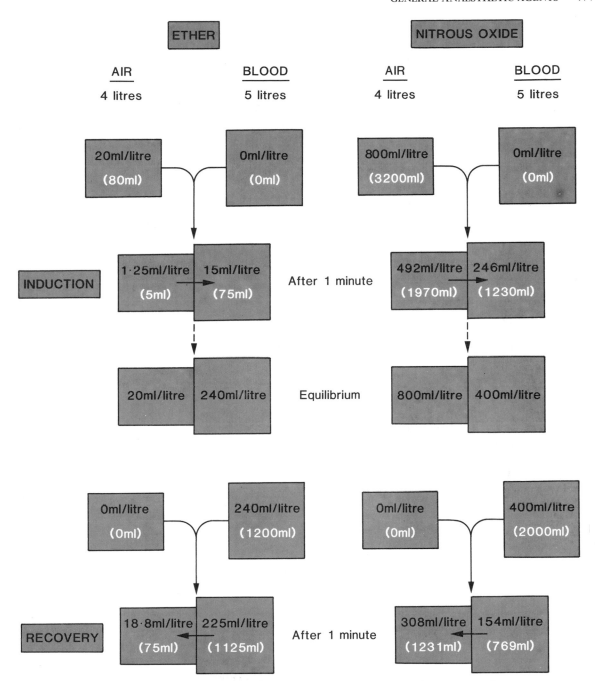

Fig. 20.2 The effect of blood:gas partition coefficient on the rate of equilibration of inhalation anaesthetics. The diagram compares agents of high water solubility (ether) and low water solubility (nitrous oxide). Black figures represent the concentration of anaesthetic; white figures represent the amount of anaesthetic that becomes redistributed between blood and alveolar air during one minute. The concentrations in the inspired air (upper diagram) are approximately those required for anaesthesia, and the redistribution of anaesthetic in the first minute between alveolar air (4 litres) and pulmonary blood (5 litres) is shown. With ether, most of the inhaled anaesthetic is extracted by the blood, and after 1 minute the blood concentration is only 15/240, or 16%, of its equilibrium value. With nitrous oxide, the proportion extracted in the first minute is much less, and the blood concentration reaches 246/400, or 62%, of its equilibrium value.

Similarly, on removing the anaesthetic from the inspired air (lower diagram), the blood ether concentration drops in one minute by only 4%, whereas that of nitrous oxide drops by 62%.

fluences the kinetics of its distribution in the body, the main effect being that high lipid solubility tends to delay recovery from the effects of anaesthesia. Values of blood:gas and oil:gas partition coefficients for some anaesthetics are given in Table 20.1.

Induction and recovery

The brain has a large blood flow, and the blood-brain barrier is freely permeable to anaesthetics. Thus, the concentration of anaesthetic in the brain remains virtually in equilibrium with the concentration in the arterial blood (i.e. with the concentration in the blood leaving the lungs). The kinetics of transfer of anaesthetic between the inspired air and the arterial blood therefore determine the kinetics of the pharmacological effect.

If an anaesthetic is added to the inspired air at a concentration which, *at equilibrium*, will produce surgical anaesthesia, the rate at which this equilibrium is approached depends mainly on the blood:gas partition coefficient, and (contrary to what one might intuitively suppose) the *lower* the solubility in blood, the *faster* the process of equilibration. Ether is a typical high-solubility anaes-

thetic (blood:gas partition coefficient = 12.09) whereas nitrous oxide is relatively insoluble (blood:gas partition coefficient = 0.5). Imagine that each is added to the inspired air at concentrations sufficient to produce the same eventual level of anaesthesia (20 ml/l for ether vapour; 800 ml/l for nitrous oxide (Fig. 20.2)). At equilibrium, the blood concentration of ether will be $20 \times 12 = 240$ ml/l, whereas for nitrous oxide it will be $800 \times 0.5 = 400$ ml/l. During the first minute of induction, suppose that the alveolar ventilation is 4 litres and the pulmonary blood flow is 5 litres, and consider the transfer of drug from air to blood that will occur when these two volumes are brought into equilibrium.

In the case of ether 80 ml of anaesthetic is delivered to the lungs in the first minute (white figures in Fig. 20.2). Of this amount 75 ml is taken up by the blood, bringing the arterial concentration to 15 ml/l, which is approximately 6% of the concentration at equilibrium, whereas with nitrous oxide the uptake in the first minute brings the arterial concentration to 246 ml/l, which is over 60% of the equilibrium concentration. Neglecting other factors, this means that with ether it would take about 30 minutes to reach 90% equilibrium, whereas with

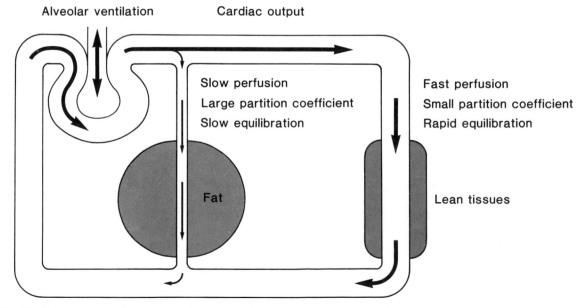

Fig. 20.3 Factors affecting the rate of equilibration of inhalation anaesthetics in the body. The body is represented as two compartments: *Lean tissues* have a large blood flow and low partition coefficient for anaesthetics, and therefore equilibrate rapidly with the blood. *Fat tissues* have a small blood flow and large partition coefficient, and therefore equilibrate slowly, acting as a reservoir of drug during the recovery phase.

nitrous oxide this would take less than 3 minutes. During recovery, when the concentration in the inspired air is reduced to zero, a similar calculation of the exchange taking place during the first minute (Fig. 20.2) shows that nitrous oxide is removed from the body much more rapidly than ether.

In discussing the exchanges between air and blood so far we have ignored the transfer of anaesthetic between blood and tissues. More elaborate models for describing the pharmacokinetics of anaesthetic drugs allow for several distinct tissue compartments, varying in their anaesthetic solubility and perfusion rate. Fig. 20.3 shows a very simple model of the circulation in which two tissue compartments are included. Body fat is particularly important, since it has a low blood flow and often a high anaesthetic solubility (see Table 20.1). Body fat constitutes about 20% of the volume of a normal

male. Thus for a drug such as halothane whose solubility in fat is about 100 times as great as its solubility in water, the amount present in the fat after *complete* equilibration would be roughly 95% of the total amount in the body. Because of the low blood flow, it takes many hours for the drug to enter and leave the fat, which results in a pronounced slow phase of equilibration following the rapid phase associated with the blood-gas exchanges (Fig. 20.4). The more fat-soluble the anaesthetic and the fatter the patient, the more pronounced this slow phase becomes.

Of the physiological factors affecting the rate of equilibrium of inhalation anaesthetics alveolar ventilation is the most important. The greater the ventilation rate, the faster is the process of equilibration particularly for drugs that have high blood:gas partition coefficients. The use of analgesic drugs,

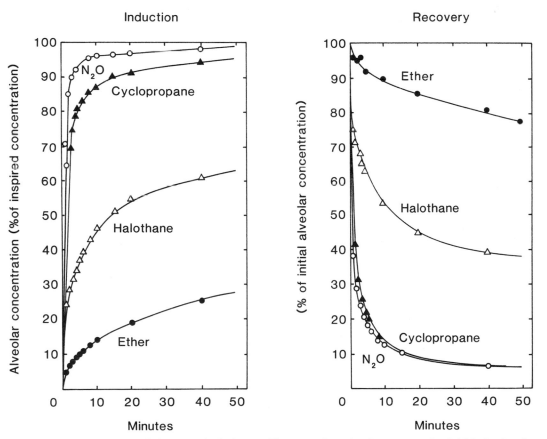

Fig. 20.4 Rate of equilibration of inhalation anaesthetics in man. The curves show alveolar concentration (which closely reflects arterial blood concentration) as a function of time during induction and recovery. The overall rate of equilibration varies with blood:gas partition coefficient (Fig. 20.2). There is also a slow phase of equilibration, most marked with highly lipid-soluble drugs (ether and halothane), due to the slow transfer between blood and fat (Fig. 20.3). (From: Papper & Kitz, 1963)

such as morphine (see Chapter 25) which reduce alveolar ventilation can thus retard recovery from anaesthesia. Changes in cardiac output produce complex effects. Increasing the cardiac output increases the rate of extraction of anaesthetic from the alveoli and thus *retards* the rise in arterial anaesthetic content, slowing down the early phase of induction. It also increases the rate of delivery of anaesthetic to the tissues, so tends to speed up the later phase of equilibration.

Recovery from anaesthesia involves the same processes as induction but in reverse (Fig. 20.4). There is a rapid decrease in arterial anaesthetic concentration, which is mirrored in the brain, followed by a slower decline as the anaesthetic is transferred from the tissues into the blood-stream. If anaesthesia with a highly fat-soluble drug has been maintained for a long time, so that the fat has had time to accumulate a substantial amount, this slow phase of recovery can become very pronounced and keep the patient in a drowsy state for some hours.

Metabolism of inhalation anaesthetics

It was originally thought that anaesthetics were too unreactive to be metabolized in the body, but it has recently been found that the metabolism of halogenated anaesthetics can be considerable (see Table 20.1), and that the resulting metabolites contribute appreciably to certain toxic effects. Only with **methoxyflurane** (approximately 50% metabolized) does metabolism contribute appreciably to the inactivation of the drug. In other cases the fraction of the absorbed drug that undergoes biotransformation is too small (20% or less) to affect its pharmacokinetic properties appreciably.

Metabolism in relation to toxicity

Certain types of anaesthetic-related toxicity, particularly **renal** and **hepatic damage**, are clearly associated with the formation of metabolites (see Chapter 36). These may be free radicals (e.g. $CCl_3^{\cdot}$ and $CCl_2^{\cdot}$ formed from chloroform in liver cells) or other products (e.g. fluoride ion and oxalate formed from methoxyflurane, which are responsible for post-operative renal damage occurring with this drug). Halothane is metabolized to bromide ion

and also to trifluoroacetic acid. The relationship of these metabolites to the occurrence of liver toxicity (see below) is not clearly established.

The problem of toxicity of low concentrations of anaesthetics inhaled over long periods by operating theatre staff has recently caused much concern, following the demonstration that such chronic low-level exposure leads to liver toxicity (associated with metabolite formation) in experimental animals. Epidemiological studies of operating theatre staff have shown increased incidence of liver disease and of certain types of leukaemia, and of spontaneous abortion and congenital malformations, compared with similar groups of subjects not exposed to anaesthetic agents. Causation has not been clearly established, but much effort has gone into measures designed to reduce the concentration of anaesthetics in the air of operating theatres.

INDIVIDUAL INHALATION ANAESTHETICS

The structures of the most important inhalation anaesthetics are shown in Figure 20.5.

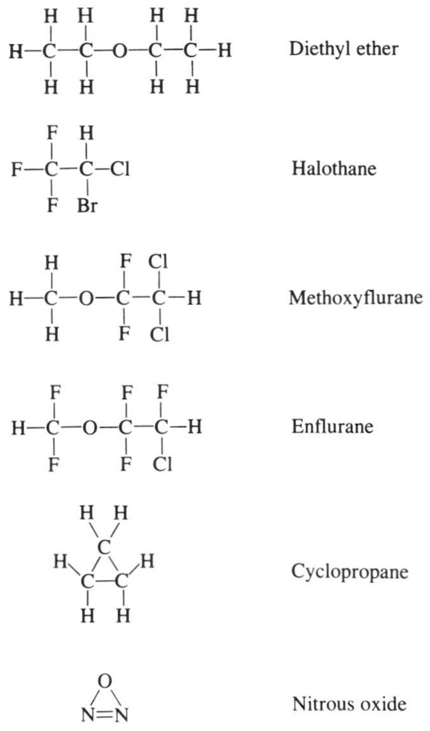

Fig. 20.5 Structures of inhalation anaesthetics.

Diethyl ether

Ether was the first anaesthetic to be used clinically, but is now very little used. It was considered a relatively safe anaesthetic in that there is considerable margin between the concentration needed for anaesthesia, and the concentration producing respiratory and cardiovascular failure. Other advantageous features are that it is an effective analgesic, has some neuromuscular blocking activity, and in anaesthetic concentrations it tends to raise blood pressure. It has serious disadvantages, however, the most important being its explosive property which necessitates considerable precautions to avoid static discharge and precludes the use of diathermy apparatus to control bleeding. It is highly irritant to the respiratory tract, and evokes a copious secretion, which is liable to cause postoperative respiratory infection. It has a relatively high blood:gas partition coefficient (see Table 20.1), so induction and recovery are slow (see previous section) resulting in a prolonged hangover, often accompanied by nausea and vomiting.

Halothane

Halothane is probably the most widely used inhalation anaesthetic. It is non-explosive and non-irritant, and induction and recovery are faster than with ether, because of its relatively low solubility in blood. It is more potent than ether (MAC 0.8% compared with 1.9% for ether; see Table 20.1) and can easily produce respiratory and cardiovascular failure. To control its concentration accurately, therefore, a special vaporization chamber is used. Even in normal anaesthetic concentrations, halothane causes a fall in blood pressure, partly due to myocardial depression and partly to vasodilatation. Halothane has a relaxant effect on the uterus, which limits its usefulness for obstetric purposes. In common with other halogenated anaesthetics, halothane tends to cause cardiac dysrhythmias, particularly ventricular extrasystoles, though this does not appear to matter much in practice.

The main adverse effect which has been attributed to halothane is liver damage. In a study of 850 000 cases involving anaesthesia with different agents, (National Halothane Study, 1966) 9 deaths

from liver failure not attributable to any other recognizable cause were reported, 7 in patients who had received halothane. Subsequent reports have suggested that the risk of liver damage is associated with *repeated* administration of halothane, and may be due to an immunological response, but this has not been fully established.

About 25% of the absorbed dose of halothane undergoes metabolism, mainly by oxidation to trifluoroacetic acid, Br^- and Cl^- ion. Trifluoroacetic acid is potentially toxic but there is no evidence to indicate whether this is clinically significant.

Nitrous oxide

Nitrous oxide is an odourless and non-explosive gas with many advantageous features for anaesthesia. It is particularly rapid in action, because of its low blood:gas partition coefficient (see Table 20.1), and is also an effective analgesic agent in concentrations too low to cause unconsciousness. It is used in this way to reduce pain during childbirth. One serious drawback of nitrous oxide is its low potency. Even at a concentration of 80% in the inspired gas mixture (the maximum possible without reducing the oxygen content) nitrous oxide does not produce surgical anaesthesia. It cannot therefore be used on its own, but is very often used in conjunction with a more powerful agent such as halothane. During recovery from nitrous oxide anaesthesia, the transfer of the gas from the blood into the alveoli can be sufficient to reduce, by dilution, the alveolar partial pressure of oxygen, producing a transient hypoxia, but this is only important in patients with respiratory disease.

Nitrous oxide was for long thought to be devoid of any serious toxic effects, but has now been shown to produce significant metabolic abnormalities, resulting from the oxidation of cobalt in vitamin B_{12} (see Nunn, 1984). Vitamin B_{12} (cobalamin; see Chapter 18) provides a co-factor required for the synthesis of methionine, and quite brief exposure to nitrous oxide causes a marked inhibition of methionine synthase activity, which takes several days to recover. Methionine functions as a methyl donor in the synthesis of DNA and many proteins. Inhibition of methionine synthesis therefore has many consequences, including inhibition of cell division, which results in anaemia and leukopenia. With a single administration of nitrous oxide, these effects are not usually detectable in man, because the bone marrow has a sufficient reserve to cope with a temporary suppression of cell division, but repeated or excessively prolonged administration are known to cause leukopenia and megaloblastic anaemia.

Prolonged exposure to very low concentrations of nitrous oxide, far below the level causing anaesthesia, affects methionine synthesis very markedly, and nitrous oxide has been implicated as one of the probable causes of the increased frequency of abortion and fetal abnormality among operating theatre staff.

Methoxyflurane

Methoxyflurane is a fluorinated ether (see Fig. 20.5) introduced in 1960 with the aim of producing a non-explosive agent without some of the drawbacks of halothane. It is exceptionally potent (MAC 0.16%; see Table 20.1) due to its very high lipid solubility. Its blood:gas partition coefficient is considerably higher than that of halothane (see Table 20.1) so induction and recovery are slower. Very high fat solubility leads to a gradual accumulation in body fat, which results in slow recovery from anaesthesia if methoxyflurane is administered for a long time.

In most respects, methoxyflurane is similar to halothane, producing a similar degree of cardiovascular and respiratory depression, and a similar likelihood of cardiac dysrhythmias. It is, however, a more effective analgesic, and produces less uterine relaxation, which may be an advantage.

The most important adverse property of methoxyflurane is its tendency to cause renal damage, which is associated with the exceptionally large proportion (50% or more) of the drug that is metabolized. Renal damage manifests itself as renal failure associated with a high urine flow and an inability to produce concentrated urine, occurring in the postoperative period. The concentration of fluoride ion in the plasma may exceed $40 \mu M$ 2–4 days postoperatively if methoxyflurane has been given for more than 1–2 hours, and this is sufficient to cause renal tubular damage. Oxalate, another metabolic product of methoxyflurane, also appears in the urine, but is not responsible for the toxic effect. Renal toxicity severely limits the usefulness of methoxyflurane for anything but brief administration, though it otherwise has many advantages.

Enflurane

Enflurane is another halogenated ether introduced in 1973, which is much faster in its actions than methoxyflurane, less liable to accumulate in body fat, and metabolized to only a very minor extent. It does not cause hepatic damage, and is much less prone than methoxyflurane to cause renal damage.

The main drawback to enflurane, which otherwise has many favourable characteristics, is that it tends to cause epilepsy-like seizures, either during induction or following recovery from anaesthesia. In this connection it is interesting that a related substance, the fluorine-substituted diethyl-ether, hexafluoroether, is a powerful convulsant agent, though the mechanism is not understood.

A variety of other inhalation anaesthetics have been introduced and gradually superseded, mainly because of their inflammable nature or because of toxicity. They include chloroform (abandoned because of hepatotoxicity) vinyl ether (explosive), cyclopropane (explosive) and trichloroethylene (chemically unstable, no special advantages). Further information is presented by Vickers et al (1984).

INTRAVENOUS ANAESTHETIC AGENTS

Even the fastest-acting inhalation anaesthetics, such as nitrous oxide, take a few minutes to act, and cause a period of excitement before anaesthesia is produced. Intravenous anaesthetics act much more rapidly, producing unconsciousness in about 20 seconds, as soon as the drug reaches the brain from its site of injection. These drugs are normally used for **induction of anaesthesia**.

Other agents (e.g. **diazepam**; see Chapter 21), which are known as **basal anaesthetics**, act rather less rapidly but can be used to produce sedation prior to anaesthesia, thus reducing the amount of the inhalation anaesthetic that is required. In general, intravenous anaesthetics are unsatisfactory for producing *maintained* anaesthesia on their own because their elimination from the body is usually much slower than that of an inhalation agent, so that they do not provide the rapid control of depth of anaesthesia that is required during surgery. However, some drugs (e.g. **thiopentone, ketamine**; see below) act for sufficiently long (10–20 minutes) that they can be used for short operations without the need for an inhalation agent.

The main drugs comprising these two groups are:

1. *Induction agents*
   a. **Thiopentone** (the most commonly used induction agent)
   b. **Althesin**
   c. Less important drugs include **propanidid** and **etomidate**
2. *Basal anaesthetics*
   a. **Ketamine**
   b. **Diazepam**

Various other combined formulations of neuroleptic drugs (see Chapter 22) and analgesics (see Chapter 25) may also be used to produce a state of deep sedation and analgesia (known as neuroleptanalgesia) in which the patient remains responsive to simple commands and questions, but does not respond to painful stimuli or retain any memory of the procedure.

Thiopentone

Thiopentone is a member of the barbiturate group of central nervous system depressants (see Chapter 21). Many of these have been produced and tested, but thiopentone is the only one of major importance in anaesthesia. Chemically it is a thiobarbiturate (Fig. 20.6) with a sulphur atom replacing oxygen in the urea residue of the barbiturate ring. The importance of this is that it confers very high lipid solubility, which is the main factor responsible for the speed and transience of its effect when it is injected intravenously (see below). The free acid is insoluble in water, so thiopentone is given as the sodium salt. This solution is strongly alkaline, and is unstable, so the drug must be dissolved immediately before it is used.

Pharmacokinetic aspects

On intravenous injection, thiopentone causes unconsciousness within about 20 seconds and lasting for 5–10 minutes. The anaesthetic effect closely parallels the concentration of thiopentone in the blood reaching the brain, because the lipid solubility of the drug is sufficiently large that it can cross the blood-brain barrier without appreciable hindrance. It is this property that makes thiopentone

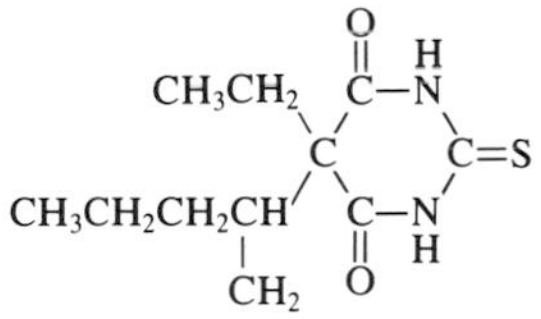

Thiopentone

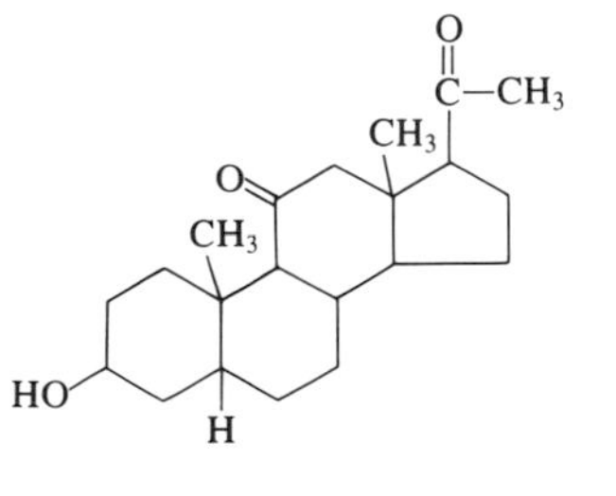

Alphaxolone (active ingredient of althesin)

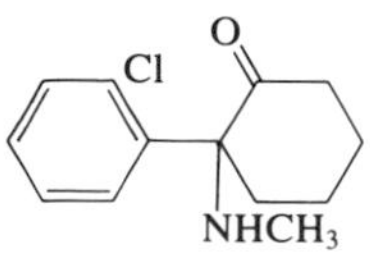

Ketamine

Fig. 20.6 Structures of intravenous anaesthetics.

different in its characteristics from most other barbiturates. With **pentobarbitone**, for example, which differs only in possessing an oxygen atom instead of sulphur attached to the ring and is less lipid-soluble, intravenous injection produces unconsciousness only after an appreciable delay (1–2 minutes), even though the concentration in the blood follows a similar time-course, because the concentration in the brain does not rise and fall nearly so quickly as with thiopentone (Fig. 20.7).

The decline in the blood concentration of thiopentone following the initial peak (Fig. 20.7) occurs because of *redistribution* of the drug, first of all to tissues with a large blood flow (liver, kidneys, brain, etc) and more slowly to muscle. Uptake into body fat, though favoured by the high lipid solubility of thiopentone, occurs only slowly, because of the low blood flow to this tissue. After several hours, however, most of the thiopentone present in the body will have accumulated in body fat, the rest having been metabolized. Recovery from the anaesthetic effect depends entirely on redistribution of

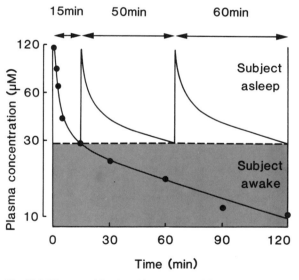

Fig. 20.7 Pharmacokinetics of intravenous thiopentone in man. Plasma concentration (logarithmic scale) following a single intravenous injection is shown as the experimental points. The concentration falls from a peak of 120 μM to 30 μM in about 15 minutes, due to redistribution of the drug into well-perfused tissues, and then falls much more slowly as it is distributed into fatty tissues.
  The curves show the predicted time course of the plasma concentration if subsequent injections are given each time the patient recovers consciousness. The duration of action becomes much longer as the slow phase of equilibration becomes more pronounced. (Data from: Brodie et al, 1950)

the drug, since very little is metabolized in the first 10 minutes after injection. The blood concentration drops rapidly from its peak, but then declines only slowly as the drug is taken up by body fat and metabolized (Fig. 20.7). This means that thiopentone produces a long-lasting 'hangover', and also that repeated intravenous doses cause progressively longer periods of anaesthesia, since this plateau in blood concentration becomes progressively more elevated as more drug accumulates in the body. For this reason, thiopentone cannot be used to maintain surgical anaesthesia, but only as an induction agent.

Thiopentone binds to plasma albumin (roughly 70% of the blood content normally being bound). The fraction bound is less in states of malnutrition, liver disease or renal disease, which affect the concentration and drug binding properties of plasma albumin, and this can appreciably reduce the dose needed for induction of anaesthesia.

Actions and side effects

The actions of thiopentone on the nervous system are very similar to those of inhalation anaesthetics, though it has no analgesic effect, and can cause profound respiratory depression even in amounts that fail to abolish reflex responses to painful stimuli. It is thus unsatisfactory as an agent for producing surgical anaesthesia and is used only for induction, prior to the administration of an inhalation anaesthetic.

Its long after effect (Fig. 20.7) associated with a slowly-declining plasma concentration means that drowsiness and some degree of respiratory depression persist for about 2 hours.

A serious danger of thiopentone injection is that it may accidentally be injected around, rather than into, the vein, or into an artery. This can cause local tissue necrosis and ulceration, or severe arterial spasm which can result in gangrene. Immediate injection, through the same needle, or a vasodilator such as phentolamine is the recommended procedure if this accident occurs. Thiopentone, like other barbiturates, can precipitate an attack of porphyria in susceptible individuals (see Chapter 4).

Althesin

The anaesthetic effects of high doses of corticosteroids such as hydrocortisone were observed nearly 50 years ago, but althesin, the first clinically useful intravenous anaesthetic incorporating a steroid structure, was not introduced until 1971.

The active substance in althesin is **alphaxolone** (see Fig. 20.6) which is combined with the acetoxy-derivative (**alphadolone**) and with a detergent (cremophor) in order to increase its solubility. On the basis of animal tests althesin has a greater therapeutic index than thiopentone. Thus, in mice the ratio of the LD_{50} to the ED_{50} is about 30 for althesin, compared with 7–8 for thiopentone and most other intravenous anaesthetics. The relationship between therapeutic index and clinical safety is, of course, questionable (see Chapter 2). Induction and recovery occur about as fast with althesin as with thiopentone, though recovery from althesin depends partly on rapid metabolic transformation in the liver, as well as on redistribution, so it produces less cumulative effect. Althesin is not appreciably protein bound, which is an advantage compared with thiopentone. The solution as injected is neutral, and no untoward effects occur if it is accidently injected into the tissues or into an artery.

The main drawback of althesin is the unpredictable, though rare, occurrence of severe hypersensitivity reactions, resulting in hypotension and bronchoconstriction. In other respects it has real advantages over thiopentone as an induction agent.

Ketamine

This drug (see Fig. 20.6) closely resembles, both chemically and pharmacologically, **phencyclidine**, which is a 'street-drug' with a pronounced effect on sensory perception (see Chapter 26). Both drugs produce a similar anaesthesia-like state, but ketamine produces considerably less euphoria and sensory distortion than phencyclidine and is thus more useful in anaesthesia.

Given intravenously, ketamine works nearly as rapidly as thiopentone, but produces a different effect, known as 'dissociative anaesthesia' in which there is a marked sensory loss and analgesia, and paralysis of movement, without actual loss of consciousness. During induction and recovery, involuntary movements and peculiar sensory experiences often occur.

Ketamine does not act simply as a depressant, and it produces cardiovascular and respiratory effects quite different from those of anaesthetics. Blood pressure and heart rate are usually increased, and respiration is unaffected by effective anaesthetic doses.

The main drawback of ketamine, in spite of the safety associated with a lack of depressant activity, is that hallucinations, and sometimes delirium and irrational behaviour, are common during recovery. These after effects are much less marked in children, but have prevented the widespread use of ketamine in adults.

REFERENCES AND FURTHER READING

Angel A 1980 Effects of anaesthetics on nervous pathways. In: Gray T C, Nunn J F, Utting J E (eds) General anaesthesia, Vol I. Butterworth, London

Franks N P, Lieb W R 1982 Molecular mechanisms of general anaesthesia. Nature 300: 487–493

Halsey M J 1980 Physicochemical properties of inhalation anaesthetics. In: Gray T C, Nunn J F, Utting J E (eds) General anaesthesia, Vol I. Butterworth, London

Miller K W, Paton W D M, Smith R A, Smith E B 1973 The pressure reversal of general anaesthesia and the critical volume hypothesis. Mol Pharmacol 9: 131–143

National halothane study (summary) 1966 JAMA 197: 775–788

Nunn J F 1984 Interaction of nitrous oxide and vitamin B_{12}. Trends in Pharmacological Sciences 5: 225–227

Richards C D 1980 The mechanism of general anaesthesia. In: Norman J, Whitwam J (eds) Topical reviews in anaesthesia, Vol I. Wright, Bristol

Vickers M D, Schnieden H, Wood-Smith F G 1984 Drugs in anaesthetic practice. Butterworth, London

Anxiolytic and hypnotic drugs

In this chapter we discuss **anxiolytic drugs** (used to treat the symptoms of anxiety) and **hypnotic drugs** (used to treat insomnia). Though the clinical objectives are different, the same drugs are often used for both purposes. This is a reflection of the fact that all drugs that relieve anxiety also cause a degree of sedation and drowsiness, which is one of the main drawbacks in the clinical use of anxiolytic drugs. Until recently, the sedatives that were in clinical use (mainly barbiturates and related compounds) were pharmacologically indistinguishable from general anaesthetics (see Chapter 20). In high doses all of these drugs cause unconsciousness, and eventually death from respiratory and cardiovascular depression. The discovery of the **benzodiazepines** in 1961 introduced a new type of anxiolytic drug whose action differed fundamentally from that of general anaesthetics, and these drugs quickly replaced most of the earlier anxiolytic and hypnotic drugs.

THE MEASUREMENT OF ANXIOLYTIC ACTIVITY

The distinction between a pathological, as opposed to a normal, state of anxiety, is hard to draw, but in spite of (or perhaps because of) this diagnostic vagueness, anxiolytic drugs are among the most frequently-prescribed substances. A recent study in Western European countries showed that the proportion of the total population using anxiolytic drugs regularly was 17% in Belgium and France, 14% in the UK and 10% in Spain.

The chief manifestations of anxiety (Dews, 1981) are:

1. Verbal complaint. The patients says that he or she is excessively anxious
2. Somatic and autonomic effects. The patient is restless and agitated, has tachycardia, increased sweating, weeping, etc
3. Interference with normal productive activities.

These are essentially human manifestations, and except for certain components of the somatic and autonomic changes, have no obvious counterpart in experimental animals. To develop new anxiolytic drugs it is essential to have animal tests that give a good guide to activity in man, and considerable effort has gone into developing and validating such tests.

Tests on animals

The use of **operant conditioning** methods (Iversen & Iversen, 1981) has provided some useful tests for anxiolytic activity. If an animal is trained to press a bar in order to receive a reward (a food pellet, say, after every 50th response) anxiolytic drugs usually increase the rate of bar-pressing somewhat, unless the dose is so large that the animal is obviously sedated. This is not a particularly discriminating test as it stands, for other kinds of drug (e.g. stimulants, such as amphetamine) have the same effect. Operant conditioning tests become more discriminative when some degree of conflict is introduced into the test protocol. For example, in a test developed by Geller & Seifter (1960) rats were trained to respond consistently under two different conditions. In one condition, the normal pattern of reward by a food pellet in response to bar pressing occurred, and the rats achieved high and consistent rates. At intervals, indicated by an auditory signal, bar pressing resulted in an occasional 'punishment' in the form of an electric shock in addition to the reward of a food pellet. Normally the rats cease pressing the bar, and thus avoid the shock, during the period when the signal is sounding. The completeness of this suppression depends on the intensity and frequency of the shocks delivered. The effect of an anxiolytic drug is to relieve this suppressive effect (Fig. 21.1) and to cause the rats to

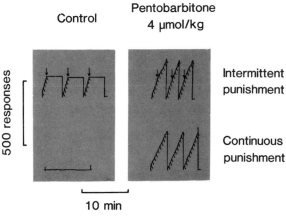

Fig. 21.1 Effect of pentobarbitone in a conflict test. Pigeons were trained to peck a key to obtain food, key-pecking being monitored by upward deflection of the trace. The rewards occurred after a fixed number of pecks, each one being signalled by a downward blip on the record.

Upper traces: After each arrow, the food reward was accompanied by electric shock. In normal animals, this completely suppressed key-pecking behaviour, but in pentobarbitone-treated animals, pecking continued almost as rapidly as before.

Lower traces: Food rewards were accompanied by electric shocks throughout the test. Normal animals did not peck the key, whereas after pentobarbitone they did so in spite of the delivery of the shock. (From: Kelleher & Morse, 1964)

continue bar-pressing for reward in spite of the 'punishment'. Surprisingly, analgesic drugs, which presumably make the punishment less painful, are ineffective in this test in animals, as are other types of psychotropic drug, and other evidence suggests that it is the behavioural response to the painful stimulus, rather than an elevation of the pain threshold that is changed by anxiolytic drugs.

Other types of behavioural test are also used to measure anxiolytic activity. Thus, aggressive behaviour can be produced experimentally by lesions of the midbrain septum, or by housing mice individually for a time and then introducing a stranger into the cage. Anxiolytic drugs reduce the amount of aggressive behaviour which can be measured, for example by observing the frequency with which the dominant mouse attacks others. They also increase the amount of social interaction occurring between pairs of rats placed in an unfamiliar environment, this being a situation in which social interaction is greatly decreased in control animals. In both this test and the Geller–Seifter test described above, the response is an increase in behavioural activity, so it is clear that the anxiolytic drugs are producing something more than a nonspecific sedation.

Tests on humans

Various 'anxiety scale' tests have been devised, in which a patient's responses to a standard battery of questions are scored, and these are widely used to assay the clinical effectiveness of anxiolytic drugs. Effects have been clearly demonstrated in tests of this kind, but it is often found that placebo treatment produces highly significant responses of a magnitude comparable to that produced by active drugs.

Other tests rely on measurement of the somatic and autonomic effects associated with anxiety. An example is the **galvanic skin response (GSR)** in which the electrical conductivity of the skin is used as a measure of sweat production. Any novel stimulus, whether pleasant or unpleasant, causes a brief reduction of resistance. This forms the basis of the lie-detector test. If an innocuous stimulus is repeated at intervals, the magnitude of the response decreases (habituation). The rate of habituation is less in anxious patients than in normal subjects, and is increased by anxiolytic drugs (Lader & Wing, 1966). GSR habituation seems to be a particularly sensitive measure, for many tests of autonomic function in anxious subjects (e.g. heart rate changes) show no clearcut change in response to anxiolytic drugs.

A human version of the Geller–Seifter punishment avoidance test described above involves the substitution of money for food pellets, and the use of graded electric shocks as punishment. As with rats, administration of diazepam increased the rate of button-pressing for money during the periods when the punishment was in operation, though the subjects reported no change in the painfulness of the electric shock. Subtler forms of torment and reward could easily be envisaged.

CLASSIFICATION OF ANXIOLYTIC AND HYPNOTIC DRUGS

The main groups of drugs are:

1. **Benzodiazepines**. The most important group clinically
2. **Barbiturates**. The major group until 20 years ago; now largely superseded by benzodiazepines
3. Miscellaneous other drugs, e.g. **chloral hydrate**, **glutethimide**, **meprobamate**, **methaqualone**, **paraldehyde**.

BENZODIAZEPINES

The first compound of this group, chlordiazepoxide (Fig. 21.2) was synthesized by accident in 1961, the unusual 7-membered ring having been produced as a result of an unplanned reaction of a heterocyclic 6-membered ring compound with methylamine, and its unusual pharmacological activity was recognized as a result of a routine screening procedure. This series of compounds quite soon became the most widely-prescribed drugs in the pharmacopoeia, and outstandingly profitable to Hoffmann la Roche, the company that discovered them—a potent reminder to advocates of rational drug design that historical examples do not always support their view.

Chemistry and structure-activity relationships

The basic chemical structure of benzodiazepines is shown in Figure 21.2. All share the same unusual ring structure, differing in the substituent groups. Thousands of compounds have been made and tested, and about 20 are available for clinical use. They are basically similar in their pharmacological actions, though some degree of selectivity has been reported. Thus it is claimed that some compounds show a greater anticonvulsant activity in relation to their sedative and anxiolytic effects, than others. Results from different laboratories, however, show wide variations, probably because of

Fig. 21.2 Structures of some benzodiazepines.

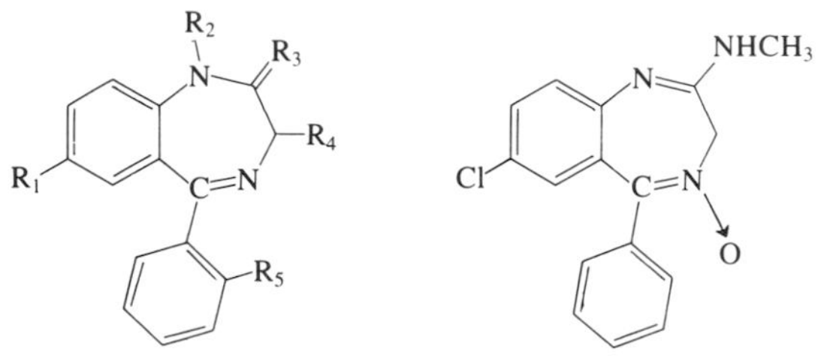

Drug	R_1	R_2	R_3	R_4	R_5
Diazepam	Cl	CH_3	=O	H_2	H
Nitrazepam	NO_2	H	=O	H_2	H
Flurazepam	Cl	$(CH_2)_2N(C_2H_5)_2$	=O	H_2	H
Flunitrazepam	NO_2	H	=O	H_2	F
Oxazepam	Cl	H	=O	OH	H
Temazepam	Cl	CH_3	=O	H_2	H
Clonazepam	NO_2	H	=O	H_2	Cl
Lorazepam	Cl	H	=O	OH	Cl
Clorazepate	Cl	H	=O	COOH	H
Nordiazepam	Cl	H	=O	H_2	H

variations in experimental methodology*. It is therefore risky to assume that the differences in pharmacological specificity that have been reported will be reflected in clinical use. From a clinical point of view, differences in pharmacokinetic behaviour among different benzodiazepines (see below) are more important than differences in pattern of activity.

Most of the clinically useful benzodiapines have the structure shown in Figure 21.2, with −Cl or −NO_2 at R_1, −H or −CH_3 at R_2, −H or −OH at R_4 and −H, −F or −Cl at R_5. Recently, drugs with a similar structure have been discovered, which specifically antagonize the effects of the benzodiazepines (see below).

Pharmacological effects

The most important effects are on the central nervous system and consist of:

1. Reduction of anxiety and aggression

---

* For example, the ED_{50} for diazepam in mice, measured by a standard laboratory test for motor coordination (the rotarod test) varied between 2.1 and 30 mg/kg in seven different laboratories (Haefely et al, 1981).

2. Sedation and induction of sleep
3. Reduction of muscle tone and coordination
4. Anticonvulsant effect.

Reduction of anxiety and aggression

The measurement of anxiolytic effects in animals and man has been discussed above. Benzodiazepines also exert a marked 'taming' effect, allowing animals to be handled much more easily. If given to the dominant member of a pair of animals (e.g. mice or monkeys) housed in the same cage, benzodiazepines reduce the number of attacks by the dominant individual and increase the number of attacks made upon him.

Sedation and induction of sleep

Benzodiazepines decrease the time taken to get to sleep, and increase the total duration of sleep, though the latter effect occurs only in subjects who normally sleep for less than about 6 hours each night. Both effects tend to decline when benzodiazepines are taken regularly for 1–2 weeks.

On the basis of EEG measurements several levels of sleep can be recognized (Kay et al, 1976). Of particular psychological importance are 'rapid eye movement' (REM) sleep, which is associated with dreaming, and 'slow wave' (SW) sleep, which corresponds to the deepest level of sleep, when the metabolic rate and adrenal steroid secretion are at their lowest and the secretion of growth hormone is at its highest (see Chapter 16). All hypnotic drugs reduce the proportion of REM sleep, though benzodiazepines affect it less than other hypnotics. Deliberate interruption of REM sleep causes irritability and anxiety, even if the total amount of sleep is not reduced, and the lost REM sleep is made up for, at the end of such an experiment, by a rebound increase. The same pattern of rebound in REM sleep is seen at the end of a period of administration of benzodiazepines or other hypnotics. It is therefore assumed that REM sleep has a function, and that the relatively slight reduction of REM sleep by benzodiazepines is a point in their favour.

The proportion of SW sleep is significantly reduced by benzodiazepines, though a recent study showed no change in growth hormone secretion.

Insomnia is subjectively unpleasant rather than

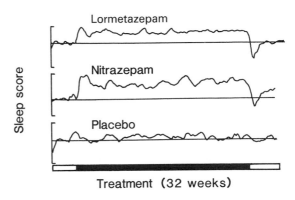

Fig. 21.3 Effects of long-term benzodiazepine treatment on sleep quality. 100 poor sleepers were given, under double-blind conditions, lormetazepam 5 mg, nitrazepam 2 mg, or placebo nightly for 24 weeks, the test period being preceded and followed by 4 weeks of placebo treatment. They were asked to assess, on a subjective rating scale, the quality of sleep during each night, and the results are expressed as a 5 day rolling average of these scores.

The improvement in sleep quality (upward deflection of line relative to control baseline) was maintained during the 24-week test period, and was followed by a 'rebound' worsening of sleep when the test period ended. (From: Oswald et al, 1982)

objectively harmful, so the best guide to the usefulness of hypnotic drugs in improving the quality of sleep may be the patient's own judgement. Figure 21.3 shows the improvement of subjective ratings of sleep quality produced by a benzodiazepine, and the rebound decrease at the end of a 32 week period of drug treatment. It is notable that, though tolerance to objective effects, such as reduced sleep latency, occurs within a few days, this is not obvious in the subjective rating of sleep quality.

Reduction of muscle tone and coordination

Benzodiazepines have been claimed to reduce muscle tone by a central action that is independent of their sedative effect. Cats are particularly sensitive to this action, and some benzodiazepines (e.g. clonazepam, flunitrazepam) reduce decerebrate rigidity in doses that are much smaller than those needed to produce behavioural effects. In other species the effect is less clear. Several tests have been devised to measure muscle tone. Mice may be suspended by their forelimbs from a horizontal wire, and the time taken for them to clamber on to the wire with their hind feet measured. Alternatively, the tension needed to detach their grip can be measured. Coordination can be tested by measuring the length of time for which they can stay on a slowly rotating horizontal plastic rod, or the time taken for them to escape from confinement by climbing up the inside of a tubular chimney. Performance in all of these acrobatic tricks is impaired by benzodiazepines and other sedatives, but it is not clear that particular drugs show selectivity in this respect in species other than the cat. Studies in man have failed to show differences between benzodiazepines.

Increased muscle tone is a common feature of anxiety states in man, and may contribute to the aches and pains, including headache (often related to increased muscle tone), which often trouble anxious patients. The relaxant effect of benzodiazepines may therefore be clinically useful. A reduction of muscle tone appears to be possible without producing appreciable impairment of coordination.

Anticonvulsant effects

All of the benzodiazepines have anticonvulsant activity in experimental animal tests. They are generally more effective against chemically-induced convulsions (leptazol, bicuculline, etc; see Chapters 24 & 26) than against electrically-induced convulsions, and are among the most potent agents known in preventing leptazol-induced convulsions. Benzodiazepines do not affect strychnine-induced convulsions in experimental animals. Both bicuculline and strychnine are believed to act by blocking the action of inhibitory transmitters in the central nervous system; strychnine exerts its effect on glycine receptors (see Chapter 26), whereas bicuculline and several other chemical convulsant agents act on GABA receptors. Since benzodiazepines enhance the action of GABA (see below), but not glycine, the selectivity of their anticonvulsant action is explicable. There is some evidence that clonazepam is relatively more effective as an anticonvulsant in relation to its behavioural effects than other benzodiazepines, and this drug is sometimes used clinically, particularly for the treatment of **absence seizures** and **myoclonic seizures** in children (see Chapter 24). Diazepam, given intravenously, is an effective way of terminating the repeated seizures that constitute status epilepticus.

Mechanism of action

Until 1977 the benzodiazepines were thought, in the absence of any clear evidence to the contrary, to be acting as non-specific depressants, much like anaesthetics (see Chapter 20). In 1977, groups in Denmark and Switzerland independently found that radioactive diazepam binds with high affinity to a distinct population of binding sites in the brain, and that other benzodiazepines competitively inhibit this binding with affinities that correlate quite closely with their pharmacological potencies. Binding to tissues other than the brain is weak or absent, and within the brain diazepam binding shows a distinct regional distribution (Young & Kuhar, 1979, 1980). Binding is highest in the cerebral cortex, less in the limbic system and midbrain, and still less in the brainstem and spinal cord. It agrees roughly but not exactly, with counts of GABA receptors, though the number of benzodiazepine sites is consistently less. The correlation between affinity for binding sites and pharmacological potency among a range of benzodiazepines is reasonable but not perfect (Fig. 21.4). The discrepancies are up to 10-fold for some compounds. This may be partly due to the fact that the pharmacological measurements were made *in vivo* so that the drugs were subject to metabolic alteration. It is known that benzodiazepines are metabolized at very variable rates, and that in some cases the metabolites are pharmacologically active. Alternatively there may be some heterogeneity among binding sites which tends to obscure a simpler correlation of overall binding with activity.

About the same time that the existence of specific benzodiazepine binding was discovered, evidence was accumulating that these drugs specifically augment the actions of GABA (Fig. 21.5), and that they oppose the effects of antagonists of GABA, such as bicuculline. This augmentation of the pharmacological effects of GABA is confined to $GABA_A$ receptors in the central nervous system, which produce an increased chloride conductance (see Chapter 19); actions produce by $GABA_B$ receptors (reduction of calcium currents and increased potassium permeability) are not affected, nor are $GABA_A$ responses in peripheral neurons (which lack benzodiazepine binding sites).

Binding studies have revealed something of the

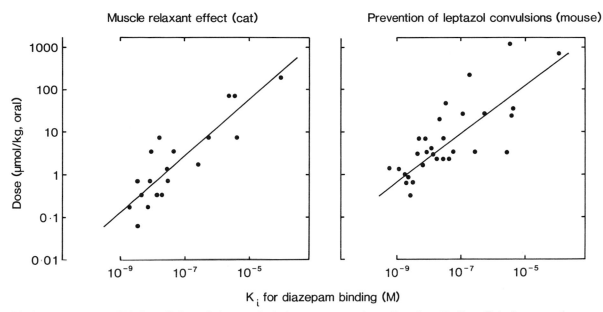

Fig. 21.4 Correlation of binding affinity and pharmacological potency among benzodiazepines. Binding affinity is expressed as an equilibrium constant, and was calculated by measuring the concentration of drug needed to inhibit the binding of ^{3}H-diazepam to brain membranes. The ordinates show equipotent doses in two biological test systems. (Data from: Braestrup & Squires, 1978)

mechanism of this interesting interaction. There is a mutual augmentation of binding between GABA and benzodiazepines. The two agents bind to independent sites on the same receptor-ion channel complex, and each increases the affinity of the sites for the other, without affecting the total number of sites. Benzodiazepines do not open chloride channels by themselves, but they act allosterically to increase the affinity of the receptors for GABA. Enhancement of the GABA effect has recently been shown by a noise analysis (see Chapter 1) to be associated with an increase in the number of channels that are opened by a given concentration of GABA, rather than with an increase in channel conductance or average open time (Fig. 21.5). There is, it need hardly be said, evidence from binding studies for more than one class of benzodiazepine receptor, but pharmacological studies have not so far confirmed the need for such a sub-classification.

Work on biochemical characterization of the benzodiazepine/GABA receptor and its associated chloride channel is proceeding rapidly, and the gene coding for the receptor has recently been isolated from rat brain DNA. On injection into toad oocytes, the complementary RNA causes the oocyte to express the protein on its surface and display sensitivity to GABA and benzodiazepines exactly like a neuron (Houamed et al, 1984). Exactly how the benzodiazepine and GABA binding sites are linked together and related to the chloride channel remains unclear. The mechanism shown in Figure 21.6 is one theoretical possibility.

Benzodiazepine antagonists and the hunt for the endogenous mediator

Recently the Hoffman la Roche group (Hunkeler et al, 1981) reported on some compounds related to benzodiazepines which acted as competitive antagonists, in both binding and functional assays. The best-known compound, Ro 15-1788, was originally reported to lack effects on behaviour or on drug-induced convulsions when given on its own, though more recent work (File, 1983) shows that it and other benzodiazepine antagonists do show some 'anxiogenic' and pro-convulsant activity. Benzodiazepine antagonists might have clinical uses in treating overdosage, or in anaesthesiology, where it would be convenient to be able to terminate benzodiazepine effects rapidly.

The existence of specific benzodiazepine receptors suggested that there might be an endogenous

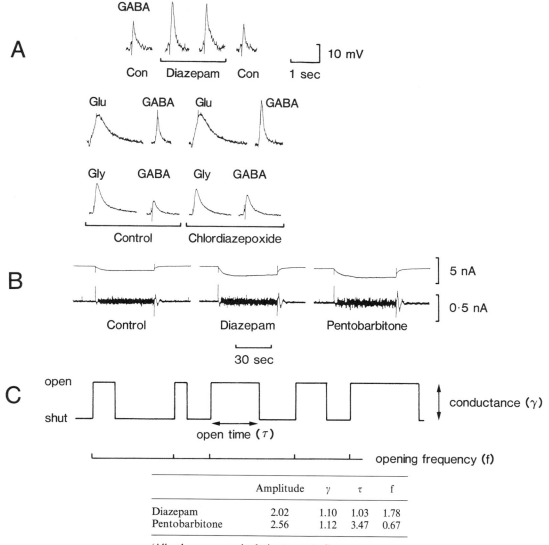

Fig. 21.5 Potentiating effect of benzodiazepines and pentobarbitone on the action of GABA in mouse spinal cord neurons grown in tissue culture. Drugs were applied by ionophoresis from micropipettes placed closed to the cells. The membrane was hyperpolarised to −90 mv and the cells were loaded with chloride ions from the recording microelectrode, so inhibitory amino-acids (GABA and glycine), as well as excitatory ones (glutamate) caused depolarizing responses.

A. The potentiating effect is restricted to GABA responses, glutamate and glycine responses being unaffected.

B. Enhancement of GABA responses by diazepam and pentobarbitone, recorded with a voltage-clamp technique. Inward current (i.e. outward flux of chloride ions) is shown as a downward deflection in the upper records. The lower records are at higher gain, and are filtered to remove the DC component, leaving the high-frequency noise signal (see Chapter 1) which was analysed to provide estimates of channel conductance, mean channel lifetime and opening frequency.

C. Schematic diagram of channel opening parameters. The table below shows the effects of diazepam and pentobarbitone. Diazepam acts mainly to increase the channel opening frequency, whereas pentobarbitone increases the mean open time. (From: MacDonald & Barker, 1978; Study & Barker, 1981)

ligand (analogous to endorphins in relation to the morphine receptor) whose function was to regulate the inhibitory effect of GABA. So far no such substance has been definitely identified. One much-touted candidate was ethyl β-caroline 3-carboxylate (βCCE), which was discovered in 1980 by assaying urine samples for activity in inhibiting benzodiazepine binding. βCCE is now known to be an

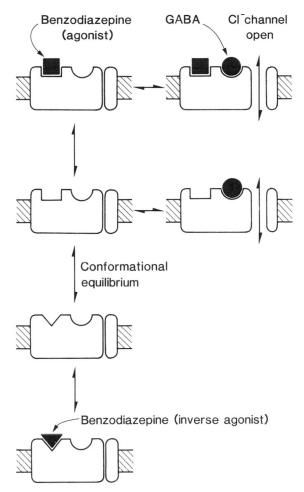

Benzodiazepine (agonist) **GABA** **Cl⁻channel open**

Conformational equilibrium

Benzodiazepine (inverse agonist)

Fig. 21.6 Model of benzodiazepine/GABA receptor interaction. Benzodiazepine agonists (e.g. diazepam) and antagonists (e.g. Ro 15-1788) are believed to bind to a site on the GABA receptor distinct from the GABA building site. A conformational equilibrium exists between states in which the benzodiazepine receptor exists in its *agonist binding* conformation (above) and in its *inverse agonist binding* conformation (below). In the latter state the GABA receptor has a much reduced affinity for GABA, so that the chloride channel remains closed.

artefact of the extraction procedure. Claims have also been made that the benzodiazepine receptor is normally occupied by a protein, called GABA-modulin, which holds the GABA receptor/chloride channel in a non-functional state. This protein is supposed to be displaced by benzodiazepines, but the theory (Costa & Guidotti, 1979) is highly contentious, and the hunt for the endogenous ligand seems, at the time of writing, to be losing the scent.

Recently, a new type of drug has been discovered—sometimes referred to as an **inverse agonist**—which binds to benzodiazepine receptors and exerts the *opposite* effect to that of conventional benzodiazepines, producing signs of increased anxiety and convulsions. It may be possible (Fig. 21.6) to explain these complexities in terms of the 2-state model discussed in Chapter 1, by postulating that the benzodiazepine receptor exists in two distinct conformations, only one of which can bind a GABA molecule and open the chloride channel. The other conformation cannot bind GABA. Normally, with no benzodiazepine receptor ligand present, there is an equilibrium between these two conformations; sensitivity to GABA is present, but submaximal. Benzodiazepine *agonists* (e.g. diazepam) are postulated to bind only to the first conformation, thus shifting the equilibrium and enhancing GABA sensitivity. *Inverse agonists* bind selectivity to the GABA-insensitive conformation, and have the opposite effect. *Competitive antagonists*, such as Ro 15-1788 bind equally to both, and consequently do not disturb the conformational equilibrium, but prevent the binding of other substances to the benzodiazepine receptor, thus antagonizing the effect of both agonists and inverse agonists

Pharmacokinetic aspects

Benzodiazepines are all completely absorbed when given orally, usually giving a peak plasma concentration in about 1 hour. Some (e.g. oxazepam, lorazepam) are absorbed more slowly. They bind strongly to plasma protein, but their high lipid solubility causes many of them to accumulate gradually in body fat. These two factors result in distribution volumes not far from 1 litre/kg body weight for most drugs. They are normally given by mouth, but can be given intravenously (e.g. diazepam in status epilepticus). Intramuscular injection often results in slow absorption.

Benzodiazepines are all inactivated by metabolic processes, and are eventually excreted as glucuronide conjugates in the urine. They vary greatly in duration of action, and can be roughly divided into short and long-acting compounds (Table 21.1). The distinction between these two categories depends on whether or not the drug forms a long-lasting pharmacologically active metabolite, such as N-desmethyldiazepam (**nordiazepam**). The half-life of

Table 21.1 Characteristics of benzodiazepines in man

Drug	Half-life of parent compound (hours)	Active metabolite	Half-life of metabolite (hours)	Category
Lorazepam	12	—		Short-acting
Oxazepam	8	—		Effective t_1 < 24 hours
Temazepam	8	—		
Diazepam	32	nordiazepam	~ 60 (40–200)	
Chlordiazepoxide	12	nordiazepam	~ 60 (40–200)	Long-acting
Flurazepam	1	desalkyl-flurazepam	~ 60 (40–200)	Effective t_1 > 24 hours
Nitrazepam	28	—		
Clonazepam	50	—		

this compound, which lies on the metabolic pathway of many of the benzodiazepines, is about 60 hours, and this accounts for the tendency of many benzodiazepines to produce cumulative effects and long hangovers when they are given at regular intervals. The short-acting compounds are those that are metabolized directly by conjugation with glucuronide. The main pathways are shown in

Adverse effects of benzodiazepines

These may be divided into:

1. Toxic effects resulting from acute overdosage
2. Unwanted effects occurring during normal therapeutic use
3. Tolerance and dependence.

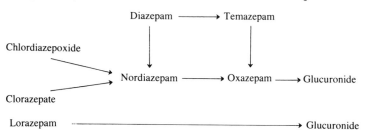

Fig. 21.7 The metabolism of benzodiazepines. The N-demethylated metabolite, nordiazepam, is formed from many benzodiapines, and is important because it is biologically active and has a very long half-life.

Figure 21.7. Figure 21.8 shows the gradual build-up, and slow disappearance, of nordiazepam from the plasma of a human subject given diazepam daily for 15 days.

Advancing age affects the rate of oxidative reactions more than that of conjugation reactions. Thus the effect of the long-acting benzodiazepines, which may be used regularly as hypnotics or anxiolytic agents for many years, tends to increase with age, and it is common for drowsiness and confusion to develop insidiously for this reason.*

Acute toxicity

Benzodiazepines in acute overdose are considerably less dangerous than other anxiolytic/hypnotic drugs (Table 21.2). Since such agents are often used in attempted suicide, this is an important advantage. The effect of an overdose is to cause prolonged sleep, with the patient normally remaining rousable, without serious depression of respiration or cardiovascular function.

Side effects during therapeutic use

The main side effects are drowsiness, confusion and impaired motor coordination, which considerably impairs manual skills such as driving performance. An interaction with alcohol is often claimed, whereby a low plasma concentration of a benzodia-

---

* At the age of 91, the gradmother of one of the authors was growing increasingly forgetful and mildly dotty, having been taking nitrazepam for insomnia regularly for years. To the author's lasting shame, it took a canny general practitioner to diagnose the problem. Cancellation of the nitrazepam prescription produced a dramatic improvement.

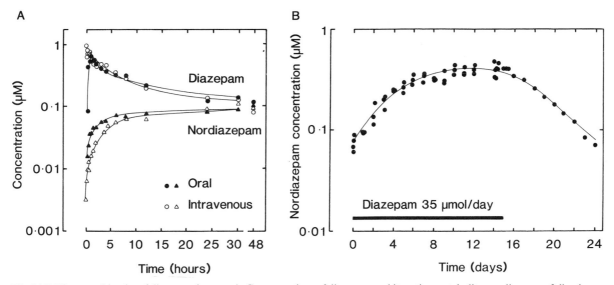

Fig. 21.8 Pharmacokinetics of diazepam in man. A. Concentrations of diazepam and its active metabolite, nordiazepam, following a single oral or intravenous dose. Note the negligible disappearance of both substances after the first 20 hours. B. Accumulation of nordiazepam during two weeks of daily administration of diazepam, and slow decline (half-life about 3 days) after cessation of diazepam administration. (Data from Kaplan et al, 1973)

zepine can enhance the depressant effect of alcohol in a more than additive way. The objective evidence for this is unconvincing. The long and unpredictable duration of action of many benzodiazepines is important in relation to side effects. Drugs such as nitrazepam that are used as hypnotics have been shown to produce a substantial day-after impairment of job performance and driving skill.

Tolerance and dependence

Benzodiazepines seem to have much the same tendency to produce dependence as do other hypnotics

Table 21.2 Therapeutic ratios of central nervous system depressants in man

Drug	Approximate effective dose (mg)	Approximate lethal dose (mg)	Ratio
Morphine	10–20	60–200	3–20
Chlorpromazine	50–100	2000	20–40
Phenobarbitone	100–200	2000–10 000	10–100
Glutethimide	250–500	10 000–40 000	20–160
Chlordiazepoxide	5–50	1400–21 000	280–4200
Diazepam	2–20	3500–35 000	175–17 500
Hexobarbitone	250–500	2000–10 000	4–40
Meprobamate	400–1200	20 000–40 000	20–100

(From: Haefely et al, 1981a)

such as barbiturates, though they are less liable to produce tolerance.

Tolerance has two components. **Pharmacokinetic tolerance** (i.e. a decrease in the plasma concentration produced by the same dose) is not important for benzodiazepines, since they have little inducing effect on hepatic microsomal enzymes. They do, however, produce some degree of **tissue tolerance**; this seems to be similar in degree to that occurring with the barbiturates, though objective measurements are few. The sleep-inducing effect shows relatively little tolerance (see Fig. 21.3). Lader (1983) found in eight normal subjects, that the euphoria associated with an intravenous injection of diazepam disappeared in subjects taking oral diazepam daily, as did the surge in growth hormone release. It is not clear whether tolerance to the anxiolytic effect is significant.

Dependence. Early claims that benzodiazepines cannot produce dependence have now been recognized as false (Lader, 1983). In human subjects and patients, stopping benzodiazepine treatment after weeks or months causes an increase in symptoms of anxiety, together with tremor and dizziness (Marks, 1978). In experimental animals, withdrawal causes nervousness, tremor, loss of appetite and sometimes convulsions. The withdrawal syndrome, in both animals and man, is generally slower in onset and less intense than with barbiturates, probably because of the long plasma half-life of most benzodiazepines. Short-acting benzodiazepines cause more abrupt withdrawal effects.

It is well recognized clinically that patients who are anxious to give up the regular taking of benzodiazepines find great difficulty in doing so.

OTHER SEDATIVE AND HYPNOTIC DRUGS

Clinically, the benzodiazepines have largely superseded other types of sedative drug, which only warrant a brief description.

Barbiturates

Since the discovery of the sleep-inducing properties of substances based on the barbituric acid structure (reputedly named after St Barbara, on whose day in

Barbiturates:

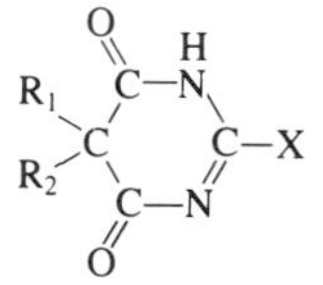

Drug	R_1	R_2	X
Phenobarbitone	Ethyl	Phenyl	—OH
Pentobarbitone	Ethyl	1-Methylbutyl	—OH
Triopentone	Ethyl	1-Methybutyl	—SNa

Other hypnotics:

$CCl_3CH(OH)_2$ CCl_3CH_2OH
Chloral hydrate   Trichlorethanol

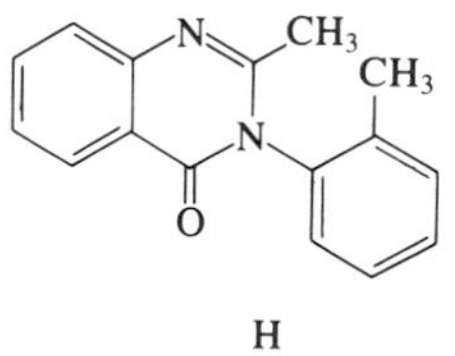

Methaqualone

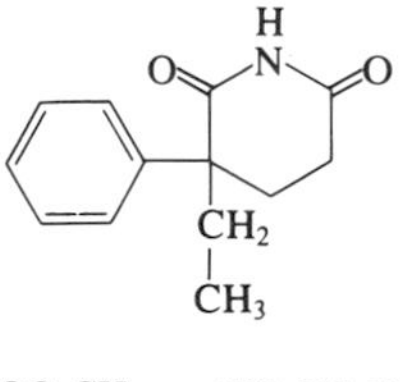

Glutethimide

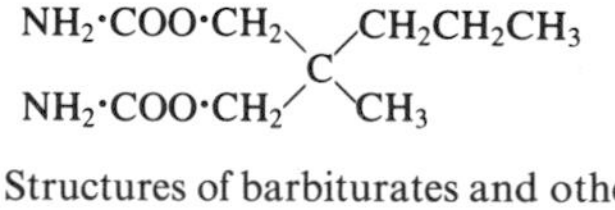

$NH_2 \cdot COO \cdot CH_2$ $CH_2CH_2CH_3$
$NH_2 \cdot COO \cdot CH_2$ CH_3

Meprobamate

Fig. 21.9 Structures of barbiturates and other sedative drugs.

1864 the synthesis was achieved), which is shown in Figure 21.9, hundreds of barbiturates have been made and tested, the main variations being achieved by substitutions at C5 of the ring. Nearly all of the compounds have depressant activity on the central nervous system, producing a gradation of effect very similar to the successive stages of anaesthesia seen with inhalation anaesthetics, and causing death from respiratory and cardiovascular depression if given in doses more than 10–100 times the clinically used dose (see Table 21.2). In addition to this overall depressant activity, some barbiturates (e.g. **phenobarbitone**) have specific anticonvulsant activity, (see Chapter 24), which does not seem to be a reflection of the non-specific central nervous system depression, and these have a continuing clinical use.

Varying the size and lipophilicity of the substituents on C5, affects the lipid solubility of barbiturates. One of the most highly lipid soluble is **thiopentone**, in which the oxygen at C1 is replaced by sulphur. This compound is widely used as an intravenous anaesthetic agent (see Chapter 20), the very short duration of action being the result of its extremely rapid passage across the blood–brain barrier.

Other barbiturates, lacking the specific anticonvulsant activity of phenobarbitone or the pharmacokinetic properties of thiopentone, have a sedative and anxiolytic effect that lasts 6–12 hours following oral administration. **Pentobarbitone** is typical of many very similar compounds, which are still occasionally used as sleeping pills and anxiolytic drugs. Their pharmacological effects are very similar to those of benzodiazepines in most animal tests, except that, in large doses, they cause much more profound central nervous system depression. They show similar activity in the Geller–Seifter test in experimental animals, supressing the inhibitory effect of punishment on the rate of responding for a reward, but are alleged to have a less marked anxiolytic effect in man. Barbiturates have no analgesic action. The mechanism of action of barbiturates is not well understood. They affect synaptic transmission rather than neuronal excitability, and there is some evidence that they produce a similar type of enhancement of GABA-mediated inhibition as the benzodiazepines. They do not, however, bind to the same site on the GABA-receptor/chloride channel

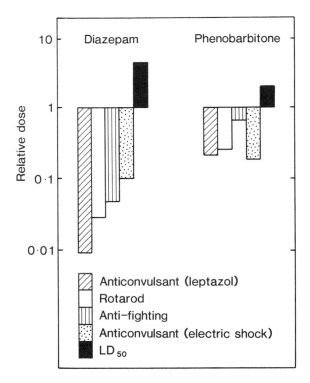

Fig. 21.10 Pharmacological profiles of diazepam and phenobarbitone. The equiactive doses of the two drugs in various tests are expressed relative to their hypnotic dose (ED_{50}) in mice. It can be seen that diazepam is relatively more effective as an anticonvulsant against leptazol-induced convulsions, and has a relatively higher lethal dose than phenobarbitone. (Data from: Schallek, 1981)

as the benzodiazepines and their action seems to be much less specific.

A comparison of the actions of phenobarbitone and diazepam in a series of screening tests in mice is shown in Figure 21.10. The dose scale has been normalised to the ED_{50} for the hypnotic effect. It can be seen that, relative to its hypnotic effect, phenobarbitone is less effective than diazepam in preventing leptazol-induced convulsion, in impairing performance on the rotarod test, and in suppressing fighting behaviour, but equally effective in suppressing electrically-induced convulsions. Phenobarbitone also has a relatively lower LD_{50}, which is also evident in Figure 21.10.

Barbiturates have several disadvantages compared with benzodiazepines. The main one is that they are lethal in overdose. Tolerance develops to a marked degree; this is partly due to **pharmacokinetic tolerance**, since barbiturates strongly induce the synthesis of hepatic cytochrome P450 and conjugating enzymes and thus the rate at which they are metabolized increases over the first few days of administration. In addition a true **tissue tolerance** develops, as with benzodiazepines. The inducing effect of barbiturates increases the rate of metabolic degradation of many other drugs, e.g. warfarin, steroids, (see Chapter 4), giving rise to a number of clinically important drug interactions. Induction of **δ-aminolaevulinic acid synthetase** results in increased porphyrin synthesis, which can initiate a severe and potentially fatal attack of acute porphyria in patients suffering from this inherited disorder (see Chapter 4). Dependence on barbiturates also develops with continued administration, though it is not clear that this is a more serious problem than with benzodiazepines. Barbiturates produce euphoria under appropriate social circumstances, as do most central nervous system depressants, and barbiturate abuse, usually by intravenous injection, is a common problem.

The action of most barbiturates is terminated by metabolic degradation, usually by oxidation to inactive metabolites that are excreted in the urine. Thiopentone (see Chapter 20) is short-acting because it is rapidly redistributed following intravenous injection. Its ultimate removal from the body depends on metabolic transformation. Phenobarbitone (plasma half-life 24–96 hours) is a long-acting drug, about 50% of which is excreted unchanged in the urine. Because, like all barbiturates, it is a weak acid, urinary excretion is greatly speeded by making the urine alkaline (see Chapter 3) which can be useful in treating phenobarbitone poisoning.

The plasma half-life of most other barbiturates in man is in the range 12–36 hours, and is rather unpredictable because of individual variation. Pronounced hangover effects have been demonstrated when barbiturates (even those that were at one time classified as 'short-acting' on the basis of studies of the duration of anaesthesia in rats) are used as hypnotics.

Meprobamate (Fig. 21.9)

This is a somewhat more selective central nervous system depressant than the barbiturates, and is claimed to produce relatively more anxiolytic and muscle relaxant effects, with less likelihood of respiratory depression, though the ratio of effective to lethal doses in man (Table 21.2) does not suggest it is much safer in practice. It does not produce anaesthesia, even in high doses, and is not an anticonvulsant. Pharmacologically, it lies somewhere between the barbiturates and the benzodiazepines (Haefely et al, 1981) with no striking clinical advantages. It has a similar tendency to cause tolerance and dependence. Following its introduction in 1955 its advantages as a tranquilizer were strongly overrated and it achieved very widespread use. In addition, it also found its way quickly on to the streets and achieved even more widespread abuse. Nothing is known about its mechanism of action.

Chloral hydrate and trichlorethanol

Trichlorethanol is a derivative of ethanol, with pronounced sedative action. Chloral hydrate is rapidly converted, by loss of a water molecule, to trichlorethanol, this being the form in which it acts. Chloral hydrate is much less irritant than trichlorethanol, and so more useful for oral administration. It appears to be a safe and effective hypnotic, whose plasma half-life (about 6 hours) is shorter than that of most other hypnotic drugs, so that it is less likely to produce a hangover.

Glutethimide and methaqualone

These closely resemble barbiturates. Glutethimide (plasma half-life 5–20 hours) is used as a hypnotic. It induces hepatic enzymes as barbiturates do, and has no clear advantages. Methaqualone is reported to have greater anxiolytic activity, but is liable to cause delirium and vivid dreaming so may not be satisfactory as a hypnotic.

REFERENCES AND FURTHER READING

Costa E C, Guidotti A 1979 Molecular mechanisms in the receptor action of benzodiazepines. Ann Rev Pharmacol Toxicol 19: 531–545
Dews P B 1981 Behavioural pharmacology of anxiolytics. Handbook Exp Pharmacol 55(II): 285–293
File S E 1983 Behavioural actions of benzodiazepine antagonists. In: Trimble M R (ed) Benzodiazepines divided. John Wiley & Sons, Chichester
Geller I, Seifter J 1960 The effects of meprobamate, barbiturates, d-amphetamine and promazine on experimentally induced conflict in the rat. Psychopharmacologia I: 482–492
Haefely W, Pieri L, Polc P, Schaffner R 1981a General pharmacology and neuropharmacology of benzodiazepine derivatives. Handbook Exp Pharmacol 55(II): 13–262
Haefely W, Schaffner R, Polc P, Pieri L 1981b General pharmacology and neuropharmacology of propanediol carbamates. Handbook Exp Pharmacol 55(II): 263–283
Houamed K M, Bilbe G, Smart T G, Constanti A, Brown D A, Barnard E A, Richards B M 1984 Expression of functional GABA, glycine and glutamate receptors in Xenopus oocytes injected with rat brain RNA. Nature 310: 318–321
Hunkeler W, Mohler H, Pieri L, Polc P, Bonetti L P, Cumin R, Schaffner R, Haefely W 1981 Selective antagonists of benzodiazepines. Nature 290: 514–516

Iversen S D, Iversen L L 1981 Behavioural pharmacology. Oxford University Press, Oxford
Kay D C, Blackburn A B, Buckingham J A, Karacan I 1976 Human pharmacology of sleep. In: Williams R L & Karacan I (eds) Pharmacology of sleep. John Wiley & Sons, New York
Lader M H 1983 Benzodiazepine withdrawal states. In: Trimble M R (ed) Benzodiazepines divided. John Wiley & Sons, Chichester
Lader M H, Wing L 1966 Physiological measurements, sedative drugs and morbid anxiety. Oxford University Press, Oxford
Marks J 1978 The benzodiazepines. Use, overuse, misuse, abuse. MTP Press, Lancaster
Study R E, Barker J L 1981 Diazepam and pentabarbital: fluctuation analysis reveals different mechanisms for potentiation of γ-aminobutyric acid response in cultured central neurons. Proc Nat Acad Sci 78: 7180–7184
Tyrer P J 1982 Drugs in psychiatric practice. Butterworth, London
Young W S, Kuhar M J 1979 Autoradiographic localization of benzodiazepine receptors in the brains of humans and animals. Nature 280: 393–395
Young W S, Kuhar M J 1980 Radiohistochemical localization of benzodiazepine receptors in rat brain. J Pharmacol Exp Ther 212: 337–346

Neuroleptic drugs

Neuroleptic drugs are also known as **antischizophrenic drugs**, **antipsychotic drugs** or **major tranquillizers** (see Chapter 19). Although originally defined in terms of their clinical usefulness in the treatment of psychotic illness and their behavioural effects in animals, these drugs have in common the pharmacological property of antagonizing the actions of dopamine, and this is responsible for most of their effects on the nervous system.

The term **psychosis** refers to a group of mental disorders which are considered to be endogenous in origin (i.e. they represent some inherent malfunction of the brain), as distinct from **neurosis**, which is regarded as an abnormal reaction to external circumstances, and results in anxiety states, phobias, etc (see Chapter 21). The most important types of psychosis are: (1) schizophrenia; (2) affective disorders (e.g. depression, mania); and (3) organic psychoses (mental disturbances caused by head injury, alcoholism, or other kinds of organic disease). Neuroleptic drugs are effective in the treatment of schizophrenia. Drugs used to treat affective disorders are discussed in Chapter 23.

THE NATURE OF SCHIZOPHRENIA

Schizophrenia (see review: Crow, 1982) is estimated to affect about 1% of the population and is one of the most important forms of psychiatric illness because it often affects people from an early age, is chronic and is highly disabling. There is a strong hereditary factor in its aetiology, which points to the possibility of a fundamental biochemical abnormality. The main clinical features of the disease are: **delusions** (often paranoid in nature); **hallucinations**, usually in the form of voices, and often exhortatory in their message; **thought disorder**, which causes the individual to draw irrational conclusions, and may be associated with the feeling that thoughts are inserted or withdrawn by an outside agency; **withdrawal** from social contacts and **flattening of emotional responses**. Most cases of schizophrenia begin in adolescence or young adult life, and, if untreated, the disease usually becomes progressively worse, though periods of remission are common. Schizophrenic patients comprise a large proportion of patients in long-stay psychiatric hospitals.

The symptoms of schizophrenia can be divided into two groups, which may have different underlying causes (see Crow, 1982). The *positive* symptoms include delusions, hallucinations, and thought disorder, while the *negative* symptoms include dementia, loss of emotional responses and loss of social interactions. It is suggested that the positive symptoms result from some specific neurochemical abnormality (see below) whereas the negative symptoms reflect brain atrophy. Recent work has shown that chronic schizophrenia patients undergo progressive shrinkage of the brain, revealed by computerized tomography (CAT scanning), so it is possible that the biochemical abnormality that causes the positive symptoms of acute schizophrenia leads also to gradual degeneration of neurons which gives rise in turn to the progressive negative symptoms.

Theories of schizophrenia

This topic has been briefly discussed in Chapter 19. The cause of schizophrenia remains mysterious (Crow, 1982). The disease shows a strong, but by no means invariable, hereditary tendency, and there is some evidence that the genetic factor may produce a predisposition to a virus infection which actually causes the disease (Crow, 1982). The search for an underlying neurochemical disorder has gone on for many years, the hope being that a biochemical understanding of the mechanism would provide the basis for rational drug treatment. In fact, it has usually happened the other way round—chance clinical observations have provided the starting point for the development of biochemical theories.

The main theories that have been proposed at various times are:

Serotonin theories

A suggestion that serotonin deficiency might be the underlying cause of schizophrenia was based on the observation that LSD, an ergot derivative synthesized in 1943 (see Chapter 26) which antagonizes some peripheral action of serotonin, produces hallucinations and sensory disturbances rather similar to those occurring in schizophrenia. Further analysis (see Chapter 26) has shown that LSD does not act simply as an antagonist at serotonin receptors in the brain. Also, the type of hallucinations produced differ in many respects from schizophrenia, and the clinical effectiveness of antischizophrenic drugs does not seem to be related to an action on serotonin receptors. These findings, coupled with the lack of biochemical evidence suggesting reduced serotonin production in schizophrenia, make the theory no longer tenable.

An alternative view is that excessive production of a serotonin metabolite, **dimethyltryptamine (DMT)**, might be responsible (Gillin et al, 1976). DMT has a hallucinogenic effect in man, similar to drugs such as LSD and mescaline (see Chapter 26). It is found in the blood and urine of normal and schizophrenic subjects, but not in significantly different quantities, and its hallucinogenic effects are not strongly blocked by neuroleptic drugs. It must be concluded that the evidence linking schizophrenia to abnormal production of DMT (or, as far as current knowledge goes, of any other endogenously produced hallucinogen) is very weak.

Noradrenaline theories (Hornykiewicz, 1982; Mason, 1983)

The noradrenaline theories are based on conflicting biochemical evidence of changes in noradrenaline and dopamine β-hydroxylase content in post-mortem schizophrenic brains (increased NA content in certain midbrain areas, with reduced dopamine β-hydroxylase) coupled with an earlier suggestion that failure of the 'reward' system associated with activity of noradrenergic neurons in the *locus coeruleus* (see Chapter 19) is a key feature of schizophrenia. There are many inconsistencies in this theory (Iversen et al, 1983). It is not clear whether the biochemical changes are produced by over- or under-activity of noradrenergic neurons, or whether they may be secondary to drug treatment. Furthermore, drugs that stimulate or block central noradrenaline receptors are not particularly effective in schizophrenia.

In 1962 much excitement was generated by the finding of an abnormal substance in the urine of schizophrenic patients which appeared as the 'pink spot' on 2-dimensional chromatograms. This was found to be a dimethoxy-derivative of a catecholamine, but the excitement declined rapidly when it was shown to be of dietary origin and present equally in the urine of normal individuals living in the same environment.

Dopamine theory

The dopamine theory, put forward by Randrup & Munkvad in 1965, is supported by a good deal of evidence though much of it is indirect. The best evidence comes from pharmacological observations in man and experimental animals. Amphetamine, which releases dopamine in the brain (see Chapter 26), produces in man a syndrome indistinguishable from the 'positive' symptoms of schizophrenia. In animals it causes behavioural disturbances (especially stereotyped behaviour) which resemble the behaviour of schizophrenic patients and which have clearly been shown to result from dopamine release. Dopamine agonists (e.g. apomorphine, bromocriptine) produce similar effects in animals, and these drugs, like amphetamine, exacerbate the symptoms of schizophrenic patients. Furthermore, dopamine antagonists, and drugs that block dopamine release (e.g. reserpine; see Chapter 7), are effective in controlling the positive symptoms of schizophrenia, and in preventing amphetamine-induced behavioural changes. The correlation be-

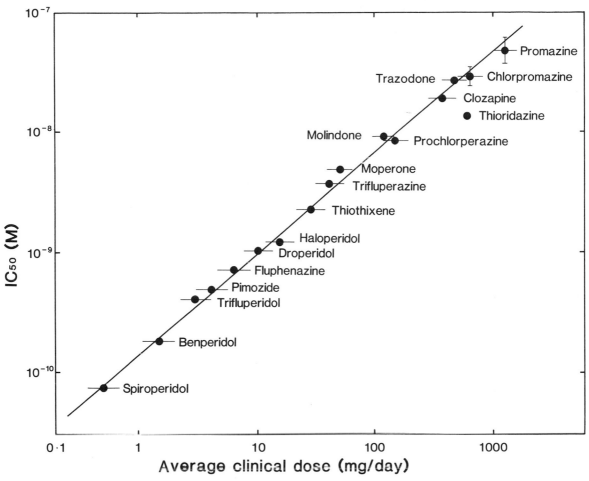

Fig. 22.1 Correlation between the clinical potency and receptor-binding activities of neuroleptic drugs. Clinical potency is expressed as the daily dose used in treating schizophrenia, and binding activity is expressed as the concentration needed to produce 50% inhibition of haloperidol binding. (From: Seeman et al, 1976)

tween clinical potency and activity in blocking D_2-receptors, measured by inhibition of specific binding of ^3H-haloperidol to brain tissue, is impressive (Fig. 22.1). On the other hand, the pharmacological evidence favouring dopamine hyper-reactivity in schizophrenia has been difficult to substantiate by direct neurochemical measurements. The amount of homovanillic acid (HVA, the main dopamine metabolite; see Chapter 19) in the CSF of schizophrenic patients is normal or low, rather than high. In post-mortem brains, many studies have failed to demonstrate either that dopamine or its metabolites are present in abnormally high concentrations, or that the activity of dopamine-metabolizing enzymes is abnormal.

One difficulty in interpreting such studies is that

nearly all schizophrenic patients are treated with drugs (e.g. chlorpromazine) that are known to affect dopamine metabolism, whereas the non-schizophrenic control group are not. In some studies it has been possible to allow for this factor, but the results are still generally negative.

A recent study (Reynolds, 1983) has, however, shown an abnormally high dopamine content post-mortem in a restricted area of the temporal lobe of schizophrenic subjects. The amygdala, which receives a dopaminergic innervation from the ventral tegmental region of the midbrain via part of the meso-limbic dopaminergic pathway was consistently richer in dopamine in schizophrenic than in control brains. The noradrenaline content was not affected. Most surprisingly the abnormally high

a.

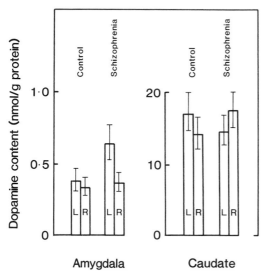

b.

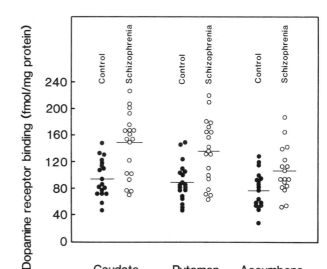

Fig. 22.2 Neurochemical changes in schizophrenia.
(a) Changes in dopamine content of brains of schizophrenic patients, measured post-mortem. There is an increased dopamine content in the amygdala on the right side but no change on the left, and no change in the caudate nucleus. (Data from: Reynolds, 1983)
(b) Dopamine receptors, measured by spiroperidol binding. There is an increase in all three brain areas, which is statistically significant, though the individual variation is large. Mean values are shown by horizontal lines.

dopamine content was confined to the left side of the brain (Fig. 22.2), which makes it most unlikely that it could have been the result of neuroleptic drug treatment. This finding accords with other evidence suggesting asymmetry in the neurological abnormality in schizophrenia (e.g. the frequent occurrence of left-sided temporal lobe epilepsy in schizophrenic patients) and is the clearest evidence so far of a primary disturbance of dopamine metabolism in schizophrenia.

Other evidence for a change in dopamine function is a small increase in the number of dopamine (D_2) receptors, measured by the binding of radioactive spiroperidol (Fig. 22.2). Most evidence suggests that the abnormality in schizophrenia is related to D_2 rather than D_1 (adenylate cyclase-linked) receptors, though the two subtypes have a very similar distribution in the brain. The increase in receptor binding appears to be confined to D_2 receptors, and the antischizophrenic effect of various drugs relates more closely to their activity on D_2 than D_1 receptors.

NEUROLEPTIC DRUGS

Chemical aspects

Neuroleptic drugs fall into three main chemical groups (Fig. 22.3), namely:

1. Phenothiazines and related tricyclic compounds
2. Butyrophenones
3. Benzamides.

The main characteristics of these drugs are summarized in Table 22.1.

Phenothiazines and related tricyclic compounds form the most important group, comprising:
a. Phenothiazines, which are further subdivided according to the nature of the side-chain into:
   (i) Aliphatic derivatives (e.g. chlorpromazine)
   (ii) Piperazine derivatives (e.g. fluphenazine)
   (iii) Piperidine derivatives (e.g. thioridazine)
The nature of the side-chain determines both the potency and the pharmacological specificity. Thus, the piperazine compounds are much more potent than aliphatic compounds, and have rela-

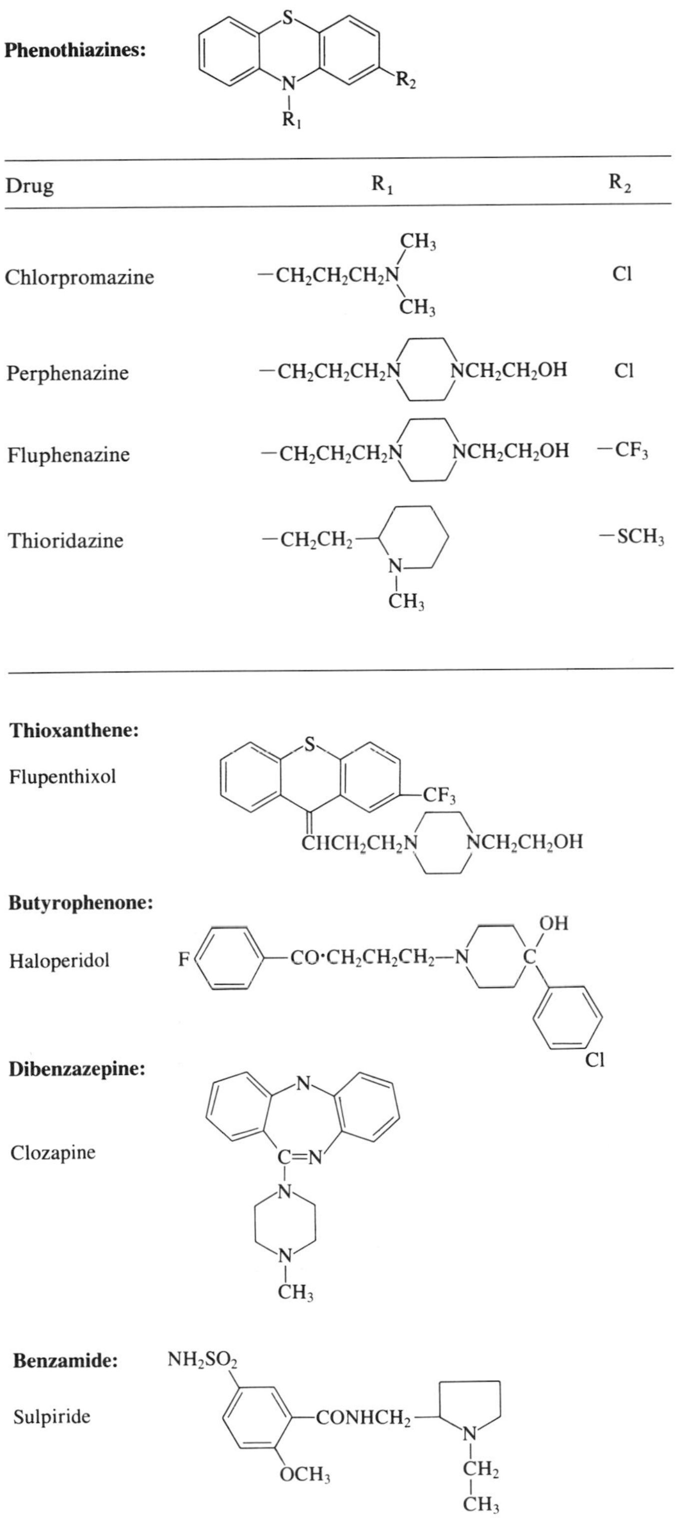

Phenothiazines:

Drug	R_1	R_2
Chlorpromazine	$-CH_2CH_2CH_2N$ with two CH_3 groups	Cl
Perphenazine	$-CH_2CH_2CH_2N$ (piperazine) NCH_2CH_2OH	Cl
Fluphenazine	$-CH_2CH_2CH_2N$ (piperazine) NCH_2CH_2OH	$-CF_3$
Thioridazine	$-CH_2CH_2-$ (piperidine, $N-CH_3$)	$-SCH_3$

Thioxanthene:

Flupenthixol

Butyrophenone:

Haloperidol

Dibenzazepine:

Clozapine

Benzamide:

Sulpiride

Fig. 22.3 Structures of neuroleptic drugs.

Table 22.1 Characteristics of neuroleptic drugs

Drug	Chemical type	Actions	Uses	Side effects/toxicity				Pharmacokinetics	Notes
				Sedation	EP*	Hyp†	Other		
All agents		Dopamine antagonism	Psychoses, esp. schizophrenia, mania				↑plasma prolactin, causing gynaecomastia, lactation, etc	Well absorbed (ex. sulpiride) Metabolites excreted in urine. Plasma, t½ 15–30 hour (ex. droperidol sulpiride)	
Chlorpromazine	Phenothiazine (aliphatic)	Antagonism at α-adrenoceptors, histamine (H₁), muscarinic, serotonin, receptors	Anti-emetic	+++	++	++	Obst. jaundice (mainly chlorpromazine), Hypothermia,		
Fluphenazine	Phenothiazine (piperazine)		Anti-emetic	+	+++	+	Dry mouth, blurred vision, etc.		Available as depot preparation.
Trifluoperazine	Phenothiazine (piperazine)		Anti-emetic	+	+++	+	Hypersensitivity		Calmodulin inhibitor
Thioridazine	Phenothiazine (piperidine)		Not anti-emetic	++	+	++			Strong muscarinic antagonist
Haloperidol	Butyrophenone	Little α-adrenoceptor or muscarinic receptor block	Anti-emetic	–	+++	+			
Droperidol	Butyrophenone		Anaesthetic premedication	–	+++	+		Short-acting	Used in neuroleptanalgesia
Flupenthixol	Thioxanthene			+	++	++	Restlessness		Available as depot preparation
Clozapine	Dibenzodiazepine	Strong muscarinic receptor block		++	++	+	Convulsions in some patients, salivation		Agranulocytosis in one study
Sulpiride	Benzamide	Selective D₂-receptor block	Anti-emetic	+	–	+		Poorly abs., t½ 5–10 hours	

* Extra-pyramidal motor disturbances.
† Postural hypotension.

tively less α-adrenoceptor blocking activity, while the piperidine group is intermediate in potency and possess more anti-muscarinic activity than chlorpromazine (see below).

b. Thioxanthenes (e.g. **flupenthixol**). These differ from phenothazines only in the substitution of carbon for nitrogen in the middle ring position. Flupenthixol is identical with fluphenazine apart from this change.

c. Dibenzodiazepines (e.g. **clozapine**). The middle ring is a 7-membered structure similar to that of the benzodiazepines (see Chapter 21).

Butyrophenones (e.g. **haloperidol**) are chemically unrelated to phenothiazines and were discovered accidentally in the course of screening a variety of compounds related to the analgesic, pethidine.

Benzamides (e.g. **sulpiride**) originated from modifications of the structure of procainamide (an antidysrhythmic drug; see Chapter 10). This led first to **metoclopramide** (see Chapter 15) a drug which reduces gastrointestinal motility and also has antidopamine effects in the periphery, as well as showing some antipsychotic activity, and then to **sulpiride**, an effective neuroleptic drug.

The therapeutic activity of chlorpromazine in schizophrenic patients was discovered by the acute observations of a French surgeon, Laborit, in 1947. He tested various substances, including promethazine, for their ability to alleviate signs of stress in patients undergoing surgery, and concluded that promethazine had a calming effect that was different from mere sedation. Elaboration of the phenothiazine structure produced chlorpromazine, whose antipsychotic effect was demonstrated, at Laborit's instigation, by Delay & Deniker in 1953. This drug was quickly found to be much more effective than any hitherto available in controlling the symptoms of psychotic patients without excessively sedating them. Thus, the clinical efficacy of phenothiazines was demonstrated long before their mechanism of action was understood.

Pharmacological investigation showed that phenothiazines blocked the actions of many different mediators, including histamine, catecholamines, acetylcholine and serotonin, and this multiplicity of actions led to the trade name Largactil for chlorpromazine. It is now clear (see Fig. 22.1) that antagonism at dopamine receptors is the main determinant of antipsychotic action.

Mechanism of action

Dopamine receptors and dopaminergic neurons

The classification of dopamine receptors in the CNS is discussed in Chapters 11 & 19 (see Table 11.3). There appear to be two distinct receptor types: D_1 which is coupled to adenylate cyclase and whose function is unknown; and D_2 which mediates the main pre- and post-synaptic actions of dopamine.* The neuroleptic drugs owe their behavioural effects to blockade of D_2-receptors. Antagonism at D_2-receptors can be measured in experimental animals by various tests, such as inhibition of amphetamine-induced stereotypic behaviour, or of apomorphine-induced turning behaviour in animals with unilateral striatal lesions (see Chapter 19), and *in vitro* by ability to inhibit the binding of a radioactive D_2 antagonist (e.g. spiroperidol) to brain membrane fragments. The main groups, phenothiazines, thioxanthenes and butyrophenones show relatively little specificity between the two main receptor types, but some newer compounds (e.g. sulpiride) are fairly specific for D_2-receptors.

The interaction between these different receptors is complex. All neuroleptic drugs have been found to increase initially the rate of production of dopamine in areas of the brain containing dopaminergic nerve terminals, such as the striatum and limbic system (see review: Creese et al, 1978). This is detectable by an increase in tyrosine hydroxylase activity, and an increase in the concentration of the dopamine metabolites, homovanillic acid and DOPAC. At the same time, electrical recording has shown that the activity of dopaminergic neurons (e.g. in the A9 and A10 areas; see Chapter 19) is increased by these drugs (Bunney et al, 1973). This increase in electrical activity and transmitter release is ascribed to two mechanisms: (a) blocking of pre-synaptic inhibitory receptors (autoreceptors)

---

* There is some evidence that the receptors mediating the pre- and post-synaptic actions of dopamine are different (Offermeier & van Rooyen, 1982), and the pre-synaptic autoreceptors are classified by some authors as D_3 (Seeman, 1980).

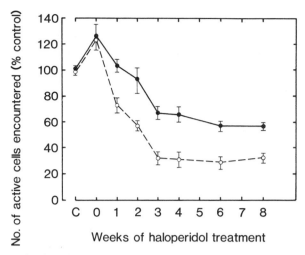

Fig. 22.4 Effect of chronic haloperidol treatment on the activity of dopaminergic neurons in the rat brain. In both A9 (solid line) and A10 (broken line) regions (see Chapter 19) the activity of dopaminergic neurons, recorded with microelectrodes from anaesthetized animals, first increases and then declines for three weeks before reaching a steady level. (From: White & Wang, 1983)

on dopaminergic nerve terminals; and (b) reduction in activity of a non-dopaminergic inhibitory feedback pathway running from the striatum back to A9 neurons in the substantia nigra. Activation of this pathway is assumed to depend on an excitatory action of dopamine in the striatum, which is blocked by neuroleptic drugs.

The increase in activity of dopaminergic neurons is not maintained when neuroleptic drugs are administered chronically. Both the biochemical and electrophysiological hyperactivity decline after about 3 weeks of treatment in rats (Fig. 22.4). The mechanism of this secondary decline is not certain, but it probably involves pre-synaptic (D_3) autoreceptors in some way, since **clozapine**, a recently introduced neuroleptic drug that is reported not to block these receptors, does not produce this effect. Another late effect, seen only when neuroleptic drugs are given chronically, is a slight proliferation of dopamine receptors, detectable as an increase in haloperidol binding (Creese et al, 1978), and also a pharmacological supersensitivity to dopamine, somewhat akin to the phenomenon of denervation supersensitivity.

These late effects of chronic neuroleptic treatment have received considerable attention, for it is well-established that some of the major beneficial and adverse clinical effects are delayed in their onset,

even though the primary action of the drugs in blocking dopamine receptors occurs immediately. At present neither the mechanism of the delayed effects, nor their relationship to the clinical response is at all well understood, A discussion of some recent ideas is given by Creese (1983).

Behavioural effects

Neuroleptic drugs produce many different behavioural effects in experimental animals, but no single test is known that distinguishes them clearly from other types of psychotropic drug. Most kinds of motor behaviour are inhibited. Thus, chlorpromazine reduces spontaneous activity and in larger doses causes **catalepsy**, a state in which the animal remains immobile though it will still respond to stimulation. Neuroleptics were shown to be particularly active in suppressing **conditioned avoidance responses**. Thus, a rat may be trained to respond to a signal (the conditioning stimulus) by behaviour (e.g. climbing a pole) that enables it to avoid an electric shock delivered a few seconds after this stimulus. Chlorpromazine will inhibit the response to the conditioning stimulus, though the animal will continue to respond when the painful shock is applied. Conditioned behaviour maintained by either reward or punishment is inhibited by neuroleptic drugs. Many of these effects are probably the result of suppression of motor activity by dopamine antagonism in the basal ganglion, but there is also evidence for behavioural effects that are not the result of overall motor inhibition. For example, in a variant of the conditioned avoidance response, a rat may be trained to respond to a stimulus by remaining immobile, thereby avoiding a painful shock, and chlorpromazine impairs this response as well as responses that demand active motor participation. Furthermore, in doses too small to reduce spontaneous motor activity, chlorpromazine reduces social interactions (grooming, mating, fighting, etc) in mice. It is also found that chlorpromazine reduces the ability of rats to discriminate between two conditioning stimuli (e.g. a red and a green light).

The antidopamine activity of neuroleptics can be revealed in tests where they are used to antagonize the behavioural effects of amphetamine, which are due mainly to dopamine release (see Chapters 19 &

26) or of apomorphine, which is a dopamine agonist. Various forms of stereotyped behaviour in rats and mice induced by amphetamine are strongly inhibited by neuroleptic drugs in doses too small to produce overt behavioural effects. Interestingly, some neuroleptics, such as clozapine and thioridazine, do not antagonize amphetamine in these tests. These particular drugs are notable in having less tendency than other neuroleptics to cause extrapyramidal side effects in man (see below), and it appears that the amphetamine tests reflect the activity of the neuroleptics mainly on the basal ganglia, whereas other behavioural tests may relate to activity elsewhere, e.g. in the limbic system.

In man, the effect of neuroleptic drugs is to produce a state of apathy and reduced initiative. The subject displays few emotions, is slow to respond to external stimuli and tends to be drowsy. He is, however, easily aroused and can respond to questions accurately, showing no obvious confusion or loss of intellectual function. Aggressive tendencies are strongly inhibited. The effects in man are quite distinct from those of hypnotic and anxiolytic drugs, which cause drowsiness and confusion, with euphoria rather than apathy.

Because of the lack of any single animal test which reliably predicts antipsychotic activity in man, the screening of potential new antipsychotic drugs requires an elaborate battery of animal tests and the construction of an 'activity profile' for each compound. The most useful tests for predicting antipsychotic activity in man are those that measure dopamine antagonism (e.g. inhibition of abnormal behaviour induced by apomorphine, enhancement of dopamine turnover).

Other effects related to dopamine antagonism

Anti-emetic activity

This is a property of many neuroleptic drugs (see Chapter 15), and seems to be partly a function of their ability to antagonize dopamine, since dopamine agonists (e.g. apomorphine) act on the chemoreceptor trigger zone in the medulla to cause nausea and vomiting, and this action is blocked by neuroleptic drugs. The possession of anti-histamine activity by many phenothiazines is probably also important, though the reason for the pharmacological correlation between H_1-receptor antagonism and anti-emetic action is not understood. The neuroleptic phenothiazines are effective in controlling nausea and vomiting produced by drugs (e.g. cancer chemotherapeutic agents) and also in conditions such as pregnancy and renal failure, but not against motion sickness, whereas antihistamines (and muscarinic antagonists) are effective in motion sickness.

Tardive dyskinesia and extrapyramidal motor disturbances

Neuroleptic drugs produce two main kinds of motor disturbance in man which are clearly related to their action as dopamine antagonists and closely resemble the syndromes that occur when patients with Parkinsonism are treated with laevodopa (see Chapter 24). The two syndromes are (a) **Parkinsonism-like symptoms** and (b) **tardive dyskinesia** (Crane, 1978). Since (see Chapter 24) Parkinsonism is the result of a deficiency of dopaminergic neurons in the nigrostriatal pathway, it is not surprising that neuroleptic drugs produce a similar syndrome, characterized by muscle rigidity, loss of mobility, tremor and oculogyric crises. Acute symptoms of this kind occur in a large proportion of patients treated with neuroleptics. The symptoms are closely related to the dose used, develop quite rapidly and are reversible.

Tardive dyskinesia is a much more puzzling and serious form of movement disorder. The syndrome consists of involuntary movements, often of the face and tongue, but also of the trunk and limbs, which can be severely disabling. The syndrome, which closely resembles the dyskinesia resulting from *prolonged* treatment of Parkinsonism patients with levodopa, appears after an interval of a few months to several years after neuroleptic treatment has been started (hence the description 'tardive') and is not usually reversible. The incidence has been estimated at over 10% of neuroleptic-treated patients, but this depends greatly on the drug dosage, the age of the patient (commonest in patients over 50) and partly on the particular drug used. Some neuroleptics (e.g. thioridazine, clozapine) have much less tendency to produce this effect; the reason for this is not clear. It may represent a selective effect on the mesolimbic dopaminergic pathway with sparing of the nigrostriatal pathway, or it may be associated with the marked antimuscarinic activity of these drugs, which tends to counteract their effects on the motor system (see Chapter 24).

Endocrine effects

There is known to be a dopaminergic pathway from the hypothalamus to the median eminence (the tubero-infundibular pathway; see Chapters 16 & 19), and dopamine is believed to act physiologically via D_2-receptors as an inhibitor of prolactin secretion, being transported from its site of release in the median eminence to the anterior pituitary gland via the hypophyseal portal system. The result of blocking D_2-receptors by neuroleptic drugs is thus to increase the serum prolactin concentration (Fig. 22.5), the main effect of which is to cause breast enlargement and lactation, in men as well as women (see Chapter 16). As can be seen from Figure 22.5, the effect continues for a long time during chronic administration, without any habituation.

Other less pronounced endocrine changes have also been reported, including a decrease of growth hormone secretion, and an increase in aldosterone secretion, leading to thirst and water retention, but these, unlike the prolactin response, are unimportant clinically.

Actions unrelated to dopamine antagonism

Phenothiazines and, to a variable extent, other neuroleptic drugs block the actions of acetylcholine (muscarinic), histamine (H_1), noradrenaline (α) and serotonin.

Blocking muscarinic receptors produces a variety of peripheral effects, including blurring of vision and increased intraocular pressure, dry mouth and eyes, constipation, urinary retention, etc (see Chapter 6). It may, however, also be important in relation to extrapyramidal side effects. Acetylcholine acts in opposition to dopamine in the basal ganglia (see Chapter 24) and concurrent blocking of both transmitters is less likely to produce symptoms of Parkinsonism than blocking dopamine receptors alone. It is possible that the relative lack of extrapyramidal side effects with clozapine and thioridazine is due to their high antimuscarinic potency.

Blocking α-adrenoceptors results in the important side effect in man of orthostatic hypotension (see Chapter 11). It may also contribute to the sedative action of many neuroleptics, but does not seem to be important for their antipsychotic action. Different neuroleptics vary greatly in their relative α-receptor and dopamine receptor blocking activity. Thus haloperidol, flupenthixol and fluphenazine have very little α-receptor blocking action, and thus lack these side effects, whereas with other drugs, such as chlorpromazine, clozapine and thioridazine, they are very pronounced.

Antihistamine (H_1) activity is a property of many phenothiazines including a number that have no antipsychotic effect, and some other neuroleptic drugs (e.g. thioridazine). All H_1 antihistamines have sedative and anti-emetic properties (see above), though the mechanism of these actions is not understood.

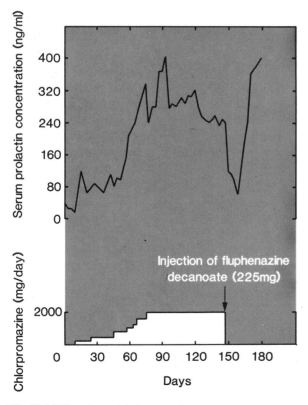

Fig. 22.5 Effect of neuroleptics on prolactin secretion in a schizophrenic patient. When daily dosage with chlorpromazine was replaced with a depot injection of fluphenazine the plasma prolactin initially dropped, because of the delay in absorption, and then returned to a high level. (From: Meltzer et al, 1978)

Side effects of neuroleptic drugs

The major side effects of neuroleptics can be inferred from their pharmacological actions, as discussed above, though individual drugs differ somewhat (see Table 22.1). Acute toxicity is not a problem in clinical practice, doses up to 100 times the therapeutic dose usually being non-fatal.

The important sides effects are:

Cardiovascular effects

Postural hypotension results partly from α-adrenoceptor block and partly from a direct vasodilator action. Many phenothiazines antagonize the action of calmodulin (see Chapter 1), which may be important in this connection.

Sedation

This tends to decrease with continued use.

Autonomic effects

In addition to α-receptor block, many neuroleptics have atropine-like actions, causing visual disturbance, dry mouth, constipation, etc.

Extrapyramidal effects (see above)

These consist of:

1. Acute, reversible effects, namely:
   a. Parkinsonian syndrome consisting of rigidity, tremor and alkinesia, tending to occur in elderly patients
   b. Motor restlessness (akathisia), the mechanism of which is not well understood; it occurs often in younger patients, and may be controlled with diazepam
2. Chronic effects. The most important is tardive dyskinesia (see above), which is similar to Huntington's chorea (see Chapter 24). It usually develops after years of treatment, tends to get worse if the neuroleptic is stopped, and, like Huntington's chorea, is unresponsive to most forms of drug treatment. It is the most serious side effect of neuroleptic drugs, and can occur at any age.

Endocrine disturbances

These result from increased prolactin secretion (gynaecomastia, lactation and painful breasts).

Idiosyncratic and hypersensitivity reactions

1. Jaundice. This occurs with chlorpromazine and other phenothiazines which are used in large doses. The introduction of drugs of much higher neuroleptic potency has virtually eliminated this problem. The jaundice is usually mild, and of obstructive origin, associated with blocking of the bile canaliculi by precipitated material rather than with parenchymal cell damage. The exact mechanism of the reaction is uncertain. The effect disappears quickly when the drug is stopped.
2. Leukopenia and agranulocytosis. As with many drugs this is a rare, but potentially fatal reaction, which can occur in the first few weeks of treatment. It probably represents a type of hypersensitivity reaction (see Chapter 36). The incidence of leukopenia (usually reversible) is less than 1 in 10 000 for chlorpromazine and is probably lower for more potent drugs. Clozapine, whose lack of extrapyramidal side effects is a major clinical advantage, was reported in 1975 to have caused 16 cases of agranulocytosis (8 of them fatal) among 2800 patients in a Finnish study. This seems to have been an isolated event, but its occurrence has limited the acceptance of clozapine for clinical use.
3. Skin reactions. Urticarial reactions are common in the first few weeks of treatment, but are not serious. Recovery may occur even if the drug is continued.

Pharmacokinetic aspects

Detailed information on the absorption and metabolism of chlorpromazine has been obtained, and it is typical of many phenothiazines. Chlorpromazine is erratically absorbed into the bloodstream after oral administration. Figure 22.6 shows the wide range of variation of the peak plasma concentration as a function of dosage in fourteen patients. At a rather high dosage level (6–8 mg/kg) the variation in peak plasma concentration was nearly 90-fold,

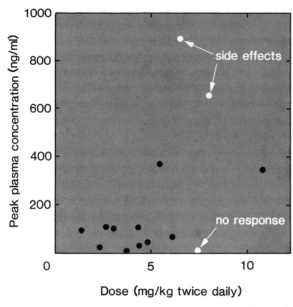

Fig. 22.6 Individual variation in the relation between dose and plasma concentration of chlorpromazine in a group of schizophrenic patients. (Data from: Curry et al, 1970)

and of the four patients, two showed marked side effects, one was correctly controlled and one showed no clinical response. It is not poor absorption from the gut lumen that accounts for the variability, for phenothiazines are highly lipid soluble and none are excreted in the faeces. Nor is it rapid first pass metabolism in the liver. It seems instead to be due to a large and variable amount of tissue binding. In accordance with this, the volume of distribution of many neuroleptics greatly exceeds the total body volume (see Table 3.2), indicative of considerable extravascular sequestration of the drug. They are bound (usually about 90%) to plasma protein.

The relationship between the plasma concentration and the clinical effect of chlorpromazine is also highly variable. It is stated that the therapeutic range of plasma concentration lies between 30 and 300 ng/ml, which is unusually wide (compare, for example, digoxin; p. 239). Several studies have failed to show significant correlation between plasma concentration and any measure of pharmacological effect, including clinical improvement, increase in CSF homovanillic acid concentration or increase in plasma prolactin concentration (Sedvall, 1981). Thus, dosage of neuroleptics has to be adjusted largely on a trial and error basis, without

useful guidance from pharmacokinetic data. Adjustment of the dose is made even more difficult by the fact that at least 40% of schizophrenic patients fail to take drugs as prescribed. It is remarkably fortunate that the acute toxicity of neuroleptic drugs is slight, given the unpredictability of the clinical response.

The half-time for removal of most neuroleptics from the plasma is 15–30 hours, clearance depending entirely on hepatic transformation by a combination of oxidative and conjugative reactions. The metabolism of phenothiazines is complex, and many different metabolites are formed. Though some of these are biologically active it is unlikely that they contribute much to the pharmacological response.

Most neuroleptic drugs can be given orally or by intramuscular injection, once or twice a day. Slow release preparations of fluphenazine are available, in which the active drug is esterified with heptanoic or decanoic acid and dissolved in oil. Given as an intramuscular injection, the drug acts for 2–4 weeks, but may produce acute side effects initially.

Clinical uses and clinical efficacy

The major use of neuroleptic drugs is in the treatment of schizophrenia. They are also useful as anti-emetics, being effective in conditions such as uraemia and iatrogenic nausea and vomiting caused by radiation, cytotoxic drugs, opioid analgesics, etc. Phenothiazines are not very effective in controlling

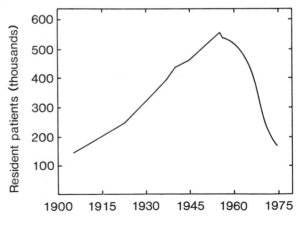

Fig. 22.7 Patient population in public mental hospitals in US. (From: Bassuk & Gerson, 1978)

motion sickness, and are considered inadvisable for use in pregnancy.

Minor uses include the treatment of Huntington's chorea (mainly haloperidol; see Chapter 24). Some of the new neuroleptics (e.g. sulpiride) have been claimed to have antidepressant actions.

The clinical efficacy of neuroleptic drugs in enabling schizophrenic patients to lead more normal lives is evident from the sharp decline in the in-patient population (mainly comprised of chronic schizophrenics) of mental hospitals since the later 1950s (Fig. 22.7). Undoubtedly the major decline between 1960 and 1970 reflects changing public and professional attitudes towards hospitalization of the mentally ill, but it is generally acknowledged that the efficacy of neuroleptics was an essential enabling factor. Many double blind trials have been carried out, which show objectively that neuroleptics reduce schizophrenic symptoms more effectively than placebo treatment (Davis & Garver, 1978). In one large multicentre trial organized by the National Institutes of Health in 1964, three pheno-thiazines were tested against a placebo over a 6 week period in a total of 344 newly admitted acutely schizophrenic patients, clinical improvement being assessed by means of standardized rating scales, covering a range of schizophrenic symptoms. Figure 22.8 summarizes the results.

Though 60% of the placebo group showed improvement, the phenothiazine group fared significantly better, 94% showing improvement. Correspondingly, 40% of the control group were unchanged or worse, whereas only 6% of the treated group failed to improve, and almost no treated patients got worse. At the end of the trial period the median rating for the placebo group was 4.5 (moderately to markedly ill) compared with 3.0 (mildly ill) for the treated group. This trial showed no differences between the three phenothiazines tested, either in the assessment of their overall

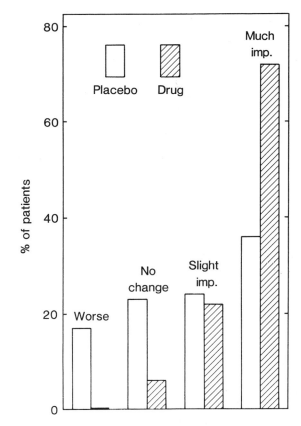

Fig. 22.8 Clinical trial of phenothiazines in acute schizophrenia. (Results of NIMH collaborative study, 1964)

efficacy, or in a more detailed analysis of their ability to control specific symptoms. Crow (1982) has, however, concluded that all neuroleptics control the 'positive' symptoms (delusions, paranoia, aggression, etc) more effectively than the 'negative' symptoms (apathy, reduction in speech).

In general, clinical trials have shown no significant differences in the therapeutic efficacy of different neuroleptics, the main difference being in the incidence and type of the major side effects.

REFERENCES AND FURTHER READING

Bunney B S, Walters J R, Roth R H, Aghajanian G K 1973 Dopaminergic neurons: effect of antipsychotic drugs and amphetamine on single cell activity. J Pharmacol Exp Ther 185: 560–571

Crane G E 1978 Tardive dyskinesia and related neurologic disorders. Handbook of Psychopharmacology 10: 165–196

Creese I 1983 Classical and atypical antipsychotic drugs: new insights. Trends in Neurosciences 6: 479–481

Creese I, Burt D R, Snyder S H 1978 Biochemical actions of neuroleptic drugs: focus on the dopamine receptor. Handbook of Psychopharmacology 10: 37–89

Creese I, Hamblin M W, Leff S E, Sibley D R 1983 CNS dopamine receptors. Handbook of Psychopharmacology 17: 81–138

Crow T J 1982 Schizophrenia. In: Crow T J (ed) Disorders of Neurohumoral Transmission. Academic Press, London

Davis J M, Garver D L 1978 Neuroleptics: clinical use in psychiatry. Handbook of Psychopharmacology 10: 129–164

Gillin J C, Kaplan J, Stillman R, Wyatt R J 1976 The psychedelic model of schizophrenia: the case for N,N-dimethyltryptamine. Am J Psychiat 133: 203–208

Hornykiewicz O 1982 Brain catecholamines in schizophrenia — a good case for noradrenaline. Nature 299: 484–486

Iversen L L, Reynolds G P, Snyder S H 1983 Pathophysiology of schizophrenia — causal role for dopamine or noradrenaline. Nature 305: 577

Mason S T 1983 Designing a non-neuroleptic antischizophrenic drug: the noradrenergic strategy. Trends in Pharmacological Sciences 4: 353–355

Offermeier J, van Rooyen J M 1982 Is it possible to integrate dopamine receptor terminology? Trends in Pharmacological Sciences 3: 327–329

Reynolds G P 1983 Increased concentrations and lateral asymmetry of amygdala dopamine in schizophrenia. Nature 305: 527–529

Sedvall G 1981 Correlations between clinical, biochemical and pharmacokinetic data in chlorpromazine-treated patients. In: Usdin E (ed) Clinical pharmacology in psychiatry. Elsevier, New York.

Seeman P 1980 Brain dopamine receptors. Pharmacol Rev 32: 230–287

Seeman P, Lee T, Cha-Wong M, Wong K 1976 Antipsychotic drug doses and neuroleptic/dopamine receptors. Nature 261: 717–719

Tyrer P J 1982 Drugs in psychiatric practice. Butterworth, London

Drugs used in affective disorders

THE NATURE OF AFFECTIVE DISORDERS

Affective disorders, which comprise a major class of psychoses, are distinct from schizophrenia, in that they are characterized by changes of mood (depression or mania) rather than by thought disturbances.

The symptoms of depression are a general feeling of misery, apathy and hopelessness; preoccupation with guilt, inadequacy and ugliness; inanition, loss of appetite, slowing of movements, and indecisiveness. Mania is in most respects exactly the opposite, with excessive exuberance, enthusiasm and self-confidence, which, as with depression, are generally inappropriate to the circumstances.

A useful distinction may be drawn between **bipolar** and **unipolar** depression. In bipolar depression, the patient oscillates between depression and mania, and there is strong evidence for an hereditary link in the condition, suggesting that a biochemical abnormality underlies the disorder. Patients with unipolar depression do not swing into bouts of mania, and there is no evidence of a genetic cause. They tend to be older than bipolar depressives when the illness first occurs, and their depression is more often mixed with symptoms of anxiety and agitation than is the case with patients with bipolar depression, who tend to be inert and apathetic during their depressive phase.

There is disagreement about whether these two clinical categories represent fundamentally different disorders. One view is that unipolar depression may be either 'reactive' in origin or 'endogenous', the former being a non-psychotic reaction to distressing circumstances, such as bereavement or poverty, while the latter is, like bipolar depression, the result of a biochemical abnormality within the brain. There is some evidence (see below) that these two types of depressive illness respond differently to antidepressant drugs. Some patients suffering from bipolar depression also show symptoms associated with schizophrenia, whereas patients with unipolar depression often show symptoms of anxiety neurosis, so the depressive illnesses appear as a broad continuum stretching from what is probably a fundamental biochemical disturbance to psychological disturbances that are initiated by external events. Depression is a very common illness. In one year in Britain roughly 1.5% of the population is treated for depressive illness by general practitioners, according to studies carried out in 1957 and 1966, and in London the lifetime probability of being admitted to hospital as a result of severe depression has been estimated at about 1%.

The monoamine theory of depression

The main biochemical theory that has been put forward is the monoamine hypothesis (Schildkraut, 1965), which states that depression is caused by a functional deficit of monoamine transmitters at certain sites in the brain, while mania results from a functional excess.

The monoamine hypothesis grew originally out of associations between the clinical effects of various drugs which cause or alleviate symptoms of depression and their known neurochemical effects on monoaminergic transmission in the brain. Initially the hypothesis was formulated in terms of noradrenaline, but subsequent work showed that most of the observations were equally consistent with serotonin being the key substance (Coppen et al, 1972). This pharmacological evidence, which is summarized below, gives general support to the

Table 23.1 Pharmacological evidence relating to the monoamine hypothesis of depression.

Drug	Principle action	Effect in depressed patients
1. Effects consistent with the hypothesis		
Tricyclic antidepressants	Block NA and serotonin reuptake	Mood ↑
MAO inhibitors	Increase stores of NA and serotonin	Mood ↑
α-methyltyrosine	Inhibits NA synthesis	Mood ↓ Calming of manic patients.
Methyldopa	Inhibits NA synthesis	Mood ↓
Reserpine	Inhibits NA and serotonin storage	Mood ↓
Electroconvulsive therapy	?Increases CNS responses to NA and serotonin	Mood ↑
2. Effects that do not support hypothesis		
Amphetamine	Releases NA and blocks reuptake	None. Euphoria in normal subjects.
Cocaine	Inhibits NA reuptake	None. Euphoria in normal subjects.
Tryptophan 5-hydroxytryptophan	Increase serotonin synthesis	Mood ?↑ in some studies.
α- and β-adrenoceptor antagonists	Block actions of NA	Mood slightly ↓ with β-antagonists. No effect on manic patients.
Methysergide	Serotonin antagonist	None
L-dopa	Increases NA synthesis	None
Iprindole	No effect on amine metabolism	Mood ↑

monoamine hypothesis, though there are several anomalies. Attempts to obtain more direct evidence, by studying monoamine metabolism in depressed patients, or by measuring changes in the number of monoamine receptors in post-mortem brain tissue, have in general provided only very equivocal support for the theory, and the interpretation of these studies is often problematical. Similarly, investigation by functional tests of the activity of known monoaminergic pathways (e.g. those controlling pituitary hormone release) in depressed patients have also given equivocal results. The evidence relating to the monoamine theory is well reviewed by Johnstone (1982), Zis & Goodwin (1982) and Baker & Dewhurst (1985).

Pharmacological evidence

Table 23.1 summarizes the main drugs that are known to affect monoamine metabolism, and compares their predicted effect on mood with the observed effect. In general there is reasonable support for the theory, though there are several examples of drugs that might have been predicted to improve or worsen depressive symptoms but fail to do so convincingly. It has to be recognized that the basis for predicting the effects of drugs on mood is, at best, very simple-minded. Thus, supplying a transmitter precursor will not actually increase the release of transmitter unless availability of the precursor is rate-limiting. Similarly, a drug that releases monoamines from normal nerve terminals may fail to do so if the nerve terminals are functionally defective. The absence of a useful antidepressant action of amphetamine is therefore not strong evidence against the monoamine theory.

More difficult to reconcile with the monoamine theory in any simple way is the fact that the biochemical actions of antidepressant drugs appear very rapidly, whereas their antidepressant effects usually take days or weeks to develop. A similar situation exists in relation to anti-schizophrenic drugs (see Chapter 22), and it strongly suggests that it may be the secondary, adaptive changes in the brain, rather than the primary drug effect, that are important in producing the clinical improvement. Where such effects have been studied in experimental animals treated chronically with antidepressant drugs, the results have generally been difficult to interpret in the context of the simple monoamine hypothesis. Thus, chronic administration of tricyclic antidepressants or of monoamine oxidase inhibitors (MAOI) causes a reduction in the activity of noradrenaline-sensitive adenylate cyclase in various brain regions. Interestingly **iprindole**, an effective antidepressant that does not inhibit noradrenaline reuptake or MAO (see below), also causes a reduction of the adenylate cyclase response to noradrenaline. The reduction of this response has been attributed to a reduction of the number of β-adrenoceptors as measured by binding studies, α-adrenoceptors remaining unchanged. In contrast to these effects on adrenoceptors, serotonin receptors are unchanged after chronic antidepressant treatment, as measured either by the number of serotonin binding sites or by the responsiveness of individual neurons to applied serotonin. It is clear that shifting our attention from the acute biochemical effects of antidepressant drugs to long-term adaptive changes leads to the appearance of serious inconsistencies with the simple monoamine theory, to the extent that some authors have suggested that excessive rather than deficient activation of β-adrenoceptors in particular parts of the brain underlies depressive illness.

Biochemical studies

The most direct way of testing the amine hypothesis is to look for biochemical abnormalities in CSF, blood or urine, or in post-mortem brain tissue, from depressed or manic patients. The major metabolites of noradrenaline, serotonin and dopamine that appear in the CSF, blood and urine (see Chapters 7 & 19) are respectively 3-methoxy 4-hydroxyphenylglycol (MHPG), 5-hydroxyindoleacetic acid (5HIAA) and homovanillic acid (HVA). There are two fundamental problems in relating changes in the concentration of these metabolites in body fluids to changes in transmitter function in the brain. One is that many secondary factors can affect their concentration, such as diet, transport between CSF, blood and urine, or release of monoamines from non-cerebral sites. The second is that psychotropic drug treatment, which most depressed patients receive, affects the metabolite concentrations markedly.

Among a variety of clinical studies, there is now a general consensus that MHPG in urine and CSF is reduced (by roughly 25% compared with normal subjects) in depression, and that it shows a cyclic change in patients who switch between depressive and manic states (see review: Johnstone, 1982). These changes do not seem to be due to variations in peripheral sympathetic activity associated with greater physical activity in the manic state, since exercise per se has little effect on the results.

Results obtained with 5HIAA are more variable.

Urinary excretion of 5HIAA does not change in depression, but several studies have shown a fall in CSF 5HIAA. In some, **probenecid** (see Chapter 14) has been used to inhibit the transport of 5HIAA from CSF to blood; the ensuing rise in 5HIAA concentration in the CSF then provides a measure of the rate of production of 5HIAA by the brain. Such studies have given highly variable results. The results of one thorough study, shown in Figure 23.1, showed an equal (50%) reduction of 5HIAA in lumbar CSF in depressed, manic and recovered depressed patients. In relation to the serotonin hypothesis, Coppen's group has also measured tryptophan (a serotonin precursor) and found the concentration to be lower than normal in CSF and

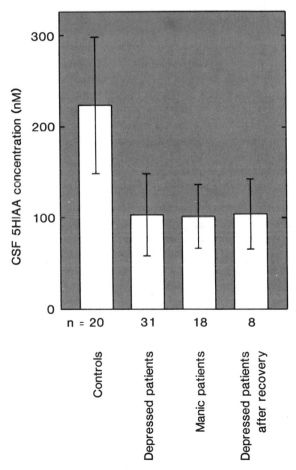

Fig. 23.1 Reduced concentration of a serotonin metabolite in CSF of patients with affective disorders. 5 hydroxyindoleacetic acid (5HIAA) is the main metabolite of serotonin found in CSF. The error bars show standard deviations, and the reduction compared with control is significant ($p < 0.001$) in all three groups.

blood (after allowance for binding to protein) from depressed patients, though others have failed to confirm this finding. Similarly the 5HIAA or serotonin content of post-mortem brain tissue has been found, in some studies, to be lower in the brains of suicide victims (assumed to be suffering from severe depression) than in the brains of victims of other forms of sudden death.

Studies on blood platelets have been widely used to study possible biochemical abnormalities underlying mental disease. This is because the platelets (which, unlike the brain, are easily studied in man) possess mechanisms for the uptake and metabolism of serotonin very similar to those found in the brain. The main results so far reported in depressed patients are that serotonin uptake by platelets is reduced in comparison to control patients (an effect not attributable to drug treatment). Platelet MAO activity, however, is not consistently altered, though there are suggestions that it is reduced in some bipolar depressive patients. The finding of an abnormality in serotonin uptake by platelets is generally consistent with the monoamine theory, though it requires some special pleading (readily forthcoming) to explain how this could lead to a deficit, rather than an enhancement, of serotoninergic transmission in the brain.

Functional studies

Various attempts have been made to test for a functional deficit of monoamine pathways in depression. Hypothalamic neurons controlling pituitary function receive noradrenergic and serotoninergic inputs, which control the discharge of these cells and thus regulate the secretion of pituitary hormones such as ACTH and growth hormone (see Chapter 16). It has been found in several studies that the plasma cortisol concentration is high in depressed patients and that it fails to respond with the normal fall when a synthetic steroid, such as dexamethasone, is given. Other hormones in plasma are also affected; e.g. growth hormone concentration is reduced, and prolactin is increased. It is difficult to assess whether or not these changes reflect deficient monoamine transmission.

In summary there is a good deal of circumstantial evidence to suggest that Schildkraut's monoamine

theory is basically correct. (Johnstone (1982) puts it more circumspectly: 'Thus the body of circumstantial evidence . . . is such that it is unlikely that the hypothesis is incorrect.') There are, however, some glaring inconsistencies, of which the most obvious are the following:

1. Neither amphetamine, cocaine or L-dopa have antidepressant actions.
2. Antidepressant drugs have a delayed therapeutic effect, which coincides with an apparent inhibition rather than facilitation of monoaminergic transmission.
3. Some clinically effective antidepressants seem to lack any actions that could enhance monoamine transmission.
4. The biochemical changes associated with depression have, in several studies, been identical with changes observed in manic patients.

Recognizing these inconsistencies, many authors (see review: Maj et al, 1984) have suggested more complicated mechanisms than a simple transmitter deficit, and have invoked dopamine, acetylcholine and peptides in delicately balanced arrays in attempts to account for all the facts. Receptor down-regulation and its counterpart, denervation super-sensitivity, as long-term effects of agents that enhance or inhibit transmitter function are also often invoked. Other actions in the brain common to many antidepressant drugs have also been recognized, such as antagonism at presynaptic α_2-receptors (see Chapter 7), antagonism at serotonin receptors and antagonism of histamine activation of adenylate cyclase (Green & Costain, 1981). It seems clear that Schildkraut's basic idea will need to be modified and elaborated, but the evidence is still too tenuous to support a more detailed model.

Animal models of depression

Progress in unravelling the neurochemical mechanisms of depression is, as in so many areas of psychopharmacology, considerably limited by the lack of good animal models of the clinical condition. There is no known animal condition corresponding to the inherited condition of depression in man, but various procedures have been described which produce behavioural states (withdrawal from social interaction, loss of appetite, reduced motor activity, etc) typical of human depression (Porsolt, 1985). For example, the delivery of repeated inescapable painful stimuli leads to a state of 'learned helplessness', in which, even when the animal is free to escape it fails to do so. Mother–infant separation in monkeys, and administration of amine-depleting drugs, such as reserpine, also produce states that superficially resemble human depression. As well as being inherently distasteful, these experiments often require elaborate and expensive experimental protocols, and there is only a limited amount of information about the similarity of these states to human depression. However, it has been reported that the learned helplessness state, and the effect of mother–infant separation, can be reversed by tricyclic antidepressants, and increased by small doses of α-methyltyrosine (which inhibits noradrenaline synthesis), suggesting a basic similarity to the human state.

ANTIDEPRESSANT DRUGS

TYPES OF ANTIDEPRESSANT DRUG

The major classes of drug that are used to treat depressive illness are:

1. Tricyclic antidepressants (TCA), e.g. imipramine, amitryptiline.
2. Monoamine oxidase inhibitors (MAOI), e.g. phenelzine, tranylcypromine.
3. 'Atypical' antidepressants. This group includes compounds that act similarly to TCA but have a different chemical structure (e.g. nomifensine) and also compounds with different pharmacological actions (e.g. mianserin, iprindole). Many of these are relatively new compounds whose clinical efficacy has not yet been fully assessed.
4. Lithium.

Mention should also be made of electroconvulsive therapy (ECT) which appears to be more effective clinically (though unpleasant for the patient) than antidepressant drugs (see later section).

Many other compounds have been suggested and tested clinically in depressed patients, producing a variety of claims and counter-claims about their effectiveness. For example, L-tryptophan, the amino-acid precursor of serotonin, has been given in large doses with the object of correcting the supposed deficit in serotonin synthesis. The results have been confusing, but it appears now that the antidepressant effect of L-tryptophan, in those patients whom it benefits, is rather short-lived and less than the effect of other drugs or ECT, so this drug has not found much clinical application.

MEASUREMENT OF ANTIDEPRESSANT ACTIVITY

The clinical effectiveness of the first MAOI and TCA drugs was discovered by chance when these drugs were given to patients for other reasons. **Iproniazid**, the first MAOI, was originally used to treat tuberculosis, being chemically related to the established anti-tuberculosis drug, isoniazid (see Chapter 30); **imipramine**, the first TCA, resembles chlorpromazine (see Chapter 22) and was first tried as an anti-schizophrenic drug. Later, the monoamine hypothesis of depression produced a kind of biochemical rationale for their antidepressant actions and suggested ways of testing new compounds biochemically as a preliminary to clinical trials. The results of such biochemical tests are successful in predicting clinical efficacy for conventional TCA and MAOI, but fail to predict efficacy among the newer group of atypical antidepressant drugs. Various behavioural tests have also been used, though there is no animal model that satisfactorily resembles depressive illness in man. Some of the most useful tests are the following:

1. Potentiation of noradrenaline effects in the periphery. Stimulation of sympathetic nerves, or administration of noradrenaline, causes contraction of smooth muscle, which is enhanced if the noradrenaline reuptake mechanism of the nerve terminal is blocked (see Chapter 7). This test gives positive results with TCA, but does not reveal MAOI or atypical antidepressant activity.
2. Potentiation of the central effects of amphetamine. Amphetamine works partly by releasing noradrenaline in the brain, and its actions are enhanced both by MAOI (which increase noradrenaline stores) and by TCA (which block reuptake). Atypical antidepressants also give a positive

response, for uncertain reasons, making it a useful test for predicting activity in man.

3. Antagonism of reserpine-induced depression. Reserpine depletes the brain of both noradrenaline and serotonin, causing various measurable effects (hypothermia, bradycardia, reduced motor activity, etc.) which are reduced by antidepressant drugs. This test also reveals activity among the atypical drugs, which do not affect MAO or transmitter reuptake in biochemical assays.

4. Block of amine uptake *in vitro*. Radioactive noradrenaline or serotonin can be used to measure neuronal uptake in the brain or peripheral tissues. If brain tissue is homogenized, the nerve terminals are broken off, but reseal spontaneously to form vesicular structures (synaptosomes) which can be separated from the rest of the cellular components by differential centrifugation. Synaptosomes can accumulate and release transmitters much like intact nerve terminals, and form a convenient preparation for measuring the effect of amine uptake inhibitors. Among TCA there is a fairly good correlation between antidepressant activity and potency in inhibiting noradrenaline or serotonin uptake, but MAOI and many atypical antidepressants have no effect.

A general point that has to be borne in mind when using *in vitro* tests to assess potential antidepressants is that many drugs (particularly TCA) are metabolized to pharmacologically active substances *in vivo*. In several cases (see below), the metabolite has a different ratio of selectivity with respect to noradrenaline and serotonin uptake, and it is often unclear whether the parent drug, or the metabolite, is actually responsible for the clinical effect.

It has recently been found (Langer et al, 1982) that the antidepressant effects of many drugs correlate closely with their ability to compete with ^3H imipramine for binding sites in the brain and on blood platelets. These binding sites do not correspond to any known neurotransmitter receptors, and are probably associated with the serotonin uptake mechanism which is common to platelets and serotoninergic nerve terminals. It is interesting that electroconvulsive therapy, as well as antidepressant drug treatment, both reduce the number of these binding sites in the brain. Some of the

'atypical' antidepressants (see later section) such as **mianserin**, do not, however, affect these binding sites, arguing against a simple unitary hypothesis of how antidepressant drugs work.

TRICYCLIC ANTIDEPRESSANTS

These drugs form the most important group of antidepressants in current clinical use, having now largely supplanted MAOI. They are, however, far from ideal in practice, and there is a considerable need for drugs which act more quickly and reliably, and produce fewer side effects.

Chemical aspects

TCA are closely related in structure to the phenothiazines (see Chapter 22) and were initially produced, in 1949, as potential neuroleptic drugs. The prototype compound, **imipramine**, differs from promazine (the corresponding phenothiazine), only in replacement of the sulphur atom by a dimethylene link to form a **dibenzazepine** structure (Fig. 23.2). The ring structure is considerably distorted by this change, and the two outer rings become twisted out of alignment so that the molecule is no longer symmetrical as are phenothiazines.

Imipramine was found to be of no use in schizophrenia, but effective in relieving depression, so other compounds were synthesized, following much the same pattern as the development of the neuroleptic drugs (Fig. 23.2). Thus, insertion of the same dimethylene bridge into the thioxanthene structure resulted in the **dibenzcycloheptene** structure (e.g. **amitriptyline**), while addition of a chlorine atom to imipramine, as in chlorpromazine, led to another useful drug **clomipramine**. All of these compounds are tertiary amines, with two methyl groups attached to the basic nitrogen atom. They are quite rapidly demethylated *in vivo* (see Fig. 23.3) to the corresponding secondary amines (**desipramine**, **nortriptyline**, etc), which are themselves active and may be administered as drugs in their own right (Fig. 23.2). Other tricyclic derivatives with slightly modified bridge structures include **protriptyline** and **doxepin**. The pharmacological differences between these drugs are not very great, and relate mainly to their side effects, which are discussed below.

1. Dibenzazepines

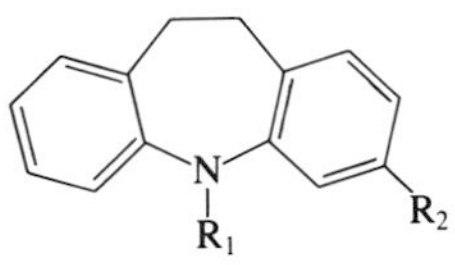

Drug	R$_1$	R$_2$
Imipramine	$-CH_2CH_2CH_2N\overset{CH_3}{\underset{CH_3}{}}$	H
Desipramine	$-CH_2CH_2CH_2NHCH_3$	H
Clomipramine	$-CH_2CH_2CH_2N\overset{CH_3}{\underset{CH_3}{}}$	Cl

2. Dibenzcycloheptenes

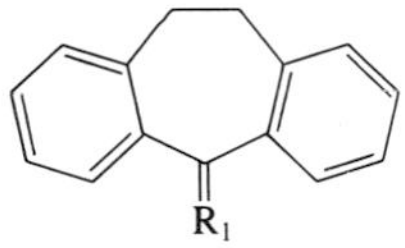

Drug	R$_1$
Amitriptyline	$=CHCH_2CH_2N\overset{CH_3}{\underset{CH_3}{}}$
Nortriptyline	$=CHCH_2CH_2NHCH_3$
Protriptyline	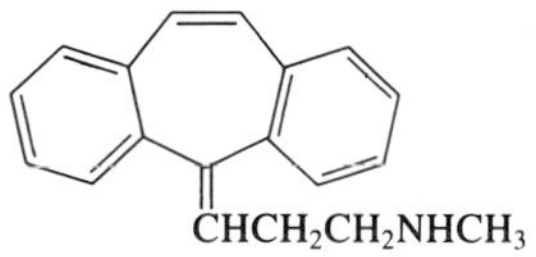 $CHCH_2CH_2NHCH_3$

Fig. 23.2 Chemical structures of tricyclic antidepressants.

Mechanism of action

As discussed above, the main effect of TCA is to block the uptake of amines by nerve terminals, probably by competition for the carrier which forms part of this membrane transport system (see Chapter 7). Synthesis of amines, storage in synaptic vesicles, and release are not directly affected, though some TCA appear to increase transmitter release indirectly by blocking presynaptic α_2-adrenoceptors. Most TCA inhibit noradrenaline and serotonin uptake by brain synaptosomes quite strongly, but have much less effect on dopamine uptake. Among the conventional TCA, there is relatively little selectivity between noradrenaline and serotonin uptake (see Fig. 23.6), and it is not at all clear which type of activity is most important in relation to their antidepressant effects. It has been suggested that improvement of mood reflects mainly an enhancement of serotonergic transmission, whereas increased motor activity ('psycho-motor stimulation') results from facilitation of noradrenergic transmission (Iversen & Mackay, 1979; Carlsson, 1984). Interpretation is made difficult by the fact that the major metabolites of TCA have considerable pharmacological activity (in some cases greater than that of the parent drug) and often differ from the parent drug in respect of their noradrenaline/serotonin selectivity (Table 23.2).

Table 23.2 Inhibition of neuronal noradrenaline and serotonin uptake by tricyclic antidepressants and their metabolites

Drug/metabolite	NA uptake	Serotonin uptake
Imipramine	+++	++
Desmethylimipramine (DMI)	++++	+
Hydroxy-DMI	+++	−
Clomipramine (CMI)	++	+++
Desmethyl-CMI	+++	+
Amitriptyline (AMI)	++	++
Nortriptyline (desmethyl-AMI)	+++	++
Hydroxy-nortriptyline	++	++

Data from: Potter et al, 1984

In addition to their effects on amine uptake, most TCA affect one or more types of neuro-transmitter receptor, including muscarinic ACh receptors, histamine receptors and serotonin receptors. The antimuscarinic effects of TCA probably do not contribute to their antidepressant effects, but are responsible for various troublesome side effects (see below). The antihistamine actions were revealed in a study of histamine-activated adenylate cyclase activity in guinea pig brain (Kanof & Greengard, 1978) which showed a close correlation between the blocking of this response (thought to be mediated by H_2-receptors; see Chapter 8) and antidepressant activity. This correlation was not confined to TCA but extended also to other groups of antidepressants. Its significance is still very uncertain.

Other studies (Sulser, 1983; Snyder & Peroutka, 1984) have suggested that down-regulation of β-adrenoceptors and 5-HT$_2$ receptors is consistently produced by antidepressant drugs and may be essential for their clinical effects, but the mechanism has not been elucidated.

Actions and side effects

In non-depressed human subjects, TCA cause sedation, confusion and motor inco-ordination. These effects occur also in depressed patients in the first few days of treatment, but tend to wear off in 1–2 weeks as the antidepressant effect develops. In experimental animals, TCA also produce sedation unless the animals have been treated with a reserpine-like drug, in which case the depressant effect of reserpine is reversed.

Side effects with normal clinical dosage

TCA produce a number of troublesome side effects, mainly due to interference with autonomic control.

Atropine-like effects include dry mouth, blurred vision, constipation and urinary retention. These effects are strong with amitriptyline, much weaker with desipramine. **Postural hypotension** occurs with TCA. This may seem anomalous for drugs which enhance noradrenergic transmission, and possibly results from an effect on adrenergic transmission in the medullary vasomotor centre (see Chapter 11). The other common side effect is **sedation** (see above). Since many depressed patients have difficulty in sleeping, this effect may actually be helpful, but the long duration of action means that daytime performance is often affected by drowsiness and difficulty in concentrating.

Interactions with other drugs (see Chapter 4). TCA are particularly likely to cause adverse effects when given in conjunction with other drugs. They are strongly bound to plasma protein, so their effects tend to be enhanced by competing drugs (e.g. aspirin, phenylbutazone). They rely on hepatic microsomal metabolism for elimination from the body, and this may be inhibited by competing drugs (e.g. neuroleptics, some steroids).

They cause a strong potentiation of the effects of

alcohol, for reasons that are not well understood, and deaths have occurred as a result of this, when severe respiratory depression has followed the drinking of a normally harmless amount of alcohol. TCA also interact with various antihypertensive drugs (see Chapter 11). Adrenergic neuron blocking drugs (e.g. guanethidine) gain access to adrenergic nerve terminals via the noradrenaline uptake system. Blocking this transport with TCA therefore prevents these antihypertensive drugs from working, and causes hypertension. A similar interaction occurs with methyldopa. With clonidine, on the other hand, TCA can cause a further sharp fall in blood pressure. Dangerous consequences can result from an excessive rise or a fall in blood pressure, so the use of TCA in patients being treated for hypertension is generally unwise.

Acute toxicity

Antidepressant drugs (most commonly TCA) are now one of the most frequently used methods for attempted suicide, so their acute toxic effects are a matter of some practical importance. The main effects are on the central nervous system and the heart.

The initial effect of TCA overdosage is to cause excitement and delirium, which may be accompanied by convulsions. This is followed by coma and respiratory depression lasting for some days before a gradual recovery. Pronounced atropine-like effects are produced, with flushing, dry mouth and skin, and inhibition of gut and bladder.

Cardiac dysrhythmias are common, usually atrial or ventricular extrasystoles, and sudden death may occur from ventricular fibrillation. The mechanism is not understood, but the dysrhythmias often fail to respond to β-receptor blocking drugs, so it is not very likely that enhanced noradrenaline effects on the heart are responsible.

One form of treatment that has been reported to control the main CNS effects is the use of the anticholinesterase, physostigmine (see Chapter 6). This suggests that the antimuscarinic effects of TCA may be partly responsible, and indeed the symptoms produced closely resemble those of atropine poisoning.

Pharmacokinetic aspects

TCA are all rapidly absorbed when given orally and bind strongly to plasma albumin, most being

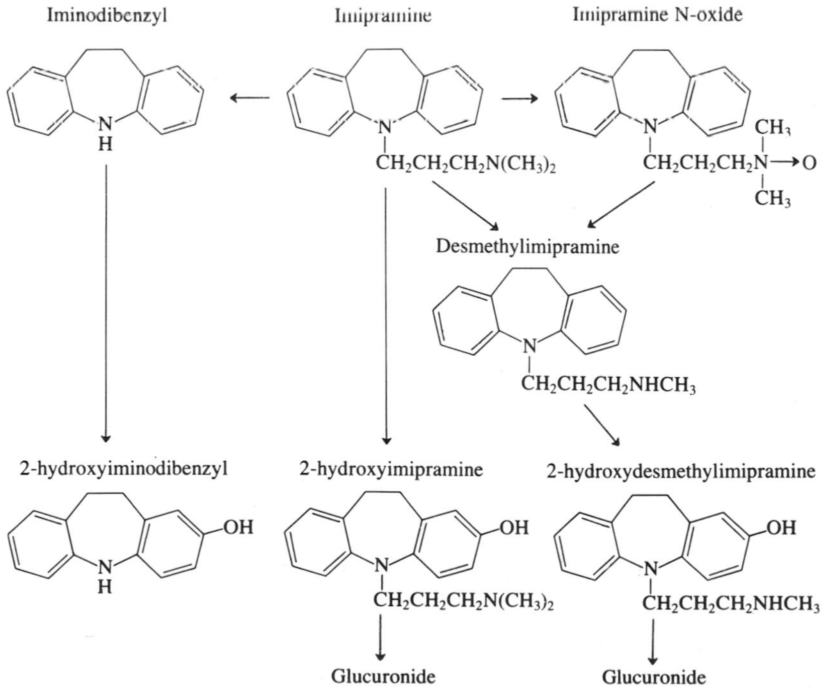

Fig. 23.3 Metabolism of imipramine, which is typical of that of other tricyclic antidepressants.

90–95% bound at therapeutic plasma concentrations. They bind to extravascular tissues, which accounts for their generally large distribution volumes (usually 10–50 l/kg) and low rates of elimination. This extravascular sequestration means that extracorporeal dialysis is rather ineffective in acute overdosage. TCA are metabolized in the liver by two main routes (see Fig. 23.3), namely **N-demethylation**, whereby tertiary amines are converted to secondary amines (e.g. imipramine → desmethylimipramine; amitriptyline → nortriptyline) and **ring hydroxylation**. Both the desmethyl and the hydroxylated metabolites commonly retain biological activity (Table 23.2). During prolonged treatment with TCA, the plasma concentration of these metabolites is usually comparable to that of the parent drug, though there is wide variation between individuals. Inactivation of the drug occurs by glucuronide conjugation of the hydroxylated metabolites, the glucuronides being excreted in the urine.

The overall half-times for elimination of TCA are generally long, ranging from 10–20 hours for imipramine and desipramine to about 80 hours for protriptyline. They are even longer in elderly patients. Thus, gradual accumulation is possible, leading to slowly-developing side effects.

MONOAMINE OXIDASE INHIBITORS (MAOI)

Drugs of this type were among the first to be introduced clinically as antidepressants, but have now been largely superseded by tricyclic and other types of antidepressant whose clinical efficacy is rather better, and whose side effects are generally less, than those of MAOI.

MAO (see Chapter 7) is found in nearly all tissues, and exists in two distinct molecular forms (Table 23.3). MAO-A has a substrate preference for noradrenaline and serotonin, and is the target for the antidepressant MAOI. MAO-B has a substrate preference for phenylethylamine, and both enzymes act on dopamine. Type B is selectively inhibited by **selegiline** (alternative name: **deprenyl**), which has been used clinically in the treatment of Parkinsonism (see Chapter 24). Most of the current antidepressant MAOI act on both forms of MAO. MAO is located intracellularly, mostly associated with mitochondria, and has two main functions. (1) Within noradrenergic and serotoninergic nerve terminals MAO has the effect of regulating the free intraneuronal concentration of noradrenaline or serotonin, and hence the releasable stores of these transmitters. It is not involved in the inactivation of released transmitter. The biochemical role of MAO in noradrenaline metabolism, and the effect of MAOI, are discussed in Chapter 7. (2) MAO is important in the inactivation of endogenous and ingested amines which would otherwise produce unwanted effects. An example is tyramine, which is a substrate for both MAO-A and MAO-B, and is important in producing some of the side effects of MAOI (see below).

Chemical aspects

Many substances similar to phenylethylamines act as weak competitive inhibitors of MAO. Amphetamine is an example, though its actions on adrenergic transmission (see Chapter 7) are not

Table **23.3** Substrates and inhibitors for Type A and Type B monoamine oxidase

	Type A	Type B
Preferred substrates	Noradrenaline Serotonin	Phenylethylamine Benzylamine
Nonspecific substrates	Dopamine Tyramine	
Specific inhibitors	Clorygyline	Selegiline
Nonspecific inhibitors	Paragyline Tranylcypromine Iproniazid	

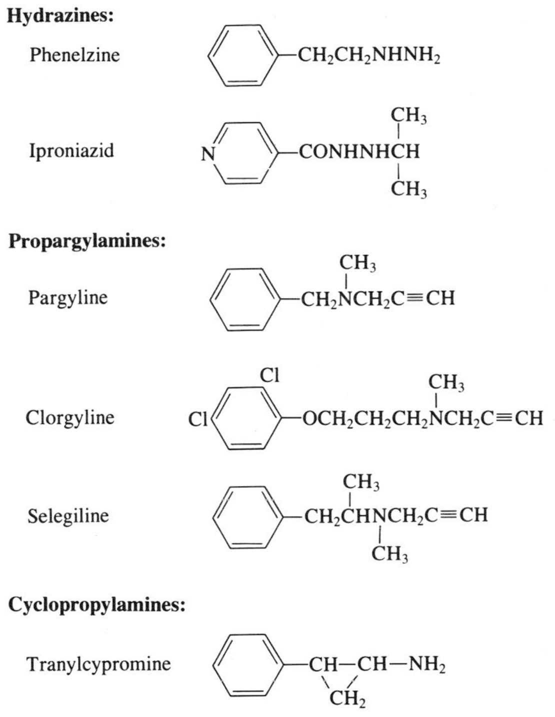

Hydrazines:

Phenelzine

$\langle\!\!\!\!\!\!\bigcirc\!\!\!\!\!\!\rangle$—CH$_2CH_2$NHNH$_2$

Iproniazid

$N\langle\!\!\!\!\!\!\bigcirc\!\!\!\!\!\!\rangle$—CONHNHCH
$\quad\quad\quad\quad\quad$ CH$_3$
$\quad\quad\quad\quad\quad$ |
$\quad\quad\quad\quad\quad$ |
$\quad\quad\quad\quad\quad$ CH$_3$

Propargylamines:

Pargyline

$\langle\!\!\!\!\!\!\bigcirc\!\!\!\!\!\!\rangle$—CH$_2NCH_2$C≡CH
$\quad\quad\quad\quad\quad$ CH$_3$

Clorgyline

Cl$\langle\!\!\!\!\!\!\bigcirc\!\!\!\!\!\!\rangle$—OCH$_2CH_2CH_2NCH_2$C≡CH
Cl$\quad\quad\quad\quad\quad\quad\quad\quad\quad\quad$ CH$_3$

Selegiline

$\langle\!\!\!\!\!\!\bigcirc\!\!\!\!\!\!\rangle$—CH$_2$CHNCH$_2$C≡CH
$\quad\quad\quad\quad\quad$ CH$_3$
$\quad\quad\quad\quad\quad\quad\quad\quad$ CH$_3$

Cyclopropylamines:

Tranylcypromine

$\langle\!\!\!\!\!\!\bigcirc\!\!\!\!\!\!\rangle$—CH—CH—NH$_2$
$\quad\quad\quad\quad\quad$ CH$_2$

Fig. 23.4 Chemical structures of monoamine oxidase inhibitors.

primarily the result of this mechanism. The clinically effective MAOI (Fig. 23.4) possess a phenylethyl-amine-like structure with a chemically reactive group attached, which enables the inhibitor to bind covalently to the enzyme, resulting in a non-competitive and longlasting inhibition. In many MAOI (e.g. **iproniazid**, **phenelzine**) this reactive moiety is a **hydrazine** group. It may also be a **propargylamine** (as in **pargyline**, **deprenyl**) or a **cyclopropylamine** (as in **tranylcypromine**). Recovery of MAO activity after inhibition takes several weeks with most drugs, but is quicker after tranylcypromine which forms a less stable bond with the enzyme.

Most of the clinically used MAOI are non-selective between MAO-A and MAO-B. Exceptions are selegiline (MAO-B specific, and not used as an antidepressant) and **clorgyline** (MAO-A specific and effective in depression).

MAOI are not particularly specific in their actions and inhibit a variety of other enzymes as well as MAO, including many enzymes involved in the metabolism of other drugs. This is responsible for some of the many clinically important drug interactions associated with MAOI.

Pharmacological effects

MAOI cause a rapid and sustained increase in the serotonin, noradrenaline and dopamine content of the brain, serotonin being affected most and dopamine least. Similar changes occur in peripheral tissues such as heart, liver and intestine, and increases in the plasma concentrations of these amines are also detectable. Although these increases in tissue amine content are largely due to accumulation within neurons, transmitter release in response to nerve activity is not increased. In contrast to the effect of TCA, MAOI do not increase the response of peripheral organs, such as the heart and blood vessels, to sympathetic nerve stimulation. The main effect of MAOI is to increase the cytoplasmic concentration of monoamines in nerve terminals, without greatly affecting the vesicular stores which form the pool that is releasable by nerve stimulation. The increased cytoplasmic pool results in an increased rate of spontaneous leakage of monoamines, and also an increased release by indirectly acting sympathomimetic amines such as amphetamine and tyramine (see Chapter 7). This occurs because these amines work by displacing noradrenaline from the vesicles into the nerve terminal cytoplasm, from which it may either leak out and produce a response, or be degraded by MAO (see Fig. 7.15). Inhibition of MAO increases the proportion that escapes, and thus enhances the response. Tyramine thus causes a much greater rise in blood pressure in MAOI-treated animals than in controls. This mechanism is important in relation to the 'cheese reaction' produced by MAOI in man (see later section).

In normal human subjects, MAOI causes an immediate increase in motor activity, and euphoria and excitement develop over the course of a few days. This is in contrast to TCA which cause only sedation and confusion when given to non-depressed subjects. Experimental animals show a similar pattern of increased motor activity, and MAOI (like TCA) are effective in reversing the behavioural effects of reserpine treatment. The effects of MAOI on amine metabolism develop rapidly, and the effect of a single dose lasts for several days. There is a clear discrepancy, as with TCA, between the rapid biochemical response and the delayed antidepressant effect.

Side effects and toxicity

Many of the unwanted effects of MAOI result directly from MAO inhibition, but some are produced by other mechanisms.

Hypotension is a common side effect; indeed pargyline was at one time used as an antihypertensive drug. At first sight it seems surprising in view of the increase in noradrenaline storage and release that occurs. One possible explanation is that amines such as dopamine or octopamine are able to accumulate within peripheral sympathetic nerve terminals and displace noradrenaline from the storage vesicles, thus reducing noradrenaline release associated with sympathetic activity.

Excessive central stimulation may cause tremors, excitement, insomnia, and, in overdose, convulsions.

Weight gain, associated with increased appetite, occurs in a proportion of patients, and can be so extreme as to require the drug to be discontinued.

Atropine-like side effects (dry mouth, blurred vision, urinary retention, etc) are common with MAOI, though they are less of a problem than with TCA.

MAOI of the hydrazine type (e.g. phenelzine, iproniazid) produce, very rarely (less than 1 in 10 000), severe **hepatotoxicity**, which seems to be due to the hydrazine moiety of the molecule. Their use in patients with liver disease is therefore unwise.

Interaction with other drugs and foods

This is the most serious problem with MAOI, and is the main factor (coupled with their uncertain clinical efficacy) that has caused their clinical use to decline.

The **'cheese reaction'** is a direct consequence of MAO inhibition, and occurs when normally inocuous amines (mainly tyramine) are ingested. Tyramine is normally metabolized by MAO in the gut wall and liver and so little dietary tyramine reaches the systemic circulation. When this is prevented, tyramine is absorbed, and moreover its sympathomimetic effect is enhanced (see above). The result is acute hypertension, giving rise to a severe throbbing headache, and occasionally even to intracranial haemorrhage. Though many foods contain some tyramine, it appears that at least 10 mg of tyramine needs to be ingested to produce such a response and the main danger is from mature cheeses and from concentrated yeast products such as Marmite. Administration of indirectly acting sympathomimetic amines (e.g. **ephedrine**, **amphetamine**) is also likely to cause severe hypertension in patients receiving MAOI; directly acting agents, such as adrenaline used in conjunction with local anaesthetic injection (see Chapter 27) are not hazardous.

Hypertensive episodes have also been reported

Table 23.4 Comparison of tricyclic antidepressants and monoamine oxidase inhibitors

	TCA	MAOI
Acute effect	Sedation, dysphoria	Euphoria
Delay in therapeutic effect	2–4 weeks	2–4 weeks
Duration of action	Days	Weeks
Main side effects	Atropine-like effects Sedation Postural hypotension Tachycardia/dysrhythmias	Atropine-like effects Insomnia Postural hypotension Weight gain Liver damage (rare)
Main interactions	CNS depressants, e.g. alcohol, anaesthetics (increased effect)	As TCA
	Adr. neuron blocking drugs (reduced effect)	Cheese reaction, i.e. hypertension after tyramine-containing foods
	Aspirin, phenylbutazone, etc. (increased effect due to competition for protein binding).	Indirectly-acting sympathomimetic amines (hypertension).

in patients given TCA and MAOI simultaneously. The probable explanation is that inhibition of noradrenaline reuptake further enhances the cardiovascular response to dietary tyramine, thus accentuating the cheese reaction. This combination of drugs can also produce excitement and hyperactivity.

MAOI interacts with some drugs to cause not merely an enhancement of their action, but an abnormal syndrome. An important example is the opioid analgesic **pethidine** (see Chapter 25) which may cause severe hyperpyrexia, with restlessness, coma and hypotension when given in combination with MAOI. The mechanism is not known for certain, but it is likely that an abnormal pethidine metabolite is produced because of inhibition of the normal demethylation pathway.

A comparison of the main characteristics of TCA and MAOI is given in Table 23.4.

'ATYPICAL' ANTIDEPRESSANTS

Uncertainty about the exact biochemical mode of action of antidepressants has meant that the development of new drugs has often been empirical. This has resulted in the introduction of a heterogeneous group of compounds, only distantly related to conventional TCA though sharing some of their biochemical actions. Many of these are claimed to have fewer side effects (e.g. sedation, anticholinergic effects) than TCA in clinical use, and in some cases they appear to act with less delay.

They can be divided into three broad categories (Fig. 23.5):

1. Non-tricyclic structures with similar noradrenaline-uptake blocking effects to TCA (e.g. **nomifensine**, **maprotiline**). These drugs are all relatively inactive against serotonin uptake (Fig. 23.6)

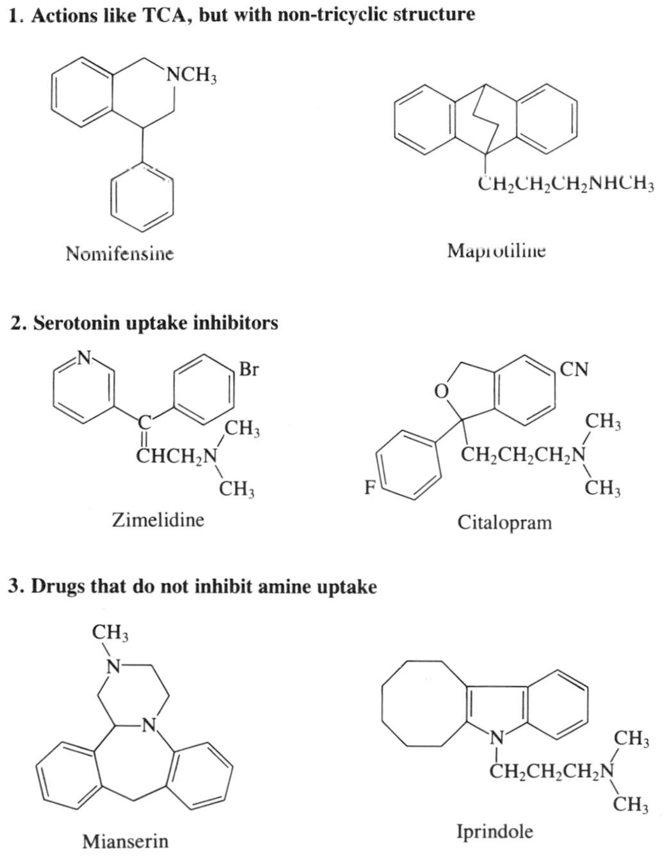

1. Actions like TCA, but with non-tricyclic structure

Nomifensine

Maprotiline

2. Serotonin uptake inhibitors

Zimelidine

Citalopram

3. Drugs that do not inhibit amine uptake

Mianserin

Iprindole

Fig. 23.5 Chemical structures of some atypical antidepressants.

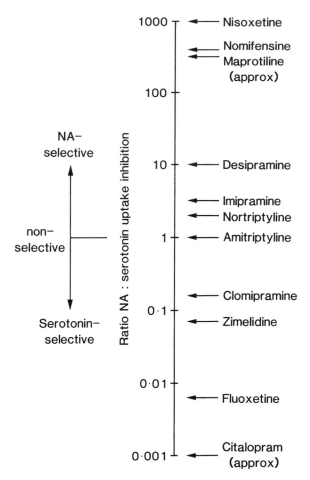

Fig. 23.6 Selectivity of inhibition of noradrenaline and serotonin uptake by various antidepressants. (Redrawn from: Iversen & Mackay, 1979)

but nomifensine is unusual in being highly active as a dopamine uptake inhibitor.

2. Drugs that selectively block serotonin uptake, with little or no effect on noradrenaline uptake (e.g. **zimelidine**, **citalopram**). These are effective antidepressants, though not significantly better in practice than imipramine. Zimelidine also has some analgesic activity, probably because it potentiates the effect of the descending serotonin inhibitory control to the nociceptive pathway (see Chapter 25).

3. Drugs that do not affect amine reuptake (e.g. **mianserin**, **iprindole**). The mechanism of action of these drugs is uncertain. One possibility is that mianserin increases noradrenaline release by blocking α_2-adrenoceptors on noradrenergic nerve terminals (see Chapter 7), thus reducing the inhibi-

tory feedback control of noradrenaline release. Iprindole does not, however, work in this way, and, tantalizingly, seems to lack every expected property of an antidepressant drug except for clinical efficacy.

ELECTROCONVULSIVE THERAPY (ECT)

A tortuous line of reasoning, namely that schizophrenia and epilepsy were considered to be mutually exclusive, led to the use of induced convulsions as therapy for psychological disorders in the 1930s, and its efficacy in treating severe depression has been repeatedly confirmed. ECT in man involves stimulation through electrodes placed on either side of the head, with the patient lightly anaesthetized and paralysed with a neuromuscular blocking drug so as to avoid physical injury. Controlled trials have shown ECT to be at least as effective as antidepressant drugs, with response rates ranging between 60 and 80% in most studies (Kiloh, 1982). The effect of ECT on experimental animals has been carefully analysed to see if it provides clues as to the mode of action of antidepressant drugs (Grahame-Smith, 1984), but the clues it gives are distinctly enigmatic. Serotonin synthesis and uptake are unaltered, and noradrenaline uptake is somewhat increased (in contrast to the effect of TCA). However, decreased noradrenaline responsiveness, both biochemical and behavioural, and increased serotonin responsiveness, are effects produced by both ECT and long-term administration of antidepressant drugs. This lends support to the view that it may be the long-term regulation of neurotransmitter sensitivity produced by antidepressant drugs, rather than their immediate effects, that underlies their clinical effectiveness.

CLINICAL EFFECTIVENESS OF ANTIDEPRESSANT TREATMENTS

Many carefully controlled clinical trials have been reported, and these have established the overall clinical efficacy of TCA, thought it is clear that a substantial proportion of patients recover spontaneously, and that some patients fail to improve

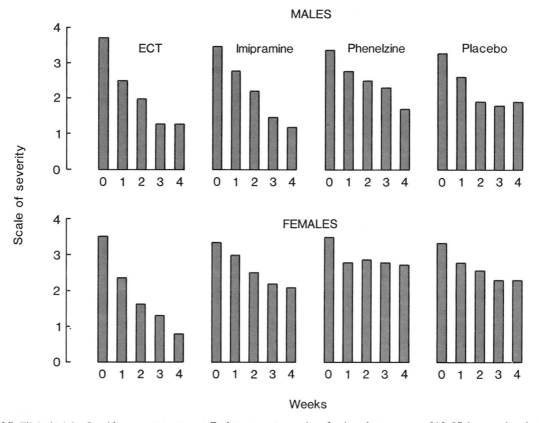

Fig. 23.7 Clinical trials of antidepressant treatment. Each treatment was given for 4 weeks to groups of 15–37 depressed patients, and the scale of severity assessed weekly. From these results, ECT appears to be the most effective treatment, whereas phenelzine was no better than placebo. (Results from: MRC Trial, 1965)

with drug treatments. The effects of the drugs are significant, but not miraculous.

The results of a Medical Research Council trial in 1965 (Fig. 23.7) showed ECT to be the most effective treatment. Imipramine also produced significant improvement, but the MAOI, phenelzine, appeared to be no better than the placebo. Subsequent trials have confirmed this result, and comparisons of other TCA and the new atypical antidepressants with imipramine have generally shown them to be about equally effective. The ineffectiveness of phenelzine reported in the Medical Research Council trial (together with the incidence of severe hypertensive episodes) caused MAOI to lose favour clinically. Subsequent trials (Nies & Robinson, 1982) showed that with larger dosage MAOI may be significantly better than TCA for patients with mild depression, particularly those with neurotic symptoms (anxiety, etc), as opposed

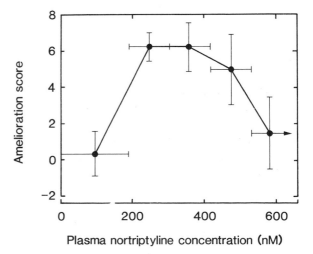

Fig. 23.8 'Therapeutic window' for nortriptyline. The amelioration of depression, determined from subjective rating scales, is optimal at plasma concentrations between 200 and 400 nM, and declines at high levels. (From: Asberg et al, 1971)

to psychotic symptoms (withdrawal, delusions, etc) where TCA appear to be more successful. Even the most favourable trials, however, show that about 30% of depressed patients fail to show improvement. Attempts to identify which patients will respond on the basis of behavioural or biochemical measurements (e.g. platelet MAO activity, MHPG excretion) have not been successful.

The relationship between plasma concentrations and the therapeutic effect may not be simple according to a recent study on nortriptyline (Fig. 23.8) which shows that too high a plasma concentration actually *reduces* the antidepressant effect, and there is quite a narrow 'therapeutic window'. Whether this is true for other antidepressant drugs is not known.

LITHIUM

Lithium is quite different in its effects from the antidepressant drugs discussed so far, in that it controls the manic phase of manic-depressive (bipolar) illness and has no effect on unipolar depression. Used prophylactically in bipolar depression, lithium is able to prevent the swings of mood and thus to control the depressive as well as the manic phases of the illness. Given in an acute attack, lithium is effective only in controlling mania and has no effect during the depressive phase. Other drugs (e.g. neuroleptics) are equally effective in controlling acute mania, and considerably safer, so the clinical use of lithium is mainly confined to prophylactic control of manic-depressive illness.

The psychotropic effect of lithium was discovered in 1949 by Cade who had predicted that urate salts should prevent the state of hyperexcitability induced by uraemia in guinea pigs. He found lithium urate to produce an effect, quickly discovered that it was due to lithium rather than urate, and went on to show that lithium produced a rapid improvement in a group of manic patients.

Pharmacological effects and mechanism of action

Lithium is clinically effective at a plasma concentration of about 1 mM, and above 2 mM produces a variety of toxic effects. In normal subjects, 1 mM lithium in plasma has no appreciable psycho-

tropic effects. It does, however, produce many detectable biochemical changes, and it is still extremely unclear how these may be related to its therapeutic effect.

Lithium is a monovalent cation, which partially mimics the effects of a variety of other cations in cellular processes. Thus, it resembles sodium in excitable tissues, being able to permeate the fast voltage-sensitive channels that are responsible for action potential generation (see Chapter 27). It is not, however, pumped out nearly so quickly as sodium by the Na/K ATPase and tends to accumulate inside excitable cells to a greater extent than sodium. This leads to a partial loss of intracellular potassium, and partial depolarization of the cell. Its effects on monoamine metabolism are complex. Given acutely, lithium increases noradrenaline and serotonin turnover in the brain, but seems to inhibit depolarization-evoked release. These changes apparently subside during long-term administration, though the drug remains clinically effective, so their significance is unclear.

Two well-defined biochemical effects have been described in isolated tissues:

1. Hormone-induced cAMP production is usually reduced (e.g. the response of renal tubular cells to ADH; see Chapter 14). This is not, however, a pronounced effect in the brain.
2. The phosphatidyl inositol (PI) pathway (see Chapter 1) is blocked at the point where inositol-1-phosphate is hydrolysed to free inositol. This step is required for the regeneration of phosphatidylinositol biphosphate (PIP_2) in the membrane after it has been hydrolysed by agonist action, as described in Chapter 1. Lithium thus causes a depletion of membrane PIP_2 and accumulation of intracellular inositol-1-phosphate.

It seems quite possible that the effects of lithium on these two important second messenger systems somehow underlie its therapeutic effect, and that its cellular selectivity depends on the uptake of lithium in varying amounts, reflecting the activity of sodium channels in different cells. This could account for its relatively selective action in the brain and kidney, even though many other tissues use the same second messengers.

Pharmacokinetic aspects and toxicity

Lithium excretion by the kidney occurs in two phases. About half of an oral dose is excreted within about 12 hours; the remainder, which presumably represents lithium taken up by cells, is excreted over the next 1–2 weeks. This slow excretion means that, with regular dosage, lithium accumulates slowly over approximately 2 weeks before a steady state is reached. The narrow therapeutic limit for the plasma concentration (approximately 0.8–1.5 mM) means that monitoring is essential. Factors such as renal disease or sodium depletion reduce the rate of excretion and thus increase the likelihood of toxicity.

The main toxic effects are:

1. Renal effects—polyuria (with resulting thirst) resulting from inhibition of the action of antiduretic hormone. At the same time there is some sodium retention, associated with increased aldosterone secretion. With prolonged treatment, serious renal tubular damage may occur, making it essential to monitor renal function regularly in lithium-treated patients.
2. Thyroid enlargement, sometimes associated with hypothyroidism.
3. Various neurological effects, progressing from nausea, vomiting, tremor and some confusion, to coma, convulsions and death as the plasma concentration increases.

REFERENCES AND FURTHER READING

Baker G B, Dewhurst W G 1985 Biochemical theories of affective disorders. In: Dewhurst W G, Baker G B (eds) Pharmacotherapy of affective disorders. Croom-Helm, Beckenham

Carlsson A 1984 Current theories on the mode of action of antidepressant drugs. Adv Biochem Psychopharmol 39: 213–221

Coppen A, Prange A J, Whybrow P C, Noguera R 1972 Abnormalities of indoleamines in affective disorders. Arch gen Psychiat 26: 474–478

Dewhurst W G, Baker G B (eds) 1985 Pharmacology of affective disorders. Croom-Helm, Beckenham

Grahame-Smith D G 1984 The neuropharmacological effects of electroconvulsive shock and their relationship to the therapeutic effect of electroconvulsive therapy in depression. In: Usdin E et al (eds) Frontiers in biochemical and pharmacological research in depression. Raven Press, New York

Green A R, Costain D W 1981 Pharmacology and biochemistry of psychiatric disorders. Wiley-Interscience, Chichester

Iversen L L, Mackay A V P 1979 Pharmacodynamics of antidepressants and antimanic drugs. In: Paykel E S, Coppen A (eds) Psychopharmacology of affective disorders. Oxford University Press, Oxford

Johnstone E C 1982 Affective disorders. In: Crow T J (ed) Disorders of neurohumoral transmission. Academic Press, London, p255–286

Kanof P D, Greengard P 1978 Brain histamine receptors as targets for antidepressant drugs. Nature 272: 329–333

Kiloh L G 1982 Electroconvulsive therapy. In: Paykel E S (ed) Handbook of affective disorders. Churchill-Livingstone, Edinburgh, p262–275

Langer S Z, Zarifian E, Briley M, Raisman R, Sechter O 1982 High affinity ^{3}H-imipramine binding: a new biological marker in depression. Pharmacopsychiatria 15: 4–10

Maj J, Przegalinski E, Mogilnicka E 1984 Hypotheses concerning the mechanism of action of antidepressant drugs. Rev Physiol Biochem Pharmacol 100: 1–74

Nies A, Robinson D S 1982 Monoamine oxidase inhibitors. In: Paykel E S (ed) Handbook of affective disorders. Churchill-Livingstone, Edinburgh, p246–261

Paykel E S (ed) 1982 Handbook of affective disorders. Churchill-Livingstone, Edinburgh, p246–261

Porsolt R D 1985 Animal models of affective disorders. In: Dewhurst W G & Baker G B (eds) Pharmacotherapy of affective disorders. Croom-Helm, Beckenham

Schildkraut J J 1965 The catecholamine hypothesis—a review of the supporting evidence. Amer J Psychiat 122: 509–522

Snyder S H, Peroutka S J 1984 Antidepressants and neurotransmitter receptors. In: Post R M, Bellenger J C (eds) Neurobiology of mood disorders. Williams & Williams, Baltimore, p686–697

Sulser F 1983 Mode of action of antidepressant drugs. J Clin Psychiat 44: 14–20

Zis A P, Goodwin F K 1982 The amine hypothesis. In: Paykel E S (ed) Handbook of affective disorders. Churchill-Livingstone, Edinburgh, p175–190

Drugs used in treating motor disorders: epilepsy, Parkinsonism and spasticity

EPILEPSY

Epilepsy is a very common disorder, affecting roughly 0.5% of the population. Usually there is no recognizable cause, though it may develop as a consequence of various kinds of brain damage, such as trauma, infection or tumour growth.

The characteristic event in epilepsy is the **seizure**, which is associated with the episodic high frequency discharge of impulses by a group of neurons in the brain. What starts as a local abnormal discharge may then spread to other areas of the brain. The site of the primary discharge and the extent of its spread determines the symptoms that are produced,

A. Normal

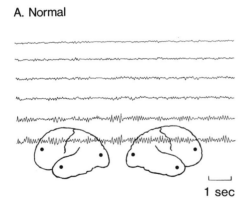

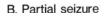
1 sec

B. Partial seizure

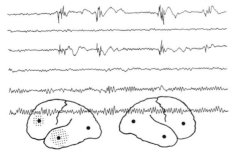

C. Generalized seizure (grand mal)

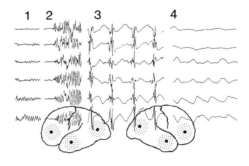

D. Generalized seizure (petit mal)

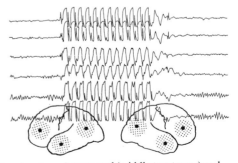

Fig. 24.1 EEG records in epilepsy. A. Normal EEG recorded from frontal (top two traces), temporal (middle two traces) and occipital (lower two traces) regions on both sides. B. Partial seizure, with synchronous abnormal discharges in left frontal and temporal regions. C. Generalized tonic-clonic (grand mal) seizure. Stretches of record show: 1. Normal EEG; 2. Onset of tonic phase; 3. Clonic phase; 4. Post-convulsive coma. D. Generalized petit mal seizure, showing sudden brief episode of 3 sec^{-1} 'spike and wave' discharge. (From: Eliasson et al, 1978)

which range from a brief lapse of attention to a full-blown convulsive fit lasting for several minutes. The particular symptoms produced depend on the function of the region of the brain that is affected. Thus involvement of the motor cortex causes convulsions, involvement of the hypothalamus causes peripheral autonomic discharge, and involvement of the reticular formation in the upper brainstem leads to loss of consciousness.

Abnormal electrical activity during a seizure can be detected by electroencephalographic (EEG) recording from electrodes distributed over the surface of the scalp. Various types of seizure can be recognized on the basis of the nature and distribution of the abnormal discharge (Fig. 24.1).

TYPES OF EPILEPSY

The agreed clinical classification of epilepsy recognizes the following major categories:

1. Partial seizures

These are seizures in which the discharge remains localized. They may produce relatively simple symptoms without loss of consciousness, such as involuntary muscle contractions, abnormal sensory experiences or autonomic discharge, or they may cause more complex effects on consciousness, mood and behaviour, often termed psychomotor epilepsy. The localized EEG discharge in this type of epilepsy is shown in Figure 24.1B.

An epileptic focus in the motor cortex results in attacks, sometimes called **Jacksonian epilepsy**, consisting of repetitive jerking of a localized muscle group, which spreads and may involve much of the body within about 2 minutes before dying out. Though the patient loses voluntary control of the affected parts of the body, he does not lose consciousness. In **psychomotor epilepsy**, which is often associated with a focus in the temporal lobe, the attack may consist of stereotyped purposive movements such as rubbing or patting movements, or much more complex behaviour such as dressing or walking or hair-combing. The seizure usually lasts for a few minutes, after which the patient recovers with no recollection of the event. The behaviour during the seizure can be bizarre and may be accompanied by a strong emotional response.

2 Generalized seizures

These seizures begin locally, but spread quickly to involve the reticular system, thus producing abnormal electrical activity throughout both hemispheres. Immediate loss of consciousness is thus characteristic of generalized seizures. The main categories are **tonic-clonic seizures** (grand mal) and **absences** (petit mal).

A tonic-clonic seizure consists of an initial strong contraction of the whole musculature, causing a rigid extensor spasm. Respiration stops and defaecation, micturition and salivation often occur. This tonic phase lasts for about 1 minute and is followed by a series of violent, synchronous jerks which gradually die out in 2–4 minutes. The patient stays unconscious for a few more minutes and then gradually recovers, feeling ill and confused, and is sometimes injured by convulsive episode. The EEG shows generalized continuous high frequency activity in the tonic phase, and an intermittent discharge in the clonic phase (Fig. 24.1C).

Absence seizures are much less dramatic but may occur more frequently (many seizures each day) than tonic-clonic seizures. The patient abruptly ceases whatever he is doing, sometimes stopping speaking in mid-sentence, and stares vacantly for a few seconds, with little or no motor disturbance. The patient is unaware of his surroundings, and recovers abruptly with no after-effects. The EEG pattern shows a characteristic synchronous discharge during the period of the seizure (Fig. 24.1D).

Pharmacologically, there is a clear distinction between drugs that are effective in absence seizures and those that are effective in other types of epilepsy, though most drugs show little selectivity with respect to the other clinical subdivisions.

CELLULAR MECHANISMS UNDERLYING EPILEPSY

The underlying neuronal abnormality in epilepsy is poorly understood. Because detailed studies are difficult or impossible to carry out on epileptic patients, many different animal models of epilepsy have been investigated. These include a variety of genetic strains that show epilepsy-like characteristics (e.g. mice that convulse briefly in response to certain sounds, and strains of beagles with a congenital abnormality that closely resembles human epilepsy). Local cortical damage (e.g. produced by applying alumina paste or crystals of a cobalt salt) results in a type of focal epilepsy. Local application of penicillin crystals has a similar effect, probably by interfering with inhibitory synaptic transmission. Convulsant drugs, such as **leptazol** (see Chapter 26) are often used, particularly in the testing of anti-convulsant agents, and seizures caused by electrical stimulation of the whole brain are used for the same purpose. It has been found empirically that activity in inhibiting leptazol-induced convulsions is a fairly good index of effectiveness against absence seizures, whereas activity against electrically-induced con-vulsions is a guide to effectiveness in controlling other types of epilepsy, such as tonic-clonic seizures.

An interesting form of experimental epilepsy is the so-called 'kindling response' (Goddard, 1983). Low intensity electrical stimulation of certain regions of the limbic system, such as the amygdala, with implanted electrodes normally produces no seizure response. If a brief period of stimulation is repeated daily for several days, however, the response gradually increases until very low levels of stimulation will evoke a full seizure. The mechanism by which this change occurs is not clear, but it may be relevant to human epilepsy. Thus it is often found that surgical removal of a damaged region of cortex fails to cure epilepsy, as though the abnormal discharge from the region of primary damage had somehow produced a secondary hyper-excitability elsewhere in the brain. A recent study (Servit & Musil, 1981) has shown that prophylactic treatment with anticonvulsant drugs for 2 years following severe head injury reduces the subsequent incidence of post-traumatic epilepsy, which suggests that a phenomenon similar to kindling may underly this form of epilepsy.

By intracellular recording techniques it was shown in 1963 that the group of neurons from which the epileptic discharge originates display an unusual type of electrical behaviour, termed the **paroxysmal depolarizing shift** (PDS) during which the membrane potential suddenly decreases by about 30 mV and remains depolarized for up to a few seconds before returning to normal. A burst of action potentials often accompanies this depolar-ization (Fig. 24.2). This event probably results from the abnormally exaggerated and prolonged action

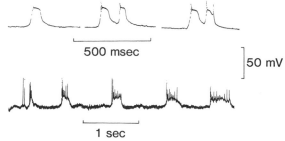

Fig. 24.2 *Upper record.* Paroxysmal depolarizing shift recorded with an intracellular microelectrode from cortical neurons of anaesthetized cats. Seizure activity was induced by topical application of penicillin.

Lower record. Intracellular recording from caudate nucleus of anaesthetized cat. The glutamate analogue, N-methyl D-aspartate was applied by ionophoresis from a nearby micropipette. Note the periodic waves of depolarization, associated with a burst of action potentials, which closely resemble the paroxysmal depolarizing shift.

(From: (Top) Matsumoto & Marsan, 1964; (Bottom) Herrling et al, 1983)

of an excitatory transmitter, and it is interesting that activation of one of the three types of glutamate receptor that are believed to occur on central neurons (see Chapter 19) produces 'plateau-shaped' depolarizing responses very similar to the PDS (Fig. 24.2). It is possible that hyperactivity of glutamate or another excitatory amino-acid is responsible for the discharge of epileptic neurons, and efforts to develop glutamate antagonists as anticonvulsant drugs appear to be promising. Various agents that block the potassium perme-ability of neurons, such as **aminopyridines** (see Chapters 6 & 27) can also produce a response pattern very similar to the PDS, so it is possible that an alteration of the potassium channels of the neuronal membrane accounts for the abnormal pattern of excitability in epilepsy.

Attempts to find a common neurochemical basis for human or experimental epilepsy have been disappointing. The quest has focused mainly on a possible deficit in inhibitory transmission, mediated by GABA, glycine or taurine, or on hyperactivity of an excitatory transmitter, such as glutamate or aspartate.

Studies on the amino-acid content of areas of cortex removed from patients with focal epilepsy (Van Gelder et al, 1972) showed that the whole cortex was deficient in both GABA and aspartate compared with normal, while the epileptic focus contained, in addition, a low content of glutamate and taurine, and a greatly raised content of glycine. Genetically susceptible animal strains show a variety of neurochemical abnormalities, but no clear-cut pattern. The abnormality could, of course, consist of altered transmitter release, or altered receptor sensitivity which would not necessarily be detected by measuring neurotransmitter content.

MECHANISM OF ACTION OF ANTICONVULSANT DRUGS

Whether or not a disturbance of excitatory or inhibitory transmission is part of the causation of epilepsy, pharmacological modification of GABA- or glutamate-mediated transmission has a strong effect on the epileptic discharge. Thus some of the clinically effective anticonvulsants enhance the inhibitory effect of GABA by affecting the function of the GABA-receptor-chloride channel complex, whereas drugs that inhibit the action of GABA (e.g. picrotoxin; see Chapter 26) act as convulsants. Similarly antagonists of excitatory amino-acids are anticonvulsant, whereas the excitatory amino-acids themselves, or agents that increase their synaptic effectiveness, act as convulsants.

In many cases the mechanism of action of anticonvulsant drugs is very poorly understood (see: Woodbury et al, 1982; Frey & Janz, 1985 for further information). **Phenobarbitone** is a barbiturate (see Chapter 21) which has a considerably greater anticonvulsant effect in relation to its sedative action than other barbiturates, such as pentobarbitone. One of its effects is to enhance the action of GABA as an inhibitory transmitter by binding to a site on the GABA-receptor-channel complex that is distinct from either the GABA or the benzodiazepine binding sites (see Chapters 19 & 21), and this is a possible explanation of its anticonvulsant properties. However, phenobarbitone is no more effective than pentobarbitone in potentiating the action of GABA, though it is much more effective as an anti-epileptic drug, so this cannot be the whole explanation. Furthermore, phenobarbitone is as effective against electrically-induced convulsions as it is against lepatazol-induced convulsions in rats or mice, whereas benzodiazepines, which are known to work by increasing the action of GABA (see Chapter 21), are without effect on electrically induced convulsions. Phenobarbitone reduces the

electrical activity of neurons within an artificially-induced epileptic focus within the cortex, whereas **diazepam** (a benzodiazepine) does not much alter the focal activity, but appears to prevent it from spreading. It is therefore unrealistic to attribute the action of phenobarbitone solely to its interaction with GABA, and there is good evidence that it can also act by inhibiting excitatory synaptic responses, though little is known about the mechanism.

Phenytoin has been studied in great detail, but its mechanism of action remains rather mysterious. It seems to work by affecting the characteristics of the membrane that control electrical excitability rather than by acting on synaptic transmission. It has some local-anaesthetic activity, blocking the increase in sodium conductance that is required for action potential initiation (see Chapter 27). This effect probably accounts for its antidysrhythmic action (see Chapter 10) and it is possible that the use-dependent nature of this blocking action, discussed in Chapter 10, is important in producing a selective block of high frequency discharges, which would obviously be relevant in epilepsy. However, phenytoin has also been reported to affect other aspects of membrane function, including inhibition of calcium entry and activation of the sodium pump. The latter effect results in an increased **post-tetanic hyperpolarization**, producing a decrease in the excitability of membrane following a burst of repetitive activity.

The rather scant information available on the mechanism of action of other anticonvulsant drugs is summarized in Table 24.1.

It is estimated that anti-epileptic drugs are fully effective in controlling seizures in 50–80% of patients, though unpleasant side effects are common (see below). There is clearly a need for more specific and effective drugs, but progress in this direction has been very slow. Phenobarbitone was introduced in 1912, and phenytoin in 1935. A number of less important drugs appeared over the next 20 years, followed by **ethosuximide** (1960), **diazepam** (1968) and **valproate** (1978). Current work is aimed mainly at developing effective GABA agonists and glutamate antagonists. In the latter category, several pharmacologically effective agents have been produced, such as **α-aminoadipic acid** and **aminophosphonovaleric acid** (APV; see Chapter 19) which have anticonvulsant properties in experi-

Table 24.1 Properties of anticonvulsant drugs

Drug	Cellular mechanism	Effect on neuronal discharge	Effect on exptl. models		Clinical uses	Main unwanted effects
			electro-shock	leptazol		
Phenobarbitone	?enhanced GABA action	↓ discharge in epileptic focus	↓	↓	All types except absence seizures	Sedation, megaloblastic anaemia. Enzyme induction. Exacerbation of porphyria } esp. phenobarbitone. Hypersensitivity reactions } esp. primidone
Primidone	?inhibition of excitatory synaptic responses					
Phenytoin	Block of Na$^+$ channels. Stimulation of Na$^+$ pump	↓ spread	↓	—	All types except absence seizures	Ataxia, vertigo, gum hyperplasia. Hirsutism, megaloblastic anaemia. Fetal malformations. Pharmacokinetic complications
Ethosuximide	Unknown	Unknown	—	↓	Absence seizures	Nausea, anorexia
Trimethadione	Enhanced pre- and post-synaptic inhibition. ?enhanced GABA action	Unknown	—	↓	Absence seizures	Severe hypersensitivity reactions, including aplastic anaemia (rare). Fetal malformations
Valproate	Inhibits GABA breakdown	Unknown	↓ or —	↓	Absence seizures and other types	Hair loss. Hepatotoxicity (rare)
Carbamazepine	Unknown. Depresses post-tetanic potentiation	↓ spread	↓	↓	All types except absence seizures. Also trigeminal neuralgia	Drowsiness, ataxia, mental impairment. Water retention. Occasional severe hypersensitivity reactions
Benzodiazepines (e.g. diazepam clonazepam)	Enhanced GABA action	↓ discharge	—	↓	All types. Especially status epilepticus	Drowsiness etc (see Chapter 21)

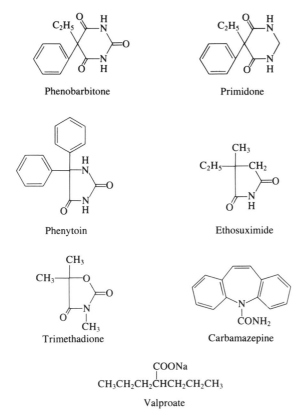

Fig. 24.3 Structures of anticonvulsant drugs.

mental animals, and it is hoped that new drugs for clinical use may be developed from these starting points.

INDIVIDUAL DRUGS

The structures of the main anticonvulsant drugs are shown in Figure 24.3 and their properties are summarized in Table 24.1.

Phenytoin

Phenytoin is the most important member of the **hydantoin** group of compounds, which are structurally related to the barbiturates. It was found to be highly effective in reducing the intensity and duration of electrically-induced convulsions in mice, though ineffective against leptazol-induced convulsions. Its mechanism of action is discussed above.

Clinically, it is effective against various forms of

partial and generalized seizures, but not against absence seizures, which may even get worse. Its uses as an antidysrhythmic drug is discussed in Chapter 10.

Phenytoin has certain pharmacokinetic peculiarities which are important to take into account when it is used clinically (Perucca & Richens 1982). It is well absorbed when given orally, and about 80–90% of the plasma content is bound to albumin. Other drugs, such as salicylates, phenylbutazone, valproate, etc, inhibit this binding competitively (see Chapter 4). This increases the free phenytoin concentration, but also increases hepatic clearance of phenytoin, so may enhance or reduce the effect of the phenytoin in an unpredictable way. Phenytoin is metabolized by the hepatic mixed function oxidase system and excreted mainly as glucuronide. It causes induction, and thus increases the rate of metabolism of other drugs (e.g. anticoagulants). The metabolism of phenytoin itself can be either enhanced, or competitively inhibited by various other drugs that share the same hepatic enzymes. Phenobarbitone produces both effects, and since competitive inhibition is immediate whereas induction takes time, it initially enhances and later reduces the pharmacological activity of phenytoin. Ethanol has a similar dual effect.

The metabolism of phenytoin shows the characteristic of saturation (see Chapter 3) which means that over the therapeutic plasma concentration range the rate of inactivation does not increase in proportion to the plasma concentration. The consequences of this are: (a) the plasma half-life (approximately 20 hours) increases as the dose is increased; and (b) the steady-state mean plasma concentration, achieved when a patient is given a constant daily dose, varies disproportionately with the dose. This can be a striking phenomenon. Figure 24.4 shows that in one patient increasing the dose by 50% caused the steady state plasma concentration to increase more than four-fold.

The range of plasma concentration over which phenytoin is effective without causing excessive side effects is approximately 40–100 μM. The very steep relationship between dose and plasma concentration, and the many interacting factors, mean that there is considerable individual variation in the plasma concentration achieved with a given dose. A simple radioimmunoassay for

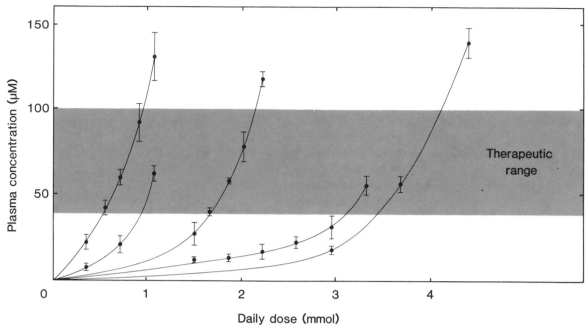

Fig. 24.4 Non-linear relationship between daily dose of phenytoin and steady-state plasma concentration in five individual human subjects. Although the therapeutic range is quite broad (40–100 μM) the daily dose required varies greatly between individuals, and for any one individual the dose has to be adjusted rather precisely to keep within the acceptable plasma concentration range. (Redrawn from: Richens & Dunlop, 1975)

phenytoin in plasma is available, and its use has helped considerably in achieving an optimal therapeutic effect. The tendency in the past has been to use complex multiple prescriptions in cases where a single drug failed to give adequate control. Now that phenytoin dosage can be monitored quite precisely, the use of polypharmacy in treating epilepsy is declining. Side effects of phenytoin begin to appear at plasma concentrations exceeding 100 μM and may be severe above about 150 μM. The milder side effects include **vertigo**, **ataxia**, **headache** and **nystagmus**, but not sedation. At higher plasma concentrations, marked **confusion** with **intellectual deterioration** occur; these effects occur acutely and are quickly reversible. **Hyperplasia of the gums**, which is disfiguring rather than harmful, often develops gradually, as does **hirsutism**, which probably results from increased androgen secretion. **Megaloblastic anaemia**, associated with a disorder of folate metabolism, sometimes occurs, and can be corrected by giving folic acid (see Chapter 18). **Hypersensitivity** reactions, mainly skin rashes, are quite common. Phenytoin has also been implicated as a cause of the increased incidence of fetal mal-

formations in children born to epileptic mothers (Janz, 1975), particularly the occurrence of cleft palate (see Chapter 36).

In spite of its many side effects and unpredictable pharmacokinetic behaviour, phenytoin is probably the most useful drug in treating most forms of epilepsy apart from absence seizures.

Phenobarbitone

Phenobarbitone was one of the first barbiturates to be developed and its anticonvulsant properties were recognized in 1912. Its mechanism of action, so far as it is understood, is discussed above. In its action against experimentally induced convulsions and clinical forms of epilepsy it closely resembles phenytoin; though it has appreciable activity against leptazol-induced seizures it is (like phenytoin) ineffective in treating absence seizures. Phenobarbitone is well absorbed and about 50% of the drug in the blood is bound to plasma albumin. It is eliminated slowly from the plasma ($t_{\frac{1}{2}}$ 50–140 hours). About 25% is excreted unchanged in the urine, its lipid solubility being sufficiently low that it is incompletely reabsorbed from the renal tubules. Since phenobarbitone is a weak acid, its ionization and hence renal elimination are increased if the urine is made alkaline (see Chapter 4). The remaining 75% is metabolized, mainly by oxidation and conjugation, by the hepatic microsomal enzymes. Phenobarbitone is a particularly effective inducer, and by this mechanism it lowers the plasma concentration of several other drugs to an extent (sometimes by 50% or more) that is clinically important (Table 24.2).

The clinical uses of phenobarbitone are virtually the same as those of phenytoin, though phenytoin is usually preferred because of the absence of sedation.

Primidone

Primidone is a close relative of phenobarbitone, and closely resembles it pharmacologically. Part of its action is due to formation of phenobarbitone as a metabolite. It has no clear-cut advantages, and

Table 24.2 Effects of phenobarbitone* on the metabolism of other drugs

Drug	Effect on plasma concentration	Consequence
Digitoxin	Decrease	Increased dose needed
Dexamethasone*	Decrease	Increased dose needed
Prednisolone*	Decrease	Increased dose needed
Chlorpromazine	Decrease	Increased dose needed
Vitamin D	Decrease	Osteomalacia
Oral contraceptives*	Decrease	Loss of effect
Warfarin	Decrease	Increased dose needed
Diazepam*	Decrease	Increased dose needed
Quinidine*	Decrease	Increased dose needed
β-blockers	Decrease	Increased dose needed
Tricyclic antidepressants	Decrease	Increased dose needed
Phenytoin	Variable (usually increase initially then decrease)	Unpredictable

* Also reported for phenytoin.
(Data from: Perruca & Richens, 1985 Handbook of Experimental Pharmacology 74: 831)

The main side effect of phenobarbitone is sedation, which often occurs at plasma concentrations within the therapeutic range for seizure control. This is a serious drawback, since the drug may have to be used for years on end. Some degree of tolerance to the sedative effect seems to occur, but objective tests of cognition and motor performance have generally shown impairment even after long-term treatment (Mattson & Cramer, 1982). Other side effects that may occur with clinical dosage include megaloblastic anaemia (similar to that caused by phenytoin), mild hypersensitivity reactions and osteomalacia. Like other barbiturates (see Chapter 20) it must not be given to patients with porphyria. In *overdose*, phenobarbitone produces coma and respiratory and circulatory failure, as do all barbiturates.

one disadvantage is that it can cause severe hypersensitivity reactions.

Ethosuximide

Ethosuximide, which belongs to the succinimide class, is yet another drug developed by modifying the barbituric acid ring structure. Pharmacologically and clinically, however, it is different from the drugs so far discussed, in that it is active against leptazol-induced convulsions in animals and against absence seizures in man, with little or no effect on other types of epilepsy, closely resembling **trimethadione** (see below) in this respect. Its mechanism of action is not understood. It is well absorbed, and metabolized and excreted much like phenobarbitone, with a plasma $t_{\frac{1}{2}}$ of about 50 hours.

Its main side effects are nausea and anorexia, sometimes lethargy and dizziness. Very rarely it can cause severe hypersensitivity reactions.

It is used clinically for its selective effect on absence seizures, being less likely to produce serious toxic effects than trimethadione, which it has largely supplanted.

Trimethadione

Trimethadione is structurally and pharmacologically similar to ethosuximide and when introduced in 1946 it was the first drug to be effective in treating absence seizures. It causes more marked sedation than ethosuximide (a serious unwanted effect, particularly since absence seizures occur often in children). It can also, though rarely, cause severe hypersensitivity reactions, including aplastic anaemia, which may be fatal. In pregnancy, trimethadione is liable to produce fetal abnormalities.

Both ethosuximide and trimethadione are said to precipitate tonic-clonic seizures in susceptible patients.

Valproate

Valproate is a simple monocarboxylic acid, chemically unrelated to any other class of anticonvulsant drug, and in 1963 it was discovered quite accidentally to have anticonvulsant properties in mice. It inhibits most kinds of experimentally-induced convulsion, and is effective in many clinical types of epilepsy. Valproate causes a significant increase in the GABA content of the brain, without affecting other amino-acids (Godin et al, 1969) which may well account for its anticonvulsant properties. It is a weak inhibitor of two enzyme systems that inactivate GABA, namely GABA-transaminase and succinic semialdehyde dehydrogenase, but *in vitro* studies suggest that these effects would be very slight at clinical dosage. Other more potent inhibitors of these enzymes also increase GABA content and have an anticonvulsant effect in experimental animals, but the precise mode of action of valproate remains uncertain (Johnston & Slater, 1982). There is some evidence that it enhances the action of GABA by a post-synaptic action.

Valproate is well absorbed orally and excreted, mainly as the glucuronide, in the urine, the plasma half-life being about 15 hours.

Compared with most anti-epileptic drugs, valproate is relatively free of unwanted effects. It causes thinning and curling of the hair in about 10% of patients. Potentially the most serious side effect is hepatotoxicity. An increase in serum glutamic oxaloacetic transaminase (SGOT), which signals liver damage of some degree, commonly occurs, but proven cases of valproate-induced hepatitis are rare. The few cases of fatal hepatitis in valproate-treated patients may well have been caused by other factors.

Valproate is used in many kinds of epilepsy, but has been particularly successful in certain types of infantile epilepsy, where its low toxicity and lack of sedative action are important.

Carbamazepine

Carbamazepine is chemically derived from the tricyclic antidepressant drugs (see Chapter 23), and was found in a routine screening test to inhibit electrically-evoked seizures in mice. Pharmacologically and clinically its actions resemble those of phenytoin (Suria & Killam, 1980), though it appears to be particularly effective in treating complex partial seizures (e.g. psychomotor epilepsy). It is also used to treat **trigeminal neuralgia**, an exceedingly painful condition which seems to result from a paroxysmal discharge of neurons associated with the trigeminal sensory pathway, which is triggered by slight sensory stimulation. Though not obviously associated with epilepsy, this condition probably involves similar neuronal mechanisms.

Carbamazepine is well absorbed. Its plasma half-life is about 30 hours when it is given as a single dose, but it is a strong inducing agent, and the plasma half-life shortens to about 15 hours when it is given repeatedly.

It produces a variety of unwanted effects, ranging from drowsiness, dizziness and ataxia (which occur in up to 50% of patients) to more severe mental and motor disturbances. It can also cause water retention, and a variety of gastrointestinal and cardiovascular side effects. Occasional dangerous or fatal bone marrow depression and other severe forms of hypersensitivity reaction have occurred. Though rare, this type of toxicity means that carbemazepine tends to be used for epilepsy only when other drugs have proved insufficient. It has a special place in the treatment of trigeminal neuralgia.

Benzodiazepines (see Chapter 20)

Diazepam, given intravenously, is used to treat **status epilepticus**, a life-threatening condition in which epileptic seizures occur almost without a break. Its sedative effect is too pronounced for it to be used prophylactically. **Clonazepam** is claimed to be relatively selective as an anticonvulsant, and is used in absence seizures and in tonic-clonic seizures in children. Sedation is the main side effect.

PARKINSONISM

Parkinsonism is a progressive disorder of movement, which occurs most commonly in the elderly. The main symptoms are:

1. **Tremor** at rest, usually starting in the hands and resulting in 'pill-rolling' movements, which tend to diminish during voluntary activity.

2. **Muscle rigidity**, which is detectable as an increased resistance in passive limb movement.

3. **Decrease in the frequency of voluntary movements** (hypokinesia) which is partly the result of muscle rigidity, but partly due to an inherent inertia

of the motor system which means that motor activity is difficult to stop as well as to initiate. Parkinsonian patients show a characteristic fast shuffling gait which takes some effort for them to begin, and once in progress they cannot quickly stop or change direction. Parkinson's disease is commonly associated with dementia, though this is probably a reflection of the same degenerative process affecting other parts of the brain, rather than a direct consequence of the damage to the basal ganglia which is responsible for the motor symptoms.

Parkinson's disease often occurs with no obvious underlying cause, but it may be the result of cerebral ischaemia (progressive arteriosclerosis or stroke), virus encephalitis, or other types of pathological damage. It can also be **drug-induced**, the main drugs that cause it being those that reduce the amount of dopamine in the brain (e.g. reserpine; see Chapter 7), or block dopamine receptors (e.g. neuroleptic drugs, such as chlorpromazine; see Chapter 22). In contrast to schizophrenia and many other neurological and behavioural disorders, Parkinsonism shows no hereditary tendency, and an environmental cause seems more likely (see below).

Parkinsonism has been known for many years to be due to a disorder of the basal ganglia, but its neurochemical origin was discovered by

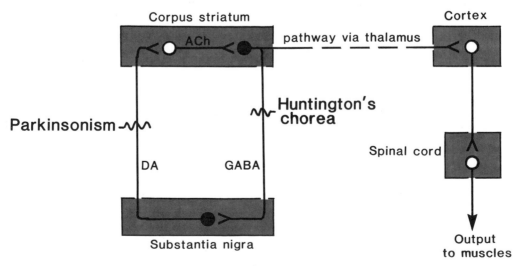

Fig. 24.5 Simplified diagram showing the organisation of the motor system, and lesions that are believed to cause Parkinsonism and Huntington's chorea. Black and white cell bodies denote inhibitory and excitatory neurons respectively.

Hornykiewicz in 1960 (see review: Hornykiewicz, 1973), who showed that the dopamine content of the substantia nigra and corpus striatum (see Chapter 19) in post-mortem brains of Parkinson's disease patients was extremely low (usually less than 10% of normal) and this was later correlated with a loss of the cell bodies of dopaminergic neurons from the substantia nigra, and degeneration of nerve terminals in the striatum (Fig. 24.5). Noradrenaline and serotonin contents were also low in these patients, but much less affected than dopamine, and other evidence showed that these cells were still alive and functioning, whereas the dopamine cells were largely absent. Further studies have shown the symptoms of Parkinsonism appear when the striatal dopamine content is reduced to 20–40% of normal (Schultz, 1982). Lesions of the nigro-striatal tract, or chemically induced depletion of dopamine in experimental animals also produce symptoms of Parkinsonism. The symptom that is most clearly related to dopamine deficiency is hypokinesia, which occurs immediately and invariably in lesioned animals. Rigidity and tremor involve more complex neurochemical disturbances of other transmitters (particularly acetylcholine, serotonin and GABA), as well as dopamine. In experimental lesions, two secondary consequences follow damage to the nigro-striatal tract, namely a hyperactivity of the remaining dopaminergic neurons, which show an increased rate of transmitter turnover, and an increase in the number of dopamine receptors, which produces a state of denervation hypersensitivity (see Chapter 5). These compensatory mechanisms presumably act to preserve transmission in the face of a declining number of neurons, and are important in relation to the therapeutic effectiveness of levodopa (see: Riederer et al, 1983 for a recent short review).

New light has recently been thrown on the possible aetiology of Parkinsonism. In 1982 a group of young drug addicts in California suddenly developed the disease, and the cause was traced to the

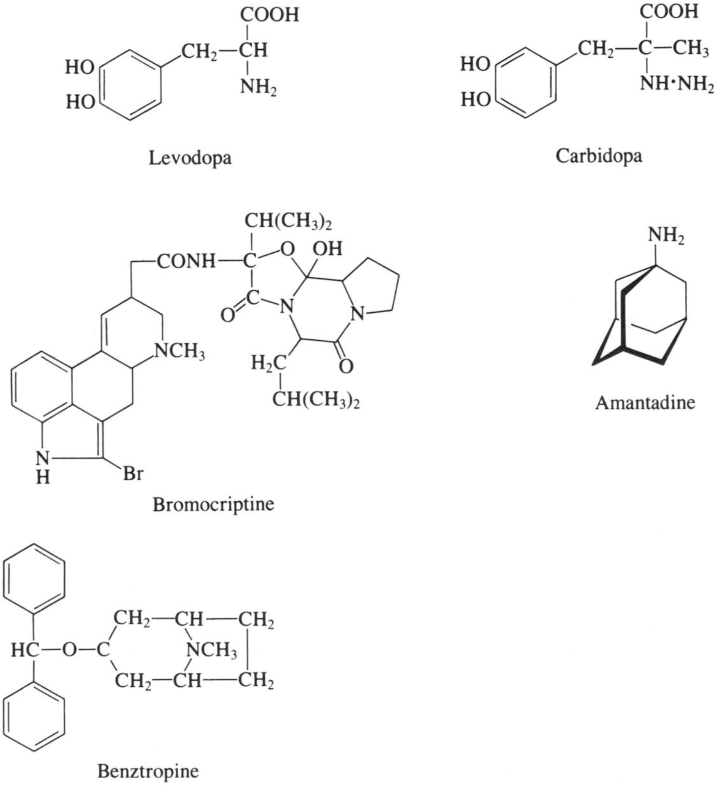

Fig. 24.6 Drugs used in treating Parkinson's disease.

compound 1-methyl 4-phenyl 1,2,3,6-tetrahydro-pyridine (MPTP), which was present in an illicitly-manufactured heroin substitute (Langston,1985). MPTP has been found to cause irreversible destruction of nigro-striatal dopaminergic neurons in various species, and to produce a Parkinsonism-like state in primates. MPTP probably acts by being converted within the neurons to a toxic metabolite, by the enzyme MAO-B (see Chapter 23) which is found in dopaminergic, but not other catecholamine-containing cells. MPTP appears to be selective in destroying nigro-striatal neurons, and does not affect dopaminergic neurons elsewhere; the reason for this is unknown. Selegiline, a selective MAO-B inhibitor, prevents MPTP-induced neurotoxicity. It is is also used in treating Parkinsonism (see below), on the basis of its ability to inhibit dopamine breakdown, and the possibility now arises that it might also be working by blocking the metabolic activation of a putative naturally-occurring MPTP-like substance, which is involved in the causation of Parkinson's disease. Whether or not this speculation proves to have any substance, MPTP is likely to be a very useful experimental tool for studying the causes and treatment of the disease.

The corpus striatum is exceptionally rich in acetylcholine as well as dopamine. Acetylcholine has excitatory effects, whereas dopamine is mainly inhibitory, and it has been suggested that the symptoms of Parkinsonism (and of Huntington's chorea (see below) result from an imbalance between these two systems (Calne, 1978)). Accordingly, drug treatment is aimed at restoring this balance. The drugs that are effective fall into four main categories (Fig. 24.6).

1. Drugs that replace dopamine (e.g. **levodopa**)
2. Drugs that mimic the action of dopamine (e.g. **bromocriptine**)
3. Drugs that release dopamine (e.g. **amantadine**)
4. Acetylcholine antagonists (e.g. **benztropine**)

Recent developments (Dunnett, 1982) suggest that it might eventually be possible to implant dopamine-rich fragments of brain tissue into the striatum of patients with Parkinson's disease, following the demonstration in rats that behavioural changes associated with a loss of dopaminergic neurons could be partly restored in this way.

Levodopa

Following the discovery that Parkinson's disease is associated with a loss of dopamine from the striatum, attempts to treat the disease by replenishment of dopamine were made. Since dopamine itself does not cross the blood-brain barrier, dopa was tried. Initial tests with the racemate, DL-dopa, were unsuccessful, with little benefit and many side effects, but the use of the pure L-isomer, levodopa, brought about a great improvement, and this drug is now the first-line treatment for Parkinsonism.

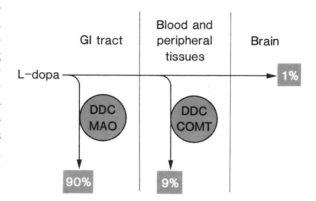

Fig. 24.7 The fate of levodopa after oral administration. DDC—dopa decarboxylase; MAO—monoamine oxidase; COMT—catechol-O-methyl transferase.

Levodopa has to be given in large and frequent doses, amounting to 3–8 g/24 hours in three or four doses. It is well absorbed from the small intestine, a process which relies on active transport, though much of it is inactivated by monoamine oxidase in the wall of the intestine (Fig. 24.7). The plasma half-life is short (about 2 hours) and about 95% of the drug is converted to dopamine in peripheral tissues, where dopa decarboxylase is widespread. Less than 1% enters the brain. Decarboxylation occurs rapidly within the brain, since dopa decarboxylase is widespread and by no means confined to neurons. It is known that the anti-Parkinson effect of levodopa depends on dopamine formation in the brain, because the effect is prevented by decarboxylase inhibitors that enter the brain, but not by those, such as carbidopa (see below), that do not. It is not certain whether the effect depends on an increased release of dopamine from the few surviving dopaminergic neurons or to a 'flooding' of the synapse with exogenous dopamine. In experimental animals with unilateral substantia nigra lesions that remove virtually all of the striatal dopaminergic nerve terminals on one side, levodopa causes turning behaviour (see Chapter 19) as effectively as a dopamine agonist such as apomorphine, so levodopa can evidently act even when no dopaminergic nerve terminals are present. On the other hand, the therapeutic effectiveness of levodopa decreases as the disease advances, so part of its action may rely on the presence of functional dopaminergic neurons.

Therapeutic effectiveness and unwanted effects of levodopa

At the beginning of treatment with levodopa, with the dose gradually built up to achieve the optimal effect, many trials have shown that about 80% of patients show improvement, particularly of rigidity and hypokinesia, and about 20% are restored virtually to normal motor function. As time progresses, the effectiveness of levodopa gradually declines. In a typical study Sweet & McDowell (1975) found that, out of 100 patients treated with levodopa for 5 years, only 34 were better than they had been at the beginning of the trial, 32 patients having died and 21 having withdrawn from the trial. It is likely that the loss of effectiveness of levodopa mainly reflects the natural progression of the disease, for there is no evidence that drug treatment can affect the underlying pathological process. Levodopa was found in the above clinical trials to improve the life expectancy of Parkinson patients, though it remained shorter than that of controls of the same age. This is probably the result of improved motor function rather than an effect on the disease. Two troublesome phenomena, however, appear to be the result of prolonged levodopa treatment rather than of the disease per se. These are:

1. The development of **involuntary choreiform movements**, which are the result of excessive activation of dopamine receptors. These movements usually affect the face and limbs, and can become very severe. They disappear if the dose of levodopa is reduced, but this causes rigidity to return. It is not known why the margin between the beneficial and the unwanted effect becomes progressively narrower.

2. Rapid fluctuations in clinical state, where

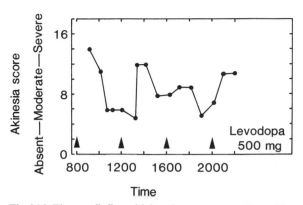

Fig. 24.8 The on-off effect with levodopa treatment. The sudden changes in clinical state occurring every few hours are unrelated to the regular 4-hourly doses of levodopa. (From: Barbeau, 1974)

hypokinesia and rigidity may suddenly worsen for anything from a few minutes to a few hours, and then improve again. This '**on-off effect**' (Fig. 24.8) is not seen in untreated Parkinsonism patients, or with other anti-Parkinson drugs. It can produce such an abrupt loss of mobility that the patient suddenly stops while walking and feels rooted to the spot, or is unable to rise from a chair in which he had sat down normally a few moments earlier. The mechanism of this remarkable effect is not understood. In some patients, rigidity and hypokinesia occur as the plasma dopa concentration falls after a dose, but often the attacks are unrelated to levodopa dosage, as in Figure 24.8.

In addition to these slowly-developing side effects, levodopa produces several acute effects, which are experienced by most patients at first, but tend to disappear after a few weeks.

a. **Nausea and anorexia**. Dopamine stimulates the vomiting centre (see Chapters 15 & 19), and about 60% of patients complain of nausea initially when taking levodopa. Circulating dopamine, which reaches the chemoreceptor trigger zone via a permeable region of the blood-brain barrier, appears to be responsible.

b. **Hypotension**. Though a precursor of noradrenaline might be expected to raise blood pressure, the opposite actually happens, though usually not to an important degree. It results partly from a central action, and partly by the vasodilator action of dopamine in the periphery (see Chapter 11). Cardiac dysrhythmias may also occur.

c. **Psychological effects**. Levodopa, by increasing

dopamine activity in the brain, can produce a schizophrenia-like syndrome (see Chapters 19 & 22) with delusions and hallucinations. A more common effect, seen in about 20% of patients, is the occurrence of confusion, disorientation, insomnia or nightmares.

Optimization of levodopa treatment

Three strategies have been devised to enhance the central effects of levodopa and minimize its peripheral effects: (a) inhibition of dopa decarboxylase in the periphery by **carbidopa**; (b) inhibition of dopamine degradation in the central nervous system by the monoamine oxidase inhibitor, selegiline; and (c) block of dopamine receptors in the periphery by **domperidone**.

Carbidopa (Fig. 24.6) is a hydrazine derivative of dopamine, which inhibits dopa decarboxylase but does not penetrate the blood-brain barrier. It therefore inhibits the formation of dopamine from levodopa peripherally but not in the brain. Combined with levodopa it enables the dose of levodopa to be reduced four to eight-fold and greatly reduces the peripheral side effects. The central side effects are not, of course, reduced, but it has been claimed that the proportion of patients showing clinical benefit is increased. A combination of carbidopa and levodopa is now used routinely in treating Parkinson's disease.

Selegiline (see Chapter 23) is a monoamine oxidase (MAO) inhibitor that is selective for the form of MAO (known as MAO-B) which predominates in dopamine-containing regions of the central nervous system. It therefore lacks the dangerous peripheral effects on non-selective MAO inhibitors and can be used on its own to facilitate dopaminergic transmission in mild cases of Parkinsonism, or as an adjunct to treatment with levodopa (Birkmayer et al, 1975).

Domperidone is a dopamine antagonist related to haloperidol (see Chapter 22) which does not penetrate the blood-brain barrier. Its usefulness as a means of reducing the side effects of levodopa is being assessed.

Other drugs used in Parkinsonism

Bromocriptine

This drug (Fig. 24.6), derived from the ergot alkaloids (see Chapter 7), is a potent agonist at dopamine receptors of the D_2 category (see Chapter 11) in the central nervous system. It has a powerful effect on the anterior pituitary gland, where dopamine is the mediator responsible for inhibition of prolactin release (see Chapter 16), and it was first introduced for the treatment of galactorrhoea and gynaecomastia. It has recently been found to be effective also in Parkinsonism (Lieberman et al, 1979). Preliminary studies suggest that it has very similar effects to levodopa, and also are very similar disadvantages. Its duration of action is longer (plasma half-life 6–8 hours) so that it does not need to be given so frequently, but it is expensive at present, and tends to be used only for patients who do not respond satisfactorily to levodopa. On-off effects are said to be less common with bromocriptine, but other side effects, including involuntary movements, are very similar. The endocrine disturbance produced by bromocriptine in Parkinsonism patients appears to be much less than in normal subjects, for reasons that are not clear.

There is some evidence that bromocriptine may be effective in patients who become refractory to levodopa because of a progressive loss of dopaminergic neurons from the corpus striatum, but this has not been firmly established.

Amantadine

Amantadine (Fig. 24.6) was introduced as an antiviral drug (see Chapter 31), and discovered by accident in 1969 to be beneficial in Parkinson's disease. Many possible mechanisms for its action have been suggested, based on neurochemical evidence of increased dopamine release, inhibition of amine uptake or a direct action on dopamine receptors. In many cases, unrealistically high concentrations were needed to produce effects; most authors now suggest, though not with much conviction, that increased dopamine release is primarily responsible for the clinical effects.

Amantadine is certainly less effective than levodopa or bromocriptine, and its action declines with time. Its side effects are considerably less severe, though qualitatively similar to those of levodopa.

Acetylcholine antagonists

Atropine and related drugs have been used for

many years in treating Parkinsonism, and were the main form of treatment before levodopa was discovered. Muscarinic acetylcholine receptors exert an excitatory effect, opposite to that of dopamine, on striatal neurons (see Fig. 24.5) and also exert a pre-synaptic inhibitory effect on dopaminergic nerve terminals. Suppression of these effects thus makes up, in part, for a lack of dopamine. The action of muscarinic antagonists is more limited than that of levodopa, and they diminish tremor more than rigidity or hypokinesia (which are more disabling in their effects). Furthermore, the side effects—dry mouth, constipation, impaired vision, urinary retention—are often troublesome, so they are used mainly as an adjunct for patients who respond poorly to levodopa alone. The drugs used for this purpose (e.g. **benztropine**; Fig. 24.6) have less peripheral effect in relation to their central effect than atropine. Drowsiness and confusion are the main side effects. Patients suffering from Parkinson's disease very often show some degree of dementia, in which loss of cortical cholinergic neurons may be involved (see Chapter 19), and further inhibition by acetylcholine antagonists would be expected to exacerbate this.

HUNTINGTON'S CHOREA

Huntington's chorea is an inherited disorder resulting in progressive brain degeneration, which usually becomes manifest in middle of life. Its effects are to produce progressive dementia and severe involuntary writhing movements which make speech and feeding progressively more difficult. The inheritance of Huntington's chorea shows it to be carried by a single autosomal dominant gene, but the nature of the primary biochemical defect remains undetermined. The effect of the disease is to cause a widespread loss of cortical cells, which is presumably responsible for producing dementia, and also loss of cells from the corpus striatum, which causes the motor disturbance. Bird & Iversen (1974), in a study of post-mortem brains from patients with Huntington's chorea, found that the dopamine content of the striatum is normal or slightly increased, while there is a 75% reduction in the activity of the GABA-synthesizing enzyme **glutamic acid decarboxylase**, and a smaller and more variable reduction in the activity of **choline acetyltransferase**, the enzyme responsible for acetylcholine synthesis.

It is believed that the loss of GABA-mediated inhibition in the striatum produces a hyperactivity of dopaminergic synapses. There is also an underactivity of cholinergic transmission, so the syndrome is in some senses a mirror image of Parkinsonism (see Fig. 24.5). The effects of drugs that influence dopaminergic transmission are correspondingly the opposite of those that are observed in Parkinsonism, dopamine antagonists being effective in reducing the involuntary movements, while anti-Parkinson drugs such as levodopa and bromocriptine make them worse. Drugs do not affect the underlying cause of the disease.

MUSCLE SPASM AND CENTRALLY-ACTING MUSCLE RELAXANTS

Many diseases of the brain and spinal cord produce an increase in muscle tone which can be painful and disabling. **Spasticity**, resulting from birth injury or cerebral vascular disease, and the paralysis produced by spinal cord lesions are examples. Local injury or inflammation, as in arthritis, can have the same effect, and chronic back pain is also often associated with local muscle spasm.

Though skeletal muscle can be relaxed by neuromuscular blocking drugs (see Chapter 6) they are too non-selective to be useful in treating muscle spasm. Instead, certain centrally-acting drugs are available which have the effect of reducing the background tone of the muscle without seriously affecting its ability to contract transiently under voluntary control. The distinction between voluntary movements and background tone is not, however, a sharp one, and the selectivity of those drugs is not complete. Postural control, for example, often requires a steady background contraction of certain muscle groups, and this is usually jeopardized by centrally-acting muscle relaxants. Furthermore, drugs that inhibit transmission in the complex polyneuronal pathways that control muscle tone are likely to produce rather widespread effects on the central nervous system, and drowsiness and confusion turn out to be very common side effects of these agents.

The main group of drugs that have been used to

control muscle tone are: (1) **Mephenesin** and related drugs; (2) **Baclofen**; and (3) **Benzodiazepines** (see Chapter 21).

Mephenesin

Mephenesin is an aromatic ether with no nitrogen atom in the molecule, which was developed in 1943 as the most active member of a series of such compounds. All of these drugs cause, in large doses, muscular paralysis, without loss of consciousness, by an action on the central nervous system. Mephenesin acts mainly on the spinal cord, causing a selective inhibition of poly-synaptic excitation of motorneurons. Thus, it strongly inhibits the flexor reflex without affecting the tendon jerk reflex, which is mono-synaptic, and it abolishes decerebrate rigidity. Its mechanism of action at the cellular level is unknown.

Mephenesin is little used clinically, though it is sometimes given as an intravenous injection to reduce acute muscle spasm resulting from injury.

Baclofen

Baclofen (see Chapter 19) is a chlorophenyl deriva-
tive of GABA, originally prepared as a lipophilic GABA-like agent in order to allow penetration of the blood-brain barrier, which GABA itself does not do. Baclofen produces many GABA-like inhibitory effects in the central nervous system, but its action differs in important ways from that of GABA (Bowery, 1982). In particular, the inhibitory effect of GABA is strongly opposed by the antagonist bicuculline, whereas that of baclofen is not (see Chapter 19). Baclofen also fails to inhibit the binding of radioactive GABA to brain membranes, which it would be expected to do if both drugs were acting on the same receptors. Bowery (1982) has suggested that baclofen acts selectively on pre-synaptic GABA$_B$ receptors, which are not sensitive to bicuculline and are not strongly labelled by radioactive GABA; the antispastic action of baclofen is exerted mainly on the spinal cord, where it inhibits both mono-synaptic and poly-synaptic activation of motoneurons (Davies, 1981). In spite of this lack of specificity, baclofen has a more powerful effect on spasticity than mephenesin, and is more effective when given orally. Careful adjustment of the dose is needed to avoid inco-ordination and loss of postural control.

REFERENCES AND FURTHER READING

Barbeau A 1974 The clinical physiology of side effects in long-term L-DOPA therapy. Adv Neurol 5: 347–365
Bird E J, Iversen L L 1974 Huntington's chorea. Post-mortem acetyltransferase and dopamine in basal ganglia. Brain 97: 457–472
Birkmayer W, Riederer P, Youdim M B H 1975 The potentiation of the anti-akinetic effect of L-dopa treatment by an inhibitor of MAO-B, deprenil. J Neurol Transm 36: 303–326
Bowery N G 1982 The kindling model of epilepsy. Trends in Pharmacological Sciences 3: 400–403
Calne D B 1978 Parkinsonism, clinical and neuropharmacological aspects. Postgrad Med 64: 82–88
Davies J 1981 Selective depression of synaptic excitation in cat spinal neurones by baclofen: an ionophoretic study. Br J Pharmac 72: 373–384
Dunnet S B, Bjorklund A, Strenevi U, Iversen S D 1982 CNS transplantation: structural and functional recovery from brain damage. Prog Brain Res 55: 431–443
Frey H H, Janz D (eds) 1985 Antiepileptic drugs. Handbook of Experimental Pharmacology, Vol 74. Springer-Verlag, Berlin
Goddard G V 1983 The kindling model of epilepsy. Trends in Neurosciences 6: 275–279
Godin Y, Heiner L, Mark J, Mandel P 1969 Effects of di-n-propylacetate, an anticonvulsive compound, on GABA metabolism. J Neurochem 16: 869–873
Hornykiewicz O 1973 Parkinson's disease: from brain homogenate to treatment. Fed Proc 32: 183–190

Janz D 1975 The teratogenic risk of anti-epileptic drugs. Epilepsia 16: 159–169
Johnston D, Slater G E 1982 Valproate mechanisms of action. In: Woodbury D M, Penry J K, Pippenger C E (eds) Antiepileptic drugs. Raven Press, New York, ch 50
Langston W J 1985 MPTP and Parkinson's disease. Trends in Neurosciences 8: 79–83
Lieberman A N, Kupersmith M D, Goprinathan G, Estey E, Goodgold A, Goldstein M 1979 Bromocriptin in Parkinson disease: further studies. Neurology 29: 363–369
Mattson R H, Cramer J A 1982 Toxicity. In: Woodbury D M, Penry J K, Pippenger C E (eds) Antiepileptic drugs. Raven Press, New York, ch 26
Perucca E, Richens A 1962 Biotransformation. In: Woodbury D M, Penry J K, Pippenger C E (eds) Antiepileptic drugs. Raven Press, New York, ch 3
Riederer P, Reynolds G P, Jellinger K 1983 The pharmacology of Parkinson's disease: L-dopa and beyond. Trends in Pharmacological Sciences 5: 25–27
Schultz W 1982 Depletion of dopamine in the striatum as an experimental model of Parkinsonism: direct effects and adaptive mechanisms. Prog Neurobiol 18: 121–166
Servit Z, Musil F 1981 Prophylactic treatment of post-traumatic epilepsy: results of a long-term follow-up in Czechoslovakia. Epilepsia 22: 15–20
Suria A, Killam E K 1980 Carbamazepine. Adv Neurol 27: 563–575
Sweet R D, McDowell F H 1975 Five year's treatment of

Parkinson's disease with levodopa. Therapeutic results and survival of 100 patients. Ann Int Med 83: 456–463

Van Gelder N M, Sherwin A L, Rasmussen T 1972 Amino acid content of epileptogenic human brain: focal versus surrounding regions. Brain Res 40: 385–393

Woodbury D M, Penry J K, Pippenger C E (eds) 1982 Antiepileptic drugs. Raven Press, New York

Analgesic drugs

The control of pain is one of the most important uses to which drugs are put. Analgesic drugs fall into four main categories:

1. Morphine-like drugs (opioids)
2. Non-steroidal anti-inflammatory drugs (aspirin and related substances; see Chapter 9)
3. Local anaesthetics (see Chapter 27)
4. Miscellaneous drugs used for specific painful conditions (e.g. migraine, trigeminal neuralgia, labour). These are discussed elsewhere in the appropriate chapters.

Morphine-like drugs, as well as most of the drugs in group 4, produce analgesia by acting on the central nervous system, whereas aspirin-like drugs and local anaesthetics act peripherally. In this chapter we consider first some physiological aspects of pain perception, and then present the pharmacology of the opioid drugs in detail.

NEURAL MECHANISMS OF PAIN SENSATION

Nociceptive afferent neurons

In many cases, though by no means all,* pain is associated with electrical activity in small diameter primary afferent fibres of peripheral nerves. These nerves have fine branching terminals in peripheral tissues, and any given afferent fibre can be activated by stimuli of various kinds (mechanical, thermal, chemical), provided the stimulus intensity is sufficiently high. Studies in which activity in single afferent fibres has been recorded in human subjects have shown that stimuli sufficient to excite these small afferent fibres also evoke a painful sensation. These afferents are known as **polymodal nociceptors**, and they are distinguished from the low threshold receptors which respond to specific stimuli such as light touch or small temperature changes.

Nociceptive information is conveyed in cutaneous nerves by fibres of the Aδ group (fine myelinated fibres conducting at 4–30 m/s, some of which are non-nociceptive) and the C group (non-myelinated fibres conducting at 2.5 m/s or less). Though there are some species differences, the majority of the C-fibres are associated with polymodal nociceptive endings. Afferents from muscle and viscera also convey nociceptive information. In the nerves from these tissues, the small myelinated fibres terminate in high threshold mechanoreceptors, while the unmyelinated fibres terminate in polymodal nocicep-

---

* Many of the most severe and intractable forms of pain have only an indirect relationship, or none at all, to the occurrence of a peripheral stimulus (Melzack & Wall, 1982). The most striking example is 'phantom-limb' pain which occurs after amputations. The pain is usually not relieved by local anaesthetic injection close to the severed nerve, implying that electrical activity in afferent fibres is not an essential component. At the other extreme, there are many well-documented reports of mystics and showmen who subject themselves to horrifying ordeals with knives, burning embers, nails and hooks without apparently suffering pain. In various clinical situations (e.g. trigeminal neuralgia) very severe pain may be triggered by a mild and innocuous stimulus to the skin. In these situations, which Melzack & Wall suggest may be typical of many chronic pain syndromes in man, the disturbance concerns the central processing mechanism rather than the afferent input, and the concept of a simple 'pain pathway' may be misleading. Much of the experimental work on pain has, for obvious reasons, concentrated on acute pain resulting from strong stimulation or tissue injury, where the sensation is clearly related to the afferent input. In general, such studies quite reliably predict the effectiveness of analgesic drugs for acute pain, but often fail to do so for chronic pain, a fact which emphasizes the limited relevance of the 'pain pathway' in chronic pain states.

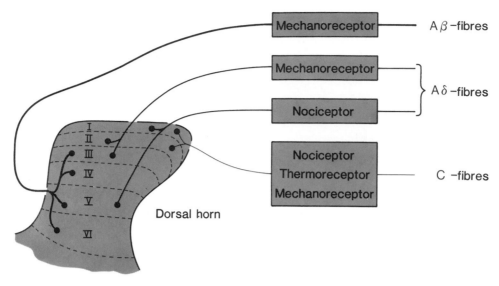

Fig. 25.1 The termination of afferent fibres in the dorsal horn of the spinal cord.

tors as in the skin. Experiments on human subjects, in which recording or stimulating electrodes are applied to cutaneous sensory nerves, have shown that activity in the $A\delta$ fibres causes a sensation of sharp, well-localized pain, whereas C-fibre activity causes a dull burning pain.

The mechanism by which a variety of different stimuli can evoke activity in nociceptive nerve terminals is only dimly understood. With many pathological conditions, tissue injury is the immediate cause of the pain, and this results in the local release of a variety of chemical agents which are assumed to act on the nerve terminals, either activating them directly or enhancing their sensitivity to other forms of stimulation. The pharmacological properties of nociceptive nerve terminals are discussed in more detail below.

The cell bodies of spinal nociceptive afferent fibres lie in dorsal root ganglia and fibres enter the spinal cord via the dorsal roots, ending in the grey matter of the dorsal horn (Fig. 25.1). Most of the nociceptive afferents terminate in the superficial region of the dorsal horn, the C-fibres and some $A\delta$ fibres innervating cell bodies in laminae I and II, while other $A\delta$ fibres penetrate deeper into the dorsal horn (lamina V). Cells in laminae I and V give rise to the main projection pathways from the dorsal horn to the thalamus.

The substantia gelatinosa and the gate control theory

Much attention has been focused on the function of lamina II (the **substantia gelatinosa, SG**) whose cells form a network of very short projections, mainly to lamina I and lamina V cells of the same segment. These cells probably act to regulate transmission between the primary afferent fibres and the spinothalamic tract neurons. Some SG neurons exert a post-synaptic excitatory effect on spinothalamic cell bodies, while others exert a pre- or post-synaptic inhibitory effect. The latter group can effectively interrupt transmission at the first synapse of the pain pathway, giving rise to the term 'gate control theory' which was first proposed by Wall & Melzack in 1965. The former group may be responsible for the marked **hyperalgesia** (increase in pain sensitivity) that occurs in the neighbourhood of a painful lesion, since they effectively reduce the threshold for transmission of afferent impulses through the first synaptic relay (see Melzack & Wall, 1982, for a recent discussion). According to this view (summarized in Fig. 25.2) the substantia gelatinosa cells respond both to the activity of afferent fibres entering the cord (thus allowing impulses in one group of afferent fibres to regulate the transmission of impulses arriving via another

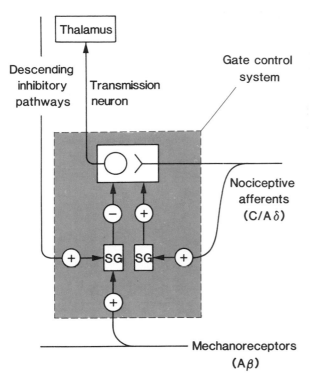

Fig. 25.2 The gate control system. This system regulates the passage of impulses from the peripheral afferent fibres to the thalamus via transmission neurons originating in the dorsal horn. Neurons in the substantia gelatinosa (SG) of the dorsal horn act to inhibit or facilitate the transmission pathway. Inhibitory interneurons are activated by descending inhibitory neurons, or by non-nociceptive afferent input. Facilitatory interneurons are activated by the nociceptive afferent fibres. This autofacilitation causes successive bursts of activity in the nonociceptive afferents to become increasingly effective in activating transmission neurons. (Melzack & Wall, 1982)

pathway) and to the activity of descending pathways (see below). The substantia gelatinosa is rich in both opioid peptides and opioid receptors and is likely to be an important site of action for morphine-like drugs (see later section).

From the spinothalamic tracts the projection fibres form synapses mainly in the ventral and medial parts of the thalamus with cells whose axons run to the somatosensory cortex. In the medial thalamus in particular, many cells respond specifically to noxious stimuli in the periphery and lesions in this area cause analgesia. Pain sensation does not require that impulses should reach the somatosensory cortex. There is no clear evidence of specifically nociceptive cells in the cortex, and lesions of the somatosensory areas do not prevent the sens-

ation of pain though they can alter its quality. It appears to be the affective, discriminatory and motivational aspects of pain, rather than the sensation itself, that depend on the cerebral cortex.

Descending inhibitory controls

As mentioned above, descending pathways constitute one of the gating mechanisms that controls impulse transmission in the dorsal horn (Lewis & Liebeskind, 1983). A key part of this descending system is the **periaqueductal grey (PAG)** area of the midbrain, a small area of grey matter surrounding the central canal. It was found in 1969 by Reynolds that electrical stimulation of this brain area in the rat causes analgesia sufficiently intense that abdominal surgery could be performed without anaesthesia and without eliciting any marked response. The loss of sensation is confined to nociceptive stimuli, other sensory modalities being unaffected.

The main neuronal pathway activated by PAG stimulation runs first to an area of the ventral medulla close to the midline, the **nucleus raphe magnus (NRM)**, and thence via fibres running in the dorso-lateral funiculus of the spinal cord, which form synaptic connections on dorsal horn interneurons. The transmitter at these synapses is serotonin, and the interneurons in turn act to inhibit the discharge of spinothalamic neurons (Fig. 25.3). Activation of this pathway inhibits transmission specifically in nociceptive pathways, with less effect on other forms of sensation. The NRM itself receives an input from spinothalamic neurons, so this descending inhibitory system may form part of a regulatory feedback loop whereby transmission of nociceptive input through the dorsal horn is controlled according to the amount of activity reaching the thalamus.

The descending inhibitory pathway is probably an important site of action for opioid analgesics (see below). Both PAG and SG are particularly rich in enkephalin-containing neurons, and there is evidence that opioid antagonists, such as **naloxone** (p. 565) can prevent electrically-induced analgesia, which would suggest that opioid peptides may function as transmitters in this system. This observation has been challenged, however, and the physiological role of opioid peptides in regulating

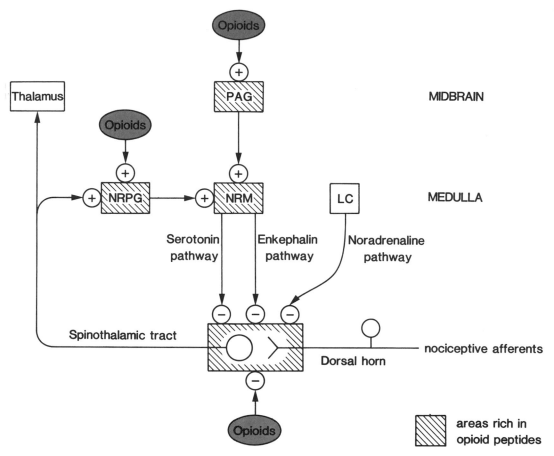

Fig. 25.3 Postulated sites of action of opioids on pain transmission. Opioids excite neurons in the peri-aqueductal grey matter (PAG) and in the nucleus reticularis paragigantocellularis (NRPG), which in turn project to the nucleus raphe magnus (NRM). From the NRM serotoninergic and enkephalinergic neurons run to the substantia gelatinosa of the dorsal horn, and exert an inhibitory influence on transmission. Opioids also act directly on the dorsal horn. The locus coeruleus (LC) sends noradrenergic neurons to the dorsal horn, which also inhibit transmission.

The pathways shown in this diagram represent a considerable oversimplification, but depict the general organization of the supraspinal control mechanisms.

pain transmission remains controversial (Fields, 1981; Lewis & Liebeskind, 1983; Woolf & Wall, 1983). There is also evidence of a noradrenergic pathway from the **locus coeruleus** (see Chapter 19) which has a similar inhibitory effect on transmission in the dorsal horn (Fig. 25.3).

Chemical mediators and the nociceptive pathway

Chemosensitivity of pain endings

In most cases stimulation of pain endings in the periphery is chemical in origin. Excessive mechanical or thermal stimuli can obviously cause acute pain, but the persistence of such pain after the stimulus had been removed, and the pain resulting from inflammatory or ischaemic changes in tissues, generally reflect a chemical stimulation of the pain afferents. A knowledge of the nature of these substances and of the mechanisms by which they stimulate sensory nerve terminals can provide an approach to the discovery of analgesic drugs. Most of our current knowledge comes from the work of Keele & Armstrong (1964) who developed a simple method for measuring the pain-producing effect of various substances which act on cutaneous nerve endings. Applying cantharidin to the skin of the forearm of human subjects causes a small blister, the base of which may be bathed in drug solutions, which gain access to the nerve terminals in the dermis. Pain is recorded subjectively, and with practice the subjects are able to achieve quite reproducible responses.

The main groups of substances that stimulate pain endings in the skin are:

1. Various neurotransmitters including **serotonin**, **histamine** and **acetylcholine**. Serotonin is the most active; histamine is much less active and tends to cause itching rather than actual pain. Both of these substances are known to be released locally in inflammation.

2. **Kinins**. The most active substances are **bradykinin** and **kallidin** (see Chapter 9), two closely related peptides produced under conditions of tissue injury by a cascade mechanism similar to the blood coagulation cascade (see Chapter 12), which results in the proteolytic cleavage of the active kinins from a precursor protein contained in the plasma. Bradykinin is the most potent pain-producing substance known at present. It can also stimulate some other types of afferent fibre, but much less powerfully than pain endings. Bradykinin also affects vascular smooth muscle (generally causing dilatation in small vessels and constriction of large vessels), visceral smooth muscle (contraction), pre-synaptic nerve terminals (increase of transmitter release by pre- and post-ganglionic autonomic nerve terminals) and the epithelium of the gastrointestinal tract (increased fluid secretion; see Chapter 15). Bradykinin causes the release of prostaglandins in many tissues, and some of its physiological effects are probably produced in this way, since they are prevented by cyclo-oxygenase inhibitors, such as indomethacin (see Chapter 9). The pain-producing effect of bradykinin appears to depend partly on prostaglandin production (see below; Fig. 25.4). It seems certain that bradykinin acts by combining with specific receptors, and much effort has gone into finding competitive antagonists, which might prove to be effective analgesic agents, so far with little success.

3. **Various metabolites and substances released from active cells**, such as lactic acid, ATP and ADP, potassium ion. These agents are mainly of interest as potential mediators of ischaemic pain (see Chapter 10), and very little is known about how they act.

4. **Prostaglandins**. Prostaglandins do not themselves cause pain, but they strongly enhance the pain-producing effect of other agents such as serotonin or bradykinin (Fig. 25.4). Prostaglandins of the E and F series are known to be released in inflammation and also during tissue ischaemia. How they act to sensitize the nerve terminals to other agents is not known at present. It is of interest that bradykinin itself causes prostaglandin release, and thus has a powerful 'self-sensitizing' effect on nociceptive nerve terminals.

5. **Capsaicin and related irritant substances**. Capsaicin is the active substance in red peppers and is responsible for their burning taste. Other spicy plants (ginger, black pepper, etc) also contain similar

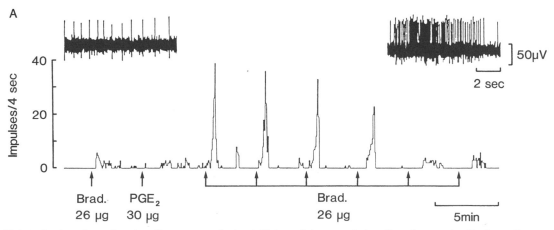

Fig. 25.4 Activation of a nociceptive afferent neuron by bradykinin, and the potentiating effect of prostaglandin. Recordings were made from a nociceptive afferent fibre supplying a muscle, and drugs were injected into the arterial supply. Bradykinin alone caused a small discharge (left hand inset trace). Prostaglandin alone produced no effect, but subsequent doses of bradykinin were greatly potentiated. The right hand inset shows the enhanced responses to bradykinin after injection of prostaglandin. (From: Mense, 1981)

agents, but capsaicin is the most potent and most thoroughly studied. It is a highly potent pain-producing substance, which stimulates nociceptive and temperature-sensitive nerve endings in tissues. It has been shown to cause depolarization of dorsal root ganglion cells associated with C-fibres (and probably also Aδ fibres) without affecting other sensory neurons.

There are several very interesting features of the action of capsaicin: (a) After a few applications the pain-producing effect disappears and nociceptive responses to other stimuli disappear as well. (b) It causes release of substance P and other peptides from afferent neurons (see below and Chapter 19), both peripherally and within the spinal cord. In adult animals the afferent neurons are depleted of substance P and take days or weeks to recover. (c) In newborn animals, capsaicin selectively destroys C-fibre neurons in the periphery, and the animals grow up with a greatly reduced response to painful and thermal stimuli. It has therefore been widely used as an experimental tool for investigating the function of C-fibre afferents.

The desensitizing effect of capsaicin has suggested that substances of this kind might be useful as analgesics. Capsaicin itself is much too toxic, but other substances acting similarly, but with lower toxicity, may eventually prove to be useful. The explanation of its selective stimulant and neurotoxic effects on nociceptive cells is not known at present.

Transmitters of primary afferent fibres

The synapse between the primary afferent neuron and the spinothalamic tract neuron is evidently a key point for regulatory influences affecting the nociceptive pathway (see Fig. 25.3), but the identity of the transmitter is still uncertain (see reviews: Jessell, 1983; Salt & Hill, 1983). Excitatory amino-acids, such as L-glutamate (see Chapter 19) are probably not involved, since glutamate antagonists fail to block activation of dorsal horn neurons by C-fibre afferents, though these drugs do block transmission from large diameter myelinated afferent fibres.

It is well established that substance P (SP, a neuropeptide; see Chapter 19) is contained in a large proportion of the C-fibres in the dorsal root, and in the terminals of these fibres both in the dorsal horn (laminae I and II) and in the periphery. Release of SP from the peripheral terminals of pain afferents probably accounts for the vasodilatation and fluid extravasation that occurs in the triple response (see Chapter 8) and in response to antidromic electrical stimulation of sensory nerves (see reviews: Lembeck, 1983; Foreman & Jordan, 1984). Substance P is believed to function as a transmitter at the spinal cord terminals as well. The release of SP from the surface of the cord in response to painful stimulation has been demonstrated (Yaksh et al, 1980), and locally applied SP causes excitation of nociceptive cell bodies in the dorsal horn. The main reason for doubting its transmitter role (Woolf & Wall, 1983) is that depletion of SP by treatment with capsaicin (see above) has only rather small and inconsistent effects on nociception. If SP is applied locally to the spinal cord it has sometimes been reported to cause hyperalgesia and sometimes analgesia, results that give only equivocal support to its transmitter function. Peptide analogues of SP have recently been discovered that antagonize its effects, presumably by competition at SP receptors (Leander et al, 1981; Rosell et al, 1983). Some of these have been found to increase nociceptive thresholds when applied to the spinal cord, but the effects have been less than might have been expected. The antagonists so far discovered, however, have relatively low potency and most are partial agonists rather than pure competitive antagonists. There is also evidence for more than one type of SP receptor; these factors make interpretation of such experiments somewhat uncertain, and the tranmitter function of SP in the dorsal horn remains unproven. Wall & Fitzgerald (1982) suggest that it may exert a longer-term regulatory function, rather than acting as a classical excitatory transmitter.

Other peptides that occur in different populations of dorsal root ganglion neurons include vasoactive intestinal peptide (VIP) cholecystokinin C-terminal octapeptide (CCK8) and somatostatin (SOM). Any or all of these could function as central transmitters, though they are present in fewer cells than SP. Adenosine triphosphate (ATP) is another potential transmitter candidate (Salt & Hill, 1983). In agreement with this, Jessell and his colleagues have recently found that some dorsal horn neurons show a fast excitatory response to ATP. Again, the lack of specific antagonists makes it difficult to obtain clear evidence for or against a transmitter role for ATP.

Modulatory systems

Transmitters that are known to play a part in the modulation of transmission in the nociceptive pathway (see Fig. 25.3) include:

1. Opioid peptides, mainly met-enkephalin and β-endorphin. Both peptides are found in the PAG, and met-enkephalin is also found in the NRM and SG.
2. Serotonin, the transmitter of inhibitory neurons running from NRM to the dorsal horn.
3. Noradrenaline, the transmitter of the inhibitory pathway from the locus coeruleus to the dorsal horn. There is also evidence that analgesia resulting from stimulation of NRPG (see Fig. 25.3) is partly mediated via a noradrenergic pathway, but the details are unclear.

Several species differences exist among these systems, so studies of analgesic action in animals may not relate directly to man.

PAIN AND NOCICEPTION

The neurophysiological mechanisms discussed above are concerned with the transmission of information about particular kinds of peripheral stimulus, which have in common the fact that they are potentially harmful. The perception of such stimuli (termed 'nociception' by Sherrington) is not the same thing as pain, which includes a strong *affective* component. The amount of pain that a particular stimulus produces depends on many factors other than the stimulus itself. A stabbing sensation in the chest will cause much more pain if it occurs spontaneously in a middle-aged man than a similar sensation produced by a two-year old attacking him with a pointed stick. The nociceptive component may be much the same, but the affective component is quite different. Animal tests of analgesic drugs almost invariably measure nociception, and involve measuring the reaction of an animal to a mildly painful stimulus. Such measures include

the tail-flick test (measuring the time taken for a rat to withdraw its tail when a standard radiant heat stimulus is applied) or the hot-plate test (measuring the time taken for a rat to start licking its feet when placed on a 55°C hot-plate). Similar tests can be used on human subjects, who simply indicate when a stimulus begins to feel painful, but the pain in these circumstances lacks the affective component.

It is recognized clinically that many analgesics, particularly those of the morphine-type, can greatly reduce the distress associated with pain even though the patient reports no great change in the intensity of the actual sensation. It is much more difficult to devise tests that measure this affective component, and important to realize that this may be at least as significant as the anti-nociceptive component in the action of these drugs.

There is often a poor correlation between the activity of analgesic drugs in animal tests (which mainly assess anti-nociceptive activity) and their clinical effectiveness. This is probably because, as stressed by Melzack & Wall (1982), many clinical pain syndromes seem to result from a derangement of the central processing of afferent information, whereby afferent input that would normally be inocuous becomes painful. This is clearly the case with **trigeminal neuralgia**, in which agonizing pain can be triggered by a light touch or temperature change, and is probably also true for many common types of back and muscle pain. In these cases the pain may be unrelated to the activity of peripheral nociceptive fibres, and the conventional animal tests for analgesia provide a poor model.

MORPHINE-LIKE DRUGS

The term **opioid** applies to any substance which produces morphine-like effects that are antagonized by naloxone; it includes various neuropeptides and synthetic analogues whose structure may be quite different from morphine. The older term, **opiate**, is more restrictive, meaning morphine-like drugs with a close structural similarity to morphine, thus excluding peptides and many synthetic analogues.

Opium is an extract of the juice of the poppy, *Papaver somniferum*, which has been used for social and medicinal purposes for thousands of years, as an agent to produce euphoria, analgesia and sleep, and to prevent diarrhoea. It was introduced in Britain at the end of the seventeenth century, usually taken orally as 'tincture of laudanum', addiction to which acquired a certain social cachet during the next two hundred years. The situation changed when the hypodermic syringe and needle was invented in the mid-nineteenth century and opiate dependence began to take on a more sinister significance.

Chemical aspects

Opium contains many alkaloids related to morphine. The structure of morphine was determined in 1902 and since then many semisynthetic compounds (produced by chemical modification of morphine) and fully synthetic analgesics have been studied. In addition to morphine-like compounds, opium also contains **papaverine**, a smooth muscle relaxant discussed in Chapter 11.

The main groups of drugs that are discussed in this section are:

1. Morphine analogues. These are compounds closely related in structure to morphine, and often synthesized from it. They may be *agonists* (e.g. **morphine**, **heroin**, **codeine**), *partial agonists* (e.g. **nalorphine**, **levallorphan**), or *antagonists* (e.g. **naloxone**).

2. Synthetic derivatives with structures unrelated to morphine.
   a. Phenylpiperidine series, e.g. **pethidine, fentanyl**.
   b. Methadone series, e.g. **methadone, dextropropoxyphene**.
   c. Benzomorphan series, e.g. **pentazocine, cyclazocine**.

Morphine analogues (Table 25.1)

Morphine is a **phenanthrene** derivative, with two planar rings (A & B) and two aliphatic ring structures (C & D) which occupy a plane roughly at right angles to the planar rings (Fig. 25.5). Variants of the morphine molecule have been produced by substitution at one or both of the hydroxyl groups (the phenolic OH at position 3 and the alcoholic OH at position 6), and by substitution at the nitrogen atom at position 17. Some of the most important analogues are shown in Table 25.1.

Table 25.1 Morphine analogues

Drug	Substituents 3	6	N	14		Receptor action
Morphine	—OH	—OH	—CH$_3$	—H		Agonist
Heroin	—OCO·CH$_3$	—OCO·CH$_3$	—CH$_3$	—H		Agonist
Codeine	—OCH$_3$	—OH	—CH$_3$	—H		Agonist
Dihydrocodeine	—OCH$_3$	—OH	—CH$_3$	—H	(lacks double bond C$_7$–C$_8$)	Agonist
Nalorphine	—OH	—OH	—CH$_2$CH=CH$_2$	—H		Partial agonist
Naloxone	—OH	O	—CH$_2$CH=CH$_2$	—HO	(lacks double bond C$_7$–C$_8$)	Antagonist
Levorphanol	—OH	—H	—CH$_3$	—H	(lacks —O— at C$_4$–C$_5$)	Agonist
Levallorphan	—OH	—H	—CH$_2$CH=CH$_2$	—H	(lacks —O— at C$_4$–C$_5$)	Partial agonist
Etorphine						Agonist

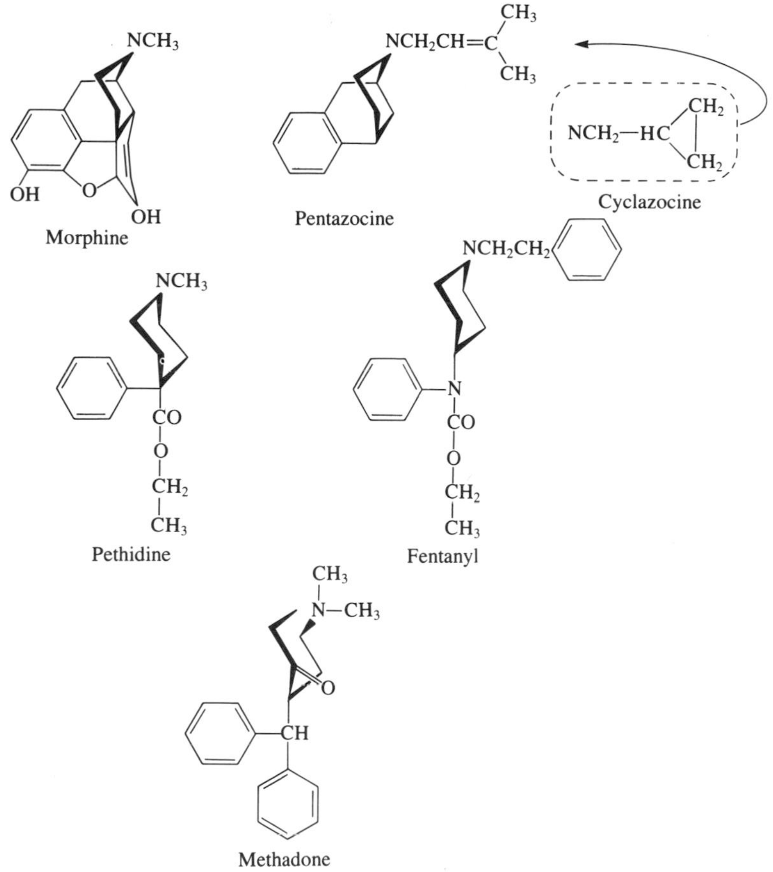

Fig. 25.5 Structures of some opiate analgesics drawn to show structural relationship to morphine.

Synthetic derivatives (Fig. 25.5)

Phenylpiperidine series. **Pethidine** (known as meperidine in USA) was discovered accidentally when new atropine-like drugs were being sought. It was the first fully synthetic morphine-like drug to be discovered and is chemically much simpler than morphine, though its pharmacological actions are very similar. **Fentanyl** is a more potent and shorter-acting derivative, which has gained favour as an adjunct to anaesthesia, rather than for the treatment of pain as such.

Methadone series. **Methadone**, though its structural formula bears no obvious chemical relationship to that of morphine, assumes a similar configuration in solution, and was designed on the basis of the common 3-dimensional structural features of morphine and pethidine. It is longer-acting than morphine, but otherwise very similar to it.

Dextropropoxyphene is very similar and used clinically for treating mild or moderate pain.

Benzomorphan series. Simplification of the morphine molecule led first to **levorphanol** (Table 25.1) in which the oxygen bridge is omitted, and then to benzomorphans, in which one of the four ring structures of morphine is also omitted. The most important members of this class are **pentazocine** and **cyclazocine**, which differ only in the nature of the substituent group attached to the N-atom. These drugs differ from morphine in the way in which they interact with their receptors (see below), and so have somewhat different actions and side effects.

Opioid receptors

The conclusion, based on pharmacological evidence of competitive antagonism of the effects of morphine by drugs such as nalorphine, that opioids produce their effects by binding to specific receptor sites, is confirmed by direct binding measurements (Snyder et al, 1973). Various pharmacological observations, however, suggested that more than one type of receptor must be involved. The original suggestion of multiple receptor types came from *in vivo* studies of the spectrum of actions (analgesia, sedation, pupillary constriction, bradycardia, etc) produced by different drugs. It was also found that some opioids, but not all, were able to relieve withdrawal symptoms in morphine-dependent animals, and this was interpreted in terms of distinct receptor subtypes. The conclusion from these and many subsequent pharmacological studies (Paterson et al, 1983; Goldstein & James, 1984; Zukin & Zukin, 1984) was that three receptors, termed μ, κ and σ, appeared to be involved in producing the main pharmacological effects in whole animals, as follows:

μ—supraspinal analgesia, respiratory depression, euphoria, physical dependence
κ—spinal analgesia, pupillary constriction, sedation
σ—dysphoria, hallucinations.

Some authors classify the σ receptor as a non-opioid receptor, since it appears that other drugs, such as phencyclidine (see Chapter 26) may also work via this receptor.

This classification was based on measurements of responses *in vivo*, and the interpretation in terms of receptor types is open to question. Subsequently Kosterlitz and others have used *in vitro* methods and a more quantitative approach. Opioids exert a pre-synaptic inhibitory effect on excitatory neurotransmission in the neuronal network of smooth muscle tissues such as the guinea pig ileum and the vas deferens of various species. Comparison of the effects of various opioids on guinea pig ileum and mouse vas deferens showed that whereas β-endorphin was equipotent on either, morphine was much more effective on the guinea pig than the mouse preparation, while met- or leu-enkephalin showed the reverse pattern of specificity. Furthermore, naloxone was about 10 times more potent in blocking opioid responses in the guinea pig than in the mouse.

These authors concluded that the receptor in the guinea pig ileum corresponded to the μ receptor,

whereas another type, christened δ, predominated in the mouse vas deferens. This conclusion probably oversimplifies the true situation, for it now appears that the guinea pig ileum has both μ and κ receptors, while the mouse vas deferens has μ, κ and δ.

Studies of the binding of various enkephalin-related peptides, and of morphine analogues, to brain homogenates have confirmed that multiple classes of receptor exist, and most studies have identified μ, κ and δ sites. So far, binding studies have failed to provide clear evidence for a separate σ receptor, and pharmacological studies have revealed no clear-cut function for the δ receptor. It is therefore mainly for the μ and κ receptors that a reasonably coherent picture has so far emerged. The isolation and molecular characterization of opioid receptors, which has recently been undertaken, will probably clarify matters considerably.

The interaction of endogenous opioid peptides (see Chapter 19) with the various receptor types has been investigated in detail (Paterson et al, 1983) and the specificity of the three main types (see Chapter 19) is summarized in Table 25.2.

Table 25.2 Affinity of opioids for μ, δ and κ binding sites

	Receptor type		
	μ	δ	κ
Opioid peptides			
β-endorphin	+++	+++	+++
leu-enkephalin	+	+++	0
met-enkephalin	++	+++	0
*Dynorphin A-(1-13) amide	++	+	+++
Opioid drugs			
Morphine	+++	+	++
Etorphine	+++	+++	+++
Pethidine	++	+	+
Phenazocine	++	++	++
Antagonists			
Nalorphine	++	++	++
Naloxone	+++	++	++

* Dynorphin A-(1-13) amide is a stable analogue of dynorphin with very similar pharmacological properties.

Agonists and antagonists

Opioids vary not only in their receptor specificity, but also in their efficacy at the different types of receptor. Thus, some agents act as agonists on one

Table 25.3 Agonist-antagonist classification of opioid drugs

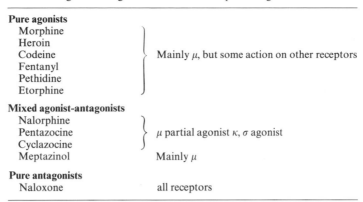

Pure agonists	
Morphine	
Heroin	
Codeine	Mainly μ, but some action on other receptors
Fentanyl	
Pethidine	
Etorphine	
Mixed agonist-antagonists	
Nalorphine	
Pentazocine	μ partial agonist κ, σ agonist
Cyclazocine	
Meptazinol	Mainly μ
Pure antagonists	
Naloxone	all receptors

type of receptor and antagonists or partial agonists at another, producing a very complicated pharmacological picture.

Three main categories may be distinguished (Table 25.3):

1. *Pure agonists*. This group includes most of the typical morphine-like drugs. They all have high affinity for μ receptors and varying affinity for δ and κ sites, and they lack appreciable activity at the putative σ receptor.

2. *Mixed agonist-antagonists*. These drugs, typified by nalorphine and pentazocine, combine a degree of morphine-like activity with the ability to antagonize some actions of morphine. Nalorphine, for example, is an agonist when tested on guinea pig ileum, but it also inhibits competitively the effect of morphine on this tissue. Whether it should be classed as a partial agonist at μ receptors or as competitive μ antagonist with agonist activity on another receptor type (e.g. κ) is not clear. *In vivo* it shows a similar mixture of agonist and antagonist actions. Most of the drugs in this group tend to cause dysphoria, rather than euphoria, an effect which may be due to an interaction with the σ receptor.

3. *Antagonists*. These drugs produce very little effect when given on their own, but block the effects of opioids. The most important is naloxone, which blocks μ receptors preferentially, but also δ, κ and σ.

Cellular mechanism of action

Most nerve cells respond to direct application of opioids by **hyperpolarization, inhibition of cell firing**, and a **pre-synaptic inhibition** of transmitter release (see reviews: Henderson, 1983; Duggan, 1983; Miller, 1984). Some neurons show excitation, but this may be due to suppression of an inhibitory pathway.

The hyperpolarizing response is due to an increase in K^+ conductance, but the mechanism by which receptor activation causes this effect is not certain. Pre-synaptic inhibition of transmitter release, which has been demonstrated at many central and peripheral synapses, including substance P release from primary afferent terminals in the spinal cord, is due partly to hyperpolarization of the nerve terminals, and partly to a reduction of the inward calcium current that occurs during the action potential. In dorsal root ganglion cells grown in tissue culture, the action potential shows a clear-cut plateau rather similar to that of cardiac muscle (see Chapter 10) which results from an inward calcium current. Opioids reduce this plateau markedly (Mudge et al, 1979), an effect which would be expected to reduce transmitter release by restricting the entry of calcium into nerve terminals.

At a biochemical level, opioid receptor activation causes inhibition of adenylate cyclase activity (reviewed by West & Miller, 1983). Reduction of the basal cAMP content in many parts of the brain has been demonstrated, and the stimulant effect of agents such as noradrenaline, dopamine and prostaglandins on cAMP production is also reduced. This effect has been extensively studied in cultured neuroblastoma cells by Klee and his colleagues. It is suggested that opioid receptor activation stimulates GTP hydrolysis by the regulatory

G-protein component of the cyclase activation system (see Chapter 1), thus accelerating the dissociation of the G protein from the cyclase. The receptor involved in this response seems to correspond in most cases to the δ receptor. Whether this biochemical response accounts for the physiological effects on neuronal function seems rather doubtful. It has not been established whether μ receptors, which seem to be responsible for many of the characteristic neurophysiological effects of opioids, are linked to cAMP synthesis.

It will be seen from this brief account that there are many gaps and areas of confusion in the classification of opioid receptors, and in the relation of these receptors (which have been recognized mainly on the basis of binding studies or *in vitro* tests on peripheral tissues) to the various pharmacological actions of opioid drugs and endogenous peptides *in vivo*. At present there are too few agonists or antagonists of sufficiently high receptor selectivity to enable the functional role of the different receptor classes to be determined unequivocally.

Pharmacological actions

Morphine derivatives produce their effects by binding to specific receptor sites in the central nervous system and elsewhere, the classification of which is discussed above. The drugs listed in Table 25.1 can be divided into agonists, partial agonists and antagonists according to the effect that they produce on the receptors. To be effective as an analgesic, a drug must possess appreciable agonist-like activity. **Morphine** will be taken as the reference compound.

The most important effects of morphine are on the central nervous system and the gastrointestinal tract, though numerous effects of less significance on many other systems have been described.

Effects on the central nervous system

1. **Analgesia**. Morphine is effective in all kinds of pain, whether acute or chronic. It undoubtedly reduces the sensation of pain (nociception) but at the same time strongly reduces the distress (affective component).

There seem to be several sites of action of morphine-like drugs in causing analgesia (see Fig. 25.3;

Duggan, 1983). Injection of morphine into the PAG region causes marked analgesia, which can be prevented by surgical interruption of the descending pathway to NRM, or by blocking serotonin synthesis pharmacologically with p-chlorophenylalanine. This latter procedure interrupts the serotininergic pathway running from NRM to the dorsal horn. Morphine also acts at spinal level, since it causes inhibition of transmission of nociceptive impulses through the dorsal horn in spinal animals, and suppresses nociceptive spinal reflexes in patients with spinal cord transection. It has been shown to inhibit substance P release in the dorsal horn *in vitro* and *in vivo* (Fig. 25.6), by exerting a pre-synaptic inhibitory effect on the central terminals of nociceptive afferent neurons. Microinjection of morphine into the SG also produces this effect.

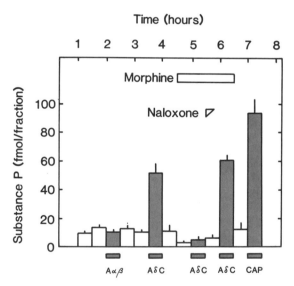

Fig. 25.6 Release of substance P from cat spinal cord. Substance P was measured by radioimmunoassay in the fluid superfusing the spinal cord. Stimulation of the sciatic nerve (grey bars) at low intensity stimulates large myelinated fibres (Aα & Aβ) only and evokes no release. Increasing the stimulus strength so as to recruit Aδ and C fibres causes SP release. The release is blocked by morphine, this effect being antagonized by naloxone. Capsaicin (CAP) added to the fluid superfusing the spinal cord also releases SP. (From: Yaksh et al, 1980)

While these effects can account for the antinociceptive action of morphine, the affective component of its analgesic effect must certainly involve other sites within the brain, possibly including the limbic system, which is probably involved in the euphoria-producing effect (Koob & Bloom, 1983). Drugs such as nalorphine and pentazocine share the antinociceptive actions of morphine but have much less effect on the psychological response to pain.

2. **Euphoria**. Morphine causes a powerful sense of contentment and well-being. This is an important component of its analgesic effect, since the agitation and anxiety associated with a painful illness or injury are thereby reduced. If morphine or heroin is given intravenously, the result is a sudden 'rush' likened to an 'abdominal orgasm'. The euphoria produced by morphine depends considerably on the circumstances. In patients who are distressed, it is a marked effect, but in patients who become accustomed to chronic pain, morphine usually causes no euphoria, though the pain is nonetheless relieved. Some patients report restlessness rather than euphoria under these circumstances.

Different opioid drugs vary greatly in the amount of euphoria that they produce. It does not occur with codeine or with pentazocine to any marked extent, and nalorphine, in doses sufficient to cause analgesia, produces dysphoria. This does not seem to be due to inhibition of tonic opioid peptide-mediated effects, since naloxone (a pure opioid antagonist) does not cause dysphoria. An action at the δ receptor is postulated.

3. **Respiratory depression**. A measurable degree of respiratory depression, resulting in increased arterial $P\mathrm{CO_2}$, occurs with a normal analgesic dose of morphine or related compounds. The two effects seem to be strictly correlated, and none of the synthetic opioids nor the endogenous opioid peptides varies significantly in the amount of respiratory depression produced at equi-analgesic doses.*

The depressant effect is associated with a decrease in the sensitivity of the respiratory centre to $P\mathrm{CO_2}$, the hypoxic stimulus to breathing from peripheral chemoreceptors being unaffected. The site and mechanism of action of opioids on respiration is not certain (McQueen, 1983). Neurons in the medullary respiratory centre itself do not appear to be directly depressed, but opioids applied to the ventral surface of the medulla in the region where CO_2 chemosensitivity is maximal, have a powerful depressant effect on respiration.

Respiratory depression by opioids is not accompanied by depression of the medullary centres controlling cardiovascular function (in contrast to the action of anaesthetics and other general depressants). This means that respiratory depression produced by opioids is much better tolerated than a similar degree of depression caused by, say, a barbiturate; nonetheless respiratory depression is the commonest cause of death in acute opioid poisoning.

4. **Depression of cough reflex**. Cough suppression, surprisingly, does not correlate closely with the analgesic and respiratory depressant actions of opioids. In general, increasing substitution on the phenolic–OH group of morphine (position 3; see Table 25.1) increases antitussive relative to analgesic activity. Thus **codeine** suppresses cough markedly in sub-analgesic doses, and is often used in cough medicines. **Pholcodeine**, with a much larger substituent group at position 3 is even more selective.

5. **Nausea and vomiting**. This side effect occurs in up to 40% of patients to whom morphine is given, and does not seem to be separable from the analgesic effect among a range of opioid analgesics. The site of action is the **area postrema (chemoreceptor trigger zone)** a region of the medulla where chemical stimuli of many kinds may initiate vomiting (see Chapter 15).

A chemically related compound, **apomorphine** (see Chapters 10 & 19) is more effective than morphine in causing vomiting, and lacks analgesic actions. The emetic effect of morphine, however, is prevented by the administration of an opioid antagonist, such as naloxone (see below) whereas that of apomorphine is not affected. On the other hand dopamine antagonists (see Chapter 24) oppose the action of apomorphine much more effectively than that of morphine.

Nausea and vomiting following morphine injection is usually transient, and disappears with repeated administration.

6. **Pupillary constriction**. This is a centrally-mediated effect, caused by stimulation of the oculomotor nucleus. Pin-point pupils are an important

---

* A recently-introduced opioid, **meptazinol**, is claimed to cause little respiratory depression at analgesic doses.

diagnostic feature in overdosage with morphine and related drugs, because most other causes of coma and respiratory depression produce pupillary dilatation.

Effects on the gastrointestinal tract

Morphine causes a marked **increase in tone and reduced motility** in many parts of the gastrointestinal system, resulting in constipation, which may be severe. There is a delay in gastric emptying, which can considerably retard the absorption of other drugs. Pressure in the biliary tract increases because of contraction of the gall bladder and constriction of the biliary sphincter. This effect is harmful in patients suffering from biliary colic due to gallstones, in whom pain may be increased rather than relieved. The rise in intrabiliary pressure can cause a transient increase in the concentration of amylase and lipase in the plasma.

The mechanism of action of morphine on visceral smooth muscle is not well understood (North & Egan, 1983). The increase in tone is reduced or abolished by atropine, suggesting an effect on intramural nerves rather than directly on smooth muscle cells. It is partly mediated by a central action of morphine, since intraventricular injection of morphine inhibits propulsive gastrointestinal movements. The local effect of morphine and other opioids on neurons of the myenteric plexus is inhibitory, the cells being hyperpolarized due to an increased potassium conductance. The receptors involved in these effects are of μ, δ and κ type, with much variation between different preparations and different species.

Other actions of opioids

Morphine releases histamine from mast cells. This can cause local effects, such as **urticaria** and **itching** at the site of the injection, or systemic effects, namely **bronchoconstriction** and **hypotension**. The bronchoconstrictor effect can have serious consequences for asthmatic patients, to whom morphine should not be given. Other opioids, except those closely related to morphine, do not release histamine.

Hypotension and bradycardia occur with large doses of most opioids, due to an action on the medulla. With morphine and similar drugs, histamine release may contribute to the hypotension.

Effects on smooth muscle other than that of the gastrointestinal tract and bronchi are slight, though spasm of the ureters, bladder and uterus sometimes occur. The Straub tail reaction, one of the more improbable phenomena in pharmacology, consists of a raising and stiffening of the tail of rats or mice given opioid drugs, and is due to spasm of a muscle at the base of the tail. It was through this effect that the analgesic action of pethidine was discovered.

Tolerance and dependence

Tolerance to opioids (i.e. an increase in the dose needed to produce a given pharmacological effect) develops rapidly, and is readily demonstrated. **Dependence** is a different phenomenon (see Chapter 35) which is much more difficult to define and measure. Morphine causes a clear-cut **physical withdrawal syndrome** (or **abstinence syndrome**), which is one factor in the genesis of dependence, and can be reproduced in experimental animals, but it also produces strong **psychological dependence** which is probably more important as a factor causing dependence in man, but is far harder to study.

Tolerance

Tolerance can be detected within 12–24 hours of morphine administration. Figure 25.7 shows the increase in the equianalgesic dose of morphine (measured by the hot-plate test) that occurred when a slow release pellet of morphine was implanted subcutaneously in mice. The pellet was removed 8 hours before the test, to allow the circulating morphine to disappear before the test was carried out. Within 3 days the equianalgesic dose increased about 5-fold. Sensitivity returned to normal within about 3 days of removing the pellet. More detailed studies have subsequently shown that a detectable level of tolerance may persist in rats for several months (Martin & Sloan, 1977). Tolerance extends to most of the pharmacological effects of morphine, including analgesia, euphoria and respiratory depression, but affects the constipating and pupil-constricting actions much less. Thus, addicts who take up to 50 times the normal analgesic dose of morphine show relatively little respiratory de-

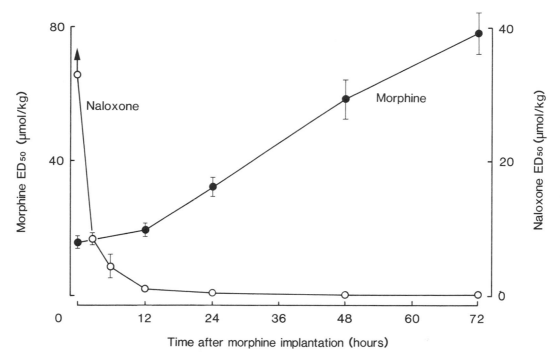

Fig. 25.7 Development of morphine tolerance in mice. The ED50 for analgesia (hot-plate test) produced by subcutaneous injection of a test dose of morphine (closed symbols) was measured at intervals after implantation of a slow-release pellet of morphine, the pellet being removed 8 hours before the assay in order to allow the circulating morphine concentration to fall to zero before the test dose was given. The ED50 increases about 5-fold after 72 hours. Simultaneously, the dose of naloxone needed to precipitate withdrawal symptoms (open circles), which can be regarded as a measure of morphine dependence, decreases very markedly. (From: Way et al, 1969)

pression, but marked constipation and pupillary constriction.

Tolerance to opioids shows considerable selectivity, in the sense that the development of tolerance to one opioid is not necessarily accompanied by tolerance to others. In general, the existence of **cross-tolerance** is taken as evidence that both opioids are acting on the same type of receptor (Wuster et al, 1983)

The mechanisms by which tolerance develops are not clear. The fact that a cross-tolerance occurs between different opioids, and that the phenomenon occurs readily *in vitro*, shows that it is not due to accelerated degradation of morphine. Binding measurements have shown no consistent change in the number of opioid receptors in brain homogenates, or in their binding characteristics, in tolerant compared with normal animals. Evidence for a cellular adaptive response comes from the work of Klee and his colleagues on cAMP production by neuroblastoma cells (Sharma et al, 1975).

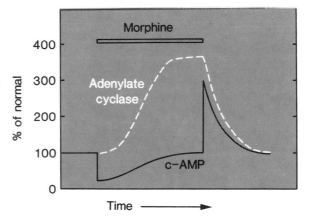

Fig. 25.8 Biochemical mechanism postulated to explain morphine tolerance and dependence. Morphine inhibits adenylate cyclase (solid line). A secondary rise in the synthesis of adenylate cyclase occurs (dotted line) so that cAMP production recovers in spite of the inhibitory effect of morphine (i.e. tolerance develops). On cessation of morphine treatment excessive cAMP production occurs, causing withdrawal symptoms, until the high level of adenylate cyclase returns to normal. (From: Sharma et al, 1975)

They found that addition of morphine to the culture dish caused a reduction in cAMP production for 2–3 days, after which it returned to normal. At this stage, if the morphine was removed, the basal cAMP production increased to about double the normal level, and the response of the cells to substances that activate adenylate cyclase (e.g. prostaglandin E_1) was similarly increased. Thus either the number or the specific activity of the cyclase molecules was increased by prolonged morphine treatment (Fig. 25.8). *In vivo* tolerance is likely to involve much more complex adaptive responses, such as suppression of activity in neuronal pathways involving opioid release, or compensatory increase in pathways that antagonize opioid effects, but hypotheses are highly speculative at present.

Physical dependence

This is characterized by a clear-cut **abstinence syndrome**. In experimental animals (for example, rats) abrupt withdrawal of morphine after chronic administration for a few days causes an increased irritability, loss of weight and a variety of abnormal behaviour patterns, such as body shakes, writhing, jumping and signs of aggression. These reactions decrease after a few days, but abnormal irritability and aggression persist for many weeks. Human addicts show a similar abstinence syndrome, somewhat resembling severe influenza, with yawning, pupillary dilatation, fever, sweating, piloerection,* nausea, diarrhoea and insomnia. Patients are extremely restless and distressed and have a strong craving for the drug. The symptoms are maximal in about 2 days and largely disappear in 8–10 days, though some residual symptoms and physiological abnormalities persist for several weeks (Martin & Sloan, 1977). Re-administration of morphine rapidly abolishes the abstinence syndrome.

Many physiological changes have been described in relation to the abstinence syndrome. For example, reflex hyperexcitability is demonstrable in the spinal cord of morphine-dependent animals, and can be produced by chronic intrathecal as well as systemic administration of morphine. The

noradrenergic pathways emanating from the **locus coeruleus** (see Chapter 19) may also play an important role in causing the abstinence syndrome. The rate of firing of locus coeruleus neurons is inhibited by opioids, and increased during the abstinence syndrome. What is interesting is that **clonidine**, an α_2-adrenoceptor agonist (see Chapter 7), also inhibits firing of locus coeruleus neurons, and is effective in suppressing the morphine abstinence syndrome (Tseng et al, 1975). Moreover, clonidine itself has analgesic activity (see later section) and cross-tolerance occurs between it and opioid analgesics (Paalzow, 1978).

Psychological dependence

This is a more complex phenomenon than physical dependence, and probably more important in the genesis of compulsive drug-taking (i.e. addiction). A degree of physical dependence is often produced when patients receive opioid analgesics in hospital for several days, but this almost never leads to addiction. On the other hand, addicts who recover fully from the abstinence syndrome are still extremely likely to revert to drug-taking later. Thus, physical dependence does not seem to be the major factor in long-term opioid abuse.

Various behavioural models have been devised to mimic psychological dependence in animals, most of them based on measurement of the potentiality of drugs to act as **reinforcers** in tests of operant conditioning. In tests on Rhesus monkeys, several drugs have been found to act as **primary reinforcers** (i.e. an animal which has not previously received the drug spontaneously learns to press a bar causing an intravenous dose to be given). These include opioids such as morphine, codeine, pethidine, methadone and pentazocine, as well as depressants, such as barbiturates or ethanol, and some stimulants (e.g. amphetamine, cocaine, nicotine). There is a close correlation between drugs that act in this way in the Rhesus monkey and drugs that lead to psychological dependence in man. Rats, on the other hand, will not spontaneously self-administer drugs in this way, but only if they are first rendered dependent. It is reasonable to infer that the primary reinforcement that occurs in monkeys is a model of psychological dependence, since it can occur with drugs that

---

* Causing goose pimples. This is the origin of the phrase 'cold turkey' used to describe the effect of morphine withdrawal.

produce no physical abstinence syndrome, whereas the self-administration behaviour seen in addicted rats is a model for physical dependence.

Rhesus monkeys spontaneously increase their rate of morphine self-administration to about 40 mg/kg per day over the course of 1–3 months (Thompson & Schuster, 1968). This rate increases if naloxone is given to the animals, and is reduced if an opioid agonist is given, suggesting that the animals regulate their dose of opioid with some precision. If the syringe is disconnected, the monkeys continue to press the lever at a high rate, and it takes months for the response to be extinguished, implying that in monkeys, as in man, the reinforcing effect of the drug long outlasts the duration of the physical abstinence syndrome.

Metabolism and pharmacokinetic aspects

The absorption of morphine congeners by mouth is variable. Morphine itself is slowly and erratically absorbed from the intestine, and is not usually given orally. In fact, when given parenterally, morphine may collect in the gastric contents by ion-trapping (see Chapter 3), and be reabsorbed later. Codeine, in contrast, is well absorbed, and normally given by mouth. Most morphine-like drugs undergo first-pass metabolism, and are therefore considerably less potent when taken orally than when injected. For therapeutic use, morphine is usually given intramuscularly (occasionally intravenously if a very rapid effect is needed), whereas less potent drugs, such as codeine, are given orally. The plasma half-life of most morphine analogues is 3–6 hours. Hepatic metabolism is the main mode of inactivation, usually by conjugation with glucuronide at the 3-OH group. Morphine glucuronide is excreted in the urine, and also in the bile. Glucuronide in the gut is hydrolysed and most of the morphine is reabsorbed (enterohepatic circulation).

Because of low conjugating capacity in neonates, morphine-like drugs have a much longer duration of action; because even a small degree of respiratory depression can be hazardous, morphine congeners should not be used in the neonatal period, nor used as analgesics during childbirth. Pethidine (see below) is a safer alternative for this purpose.

Analogues that have no free —OH in the 3-position (i.e. heroin, codeine) are metabolized to morphine, which accounts for at least part of their pharmacological activity.

Morphine produces very effective analgesia when administered intrathecally, and is being increasingly used in this way by anaesthetists, the advantage being that the sedative and respiratory depressant effects are reduced, though not completely avoided. Trials have recently been reported of opioids used 'on demand' by postoperative patients. The patients are provided with an infusion pump which they control, the maximum possible rate of administration being limited to avoid acute toxicity. Contrary to fears, patients show little tendency to use excessively large doses and become dependent; instead the dose is adjusted to achieve analgesia without excessive sedation, and is reduced as the pain subsides.

Unwanted effects

The main unwanted effects of morphine, which have been mentioned in the description of its pharmacological actions, are as follows:

1. Respiratory depression and sedation
2. Physical and psychological dependence
3. Reduced gastrointestinal motility and smooth muscle spasm, leading to constipation and sometimes biliary or ureteric spasm
4. Nausea and vomiting
5. Histamine release, leading to bronchoconstriction and itching, and sometimes hypotension.

Acute overdosage with morphine results in coma and respiratory depression, with characteristically constricted pupils. It is treated by giving naloxone intravenously. This also serves as a diagnostic test, for failure to respond to naloxone indicates a cause other than opioid poisoning for the comatose state. There is a danger of precipitating a severe withdrawal syndrome with naloxone, since opioid poisoning occurs mainly in addicts.

Other opioid analgesics

Heroin (diacetylmorphine) is produced from morphine by acetylation of both hydroxyl groups. A strong smell of vinegar commonly provides the lead to illicit heroin producers. It is pharmacologically very similar to morphine, and is converted to morphine in the body, though heroin itself is about three times as active than morphine. Because of its greater lipid solubility it crosses the blood-brain barrier more rapidly than morphine, and gives a greater 'rush' when injected intravenously. It is said to be less emetic than morphine, but the evidence for this is slight. It is still available in Britain for clinical use as an analgesic though its manufacture is banned in many countries. There is no evidence that heroin differs from morphine in either its respiratory depressant effect, or in its liability to cause dependence. Its duration of action (about 2 hours) is shorter than that of morphine.

Codeine (3-methylmorphine) is also made commercially from morphine. It is less polar, and therefore more reliably absorbed by mouth than morphine, but has only about one-sixth of the analgesic potency. Furthermore, its analgesic effect does not increase appreciably at higher dose levels (Lasagna, 1964). It is therefore used mainly as an oral analgesic for mild types of pain (headache, backache, etc). An important difference from morphine is that it causes little or no euphoria, and is rarely addictive, so is available freely without prescription. It is very frequently combined with aspirin-like drugs in proprietary analgesic preparations, but there is no evidence of any advantageous synergistic interaction between the two components.

In relation to its analgesic effect, codeine produces the same degree of respiratory depression as morphine, but the limited response even at high doses means that it is seldom a problem in practice. It does, however, cause constipation. Codeine is an antitussive agent and is often used in cough mixtures.

Dihydrocodeine is identical with codeine apart from saturation at the 7–8 double bond (Table 25.1) and is pharmacologically very similar, having no substantial advantages or disadvantages (apart from cost) over codeine.

Pethidine is virtually identical with morphine in its pharmacological effects, but with about one-tenth of the analgesic potency. It also has an antimuscarinic action which may cause dry mouth and blurring of vision as side effects. It also has relatively less antitussive effect. It produces a very similar euphoric effect, and is equally liable to cause dependence. Its duration of action is appreciably shorter than that of morphine, and the route of

metabolic degradation is different. Pethidine is partly N-demethylated in the liver to norpethidine, which has a hallucinogenic and convulsant effect. This becomes significant with large oral doses of pethidine, producing an overdose syndrome rather different from that of morphine. Pethidine is preferred to morphine for analgesia during labour, because it is shorter acting. The difference in the duration of action of morphine and pethidine is particularly marked in the neonate. This is because the conjugation reactions, on which morphine inactivation depends, are deficient in the newborn: pethidine does not rely on conjugation to be inactivated, and any drug transferred from the maternal circulation is, in contrast to morphine, fairly quickly inactivated.

Severe reactions, consisting of excitement, hyperthermia and convulsions, have been reported when pethidine is given to patients receiving monoamine oxidase inhibitors. This seems to be due to inhibition of an alternative metabolic pathway, leading to increased norpethidine formation, but the details are not known.

Fentanyl is a much more potent phenylpiperidine derivative than pethidine. Its actions are very similar, but short-lasting. Its main use has been in anaesthesia, where it is often given in conjugation with a neuroleptic, droperidol, to produce neuroleptanalgesia (see Chapter 20), a state in which surgery can be performed without the patient being rendered fully unconscious.

Etorphine is a morphine analogue of remarkable potency, more than 1000 times that of morphine, but otherwise very similar in its actions. Its high potency confers no particular clinical advantage, but it is used successfully to immobilize wild animals for trapping and research purposes, where the required dose is small enough to be incorporated into a dart or pellet.

Methadone is also pharmacologically similar to morphine, and has similar potency, the main difference being that its duration of action is considerably longer and it is claimed to have less sedative action. The increased duration seems to occur because the drug is bound in the extravascular compartment, and slowly released, thus maintaining a low plasma concentration for many hours. The half-life is 15–20 hours. One consequence is that the physical abstinence syndrome is less acute than with morphine or other short-acting drugs, though the psychological dependence is no less pronounced. For this reason, methadone is widely used as a means of treating morphine and heroin addiction. In the presence of methadone, an injection of morphine does not cause the normal euphoria, nor is there a physical abstinence syndrome, so it is often possible to wean addicts from morphine or heroin by giving regular oral doses of methadone—an improvement if not a cure.

Pentazocine is a mixed agonist-antagonist (p. 557). In low doses its potency and effects are very similar to those of morphine, but increasing the dose does not cause a corresponding increase in the effects produced. Thus, at high doses, pentazocine causes only slight respiratory depression, and it causes marked dysphoria, with nightmares and hallucinations, rather than euphoria. It also tends to raise, rather than lower, arterial blood pressure. These differences mean that pentazocine has very little tendency to cause dependence, and its acute toxicity is much less than that of morphine. Its antagonist activity is apparent in the fact that, given concurrently with morphine, pentazocine actually reduces the analgesic and other actions of morphine, and can even precipitate an abstinence syndrome in morphine addicts. Binding studies show that it has a higher affinity for κ receptors than for μ receptors, and on behavioural criteria it is postulated to act on σ receptors, this spectrum being somewhat different from that of conventional opioid drugs.

Though clearly much less addictive than the conventional opioids, pentazocine has an appreciable tendency to cause dependence, particularly if given by injection and is not quite the ideal morphine substitute that it was originally thought to be.

Opioid antagonists

Nalorphine (see Table 25.1) is closely related in structure to morphine, and was the first specific antagonist to be discovered. This was an important development, for it was the first clear evidence in favour of a specific receptor for morphine, recognition of which led to the successful search for endogenous mediators.

Nalorphine has, in fact, a more complicated action than that of a simple competitive antagonist.

It antagonizes most actions of morphine in whole animals or isolated tissues (e.g. analgesia, respiratory depression, inhibition of electrically-evoked contractions of guinea-pig ileum), and at low concentrations of nalorphine this interaction appears to be competitive. Higher concentrations of nalorphine, when tested alone, however, *mimic* these actions of morphine. It should therefore be regarded as a partial agonist at μ receptors rather than a pure competitive antagonist. Unlike morphine, however, it causes dysphoria, which is similar to the effect of large doses of pentazocine, and this has prevented its general use as an analgesic. Nalorphine can itself produce physical dependence, but can also, in small doses, precipitate a withdrawal syndrome in morphine or heroin addicts. Nalorphine now has few clinical uses. At one time it was the most effective antidote available in cases of acute morphine or heroin overdosage, but had the disadvantage that, if large doses are needed, nalorphine itself causes respiratory depression. It has therefore been superseded by naloxone which has no such effect.

Furthermore, nalorphine does not effectively antagonize the actions of other partial agonists, such as pentazocine, and is no use in treating overdosage with such drugs.

Naloxone, which was first synthesized in 1960, is a pure opioid antagonist. On the basis of binding studies it appears to have a high affinity for μ receptors, and an appreciable but lower affinity for δ and κ receptors. Pharmacological studies show that it also blocks effects associated with σ receptors. Naloxone blocks the actions of endogenous opioid peptides as well as those of morphine-like drugs, and has been extensively used as an experimental tool to determine the physiological role of these peptides, particularly in the pain pathway.

Given on its own, naloxone produces very little effect, but produces a rapid reversal of the effects of morphine and other opioids, including partial agonists such as pentazocine and nalorphine. Its effects on nociception, which might be expected if opioid peptides have an important physiological regulatory function in the pain pathway, are not at all clear-cut (Woolf & Wall, 1983). Some reports have claimed that naloxone causes hyperalgesia in normal subjects but others find no effect. There is rather more agreement that naloxone inhibits acupuncture analgesia, which is known to be associated with the release of opioid peptides within the central nervous system. Analgesia produced by PAG stimulation is more reliably prevented by naloxone.

Thus, most reports suggest that naloxone can prevent analgesia produced by various manipulations, without affecting pain sensation under physiological conditions.

Naloxone is used to treat respiratory depression caused by opioid overdosage, and occasionally to reverse the effect of opioid analgesics, used during labour, on the respiration of the newborn baby.

Naloxone is usually given intravenously and its effects are produced immediately. It is rapidly metabolized by the liver, and its effect lasts only 2–4 hours, which is considerably shorter than that of most morphine-like drugs. Thus it may have to be given repeatedly.

Naloxone has no important side effects of its own, but precipitates withdrawal symptoms in addicts. It can be used to detect opioid addiction.

Naltrexone is a recently-introduced drug very similar to naloxone but with a much longer duration of action (half-time about 10 hours). Unlike naloxone, it has appreciable agonist activity.

REFERENCES AND FURTHER READING

Duggan A W 1983 Electrophysiology of opioid peptides and sensory systems. Br Med Bull 39: 65–70

Fields H L 1981 Pain: new approaches to therapy. Ann Neurol 9: 101–106

Foreman J C, Jordan C C 1984 Neurogenic inflammation. Trends in Pharmacological Sciences 5: 116–119

Goldstein A, James I F 1984 Multiple opioid receptors: criteria for identification and classification. Trends in Pharmacological Sciences 5: 503–505

Henderson G 1983 Electrophysiological analysis of opioid action in the central nervous system. Br Med Bull 39: 59–64

Jessell T M 1983 Substance P in the nervous system. Handbook of Psychopharmacology 16: 1–105

Keele C A, Armstrong D M 1964 Substances causing pain and itch. Edward Arnold, London

Koob G F, Bloom F E 1983 Behavioural effects of opioid peptides. Br Med Bull 39: 89–94

Lasagna L 1964 The clinical value of morphine and its substitutes as analgesics. Pharm Rev 16: 47–83

Leander S, Hakanson R, Rosell S, Folkers K, Sundler F, Tornqrist K 1981 A specific substance P antagonist blocks smooth muscle contraction induced by non-cholinergic, non-adrenergic nerve stimulation. Nature 294: 467–469

Leeman S E 1980 Intrathecal morphine inhibits substance P release from mammalian spinal cord in vivo. Nature 286: 155–157

Lembeck F 1983 Sir Thomas Lewis's nocifensor system, histamine and substance-P-containing primary afferent nerves. Trends in Neurosciences 6: 106–108.

Lewis J W, Liebeskind J C 1983 Pain suppressive systems of the brain. Trends in Pharmacological Sciences 4: 73–75

McQueen D S 1983 Opioid peptide interactions with respiratory and circulatory systems. Brit Med Bull 39: 77–82

Martin W R, Sloan J W 1977 Neuropharmacology and neurochemistry of subjective effects, analgesia, tolerance and dependence produced by narcotic analgesics. Handb Exp Pharmacol 45 Part 1: 43–158

Melzack R, Wall P D 1982 The challenge of pain. Penguin, London

Miller R J 1984 How do opiates act? Trends in Neurosciences 7: 184–185

Morland J S 1982 Pain pathways: potential sites for analgesic action. In: Lednicer D (ed) Central Analgesics. Wiley, New York

Mudge A W, Leeman S E, Fishbach G D 1979 Enkephalin inhibits release of substance P from sensory neurons in culture and decreases action potential duration. Proc Natn Acad Sci USA 76: 526–530

North R A, Egan T M 1983 Actions and distributions of opioid peptides in peripheral tissues. Br Med Bull 39: 71–75

Paalzow G 1978 Development of tolerance to the analgesic effect of clonidine in rats. Cross-tolerance to morphine. Arch Pharmacol 304: 1–4

Parkhouse J, Pleuvry B J, Rees J M H 1979 Analgesic drugs. Blackwell, Oxford

Paterson S J, Robson L E, Kosterlitz H W 1983 Classification of opioid receptors. Br Med Bull 39: 31–36

Rosell S, Folkers K 1982 Substance P antagonists; a new type of pharmacological tool. Trends in Pharmacological Sciences 5: 211–212

Rosell S, Bjorkroth U, Xu J-C, Folkers K 1983 The pharmacological profile of a substance P (SP) antagonist. Evidence for the existence of subpopulations of SP receptors. Acta Physiol Scand 117: 445–449

Salt T E, Hill R G 1983 Neurotransmitter candidates of somatosensory primary afferent fibres. Neuroscience 10: 1083–1103

Sharma S K, Klee W A, Nirenberg M 1975 Dual regulation of adenylate cyclase accounts for narcotic dependence and tolerance. Proc Natn Acad Sci 72: 3092–3096

Snyder S H, Pasternak G W, Pert C 1973 In: Synaptic modulators Iversen L L, Iversen S D, Snyder S H (eds) Handbook of Psychopharmacology 5: 329–360

Thompson T, Schuster C R 1968 Behavioural Pharmacology. Prentice-Hall, New Jersey

Tseng L F, Loh H H, Wei E T 1975 Effects of clonidine on morphine withdrawal signs in the rat. Eur J Pharmacol 30: 93–99

Wall P D, Fitzgerald M 1982 If substance P fails to fulfil the criteria as a neurotransmitter in somatosensory afferents, what might its role be? Ciba Foundation Symposium 91: 249–266

Way E L, Loh H H, Shen F H 1969 Simultaneous quantitative measurement of morphine tolerance and physical dependence.

J Pharmacol Exp Ther 167: 1–8

West R E, Miller R J 1983 Opiates, second messengers and cell response. Br Med Bull 39: 53–58

Woolf C J, Wall P D 1983 Endogenous opioids, peptides and pain mechanisms: a complex relationship. Nature 306: 739–740

Wuster M, Schutz R, Herz A 1983 A subclassification of multiple opiate receptors by means of selective tolerance development. J Receptor Res 3: 199–214

Yaksh T L, Jessell T M, Gamse R, Mudge A W, Leeman S E 1980 Intrathecal morphine inhibits substance P release from mammalian spinal cord in vivo. Nature 286: 155–157

Zukin R S, Zukin S R 1984 The case for multiple opiate receptors. Trends in Neurosciences 7: 160–164

Central nervous system stimulants and psychotomimetic drugs

Drugs that have a predominantly stimulant effect on the central nervous system fall into three broad categories:

1. Convulsants and respiratory stimulants
2. Psychomotor stimulants
3. Psychotomimetic drugs.

Drugs in the first category (e.g. **doxapram**, **niketh-amide**, **leptazol**, **strychnine**) have relatively little effect on mental function, and appear to act mainly on the brainstem and spinal cord, producing exaggerated reflex excitability, an increase in activity of the respiratory and vasomotor centres, and, with higher dosage, convulsions.

Drugs in the second category (e.g. **amphetamine**, **caffeine**, **cocaine**) have a marked effect on mental function and behaviour, producing excitement and euphoria, reduced sensation of fatigue, and an increase in motor activity.

Drugs in the third category (e.g. **lysergic acid diethylamide**, **cannabis**) mainly affect thought patterns, perception and mood, producing effects that superficially resemble the changes seen in schizophrenia.

The distinctions between these three categories are not completely clear-cut. Amphetamine, for example, can produce thought disturbances resembling schizophrenia, as well as affecting motor behaviour, so it does not fit unequivocally into the category of psychomotor stimulants. Table 26.1 summarizes the classification of the drugs that are discussed in this chapter.

The actions of cannabis are predominantly depressant rather than stimulant, though it shares certain subjective effects with lysergic acid diethylamide (LSD) and other psychotomimetics. It is discussed in Chapter 35.

CONVULSANTS AND RESPIRATORY STIMULANTS

This group comprises chemically diverse substances, whose mechanism of action is, with some exceptions, not well understood. Their structures are shown in Figure 26.1. Some of these drugs were at one time called **analeptics** and were regarded as useful drugs with which to treat patients in coma or with severe respiratory failure. Objective trials, however, showed that although some restoration of function could be achieved for a time, the use of analeptic drugs did not reduce mortality, and carried a considerable risk of causing convulsions, which left the patient more deeply comatose than before. There remains a very limited clinical use for respiratory stimulants in treating acute ventilatory failure (see Chapter 13), **amiphenazole** and **dox-apram** (Table 26.1) being most commonly used, since these drugs carry less risk of causing convulsions than earlier compounds.

Also included in this group are various compounds, such as **strychnine**, **picrotoxinin** and **leptazol**, which are of interest mainly as experimental tools and have no clinical uses.

Strychnine is an alkaloid found in the seeds of an Indian tree, which has been used for centuries as a poison (mainly vermin, but also human; it is much favoured in detective stories). It is a powerful convulsant, and acts throughout the central nervous system, but particularly on the spinal cord, causing violent extensor spasms that are triggered by minor sensory stimuli, the head being thrown back and the face fixed, we are told, in a hideous grin. These effects result from blocking the action of glycine, which is the main inhibitory transmitter acting on motoneurons. Strychnine is believed to act by com-

Table 26.1 Central nervous system stimulants and psychotomimetic drugs

Category	Examples	Mode of action	Clinical significance
Convulsants and respiratory stimulants (analeptics)			
Respiratory stimulants	Amiphenazole	Not known	Occasionally used as respiratory stimulant. Risk of convulsions less than with nikethamide.
	Doxapram	Not known	Short-acting respiratory stimulant sometimes given by intravenous infusion to treat acute respiratory failure.
Miscellaneous convulsants	Strychnine	Antagonist of glycine Main action is to increase reflex excitability of spinal cord	No clinical uses
	Bicuculline	Competitive antagonist of GABA	No clinical uses
	Picrotoxinin	Non-competitive antagonist of GABA	Clinical use as respiratory stimulant now obsolete.
	Nikethamide	Not known	Risk of convulsions
	Leptazol	Not known	No clinical use. Convulsant activity in experimental animals provides a useful model for testing anticonvulsant drugs (see Chapter 24).
Psychomotor stimulants			
	Amphetamine and related compounds eg: dexamphetamine methylamphetamine methylphenidate fenfluramine	Release of catecholamines. Inhibition of catecholamine uptake	Very limited clinical use owing to dependence liability and risk of peripheral sympathomimetic effects. Some agents used as appetite suppressants. Mainly important as drugs of abuse.
	Cocaine	Inhibition of catecholamine uptake Local anaesthetic	Important as drug of abuse Occasionally used for ophthalmic anaesthesia (see Chapter 27)
	Methylxanthines eg: caffeine theophylline	Inhibition of phosphodiesterase Antagonism of adenosine (relevance of these actions to central effects is not clear)	Clinical uses related to stimulant activity, though caffeine is included in various 'tonics'. Theophylline used for action on cardiac and bronchial muscle. Constituents of beverages.
Psychotomimetic drugs (hallucinogens)			
	Lysergic acid diethylamide (LSD)	Mixed agonist/antagonist of serotonin receptors	No clinical use Important as drug of abuse
	Mescaline	Not known. Chemically similar to amphetamine	
	Psilocin	Chemically related to serotonin. Probably acts on serotonin receptors	
	Cannabis	Acts as CNS depressant with mild psychotomimetic effects	No established clinical use See Chapter 35
	Phencyclidine	Chemically similar to ketamine (see Chapter 20). Mechanism of action not known, but evidence of specific receptor binding.	Originally proposed as an anaesthetic, now important as drug of abuse

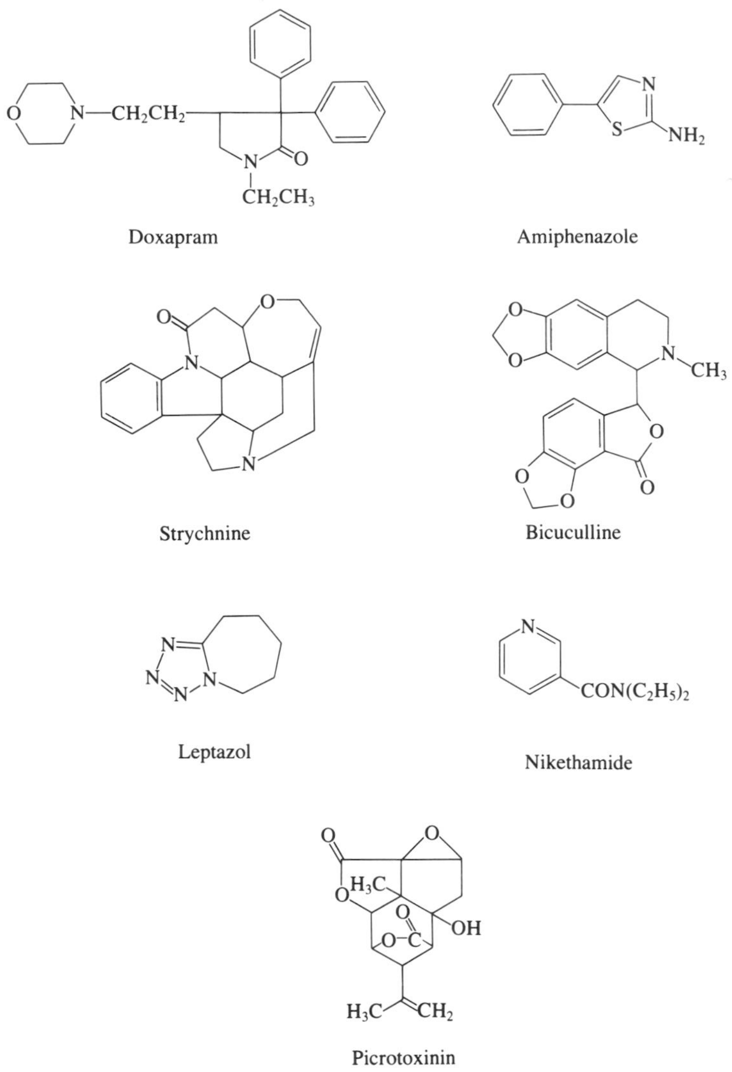

Fig. 26.1 Structures of convulsants and respiratory stimulants

petition at glycine receptors. The action of strychnine superficially resembles that of **tetanus toxin**, a protein neurotoxin produced by the anaerobic bacterium *Clostridium tetani*. Tetanus toxin reaches the spinal cord from a site of infection by being transported along the axons of sensory neurons. Its action on the inhibitory interneurons is to block the release of glycine. This is very similar to the action of a closely related toxin, botulinum toxin (see Chapter 6), which is produced by another bacterium of the *Clostridium* genus, and acts selectively to block transmitter release from cholinergic nerve terminals. In small doses strychnine causes a

measurable improvement in visual and auditory acuity; it was until quite recently included in various 'tonics', on the basis that CNS stimulation should restore the weary brain.

Bicuculline is another plant alkaloid, which somewhat resembles strychnine in its effects, but it acts by blocking the action of GABA rather than of glycine, probably also competitively. Its action is confined to $GABA_A$ receptors, which control chloride permeability, and it does not affect $GABA_B$ receptors (see Chapter 19). The main effects are on the brain rather than the spinal cord, and it has a different pattern of convulsant activity from that of strychnine. It is a useful experimental tool for studying GABA-mediated transmission, but has no clinical uses.

Picrotoxin (literally 'fish poison') is also a plant toxin. The active substance, **picrotoxinin**, acts similarly to bicuculline in that it blocks the action of GABA on chloride channels, though not competitively. Its name reflects its use as a means of incapacitating fish by throwing berries into the water. Picrotoxin, like bicuculline, causes convulsions and has no clinical uses, its use in treating barbiturate overdose having been discontinued.

Nikethamide and **leptazol** are pharmacologically very·similar, though their mode of action is unknown. They cause initial respiratory stimulation, and also raise blood pressure by acting on the brainstem, at doses somewhat lower than those which cause convulsions. Respiratory stimulation is short-lasting, and is followed by a period of depression. Inhibition of leptazol-induced convulsions by anticonvulsant drugs (see Chapter 24) correlates quite well with their effectiveness against petit mal epilepsy, and leptazol has occasionally been used diagnostically in man, since it can precipitate the typical EEG pattern of petit mal in susceptible patients.

Amiphenazole and **doxapram** are similar to the above drugs, but are claimed to have a bigger margin of safety between respiratory stimulation and convulsions. With doxapram this advantage is well established, but it nevertheless causes nausea, coughing and restlessness, which limit its usefulness. The action of doxapram is very brief, and it is normally given as an intravenous infusion, which allows the level of respiratory stimulation to be regulated continuously.

PSYCHOMOTOR STIMULANTS

Amphetamines and related drugs

Amphetamine, and its active dextro-isomer **dextroamphetamine** together with **methylamphetamine** and **methylphenidate** are a group of drugs with very similar pharmacological properties (Fig. 26.2). **Fenfluramine**, though chemically similar, has slightly different pharmacological effects. All of these drugs appear to act by releasing monoamines from nerve terminals in the brain. Noradrenaline and

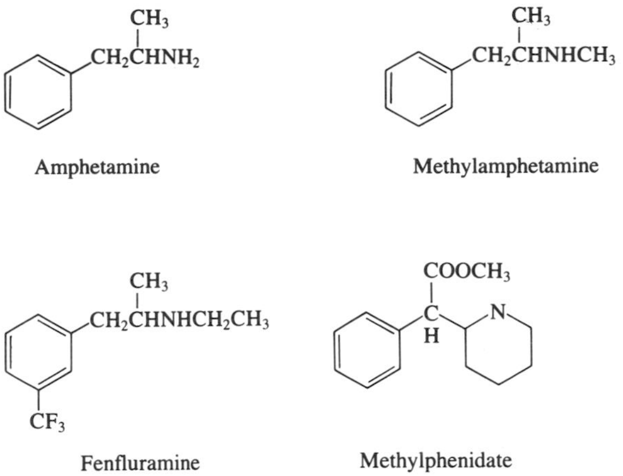

Fig. 26.2 Structures of amphetamines

dopamine are the most important mediators in this connection, but serotonin release may also play some part.

Pharmacological effects

The main central effects of amphetamine-like drugs are:

1. Locomotor stimulation
2. Alertness and euphoria.
3. Stereotyped behaviour
4. Anorexia.

In addition, amphetamines have peripheral sympathomimetic actions, manifest mainly as a rise in blood pressure and inhibition of gastrointestinal motility.

In experimental animals, amphetamines cause increased alertness and locomotor activity and increased grooming, and they also increase aggressive activity. On the other hand, systematic exploration of novel objects by unrestrained rats is reduced by amphetamine. The animals run around more, but appear less attentive to their surroundings. Studies of conditioned responses suggest that amphetamines increase the overall rate of responding without affecting the training process markedly. Thus, in a fixed interval schedule, where a reward for lever pressing is forthcoming only after a fixed interval (say 10 minutes) following the last reward, trained animals normally press the lever very infrequently in the first few minutes after the reward, and increase the rate towards the end of the 10 minutes interval when another reward is due. The effect of amphetamine is to increase the rate of unrewarded responses at the beginning of the 10 minute interval without affecting (or even reducing) the rate towards the end of the period. The effects of amphetamine on more sophisticated types of conditioned response, for example those involving discriminative tasks, are not clear-cut, and there is no clear evidence that either the rate of learning of such tasks, or the final level of performance that can be achieved, are affected by the drug. Crudely, it might be said that amphetamine tends to make animals busier rather than brighter.

With large doses of amphetamines, stereotyped behaviour occurs. This consists of repeated actions, such as licking, gnawing, rearing or repeated movements of the head and limbs. These activities are generally inappropriate to the environment, and with increasing doses of amphetamine they take over more and more of the behaviour of the animal, and the repertoire of stereotyped behaviour becomes at the same time more limited.

There is considerable evidence that these behavioural effects are produced by the release of catecholamines in the brain. Thus, treatment of newborn animals with 6-hydroxydopamine, which greatly depletes the brain of both noradrenaline and dopamine, abolishes the effect of amphetamine, as does pretreatment with α-methyltyrosine, an inhibitor of catecholamine biosynthesis (see Chapter 7). Tricyclic antidepressants (see Chapter 23) potentiate the effects of amphetamine, presumably by blocking noradrenaline reuptake. MAO inhibitors have a similar effect, resulting from an increase in the catecholamine content of the nerve terminals. Interestingly, reserpine, which inhibits vesicular storage of catecholamines and thus depletes nerve terminals of their catecholamine stores very markedly (see Chapter 7), does not block the behavioural effects of amphetamine. This is probably because amphetamine releases cytosolic rather than vesicular catecholamines (see Chapter 7). The behavioural effects of amphetamine are probably due mainly to release of dopamine rather than noradrenaline. The evidence for this is that destruction of the central noradrenergic bundle does not affect locomotor stimulation produced by amphetamine, whereas destruction of the dopamine-containing nucleus accumbens (see Chapter

19), or administration of neuroleptic drugs which antagonize dopamine (see Chapter 22), inhibits this response.

Amphetamine-like drugs cause marked anorexia, but with continued administration this effect wears off in a few days and food intake returns to normal. Amphetamine-like drugs differ in their relative activity in causing locomotor stimulation and in causing anorexia (Table 26.2). Fenfluramine, in particular, causes anorexia without stimulation (actually being somewhat sedative) and pharmacological studies suggest that this action may depend more on serotonin release than on release of noradrenaline or dopamine. The effect can be produced by local injection of amphetamine into the lateral hypothalamus.

In man, amphetamine causes euphoria; with intravenous injection, this can be so intense as to be described as 'orgasmic'. Subjects become confident, hyperactive and talkative, and sex drive is generally enhanced. Fatigue, both physical and mental, is reduced by amphetamine, and many studies have shown improvement of both mental and physical performance in fatigued, though not in well-rested subjects. Mental performance is improved for simple tedious tasks much more than for difficult tasks, and amphetamines have been used to improve the performance of soldiers, military pilots and others who need to remain alert under extremely fatiguing conditions. It has also been in vogue as a means of helping students to concentrate before and during examinations, but it is likely that the improvement caused by reduction of fatigue is offset by the mistakes of over-confidence. Amphetamine-like drugs bring about a measurable improvement of athletic performance, particularly in endurance events, and their illicit use in competitive athletics poses a considerable problem. Fortunately, most amphetamines are excreted in the urine, and are easily detected.

Table 26.2 Behavioural effects of amphetamines

	Locomotor stimulation	Sterotyped behaviour	Anorexia
Amphetamine	+ + +	+ + +	+ + +
Methylphenidate	+ + +	+ + +	+
Fenfluramine	—	—	+ + +

As appetite suppressants in man, for use in treating obesity, amphetamine derivatives have not been successful, mainly because their effectiveness is too short-lived, and the risk of producing dependence is too great. In any case, the cause of over-eating is usually psychological, and not simply a matter of continuing hunger, and is not readily amenable to drug treatment. Even fenfluramine, which does not readily cause dependence, is no longer used.

Tolerance and dependence

If amphetamine is taken repeatedly over the course of a few days, which occurs when users seek to maintain the euphoric 'high' that a single dose produces, a state of 'amphetamine psychosis' may develop, which is almost indistinguishable from an acute schizophrenia attack (see Chapter 22). Visual and auditory hallucinations occur, accompanied by paranoid symptoms and aggressive behaviour. At the same time, repetitive stereotyped behaviour may develop (e.g. polishing shoes, stringing beads). The close similarity of this condition to acute paranoid schizophrenia, and the effectiveness of neuroleptic drugs in controlling it, is consistent with the dopamine theory of schizophrenia discussed in Chapter 22. When the drug is stopped after a few days, there is usually a period of deep sleep, and on awakening the subject feels extremely lethargic, depressed and anxious (sometimes even suicidal), and is often very hungry. Even a single dose of amphetamine, which produces euphoria rather than acute psychotic symptoms, usually leaves the subject feeling tired and depressed. These after-effects may well be the result of depletion of the normal stores of noradrenaline and dopamine, but the evidence for this is not clearcut. A state of amphetamine-dependence can be produced in experimental animals; thus, rats quickly learn to press a lever in order to obtain a dose of amphetamine, and they also become inactive and irritable in the withdrawal phase. These effects do not occur with fenfluramine.

Tolerance develops rapidly to the peripheral sympathomimetic effects of amphetamine, and to its anorectic effect, but much more slowly to the other effects (locomotor stimulation and stereotyped behaviour). Dependence on amphetamine appears to be a consequence of the unpleasant after-effect that it produces, which leads to a desire for a repeat dose. There is no clearcut physical withdrawal syndrome such as occurs with opiates.

Pharmacokinetic aspects

Amphetamine is readily absorbed from the gastro-intestinal tract, and freely penetrates the blood-brain barrier. It does this more readily than other indirectly acting sympathomimetic amines such as ephedrine or tyramine (see Chapter 7), which probably explains why it produces more marked central effects than those drugs. Amphetamine is mainly excreted unchanged in the urine, and the rate of excretion is increased when the urine is made more acidic (see Fig. 3.16). Methylamphetamine is partly converted to amphetamine by hepatic metabolism. The plasma half-life of amphetamine varies from about 5 hours to 20–30 hours depending on urine flow and urinary pH.

Uses and unwanted effects

The uses of amphetamines are very few. Extensive trials have shown them to be ineffective in treating depression or obesity. One paradoxical use is in the treatment of **hyperkinetic children**, who are calmed by amphetamine and by methylphenidate. The mechanism by which this happens is unknown, but the use of amphetamines for treating so-called **minimal brain dysfunction** in children is widespread in some countries.

Narcolepsy is a disabling condition, probably a form of epilepsy, in which the patient suddenly and unpredictably falls asleep at frequent intervals during the day. Amphetamine is helpful but not completely effective.

The limited clinical usefulness of amphetamine is offset by its many unwanted effects, including hypertension, insomnia, tremors, risk of exacerbating schizophrenia and risk of dependence.

Cocaine

Cocaine is found in the leaves of a South American shrub, coca (unrelated to the cocoa plant). These leaves are used for their stimulant properties by natives of South America, particularly those living at high altitude in the Andes. It appears that cocaine improves their ability to work at high altitude without excessive fatigue. Considerable mystical significance was attached to the powers of cocaine to boost the flagging human spirit, and Freud experimented with it on his patients. As a result of Freud's experiments with cocaine, his ophthalmologist colleague, Koller, obtained supplies of the drug and discovered its local anaesthetic action (see Chapter 27), but the psychostimulant effects of cocaine have not proved to be clinically useful.

Cocaine is a potent inhibitor of catecholamine uptake by noradrenergic nerve terminals (Uptake 1; see Chapter 7), and strongly enhances the effects of sympathetic nerve activity. This occurs also in the brain, and it is likely that its psychomotor stimulant effect depends on this mechanism. The effect of cocaine closely resembles that of amphetamine, causing euphoria, garrulousness and increased motor activity. With excessive dosage, tremors and convulsions, followed by respiratory and vasomotor depression, may occur, but cocaine does not cause stereotyped behaviour or produce delusions, hallucinations and paranoia in the same way as amphetamines. The peripheral sympathomimetic actions lead to tachycardia, vasoconstriction and an increase in blood pressure. Body temperature may increase, owing to the increased motor activity coupled with reduced heat loss. Like amphetamine, cocaine produces no clear-cut physical dependence syndrome, but tends to cause depression and dysphoria following the initial stimulant effect, which can result in a considerable degree of psychological dependence. The duration of action of cocaine (about 30 minutes when given intravenously) is much shorter than that of amphetamine.

Cocaine is still used topically as a local anaesthetic, mainly in ophthalmology, but has no other clinical uses. It is a valuable pharmacological tool for the study of catecholamine release and reuptake, because of its relatively specific action in blocking Uptake 1. Cocaine has been used for centuries for its psychomotor stimulant effects, the usual route of administration being nasal inhalation. This can result in necrosis of the nasal septum, due to the prolonged vasoconstriction. In recent years the use of cocaine by the drug subculture of the Western world has increased sharply.

Methylxanthines

Various beverages, particularly tea, coffee and cocoa, contain methylxanthines to which they owe their mild central stimulant effects. The main compounds responsible are **caffeine** and **theophylline** (see Fig. 13.3). The nuts of the cola plant also contain caffeine, which is present in cola-flavoured soft drinks. By far the most important sources, however, are coffee and tea, which account for more than 90% of caffeine consumption. Among adults in tea and coffee drinking countries the average daily caffeine consumption is about 200 mg. Further information on the pharmacology and toxicology of caffeine is presented by Dews (1984).

Pharmacological effects

Methylxanthines have the following major pharmacological actions:

1. CNS stimulation
2. Diuresis (see Chapter 14)
3. Stimulation of cardiac muscle (see Chapter 10)
4. Relaxation of smooth muscle, especially bronchial muscle (see Chapter 13).

The latter two effects resemble those of β-adrenoceptor stimulation (see Chapter 7). This is thought to be because methylxanthines (especially theophylline) inhibit the enzyme, phosphodiesterase, which is responsible for the intercellular metabolism of cAMP. They thus increase intracellular cAMP and produce effects that, in general, mimic those of mediators that stimulate adenylate cyclase. Theophylline also antagonizes some of the effects of adenosine (see Chapter 11), and it is possible, but unproven, that some of its effects result from this mechanism (Snyder, 1984). However, its bronchodilator effect in asthma may not be due to either of these mechanisms (see Chapter 13). The diuretic effect probably also results from vasodilation of the afferent glomerular arteriole, causing an increased glomerular filtration rate.

Caffeine and theophylline have very similar stimulant effects on the central nervous system. Human subjects experience a reduction of fatigue, leading to insomnia, with improved concentration and a clearer flow of thought. This is confirmed by objective studies which have shown that caffeine reduces reaction time, and produces an increase in the speed at which simple calculations can be performed (though without much improvement in accuracy). Performance at motor tasks, such as typing and simulated driving, is also improved, particularly in fatigued subjects. Mental tasks, such as syllable-learning, association tests, etc, are also facilitated by moderate doses (up to about 200 mg caffeine, or about 3 cups of coffee) but inhibited by larger doses. By comparison with amphetamines, methylxanthines produce less locomotor stimulation, and do not induce euphoria, stereotyped behaviour patterns, or a psychotic state, but their effects on fatigue and mental function are rather similar.

Tolerance and habituation develop to a small extent, but much less than with amphetamines.

Uses and unwanted effects

There are few clinical uses for caffeine. It is included with aspirin in some preparations for treating headaches and other aches and pains, and with ergotamine in some anti-migraine preparations, the object being to produce a mildly agreeable sense of alertness. Theophylline is used mainly as a bronchodilator in treating severe asthmatic attacks (see Chapter 13).

Caffeine has few unwanted side effects, and is safe even in very large doses. *In vitro* tests show that it has a slight mutagenic effect, and there is evidence that large doses are teratogenic in animals, but so far epidemiological studies have not revealed any carcinogenic or teratogenic effect of tea or coffee drinking in man (Haynes & Collins, 1984; Leviton, 1984).

PSYCHOTOMIMETIC DRUGS

Psychotomimetic drugs (also referred to as **psychodelic** or **hallucinogenic** drugs) are characterized by the fact that they affect thought, perception and mood, without causing marked psychomotor stimulation or depression. Thoughts and per-

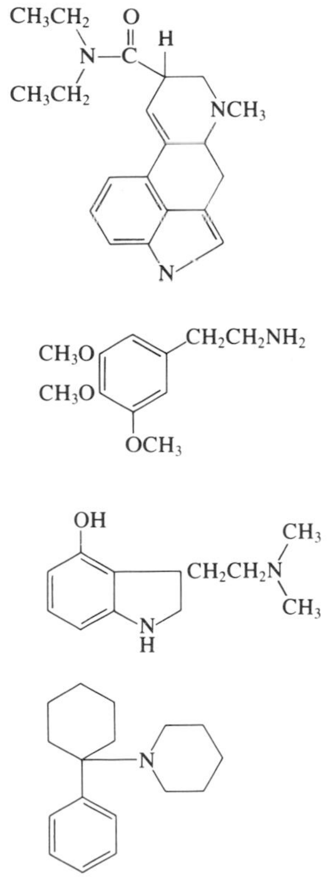

Lysergic acid diethylamide (LSD)

Mescaline

Psilocin

Phencyclidine

Fig. 26.3 Structures of some psychotomimetic drugs

ceptions tend to become distorted and dream-like, rather than being merely sharpened or dulled, and the change in mood is likewise more complex than a simple shift in the direction of euphoria or depression. Not surprisingly, the categorization of these drugs is very imprecise, and there is no sharp dividing line between the effects of, say, cocaine and those of LSD or cannabis.

Psychotomimetic drugs fall broadly into two groups (Fig. 26.3):

1. Those with a chemical resemblance to known neurotransmitters (catecholamines or serotonin). These include **LSD**, **psilocin** and **bufotenin**, which are related to serotonin; and **mescaline**, which is similar in structure to amphetamine.
2. Drugs unrelated to monoamine neurotransmitters, e.g. **cannabis**, **phenycyclidine**.

LSD, psilocin and mescaline

LSD is an exceptionally potent psychotomimetic drug, capable of producing very marked effects in man in doses less than $1\,\mu g/kg$. It is a chemical derivative of lysergic acid, which occurs in the cereal fungus, ergot (see Chapter 7), and was first synthesized by Hoffman in 1943. Hoffman deliberately swallowed about $250\,\mu g$ of LSD, and wrote 30 years later of the experience: 'the faces of those around me appeared as grotesque coloured masks...marked motoric unrest, alternating with paralysis...heavy feeling in the head, limbs and entire body, as if they were filled with lead...clear recognition of my condition, in which state I sometimes observed, in the manner of an independent observer, that I shouted half insanely'. These effects lasted for a few hours, after which Hoffman fell asleep 'and awoke next morning feeling perfectly well'. In spite of its dramatic psychological effects, LSD has few other actions, and is remarkably non-toxic, though it may have serious long-term psychological effects (see below). Mescaline, which is derived from a Mexican cactus and has been known as a hallucinogenic agent for many centuries, was made famous by Aldous Huxley in 'The Doors of Perception'. Psilocin comes from a fungus (in the form of the free acid and the phosphate ester, **psilocybin**), and has very similar properties. Both have basically similar effects to LSD but are much less potent.

The main effects of these drugs are on mental function, most notably an alteration of perception in such a way that sights and sounds appear distorted and fantastic. Hallucinations—visual, auditory, tactile or olfactory—also occur, and sensory modalities may become confused, so that sounds are perceived as visions. Thought processes tend to become illogical and disconnected, but subjects generally retain insight into the fact that their disturbance is drug-induced. Occasionally, LSD produces a syndrome that is extremely disturbing to the subject (the 'bad trip') in which the hallucinatory experience takes on a menacing quality, and may be accompanied by paranoid delusions. This sometimes goes so far as to produce homicide or suicide attempts, and in many respects, the state has much in common with acute schizophrenic illness. The main effects of psychotomimetic drugs are subjective, so it is not surprising that animal tests which reliably predict psychotomimetic activity in man have not been devised. Attempts to measure changes in perception by behavioural conditioning studies have given variable results, but some authors have claimed that effects consistent with increased sensory 'generalization' (i.e. a tendency to respond similarly to any sensory stimulus) can be detected in this way. One of the more bizarre tests involves disorganization of web-spinning patterns in spiders, whose normal elegantly symmetrical webs become jumbled and erratic if the animals are treated with LSD.

Neither LSD nor other psychotomimetic agents (except for phencyclidine; see below) are self-administered by animals under conditions where the animals can control the injection by pressing a lever. Indeed, they can be shown to have aversive rather than reinforcing properties in behavioural tests, which stands in marked contrast to most of the drugs that are widely abused by humans. Tolerance to the effects of LSD develops quite quickly, and there is cross-tolerance between it and most other psychotomimetics. There is no physical withdrawal syndrome in animals or man.

In peripheral tissues, LSD acts as an antagonist at serotonin receptors, but in the central nervous system it is believed to work mainly as an agonist.

Neurophysiological studies (Aghajanian, 1981)

show that LSD directly inhibits the firing of serotonin-containing neurons in the raphe nuclei (see Chapter 19), apparently by acting as a serotonin-like agonist on the inhibitory auto-receptors of these cells. The action of mescaline is apparently different, however, and exerted mainly on noradrenergic neurons; it is still quite unclear how changes in cell firing rates might be related to the psychotomimetic action of these drugs.

There has been much concern over reports that LSD and other psychotomimetic drugs, as well as causing potentially dangerous 'bad trips', can lead to more persistent mental disorder. There are recorded instances in which altered perception and hallucinations have lasted for up to 3 weeks following a single dose of LSD, and also reports of a persistent state resembling paranoid schizophrenia, which responds to antipsychotic drugs but may recur later. It is not at all clear whether this is due to a long-term effect of LSD, or whether LSD-taking is more likely in subjects destined to develop schizophrenia. The cautious view must be that LSD is causative. This, coupled with the fact that the occasional 'bad trip' can result in severe injury through violent behaviour, means that LSD and other psychotomimetics must be regarded as highly dangerous drugs, far removed from the image of peaceful 'experience enhancers' that the hippy subculture of the 1960s so enthusiastically espoused.

Phencyclidine

Phencyclidine (see Fig. 26.4) was originally synthesized as a possible intravenous anaesthetic agent, but was found to produce in many patients a period of disorientation and hallucinations following recovery of consciousness. Ketamine (see Chapter 20), which is a close chemical relative of phenycyclidine, is better as an anaesthetic, though it too can cause symptoms of disorientation. Phencyclidine is now of interest mainly because of its popularity (particularly in USA) as a drug of abuse, and because of some intriguing problems raised by its mode of action and possible relationship to schizophrenia (Henderson, 1982).

The effects of phencyclidine are generally very similar to those of other psychotomimetic drugs, but also include analgesia, which was one of the reasons for its introduction as an anaesthetic agent. It has the same reported tendency as LSD to cause occasional 'bad trips' and to lead to recurrent psychotic episodes. Its mode of action at a cellular level is not understood, but binding studies with radio-labelled phencyclidine suggest that specific high affinity binding sites occur on neuronal membranes, particularly in the frontal cortex and hippocampus. It is possible that this binding site is identical to the σ opiate receptor (see Chapter 25), which is believed by some authors to mediate the effects of dysphoria and hallucinations produced by certain opiates. Since phencyclidine, unlike LSD and other psychotomimetics, does not seem to act directly on monoamine-mediated transmission, the question arises whether there may be an endogenous ligand for the phencyclidine binding site, and whether such a substance might be involved in the causation of schizophrenia.

REFERENCES AND FURTHER READING

Aghajanian G K 1981 Neurophysiologic properties of psychotomimetics. In: Hoffmeister R, Stille G (eds) Handbook of Experimental Pharmacology 55(2): 89–110

Appel J B, Poling A D, Kuhn D M 1981 Psychotomimetics: behavioural pharmacology. In: Hoffmeister R, Stille G (eds) Handbook of Experimental Pharmacology 55 (3): 46–56

Dews P B (ed) 1984 Caffeine. Springer, Berlin

Estler C-J 1981 Caffeine. In: Hoffmeister R, Stille G (eds) Handbook of Experimental Pharmacology 55 (3): 369–390

Freedman D X, Boggan W O 1981 Biochemical pharmacology of psychotomimetics. In: Hoffmeister R, Stille G (eds) Handbook of Experimental Pharmacology 55 (3): 57–88

Garattini S, Samanin R 1981 The pharmacological profile of some psychomotor stimulant drugs, including chemical, neurophysiological biochemical and toxicological aspects. In: Hoffmeister R, Stille G (eds) Handbook of Experimental Pharmacology 55 (2): 545–586

Haynes R H, Collins J D B 1984 The mutagenic potential of caffeine. In: Dews P B (ed) Caffeine. Springer, Berlin

Henderson G 1982 Phenylcyclidine, a widely used but little understood psychotomimetic agent. TIPS 3: 248–250

Hofmann A 1983 A Handbook of Drug and Alcohol Abuse, 2nd Ed. Oxford University Press, New York

Hollister L E 1981 Pharmacology and toxicology of psychotomimetics. In: Hoffmeister R, Stille G (eds) Handbook of Experimental Pharmacology 55 (3): 31–44

Leviton A 1984 Epidemiologic studies of birth defects. In: Dews P B (ed) Caffeine. Springer, Berlin

Schuster C R 1981 The behavioural pharmacology of psychomotor stimulant drugs. In: Hoffmeister R, Stille G (eds) Handbook of Experimental Pharmacology 55 (2): 587–606

Snyder S H 1984 Adenosine as a mediator of the behavioral effects of xanthines. In: Dews P B (ed) Caffeine. Springer, Berlin

Local anaesthetics and other drugs that affect excitable membranes

The property of electrical excitability is what enables the membranes of nerve and muscle cells to generate propagated action potentials, which are essential for communication in the nervous system, and for the initiation of mechanical activity in cardiac and striated muscle. Electrical excitability depends on the existence of voltage-dependent ion channels in the cell membrane, most importantly on Na^+ channels that are gated in such a way that they open, and the membrane becomes selectively permeable to Na^+, when the membrane is depolarized. Of somewhat less importance are the voltage-dependent K^+ channels, which function in basically the same way, but whose properties vary considerably among different types of cell.

It is known from patch clamp recordings (see Chapter 1) that the channels are discrete structures which switch rapidly between the open and closed states, much like the receptor-operated channels discussed in Chapter 1. The difference is that the gating of the channels of excitable membranes is controlled by membrane potential rather than by binding of a transmitter molecule to a receptor.

In this chapter we discuss the various ways in which drugs and other agents can affect the functioning of these ion channels. There are, broadly speaking, two ways in which channel function may be modified, namely **block** of the channels and **modification of gating behaviour**. Either mechanism can cause an increase or a decrease of electrical excitability. Thus, blocking Na^+ channels reduces excitability, whereas block of K^+ channels tends to increase it. Similarly, an agent that affects Na^+ channel gating in such a way as to increase the probability of a channel being open will tend to increase excitability, and *vice versa*.

The most important group of drugs discussed in this chapter are the **local anaesthetics**, which act mainly by blocking Na^+ channels (though they secondarily modify Na^+ channel gating; see below). Also in the category of Na^+ channel blockers are the **class I antidysrhythmic drugs** (see Chapter 10), certain anticonvulsants, such as **phenytoin** (see Chapter 24) and two neurotoxins, **tetrodotoxin** and **saxitoxin**, which are extremely potent and selective Na^+ channel blocking agents.

The only important drugs known to affect K^+ channel function do so by blocking the channels. One of thesse agents, **4-aminopyridine**, has limited clinical use because of its facilitatory action on neuromuscular transmission.

In this chapter a brief discussion of the function of Na^+ and K^+ channels in excitable membranes is presented, followed by descriptions of individual drugs, with the main emphasis being given to local anaesthetics.

Na^+ AND K^+ CHANNELS OF EXCITABLE MEMBRANES

Our present understanding of the mechanism of electrical excitability, by which is meant the ability of a cell to generate a short-lasting, all-or-nothing depolarization (known as an action potential) in response to electrical stimulation, rests firmly on the work of Hodgkin, Huxley & Katz published in 1949–52. Before then it had been recognized that the resting cell membrane was selectively permeable to K^+, that the potential of the interior of the cell at rest was negative to the outside by some 60–90 mV, and that the action potential was associated with a large increase in membrane conductance. Hodgkin and his colleagues, in a remarkable tour de force (at a time when valve-operated amplifiers, and even oscilloscopes, had to be painstakingly designed and built, powered often by banks of car batteries to provide adequate electrical stability) devised the voltage clamp technique and applied it successfully to study the mechanism of action potential generation in the squid giant axon. Many excellent accounts of these experiments and their outcome are available (Katz, 1966; Hodgkin, 1967; Kuffler et al, 1984; Hille, 1984). Briefly, their analysis showed that the action potential is generated by the interplay of two separate ionic permeability changes: an increase in Na^+ permeability, which occurs rapidly but transiently when the membrane is depolarized beyond about $-50\,mV$; and an increase in K^+ permeability which develops more slowly but is sustained. Because of the inequality of Na^+ and K^+ concentrations on the two sides of the membrane, an increase in Na^+ permeability causes an inward current of Na^+ ions, whereas an increase in K^+ permeability causes an outward current. The sepa-

rate nature of these two currents was established by Hodgkin & Huxley by ion-substitution experiments, but can be most clearly demonstrated by the use of Na^+ and K^+ channel blocking drugs, as shown in Figure 27.1. The records in Figure 27.1 show the currents that flow through the membrane of a single node of Ranvier of a frog axon when the membrane potential is suddenly stepped from $-120\,mV$ to a more depolarized level. Stepping to $-45\,mV$ produces a transient inward current which decays in about 10 ms. With larger depolarizations, this inward current gets smaller, and a later, sustained outward current is seen. If the membrane is depolarized even further, the transient current reverses in direction. This happens when the internal potential is made positive to the sodium equilibrium potential (E_{Na}), which is a function of the intracellular and extracellular Na concentrations, and is about $+40\,mV$ under normal conditions. The explanation for this behaviour is that the sodium current at any moment depends on two

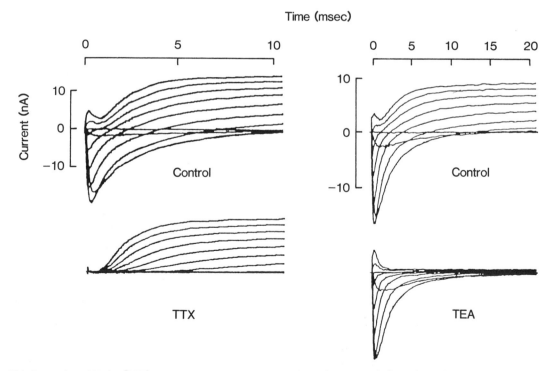

Fig. 27.1 Separation of Na^+ and K^+ currents in nerve membrane. Voltage clamp records from the node of Ranvier of a single frog nerve fibre. At time 0 the membrane potential was stepped to a depolarized level, ranging from $-60\,mV$ (lower trace in each series) to $+60\,mV$ (upper trace in each series) in 15 mV steps. Inward current is shown as a downward deflection.
   Top panels. Control records from two fibres. *Bottom panels.* Left: Effect of TTX—abolition of Na^+ currents: Right: Effect of TEA—abolition of K^+ currents. (From: Hille, 1970)

factors: (a) the state of **activation** of the channels (i.e. the fraction of channels that is open), which is a function of both membrane potential and time; and (b) the **driving force for Na$^+$ ions** (which is equal to $E_m - E_{Na}$). At potentials negative to about -60 mV no channels are activated, so no current flows. Between about -50 mV and -30 mV (the activation range for Na$^+$ channels) the channels change from zero to 100% open. With further depolarization, the peak current decreases because, though activation is 100%, $E_m - E_{Na}$ decreases. When the membrane is made more positive than E_{Na} (normally about $+40$ mV) the driving force changes in direction and the current flows outward. The Na$^+$ current can be seen uncontaminated by K$^+$ current (Fig. 27.1) if the K$^+$ channels are blocked with **tetraethylammonium** (see below). The Na$^+$ current is transient, even if the membrane depolarization is sustained, and decays to zero in

5–10 ms. This spontaneous closure of the channels is known as **inactivation**, and it is an important property of the Na channel. In the initiation or propagation of a nerve impulse (Fig. 27.2), the first event is a small depolarization of the membrane, which may be produced by transmitter action or by the approach of an action potential passing along the axon. This causes activation of the Na$^+$ channels, allowing an inward current of Na$^+$ ions to flow, which depolarizes the membrane still further. The process is thus a regenerative one, and the increase in Na$^+$ permeability is enough to bring the membrane potential close to E_{Na}. This depolarization is short-lasting because of the rapid inactivation of the Na$^+$ channels, which causes the inward current to decrease and the membrane potential to return to normal. Hodgkin & Huxley interpreted this behaviour of the Na$^+$ channels by postulating two kinds of gate controlling the chan-

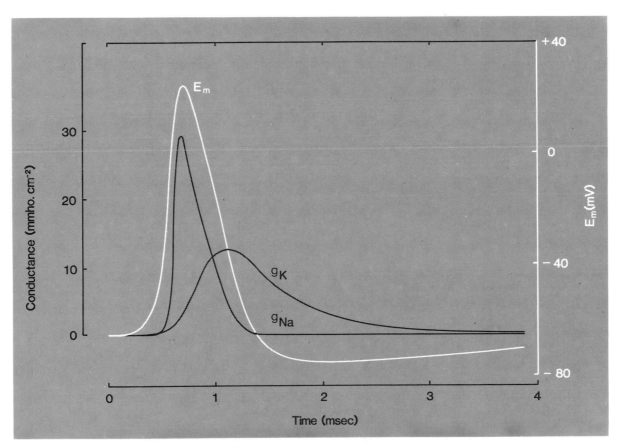

Fig. 27.2 Behaviour of Na$^+$ and K$^+$ channels during a conducted action potential. Rapid opening of Na$^+$ channels occurs during the action potential upstroke. Delayed opening of K$^+$ channels, and inactivation of Na$^+$ channels, causes repolarization.

nel, termed *m* and *h* gates. At the resting potential the *m* gates are all closed, and the *h* gates mainly open. On depolarization the *m* gates open rapidly, so that the channel conducts, and the *h* gates close, but more slowly, causing the channel to close again. On repolarization the *m* gates quickly close, and the *h* gates more slowly open. It is only after the *h* gates have re-opened that the channel is once more available for activation by depolarization and the time that this takes accounts for the refractory period of the nerve or muscle cell.

The voltage-sensitivity of these gates is due to the presence of charged regions of the channel protein, which has recently been purified and fully sequenced by gene cloning (see Catterall, 1985). Because the membrane is very thin, the membrane potential produces a very large electric field within the membrane, and changes in the strength of this field cause charged regions of the channel protein to move. This charge movement can be recorded directly, as **gating currents** (see review: Armstrong, 1981) if the ionic currents through the channel, which are much larger, are suppressed.

In many types of cell, including most nerve cells, the process of repolarization is assisted by the opening of voltage-dependent K^+ channels. These function in much the same way as Na^+ channels (i.e. they open when the cell is depolarized) but differ in two important ways. Firstly their activation kinetics are about 10 times slower; secondly, they do not inactivate appreciably. This means that the K^+ channels open later than the Na^+ channels (Fig. 27.2). Owing to the high intracellular and low extracellular K^+ concentrations, E_K is about $-100\,mV$, so that opening K^+ channels causes an outward (repolarizing) current, which occurs later than the Na^{++} current, and contributes to the rapid termination of the action potential. The behaviour of the Na^+ and K^+ channels during an action potential is shown in Figure 27.2, and an overall scheme showing the various regulatory processes and sites of drug action is shown in Figure 27.3.

Drugs that affect Na^+ channels

Many drugs are known that block voltage-sensitive Na^+ channels and thereby make it more difficult, or impossible, for an action potential to be produced. The most important group of drugs in this category are the local anaesthetics. In addition, various anti-

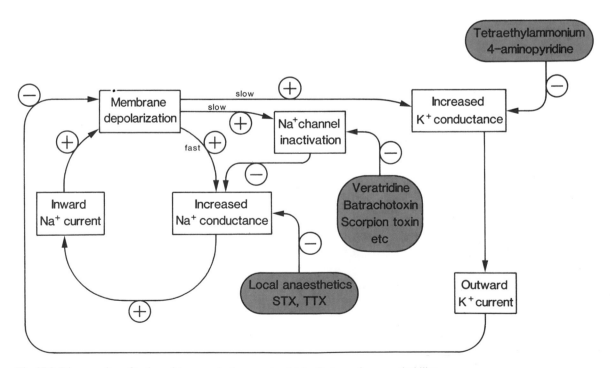

Fig. 27.3 Diagram sites of action of drugs and other agents which affect membrane excitability.

convulsant drugs (see Chapter 24) and anti-dys-rhythmic drugs (namely those belonging to class I; see Chapter 10) also work by blocking Na^+ channels. There is also a group of **neurotoxins**, exemplified by **tetrodotoxin (TTX)** and **saxitoxin (STX)** which are the most potent agents known for blocking these channels.

The second way in which drugs and toxins may affect Na^+ channel function is by modifying gating. The aspect of gating that is most susceptible to drug-induced modification is inactivation (the process whereby the Na^+ channels close, having initi-

ally opened, when the membrane is depolarized; see previous section). Various agents prevent or retard this process, and thereby cause the membrane to become hyperexcitable, so that spontaneous action potentials may be generated, or a single stimulus may produce a long train of action potentials.

Local anaesthetics

History

Though coca leaves have been consumed by South

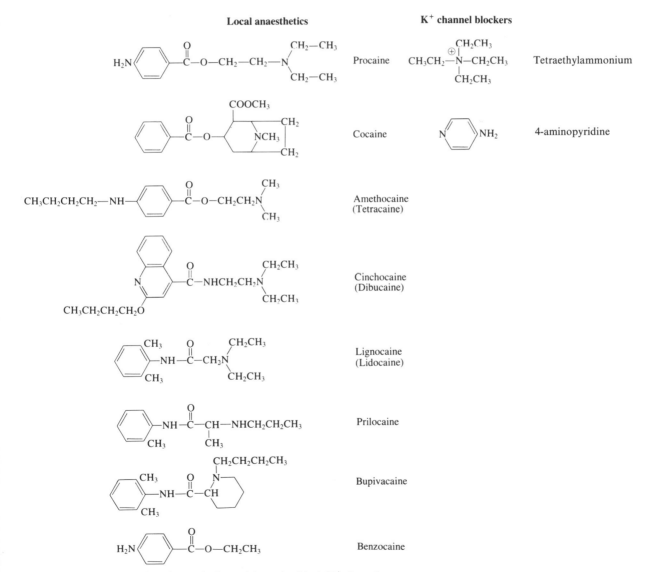

Fig. 27.4 Structures of local anaesthetics and drugs that block K^+ channels.

American Indians for thousands of years, and the numbing effect of chewing these leaves on the mouth and tongue was well known, it was not until 1884 that cocaine was proposed as a local anaesthetic for surgical procedures. Cocaine was isolated from coca leaves in 1860, and was shown to block the effects of sensory stimulation in frogs. Anrep in 1880 reported that cocaine injected under the skin caused a reversible loss of sensation, and suggested that this could be clinically useful, but the idea was not then taken up. Sigmund Freud sought to make use of its 'psychic energizing' power, reported by the users of coca leaves in the Andes (see Chapter 26), for psychiatric purposes. This was not a success, but his friend and ophthalmologist colleague in Vienna, Carl Koller, obtained some cocaine from Freud and showed in 1884 that reversible corneal anaesthesia could be produced by dropping cocaine into the eye. This time the idea was rapidly taken up, and within a few years cocaine anaesthesia was introduced into dentistry and general surgery. Efforts to find a synthetic substitute produced procaine in 1905, and many other useful compounds since then.

Chemical aspects

Local anaesthetic molecules are built on a simple chemical plan, consisting of an aromatic part linked by an ester or amide bond to a basic side-chain (Fig. 27.4). The only exception is **benzocaine**, a rather unusual local anaesthetic which has no basic group. All other local anaesthetics are weak bases, with pK_a values mainly in the range 8–9, so that they are mainly, but not completely, ionized at physiological pH. This is important in relation to their ability to penetrate the nerve sheath and axon membrane, and quaternary derivatives, which are fully ionized irrespective of pH, are ineffective as local anaesthetics (see below). Because local anaesthetic molecules consist of a hydrophobic aromatic group linked to a hydrophilic basic group they tend to accumulate at aqueous/non-aqueous interfaces (i.e. they show surface-tension lowering activity). It has been proposed that this is important for their biological activity (Skou, 1961), and that these drugs act in a similar way to volatile general anaesthetics (see Chapter 20) by expanding the volume of the cell membrane and interfering non-specifically with ion channel function. Recent evidence, however, sug-

gests a more specific interaction with Na^+ channels (see below).

The presence of the ester or amide bond in local anaesthetic molecules is important because of its susceptibility to metabolic hydrolysis. The ester-containing compounds are usually inactivated in the plasma and tissues (mainly liver) by non-specific esterases. Amides are much more stable, and these anaesthetics generally have longer plasma half-lives.

Mechanism of action

Local anaesthetics block the initiation and propagation of action potentials by preventing the voltage-dependent increase in Na^+ conductance (see Fig. 27.3). They appear to act in two main ways: (1) by acting non-specifically on membranes by virtue of their surface activity, somewhat in the manner of volatile anaesthetics; and (2) by specifically plugging Na^+ channels.

The evidence for the former mechanism comes mainly from structure-activity relationships, which suggest that surface activity is an important determinant of biological activity; from evidence that local anaesthetics (in sufficient concentration) affect various membrane functions, not only Na^+ conductance; and from the observation that local anaesthesia can be partly reversed by raising the hydrostatic pressure (as with volatile anaesthetics; see Chapter 20)—which can be interpreted to mean that volume expansion of the membrane plays a part in affecting function. It seems likely that this type of non-specific effect is significant for some local anaesthetics (especially benzocaine) but that Na^+ channel block is predominant for most. In favour of the Na^+ channel hypothesis is a considerable body of voltage clamp data on vertebrate and squid nerve (Hille, 1984). Understanding was held up for many years by the observation that local anaesthetic activity is strongly pH-dependent, being increased at alkaline pH (i.e. when the proportion of ionized molecules is low) and vice versa. This was first taken to mean that the uncharged molecule was the biologically active species, but it was later shown (Ritchie & Greengard, 1966) that this pH-dependence was reversed if the connective tissue sheath surrounding the nerve fibres was removed, implying that the uncharged species was required to penetrate the sheath, but that the cationic species might be the biologically active one. This seemed plausible, except for the fact that, even on desheathed preparations, quaternary derivatives of local anaesthetics, which are obligatorily charged, are inactive. Studies on squid axons, which can be perfused *internally* with drug solutions, as well as being exposed to them externally (Narahashi & Frazier, 1971) resolved the problem by showing that it is indeed the cationic species that is active, but that it works from the inner, rather than the outer, surface of the membrane. Thus quaternary local anaesthetics are extremely effective when applied from the inside, but ineffective from the outside because they do not penetrate the membrane. Conventional local anaesthetics, which are tertiary or secondary amines, penetrate the sheath and the axonal membrane in the uncharged form, but act from the inner surface of the axonal membrane in the cationic form (Fig. 27.5).

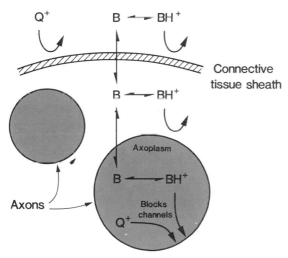

Fig. 27.5 Tissue penetration and action of local anaesthetics. A typical local anaesthetic is a weak base, of which the uncharged species (B) penetrates the nerve sheath and the axonal membrane to reach the Na$^+$ channels, which are blocked by the charged species (BH$^+$). Since BH$^+$ itself cannot cross these barriers, increasing the acidity of the external solution, which favours ionization, reduces the effectiveness of the drug. Quaternary derivatives of local anaesthetics (Q$^+$), which can exist only as cations, do not work when applied from outside the nerve fibre, but can block channels if, under experimental conditions, they are introduced directly into the axoplasm.

Further analysis of local anaesthetic action (Strichartz, 1973; Hille, 1977) has shown that many drugs show the property of 'use-dependent' block of

Na$^+$ channels, as well as affecting, to some extent, the gating of the channels. Use dependence means that the more the channels are opened, the greater the block becomes. It is a prominent feature of the action of many class I antidysrhythmic drugs (see Chapter 10), and occurs because the blocking molecule reaches its site of action within the channel only, or much more readily, when the channel is open. With quaternary local anaesthetics applied to the inside of the membrane, Strichartz showed clearly that the channels had to be cycled through their open state a few times before the blocking effect appeared. With tertiary local anaesthetics, on the other hand, block can develop even if the channels are not open, and it is likely that the blocking molecule (uncharged) can enter the channel directly from the membrane phase without having to enter the cell and enter the channel via the open gate (Fig. 27.6). The relative importance of thse two blocking pathways—the hydrophobic pathway via the membrane, and the hydrophilic pathway via the inner mouth of the channel—varies according to the lipid solubility of the drug, and the amount of use-dependence varies correspondingly.

As discussed earlier, the channel can exist in three functional states—resting, open and inactivated—defined by the states of the *m* and *h* gates. Hille has shown that many local anaesthetics bind most strongly to the inactivated state of the channel. Thus, in the presence of the drug there will be, at any given membrane potential, a larger proportion of channels which will be inactivated than would be the case normally, and this factor —modification of the gating of the channel —contributes to the overall blocking effect.

In general, local anaesthetics block conduction in small diameter nerve fibres more readily than in large fibres. However, the smallest fibres in peripheral nerve are unmyelinated C-fibres and these are rather less susceptible than the smallest myelinated (Aδ) fibres. Since nociceptive impulses are carried by Aδ- and C-fibres, pain sensation is blocked more readily than other sensory modalities (touch, proprioception etc). Motoneuron axons, being large in diameter, are also relatively resistant. The differences in sensitivity among different nerve fibres, though easily measured experimentally, is not large enough to be of much practical importance, and it is rarely possible to produce a block of

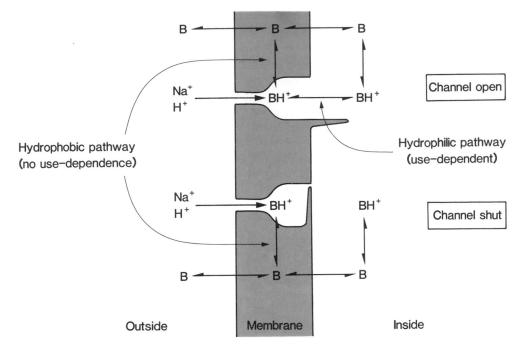

Fig. 27.6 Interaction of local anaesthetics with Na^+ channels. The blocking site within the channel can be reached via the open channel gate on the inner surface of the membrane by the charged species, BH^+ (hydrophilic pathway), or directly from the membrane by the uncharged species, B (hydrophobic pathway).

pain sensation without affecting other modalities. There is no inherent difference between the susceptibility of motor and sensory nerves to local anaesthetics.

Effects of local anaesthetics on other physiological systems

The main systems affected, apart from peripheral nerve, are the central nervous and cardiovascular systems, and these effects are important because they constitute the main source of hazard when local anaesthetics are used clinically.

The effect of all local anaesthetics on the central nervous system is, paradoxically, to cause stimulation. This produces restlessness and tremor, with subjective effects ranging from euphoria to extreme agitation. The tremor can progress to actual convulsions, which are followed by a period of central nervous system depression. The main threat to life comes from respiratory depression in this post-convulsive phase. Different local anaesthetics vary somewhat in their effects on the central nervous system. Thus, **cocaine** (see Chapter 26) produces marked euphoria at doses well below those that cause convulsions; this is probably because of its specific effect on monoamine uptake, which is not shared by other local anaesthetics. **Procaine** is particularly liable to produce unwanted central effects, which is one reason for its replacement in clinical use by agents such as **lignocaine** and **prilocaine**, whose central effects are much less pronounced.

The cardiovascular effects of local anaesthetics are due mainly to myocardial depression and vasodilatation. Reduction of myocardial contractility probably results indirectly from a partial inhibition of the Na^+ current in cardiac muscle (see Chapter 10). Reduced Na^+ entry, by blocking Na^+ channels, leads to a decrease of $[Na]_i$, which in turn reduces intracellular Ca^{++} stores (the opposite of the effect of cardiac glycosides; see Chapter 10), and this reduces the force of contraction. The antidysrhythmic effect of some local anaesthetics (especially lignocaine) is clinically useful.

Vasodilatation is due partly to a direct effect on vascular smooth muscle, and partly to inhibition of the sympathetic nervous system, both centrally and at the ganglionic level. It affects mainly arterioles. The combined effect of myocardial depression and vasodilatation is to cause a fall in blood pressure, which may be sudden and life-threatening. Cocaine is an exception in respect of its cardiovascular effects because of its ability to inhibit noradrenaline reuptake (see Chapter 7). This produces an enhancement of sympathetic activity, leading to tachycardia, increased cardiac output, vasoconstriction and increased arterial pressure.

Unwanted effects

Though local anaesthetics are usually administered in such a way as to minimise their spread to other parts of the body, they are ultimately absorbed into the systemic circulation. They may also be injected into veins or arteries by accident. The most dangerous unwanted effects result from actions on the central nervous and cardiovascular systems discussed above, namely **restlessness** and **convulsions** followed by **respiratory depression**, and **hypotension** or even **cardiac arrest**.

Hypersensitivity reactions occur, though rarely, with local anaesthetics, usually taking the form of allergic dermatitis, but occasionally causing an acute anaphylactic reaction.

Other unwanted effects that are specific to particular drugs include **mucosal irritation** (cocaine, dibucaine) and **methaemoglobinaemia** (which occurs after large doses of prilocaine, because of the production of a toxic metabolite).

Pharmacokinetic aspects

Local anaesthetics vary a good deal in the rapidity with which they penetrate tissues, and this affects the rate at which they cause nerve block when injected into tissues and the rate of onset of, and recovery from, anaesthesia. It also affects their usefulness as surface anaesthetics for application to mucous membranes. Procaine, for example, penetrates tissues poorly and is unsuitable for surface anaesthesia.

Most of the ester-linked local anaesthetics (e.g. procaine, amethocaine) are rapidly hydrolysed by plasma cholinesterase so their plasma half-life is short. Procaine is hydrolysed to p-aminobenzoic acid, a folate precursor which interferes with the anti-bacterial effect of sulphonamides (see Chapter 30), a fact which may occasionally be of clinical significance. The amide-linked drugs (e.g. lignocaine, prilocaine) are metabolised mainly in the liver, usually by N-dealkylation rather than cleavage of the amide bond, and the metabolites are often pharmacologically active.

Benzocaine is an unusual local anaesthetic of very low solubility, which is used as a dry powder to dress painful skin ulcers etc. The drug is slowly released and produces long-lasting surface anaesthesia.

The rate of onset and duration of action of some injectable local anaesthetics is shown in Table 27.1.

Table 27.1 Pharmacokinetic properties of local anaesthetics

Drug	Rate of onset	Duration	Tissue penetration	Plasma $t_{\frac{1}{2}}$ (approx)
Procaine	Moderate	Short	Slow	30 min
Lignocaine	Rapid	Moderate	Rapid	2 h
Amethocaine	Slow	Long	Moderate	1 h
Dibucaine	Moderate	Long	Moderate	3 h
Bupivacaine	Slow	Long	Moderate	3 h
Prilocaine	Moderate	Moderate	Moderate	2 h

Methods of administration

Surface anaesthesia. The local anaesthetic solution is applied directly to the mucosal surface in areas such as the nose and mouth, bronchial tree, oesophagus or genitourinary tract. It must be able to penetrate tissues readily (e.g. cocaine, lignocaine). Relatively high concentrations are often used, and systemic toxicity is not uncommon when large areas (e.g. the bronchial tree) are anaesthetised in this way.

Surface anaesthesia does not work well on the skin, except if a drug such as benzocaine is left on the skin for a long time.

To retard absorption, and prolong the anaesthetic effect, a vasoconstrictor, such as phenylephrine, may be added. Cocaine itself causes vasoconstriction, so no such addition is needed.

Infiltration anaesthesia. Anaesthetic is injected directly into the tissues to reach fine nerve branches and sensory nerve terminals. Adrenaline is often added as a vasoconstrictor, but must be avoided when extremities such as fingers or toes are being anaesthetised for fear of causing ischaemic tissue damage.

It can only be used for fairly small areas, otherwise there is a serious risk of systemic toxicity.

Nerve block anaesthesia. The anaesthetic is injected close to the appropriate sensory nerves, to produce a loss of sensation peripherally. It is a widely used method, because usually much less anaesthetic is needed than for infiltration anaesthesia. Accurate placement of the needle is important, and the onset of anaesthesia may be slow, depending on the anatomical barriers that the drug has to penetrate. The duration of anaesthesia also varies, but it may be increased by addition of adrenaline.

Intravenous regional anaesthesia is used mainly for the upper limb. The limb is first emptied of blood by applying a pressure bandage. A cuff is then applied to the upper arm and inflated above arterial pressure, thus isolating the limb vasculature. Lignocaine is injected intravenously distal to the cuff, so that it fills the vascular systems and causes anaesthesia within a few minutes. It is essential not to release the arterial cuff accidentally or too soon, since a potentially lethal bolus of drug could be released into the systemic circulation. Within a few minutes of injection the anaesthetic normally becomes dispersed in the tissues so that the cuff may be released without too sudden a systemic effect being produced. Nevertheless, it is a potentially dangerous procedure, which has caused a number of deaths.

Spinal and epidural anaesthesia. Local anaesthetic solutions may be injected into the suparachnoid space which contains cerebrospinal fluid and lies within the tough dural sheath (spinal anaesthesia) or just outside the dura, into a narrow space between the dura and the bony spinal canal, containing fat and connective tissue (epidural anaesthesia). In both cases the anaesthetic works mainly on the spinal roots as they emerge from the cord rather than on the cord itself.

Injection into the subarachnoid space produces a more extensive spread of the anaesthetic than epidural injection. The specific gravity of the saline solution in which the drug is dissolved is often increased by addition of glucose so that its spread can be partially controlled by tilting the patient. With epidural anaesthesia, this is less useful, and the spread is, in any case, less extensive.

The advantage of this form of local anaesthesia is that relatively small doses are needed, reducing the risk of systemic toxicity. The main side effects result from block of the pre-ganglionic sympathetic fibres. These are very small myelinated fibres, which are particularly sensitive to local anaesthetics (see earlier section), and the caudal and rostral extent of sympathetic block is usually greater than that of the sensory block, resulting in vasodilatation, bradycardia and a marked fall in arterial pressure. Hypotension is usually less severe with epidural block, though local vasodilatation still occurs. With spinal anaesthesia, rostral spread may cause respiratory depression if the drug reaches the intercostal and phrenic nerve roots. Block of the sympathetic supply to the intestine may occur, causing increased intestinal motility. One advantage of epidural block is that if the drug is injected in the lumbar region, the sacral parasympathetic outflow is usually unaffected, because the drug does not spread so far caudally, whereas urinary retention, caused by sacral parasympathetic block is common after spinal anaesthesia.

Both of these techniques are commonly used for surgery to the abdomen, pelvis and lower limbs in patients unsuitable for general anaesthesia. Epidural anaesthesia is also in frequent use for painless childbirth.

Tetrodotoxin and saxitoxin

We should not be surprised that nature, rather than medicinal chemistry, has provided the most potent and selective agents that act on Na^+ channels of excitable tissues. Tetrodotoxin (TTX) is produced in the tissues of a poisonous Pacific fish, the puffer fish, so called because when alarmed it inflates itself to an almost spherical spiny ball. It is evidently a species highly preoccupied with defence, but the Japanese are not easily put off, and the puffer fish is regarded by them as a special delicacy. To serve it in public restaurants, however, the chef must be registered as sufficiently skilled in removing the toxic organs (especially liver and ovaries) so as to make the flesh safe to eat. Accidental tetrodotoxin poisoning is quite common, nontheless; records of long sea-voyages often contained reference to attacks of severe weakness, progressing to complete

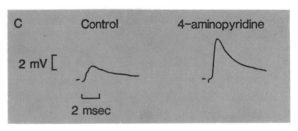

Tetrodotoxin

Saxitoxin

Fig. 27.7 Structure of tetrodotoxin and saxitoxin.

Agents that affect Na$^+$ channel gating

There are various highly lipid-soluble substances, most of them of high molecular weight and of a Baroque molecular complexity, that modify Na$^+$ channel gating in such a way as to increase the probability of opening of the channels (Hille, 1984). In addition, certain polypeptide toxins, most of them derived from scorpion or sea anemone

paralysis and death, caused by eating puffer fish. The same toxin is produced by a poisonous newt, a remarkable example of convergent evolution.

Saxitoxin (STX) is chemically different from TTX (Fig. 27.7) and is produced by a marine microorganism. This sometimes proliferates in very large numbers, and even colours the sea, giving the 'red tide' phenomenon. At such times, marine shellfish can accumulate the toxin and become poisonous to humans. TTX and STX are complex molecules, but both possess the guanidinium moiety (Fig. 27.7).

These toxins, unlike the loca anaesthetics, act exclusively from the outside of the membrane. The guanidinium ion is able to enter cells via the voltage-sensitive Na$^+$ channels, and it is likely that this part of the TTX or STX molecule lodges in the channel, leaving the rest of the molecule blocking its outer mouth. In contrast to the local anaesthetics, there is no interaction between the gating and blocking reactions with TTX or STX—their association and dissociation are independent of whether the channel is open or closed.

TTX and STX are quite unsuitable for clinical use, being expensive to obtain from their exotic sources, and very poor at penetrating tissues because of their very low lipid solubility. They have, however, been important as experimental tools for the study of Na$^+$ channels. The use of labelled TTX and STX has enabled the Na$^+$ channel protein to be isolated and purified (Barchi, 1982), and now sequenced by gene cloning (Noda et al, 1984).

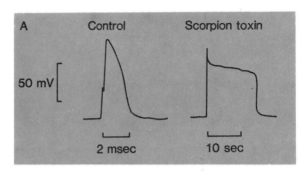

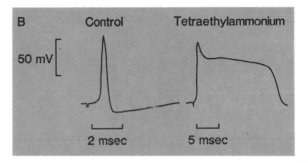

Fig. 27.8 Effects of scorpion toxin and K$^+$ channel blocking drugs on action potential configuration.

A. Scorpion toxin on the frog node of Ranvier. Scorpion toxin impedes Na$^+$ channel inactivation (see Fig. 27.3) and prolongs the action potential from 2 msec to nearly 15 sec.

B. Tetraethylammonium on squid axon. TEA blocks K$^+$ channels, and thus delays membrane repolarization.

C. 4-aminopyridine on the endplate potential in frog muscle. Enhancement of the endplate potential is due to an increase in the amount of acetylcholine released from the nerve terminals, which results mainly from the increased action potential duration in the terminals.

(From: (A) Schmitt & Schmitt, 1972; (B) Tasaki & Hagiwara, 1957; (C) Molgo et al, 1977)

venoms, act similarly. Substances in the first group include **veratridine**, **batrachotoxin**, **aconitine** and the insecticides, **DDT** and the **pyrethrins**. They affect Na^+ channel activation by shifting its voltage-dependence so that Na^+ channels open at the normal resting potential; they also inhibit inactivation, so that the channels do not close if the membrane remains depolarized (Fig. 27.3). The polypeptide venoms act mainly by the latter mechanism. In either case the cells initially become hyperexcitable, and the action potential is prolonged (Fig. 27.8). Spontaneous discharges occur at first, but the cells eventually become permanently depolarized and inexcitable. All of these substances affect the heart, producing extrasystoles and other dysrhythmias, culminating in fibrillation; they also cause spontaneous discharges in nerve and muscle, leading to twitching and convulsions. Veratridine was at one time used as an antihypertensive drug. It appears to increase baroreceptor and chemoreceptor discharge in doses lower than those needed to affect other excitable cells, and this causes a reflex fall in blood pressure. The side effects (especially nausea) are, however, severe, and veratridine is no longer used clinically. Drugs in this class are useful as experimental tools for studying Na^+ channels, but have no clinical uses.

AGENTS THAT AFFECT K^+ CHANNELS

A variety of substances are known that block voltage-sensitive K^+ channels of excitable membranes, which has the effect of prolonging the action potential (Fig. 27.8), since the delayed increase in K^+ conductance in response to depolarization (see Figs. 27.1 & 27.3) is one of the mechanisms that causes the membrane to repolarize following the action potential*. Repetitive firing can also occur, the overall effect being similar to that of drugs that block Na^+ channel inactivation. Drugs that have this effect include **tetraethylammonium (TEA)** and **4-aminopyridine (4AP)**. Their effects on nerve conduction, though much studied, and revealing

in relation to the mode of gating of K^+ channels, are not of much clinical use. 4AP was recently tested in multiple sclerosis, a demyelinating disease of the central nervous system in which conduction fails because of the loss of myelin. It was hoped that blocking K^+ channels would enable action potentials to propagate successfully through the demyelinated segments of affected axons, but the side effects (nausea and convulsions) were too troublesome for the drug to be useful in practice.

The most striking effect seen with K^+ channel blockers is an enhancement of transmitter release at many central and peripheral synapses (see Chapter 6). This can be a very large effect (Fig. 27.8) and it probably results mainly from prolongation of the action potential in the nerve terminals. This does not seem to be the only mechanism, however, for if action potentials are blocked with TTX and transmitter release is evoked directly by electrical depolarization of the nerve terminals, 4AP can still enhance release. It is suggested that it may increase Ca^{++} entry by affecting Ca^{++} channel gating in addition to blocking K^+ channels. 4AP has limited clinical use for restoring neuromuscular transmission following the use of neuromuscular blocking agents (see Chapter 6) or in disorders of neuromuscular transmission such as myasthenia gravis.

Other kinds of K^+ channels exist in different cells, and some of these are also susceptible to drug effects. Brown and his colleagues (Adams et al, 1982) have recently described the M current in various central and peripheral neurons. This is a voltage-sensitive K^+ current which acts to inhibit repetitive firing of neurons under conditions of continuing excitation. The M current is inhibited by many different neurotransmitters and modulators, including acetylcholine and various peptides. By blocking the M current, these agents encourage the cell to fire repetitively, without themselves directly causing excitation. Many cells also possess K^+ channels that are opened by an increase in intracellular Ca^{++} concentration. **Apamin**, a peptide from bee venom, which causes convulsions when injected into the brain, blocks this Ca^{++}-sensitive K^+ channel in some cells.

It is evident that the great variety of K^+ channel types in different cells offers considerable scope for developing new drugs, but the possibilities are only just beginning to be explored.

---

* Recent work by Ritchie and his colleagues has shown, rather surprisingly, that K^+ channels are not present in the nodal membrane of mammalian myelinated nerve fibres, and that K^+ channel blocking agents have little effect on the action potential. They do affect mammalian nerve terminals, however.

REFERENCES AND FURTHER READING

Adams P R, Brown D A, Constanti A 1982 Pharmacological inhibition of the M-current. J Physiol 332: 223–262

Armstrong C M 1981 Sodium channels and gating currents. Physiol Rev 61: 644–683

Barchi R L 1982 Biochemical studies of the excitable membrane sodium channel. Int Rev Neurobiol 263: 69–101

Catterall W A 1985 The electroplax sodium channel revealed. Trends in Neurosciences 8: 39–41

Hille B 1977 Local anaesthetics: hydrophilic and hydrophobic pathways for the drug-receptor interaction. J Gen Physiol 69: 497–515

Hille B 1984 Ionic channels of excitable membranes. Sinauer, Sunderland MA

Hodgkin A L 1967 The conduction of the nervous impulse. Liverpool University Press, Liverpool

Katz B 1966 Nerve, muscle and synapse. McGraw Hill, New York

Kuffler S W, Nicholls J G, Martin R 1984 From neurone to brain. Sinauer, Sunderland MA

Narahashi T, Frazier D T 1971 Site of action and active form of local anaesthetics. Neurosci Res 4: 65

Noda M, Shimizu S, Tanabe T, Takai T, Kayano T, Ikeda T et al 1984 Primary structure of electrophorus electricus sodium channel deduced from cDNA sequence. Nature 312: 121–127

Ritchie J M, Greengard P 1966 On the mode of action of local anaesthetics. Ann Rev Pharmac 6: 405–430

Skou J C 1961 The effect of drugs on cell membranes with special reference to local anaesthetics. J Pharm Pharmacol 13: 204–217

Strichartz G R 1973 The inhibition of sodium currents in myelinated nerve by quaternary derivatives of lidocaine. J Gen Physiol 62: 35–57

Chemotherapy

28

Basic principles of chemotherapy

The development of chemotherapy during the past half-century constitutes one of the most important therapeutic advances in the history of medicine.

The term '**chemotherapy**' was coined by Ehrlich at the beginning of the century to describe the use of synthetic chemicals to destroy infective agents. In recent years the definition of the term has been broadened to include '**antibiotics**'—substances produced by some microorganisms which kill or inhibit the growth of other microorganisms. The term chemotherapy is now also applied to the use of chemicals (either natural or synthetic) used to inhibit the growth of malignant or cancerous cells within the body. Ehrlich had assumed that the development of completely selective agents was an unobtainable goal and that the most that could be hoped for was the production of substances that were maximally 'parasitotropic' and minimally 'organotropic'. This view has turned out to be rather more pessimistic than was warranted because some totally selective antibacterial agents have been produced.

THE MOLECULAR BASIS OF CHEMOTHERAPY

Chemotherapeutic agents are chemicals which are intended to be toxic for the parasitic cell or cells but innocuous for the host. The feasibility of such selective toxicity depends on the existence of biochemical differences between the parasite and the host cell. The extent of this difference depends mainly on how far apart host and parasite are in terms of evolutionary development. Parasitic cells may be prokaryotes (cells *without* nuclei)—the **bacteria**, or eukaryotes (cells *with* nuclei). This second

category of parasites includes both some single-celled organisms (e.g. **fungi**, **protozoa**) and multicellular organisms (e.g. **helminths**). In general the cells of these latter organisms are likely to be more similar biochemically to the cells of the host—which are also, of course, eukaryotic.

In a separate category are the **viruses**, which are not, properly speaking, cells at all because they do not have their own biochemical machinery for generating energy or for any sort of synthesis. Viruses need to utilize the metabolic machinery of the host cell and they thus present a particular kind of problem for chemotherapeutic attack.

In yet another category are **cancer** cells—host cells which have become malignant, i.e. they have escaped from the regulating devices which control normal cells. Cancer cells can be considered to be, in a special sense, 'foreign' or 'parasitic', but are clearly more similar to normal host cells than any of the categories considered above and constitute an especially difficult problem for selective toxicity.

In approaching the question of chemotherapy and the biochemical differences between parasite and host cell, it is easier, for simplicity, to start with a bacterial cell and to ask what such a cell has to do in order to grow and divide. Figure 28.1a shows in simplified diagrammatic form the main structure and functions of a 'generalized' bacterial cell. Surrounding the cell is the **cell wall** which characteristically contains **peptidoglycan** in all forms of bacteria except mycoplasma. Peptidoglycan is *unique* to prokaryotic cells and has no counterpart in eukaryotes. Within the cell wall is the **plasma membrane**, which is similar to that of the eukaryotic cell, consisting of a phospholipid bilayer and proteins. However, in bacteria the plasma membrane does not contain any sterols and this may result in differen-

(a)

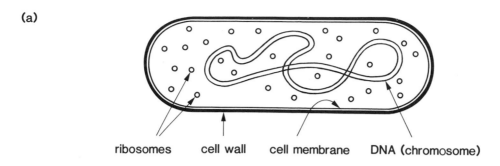

ribosomes   cell wall   cell membrane   DNA (chromosome)

(b)

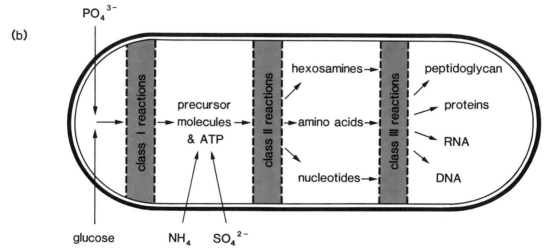

Fig. 28.1 a. Diagrammatic representation of a baeterial cell. b. Flow diagram showing the synthesis of the main types of macromolecules of a bacterial cell. Class I reactions result in the synthesis of the precursor molecules necessary for Class II reactions, which result in the synthesis of the basic molecules, which in turn are assembled into macromolecules by Class III reactions. (Modified from: Mandelstam et al, 1982)

tial penetration of chemicals. It functions as a semipermeable membrane with specific transport mechanisms for various types of nutrients. The function of the cell wall is to support this underlying plasma membrane, which is subject to an internal osmotic pressure of about 5 atmospheres, in Gram-negative organisms, and about 20 atmospheres in Gram-positive organisms.* The plasma membrane and cell wall together comprise the '**envelope**'.

Within the plasma membrane is the **cytoplasm**.

As in eukaryotes, this contains all the soluble proteins (most having enzymic functions), the ribosomes involved in protein synthesis, all the small molecule intermediates involved in metabolism and all the inorganic ions. However, the cytoplasm of the bacterium, unlike that of eukaryotes, also contains the genetic material, in the form of a single chromosome which holds all the genetic information of the cell. In further contrast to eukaryotic cells the chromosome of the bacterial cell contains no histones.

These, then, are the essential structures of the generalized bacterial cell. Some bacteria have additional components such as a capsule and/or one or more flagella, but the only additional structure with relevance for chemotherapy is the **outer membrane**, *outside* the cell wall, which is found in Gram-

---

* The terms Gram-positive and Gram-negative refer to whether or not the cell stains with a particular combination of dyes. More detail of the difference between Gram-positive and Gram-negative organisms is given in Chapter 30 (p. 626).

negative bacteria and which may prevent penetration of antibacterial agents. It also prevents easy access of lysozyme (an enzyme which can break down cell wall structures and which is found in white blood cells and tissue fluids) to the peptidoglycan of the cell wall.

Having outlined the essential structures of the bacterial cell, the next step is to consider the biochemical reactions involved in their formation (Fig. 28.1b). One can classify these reactions into three general categories:

Class I   The utilization of glucose for the generation of energy (ATP) and of simple carbon compounds (such as the intermediates of the citric acid cycle) which are used as precursors in the next class of reactions.

Class II   The utilization of the energy and precursors to make all the necessary small molecules: amino-acids, nucleotides, phospholipids, amino-sugars, carbohydrates and growth factors.

Class III   Assembly of the small molecules into macromolecules: proteins, RNA, DNA, polysaccharides and peptidoglycan.

These reactions constitute potential targets for attack by chemotherapeutic agents. Other potential targets are the formed structures of the cell, e.g. the cell membrane, or, in higher organisms, the microtubules (targets in fungi and cancer cells). Specific types of cells may be targets in some higher organisms (e.g. muscle tissue in helminths).

In considering these targets, emphasis will be placed on bacteria, but reference will also be made to protozoa, helminths, fungi, cancer cells and, where possible, viruses.

BIOCHEMICAL REACTIONS AS POTENTIAL TARGETS

Class I reactions

These reactions do not constitute a promising target, for two reasons. Firstly, there is no very marked difference between bacteria and human cells in the mechanism for obtaining energy from glucose, since both use the Embden–Meyerhof pathway and the TCA cycle. Secondly, even if the glucose pathways were to be blocked, a large variety of other compounds (amino-acids, lipids, etc) could be used by bacteria as alternatives.

Class II reactions

These reactions constitute a better target since some pathways involved in class II reactions exist in parasitic but not in human cells. For instance, human cells have in the course of evolution lost the ability to synthesize some amino-acids—the so-called 'essential' amino-acids—and also the growth factors or vitamins. Any such difference represents a potential target. A second type of target may occur even when a pathway is *apparently* identical in both bacteria and man. Examples of both occur in the synthesis of thymidylate, which requires folate. The *synthesis* of folate is an example of a metabolic pathway found in bacteria but not in man. Folate is required for DNA synthesis in both bacteria and in man (see Chapters 18 & 29). Man obtains it from the diet and has evolved a transport mechanism for taking it up into the cells. Man does not need to synthesize it and indeed cannot do so. Most species of bacteria, however, as well as the asexual forms of malarial protozoa must, of necessity, synthesize their own folate. Furthermore, they cannot make use of the preformed folate in human tissues or elsewhere because they have not evolved the necessary transport mechanism. This difference has proved to be useful for chemotherapy. **Sulphonamides** contain the sulphanilamide moiety—a structural analogue of p-aminobenzoic acid (pABA), which is essential in the synthesis of folate (see Figs. 18.4 & 30.1). Sulphonamides compete with pABA for the enzyme involved in folate synthesis and thus inhibit the metabolism of the bacteria. They are consequently *bacteriostatic* not *bactericidal* and are therefore only really effective in the presence of adequate host defences (which are discussed in Chapter 8).

The *utilization* of folate, in the form of tetrahydrofolate, as a co-factor in thymidylate synthesis (see Figs. 18.7 & 29.6) is an example of a pathway in which there is differential sensitivity of human and bacterial enzymes to chemicals (Table 28.1). This pathway is virtually identical in microorganisms and man, but one of the key enzymes,

Table 28.1 Specificity of inhibitors of dihydrofolate reductase

| Inhibitor | IC_{50} (μM) for FH_2 reductase | | |
	human	protozoal	bacterial
Trimethoprim	260	0.07	0.005
Pyrimethamine	0.7	0.0005	2.5
Methotrexate	0.001	approx. 0.1*	Inactive

* Tested on *P. berghei*, a rodent malaria.

dihydrofolate reductase, which reduces dihydrofolate to tetrahydrofolate, is many times more sensitive to the folate antagonist, **trimethoprim**, in bacteria than in man. In some malarial protozoa this enzyme is somewhat less sensitive to trimethoprim than the bacterial enzyme. The relative IC_{50} values (the concentration causing 50% inhibition) for bacterial, malarial, protozoal and mammalian enzymes are given in Table 28.1, as are those for a comparable but primarily antimalarial agent **pyrimethamine**. Another antimalarial drug which inhibits the protozoal enzyme specifically is **proguanil**. The human enzyme on the other hand is very sensitive to the effect of the folate analogue **methotrexate** (Table 28.1), and this compound is used in the chemotherapy of certain cancers (see Chapter 29). Methotrexate is inactive in bacteria because, being very similar in structure to folate, it requires active uptake by cells. Trimethoprim and pyrimethamine on the other hand enter the cells by diffusion.

The use of sequential blockade with a combination of two drugs which, in parasite cells affect the same pathway at different points (e.g. sulphonamides and the folate antagonists), is considerably more successful than the use of either alone. Furthermore, lower concentrations of each drug are effective when the two are used together. A formulation which contains both a sulphonamide and trimethoprim is **co-trimoxazole**.

Class III reactions

These constitute a particularly good target for selective toxicity because every cell *has* to make its own macromolecules—these cannot be picked up from the environment—and there are very distinct differences between mammalian cells and parasitic cells in the pathways involved in Class III reactions.

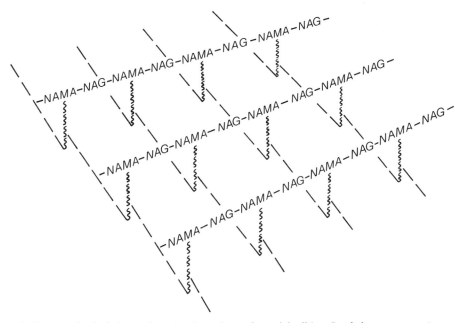

Fig. 28.2 Schematic diagram of a single layer of peptidoglycan from a bacterial cell (e.g. *Staphylococcus aureus*).
   NAMA = N-acetylmuramic acid; NAG = N-acetylglucosamine
   ⌇⌇⌇ = The amino-acid residues in the tetrapeptide side chain attached to the muramic acid
   – – – = The peptide cross-links between the side chains. In *Staph. aureus* these links consist of 5 glycine residues.
        Gram-positive bacteria have several layers of peptidoglycan.

The synthesis of peptidoglycan

This substance constitutes the cell wall of bacteria and does not occur in eukaryotes. It is the equivalent of a non-stretchable string bag enclosing the whole bacterium. For some bacteria (the Gram-negative organisms), the bag consists of a single thickness, but for others (Gram-positive organisms), the bag is several layers thick. Each layer consists of multiple backbones of amino-sugars—alternating N-acetylglucosamine and N-acetylmuramic acid residues (Fig. 28.2)—the latter having short peptide side-chains which are cross-linked to form a latticework. The cross-links differ in different species. In staphylococci they consist of 5 glycine residues (Fig. 28.2). This cross-linking is

responsible for the strength that allows the cell wall to resist the high internal osmotic pressure. The peptidoglycan is in fact one gigantic molecule with a molecular weight of many millions, constituting up to 10–15% of the dry weight of the cell.

In synthesizing the peptidoglycan layer the cell has the problem of using cytoplasmic components to build up this very large insoluble structure on the outside of the cell membrane. To do this it is necessary to transport the components, which are synthesized within the cell, and are individually hydrophilic, through the hydrophobic cell membrane. This is accomplished by linking the components to a very large lipid carrier, comprising 55 carbon atoms, which 'tows' them across the membrane. The process of synthesis of peptidoglycan is out-

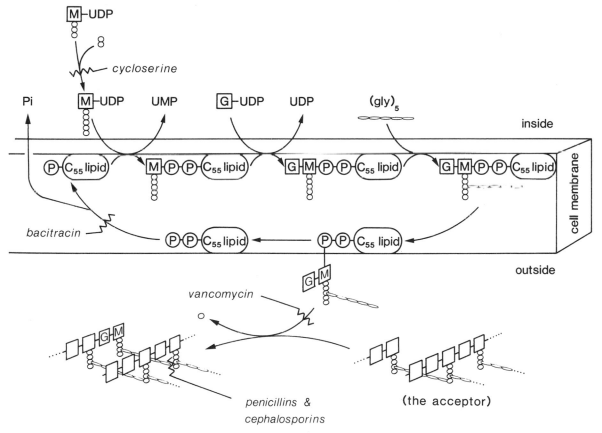

Fig. 28.3 Schematic diagram of the biosynthesis of peptidoglycan in a bacterial cell (e.g. *Staph. aureus*) with the sites of action of various antibiotics. M = N-acetylmuramic acid; G = N-acetylglucosamine. $\infty\infty\infty$ = glycine (gly) residues. $\infty\infty$ = the amino-acids of the peptide side chain on muramic acid. The hydrophilic disaccharide-pentapeptide is transferred across the lipid cell membrane attached to a large lipid (C_{55} lipid) by a pyrophosphate bridge (—P—P—). On the outside, it is enzymically attached to the 'acceptor' (the growing peptidoglycan layer). The final reaction is a transpeptidation, in which the loose end of the (gly)5 chain is attached to a peptide side chain of an M in the acceptor and during which the terminal amino-acid (alanine) is lost. The lipid is regenerated by loss of a phosphate group (Pi) before functioning again as a carrier.

lined in Figure 28.3. First N-acetylmuramic acid, which has attached to it both UDP and a pentapeptide, is transferred to the C_{55} lipid carrier in the membrane, with the release of UMP. This is followed by a reaction with UDP-N-acetylglucosamine, resulting in the formation of a disaccharide carrying the pentapeptide and attached to the carrier. This disaccharide with peptide attached is the basic building block of the peptidoglycan. In staphylococci, the five glycine residues are attached to the peptide chain at this stage, as is shown in Figure 28.3. The 'building block' is now transported to the outside of the cell and added to the growing end of the peptidoglycan, the 'acceptor', with the release of the C_{55} lipid which still has two phosphates attached. The lipid then loses one phosphate group and thus becomes available for another cycle. Cross-linking between the peptide side-chains of the sugar residues in the peptidoglycan layer then occurs, the hydrolytic removal of the terminal alanine supplying the requisite energy.

This synthesis of petidoglycan can be blocked at several different points by antibiotics (Fig. 28.3). **Cycloserine**, which is a structural analogue of D-alanine, prevents the addition of the two terminal alanines to the initial tripeptide side-chain on N-acetylmuramic acid, by competitive inhibition. **Vancomycin** inhibits the release of the building block unit from the carrier thus preventing its addition to the growing end of the peptidoglycan. **Bacitracin** interferes with the regeneration of the lipid carrier by blocking its dephosphorylation. **Penicillins** and **cephalosporins** inhibit the final transpeptidation which establishes the cross-links.

Protein synthesis

The ribosomes are cytoplasmic nucleoprotein structures which are the basic unit of machinery for the synthesis of proteins on messenger RNA templates. They are different in eukaryotes and prokaryotes and this provides the basis for the selective antimicrobial action of some antibiotics. The bacterial ribosome consists of a 50S subunit and a 30S subunit (Fig. 28.4). In this respect it differs from the mammalian ribosome which has a 60S and a 40S subunit.

A simplified version of protein synthesis in bacteria is as follows:

1. Messenger RNA (mRNA) which is transcribed from DNA (see below), becomes attached to the 30S subunit of the ribosome, which moves along the mRNA so that successive codons of the messenger pass through the ribosome from the right, the A position, to the left, the P position—as shown in Figure 28.4. (A codon is a triplet consisting of three nucleotides which codes for a specific amino-acid.)
2. The 'P site' contains the growing peptide chain attached to a transfer RNA (tRNA). An amino-acid residue linked to its specific tRNA, which carries its distinctive anticodon, moves into the A site, being bound to the site by a codon:anticodon recognition, which occurs by complementary base-pairing. (Fig. 28.4a & b)
3. A transpeptidation reaction occurs which links the peptide chain on the tRNA at the P site to the amino-acid on the incoming tRNA at the A site. (Fig. 28.4c)
4. The tRNA from which the peptide chain has been removed, is now ejected from the P site. (Fig. 28.4d)
5. The tRNA at the A site is translocated to the P site, and the ribosome moves on one codon, relative to the messenger. (Fig. 28.4d)
6. A new tRNA, with amino-acid attached and with the relevant anticodon, now moves into the A site, and the whole process is repeated.

Antibiotics may affect protein synthesis at any one of the above stages.

Some antibiotics prevent the binding of the charged tRNA, by competing with it for the A site. This is the mode of action of the **tetracyclines**. These agents affect protein synthesis in both eukaryotic and prokaryotic cells. The latter are more susceptible but selectivity is largely due to selective uptake by active transport into prokaryotic cells.

Some antibiotics cause an abnormality in codon:anticodon recognition, resulting in 'misreading' of the message on the messenger. Polypeptides continue to be assembled on the ribosome, but with the wrong sequence of amino-acids. The protein thus formed will be non-functional. Antibiotics with this action include **streptomycin**, **kanamycin**, **neomycin**, and **gentamycin**.

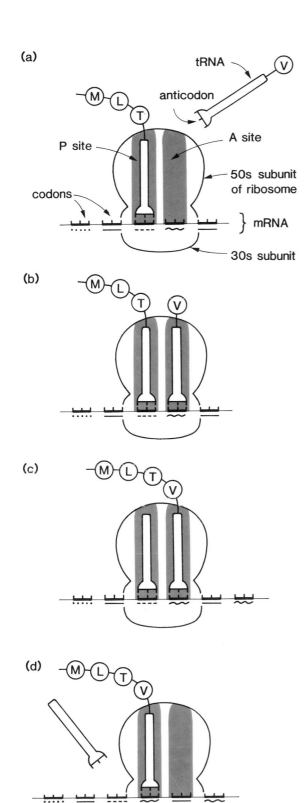

(a)

tRNA

anticodon

M L T

P site

A site

50s subunit
of ribosome

codons

mRNA

30s subunit

(b)

M L T V

(c)

M L T V

(d)

M L T V

Some antibiotics inhibit transpeptidation and the growth of the peptide chain. **Chloramphenicol**, **clindamycin** and **lincomycin** inhibit peptidyl transferase, the enzyme responsible for transpeptidation.

Some cause premature termination of the peptide chain. **Puromycin** resembles the amino-acid end of tRNA; a peptide bond is formed between puromycin and the peptide chain on the tRNA in the P site, but no further peptide bond formation is possible and the chain terminates. This antibiotic affects mammalian as well as bacterial cells; it is used as an experimental tool but not in chemotherapy.

Some antibiotics inhibit translocation. This is the mode of action of **erythromycin** which acts at the P site and causes the peptidyl tRNA to remain in the A site. Other antibiotics which inhibit translocation are **spectinomycin** and **fusidic acid**.

Nucleic acid synthesis

The nucleic acids of the cell are DNA and RNA. There are three types of RNA: messenger RNA (mRNA), transfer RNA (tRNA) and ribosomal RNA (rRNA). (The ribosomal RNA is an integral part of the ribosome, being necessary for its assembly and having a role in the binding of mRNA.) All are involved in protein synthesis (see above).

DNA is the template for the synthesis of both DNA and RNA. It exists in the cell as a double helix. Each chain or strand is a linear polymer of nucleotides. Each nucleotide consists of a base linked to a sugar (deoxyribose) and a phosphate. The bases are adenine (A), cytosine (C), guanine (G) or thymine (T). The chain is made up of alternating

Fig. 28.4 a. Ribosome with messenger RNA. (mRNA). The different mRNA codons (triplets of 3 nucleotides which code for specific amino-acids) are represented by dots, dashes and straight or wavy lines. A transfer RNA with peptide chain met, leu, trp (MLT) attached, is in the P site, bound by codon-anticodon recognition (i.e. by complementary base-pairing). The incoming transfer RNA (tRNA) carries valine (V), covalently linked.

b. The incoming tRNA binds to the A site by complementary base-pairing.

c. Transpeptidation occurs. The peptide chain attached to the tRNA in the A site now consists of met, leu, trp, val. (MLTV). The tRNA in the P site has been 'discharged', i.e. has lost its peptide.

d. The discharged tRNA is ejected from the P site. The tRNA with the peptide chain attached is translocated from the A to the P site leaving the A site free for the next tRNA. The ribosome moves to the next codon on the mRNA.

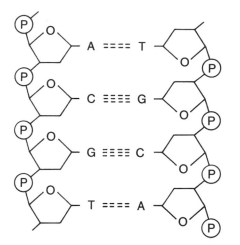

Fig. 28.5 Each strand of DNA consists of a sugar-phosphate backbone with purine or pyrimidine bases attacked. The purines are adenine (A) or guanine (G) and the pyrimidines, cytosine (C) or thymine (T). The sugar, deoxyribose, is indicated by $\langle\!\!\!\begin{array}{c}O\end{array}\!\!\!\rangle$ and the phosphate by (P) Complementarity between the two strands of DNA is maintained by hydrogen bonds between bases, either 2 or 3 (indicated by $==$ or $\equiv\equiv\equiv$).

sugar and phosphate groups with the bases attached rather like beads on a necklace. Specific hydrogen bonding between G and C and between A and T on each strand (i.e. complementary base-pairing) is the basis of the double strand structure of DNA (Fig. 28.5). The DNA helix is itself twisted,

resulting in 'supercoiling' (Fig. 28.6), and as explained above, the whole DNA molecule in a bacterium forms a single covalently closed chromosome (see Fig. 28.1).

The units, which pair with the complementary residues in the template, consist of a base linked to a sugar and three phosphate groups. Condensation occurs with the elimination of two of the phosphate groups, the enzyme responsible being DNA polymerase (Fig. 28.7).

Initiation of DNA synthesis necessitates the prior activity of an enzyme which produces local unwinding of the 'supercoil'. This enzyme is DNA gyrase (also called topoisomerase II).

RNA, like DNA, is a polymer of purine and pyrimidine nucleotides, but it exists as a single, not a double strand. The sugar moiety is ribose, and the resulting nucleotides are ribonucleotides. The bases are adenine, guanine, cytosine and uracil (U).

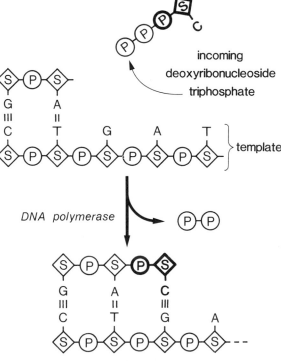

Fig. 28.7 In DNA replication, nucleotides are added, one at a time, by base-pairing to an exposed template strand and are then covalently joined together in a reaction catalysed by DNA polymerase. The units which pair with the complementary residues in the template consist of a base linked to a sugar and three phosphate groups. Condensation occurs with the elimination of two phosphates. P = phosphate, S = sugar, A = adenine, T = thymine, G = guanine, C = cytosine.

(a)   (b)

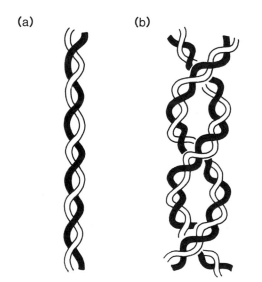

Fig. 28.6 Schematic diagram of: (a) The double helix; and (b) The double helix in supercoiled form.

It is possible to interfere with nucleic acid synthesis in five different ways:

1. *By inhibiting the synthesis of the nucleotides.* This can be accomplished by an effect on reactions earlier in the metabolic pathway. Examples of such agents which have antibacterial action are the **sulphonamides** and **folate antagonists** described under Class II reactions. Agents with a somewhat similar mechanism of action used in cancer chemotherapy are the pyrimidine analogues, e.g. **fluorouracil**, and the purine analogues, **mercaptopurine** and **thioguanine**. **Flucytosine**, an antifungal drug, is deaminated to 5-fluorouracil within the cell; selectivity for fungal cells is due to the fact that this deamination occurs to a much lesser extent in man. A pyrimidine analogue which inhibits replication of some DNA viruses is **idoxuridine**.

2. *By altering the base-pairing properties of the template.* Agents which intercalate in the DNA have this effect. Examples are the acridines (**proflavine**, **acriflavine**), which are used topically as antiseptics, and **chloroquine** which is an antimalarial drug. The acridines double the distance between adjacent base-pairs and cause a *frame-shift* mutation (Fig. 28.8). Some purine and pyrimidine analogues cause mispairing. One example is the anti-viral drug **adenine arabinoside**.

mRNA (normal)	UUU phe	CUU leu	AUU ile	GUU val	UCU..... ser
mRNA (mutant)	UUG leu	UCU ser	UAU tyr	UGU cys	UUC..... phe

Fig. 28.8 An example of a frame-shift mutation—a mutation which involves an *insertion* of an extra base (C in this example) in the DNA, so that when messenger RNA is formed, it has an additional G, as indicated above (in bold). The effect is to alter that codon and all the succeeding ones so that a completely different protein is synthesized as indicated by the different amino-acids (leu instead of phe, ser instead of leu etc). G = guanine, C = cytosine, A = adenine, U = uracil.

3. *By inhibiting either DNA or RNA polymerase.* **Actinomycin D** binds to the guanine residues in DNA and blocks the movement of RNA polymerase thus preventing transcription and consequently inhibiting protein synthesis. It is used in cancer chemotherapy in man and as an experimental tool, but not as an antibacterial agent. Specific inhibitors of bacterial RNA polymerases which act by binding to this enzyme in prokaryotic but not in eukaryotic cells include **rifamycin** and **rifampicin**, which are active, in particular, against the tubercle bacillus. **Acyclovir** (an analogue of guanine; see Fig. 31.1) is phosphorylated in herpes virus-infected cells to acyclovir triphosphate which has a relatively selective inhibitory action on the DNA polymerase of the herpes virus. **Cytarabine** (cytosine arabinoside) is used in cancer chemotherapy. Its triphosphate derivative is a potent inhibitor of DNA polymerase in mammalian cells. **Hycanthone** intercalates in DNA in schistosomes, preventing transcription and the synthesis of essential enzymes.

4. *By inhibiting DNA gyrase.* This is the mechanism of action of **nalidixic acid** and **oxolinic acid**—chemotherapeutic agents used in urinary tract infections with Gram-negative organisms.

5. *By direct effects on DNA itself.* **Alkylating agents** form covalent bonds with bases in the DNA and prevent replication. Compounds with this action are used only in cancer chemotherapy and include **mitomycin**, **nitrogen mustard derivatives** and **nitrosoureas**. No antibacterial agents work by these mechanisms.

THE FORMED STRUCTURES OF THE CELL AND/OR SPECIALIZED CELL TYPES AS POTENTIAL TARGETS

The membrane

The plasma membrane of bacterial cells is fairly similar to that in mammalian cells in that it consists of a phospholipid bilayer in which proteins are embedded. Nevertheless, this structure can be more easily disrupted in certain bacteria and some fungi than in mammalian cells.

Polymixins are cationic detergent antibiotics which have a preferential effect on bacterial cell membranes. They are peptides which contain both hydrophilic and lipophilic groups separated within the molecule. They interact with the phospholipids of the cell membrane and disrupt its structure. **Polyene antibiotics** (e.g. **nystatin** and **amphotericin**) are active against some fungi and protozoa but have little action on mammalian cells and no action on bacteria. This is because of the different overall membrane organization of the plasma membrane of the protozoal and fungal cells and because the membrane of these cells contains large amounts of ergosterol which facilitates the attachment and the subsequent effect of the polyenes. These antibiotics act as ionophores and cause leakage of cations. **Imidazoles**, such as miconazole, have antifungal action and also affect Gram-positive bacteria, their selectivity being associated with the presence of high levels of free fatty acids in the membrane of susceptible organisms.

DNA

Bleomycin, an anti-cancer antibiotic, causes fragmentation of the DNA strands following free radical formation.

Microtubules and/or microfilaments

Griseofulvin in high doses interferes with microtubule function in mammalian cells and thus with mitosis and cell division. This may be the basis for its antifungal action.

Colchicine and the vinca alkaloids, **vinblastine** and **vincristine**, are anti-cancer agents whose mode of action is interference with the function of microtubules during cell division. (Colchicine is also used in gout: see Chapter 9).

Muscle fibres

Some antihelminthic drugs have a selective-action on muscle cells in helminths. **Piperazine** hyperpolarizes muscle fibre membranes and paralyses the worm. **Levamisole** has a nicotinic-like action on the muscle, causing contraction followed by paralysis.

RESISTANCE TO ANTIOBIOTICS

During the last 40 years or so the development of effective and safe drugs to deal with bacterial infections has revolutionized medical treatment, and the morbidity and mortality from microbial disease has been dramatically reduced. Unfortunately, along with the development of man's chemotherapeutic defences against bacteria has gone the development of bacterial defences against chemotherapeutic agents, resulting in the emergence of **resistance**. This is not unexpected, it being an evolutionary principle that organisms adapt genetically to changes in their environment. Since the doubling time of bacteria can be as short as 20 min, there will be many generations in even a few hours and thus plenty of opportunity for evolutionary adaptation. The phenomenon of resistance can impose serious constraints on the options available for the medical treatment of many bacterial infections. Resistance to chemotherapeutic agents can also develop in protozoa, in multicellular parasites and in populations of malignant cells. However, in this chapter, discussion will be confined mainly to the mechanisms of resistance in bacteria.

Antibiotic resistance in bacteria spreads at three levels: carried on transposons between plasmids (explained below), by plasmids between bacteria and by bacteria between host organisms. Understanding the mechanisms involved in antibiotic resistance is of importance both for the sensible use of these drugs in clinical practice and for the development of new antibacterial drugs to circumvent resistance. One result of the studies of resistance, R-plasmids and resistance genes, has been the development of new techniques for the cloning of foreign DNA. This cloning has been used rewardingly in many branches of biology and also in the production by bacteria of biologically active peptides such as mammalian hormones.

GENETIC DETERMINANTS OF ANTIBIOTIC RESISTANCE

Chromosomal determinants

The spontaneous mutation rate for any particular gene is very low in bacterial populations—about one per 10^6–10^8 cells per generation, i.e. the probability is that one cell in say 10 million will, on division, give rise to a daughter cell containing a mutation in a particular gene. However, since in an infection there are likely to be very many more cells than this, the probability of a mutation causing a change from drug sensitivity to drug resistance may be quite high with some species of bacteria and with some drugs. Fortunately with most infective species and with most antibiotics, a single mutation is insufficient to produce resistance; if it were, the problem of resistance would be even more widespread than it is already. If such an infection is treated with a drug to which the mutant organism is resistant, the mutants will have an enormous selective advantage. Luckily in most cases, the drastic reduction of the population by the antibiotic enables the host's natural defences (see Chapter 8) to deal effectively with the invading pathogens. However, this will not occur if the infection is caused by microorganisms which are already resistant to the drug. For most organisms, resistance due to chromosomal mutation is not of great clinical relevance, possibly because the mutants often have reduced pathogenicity. Nevertheless, it is important in mycobacterial infections, particularly tuberculosis, and it is also a significant factor in leprosy.

Extrachromosomal determinants—plasmids

Many species of bacteria contain, in addition to the chromosome, extrachromosomal genetic elements called plasmids which exist free in the cytoplasms. These are covalently closed loops of DNA about 1–3% of the size of the chromosome. There may be 1–40 copies of a particular plasmid present, depending on the type, and there may be more than one type of plasmid in each bacterial cell. Plasmids that carry genes for resistance to antibiotics ('r genes') are referred to as R-plasmids. Much of the drug-resistance encountered in clinical medicines is plasmid-determined. It is not known how the r genes arose.

THE TRANSFER OF RESISTANCE GENES BETWEEN GENETIC ELEMENTS WITHIN THE BACTERIUM

Some stretches of DNA can be fairly readily transposed from one plasmid to another and also from plasmid to chromosome or vice versa. This is because integration of these bits of DNA, which are called *transposons*, into the acceptor DNA can occur independently of the normal mechanisms of genetic recombination (i.e. cross-over). During the process of integration the transposon replicates and this results in a copy in both the donor and the acceptor DNA molecules. Transposons may carry one or more resistance genes and probably account for the widespread distribution of certain of these genes on different R-plasmids and among unrelated

bacteria. Transposons are found mostly in Gram-negative bacteria.

THE TRANSFER OF RESISTANCE GENES BETWEEN BACTERIA

The transfer of resistance genes between bacteria of the same species and of different species is of fundamental importance in the spread of resistance to antibiotics. There are three mechanisms for gene transfer: conjugation, transduction and transformation.

Conjugation

This is a process involving cell to cell contact during which extrachromosomal DNA is transferred from one bacterium to another. It is the main mechanism for the spread of resistance. The ability to conjugate is encoded in *conjugative plasmids*. These are plasmids that contain *transfer genes* which code for the production of surface tubules of protein which connect the two cells—'sex pili'. Many R-plasmids are conjugative*. Many Gram-negative and some Gram-positive bacteria can conjugate. The transfer of resistance by conjugation is significant in bacteria which are normally found at high population density, as in the gut.

Transduction

This is a process by which plasmid DNA is enclosed in a bacterial virus (or phage) and transferred to another bacterium of the same species. It is a relatively ineffective means of transfer of genetic material but there is evidence that it is clinically important in the transmission of resistance genes between strains of staphylococci, and between strains of streptococci.

Transformation

This is a process whereby a bacterium takes up

---

* The combination of resistance genes with the stretch of DNA which codes for the sex pilus, which is often referred to as the 'resistance transfer factor' or 'RTF', is sometimes called the 'R factor'.

naked DNA from its environment and incorporates it into its genome. Transformation is probably not of any great importance to the clinical problem of drug-resistance.

BIOCHEMICAL MECHANISMS OF RESISTANCE TO ANTIBIOTICS

The production of an enzyme which inactivates the drug

Inactivation of β-lactam antibiotics

This is the most important example of resistance due to inactivation. The enzymes concerned are β-lactamases which cleave the β-lactam ring of penicillins and cephalosporins (see Chapter 30). Cross-resistance between the two classes of antibiotic is not complete because some lactamases have a preference for penicillins and some for cephalosporins.

Staphylococci are the principal β-lactamase-producing bacteria, and the genes which code for the enzymes are on plasmids which are transferred by transduction. In staphyloccoci the enzyme is inducible—its synthesis is very low in the absence of the drug, but minute, sub-inhibitory, concentrations derepress the gene and result in a 50–80-fold increase in production. The enzyme may diffuse through the envelope and inactivate antibiotic molecules in the surrounding medium. The potentially serious clinical problem posed by the staphylococci whose resistance is due to β-lactamase production has been solved by the development of semisynthetic penicillins (such as methicillin) which are not susceptible, and cephalosporins (such as cephamandole) which are less susceptible to inactivation by these enzymes.

Gram-negative organisms can also produce β-lactamases, which are a significant factor in their resistance to the semi-synthetic broad spectrum β-lactam antibiotics. In these organisms, the enzymes may be determined by either chromosomal genes or by plasmid genes. In the former case, the enzymes may be inducible, in the latter they are produced constitutively (i.e. they are synthesized even when the substrate is absent) and remain attached to sites

in the cell wall, preventing access of the drug to the membrane-associated target site; they do not inactivate it in the surrounding medium. Many of these β-lactamases are encoded by transposons, some of which also carry resistance determinants to several other antibiotics.

Inactivation of chloramphenicol

This is brought about by chloramphenicol acetyltransferase produced by resistant strains of both Gram-positive and Gram-negative organisms, the resistance gene being plasmid-borne. In Gram-negative bacteria the enzyme is produced constitutively which results in levels of resistance 5-fold higher than in Gram-positive bacteria, in which the enzyme is inducible.

Inactivation of aminoglycosides

This may be brought about by phosphorylation, adenylation or acetylation and the requisite enzymes have been found in both Gram-negative and Gram-positive organisms. The resistance genes are carried on plasmids and several are found on transposons.

Alteration of drug-sensitive site

The protein on the 30S subunit of the ribosome which is the binding site for aminoglycosides may be altered, as the result of a chromosomal mutation. A plasmid-mediated alteration of the binding site protein on the 50S subunit underlies resistance to erythromycin. An altered DNA-dependent RNA polymerase determined by a chromosomal mutation is the basis for resistance to rifampicin.

Decreased drug accumulation in the bacterium

An important example of this is the plasmid-mediated resistance to tetracyclines in both Gram-positive and Gram-negative bacteria. The resistance genes in the plasmid code for inducible 'resistance' proteins in the membrane which promote energy-dependent efflux of the tetracyclines and hence resistance. This type of resistance is common and has reduced the value of the tetracyclines in human and veterinary medicine. There is also recent evidence for a potentially disturbing type of resistance, involving plasmid-determined inhibition of 'porin' synthesis, which could affect those antibiotics which enter the bacterium by these channels in the outer membrane.

Altered permeability due to chromosomal mutations involving the polysaccharide components of the outer membrane of Gram-negative organisms may confer enhanced resistance to ampicillin.

Mutations affecting envelope components have been reported to affect the accumulation of aminoglycosides, β-lactams, chloramphenicol, peptide antibiotics and tetracycline.

The development of an alternative pathway that by-passes the reaction inhibited by the antibiotic

Trimethoprim-resistance due to plasmid-directed synthesis of a dihydrofolate reductase with low or zero affinity for trimethoprim has developed recently. It is transferred by transduction and may be spread on transposons.

Sulphonamide-resistance in many bacteria is plasmid-mediated and is due to the production of a form of dihydropteroate synthetase with a low affinity for sulphonamides but no change in affinity for pABA. Disturbingly, bacteria causing serious infections have recently been found to carry plasmids with resistance genes to both sulphonamides and trimethoprim.

REFERENCES AND FURTHER READING

Datta N (ed) 1984 Antibiotic resistance in bacteria. Brit Med Bull 40 (1): 1–106
Franklin T J, Snow G A 1981 Biochemistry of antimicrobial action, 3rd Edn. Chapman Hall, London

Mandelstam J, McQuillen K, Dawes I (eds) 1982 Biochemistry of bacterial growth (especially Part I, written by Editors), 3rd Ed. Blackwell Scientific, Oxford

29

Cancer chemotherapy

Cancer, can be defined very broadly as a disease in which there is uncontrolled multiplication and spread within the body of abnormal forms of the body's own cells. It is one of the major causes of death in the developed nations—one in five of the population of Europe and North America can expect to die of cancer. Figures for the last hundred years or so give the impression that the disease is increasing in these countries, but allowance has to be made for the fact that cancer is largely a disease of the later age groups, and with the advances in public health and medical science during this time many more people live to the age where they are likely to get cancer.

There are three main approaches to dealing with established cancer—surgical excision, irradiation, and chemotherapy—and the role of each of these depends on the type of tumour and the stage of its development. Chemotherapy with cytotoxic drugs is the main method of treatment for only a few relatively rare cancers but it is increasingly used as an adjuvant to surgery or irradiation in a range of common types of tumour.

Compared with chemotherapy of bacterial diseases, chemotherapy of cancer presents a difficult problem. It has proved possible to find agents with selective toxicity for many microorganisms because in addition to being quantitatively different in biochemical terms from human cells, they are also qualitatively different; but although cancer cells are abnormal, there is at present no *exploitable* qualitative biochemical difference between them and normal body cells. It is possible, however, that advances in molecular biology will change this state of affairs in the not too distant future.

Cancer cells differ from normal cells in *behaviour*, in that they manifest three characteristics not seen in normal cells; **uncontrolled proliferation**, **invasiveness**, and the **capacity to metastasize**.*

Uncontrolled proliferation. Some normal cells (such as neurons) have little or no capacity to divide and proliferate. Others, for example in the bone marrow and the epithelium of the gastrointestinal tract, have the property of continuous rapid division. Some cancer cells multiply slowly (e.g. those in plasma cell tumours) and some fast (e.g. the cells of Burkitt's lymphoma). It is therefore not generally true that cancer cells proliferate faster than normal cells—the significant difference is that their proliferation is not controlled by the processes which regulate normal tissue or organ growth. Consider, for example, the cells of the liver. Under normal conditions only a very small proportion of these are undergoing division at any one time. However, if two-thirds of the liver is removed, the remaining cells will divide fast and continuously until (in 2 weeks in the rat) the liver regains its original size. Growth then stops, because it is controlled by regulatory processes which are as yet ill-understood. The important thing about cancer cells is that their proliferation is not subject to these regulatory processes.

Invasiveness. Normal cells during differentiation

---

* Strictly speaking one should use the term 'neoplasia' (new growth) rather than the term 'cancer'. Neoplasms which have only the characteristic of localized growth are classified as *benign*. Neoplasms with the characteristics of invasiveness and/or the capacity to metastasize are classified as *malignant*. The term 'cancer' is usually applied only to this latter type of growth. The word 'tumour', though in reality meaning 'a local swelling', is also often used interchangeably with 'cancer' and will be so used here. In this chapter we shall be concerned only with the therapy of malignant neoplasia or cancer.

and during the growth of tissues and organs develop certain spatial relationships with respect to each other, and these are continuously maintained even when the cells are involved in repair processes. Thus, although the cells of the normal mucosal epithelium of the rectum proliferate continuously with a turnover time of about 2 hours, they remain as a lining epithelium. A cancer of the rectal mucosa on the other hand invades the tissues in the other layers of the rectum and may invade the tissues of other pelvic organs.

Metastases. These are secondary tumours formed by cells which have been released from the initial or primary tumour and have reached other sites through blood vessels or lymphatics, or as a result of being shed into body cavities. The cells which give rise to metastases, result from the selective growth of specialized sub-populations in the primary tumour.

GENERAL PRINCIPLES OF ACTION OF ANTICANCER DRUGS

In experiments with rapidly growing transplantable leukemias in mice it has been found that a given therapeutic dose of a cytotoxic drug destroys a constant fraction rather than a constant number of cells. Thus a dose which kills 99.99% of cells, if used to treat a tumour with 10^{11} cells, will still leave ten million viable cells. As it is probable that the same principle holds for similar tumours in man, schedules of chemotherapy of these tumours are therefore necessarily aimed at producing as near total cell kill as possible, because in contrast to the situation with chemotherapy against microorganisms, very little reliance can be placed on the host's immunological defence mechanisms against cancer cells.

One of the major difficulties in the use of anticancer therapy is that a tumour is usually far advanced before it is diagnosed. Let us suppose that a tumour arises from a single cell and that the growth is exponential—as it may well be in the initial stages of the life of the tumour. Doubling times vary with different tumours, for example being, very roughly, 24 hours with Burkitt's lymphoma, 2 weeks with some leukemias, and 3 months with mammary cancers. Approximately 30 doublings would be required to produce a cell mass with a diameter of 2 cm, containing 10^9 cells. A tumour that size is within the limits of diagnostic procedures, though it might be unnoticed in many organs, such as the liver. Another ten doublings would produce 10^{12} cells—a tumour mass which is likely to be lethal, and which would measure 20 cm or 8 inches in diameter if it were all in one clump. The neoplasm would therefore be silent for the first three-quarters or more of its existence and the problem of stopping its development after diagnosis, when there are large numbers of malignant cells, would be considerable.

However, exponential growth of this sort does not usually occur. With most solid tumours (for example, of lung, stomach, uterus, etc, as opposed to leukemias—the tumours of white blood cells) the growth rate falls as the neoplasm gets larger. This is partly because it tends to outgrow its blood supply with resultant necrosis or death of part of its bulk, and partly because not all the cells proliferate continuously. The cells of a solid tumour can be considered as belonging to three compartments: compartment A consists of dividing cells, possibly being continuously in cell cycle (Fig. 29.1); compartment B consists of resting cells (in G_0

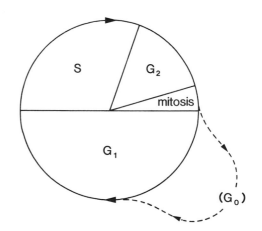

Fig. 29.1 The cell cycle. S = Synthesis of DNA, separated from MITOSIS by two gaps: G_1, a pre-DNA synthesis phase, and G_2, a post-DNA synthesis phase. Once S phase starts the cell is committed to mitosis. G_0 represents a phase in which cells are not dividing but can re-enter the cell cycle. Cells in G_0 phase are less sensitive to most anticancer agents.

phase)—cells which, though not dividing, are potentially able to do so; and compartment C consists of cells which are no longer able to divide but which contribute to the tumour volume. Essentially only cells in compartment A, which may form as little as 5% of the tumour, are susceptible to the main currently available drugs, as is explained below. The cells in compartment C do not constitute a problem—it is the existence of cells in compartment B which makes cancer chemotherapy difficult, because these cells are not very sensitive to cytotoxic drugs, but are liable to re-enter compartment A following a course of chemotherapy.

Most anticancer drugs, in particular those which are 'cytotoxic' (see below) affect only the first of the characteristics of cancer cells outlined previously— the process of cell division, i.e. they are anti-proliferative. They will therefore not only have no specific effect on invasiveness and the tendency to metastasize, but they will affect rapidly dividing normal tissues. Thus, they are likely to have, to a greater or lesser extent, the following general toxic effects: **bone marrow depression** with resultant decreased resistance to infection, **impaired wound healing**, **depression of growth** in children, **sterility**, **teratogenicity** and **loss of hair** (alopecia). They may also, themselves, cause cancer (i.e. they may be 'carcinogenic'). If there is rapid cell destruction with extensive purine catabolism, urates may precipitate in the kidney tubules and cause damage. In addition, virtually all cytotoxic drugs produce **severe nausea and vomiting**, which has been called 'the inbuilt deterrent' to patient compliance in completing a course of treatment with these agents. Some compounds have particular toxic effects which are specific for them. These will be dealt with under the individual drugs.

DRUGS USED IN CANCER CHEMOTHERAPY

The term 'cytotoxic drug' applies in principle to any drug that can damage or kill cells. In practice, it is often used more restrictively to mean drugs that inhibit cell division and are potentially useful in cancer chemotherapy. In addition to cytotoxic drugs, various types of hormone therapy are useful in suppressing the growth of particular tumours.

The main anticancer drugs can thus be divided into:

1. Cytotoxic drugs
   a. Alkylating agents, which act by forming covalent bonds with DNA and thus impeding DNA replication
   b. Anti-metabolites, which block or subvert one or more of the metabolic pathways involved in DNA synthesis
   c. Cytotoxic antibiotics, i.e. substances of microbial origin which prevent eukaryotic cell division
   d. Vinca alkaloids, which are substances of plant origin which specifically affect microtubule function and hence the formation of the mitotic spindle.

The mechanism of action of these drugs is discussed more fully below and summarized in Figure 29.2.

2. Hormones, of which the most important are steroids, namely glucocorticoids, oestrogens and androgens.

These categories do not exhaust the list of drugs used in treating cancer, and some further examples are given briefly under the heading 'miscellaneous agents'.

ALKYLATING AGENTS

These are compounds which have the property of forming covalent bonds with suitable nucleophilic substances in the cell. The main step is probably the formation of a carbonium ion—a carbon atom with only six electrons in its outer shell. Such an ion has no real independent existence—it reacts avidly and instantaneously with an electron donor such as an amine, —OH or —SH. Although alkylating agents can and probably do react with many cell constituents, it is their effect on DNA which is of significance in the treatment of cancer and most of the compounds used for this purpose are bifunctional, i.e. they have two alkylating groups. The N_7 of guanine, being strongly nucleophilic, is probably the main molecular target for alkylation in DNA, although N_1 and N_3 of adenine and N_3 of cytosine may also be affected. A bifunctional agent is able to react with two groups and can cause intra- or inter-

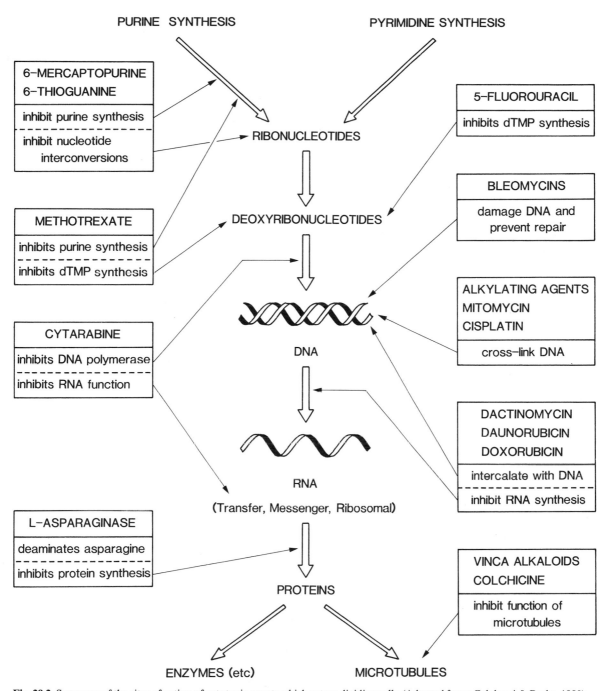

Fig. 29.2 Summary of the sites of action of cytotoxic agents which act on dividing cells. (Adapted from: Calabresi & Parks, 1980)

chain crosslinking (Figs. 29.3 & 29.4). This can interfere not only with transcription but with replication, and this is probably the critical effect of anticancer alkylating agents. Other effects of alkylation at guanine N_7 are excision of the guanine base with main chain scission, or pairing of the alkylated guanine with thymine instead of cytosine and eventual substitution of the GC pair with an AT pair. These latter two effects can also occur with monofunctional alkylating agents which are, on

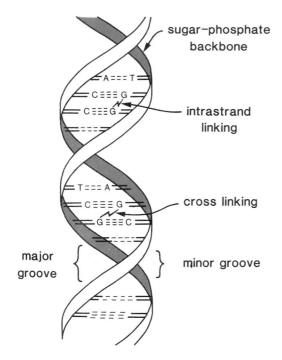

Fig. 29.3 Diagram to show intra-strand linking and cross-linking in DNA by bifunctional alkylating agents. (G = guanine, C = cytosine, A = adenine, T = thymine)

the whole, more mutagenic and carcinogenic than cytotoxic.

Although the drugs are able to act on cells in any stage of the cell cycle, they are most likely to have their effect during replication, when some parts of the DNA are unpaired and more susceptible to alkylation. But, at whatever stage of the cycle the reaction occurs, the effects are usually made manifest during S phase, resulting in a block at G_2, and subsequent cell death.

All alkylating agents depress the bone marrow and cause gastrointestinal disturbances. Two techniques have been developed which have proved relatively effective in ameliorating these toxic effects of alkylating agents: the use of small priming doses of the drugs to decrease the myelodepressive and gastrointestinal effects of subsequent large doses; and the removal of some of the patient's bone marrow before therapy followed by later reimplantation to hasten haematological recovery.

A large number of alkylating agents are available for use in cancer chemotherapy. Only a few commonly used ones will be dealt with here.

Nitrogen mustards

These drugs are related to sulphur mustard, the 'mustard gas' used during the First World War, and their basic formula is R-N-bis-(2-chloroethyl). Examples are given in Figure 29.5. In the body, each 2-chloroethyl side chain undergoes an intra-molecular cyclization with the release of a chloride ion. The highly reactive ethylene immonium derivative so formed can interact with DNA (see Fig. 29.4) and other molecules.

Mustine is the prototype nitrogen mustard in which R = CH_3. It is vesicant and has to be given into the tubing of a fast-flowing intravenous infusion. It reacts extremely rapidly with water as well as cellular constituents and is itself inactivated within minutes of administration. Apart from its use in Hodgkin's disease it has been superseded by other drugs in this group.

Cyclophosphamide is probably the most commonly used alkylating agent. It is inactive until metabolized in the liver by the P-450 mixed function oxidases to 4-hydroxycyclophosphamide, which forms aldophosphamide reversibly. Aldophosphamide is conveyed to other tissues, where it is converted to phosphoramide mustard (the actual cytotoxic molecule) and acrolein (Fig. 29.6). Cyclophosphamide has a pronounced effect on lymphocytes and is used as an immunosuppressant (see Chapter 9). It is usually given orally or by intravenous injection but may also be given intramuscularly or into the pleural or peritoneal cavities. Specific toxic effects are alopecia and haemorrhagic cystitis. This latter effect is due to acrolein and can be ameliorated by increasing fluid intake and infusing compounds which are sulphydryl donors, such as N-acetylcysteine or mesna (sodium-2-mercaptoethane sulphonate), directly into the bladder by irrigation. These agents interact specifically with acrolein forming a non-toxic compound.

Other nitrogen mustards used are **melphalan** and **chlorambucil**.

Nitrosoureas

These drugs are effective against a wide range of tumours, acting both by alkylation and by other as yet ill-understood mechanisms. The active moieties are probably alkylating and carbamoy-

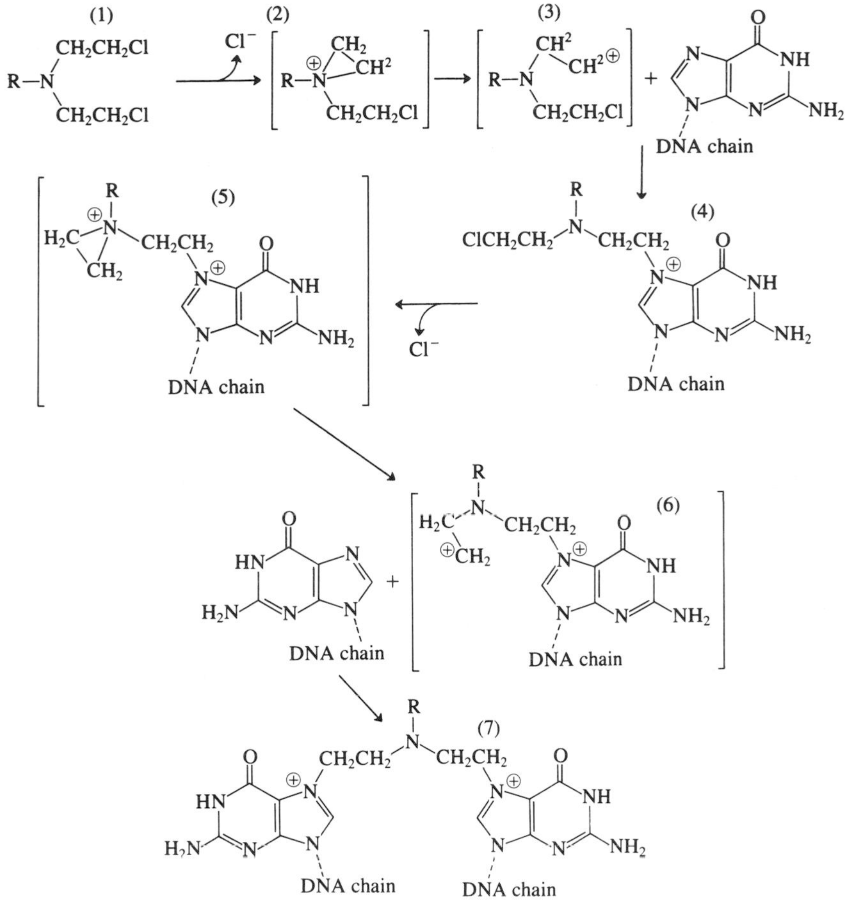

Fig. 29.4 An example of alkylation and cross-linking of DNA by a nitrogen mustard. A bis(chloroethyl)amine, (1), undergoes intramolecular cyclization forming an unstable ethylene immonium cation and releasing a chloride ion (2), the tertiary amine being transformed to a quaternary ammonium compound. The strained ring of the ethylene immonium intermediate opens to form a reactive carbonium ion (3), which reacts immediately with N-7 of guanine to give 7,alkylguanine, the N-7 being converted to a quaternary ammonium nitrogen. A bifunctional alkylating agent may undergo a second cyclization, (5), with carbonium ion formation (6), and interact with another guanine residue thus cross-linking two bases (7).

lating derivatives which are formed by spontaneous, nonenzymatic degradation. Examples are the chloroethylnitrosoureas, **lomustine** and **carmustine** (see Fig. 29.5) which, because they are lipid-soluble and can thus cross the blood-brain-barrier, may be used against tumours of the brain and meninges. However, most nitrosoureas have a severe cumulative depressive effect on the bone marrow which starts 3–6 weeks after initiation of treatment. An exception is **streptozotocin**, a methylnitrosourea. This is an antibiotic, in which the methylnitrosourea group is attached to glucose. This compound was originally used as an experimental

diabetogenic tool because of its selective toxic effect on β cells in the islets of Langerhans. It is not only useful therapeutically for tumours of these cells but also for other neoplasms. However, it has a significant toxic effect on the kidney.

Chlorozotocin, in which chloronitrosourea is attached to glucose, is undergoing trials and has proved to have much less toxicity for the bone marrow than lomustine and carmustine. It is possible that the combination of glucose with the nitrosourea group decreases the liberation from the nitrosourea of the organic isocyanates which carbamoylate lysine residues in proteins. As it is

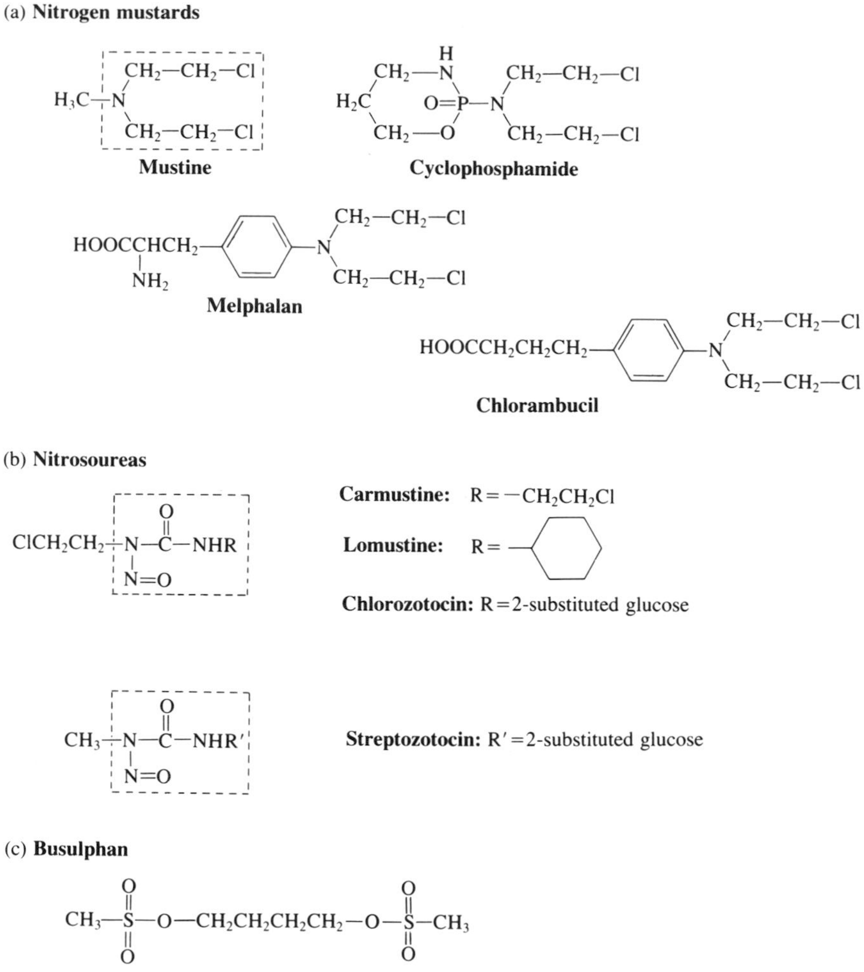

(a) **Nitrogen mustards**

Mustine

Cyclophosphamide

Melphalan

Chlorambucil

(b) **Nitrosoureas**

Carmustine: R = —CH$_2$CH$_2$Cl

Lomustine: R = —⟨hexane ring⟩

Chlorozotocin: R = 2-substituted glucose

Streptozotocin: R' = 2-substituted glucose

(c) **Busulphan**

Fig. 29.5 Alkylating agents used in anticancer therapy: (a) Nitrogen mustards; the portion of the molecule within the dotted lines is the nitrogen mustard group; (b) Nitrosoureas; the portion within the dotted lines is the nitrosourea group; (c) Busulphan (an alkylsulphonate).

believed that this carbamoylation reaction affects some of the DNA repair enzymes and may be responsible for the myelotoxicity, additional combinations of a nitrosourea group with other carrier molecules are being explored.

This line of development of anti-cancer agents may yield further useful drugs.

Busulphan

This drug has a selective effect on the bone marrow, depressing the formation of granulocytes and platelets in low dosage and red cells in higher dosage. It has little or no effect on lymphoid tissue or the gastrointestinal tract. It is accordingly used in chronic granulocytic leukemia, in which it may increase the very short life expectancy by about 9 months, the thrombocytopenia constituting a hazardous toxic effect.

Other alkylating agents are **chlorambucil, estramustine phosphate, ethoglucid, ifosfamide, melphalan, mitobronitol, thiotepa** and **treosulfan**.

ANTIMETABOLITES

Folate antagonists

The main drug in this group is **methotrexate** and it

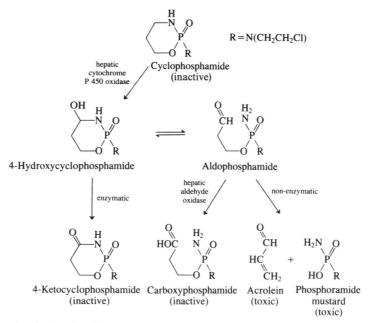

Fig. 29.6 The metabolism of cyclophosphamide.

is the most widely used antimetabolite in cancer chemotherapy.

Folates are essential for the synthesis of purine nucleotides and thymidylate, which in turn are essential for DNA synthesis and cell division. This topic is also dealt with in Chapters 18, 28 & 33. In structure folates consist of three elements: a hetero-bicyclic pteridine, para-amino benzoic acid and glutamic acid (Fig. 29.7). Folates in the blood have a single glutamate residue, but most intracellular folates are converted to polyglutamates, the multiple glutamate groups being linked by unusual gamma-

peptide bonds. These polyglutamates are preferentially retained within the cells. In order to act as co-enzymes, folates must be reduced to tetrahydro-folate (FH_4). This reaction is catalysed by **di-hydrofolate reductase** and occurs in 2 steps, first to dihydrofolate (FH_2), then to FH_4 (Fig. 29.8). Folate polyglutamates have a much higher affinity for dihydrofolate reductase than does folate mono-glutamate. FH_4 functions as a co-factor in the transfer of one-carbon units, a process which is essential for the methylation of uracil in 2-deoxyuridylate (dUMP) to form thymidylate (dTMP) and thus for

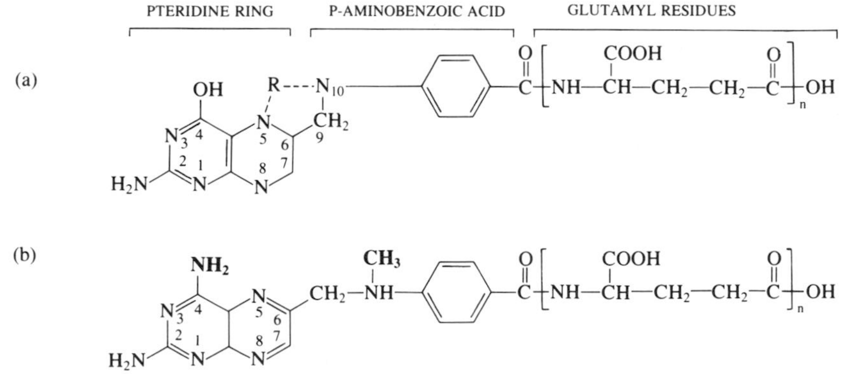

Fig. 29.7 Structure of (a) tetrahydrofolate and (b) methotrexate polyglutamates. In tetrahydrofolate, one-carbon groups (R) are transported on N-5 or N-10 or both (see Chapter 18).

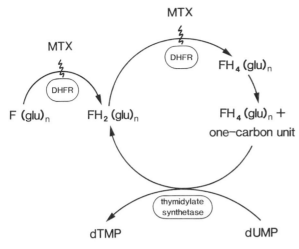

Fig. 29.8 Simplified diagram of action of methotrexate on thymidylate synthesis. Tetrahydrofolate polyglutamate [$FH_4(glu)_n$] functions as a carrier of a one-carbon unit, providing the methyl group necessary for the conversion of 2′deoxyuridylate (dUMP) to 2′deoxythymidylate (dTMP) by thymidylate synthetase. This one-carbon transfer results in the oxidation of $FH_4(glu)_n$ to $FH_2(glu)_n$. Both the subsequent regeneration of $FH_4(glu)_n$ from $FH_2(glu)_n$ by dihydrofolate reductase (DHFR) and the initial reduction of folate polyglutamate [$F(glu)_n$] to $FH_2(glu)_n$ are inhibited by methotrexate (MTX) and the polyglutamate forms of methotrexate (not shown). The reduction of $FH_2(glu)_n$ to $FH_4(glu)_n$ is probably the more important site of action of the folate antagonists.

the synthesis of DNA, and also for the de novo synthesis of purines (see also p. 439). During the formation of dTMP from dUMP, FH_4 is converted back to FH_2 (Fig. 29.8). Dihydrofolate reductase has a crucial role in maintaining the level of intracellular FH_4 by reducing the FH_2 produced from folate reduction and that generated during thymidylate synthesis. Methotrexate inhibits dihydrofolate reductase and depletes intracellular FH_4 (Fig. 29.8). Methotrexate is an analogue of folate (see Fig. 29.7) and has a higher affinity for the enzyme than FH_2, the equilibrium dissociation constant for methotrexate being approximately 1 nM. It appears that the binding of methotrexate to dihydrofolate reductase involves an additional hydrogen bond or ionic bond not present when FH_2 binds. The reaction most sensitive to FH_4 depletion is thymidylate synthesis, which is inhibited at a methotrexate concentration of 1 nM, whereas inhibition of purine synthesis requires ten times this concentration.

Pharmacokinetic aspects

Though it is ionized at neutral pH and has low lipid solubility, methotrexate is absorbed from the gastrointestinal tract, probably via a folate carrier system, but the rate and extent of absorption varies between patients. With optimal absorption, the peak blood concentration occurs between 1 and 5 hours after administration and remains high for about 6 hours. Increasing the dose above a certain level does not necessarily increase the absorption from the gastrointestinal tract, presumably because the carrier becomes saturated. Methotrexate may also be given intravenously or intrathecally.

About 50% of the drug is bound to plasma protein. It is distributed throughout the body fluids, including exudates and effusions, resulting in the first of 3 phases of decrease in plasma concentration. This phase has a $t_{\frac{1}{2}}$ of 45 minutes. Being a weak organic acid, negatively charged at body pH, it has low lipid solubility; its diffusion across physiologic membranes is thus very slow and it does not readily cross the blood-brain-barrier. It is actively taken up into cells by the transport system used by folate, the rate of uptake of methotrexate being higher than that of the endogenous substance. A second uptake system, which probably involves diffusion, comes into play at high blood levels of the drug (in excess of $20 \mu M$)—and this may be important in overcoming that mechanism of resistance to methotrexate which involves decreased active transport (see later section). Inside the cell, as has been stated above, methotrexate is metabolized to polyglutamate derivatives. The synthesis of these conjugates and the length of the polyglutamate chains increases with increasing drug concentration and duration of exposure. These polyglutamates dissociate from the enzyme more slowly than the monoglutamate and, unlike the parent compound, are retained in the cell for some time (weeks or months in some tissues) in the absence of extracellular drug. Retention is influenced by chain length, longer chains being retained for longer times.

Nearly half of a small dose and about 90% of a large dose is excreted unchanged in the urine, mostly within 8 hours. This results in a second phase of decrease in the plasma concentration—this phase having a $t_{\frac{1}{2}}$ of 2–3 hours. Renal excretion involves both glomerular filtration and tubular excretion.

The third phase, with a $t_\frac{1}{2}$ of 10 hours, commences after the plasma concentration has fallen below 100 nM.

Resistance to methotrexate may develop in tumour cells, a variety of mechanisms being involved: decreased membrane transport, an alteration in dihydrofolate reductase such that it has decreased affinity for the drug, increased amounts of the enzyme, and, possibly, decreased polyglutamation of the drug.

Toxic effects may occur and are mainly those to be expected with a drug which inhibits DNA synthesis—depression of the bone marrow and damage to the epithelium of the gastrointestinal tract. In addition, when high doses are used, there may be nephrotoxicity, which is probably due to precipitation of the drug or a metabolite of the drug in the renal tubules.

Clinical usage of methotrexate

Methotrexate is usually used in combination chemotherapy regimes. Either standard doses or high-dose therapy (which may involve doses ten times greater than the standard doses) may be employed. Theoretical considerations of cytotoxicity and drug resistance support the use of high plasma concentration (10–100 µM) for prolonged periods of 12–36 hours. This procedure could be lethal and must therefore be followed by 'rescue' with folinic acid (a form of tetrahydrofolate). The rationale for this procedure is that folinic acid 'rescues' normal cells more effectively than tumour cells. This latter treatment regime necessitates careful measurement of methotrexate and folinic acid concentrations in the plasma and also the use of alkaline diuresis during the methotrexate administration, to reduce nephrotoxicity.

Pyrimidine antagonists

Fluorouracil interferes with thymidylate synthesis and therefore with synthesis of DNA. Its structure is given in Figure 29.9 It is converted into a 'fraudulent' nucleotide—fluoro-deoxyuridine-monophosphate (FdUMP). This interacts with thymidylate synthetase and the folate co-factors,

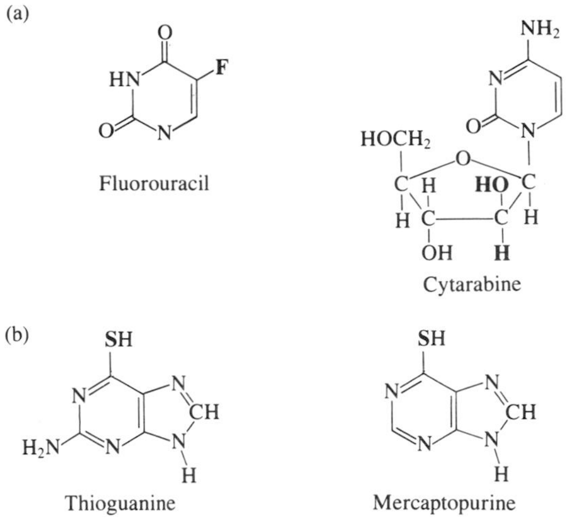

Fig. 29.9 Structural formulae of some cytotoxic antimetabolites: (a) Pyrimidine analogues; (b) Purine analogues.

but cannot be converted into thymidylate because in FdUMP, fluorine has replaced hydrogen at C_5 where methylation would take place and this carbon-fluorine bond is less susceptible to enzymic cleavage than the carbon-hydrogen bond. The result is inhibition of DNA synthesis but not RNA and protein synthesis.

Fluorouracil may be given orally or intravenously. After absorption it is rapidly distributed throughout the body water and it readily crosses the blood-brain barrier. It undergoes rapid metabolism in the liver, only 20% of a dose being excreted in the urine. Its main toxic effect is suppression of the bone marrow but an additional toxic action, disturbance of consciousness, may be seen at high doses.

Cytarabine (cytosine arabinoside; Fig. 29.9) is an analogue of the naturally occurring nucleoside, 2'deoxycytidine. It differs from cytidine only in that, on the 2' carbon of the pentose, the hydroxyl group is in the opposite configuration, giving arabinose instead of ribose. The drug is incorporated into both RNA and DNA to a limited extent, but its main cytotoxic action is the inhibition of DNA polymerase by cytosine arabinoside triphosphate. The DNA polymerases require the triphosphates of the four deoxyribonucleosides of adenine, guanine, cytosine and thymine for DNA synthesis (illustrated in Fig. 28.7). Both replication and repair synthesis are inhibited by cytosine arabinoside triphosphate, the former more than the latter. Cytarabine enters the target cell and undergoes the same phosphorylation reactions as the physiological nucleoside, to give the triphosphate.

Cytarabine is given by intravenous or subcutaneous injection. It is metabolized in the liver and has a half-life of 30 minutes. It is able to cross the blood-brain-barrier with moderate efficiency, giving CSF levels which are 40% of the plasma concentration and it can also be given intrathecally. The main toxic effects are on the bone marrow and the gastrointestinal tract.

Purine analogues

The main purine analogues used are **mercaptopurine** and **thioguanine** (Fig. 29.9). They are the 6-thiol analogues of the endogenous 6–OH purine bases, hypoxanthine and guanine respectively. They are converted, in the cell, to the ribonucleotides: 6 thioguanosine-5'-phosphate and 6 thioinosine-5'-phosphate. These 'fraudulent' nucleotides probably produce their cytotoxic actions by many different mechanisms. They have several inhibitory actions on de novo purine synthesis and they may themselves be incorporated into DNA.

Mercaptopurine is well absorbed when given orally. It is metabolized by xanthine oxidase and the products excreted in the urine. Thioguanine absorption from the gastrointestinal tract is erratic and it may be given intravenously. In addition to the expected myelotoxicity (damage to the bone marrow) both agents produce a reversible toxic effect on the liver.

Other purine analogues—the immunosuppressant **azathioprine** (which gives rise to mercaptopurine *in vivo* (see Fig. 9.14) and the xanthine oxidase inhibitor **allopurinol** (see Chapter 9)—are used for non-malignant conditions. Allopurinol inhibits the breakdown of mercaptopurine and increases both its effect and its toxicity.

CYTOTOXIC ANTIBIOTICS

Antitumour antibiotics produce their effects mainly by direct action on DNA.

Actinomycin D is one of a series of antibiotics obtained from *Streptomyces* micro-organisms. It intercalates, in the minor groove, between adjacent guanosine-cytosine pairs in DNA, interfering with the movement of RNA polymerase along the gene and thus preventing transcription. It has effects on cells in all phases of the cell cycle, but is particularly potent on rapidly proliferating cells. It can have all the toxic effects outlined previously at the beginning of this chapter. It is usually given by injection and rapidly disappears from the plasma, but it does not cross the blood-brain-barrier.

Anthracycline antibiotics, **doxorubicin** and **daunorubicin** produce a variety of effects that could be implicated in their cytotoxic action. They bind to DNA and inhibit both DNA and RNA synthesis, but do not have much effect on protein synthesis. The generation of free radicals may be involved in their effects. Both agents are given intravenously and are rapidly taken up by most tissues, but do not cross the blood-brain-barrier. Extravasation at the injection site can cause local necrosis of tissue. In addition to the general toxic effects outlined previously, both drugs have an unusual toxic effect on the heart and may cause dysrhythmias, hypotension and cardiac failure.

The **bleomycins** are a group of metal-chelating glycopeptide antibiotics which degrade preformed DNA, causing chain fragmentation and release of free bases. Their action on DNA is thought to involve chelation of ferrous iron and interaction with oxygen, resulting in the oxidation of the iron and generation of superoxide and/or hydroxyl radicals. Bleomycin is most effective in the G_2 phase of the cell cycle and mitosis, but is also very active against non-dividing cells. It is given by injection, is rapidly distributed and is cleared by renal excretion with a half-life of 120 minutes. In contrast to most anticancer drugs bleomycin causes little myelosuppression. Its most series toxic effect is pulmonary fibrosis which may occur in 10% of patients treated and be fatal in 1%. About half the patients manifest mucocutaneous reactions and many may develop hyperpyrexia.

Mitomycin, after enzymic activation in the cells, functions as a bifunctional alkylating agent, alkylating preferentially at O_6 of guanosine. It crosslinks DNA and may also degrade DNA through the generation of free radicals. It is given intravenously, is widely distributed in the body and is metabolized in the liver. It causes marked myelo-suppression.

VINCA ALKALOIDS

These agents are derived from the periwinkle plant, the main alkaloids being **vincristine** and **vinblastine** though others such as **vindesine** are on trial. They act by binding to tubulin and inhibit its polymerization into microtubules (see Chapter 2). This prevents spindle formation in mitosing cells, resulting in arrest at metaphase. The alkaloids can, in fact, affect tubulin at any stage of the cell cycle of dividing cells, but their effects will only become manifest during mitosis. They will also inhibit other cellular activities which involve the microtubules such as phagocytosis, chemotaxis and some cellular functions in the CNS. (Colchicine has a similar action on tubulin. It is not useful in cancer chemotherapy but is used to treat gout: see Chapter 9).

They are all given by injection and, as with the anthracycline antibiotics, (see above) extravasation may cause local damage. The drugs are rapidly sequestered in cells, particularly the white blood cells and platelets, which together may contain nearly half of the drug content of the blood. Vincristine has a longer half-life than the other two alkaloids—at 48 hours the tissues still contain more than 50% of the administered drug. Excretion of breakdown products is primarily into the bile.

The vinca alkaloids are relatively non-toxic: vincristine has very mild myelosuppressive activity, but causes neuromuscular abnormalities fairly frequently; vinblastine is less neurotoxic but causes leucopenia; vindesine has both moderate myelotoxicity and neurotoxicity.

CISPLATIN

This is a water-soluble square planar co-ordination complex containing a central platinum atom surrounded by two chloride atoms and two ammonia groups (Fig. 29.10). In the 'cis' configuration the two chloride atoms are on one side and the two ammonia molecules on the other. The exact details of the mechanism of action are not known, but it seems probable that its action is analogous to that of the alkylating agents. When it enters the cell, the chloride ions dissociate leaving a reactive diamine platinum complex which reacts with water and then interacts with DNA. It is thought that it causes intrastrand cross-linking—probably between N_7 and O_6 of adjacent guanine molecules—which results in the breaking of the hydrogen bonds between the guanine and cytosine bases and thus local denaturation of the DNA chain.

Cisplatin is given by slow intravenous injection or infusion. After 3 hours it is concentrated in the kidney, and at 40 hours in the liver and intestine as well. In the plasma most of it is bound to protein. Its clearance from the plasma is biphasic, with a half-life of minutes for the first phase and days for the second phase. It is seriously nephrotoxic unless regimes of hydration and diuresis are instituted. It has low myelotoxicity but causes severe nausea and vomiting. Tinnitus and hearing loss in the high frequency range may occur, as may peripheral neuropathies, hyperuricacmia and anaphylactic reactions.

HORMONES

Tumours derived from hormone-sensitive tissues may be hormone-dependent. Their growth can be

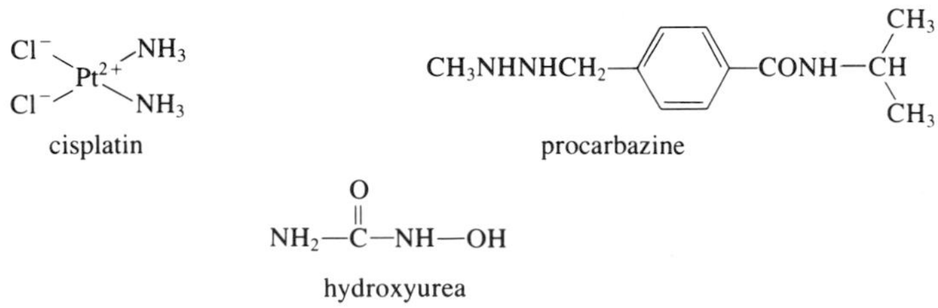

Fig. 29.10 The chemical structures of cisplatin, procarbazine and hydroxyurea.

inhibited by other hormones or hormone antagonists.

Glucocorticoids have inhibitory effects on lymphocyte proliferation (see Chapter 9) and are used in leukemias and lymphomas. The **sex hormones** (see Chapter 17) may also be used. **Oestrogens** block the effect of androgens in androgen-dependent prostatic tumours and may also be used in some cases of mammary cancer, especially in males. **Antioestrogens** such as tamoxifen are often effective in hormone-dependent mammary cancer in postmenopausal women. **Progestogens** have been useful in endometrial neoplasms and carcinomas of the prostate and breast. **Androgens** may also have a place in the treatment of breast cancer.

The hormone-dependency of tumours is related to the presence of steroid receptors in the tumour cells. The number of receptors can be estimated in biopsy specimens and this provides a guide to the potential efficacy of hormone therapy.

RADIOACTIVE ISOTOPES

These have a place in the therapy of tumours —radiophosphorus for polycythaemia vera and radio-gold for abdominal tumours. Radioactive iodine (^{131}I) used in treating thyroid tumours, is discussed in Chapter 16.

MISCELLANEOUS AGENTS

Procarbazine is a methylhydrazine derivation (Fig. 29.10). It was originally synthesized as a potential inhibitor of monoamine oxidase, but has proved to be a first line drug for the treatment of Hodgkin's disease. Its mechanism of action is not fully understood. It can be shown to inhibit DNA and RNA synthesis and to interfere with mitosis at interphase. Its effects may be due to the production of active metabolites.

It has been reported to be leukaemogenic, carcinogenic and teratogenic in experimental animals. It interacts with some agents: it causes disulfiram-like actions with alcohol, exacerbates the effects of CNS depressants and, because it is a weak monoamine oxidase inhibitor, may produce hypertension if given with certain sympathomimetic agents.

Hydroxyurea is a urea analogue (Fig. 29.10) which inhibits ribonucleotide reductase, thus interfering with the conversion of ribonucleotides to deoxyribonucleotides.

Etoposide is a semisynthetic derivative of podophyllotoxin, an extract of mandrake root. It inhibits the late stage of DNA synthesis in the cell cycle and is believed to cause breakdown of the DNA. It may also interfere with the electron transport chain in mitochondria. It may be given orally or intravenously, and is distributed throughout the body, but does not cross the blood-brain barrier.

Asparaginase is an enzyme which breaks down asparagine to aspartic acid and ammonia. It is active against tumour cells which, having lost the capacity to synthesize asparagine, require an exogenous source of this substance. Most normal body cells are able to synthesize asparagine and the drug thus has a fairly selective action on certain tumours. It has very little suppressive effect on the bone marrow, or the mucosa of the gastrointestinal tract or hair follicles. However, about half the patients treated show evidence of interference with liver function. Approximately one in twenty individuals develop acute pancreatitis which, in some cases, has proved fatal. Dysfunction of the blood coagulation mechanisms and depression of CNS function have also been reported. Asparagine can inhibit both T lymphocyte and B lymphocyte mediated immune responses. It is derived from bacteria and is itself antigenic and may elicit hypersensitivity reactions. It is used in combination chemotherapy regimes for some types of acute leukemia in children.

Mitotane is related to the insecticide DDT. It interferes with the synthesis of adrenocortical steroids (p. 395) having eventually a cytotoxic action on cells in the adrenal cortex. It is used solely for tumours of adrenal cortical cells. It is given orally and less than half is absorbed from the intestine. The drug tends to accumulate in fatty tissue, from which it is released slowly.

DRUG RESISTANCE

Neoplastic cells may manifest resistance to cytotoxic drugs, which may be primary (present when the drug is first given) or acquired (developing during treatment with the drug). Acquired resistance may be due either to adaptation of the tumour cells or to mutation, with the emergence of cells which are less affected or unaffected by the drug and which consequently have a selective advantage over the sensitive cells. Examples of various mechanisms of resistance are:

1. A decrease in amount of drug taken up by the cell (methotrexate, daunomycin)
2. Insufficient activation of the drug (mercaptopurine, fluorouracil, cytarabine). By this is meant that there may be decreased metabolism of these agents so that they do not enter the pathways where they would normally exert their effects. Thus fluoruracil may not be converted to FdUMP, cytarabine may not undergo phosphorylation, mercaptopurine may not be converted into a 'fraudulent' nucleotide
3. Increase in inactivation (cytarabine, mercaptopurine)
4. Increased concentration of target enzyme (methotrexate)
5. Decreased requirement for substrate (asparaginase)
6. Increased utilization of alternative metabolic pathways (anti-metabolites)
7. Rapid repair of drug-induced lesion (alkylating agents).

CELL CYCLE: DRUG EFFECTS AND THEIR POSSIBLE CLINICAL APPLICATIONS

The mitotic cycle of dividing cells can be considered to consist of four phases: an 'S-phase' of DNA synthesis, separated from *mitosis* by two gaps—G_1, which is a pre-DNA synthesis phase, and G_2 which is a post-DNA-synthesis phase (see Fig. 29.1). Cells which are not dividing but which can re-enter the cell cycle may be considered as being in resting or G_0 phase. The cells which are constantly in cell cycle constitute the 'growth fraction' of the tumour.

Anticancer drugs can be classified in terms of their actions on the cycle as:

1. *Phase-specific agents*, i.e. acting at a specific phase of the cell cycle. The vinca alkaloids act in mitosis. Cytarabine, hydroxyurea, thiouracil,

methotrexate and mercaptopurine act in S-phase. Some of these compounds have some action during G_1 phase and thus may slow the entry of a cell into S-phase where it would be more susceptible to the drug.

2. *Cycle-specific agents*, i.e. acting at all stages of the cell cycle and not having much effect on cells out of cycle: alkylating agents; actinomycin D, doxorubicin, daunomycin, cisplatin.

3. *Cycle non-specific agents*, i.e. acting on cells whether in cycle or not: bleomycins and nitrosoureas.

It has been proposed that this information could be of value in selecting agents for clinical use. Tumours with a high growth fraction should respond to phase-specific and cycle-specific agents. For tumours with a small growth fraction or large tumours in which growth has reached a plateau, attempts to decrease tumour size by the use of cycle-non-specific agents (together with surgery or X-ray) could be considered. It is also suggested that combinations of cytotoxic drugs should be based on the above classification. One possible application proposed is the use, first, of a drug acting in mitosis, such as vincristine, which would arrest cells in metaphase. When the cells which survive this move on in the cell cycle they should be synchronized, and the subsequent use of a drug specific for S-phase would be more effective because the timing could be adjusted to coincide with the occurrence of the S phase of the surviving cells. Inevitably, however, synchronization of normal as well as tumour cells occurs, and it is not clearly established that treatment schedules based on these principles are better than purely empirical schedules.

TREATMENT SCHEDULES

Treatment with combinations of several anticancer agents may increase the cytotoxicity against cancer cells without necessarily increasing the general toxicity and may also decrease the possibility of the development of resistance to individual agents. Detailed consideration of the combination schedules used in the clinic is beyond the scope of this book. Drugs are often given in large doses intermittently rather than in small doses continuously. This is because: (a) such a regime permits the bone marrow to regenerate during the intervals; and (b) it has been shown that the same total dose of an agent is more effective when given in one or two large doses than in multiple small doses.

POSSIBLE FUTURE STRATEGIES FOR CANCER CHEMOTHERAPY

Two of the main drawbacks of the current chemotherapy of cancer are: (a) the lack of selectivity of the drugs against tumour cells as compared to normal cells; and (b) the fact that, with many tumours, total elimination of malignant cells is not possible with therapeutic doses and the host's immune response is often not adequate to deal with the remaining cells. Attempts are being made to overcome these two problems—the first, by using selective targeting of anticancer compounds and the second, by boosting or augmenting the host's immune responses to the tumour. Other possible approaches may arise in the future from an understanding of the role of oncogenes and growth factors in cancer development, and the mode of action of tumour promoters.

THE TARGETING OF TOXINS AGAINST CANCER CELLS

In those instances where tumour-specific antigens can be identified, it might be possible to raise **mono-clonal antibodies** against the antigens. These antibodies would not necessarily be toxic for the tumour themselves but could be used to direct radioactive isotopes or toxic molecules, such as **ricin**, specifically to the malignant cells. Ricin is a very potent protein toxin derived from a plant *Ricinus communis*. It consists of two polypeptide chains, A and B, joined by a single disulphide bond. The toxin can attach to cells by means of the B chain, which binds to galactose sugars in the membrane. The A chain is then taken up by endocytosis and kills the cell. Attempts are being made to disrupt the galactose binding sites on the B chain and then to attach the whole molecule to a monoclonal antibody which is specific for a particular tumour.

Other toxins are also being investigated. Complexes of toxins and monoclonal antibodies may be used in future in the therapy of cancer.

Another use of monoclonal antibodies with bound toxins is to purge tumour cells from bone marrow taken from a patient, prior to the use of radiation and/or megadose chemotherapy regimes. Purging can also be accomplished by the use of complement after adding monoclonal antibodies against tumour cell antigens to the marrow *in vitro*. The purged marrow is then re-injected to reconstitute the bone marrow of the patient.

A major problem for the development of this approach is that most human tumours appear to be caused by environmental carcinogens; and experimental work on animals has shown that while most, if not all, tumours induced by a particular virus have common, tumour-specific antigens, this is not necessarily so for chemically-induced tumours. Furthermore, for the approach to be successful the antigen must not only be specific for the tumour and not present in normal cells, but it must be expressed on the *outside* of the cell membrane. An additional problem is that in some tumours, some of the malignant cells may undergo further mutations and thus, when the tumour is detected clinically, it may consist of several clones of malignant cells with different surface antigens.

ENHANCEMENT AND/OR AUGMENTATION OF THE HOST'S IMMUNE RESPONSE

It was postulated many years ago, by Thomas and later Burnet, that the immunologically-mediated rejection of tissue allografts was the expression of a response which had really been evolved for the rejection of a different sort of 'foreign' tissue— malignant tumours. It was considered by many, at the time, that 'immunotherapy' of tumours was just around the corner. However, early attempts at immunotherapy (such as boosting cell-mediated responses with BCG, the 'bacillus of Calmette and Guerin' which can be used to immunize against tuberculosis) proved to be unsuccessful and it has since become obvious that the immune response is very much more complex than was realized at the time. With recent advances in the understanding of immune reactions and recent technological developments, has come a reawakening of interest in the possibility of a modified form of immunotherapy of cancer.

γ-**Interferon**, which can be derived from mammalian cells (p. 650) or, by recombinant DNA techniques, from bacterial cells, has shown activity against certain human tumours. Interferon has anti-proliferative as well as immunoregulatory effects and this in addition to stimulating a response ab initio, can augment an existing response. Two other lymphokines, which may in the future have a similar effect in augmenting the host's response to tumour, are **lymphotoxin** and **tumour necrosis factor**. Both kill tumour cells in experimental systems and the recombinant DNA cloning of both has been achieved.

Another major mediator of the immune response, **interleukin-2** (p. 184), may prove to be effective in enhancing the host's reaction against tumour cells. Recombinant human interleukin 2 is available for testing and has shown beneficial effects against metastatic tumours in mice. Trials in cancer patients are under way. The possible therapeutic effect of **thymic hormones**—peptides isolated from the thymus, which have immunoregulatory activity—is also being tested in cancer patients.

MODIFICATION OF THE EFFECT OF ONCOGENE PRODUCTS

Although this approach has no immediate therapeutic significance it is likely to be of immense importance in cancer treatment in the future. It will therefore be considered here.

A major reason why cancer cells manifest uncontrolled proliferation appears to be that they have developed the ability both to produce and to respond to their own 'growth factors'—proteins which stimulate DNA synthesis and cell proliferation. The basis for this ability appears to be the presence in the DNA of the cancer cell of an 'oncogene' or 'oncogenes'. These genes (which confer malignancy on a cell) were originally shown to be due to the insinuation of viral genetic material into the host cell. It is now known that the host's own genes can promote malignancy when suitably activated. These 'proto-oncogenes' are almost cer-

tainly those genes which normally control cell proliferation. They can be converted into active oncogenes not only by certain viruses but also as a result of somatic mutation caused by chemical carcinogens (see Chapter 36). It is now considered that the phenotypic abnormality of the cancer cell can be traced back to a few central growth regulator genes whose function has been distorted.

Cells in multicellular organisms grow in response to (a) *extracellular signals* (growth factors) which act on (b) *cell surface receptors*, which in turn trigger (c) *intracellular transduction events* (stimulus-activation coupling events) which result in cell

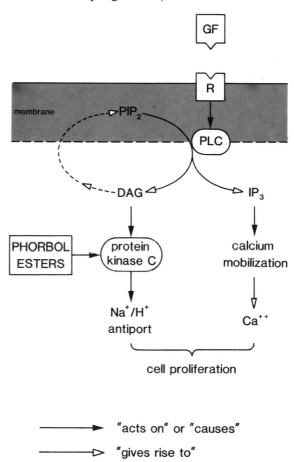

Fig. 29.11 Simplified diagram of some stimulus-activation coupling mechanisms which are relevant for the action of tumour promoters and oncogenes. See text for details. PIP_2 = phosphatidylinositol biphosphate; PLC = phospholipase C; IP_3 = inositol trisphosphate; DAG = diacylglycerol; R = receptor; GF = growth factor. The turnover of polyphosphoinositides is represented by the dashed lines from DAG to PIP_2 and probably takes place within the membrane.

proliferation. One of the main intracellular transduction events during cell proliferation in response to the action of growth factors on their receptors is the breakdown of phosphatidylinositol biphosphate by phospholipase C (see Fig. 29.11 & Chapter 1). This generates two intracellular messengers—diacylglycerol, (which activates protein kinase C) and inositol trisphosphate (which increases free intracellular Ca^{++}). Protein kinase C is believed to activate a Na^+/H^+ exchange carrier which causes Na^+ influx and H^+ efflux and decreases intracellular pH—events which are important in stimulus/activation coupling for cell proliferation.

Oncogenes can confer autonomy of growth on cells by affecting one or more of the three main elements in the growth control pathway cited above.

1. By coding for the production of growth factor(s)

Certain viruses induce cells to produce growth factors which are related to normal cell products. One such product is *platelet-derived growth factor* (PDGF) which is normally released from stimulated platelets and thought to be important in the repair of blood vessels as well as in the pathogenesis of atherosclerosis. PGDF is known to stimulate polyphosphoinositide metabolism. It is closely related to the oncogene product of simian sarcoma virus. Human osteosaceoma cells, human bladder cancer cells and various experimentally produced tumours also produce PDGF-like molecules.

Some human lung cancers produce *bombesin*, a tetradecapeptide which stimulates gastric secretion (see Chapter 15) and cells of these tumours can be stimulated to proliferate by bombesin. Monoclonal antibodies against the C-terminal portion of bombesin inhibits the growth of xenografts of this tumour in nude mice (mice which lack T cells and which therefore cannot reject the tumour).

2. By coding for an altered form of, or increased number of the receptors for the growth factors

For example, the growth of normal fibroblasts, (which is important in normal repair processes) requires *epidermal growth factor* (EGF). The cells of human head and neck cancers contain very large numbers of receptors for EGF, while other tumours contain receptors with extremely high affinity for EGF. Monoclonal antibodies to EGF inhibit the growth of these tumours in nude mice. Some tumour cells express a modified form of the EGF receptor which lacks that portion of the receptor responsible for binding EGF. It appears that this truncated form of the receptor is able to generate a mitogenic signal, in the absence of growth factors, causing the cell to divide.

3. By coding for products which modify the stimulus/activation coupling mechanisms in the cell

Some oncogenes code for the kinases which produce phosphatidylinositol biphosphate (PIP_2) from phosphatidyl inositol (Fig. 29.11). One oncogene (the c-ras gene, the first human oncogene to be identified) appears to cause uncontrolled stimulation on the phospholipase C which breaks down PIP_2. This may be through the modification of the action of a guanine nucleotide regulatory protein associated with ligand/receptor activation, the modification resulting in GTPase activity being lost and thus the mechanism for switching off cell activation being lost.

Some peptides encoded by oncogenes are localized in the nucleus and there is evidence that they function as regulators of transcription. They are thought to be involved in the signalling pathways for growth factors. Others appear to act by modifying cytoskeletal proteins.

At least 18 cellular oncogenes are known in addition to the 12 or more carried by various DNA tumour viruses, and it is thought that cooperation between several oncogenes may be required for the expression of malignancy.

At present there are no clinically available compounds which inhibit cancer cells by modifying the events just described. However the fact that monoclonal antibodies against specific growth factors or their receptors can interfere with tumour growth in experimental systems, holds out hope for the future. The development of peptide analogues designed to compete with growth factors or with the substrates of growth factor-activated enzymes might also be a fruitful future approach to the control of malignant cell growth. Another, possibly fruitful approach might be the exploitation of the fact that one of the growth factors necessary for the development of granulocytes and macrophages (granulocyte colony stimulating factor) has been shown *in vitro* to manifest a remarkable capacity to induce differentiation of myeloid leukemic cells and thus suppress the leukemia.

THE MODIFICATION OF THE EFFECTS OF TUMOUR PROMOTERS

In the production of cancer, the effect of agents known as 'tumour promoters' are believed by many to be as important as the effect of the actual chemical carcinogen (cancer-producing agent) which causes the mutation in the DNA. It is possible that in many instances the genetic changes produced by a chemical carcinogen may not be expressed as overt cancer in the absence of tumour promoter activity. Recent work has led to an understanding of the main mode of action of one of the major classes of tumour promoters—the phorbol esters (substances derived from croton oil). These agents, which are powerful stimulants of many different types of cell, are now known to activate protein kinase C—an important enzyme in the stimulus-activation coupling mechanisms in the cells concerned (Fig. 29.11). They act as analogues of diacylglycerol which is the endogenous activator of the kinase. However, unlike diacylglycerol, they are not rapidly metabolized but remain in the membrane, stimulating the enzyme for prolonged periods. This effect is thought to underly their propensity to stimulate proliferation of cells and may explain their tumour promoting action. **Retinoids**, derivatives of vitamin A, can be shown to inhibit the action of phorbol esters in some experimental systems. The possible role of these agents in blocking the progression of certain premalignant conditions to invasive cancer is under test.

Further unravelling of the role of tumour promoters in proliferating cells may well, in the future, lead to new approaches in the pharmacological attack on cancer.

REFERENCES AND FURTHER READING

Cairns J 1980 Conclusions and perspectives. In: Hecker E, Fusenig N E, Kunz W, Marks F, Thielmann H W (eds) Cocarcinogenesis and biological effects of tumor promoters. Raven Press, New York 647–651

Chabner B A, Pinedo H M (eds) 1984 The cancer pharmacology annual 2. Elsevier Science, Amsterdam

Davy P, Tudhope G R 1983 Anticancer chemotherapy. Brit Med J 287: 110–113

Hall A 1984 Oncogenes—implications for human cancer—a review. J Roy Soc Med 77: 410–416

Jolivet J, Cowan K H, Curt G A, Clendeninn N J, Chabner B A 1983 The pharmacology and clinical use of methotrexate. New Eng J Med 309: 1094–1104

Metcalf D 1985 The granulocyte-macrophage colony-stimulating factors. Science 229: 16–22

Neidle S, Waring M J (eds) 1983 Molecular aspects of anti-cancer drug action. MacMillan, New York

Sporn M B, Roberts A B 1985 Autocrine growth factors and cancer. Nature 313: 745–747

Steel G G, Stephens T C 1979 The relationship of cell kinetics to cancer chemotherapy. Adv Pharm Ther 10: 137–145

Weinberg R A 1984 Cellular oncogenes. Trends in Biochem Sci 9: 131–133

30

Antibacterial agents

A detailed classification of the bacteria of medical importance is beyond the scope of this book and the reader in search of fuller information should consult a textbook of medical microbiology. However, a short list of the commoner and/or more important microorganisms which cause disease is given in Table 30.1. Individual chemotherapeutic agents are dealt with briefly in this chapter and a general indication of their main antibacterial actions is given in Table 30.1. Some of the types of disease that may be caused by the organisms are included in the table but it should be understood that most of the organisms may, on occasion, produce other types of infection.

It will be seen from the table that many of the organisms cited are classified as either Gram-positive or Gram-negative. This classification is based on whether the organisms do or do not stain with Gram's stain, but has a significance far beyond that of an empirical staining reaction. Gram-positive and Gram-negative organisms are different in several respects, not least in the structure of the

Table 30.1 General outline of the action of antibiotics against common or important microorganisms. This is not meant to be a definitive guide for clinical treatment, but a general indication of the main antimicrobial actions and thus of the overall usefulness of commonly used antibiotics. The selection of antibiotic to treat an infection will change as resistance occurs and as new agents are introduced. Susceptibility tests should be performed if possible.

Microorganism	Antiobiotics	
	1st choice	2nd choice
GRAM POSITIVE COCCI		
Staphylococcus (infections of wounds, boils etc)		
non β-lactamase-producing	penicillin G or V	a cephalosporin vancomycin
β-lactamase-producing	a β-lactamase-resistant penicillin	a cephalosporin vancomycin
methicillin-resistant	vancomycin	cotrimoxazole erythromycin rifampicin
Streptococcus (septic infections) (haemolytic)	penicillin G or V + or − an aminoglycoside	a cephalosporin erythromycin vancomycin
Pneumococcus (pneumonia)	penicillin G or V	a cephalosporin erythromycin
GRAM NEGATIVE COCCI		
Gonococcus (gonorrhea)	penicillin G ampicillin a tetracycline	erythromycin spectinomycin cefoxitin
Meningococcus (meningitis)	penicillin G	chloramphenicol

Table 30.1—Continued

Microorganism	Antiobiotics	
	1st choice	2nd choice
GRAM POSITIVE BACILLI		
Corynebacterium (diphtheria)	erythromycin	penicillin G
Clostridium (tetanus, gangrene)	penicillin G	a tetracycline
Listeria	ampicillin + or − an aminoglycoside	a tetracycline
GRAM NEGATIVE BACILLI		
Coliform organisms *E. coli, Enterobacter,* *Klebsiella*; (infections of gut or urinary tract)	an aminoglycoside a third generation cephalosporin	cotrimoxazole carbenicillin chloramphenicol
Shigella (dysentery)	ampicillin cotrimoxazole	chloramphenicol
Salmonella (typhoid, paratyphoid)	chloramphenicol	cotrimoxazole ampicillin
Haemophilus	chloramphenicol	ampicillin, cotrimoxazole, a third generation cephalosporin
Bordetella (whooping cough)	erythromycin	ampicillin
Brucella	a tetracycline + or − streptomycin	streptomycin a sulphonamide cotrimoxazole
Yersinia (plague)	streptomycin + or − a tetracycline	chloramphenicol
Vibrio (cholera)	a tetracycline	cotrimoxazole
Legionella (pneumonia)	erythromycin	rifampicin a tetracycline
Pseudomonas aeruginosa (infection of burns etc)	carbenicillin + an aminoglycoside	aminoglycoside a cephalosporin
Bacteroides fragilis	chloramphenicol clindamycin metronidazole	cefoxtin
Gram-negative anaerobic bacilli other than *B fragilis*	penicillin G	clindamycin tetracycline a cephalosporin
SPIROCHAETES Organisms causing syphilis	penicillin G	erythromycin a tetracycline
RICKETTSIAE (typhus, Q fever etc)	a tetracycline	chloramphenicol
OTHER ORGANISMS *Mycoplasma pneumoniae*	a tetracycline	erythromycin
Chlamydia	a tetracycline	chloramphenicol erythromycin
MYCOBACTERIA (see text for details)		

cell wall. This latter factor has implications for the action of antibiotics and so will be considered briefly here.

The cell wall of Gram-positive organisms is a relatively simple structure 15–50 nm thick and in contrast to that of Gram-negative organisms it can be readily separated from the plasma membrane by mechanical means. It consists of about 50% peptidoglycan (see p. 599), about 40–45% acidic polymer (often techoic acid) which results in the cell surface being highly polar and carrying a negative charge, and about 5–10% proteins and polysaccharides. The strongly polar polymer layer influences the penetration of ionized molecules, and favours the penetration of positively charged compounds such as streptomycin into the cell.

The cell wall of Gram-negative organisms is much more complex. From the plasma membrane outwards it consists of:

1. A periplasmic space containing enzymes and other components
2. A peptidoglycan layer 2 nm in thickness and comprising 5% of the cell wall mass; this is often linked to lipoprotein molecules which project outwards
3. An outer membrane consisting of a lipid bilayer similar in some respects to the plasma membrane. It contains protein molecules and on its inner aspect has lipoprotein which is linked to the peptidoglycan. Complex polysaccharides are important components on its outer surface. They are different in different strains of bacteria and are the main determinants of the antigenicity of the organism. They constitute the 'endotoxins' which, *in vivo*, trigger various aspects of the inflammatory reaction—activating complement, causing fever etc (see Chapter 8). Recent studies have shown that there are proteins in the outer membrane which form transmembrane water-filled channels, termed 'porins', through which hydrophilic antibiotics may move freely.

Difficulty in penetrating this complex outer layer is probably the reason why some antibiotics are less active against Gram-negative than Gram-positive bacteria. This is of particular relevance in determining the extraordinary insusceptibility to antibiotic drugs of *Pseudomonas aeruginosa*—a pathogen which can cause life-threatening infections of burns and wounds. Antibiotics for which penetration is a problem include penicillin G, methicillin, the macrolides, rifampicin, fusidic acid, vancomycin, bacitracin and novobiocin (see below). There is evidence that it is the lipopolysaccharide of the cell wall which is the major barrier to penetration.

SULPHONAMIDES

In the 1930s it was demonstrated for the first time by Domagk, that a chemotherapeutic agent could influence the course of a bacterial infection. The drug was **prontosil**, a dye, and it was shown not only to protect mice against several thousand times the lethal dose of haemolytic streptococci but also to be effective in similar infections in man. However, prontosil proved to be a pro-drug, inactive *in vitro* and needing to be metabolized *in vivo* to give the active product—a sulphanilamide (Fig. 30.1). A large number of sulphonamides have been developed since, and although their therapeutic importance has declined somewhat they are still useful drugs. Furthermore, they are of considerable historical and theoretical interest, not least because chemical modification of the sulphonamide structure has given rise to several important groups of drugs, especially diuretics (acetazolamide and the thiazides; see Chapter 14) tuberculostatic and antileprotic agents (the sulphones; see below) and oral hypoglycaemic drugs (sulphonylureas; see Chapter 16).

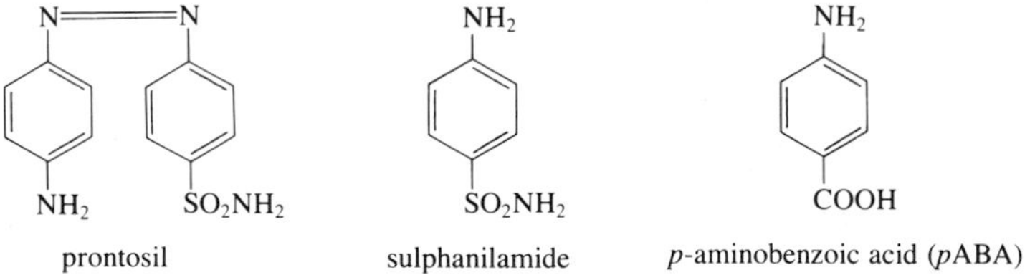

Fig. 30.1 Prontosil, sulphanilamide and p-aminobenzoic acid.

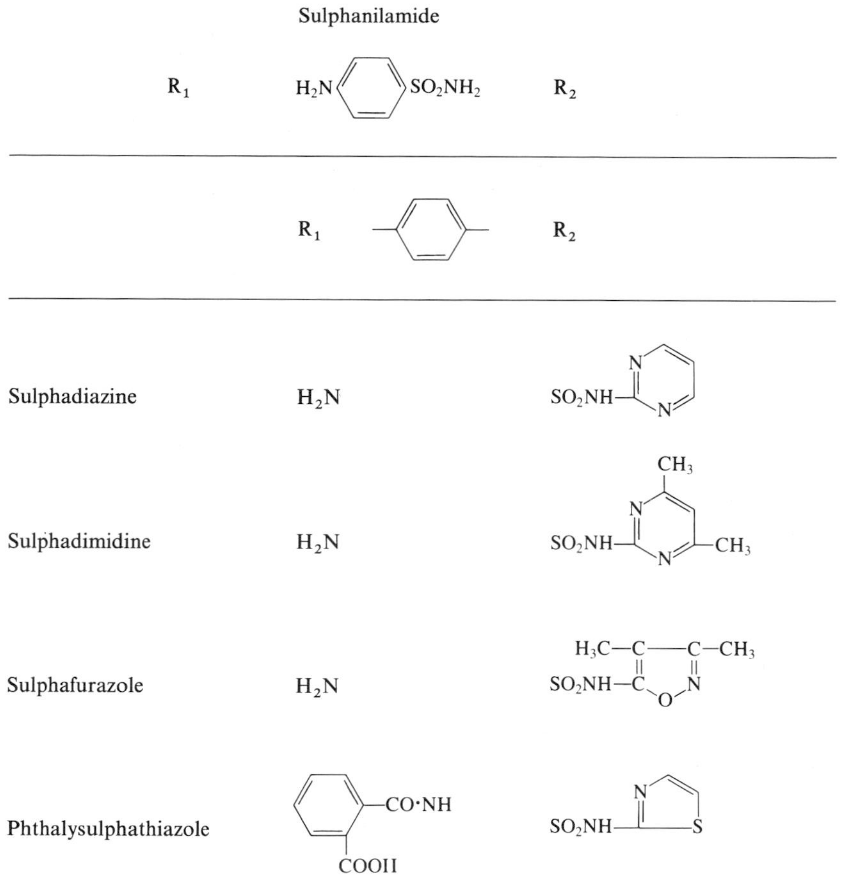

Sulphanilamide

R₁ H_2N⟨benzene⟩SO_2NH_2 R₂

R₁   ⟨benzene ring⟩   R₂

Sulphadiazine	H_2N	SO_2NH—⟨pyrimidine⟩
Sulphadimidine	H_2N	SO_2NH—⟨dimethylpyrimidine, CH_3, CH_3⟩
Sulphafurazole	H_2N	H_3C—C C—CH_3 / SO_2NH—C, O, N ⟨isoxazole⟩
Phthalylsulphathiazole	⟨benzene⟩—CO·NH / COOH	SO_2NH—⟨thiazole⟩

Fig. 30.2 Structural formulae of some sulphonamide drugs.

Chemistry of the sulphonamides

The chemical structures of some of the more commonly used sulphonamides are shown in Figure 30.2. Either the amide moiety (SO_2NH_2) or the amino group (NH_2) of sulphanilamide can be substituted. The most active drugs are those in which the former substitution has been made. These include **sulphadiazine**, **sulphadimidine** and **sulphafurazole** (sulphisoxazole).

Compounds in which the amino group has been substituted are pro-drugs which must be activated in the body since a free amino group is necessary for antimicrobial activity. An example is **phthalylsulphathiazole** (Fig. 30.2), which is activated in the intestine where the phthalyl group is slowly removed by hydrolysis to give the active agent. This drug is not absorbed and is used mainly for its action within the gastrointestinal tract.

The sulphonamides are usually used as their sodium salts which are readily soluble in water. The solutions of most sulphonamides are alkaline, except for that of sulphacetamide which is near neutral and can thus be used on mucous membranes and in the eye.

Mechanism of action

Sulphanilamide is a structural analogue of p-aminobenzoic acid (see Fig. 30.1) which is essential for the synthesis of folic acid in bacteria. As explained in Chapter 28, folate is required for DNA and RNA synthesis in both bacteria and mammals, but mammals obtain their folic acid in their diet and do not need to synthesize it, whereas bacteria do. The main mechanism of antibacterial action of the sulphonamides then, is by competing with p-aminobenzoic acid (pABA) for the enzyme *dihydropteroate synthetase*, and the effect of the sulphonamide may be overcome by adding excess pABA. The action of a sulphonamide is to inhibit growth of the bacteria not to kill them, i.e. it is *bacteriostatic* rather than *bactericidal*. Resistance is common. It is plasmid-mediated and due to the synthesis of an enzyme resistant to inhibition by the drug.

Pharmacokinetic aspects

Because the action of sulphonamides is bacteriostatic, successful treatment necessitates maintaining an adequate concentration for long enough to allow cellular defence mechanisms (see Chapter 8) to destroy the pathogenic bacteria. Most sulphonamides are readily absorbed in the gastrointestinal tract and reach maximum concentrations in the plasma in 4–6 hours. Exceptions are those poorly absorbed compounds, exemplified by phthalylsulphathiazole, which are specifically intended for antibacterial action within the gastrointestinal tract.

Apart from the use of sulphacetamide in the eye, sulphonamides are usually not given topically, mainly because of the risk of sensitization and allergic reactions.

Distribution depends partly on plasma protein binding, which varies with different compounds, being 60–80% for sulphadimidine, 22–55% for sulphadiazine and 25% for sulphafurazole. Sulphadiazine is distributed throughout the body water whereas sulphafurazole remains in the extracellular space. The drugs pass into inflammatory exudates, cross the placental barrier and reach an effective concentration in the CSF.

They are metabolized mainly in the liver, the major product being an acetylated derivative which lacks antibacterial action.

Unwanted effects

Mild to moderate toxic effects, which do not necessarily warrant withdrawal of the drug, are nausea and vomiting, headache and mental depression. Cyanosis due to methaemoglobinaemia may occur and is a lot less alarming than it looks. Serious toxic effects which necessitate cessation of therapy include hypersensitivity reactions, bone marrow depression and crystalluria. This last results from the precipitation of the acetylated metabolites in the urine. It can be prevented by giving plenty of fluids, and keeping the urine alkaline, and is less likely to occur with the more water-soluble preparations such as sulphafurazole.

Clinical use

Sulphonamides have largely been superseded by other antibacterial agents for the therapy of gonococcal, staphylococcal, streptococcal and shigella infections because many strains of these organisms have developed sulphonamide resistance. In the absence of resistance, sulphonamides are not only effective but are cheap and have the advantage of not producing a disturbance of gut flora, as may happen with broad spectrum antibiotics (see below).

The more water soluble sulphonamides are among the drugs of choice for acute urinary tract infections, and they are also drugs of first choice for the treatment of infections with *Nocardia*. They may be drugs of second choice in a variety of infections.

One particular sulphonamide, **sulphamethoxazole**, is often given together with trimethoprim, the combination constituting **cotrimoxazole** (see below).

TRIMETHOPRIM

In structure, trimethoprim (Fig. 30.3) has some

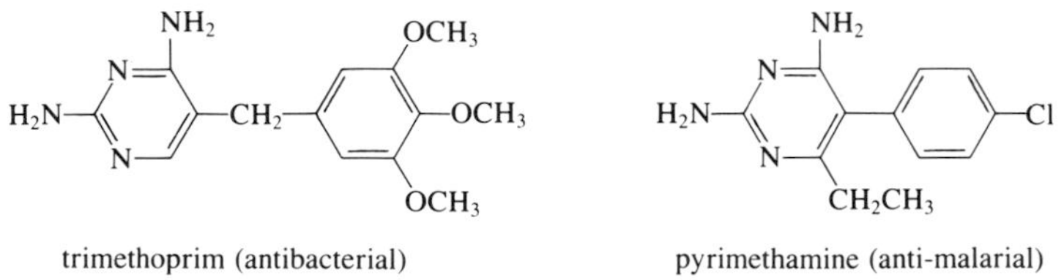

trimethoprim (antibacterial)

pyrimethamine (anti-malarial)

Fig. 30.3 Trimethoprim and pyrimethamine.

resemblance to folate. It is chemically related to the antimalarial drug, pyrimethamine, and, like it, is a *folate antagonist*. The metabolic importance of folate has been outlined in Chapters 18 & 29, and, as explained in Chapter 28, one of the key enzymes in folate metabolism, dihydrofolate reductase, is many times more sensitive to trimethoprim in bacteria than in man.

Trimethoprim is active against most common bacterial pathogens, and it is bacteriostatic rather than bactericidal. It is usually given as a mixture with a sulphonamide, sulphamethoxazole. This is called **cotrimoxazole**. Since sulphonamides affect an earlier stage in the same metabolic pathway in bacteria, i.e. folate synthesis, they strongly potentiate the action of trimethoprim. When given in combination, trimethoprim and sulphonamides are effective at doses one-tenth or less of what would be needed if either drug were used on its own, so the use of cotrimoxazole greatly reduces the incidence of unwanted effects.

Pharmacokinetic aspects

Trimethoprim is fully absorbed in the gastrointestinal tract and is widely distributed throughout the tissues and body fluids. It reaches high concentrations in the lungs and the kidneys and relatively high concentrations in the CSF. When given with sulphamethoxazole, about two-thirds of each is protein bound and about half of each is excreted within 24 hours. Since trimethoprim is a weak base, its elimination by the kidney increases with decreasing urinary pH.

Unwanted effects

These include nausea, vomiting and skin rashes. A 'toxic' effect which is related to its pharmacological action, folate deficiency, with resultant megaloblastic anaemia (see Chapter 18) can be prevented by giving folinic acid.

Clinical uses

Trimethoprim is used on its own in acute urinary tract infections. Cotrimoxazole is effective in a variety of infections, being active particularly against many types of Gram-negative organisms.

PENICILLIN

In 1928 Fleming, working at St Mary's Hospital in London, observed that a culture plate on which staphylocci were being grown, had become contaminated with a mould of the genus *Penicillium*, and that bacterial growth in the vicinity of the mould had been inhibited. He isolated the mould in pure culture and demonstrated that it produced an antibacterial substance which he called **penicillin**. This substance was subsequently extracted and its antibacterial effects analysed by Florey & Chain and their colleagues at Oxford in 1940. They showed that it had powerful chemotherapeutic properties in infected mice and that it was non-toxic. Its remarkable antibacterial effects in man were demonstrated in 1941. The penicillins are extremely effective antibiotics and are very widely used.

Chemistry of penicillin

The general formula of penicillin is shown in Fig. 30.4. The basic nucleus is 6-aminopenicillanic acid, which consists of a thiazolidine ring (A) linked to a β-lactam ring (B). This latter ring carries a secondary amino group. In different penicillins different acyl groups are attached to the amino group

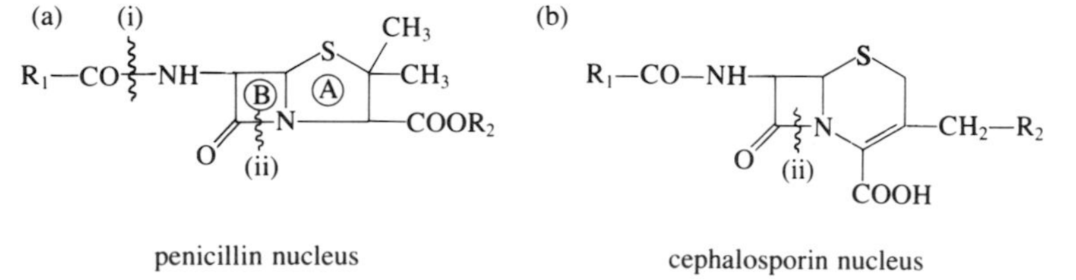

penicillin nucleus   cephalosporin nucleus

Fig. 30.4 (a) General structure of the penicillins **A**: thiazolidine ring, **B**: β-lactam ring; (b) General structure of the cephalosporins and cephamycins: (i) site of action of amidases, (ii) site of action of β-lactamases (penicillinases).

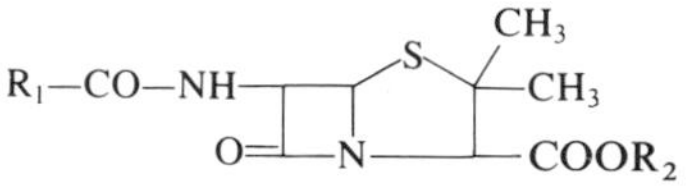

$$R_1-CO-NH \underset{O=}{\overset{}{\rule{0pt}{0pt}}} \text{—} \quad \overset{S}{\underset{N}{\bigsqcup}} \overset{CH_3}{\underset{COOR_2}{\rule{0pt}{0pt}}}$$

R_1	Name	R_2	Important Properties
(phenyl)—CH_2—	Benzylpenicillin (Penicillin G)	Na or K	Best given by injection
	Procaine penicillin	Procaine	Given by injection
	Benzathine penicillin	Benzathine	
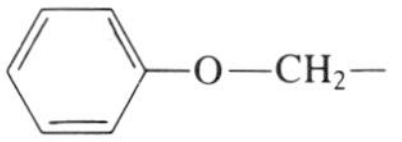 (phenyl)—O—CH_2—	Phenoxymethylpenicillin (Penicillin V)	H, K or Ca	Can be given orally
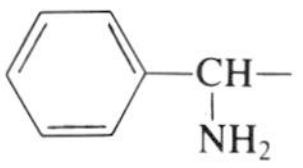 (phenyl)—CH— with NH_2	Ampicillin	H or Na	Can be given orally. Broad spectrum
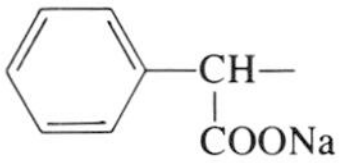 (phenyl)—CH— with COONa	Carbenicillin	Na	Broad spectrum
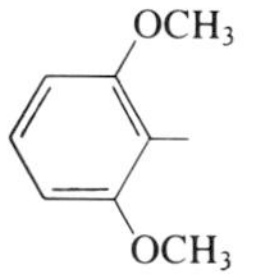 (phenyl with OCH₃, OCH₃) Methicillin ring	Methicillin	Na	β-lactamase-resistant
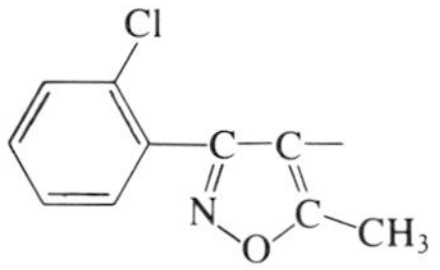 (chlorophenyl-isoxazole)	Cloxacillin	Na	β-lactamase-resistant. Can be given orally
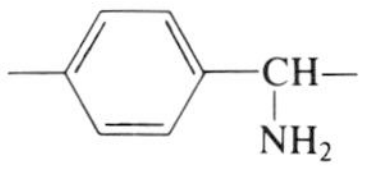 (phenyl)—CH— with NH_2	Amoxycillin	Na	Broad spectrum. Can be given orally

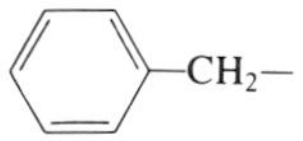

Fig. 30.5 Structures and important properties of some penicillins.

with an amide linkage. Semisynthetic penicillins are made by the addition of particular side-chains to naturally produced molecules (Fig. 30.5).

Penicillins may be destroyed by enzymes—amidases which act at site (i), and β-lactamases (penicillinases) which act at site (ii), cleaving the β-lactam ring (see Fig. 30.4).

Mechanisms of action

Penicillins interfere with the synthesis of the bacterial cell wall peptidoglycan (see Chapter 28). After attachment to binding sites on the bacterium, they inhibit the transpeptidation enzyme which cross-links the peptide chains attached to the backbone of the peptidoglycan (see Fig. 28.3). The final result is lysis of the bacterium.

Resistance to penicillin may be due to different causes, the main ones being:

1. The production of β-lactamases. This process is genetically controlled, the gene residing in a plasmid which can be transferred from one bacterium to another even across the boundaries of species. β-lactamase production is particularly important in staphylocci; streptococci do not produce these enzymes. Since the introduction of penicillin, staphylococcal resistance due to β-lactamase production has advanced progressively, occurring first in staphylococcal strains in hospitals and then in strains in the community at large. At the present

time, in developed countries, at least 80% of staphylococci produce β-lactamase. One possible future solution to the problem of the susceptibility of penicillin to β-lactamase could be the concomitant use of β-lactamase inhibitors. One such is clavulanic acid, which was isolated from a strain of Streptomyces. Clavulanic acid, a natural inhibitor of the enzyme, contains a β-lactam ring and is thought to bind covalently to the enzyme at or near its active site, the complex being cleaved only very slowly to release active enzyme—protecting the penicillin from the enzyme meanwhile.

2. The inability of the drug to penetrate to the site. This occurs particularly with Gram-negative organisms which have an outer membrane that limits the penetration of hydrophilic antibiotics.

Types of penicillin and their antimicrobial activity

Benzylpenicillin (penicillin G) and congeners

These early penicillins were found to be very active against Gram-positive cocci but much less active against Gram-negative bacilli.

Benzylpenicillin is the only naturally occurring penicillin in clinical use. It is destroyed by β-lactamase. It is the drug of choice for infections caused by streptococci, pneumococci, meningococci, gonococci and non-penicillinase-producing staphylococci (see Table 30.1). It is also the first line of treatment for diphtheria, syphilis, tetanus, gas-gangrene and actinomycosis. If given orally, its absorption is irregular and poor, due to destruction by gastric acid and adsorption on food. It is usually given by injection and its effects last for 4–6 hours.

Procaine penicillin is a salt of benzylpenicillin which has low solubility and is slowly absorbed. It can be used in intramuscular depot preparations which result in therapeutic concentrations within 2 hours, lasting for up to 24 hours.

Benzathine penicillin and **benethamine penicillin** are salts of benzylpenicillin which are only sparingly soluble. Their action lasts for up to 10 days, though the plasma concentration is fairly low. These preparations have rather limited and specific clinical indications, being used particularly for the prevention of some types of streptococcal infections.

Phenoxymethylpenicillin (penicillin V) is closely related to benzylpenicillin and has a similar spectrum of antimicrobial activity, but is less potent. It is acid-stable and can be given by mouth. However, its absorption and thus plasma concentration, is variable and unpredictable and it is therefore not used for serious infections.

β-lactamase-resistant penicillins

These are relatively resistant to the action of the enzymes which cleave the β-lactam ring. They are not as potent as benzylpenicillin. They have a narrow spectrum of activity, being effective almost exclusively against Gram-positive organisms and thus their main clinical use is against infections caused by β-lactamase-producing staphylococci. This class includes **cloxacillin**, **flucloxacillin**, **dicloxacillin** and **nafcillin**. All of these are sufficiently acid-stable to be given orally. They are rapidly but incompletely absorbed from the gut and maximum plasma concentrations are reached within 1 hour. They can also be given parenterally. They are eliminated mainly by the kidney, though there is some excretion in the bile. The plasma half-life for each drug is 30–60 mins. **Methicillin** is a β-lactamase-resistant antibiotic which is not acid-stable and which has to be given by injection.

Broad-spectrum penicillins

This group of antibiotics has a broader spectrum of antibacterial activity than benzylpenicillin in that they have greater activity against Gram-negative organisms. They are all destroyed by β-lactamase and are somewhat less potent than benzylpenicillin against many Gram-positive cocci.

Ampicillin is acid-resistant, can be given orally as well as parenterally, and is one of the most widely used antibiotics. **Talampicillin** and **amoxycillin** are related compounds with even more complete absorption in the gastrointestinal tract. **Carbenicillin** is a broad-spectrum penicillin which has to be given parenterally and is used mainly for infections with pseudomonads. In **mecillinam** the anti-bacterial spectrum has been reversed and this antibiotic is much more potent against Gram-negative than against Gram-positive organisms. It is useful in typhoid fever.

Pharmacokinetic aspects

When given orally, different penicillins are absorbed to differing degrees (see below) depending on their stability in acid and their protein binding. Parenteral administration can be intramuscular, subcutaneous or intravenous. Intrathecal administration is inadvisable as convulsions may ensue. After intramuscular injection, absorption is rapid and maximum plasma concentrations are reached within 15 minutes. The drugs are widely distributed in the body fluids, passing into joints, into pleural and pericardial cavities, into the bile, the saliva and the milk and across the placenta. Penicillins do not readily cross the blood-brain barrier unless the meninges are inflamed, in which case they may reach therapeutically effective concentrations in the CSF.

Elimination is mainly renal and occurs rapidly, usually on one transit through the kidney, 90% of it being by tubular secretion. The short plasma half-life (about 1 hour) is one of the main problems in the clinical use of penicillins, which has to be overcome either by frequent dosage or by the use of a slow-release preparation, such as procaine penicillin. Alternatively, tubular secretion can be partially blocked by **probenecid**, which raises the plasma concentration and prolongs the action of penicillins (see Chapters 5 & 14). A large proportion of penicillin is excreted unchanged in the urine. When first tested clinically, in 1940, on an Oxford policeman, the drug was so scarce that the patient's urine was collected, and the drug extracted for re-use.

Unwanted effects

One of the remarkable features of the penicillins is their relative freedom from toxic effects. However, *hypersensitivity* reactions occur, the basis of which appears to be the fact that degradation products of penicillin combine with host protein and become antigenic. There are cross-reactions between various types of penicillin. *Skin rashes* of various sorts and fever are the most common manifestations of hypersensitivity; much more serious is *acute anaphylactic shock*, with circulatory collapse and obstruction of breathing due to oedema and spasm of the bronchi. This may, in some cases, be fatal but fortunately is very rare. A less sudden manifestation of hypersensitivity, coming on after 1–2 weeks' treatment, is a type of *serum sickness* with fever, urticarial skin eruptions and, in severe cases, generalized oedema, multiple joint effusions and enlargement of spleen and lymph glands. This syndrome is also rare. Other hypersensitivity reactions seen occasionally are *vasculitis, interstitial nephritis* and various *haematologic disturbances.*

The occurrence of these allergic reactions is unpredictable, but in general if an individual does not react to penicillin when first given it, the chance of reacting to subsequent administration is low—the incidence being less than 1%. Furthermore, only 10–15% of individuals who have had a reaction to penicillin will react if given penicillin again. However, if there is a history of a previous hypersensitivity reaction, an alternative treatment should be considered.

A side effect of the penicillins, particularly the broad-spectrum type given orally, is alteration of the bacterial flora in the gut. This may be associated with gastrointestinal disturbances and, in some cases, with suprainfection with microorganisms not sensitive to penicillin.

CEPHALOSPORINS AND CEPHAMYCINS

Cultures of a *Cephalosporium* fungus obtained from the sea near a sewer outlet in Sardinia were found to yield extracts which inhibited the growth of *Staphylococcus aureus*. Subsequent work by Abraham and Newton in Oxford resulted in the identification of three distinct antibiotics, cephalosporins N and C, which are chemically related to penicillin, and cephalosporin P—a steroid antibiotic which resembles fusidic acid (see below).

The nucleus of cephalosporin C, (see Figs. 30.4 & 30.6) has been isolated and a large number of semi-synthetic broad-spectrum cephalosporins have been produced by the addition to this nucleus of different side-chains (Fig. 30.6). These agents are water soluble and relatively acid-stable. They vary in susceptibility to β-lactamases. Cephalosporins in clinical use include the 'first generation' compounds **cephradine** and **cephazolin**, and the 'second generation' compounds **cefuroxime** and **cephamandole**. 'Third generation' compounds include **cefoperazone** and **cefotaxime**.

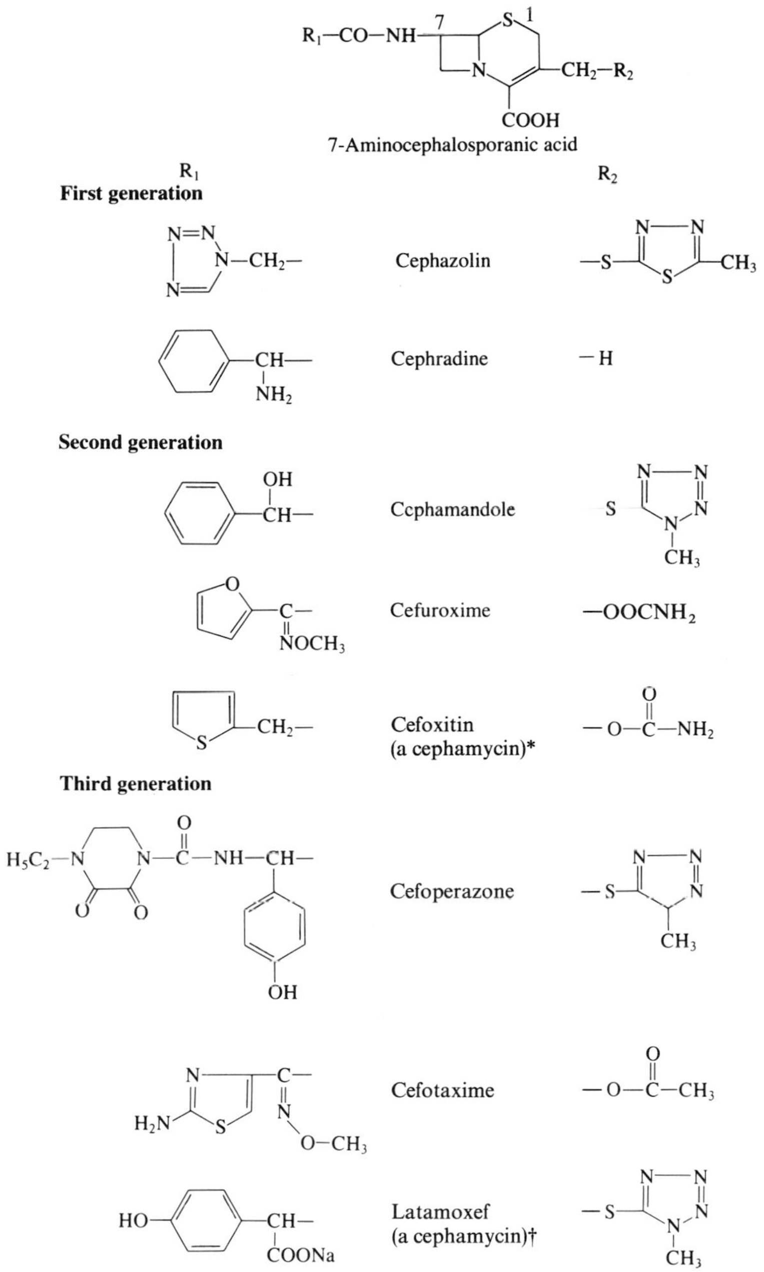

Fig. 30.6 Structures of some cephalosporins and cephamycins.
 * In cefoxitin there is $-OCH_3$ at position 7.
 † In latamoxef there is $-OCH_3$ at position 7 and oxygen instead of sulphur at position 1.

The cephamycins (e.g. **cefoxitin**) are β-lactam antibiotics produced by *Streptomyces* organisms and they are closely related to the cephalosporins, differing only in having an additional methoxy group (CH_3O-) attached to the β-lactam ring. **Latamoxef** is a synthetic cephamycin compound.

Mechanism of action

The mechanism of action of these agents is the same as that of the penicillins—interference with peptidoglycan synthesis. This is described in Chapter 28 and illustrated in Figure 28.3. As with the penicillins, resistance occurs if an organism generates enzymes which cleave the β-lactam ring (although penicillinase-producing staphylococci may be susceptible to cephalosporins) or if it has an outer membrane which prevents penetration of the drug. Cefotoxin and the cephalosporins are not readily attacked by the plasmid-encoded β-lactamases, but there are reports of resistance due to mutations involving the binding-site proteins.

The *antibacterial spectrum* of these agents is broad and is similar for most of the cephalosporins. It includes a variety of Gram-positive cocci (including some which are penicillin-resistant) and several Gram-negative organisms. Cefotaxime, cefuroxime and latamoxef have a broader spectrum of antibiotic activity than the compounds developed first, but are less active against Gram-positive organisms.

Pharmacokinetic aspects

Some cephalosporins, such as cephradine, may be given orally but most are given parenterally, intramuscularly (which may be painful with some agents) or intravenously.

After absorption they are widely distributed into the body, passing into the pleural, pericardial and joint fluids and across the placenta. Some, such as cefoperazone and latamoxef also cross the blood-brain barrier. Elimination is mainly via the kidney by both tubular secretion and glomerular filtration, though high concentrations are also found in the bile.

Unwanted effects

Hypersensitivity reactions, very similar to those found with penicillin, may be seen. Some cross-reactions occur; about 10% of penicillin-sensitive individuals will have allergic reactions to cephalosporins.

TETRACYCLINES

These are broad-spectrum antibiotics which have a polycyclic structure (Fig. 30.7). The first tetracyclines used, **chlortetracycline** (now superseded), **oxytetracycline**, and **demeclocycline** were derived

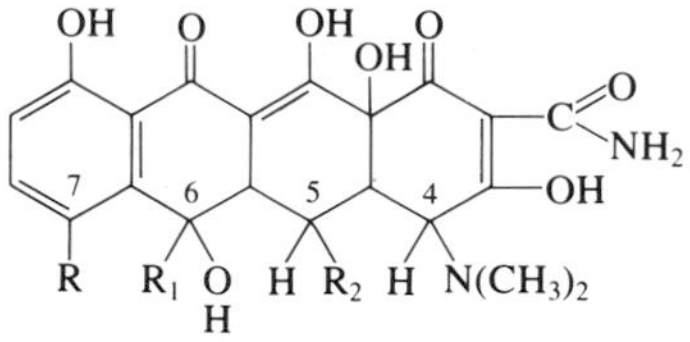

	R	R_1	R_2	Renal Clearance (ml/min)
Chlortetracycline	—Cl	—CH_3	—H	35
Oxytetracycline	—H	—CH_3	—OH	90
Tetracycline	—H	—CH_3	—H	65
Demeclocycline	—Cl	—H	—H	35
Methacycline	—H	=CH_2*	—OH	31
Doxycycline	—H	—CH_3*	—OH	16
Minocycline	—N(CH_3)$_2$	—H	—H	10

*There is no —OH at position 6 on methacycline and doxycycline.

Fig. 30.7 Structural formulae of tetracycline drugs.

from cultures of *Streptomyces*. More recently developed compounds, **tetracycline**, **methacycline**, **doxycycline** and **minocycline** are synthetic or semi-synthetic.

Mechanism of action

The mechanism of action of these agents is inhibition of protein synthesis after uptake into susceptible organisms by active transport. This action is described in Chapter 28 (p. 600). The tetracyclines are bacteriostatic, not bactericidal.

Their *spectrum of antibacterial activity* is very wide and includes a variety of microorganisms such as Gram-positive and Gram-negative bacteria, *Mycoplasma*, *Rickettsia*, *Chlamydia*, *Brucella* and some protozoa (e.g. amoebae). Minocycline is also effective against *Neisseria meningitidis*. However, some strains of organisms have become resistant, decreasing the usefulness of these agents. Resistance is transmitted by plasmids and since the genes controlling resistance to tetracyclines are closely associated with genes for resistance to other antibiotics, organisms may become resistant to many drugs simultaneously. The basis of resistance in most bacteria is the synthesis of 'resistance' proteins which transport the tetracyclines out of the bacterium.

Pharmacokinetic aspects

The tetracyclines are usually given orally but may be

given parenterally. The absorption of most preparations from the gut is irregular and incomplete, and is improved in the absence of food. Minocycline and doxycycline are virtually completely absorbed. Since tetracyclines chelate metal ions (calcium, magnesium, iron, aluminium), forming non-absorbable complexes, absorption is decreased in the presence of milk, certain antacids and iron preparations (see Chapter 5). The drugs have a wide distribution, entering most fluid compartments, crossing the placenta to the foetus and appearing in the milk. Minocycline is found in high concentration in tears and saliva. Excretion of most tetracyclines is by two routes—*via* the bile and *via* the kidney by glomerular filtration. Most tetracylines will accumulate if renal function is impaired and this may exacerbate renal failure. Doxycycline is an exception, being excreted largely into the gastrointestinal tract. Minocycline is partly metabolized.

Unwanted effects

The commonest are gastrointestinal disturbances, due initially to direct irritation and later to modification of the gut flora. Suprainfection may occur.

Because they chelate calcium, tetracyclines are deposited in growing bones and teeth, causing staining and sometimes dental hypoplasia and bone deformities. They should therefore never be given to children, pregnant women or nursing mothers.

Phototoxicity (sensitization to sunlight) has been seen, more particularly with demeclocycline. Minocycline may produce vestibular disturbances (dizziness and nausea), the frequency of these reactions being dose-related. High doses of tetracyclines may decrease protein synthesis in most cells and long-term therapy may cause disturbances of the bone marrow.

Clinical use

Because of their broad spectrum of activity they may be employed in a variety of infections. They are the drugs of choice in rickettsial, mycoplasma and chlamydial infections, and are drugs of second choice for infections with several different organisms (see Table 30.1) and are useful in mixed infections of the respiratory tract.

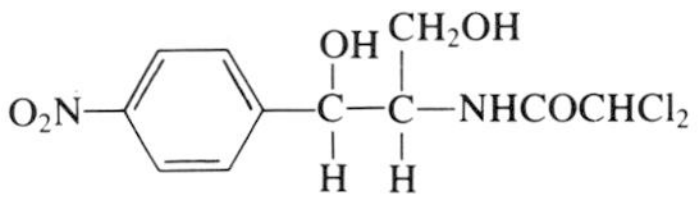

Fig. 30.8 Chloramphenicol.

CHLORAMPHENICOL

This was originally isolated from cultures of *Streptomyces* but is now synthesized commercially for clinical use. Its structure is illustrated in Figure 30.8. Its salts are very soluble in water and, when hydrolysed in the tissues, release free chloramphenicol which has relatively high lipid solubility.

Its *mechanism of action* is by inhibition of protein synthesis as described in Chapter 28 (p. 601). Chloramphenicol binds to the 50S subunit of the bacterial ribosome at the same site as erythromycin and clindamycin. The three drugs may compete and thus interfere with each others' actions if given concurrently.

Like the tetracycline drugs, chloramphenicol has a wide spectrum of antimicrobial activity, including Gram-negative and Gram-positive organisms and rickettsiae. It is bacteriostatic for most organisms but bactericidal to *Haemophilus influenzae*.

Resistance may occur. Mutants may be found but they are usually only slightly more resistant than the parent cells and resistance will thus develop rather slowly during treatment.

R-plasmids containing determinants for multiple drug resistance for chloramphenicol, streptomycin, tetracycline etc. may be transferred from one bacterial species to another by transduction. The R genes code for chloramphenicol acetyl-transferase and may occur on transposons (p. 605). New derivatives of chloramphenicol with the terminal OH on the side chain replaced by fluorine are reported not to be susceptible to acetylation and thus to retain antibacterial activity.

Pharmacokinetic aspects

Given orally, chloramphenicol is rapidly and completely absorbed and reaches its maximum concentration in the plasma within 2 hours; it can also be given parenterally. As might be expected from its lipid solubility it is widely distributed throughout the tissues and body fluids including the CSF, in which its concentration may be as high as that in the blood. In the plasma it is 30–50% protein-bound and its half-life is $1\frac{1}{2}$–$3\frac{1}{2}$ hours. Therapeutically useful plasma concentrations are found for up to 6 hours after an average oral dose. About 10% is excreted unchanged in the urine, and the remainder is inactivated in the liver either by conjugation with glucuronic acid or by reduction to inactive amines prior to renal excretion.

Unwanted effects

The most important of these is depression of the bone marrow—an effect which may occur even with very low doses in some individuals. A disturbance in red cell maturation sometimes associated with some degree of leucopenia and/or thrombocytopenia occurs in many individuals taking chloramphenicol for 2 weeks or more. It disappears when treatment is stopped. In a small proportion of patients aplastic anaemia may occur, the incidence being approximately 1 in 30 000 of those on chloramphenicol. If the aplasia is severe it is very likely to result in death. Patients who recover have a high incidence of leukemia. Bone marrow aplasia is thought not to occur with newer analogues of chloramphenicol.

Chloramphenicol must not be used in the newborn because inadequate inactivation and excretion of the drug (see Chapter 4) may result in the 'grey baby syndrome'—vomiting, diarrhoea, flaccidity, low temperature and an ashen-grey colour—which carries a 40% mortality.

Hypersensitivity reactions may occur, as may gastrointestinal disturbances and other sequelae of alteration of microbial flora.

Clinical use

Clinical use of chloramphenicol should be reserved for serious infections in which the benefit of the drug is greater than the risk of toxicity. These include typhoid fever, infections caused by *Haemophilus influenzae* and *Bacteroides fragilis* and meningitis in patients in whom penicillin cannot be used.

AMINOGLYCOSIDES

The aminoglycosides are a group of antibiotics of

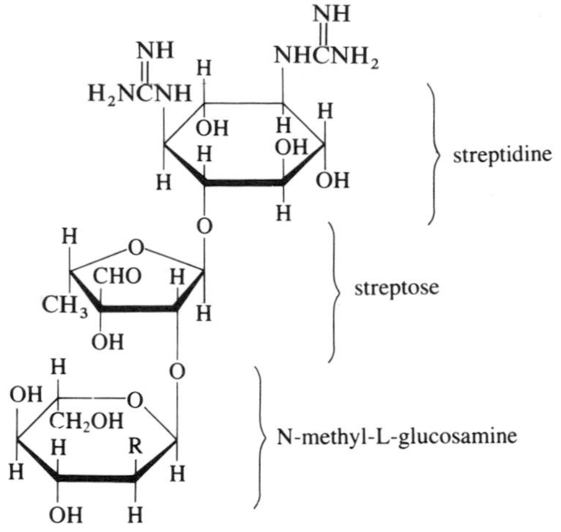

Fig. 30.9 Structure of streptomycin (R=CH$_3$NH).

similar chemical structure, antimicrobial activity, pharmacokinetic characteristics and toxicity. The main agents are **streptomycin, gentamycin, amikacin, kanamycin, tobramycin, netilmycin, neomycin** and **framycetin**. The structure of streptomycin is given in Figure 30.9. Other aminoglycosides consist similarly of two or more amino sugars attached by glycosidic linkage to a hexose nucleus, (which is deoxystreptamine rather than streptidine, as in streptomycin), with variations in the structures of the substituent groups.

Mechanism of action

All bind to a non-enzymic site on the 30S subunit of the bacterial ribosome which causes an alteration in codon:anticodon recognition. This results in misreading of the messenger RNA and hence in the production of defective bacterial proteins (p. 600). Their penetration through the cell membrane of the bacterium depends partly on oxygen-dependent active transport by a polyamine carrier system and they have minimal action against anaerobic organisms. Their effect is bactericidal and is enhanced by agents which interfere with cell wall synthesis.

Resistance

This may occur by several different mechanisms (p. 604), the most important being inactivation by microbial enzymes, the genes for which are carried on plasmids. There are nine or more of these inactivating enzymes and they are situated in the plasma membrane in the region of the carriers for the drugs. The inactivated drug is not well taken up by the transport mechanism and does not interfere with protein synthesis. (Netilmicin and amikacin are not affected by these inactivating enzymes.) Other mechanisms of resistance include failure of penetration (this can be largely overcome by the concomitant use of penicillin) and lack of binding of the drugs to the ribosome due to a mutation which alters the binding-site on the 30S subunit. This last affects mainly streptomycin and is a rare reason for resistance.

Spectrum of antibacterial activity

The aminoglycosides are effective against many aerobic Gram-negative and some Gram-positive organisms. Streptomycin and kanamycin are also active against *Mycobacterium tuberculosis* (see below).

Pharmacokinetic aspects

The aminoglysides are polycations and highly polar. They are not absorbed in the gastrointestinal tract but are rapidly absorbed after intramuscular or subcutaneous injection. They can also be given intravenously or intrathecally. Binding to plasma proteins is minimal, being about 10%. They do not enter cells, nor do they cross the blood-brain barrier into the CNS, penetrate the eye or reach high concentrations in secretions and body fluids. They may, however, cross the placenta. Tissue levels are low except in the cortex of the kidney. The plasma half-life is 2–3 hours. Elimination is virtually entirely by glomerular filtration in the kidney, 50–60% of a dose being excreted unchanged within 24 hours. If renal function is impaired, accumulation occurs with a resultant increase in those toxic effects (such as oto- and nephrotoxicity) which are dose-related.

Unwanted effects

Toxicity limits the usefulness of these agents, the main hazards being ototoxicity and nephrotoxicity.

Ototoxicity involves progressive damage and destruction of the sensory cells in the cochlea and vestibular organ of the ear. The result may be vertigo, ataxia and loss of balance in the case of vestibular damage, and auditory disturbances, including deafness, in the case of cochlear damage. Any aminoglycoside may produce both types of effect, but streptomycin and gentamycin are more likely to interfere with vestibular function whereas with kanamycin, neomycin and amikacin the side effects are mostly on hearing. The incidence of these toxic effects on hearing and balance when short-term therapy is employed, is 3% for amikacin, 2% for gentamycin and 1% for streptomycin, kanamycin and tobramycin. A higher incidence occurs with long-term use or if there is accumulation.

The *nephrotoxicity* consists of damage to the kidney tubules and can be reversed if the use of the drugs is stopped. Nephrotoxicity is more likely to occur in the elderly and in patients with pre-existing renal disease or in conditions in which urine volume is reduced. In these cases plasma concentrations of the drugs must be monitored.

A rare toxic reaction is paralysis due to neuromuscular blockade, usually only seen if the agents are given concurrently with neuromuscular blocking agents. It is due to inhibition of the calcium uptake necessary for the exocytotic release of acetylcholine (see Chapter 6).

Clinical use

Aminoglycosides are most widely used against Gram-negative enteric organisms. They may also be given together with a penicillin in infections caused by *Streptococcus*, *Pseudomonas* or *Listeria* (see Table 30.1).

Gentamycin is the aminoglycoside most commonly used. Tobramycin and the recently-introduced netilmicin are similar in antibacterial activity to gentamycin, and are reputed to be less toxic. Amikacin is a semisynthetic drug which is resistant to most of the aminoglycoside inactivating enzymes. Neomycin and framycetin are too toxic for parenteral use and are only used topically and to reduce the bacterial flora of the gut prior to surgery. Streptomycin is virtually entirely reserved for the treatment of tuberculosis but may be used with a tetracycline to treat plague or brucellosis.

Spectinomycin

This antiobiotic is related to the aminoglycosides in

structure. Its use is confined to the treatment of gonorrhoea in patients allergic to penicillin or those whose infections are caused by penicillin-resistant gonococci.

MACROLIDES

This group of antibiotics is so-named because they possess a macrocyclic lactone-ring (Fig. 30.10), the ring being linked with amino sugars through glycosidic bonds. The main agent is **erythromycin**.

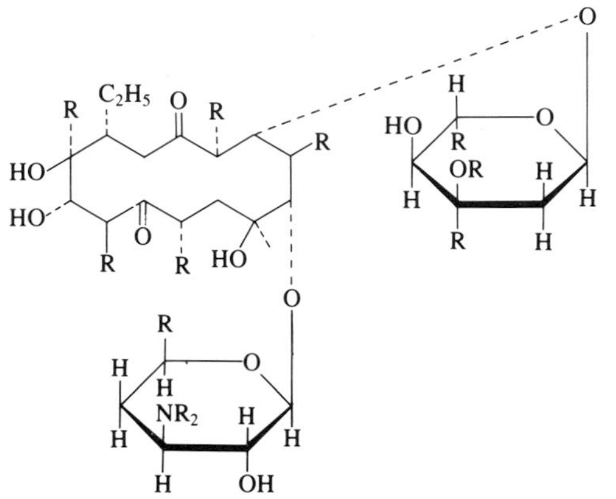

Fig. 30.10 Structure of erythromycin (R=CH$_3$).

Mechanism of action

The *mechanism of action* is inhibition of protein synthesis in bacteria by an effect on translocation (p. 601). The drug may be bactericidal or bacteriostatic, the effect depending on its concentration and on the type of the microorganism. It is bound to the 50S subunit of the bacterial ribosome. Its binding site appears to be the same as that of chloramphenicol and clindamycin and the three agents could compete, if given concurrently.

The *antimicrobial spectrum* is very similar to that of penicillin. Erythromycin is effective against Gram-positive bacteria and spirochaetes but not against most Gram-negative organisms, exceptions being gonococci and, to a lesser extent, *Haemophilus influenza*. *Mycoplasma*, *Legionella* and some chlamydial organisms are also suceptible.

Resistance may occur and is due to a plasmid-controlled alteration of the receptor for erythromycin on the bacterial ribosome.

Pharmacokinetic aspects

Erythromycin may be administered orally or parenterally. It is inactivated by gastric juice unless given as acid-resistant coated tablets. Intramuscular injections may cause pain and intravenous injections may be followed by local thrombophlebitis. Erythromycin is reasonably well absorbed in the intestine. It diffuses readily into most tissues, including prostatic fluid and the placenta, but does not cross the blood-brain barrier. About 70% or more is bound to plasma protein and its plasma half-life is about 90 minutes. It is concentrated in the liver where some is inactivated and some excreted, in active form, in the bile.

Unwanted effects

These are rare. One particular preparation, erythromycin estolate, may cause cholestatic hepatitis, with jaundice, if used for more than 14 days. Hypersensitivity reactions such as skin rashes and fever may occasionally occur, as may gastrointestinal disturbances.

Clinical use

Erythromycin is a drug of choice in infections with *Corynebacteria* and some infections with *Chlamydia*, *Mycoplasma* and *Legionella*. It may also be used as an alternative to penicillin in patients with penicillin allergy.

LINCOSAMIDES

Clindamycin is a semisynthetic modification of lincomycin, an antibiotic isolated from *Streptomyces lincolnensis*. Lincomycin itself is not much used.

Mechanism of action

This involves inhibition of protein synthesis and is similar to that of erythromycin and chloramphenicol (p. 601). All three types of antibiotic bind to the 50S subunit and may compete for the binding site if given concurrently.

The *antibacterial spectrum* of clindamycin includes Gram-positive cocci, including penicillin-resistant staphylococci, and anaerobic Gram-negative bacteria.

Pharmacokinetic factors

Clindamycin may be given orally or parenterally and is widely distributed in tissues (including bone) and in body fluids. It diffuses across the placenta but does not cross the blood-brain barrier. About 90% or more is protein-bound and its half-life in the plasma is $2\frac{1}{2}$ hours. It is inactivated in the liver and its metabolites are excreted in the urine along with 10% of the unaltered drug.

Unwanted effects

These consist mainly of gastrointestinal disturbances, the incidence varying between 2 and 20%. A potentially lethal condition, *pseudomembranous colitis*, may occur, and is due to a necrotizing toxin produced by a clindamycin-resistant organism which may be part of the normal faecal flora. Vancomycin (see below) is effective in the treatment of this condition.

Its main *clinical use* is in infections caused by *Bacteroides* organisms.

VANCOMYCIN

This is a glycopeptide antibiotic which inhibits cell wall synthesis (see Fig. 28.3) and it is bactericidal. It is effective mainly against Gram-positive bacteria including methicillin-resistant staphylococci. Resistant mutants are rare and resistance occurs slowly. There is no cross-resistance with other antimicrobial agents. It synergizes with some aminoglycoside antibiotics against some organisms which it, on its own, does not kill.

It is not absorbed from the gut and is given by the oral route only, for treatment of gastrointestinal infections. For parenteral use it is given intravenously. It is widely distributed and will penetrate the CSF if the meninges are inflamed. Only 10% is bound to plasma protein. Elimination is virtually entirely by glomerular filtration into the urine and thus it could cumulate if renal function is impaired. Its plasma half-life is about 6 hours.

Unwanted effects

Chills and fever may occur, as may local phlebitis at the site of injection. Ototoxicity has been reported, associated with very high plasma concentrations of the drug. Hypersensitivity reactions are seen occasionally.

Clinical use

The clinical use of vancomycin is limited mainly to pseudomembranous colitis (see above) and the treatment of some methicillin-resistant staphylococcal infections. It is also valuable in severe staphylococcal infections in patients allergic to penicillins and cephalosporins and in some forms of streptococcal endocarditis.

POLYMIXIN ANTIBIOTICS

These are a group of antibiotics isolated from *Bacillus polymixa*. The agents in use are **polymixin B** and **colistin** (Polymixin E).

The polymixins are simple basic peptides joined to long chain fatty acids; they have cationic detergent properties. Their *mechanism of action* involves interaction with the phospholipids of the cell membrane and disruption of its structure. They have a selective action against Gram-negative bacilli, especially pseudomonads and coliform organisms. The drugs are rapidly bactericidal and resistance is rare.

Pharmacokinetic aspects

The polymixins are not absorbed from the gastrointestinal tract. They can be given orally for infections in the gut and may also be applied topically. Intramuscular injection is painful and is to be avoided. Polymixin B sulphate may be given by slow intravenous infusion or, in meningitis due to *Pseudomonas*, by intrathecal injection.

Unwanted effects

These may be serious and include neurotoxicity and nephrotoxicity. Hypersensitivity reactions are rare.

Clinical use

The use of the polymixins is limited by their toxicity and is confined largely to severe infections caused by pseudomonads and other Gram-negative organisms not susceptible to other antibiotics. They may be used systemically for these conditions in conjunction with trimethoprim, and topically with neomycin or bacitracin in the treatment of ear, eye or skin infections caused by susceptible organisms.

FUSIDIC ACID

This is a narrow spectrum steroid antibiotic active mainly against Gram-positive bacteria but it antagonizes the action of some penicillins against staphylococci. It acts by inhibiting protein synthesis (p. 601).

Sodium fusidate is well absorbed from the gut and distributed widely in the tissues. It does not cross the blood-brain barrier. Some is excreted in the bile and some metabolized.

Unwanted effects such as gastrointestinal disturbances are fairly common. Skin eruptions and jaundice may occur. It is used mainly for infections caused by penicillin-resistant staphylococci, especially osteomyelitis, since sodium fusidate is concentrated in bone. A second agent with anti-staphylococcal activity is usually necessary.

BACITRACIN

This is an antibiotic isolated from a strain of *Bacillus subtilis*. It is a polypeptide with a range of activity similar to that of penicillin, being most active against Gram-positive organisms including β-lactamase-producing staphylococci. Its mechanism of action involves inhibition of cell-wall formation (see Chapter 28). It is less liable to produce resistance than penicillin and cross-resistance is rare.

It is not readily absorbed from the gut or from skin or mucous membrane.

Bacitracin has serious toxic effects on the kidney and is not therefore used systemically. It is used topically for infections of mouth, nose, eye and skin and is much less likely to cause hypersensitivity reactions than penicillin.

METRONIDAZOLE

This is primarily an antiprotozoal agent (p. 642) but is also active against anaerobic bacteria such as *Bacteroides*, *Clostridia* and some streptococci.

NITROFURANTOIN

This is a synthetic compound (Fig. 30.11) active against a range of Gram-positive and Gram-negative organisms. The development of resistance in susceptible organisms is rare and there is no cross resistance. Its mechanism of action is not known, but its effect is more marked in acid urine.

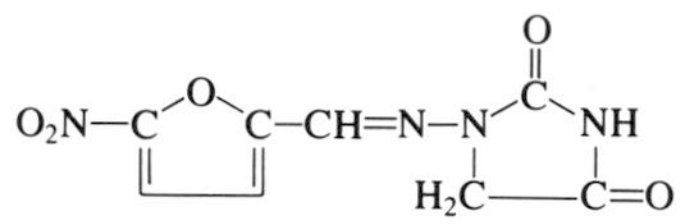

Fig. 30.11 Nitrofurantoin.

It is given orally and is rapidly and totally absorbed from the gastrointestinal tract and very rapidly excreted by the kidney by both glomerular filtration and tubular secretion; thus it reaches antibacterial concentrations in the urine but not in the plasma. In renal failure, toxic blood levels ensue.

Unwanted effects

Gastrointestinal disturbances are relatively common and hypersensitivity reactions involving the skin and the bone marrow (e.g. leukopenia) may occur. Hepatotoxicity and peripheral neuropathy have been reported.

The *clinical use* of nitrofurantoin is confined to the treatment of urinary tract infections.

NALIDIXIC ACID

This is a synthetic compound (Fig. 30.12) active

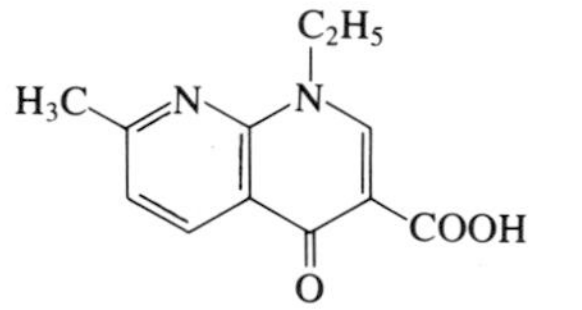

Fig. 30.12 Nalidixic acid.

against Gram-negative organisms in the urinary tract. It acts by inhibiting DNA synthesis (p. 603) and possibly also by lowering the pH of the urine. Resistant mutants may emerge rapidly during therapy but the resistance is not transferable.

The drug is rapidly absorbed in the gastro-intestinal tract, partly metabolized in the body and excreted in the urine—some in unchanged form and some as an active metabolite. Its plasma half-life is about 8 hours.

Unwanted effects include gastrointestinal disturbances, and allergic skin reactions (sometimes associated with photosensitivity). Effects on the central nervous system (visual disturbances, hallucinations) have been reported.

Clinical use of nalidixic acid is confined to the treatment of urinary tract infections due to coliform organisms.

Cinoxacin is related to nalidixic acid and has similar uses.

ANTIMYCOBACTERIAL AGENTS

The main mycobacterial infections in man are **tuberculosis** and **leprosy**—both typically chronic infections, caused respectively by *Mycobacterium tuberculosis* and *Mycobacterium leprae*. A particular problem with both these conditions is that after phagocytosis, the microorganisms can survive *inside* macrophages, unless these are 'activated' by T cell lymphokines (see Chapter 8).

DRUGS USED TO TREAT TUBERCULOSIS

The *first line drugs* used in the treatment of tuberculosis are **streptomycin** (see above), **isoniazid**, **rifampicin** and **ethambutol**. The *second line drugs* available are **pyrazinamide**, **capreomycin** and **cyclo-serine**. These latter drugs are used for infections with tubercle bacilli resistant to first-line drugs or when the first-line agents have to be abandoned due to unwanted reactions.

Because of the possibility of emergence of resistant organisms (an especial problem with streptomycin), compound drug therapy is employed, involving an *initial* phase in which at least three drugs

are used, and a *continuation* phase in which two drugs are used. Depending on the type of tuberculosis and the combination of agents employed, treatment may take 6–18 months.

ISONIAZID (ISONICOTINIC ACID HYDRAZIDE; INH)

This synthetic compound is one of the most important drugs for the treatment of tuberculosis because of its effectiveness, low cost and relative lack of toxicity. It has a simple chemical structure (Fig. 30.13) and is readily soluble in water. It is related to iproniazid, a monoamine oxidase inhibitor (see Chapter 23), which is no longer used in man due to its toxicity.

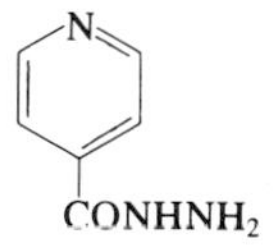

Fig. 30.13 Isoniazid.

The antibacterial activity of isoniazid is limited almost entirely to mycobacteria. It is bacteriostatic for 'resting' organisms and bactericidal for actively growing organisms. It passes freely into cells and is thus effective against intracellular organisms and it is actively taken up by tubercle bacilli. The mechanism of its action is not clearly known. There is evidence that it inhibits the synthesis of mycolic acids—important constituents of the cell wall and peculiar to mycobacteria. It is also reported to combine with an enzyme which is uniquely found in isoniazid-sensitive strains of mycobacteria, resulting in disorganization of the metabolism of the cell.

Pharmacokinetic aspects

Isoniazid is readily absorbed from the gastro-intestinal tract or after parenteral injection and is widely distributed throughout the tissues and body fluids, including the cerebrospinal fluid, where it reaches about one-fifth of the plasma concentration. An important point is that it penetrates well into 'caseous' tuberculous lesions (i.e. necrotic lesions, with a 'cheese-like' consistency). Metabolism, which involves largely acetylation, depends on genetic factors which determine whether a person is a 'slow' or a 'rapid' inactivator of the drug (see Chapter 4), slow inactivators having a better therapeutic response.

The half-life in slow inactivators is 3 hours and in rapid inactivators, 1½ hours. INH is excreted in the urine partly as unchanged drug, partly in the acetylated or otherwise inactivated form, the proportions depending on whether the individual is a slow or rapid inactivator.

Unwanted effects

These depend on the dosage and occur in about 1 in 20 individuals, the commonest being allergic skin eruptions. A variety of other adverse reactions have been reported, including hepatotoxicity, haematological changes, arthritic symptoms and vasculitis. Toxic effects involving the central or peripheral nervous systems are largely due to a deficiency of pyridoxine and are common unless prevented by administration of this substance. (INH is a structural analogue of pyridoxine and increases its excretion.) INH may cause haemolytic anaemia in individuals with glucose-6-phosphate deficiency and it decreases the metabolism of the antiepileptic agent, phenytoin, resulting in an increase in plasma concentration and toxicity of this drug.

RIFAMPICIN

This drug is a semisynthetic derivative of the antibiotic rifamycin obtained from a streptomyces organism. It acts by binding to, and inhibiting, DNA-dependent RNA polymerase, in prokaryotic but not eukaryotic cells (p. 603). It is one of the most active antituberculosis agents known. It is also active against most other Gram-positive bacteria as well as many Gram-negative species. Resistance can develop rapidly in a one-step process and is thought to be due to chemical modification of microbial RNA polymerase, resulting from a chromosal mutation.

Pharmacokinetic aspects

Rifampicin is given orally and is widely distributed in the tissues and body fluids (including the cerebrospinal fluid) giving an orange tinge to saliva,

sputum, tears and sweat. It is excreted in the bile, some being reabsorbed and re-excreted. There is progressive metabolism of the drug by deacetylation during its repeated passages through the liver. The metabolite retains antibacterial activity but is less well absorbed from the gastrointestinal tract.

Unwanted effects

These are relatively infrequent, occurring in fewer than 4% of individuals. The commonest are skin eruptions, fever and gastrointestinal disturbances. Liver damage with jaundice has been reported and has proved fatal in a very small proportion of cases, the incidence being approximately 1 in 3000 treated patients and being mainly associated with prior liver disease. A variety of symptoms of CNS disturbances have been recorded (dizziness, tiredness and confusion), as have various allergic manifestations such as urticaria and haemolysis. Drug interactions which may occur include an increase in the degradation of oestrogens and glucocorticoids, the former leading to a decreased efficacy of oral contraceptives.

ETHAMBUTOL

The chemical structure of ethambutol is shown in Figure 30.14. Only the dextrorotatory isomer has antituberculosis activity, and the drug has no effect on organisms other than mycobacteria. Ethambutol is taken up by the bacteria and after a period of 24 hours it inhibits their growth. The mechanism of action is unknown. Resistance will emerge rapidly if the drug is used on its own.

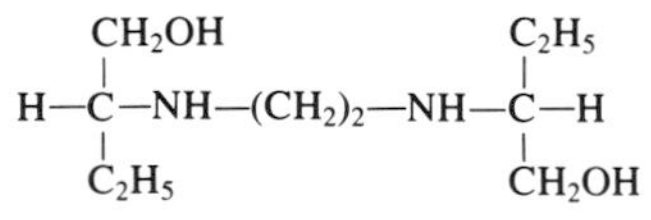

$$H-\underset{\underset{C_2H_5}{|}}{\overset{\overset{CH_2OH}{|}}{C}}-NH-(CH_2)_2-NH-\underset{\underset{CH_2OH}{|}}{\overset{\overset{C_2H_5}{|}}{C}}-H$$

Fig. 30.14 Ethambutol.

The drug is given orally and is well absorbed, reaching therapeutic plasma concentrations within 4 hours. It is partly metabolized and is excreted in the urine (50% of a dose as unchanged drug and 15% as metabolites). 20% appears in the faeces. The half-life is 3–4 hours.

Unwanted effects

These are uncommon, the most important being optic neuritis which results in visual disturbances such as a decrease in visual acuity and inability to see the colour green. This effect is dose-related, occurring in 15% of patients on high doses and 10% of patients on low doses.

PYRAZINAMIDE

This is related to nicotinamide and its chemical structure is indicated in Figure 30.15. It is inactive at neutral pH but tuberculostatic at acid pH. It is effective against the intracellular organisms in macrophages, since, after phagocytosis, the organisms will be contained in phagolysosomes in which the pH is low. Resistance is rather readily developed but cross-resistance with isoniazid does not occur.

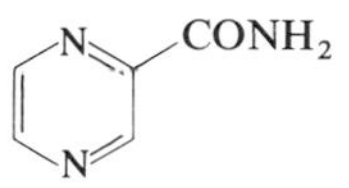

Fig. 30.15 Pyrazinamide.

The drug is well absorbed after oral administration, and is widely distributed, penetrating well into the meninges. It is excreted through the kidney, mainly by glomerular filtration.

Unwanted effects

Hepatic damage occurs in about 15% of patients and may, in rare instances, result in death from hepatic necrosis. Because of this serious toxic effect, this agent is not usually considered as a first-line drug, but is particularly useful for tuberculous meningitis.

CAPREOMYCIN

This is a peptide antibiotic given by intramuscular injection. There is some cross-reaction with kanamycin.

Unwanted effects are kidney damage and injury to the eighth nerve with deafness and ataxia. (This drug should not be given at the same time as streptomycin or other drugs which may damage the eighth nerve.)

CYCLOSERINE

This drug is a broad-spectrum antibiotic inhibiting many bacteria including coliforms and mycobacteria. It is water-soluble and destroyed at acid pH. It is a structural analogue of D-alanine (Fig. 30.16)

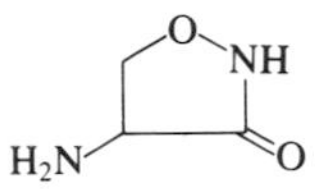

Fig. 30.16 Cycloserine.

and inhibits cell wall synthesis by preventing the addition of the two terminal alanine residues to the initial tripeptide side chain on N-acetylmuramic acid, thus preventing the synthesis of the basic building block of peptidoglycan (see Chapter 28 & Fig. 28.3). After being given orally it is rapidly absorbed and reaches peak concentrations within 4 hours. It is distributed throughout the tissues and body fluids, concentrations in the cerebrospinal fluid being equivalent to the concentration in the blood. Most of the drug is eliminated in active form in the urine, but some (approximately 35%) is metabolized.

Unwanted effects

These affect mainly the central nervous system and a wide variety of disturbances may occur ranging from headache and irritability to depression, convulsions and psychotic states.

In addition to its use in tuberculosis which is resistant to first-line drugs, it may be used in urinary tract infections.

DRUGS USED TO TREAT LEPROSY

Some anti-tuberculosis drugs such as **rifampicin** (see above) have striking antileprotic activity. Other drugs used to treat leprosy are **dapsone** and **clofazimine.**

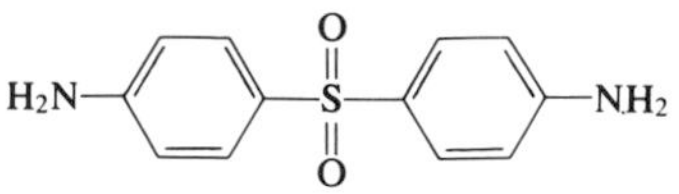

Fig. 30.17 Dapsone.

Dapsone

Dapsone is diaminodiphenyl sulphone (Fig. 30.17). It is chemically related to the sulphonamides and, since its action is antagonized by pABA, probably acts by inhibition of folate synthesis.

Resistance to dapsone is increasing and treatment with combinations of drugs is now recommended.

Dapsone is given orally and is well absorbed and widely distributed through the body water and all tissues. Peak plasma concentrations are reached within 1–3 hours. The plasma half-life is 24–48 hours but some dapsone remains in certain tissues (liver and kidney and also, to some extent, skin and muscle) for much longer periods. There is enterohepatic recycling of the drug but some is acetylated and excreted in the urine.

Unwanted reactions occur fairly frequently. Haemolysis of red cells may occur but is not usually severe enough to lead to frank anaemia. Methaemoglobinaemia is commonly seen. Anorexia, nausea and vomiting may occur, as may fever, allergic dermatitis and neuropathy. Lepra reactions (an exacerbation of lepromatous lesions) are reported and a syndrome resembling infectious mononucleosis (but which can be fatal) has occasionally been seen.

Clofazimine

This drug is a phenazine (Fig. 30.18) which is used to treat patients whose leprosy is resistant to dapsone. The drug has anti-inflammatory activity and

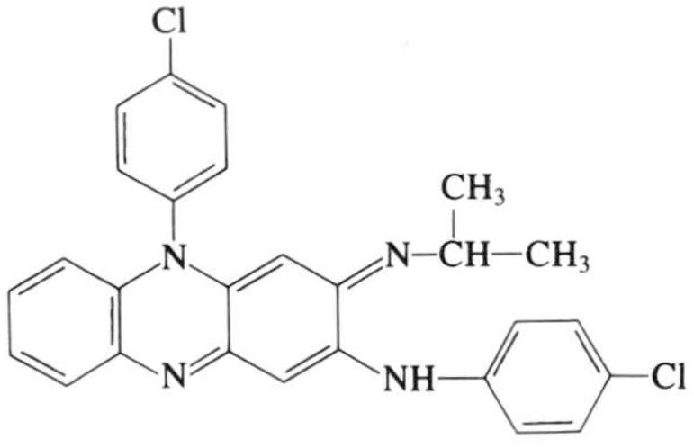

Fig. 30.18 Clofazimine.

is also therefore useful in patients in whom dapsone causes inflammatory side effects. Its mechanism of action against leprosy bacilli may involve an action on DNA.

Clofazimine is given orally and tends to cumulate in the body, being sequestered in the mononuclear phagocyte system. The anti-leprotic effect is delayed and is usually not seen for 6–7 weeks. The plasma half-life may be as long as 8 weeks.

Unwanted effects may be related to the fact that clofazimine is a dye. Thus the skin and urine can develop a reddish colour and the lesions a blue-black discoloration. Nausea, giddiness, headache and diarrhoea may also occur.

REFERENCES AND FURTHER READING

Denver Russell A, Quesnel L B 1983 (Eds) Antibiotics: assessment of antimicrobial activity and resistance. The Society for Applied Bacteriology Technical Series No. 18. Academic Press, New York
Franklin T J, Snow G A 1981 Biochemistry of antimicrobial action, 3rd edn. Chapman & Hall, London
Ristuccia A M, Cunha B A (eds) 1984 Antimicrobial therapy. Handbook of therapeutic drug monitoring series. Raven Press, New York

31

Antiviral drugs

Viruses are the simplest living organisms, consisting essentially of nucleic acid (either RNA or DNA) enclosed in a protein coat. They depend for replication on the metabolic processes of a living plant, animal or bacterial cell. They attach to the host cell, in many cases to specific receptors, and enter it by a type of phagocytosis during which the virus coat is removed. The nucleic acid of the virus then takes control of the cell's machinery for synthesizing nucleic acid and protein and switches it to the manufacture of new virus particles. This process involves DNA or RNA synthesis, synthesis of viral proteins and glycosylation. The virus particles may be released from the cell gradually, by budding, or suddenly, by the rupture of the cell.

Because viruses share many of the metabolic processes of the host cell it is difficult to find agents which are selective for the pathogen. Most antiviral agents are only effective while the virus is replicating. An additional problem is that by the time a viral infection becomes clinically detectable, the process of viral replication is very far advanced and chemotherapeutic intervention is very difficult.

There are very few antiviral agents and in general they are only effective in some herpes virus diseases and related DNA virus infections, the exception being the prophylactic use of amantadine in influenza A infections.

INHIBITION OF ATTACHMENT TO OR PENETRATION OF HOST CELLS

Amantadine

Amantadine (Fig. 31.1) is a tricyclic primary amine which is active against influenza A virus. It may also be effective in herpes zoster (shingles) and rubella (German measles). It has no action against influenza B virus. **Rimantadine** is similar in its effects.

Mechanism of action

The mechanism of action of amantadine is not fully understood. Early studies indicated that amantadine had an inhibitory effect on an early stage of influenza A virus infection. Recent evidence suggests that viruses enter cells in coated vesicles or phagosomes which subsequently fuse with lysosomes, and that the uncoating of the viral nucleic acid is accomplished by the fusion of the viral envelope with the membrane of the vacuole. Essential to this process is the low pH of the lysosomes. Amantadine, which is a weak base, is thought to prevent the uncoating and thus the transfer of free viral nucleic acids into the cell, possibly partly by increasing the intralysosomal pH. It may interfere with the primary transcription of viral RNA.

Resistant mutants can be generated in the laboratory but have been rarely reported in naturally occurring human influenza.

Pharmacokinetic aspects

Given orally, amantadine is well absorbed, reaches high levels in secretions (e.g. saliva) and most is excreted unchanged *via* the kidney. Its plasma half-life is about 15 hours and that of rimantadine, 30 hours. Aerosol administration is also feasible.

Unwanted effects

These are relatively infrequent, occurring in 5–10%

of patients, and are not serious. Dizziness, insomnia and slurred speech are the most commonly seen side effects.

Clinical use

Amantadine has proved to be relatively effective when used prophylactically in patients at risk of infection with viruses susceptible to the drug (e.g. influenza A virus)—giving about 50–80% protection. It may also have an effect on an established infection if therapy is started within 18 hours of the onset of symptoms.

Amantadine is also efficacious in some cases of Parkinsonism (see Chapter 24).

Gamma globulin

Pooled gamma globulin which contains antibodies against the virus envelope may 'neutralize' the organisms and prevent their attachment to host cells. If used before the onset of signs and symptoms it may attenuate or prevent measles, hepatitis, rabies and poliomyelitis.

INHIBITION OF NUCLEIC ACID SYNTHESIS

Vidarabine

Vidarabine (adenine arabinoside) is a purine nucleoside analogue (Fig. 31.1) with activity against all human herpes viruses, including herpes simplex (types 1 and 2), varicella-zoster virus, cytomegalovirus and Epstein-Barr virus.

Mechanism of action

Vidarabine is phosphorylated by cellular kinases to the triphosphate which acts as a relatively selective inhibitor of viral DNA polymerase (see Fig. 28.7). It is also suggested that it may be incorporated into viral DNA and cause chain termination, and that it may inhibit virus-specific ribonucleotide reductase. It inhibits viral nucleic acid synthesis at concentrations below those required to inhibit mammalian DNA or RNA synthesis.

Pharmacokinetic aspects

It is relatively insoluble and must be given in a large

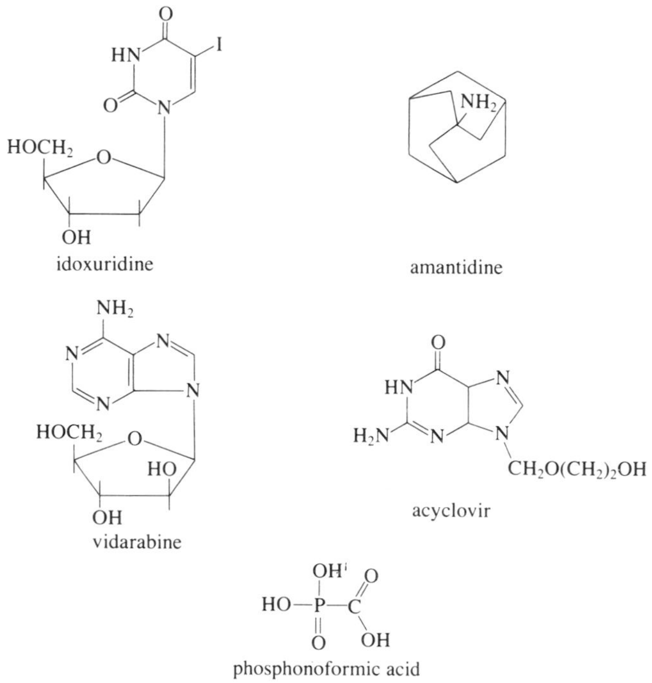

Fig. 31.1 Structures of some antiviral agents.

volume by slow intravenous infusion. It is widely distributed in the body and the CSF concentration is about one third to half that in the plasma. It is deaminated to arabinosyl hypoxanthine which has less antiviral activity than the parent drug, but may act synergistically with it. It is excreted mainly in the urine, mostly as the deaminated metabolite. Its plasma half-life is 3–4 hours.

Unwanted effects

These include nausea, vomiting and diarrhoea. Neurotoxicity (tremors, ataxia, paraesthesias, hallucinations, convulsions) may occur late in therapy with high doses, and is usually reversible. Bone marrow disturbances (leucopenia, thrombocytopenia, and megaloblastic anaemia) have been reported after high doses. Vidarabine can be mutagenic and carcinogenic.

Clinical uses

These include varicella zoster infections in immunosuppressed patients and other serious varicella zoster infections in which the benefits of the drug outweigh its risks. Used topically it is effective in herpes simplex infections in the eye. It has also been of value in treating herpes simplex encephalitis, reducing the mortality, in one study, from 70% to 28% when compared with placebo.

Idoxuridine

This is an analogue of thymidine (Fig. 31.1) which inhibits replication of DNA viruses. It is phosphorylated by cellular kinases and the triphosphate is incorporated into both viral and host DNA. It is only very slightly soluble in water and furthermore is too toxic for systemic use. It is therefore only used topically.

Its main use is in the treatment of herpes simplex and varicella zoster infections in the eye, particularly in the cornea—which is avascular. It is less effective in conjunctival infections. Dissolved in dimethylsulfoxide (DMSO) and applied topically, idoxuridine will penetrate the skin and has proved useful in recurrent herpes simplex and uncomplicated zoster. DMSO is bacteriostatic and will thus tend to prevent the secondary bacterial infection which

may occur with zoster, but it causes reddening due to histamine release. It may cause contact dermatitis.

Resistance has been reported.

Acyclovir

This agent is a guanine derivative (Fig. 31.1) with a high specificity for herpes simplex and varicella zoster viruses, herpes simplex Type 1 being more susceptible than either Type 2 and varicella zoster. (Varicella or chicken pox is caused by the same virus that causes shingles, i.e. herpes zoster.) Epstein-Barr virus (a herpes virus which causes infectious mononucleosis) can also be inhibited by fairly high plasma levels.

Mechanism of action

Acyclovir is converted to the monophosphate by thymidine kinase—the virus-specified form of this enzyme being very much more effective in carrying out the phosphorylation than the host cell's thymidine kinase—and subsequently converted to the triphosphate by the host cell kinases. It is therefore only adequately activated in infected cells. Acyclovir triphosphate inhibits viral DNA-polymerase (see Fig. 28.7) to a much greater extent than the host enzyme. It is possible for resistance to occur as a result of changes in the viral genes coding for either DNA-polymerase or thymidine kinase but the clinical significance of this is not yet clear.

Pharmacokinetic aspects

Although acyclovir is not very soluble it may be given orally and reaches peak plasma concentration in 1–2 hours. However only 20% of an oral dose is absorbed. The sodium salt may be used for intravenous infusion, after which the plasma concentration is 10–20 fold higher than with oral administration. The drug is widely distributed, reaching concentrations in the CSF which are 50% of those in the plasma. It is excreted by the kidneys partly by glomerular filtration and partly by tubular secretion. An ophthalmic ointment preparation of acyclovir is used for herpes simplex infections in the eye.

Topical application to the skin is less desirable

since it is thought that this will encourage the emergence of resistant strains of the virus.

Unwanted effects are minimal. Local inflammation may occur during intravenous injection if there is extravasation of the solution because it is very alkaline (pH 10–11).

Clinical use

This drug may be used *prophylactically* in patients who are to be treated with immunosuppressant drugs or radiotherapy and who are at risk of herpes virus infection due to reactivation of a latent virus. Given intravenously, it has also proved effective in the treatment of herpes zoster in immunocompromized patients. Oral acyclovir has been effective in the treatment of genital herpes. 'Maintenance' therapy with acyclovir reduces recurrence of this condition, though there is a possibility of the emergence of resistant strains.

Phosphonoformate

Phosphonoformate (Fig. 31.1) is a member of a new class of antiviral compounds which manifest potent inhibition of replication of herpes virus *in vitro*. Phosphonoformate acts by non-competitive inhibition of herpes-virus-induced DNA polymerase interaction with the site on the enzyme which binds the pyrophosphate (see Fig. 28.7). Clinical trials are under way.

INTERFERON

Interferons are a family of inducible proteins synthesized by many different kinds of mammalian cells in response to viral and other stimuli. Classical or type I interferon was discovered by Isaacs & Lindeman in 1957. They observed that when chicken chorio-allantoic membrane was inoculated with inactivated influenza virus, antiviral activity could be detected in the medium in which the membrane was suspended. Since then, several different types of interferon from several sources, have been described. Order was brought to the developing confusion in nomenclature by a Committee on Interferon Nomenclature in 1980 (Table 31.1). This committee also put forward the following proposal: 'That to qualify as an interferon ('IFN') a factor must be a protein which exerts virus nonspecific antiviral activity at least in homologous cells, through cellular metabolic processes involving synthesis of both RNA and protein'.

There are at least three families of interferons, and these are antigenically distinct. The α-family consists of at least eight proteins and the β-family two to three proteins. The γ-interferon is a lymphokine produced by T lymphocytes and is dealt with briefly in Chapter 8.

Interferons are produced by a variety of different cells, particularly B and T lymphocytes, macrophages and fibroblasts. In addition to viruses, which are strong inducers, there are a host of other, weaker, inducing agents. These include bacteria

Table 31.1 Nomenclature of human interferons. (Classification on the basis of antigenic specificities; based on the report of the Committee on Interferon Nomenclature, 1980).

New term	Old terms	Origin and characteristics
IFN-α (α-interferon)	Le(leucocyte) interferon Type I	pH 2 stable; induced by viruses, other microorganisms, bacterial products and various polymeric chemicals
IFN-β (β-interferon)	F(fibroblast) interferon Type I	
IFN-γ (γ-interferon)	IIF(immune); Type II, T interferon	pH 2 labile; virus-induced; antigen-induced; mitogen-induced; may be identical with 'macrophage activating factor'.

and their products, rickettsiae, protozoa, fungal polysaccharides and a range of polymeric chemicals.

Mechanism of antiviral action of interferons

Interferons work by inducing in the ribosomes of the host's cells, the production of enzymes which inhibit the translation of viral mRNA into viral proteins, and thus stop the reproduction of the viruses. Interferons bind to specific receptors on cell membranes, which may be gangliosides. The interaction leads to the production of a new messenger RNA which directs the synthesis by the host's ribosomes of antiviral proteins. These include at least three new enzymes:

1. Oligoadenylate synthetase, which synthesizes several oligonucleotides with $2'$-$5'$phosphodiester bonds and leads eventually to activation of an RNAase and degradation of viral mRNA
2. A protein kinase which leads to phosphorylation of elongation factor 2 and causes inhibition of viral peptide chain initiation
3. A phosphodiesterase which degrades the terminal nucleotides of tRNA resulting in inhibition of viral peptide chain elongation.

There appears to be marked species specificity in the action of interferons—they act only in the species in which they are produced.

Pharmacokinetic aspects

Human interferon can be produced both from human cells (pooled blood leucocytes, cultures of fibroblasts) and from bacteria (recombinant DNA techniques), and various types of interferon are available. If given intravenously they have a half-life of 2–4 hours. With intramuscular injections, peak blood concentrations are reached in 5–8 hours. They do not cross the blood brain barrier. Fibroblast interferon (IFN-β) has to be given intravenously because it appears to be either bound or inactivated at the site of intramuscular injection.

Unwanted effects are common and include fever, lassitude, headache and myalgia. Repeated injections cause chronic malaise. Bone marrow depression and alopecia may also occur.

Clinical use

The place of interferon in the treatment of viral infections remains to be established. At present the most likely use of these agents appears to be in combination with nucleoside analogues for herpes virus infections and for the prevention of respiratory virus infections.

The possibility that interferons could be useful adjuncts in cancer chemotherapy is being explored.

In both antiviral and anticancer chemotherapy interferons, especially γ-interferon, may act partly by augmenting the host's immune response (see Chapter 8).

REFERENCES AND FURTHER READING

Dolin R 1985 Antiviral chemotherapy and chemoprophylaxis. Science 227: 1296–1303
Jeffries D J 1985 Clinical use of acyclovir. Brit Med J 190 (i): 177–178
Koch-Weser J 1983 Treatment of herpes virus infections. N Engl J Med 309: 963–970 & 1034–1039
Moore M 1984 Interferon. In: Dale M M, Foreman J C (eds) Textbook of Immunopharmacology. Blackwell Scientific Publications, Oxford, Ch 28, p 347–370

Smith R A, Sidwell R W, Robins R K 1980 Antiviral mechanisms of action. Ann Rev Pharmacol Toxicol 20: 259–284
Stewart J C M, Ferguson J, Davey P 1983 New antifungal and antiviral chemotherapy. Brit Med J 286 (ii): 1802–1805
Straus S E et al 1984 Suppression of frequently occurring genital herpes. N Engl J Med 310: 1545–1550
Stuart-Harris C H, Oxford J 1983 (eds) Problems of antiviral therapy. Academic Press, New York

32

Antifungal drugs

Fungal infections are termed *mycoses* and in general can be divided into superficial infections affecting skin, nails, hair or mucous membranes, and systemic infections affecting deeper tissues and organs. Many of the fungi which can cause mycoses live in association with man as commensals or are present in his environment, but until recently, superficial infections were relatively uncommon and systemic infections very uncommon indeed, in cool and temperate climatic zones.

In the last 20–30 years there has been a steady increase in systemic fungal infections, not only by known pathogenic fungi but by fungi previously thought to be innocuous (opportunistic infections). One factor in this increase has been the widespread use and abuse in man of broad-spectrum antibiotics which eliminate or decrease the bacterial popula-

tions which normally compete with fungi. Opportunistic infections are seen mainly in patients with a deficient host response. The increasing use of immunosuppressant drugs (see Chapter 9) is one reason for the increased incidence of these diseases; patients with neutropenia, of any cause, are particularly at risk, as are patients with the acquired immune deficiency syndrome (AIDS).

In the UK the commonest **systemic** fungal infection is systemic candidiasis. Other, more rare fungal infections, are cryprococcus meningitis or endocarditis, pulmonary or cerebral aspergillosis, and rhino-cerebral mucormycosis. In the world at large the commonest systemic fungal infections are blastomycosis, histoplasmosis, coccidiomycosis and paracoccidiomycosis.

Superficial fungal infections can be classified into

Table 32.1 Outline of the uses of antifungal drugs

Disease	Drugs used
Systemic infections	
Systemic candidiasis	Amphotericin and/or flucytosine
Cryptococcosis (meningitis)	Amphotericin + flucytosine,* miconazole
Systemic aspergillosis	Amphotericin,* and/or flucytosine
Mucormycosis (rhinocerebral)	Amphotericin,* and/or flucytosine
Blastomycosis	Amphotericin
Histoplasmosis	Amphotericin,* miconazole
Coccidiomycosis	Amphotericin,* ketoconazole
Paracoccidiomycosis	Amphotericin,* ketoconazole
Superficial infections	
1. Dermatomycoses	Clotrimazole or miconazole or econazole. All used topically
(*T. pedis, T. capitis, T. corporis* etc)	
Severe tinea infections	Oral griseofulvin, oral ketoconazole
2. Candidiasis	
of the mouth	Amphotericin* or miconazole, or nystatin. All used topically
of the skin	An imidazole, or amphotericin or nystatin. All used topically
of the vagina	An imidazole or nystatin used topically
Severe infections not responding to topical therapy	Oral ketoconazole

* Indicates a drug of first choice

the *dermatomycoses* and *candidiasis*. Dermatomycoses are infections of the skin, hair and nails, caused by dermatophytes. The commonest are due to *tinea* organisms which cause various types of 'ringworm'. *Tinea capitis* affects the scalp, *Tinea cruris*, the groin, *Tinea pedis* the feet (causing 'athlete's foot'), and *Tinea corporis*, the body.

Candidiasis is an infection with a yeast-like organism which affects the mucous membranes of the mouth ('thrush'), vagina or skin. The drugs used in fungal injections are described briefly below and their clinical use is outlined in Table 32.1.

AMPHOTERICIN

Amphotericin (Fig. 32.1) is an amphoteric polyene antibiotic characterized by a macrolide ring of carbon atoms which is closed by the formation of an internal ester or lactone. It is insoluble in water and unstable at 37°C.

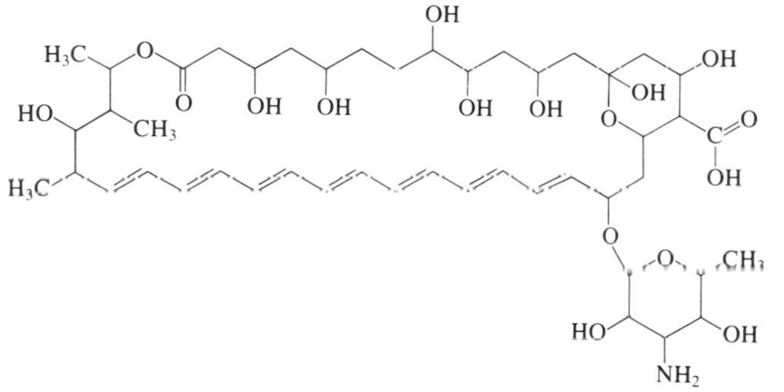

for fungi may be due to the drug's greater avidity for ergosterol (the fungal membrane sterol) than for cholesterol, the main sterol in the plasma membrane of animal cells. However, experimental work showing that the drug has some effect on sterol-free model membranes implies that factors other than sterol content may be involved. Thus the type of phospholipid, and the sterol/phospholipid ratio in particular domains also appear to be significant for amphotericin action. It seems possible that the overall membrane organization (including the factor of sterol content) is important rather than the amount of one single component.

Amphotericin enhances the antifungal effect of flucytosine (see below) and may confer antifungal activity on rifampicin, an antibacterial antibiotic which does not otherwise have antifungal properties.

There is also some complex evidence which suggests that amphotericin increases the host's response to the parasite by an immuno-stimulant effect.

Fig. 32.1 The structure of amphotericin.

Mechanism of action

The drug binds to cell membranes (like other polyene antibiotics; see Chapter 28) and interferes with permeability and with transport functions. It forms a pore in the membrane, the hydrophilic core of the molecule creating a transmembrane ion channel. One of the repercussions of this is a decrease in intracellular K^+ ions. Amphotericin has a selective action, binding avidly to the membranes of fungi and some protozoa, less avidly to mammalian cells and not at all to bacteria. There is evidence that this is because of the presence of sterols in those membranes which bind amphotericin and their absence in the others. The relative specificity

Pharmacokinetic aspects

Given orally, the drug is poorly absorbed, and it is therefore only given by this route for fungal infections of the gastrointestinal tract. For systemic infections it is given by slow intravenous injection, or, in the case of fungal meningitis, intrathecally. It can also be given topically. It is very highly protein bound and is found in fairly high concentrations in inflammatory exudates, but does not cross the blood-brain barrier. It cannot be easily removed by haemodialysis. It appears to be sequestered in the body, possibly bound to membrane cholesterol in various cells, and is excreted very slowly via the kidney, traces of the drug being found in the urine for 2 months or more after administration has ceased.

Unwanted effects

The commonest and most serious of these is renal toxicity. Some degree of reduction of renal function will occur in more than four-fifths of patients receiving the drug, and though this is generally reversed after treatment is stopped, some impairment of glomerular filtration remains, the degree being dependent on the total amount of amphotericin taken. Hypokalaemia occurs in 25% of patients and will require potassium chloride supplementation. Less frequently, hepatic function may be impaired and there may be anaemia. The process of injection frequently results initially in chills, fever, tinnitus and headache, and about one in five patients vomit. As therapy continues these reactions usually decrease. However, the drug is irritant to the endothelium of the veins and local thrombophlebitis may occur. Other unwanted effects are anaphylaxis, and thrombocytopenia. Intrathecal injections may cause neurotoxicity and topical applications, a skin rash.

NYSTATIN

Nystatin is a polyene macrolide antibiotic similar in structure to amphotericin and with the same mechanism of action. There is virtually no absorption from the mucous membranes of the body or from skin and its use is limited to fungal infections of the skin and the gastrointestinal tract.

FLUCYTOSINE

Flucytosine (Fig. 32.2) is a synthetic antifungal agent which, given orally, is active against some systemic fungal injections, especially those caused by yeast.

Mechanism of action

Its mechanism of action as an antimycotic is attributed to its conversion to 5,fluorouracil—an antimetabolite which inhibits thymidylate synthetase

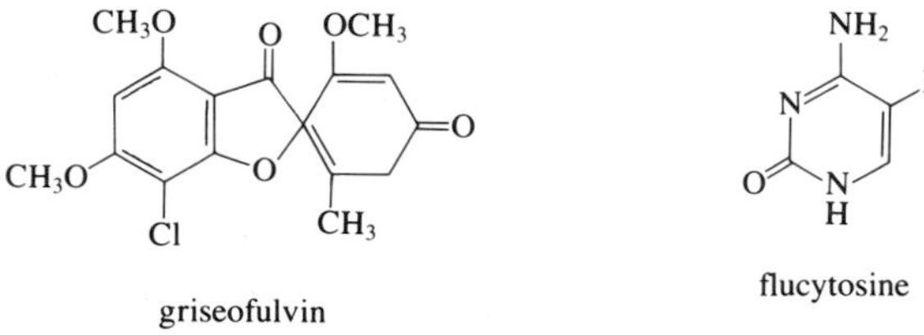

Fig. 32.2 Griseofulvin and flucytosine.

and thus DNA synthesis (see Chapters 28 & 29). Its toxicity for fungal as compared to mammalian cells is due to the fact that in the latter there is very little of the enzyme activity required for the conversion of the drug to its active metabolite. Some yeasts are naturally resistant to the drug, and among sensitive strains resistant mutants may emerge rapidly. There is a body of opinion which holds that because of the potential for the development of resistant strains, this drug should virtually never be used alone.

Pharmacokinetic aspects

Given orally, it is rapidly and almost completely absorbed, and is widely distributed throughout the body fluids including the CSF. About 85% is excreted unchanged via the kidneys and the plasma half-life is 3–5 hours. The dosage should be reduced if renal function is impaired. The drug is 20% protein bound and it can be removed by haemodialysis.

Unwanted effects

These are infrequent and the drug has been well tolerated even when given in high dosage for a prolonged period. Such toxic effects as there are, may be due to the active metabolite—5,fluorouracil. Gastrointestinal disturbances, neutropenia, thrombocytopenia and alopecia have occurred but these are usually mild and are reversed when therapy ceases. Uracil is reported to decrease the toxic effects on the bone marrow without impairing the antimycotic action.

IMIDAZOLES

The imidazoles are a group of synthetic antimycotic agents with a broad spectrum of activity. The drugs

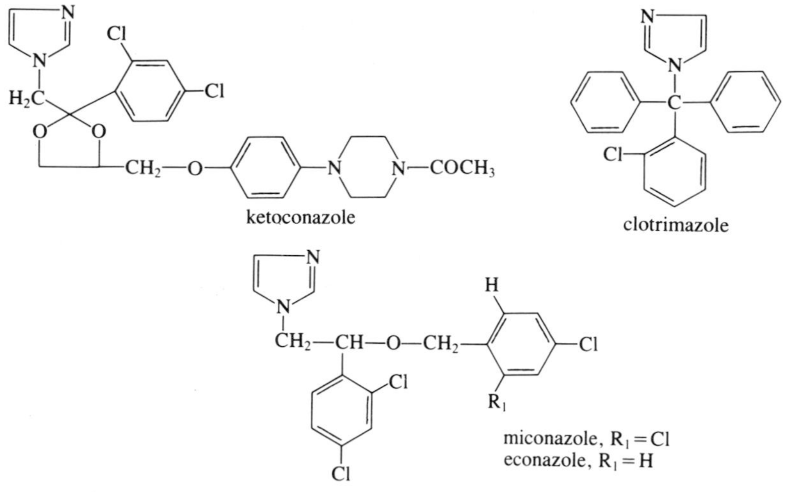

Fig. 32.3 Chemical structures of some imidazole antifungal agents.

available are **ketoconazole, miconazole, econazole** and **clotrimazole** (Fig. 32.3). The latter two are only used topically. Ketoconazole and miconazole will be described here.

Mechanism of action of the imidazoles

These agents block the synthesis of ergosterol in fungi, by interfering with C-14 demethylation. Inhibitory actions on both cytochrome P450 and cytochrome c oxidase has been reported, either or both of which may be the basis of the effect on ergosterol synthesis, since oxidation is required for the C-14 demethylation. A further action is the inhibition of the transformation of candidal yeast cells into hyphae—the invasive and pathogenic form of the parasite.

Ketoconazole

This is a relatively new drug and is the only antimycotic imidazole compound which can be given orally. It is soluble in water, and is well absorbed from the gastrointestinal tract. It is a basic drug and will be best absorbed in conditions of low pH. Antacids will reduce absorption. It is distributed widely throughout the tissues and tissue fluids but does not reach therapeutic concentrations in the CNS unless high doses are given. It is

inactivated in the liver and excreted in bile and in urine.

Unwanted effects

Liver toxicity has been reported infrequently but has proved fatal in a few cases. Other side effects which occur are gastrointestinal disturbances and pruritis. Inhibition of steroid and testosterone synthesis with resultant gynaecomastia has been recorded.

Miconazole

This is too poorly absorbed to be given orally, and for systemic infections it is given intravenously. It has a very short half-life and needs to be given every 8 hours. It reaches therapeutic concentrations in bone, joints, and lung tissue but not in the CNS. For fungal infections in the CNS it has to be given intrathecally. It is inactivated in the liver. Unwanted effects are relatively infrequent, those most commonly seen being gastrointestinal disturbances, but pruritus, anaemia and hyponatraemia are also reported. Leucopenia and thrombocytopenia are rare toxic effects. There may be problems during the process of injection—the occurrence of anaphylactic reactions, dysrhythmias, chills and fevers. The drug can have an irritant action on the venous endothelium.

Clotrimazole and econazole

Clotrimazole and econazole are imidazole antifungal agents used only for topical application. Clotrimazole interferes with amino-acid transport into the organism by an action on the cell membrane. It is active against a wide range of fungi, including candida organisms.

TOLNAFTATE

Tolnaftate is a synthetic drug used topically to treat dermatophytoses. It is active only against growing cells; it does not affect candida species.

GRISEOFULVIN

Griseofulvin is a narrow-spectrum antifungal agent isolated from cultures of *Penicillium griseofulvum* in 1939. Its structure is given in Figure 32.2. It is fungistatic and its mechanism of action involves an interaction with microtubules. This results in interference with spindle formation in dividing cells and therefore with mitosis. Impairment of the function of cytoplasmic microtubules would also interfere with the transport of material through the cytoplasm to the periphery and this action is thought to be the basis of the inhibition of hyphal cell wall synthesis. In addition there is evidence that the drug binds to RNA and also that it inhibits nucleic acid synthesis. Resistance can be shown experimentally but has not been a problem in the clinic.

Pharmacokinetic aspects

Griseofulvin is given orally. It is not very soluble in water and absorption may vary with the type of preparation, in particular with particle size. Peak plasma concentrations are reached in about 5 hours. It is taken up selectively by newly formed skin where it exerts its antimycotic effect. The plasma half-life is 24 hours but it is retained in the skin for much longer.

REFERENCES AND FURTHER READING

Borgers M 1980 Mechanism of action of antifungal drugs. Rev of Infectious Diseases 2: 520–534

Hay R J 1985 Ketoconazole: a reappraisal. Br Med J 290 (i): 260–261

Holt R J 1980 Progress in antimycotic chemotherapy 1945–1980. Infection 8 (3): 284–287

Medoff G, Braitburg J, Kobayashi G S 1983 Antifungal agents useful in the therapy of systemic fungal infections. Ann Rev Pharmacol Toxicol 23: 303–330

Stewart J C M, Ferguson J, Davey P 1983 New antifungal and antiviral chemotherapy. Br Med J 286 (i): 1802–1805

Symposium on Antifungal Therapy 1979 Postgraduate Medical Journal 55: 587–700

33

Antiprotozoal drugs

The main protozoa which produce disease in man are those causing malaria, amoebiasis, leishmaniasis, trypanosomiasis and trichomoniasis.

MALARIA

Malaria is mosquito-borne and is one of the major killer diseases of the world, currently causing an estimated one million deaths annually. It is also responsible for a staggering amount of chronic ill health. In some parts of Africa 10% of the deaths of children under 5 years are due to the direct effects of malaria and its contribution to the mortality from other diseases cannot be computed. During the 1950s and 1960s the World Health Organization attempted to eradicate malaria from most of the areas where it had been prevalent (tropical Africa was not included for logistical and other reasons). The programme was based on the use of the powerful 'residual' insecticides and the highly effective antimalarial drugs which had become available, and the aim was to interrupt the man–mosquito cycle for long enough to let the malarial reservoir disappear. At the start of the programme the incidence of this disease was estimated to be approximately 250 million cases per year. By the end of the 1950s the incidence of malaria had dropped dramatically. However by the late 1970s it was clear that although 36 of the countries in which the programme had been implemented, had remained malaria-free, the parasite had returned to large areas from which it had been virtually eradicated (India, Pakistan, Bangladesh, Sri Lanka and Turkey) and the incidence in many tropical countries was rising.

The reasons for the failure of the programme were many and various and most were due to economic and administrative factors. Some countries thought the problem was solved and ceased the antimalarial measures; some transferred the effort to their general health services, which were unable to cope with the task; some were just not able to afford to continue the necessary measures. In others, civil unrest, uncontrollable movements of large numbers of people and the inaccessibility of some areas led to the measures being either inapplicable or ineffective. Specific biological factors such as the increasing resistance of the mosquito to the insecticides and of the malarial parasite to the drugs were significant contributory factors to the failure of the programme. During the 1970s it became clear that the attempt at eradication had failed and in 1978 the recorded figures for malaria outside tropical Africa reached a new peak of nearly nine million cases. When the malarial reservoir in tropical Africa was included, the 1983 estimate of the number of new malaria infections annually throughout the world was 210–220 million, most of these (85%) being 'malignant' malaria caused by the most dangerous of all the malaria parasites, *Plasmodium falciparum*. At present about 46% of mankind are at risk from malaria because they live in malarious areas. Sporadic cases—the result of present-day extensive air travel—are seen even in areas such as Western Europe and the USA, where the risk of transmission is negligible.

THE LIFE-CYCLE OF THE MALARIAL PARASITE

The life-cycle consists of a sexual cycle which takes

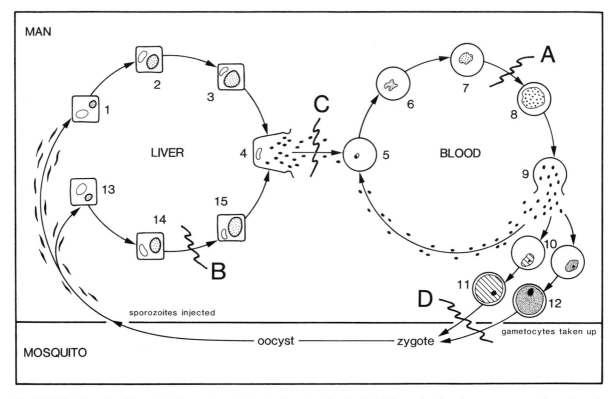

Fig. 33.1 The life cycle of the malarial parasite and the site of action of antimalarial drugs showing the pre- or exo-erythrocytic cycle in the liver and the erythrocytic cycle in the blood:

1. Entry of sporozoite or merozoite into liver cell (the parasite is shown with dots); 2 & 3. Development of the schizont in liver cell; 4. Rupture of liver cells with release of merozoites (which may enter liver cell to give a resting form of the parasite, a hypnozoite); 5. Entry of merozoite into red cell; 6. Trophozoite in red cell; 7 & 8. Development of schizont in red cell; 9. Rupture of red cell with release of merozoites; 10, 11 & 12. Entry of merozoites into red cells and development of male and female gametocytes; 13. Resting form of parasite in liver (hypnozoite); 14 & 15. Growth and multiplication of hypnozoites.

Sites of drug action: A. Drugs which cure the clinical attack; B. Drugs which affect exoerythrocytic hypnozoites and result in radical cure of *P. vivax* and *P. ovale*; C. Drugs which suppress *P. vivax* and *P. ovale* and effect radical cure of *P. falciparum*; D. Drugs which prevent transmission.

place in the female anopheline mosquito, and an asexual cycle which occurs in man (Fig. 33.1). With the bite of an infected female mosquito, *sporozoites* are injected and reach the blood stream. Within an hour they disappear from the blood into the parenchymal cells of the liver, where, during the next 10–14 days they undergo a *pre-erythrocytic* stage of development and multiplication. At the end of this stage the liver cells rupture and *merozoites* are released. These enter the red cells of the blood and form motile intracellular parasites termed *trophozoites*. The development and multiplication of the plasmodia within these cells constitutes the *erythrocytic* stage. Following mitotic replication of the nucleus, the parasite in the red cell is called a *schizont* and its growth and division, *schizogony*,

which results in the release of further merozoites when the red cell ruptures.

In certain forms of malaria, some sporozoites on entering the liver cells form *hypnozoites*, or resting forms of the parasite, which can be reactivated to continue an *exo-erythrocytic* cycle of multiplication.

Malaria parasites can multiply in the body at a phenomenal rate—a single parasite of *Plasmodium vivax* being capable of giving rise to 250 million merozoites in 14 days. In terms of the action required of an antimalarial drug, it should be appreciated that destruction of 94% of the parasites every 48 hours will only *maintain* equilibrium and will not reduce their number, or their propensity for proliferation.

Some merozoites, on entering red cells, differentiate into male and female forms of the parasite, called *gametocytes*. These can only complete their cycle when taken up by the mosquito, when it sucks the blood of an infected host.

The cycle in the mosquito involves fertilization of the female gametocyte by the male gametocyte with the formation of a zygote which develops into an *oocyst* (sporocyst). A further stage of division and multiplication takes place leading to rupture of the sporocyst with release of sporozoites, which then migrate to the mosquito salivary glands and enter another human host with the mosquito's bite.

The periodic episodes of fever which characterize malaria are due to the periodic rupture of red cells with release of merozoites and cell debris.

Relapses of malaria are likely to occur with those forms of malaria which have an exoerythrocytic cycle (Fig. 33.2). The parasite may exist in a dormant hypnozoite form in the liver and emerge after an interval of weeks or months to start the infection again.

The chief species of human malaria parasites are:

1. *Plasmodium falciparum* which has an erythrocytic cycle of 48 hours in man and produces *malignant tertian malaria*. The word 'tertian' refers to the fact that the fever recurs every third day, and it is called 'malignant' because clinically it is the most severe form of the disease seen and may be fatal. *P. falciparum* does not have a significant exoerythrocytic stage, so that if the erythrocytic stage is eradicated, relapses do not occur.

2. *Plasmodium vivax* which has an erythrocytic cycle of 48 hours and produces *benign tertian*

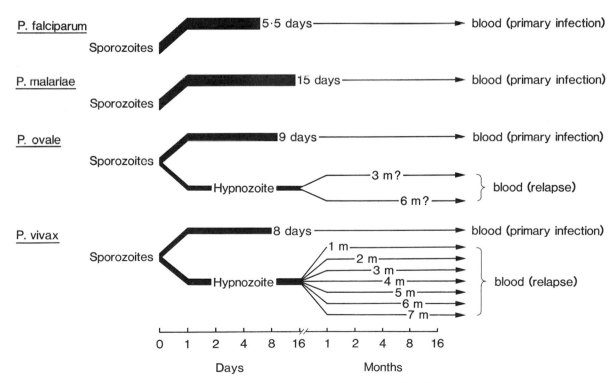

Fig. 33.2 Schematic diagram of forms of malaria with the four main species of plasmodia which infect man. The thickness of the lines indicates the proportion of the sporozoites which either differentiate into schizonts immediately (upper line) or which form the dormant 'hypnozoites'. Note that the pattern given for vivax is that seen with some strains only—other strains may have fewer relapses. m = months. (Adapted from: Bray & Garnham, 1982)

malaria, so-called because it is less severe and rarely fatal. Exoerythrocytic forms may persist for years and cause relapses.

3. *Plasmodium ovale* which has a 48 hour cycle, is the cause of a rare form of malaria. An exoerythrocytic stage occurs.

4. *Plasmodium malariae* which has a 72 hour cycle, causes *quartan* malaria. There is no exoerythrocytic cycle.

Immunity to malaria is known to occur and protects many individuals living in malarious areas, but little is known, for certain, of the immune mechanisms involved. The immunity is lost if the individual is absent from the area for more than 6 months. B lymphocytes and antibody production are clearly important since monoclonal antibodies against sporozoite antigens can confer passive immunity. Active immunization with a small number of attenuated sporozoites has been shown, experimentally, to provide protection following challenge.

Recombinant DNA techniques have been applied to this problem and have resulted in the cloning of the gene for the principal antigen of the sporozoite form of one strain of the malignant malaria caused by *Plasmodium falciparum*. The gene is in three sections, the middle section consisting of 41 four-codon repeats, corresponding to the amino-acid sequence, asparagine–alanine–asparagine–proline. Quite small portions of the antigenic proteins of sporozoites, as few as a dozen amino-acids, are known to be antigenic. A great many problems have yet to be solved (there is for example considerable interstrain variability) but it seems that it may be possible at some time in the future to make synthetic peptide vaccines for immunization against malaria.

ANTIMALARIAL DRUGS

These are usually classified in terms of the action against the different stages of the life cycle of the parasite (Fig. 33.1).

1. *Drugs used for clinical cure.* These are blood schizonticidal agents (Fig. 33.1, site A) which are effective against the erythrocytic forms of the plasmodial organism and are used to cure the clinical attack of malaria. This group of drugs includes quinoline-methanols (e.g. quinine and mefloquin); various 4-aminoquinolines (e.g. chloroquine) and agents which interfere with the synthesis of folate (e.g. sulphonamides, sulphones) or with its action (e.g. pyrimethamine). Combinations of these agents are frequently used. Some antibiotics, such as tetracycline and clindamycin, have proved useful when combined with the above agents.

2. *Drugs which effect radical cure.* These are tissue schizonticidal agents which are effective against the parasites in the liver (Fig. 33.1, site B). Only the 8-aminoquinolines (e.g. primaquine) have this action. These drugs also destroy gametocytes and thus reduce the spread of infection.

3. *Drugs used for suppressive prophylaxis.* These are drugs which prevent the development of malarial attacks. Note that true, causal prophylaxis—the prevention of infection by the killing of the sporozoites on entry into the host—is not feasible with the drugs at present in use, though it may be achieved in the future with vaccines (see above) or with drugs yet to be developed. Prevention of the development of clinical attacks can however be effected by drugs which kill the parasites when they emerge from the liver after the pre-erythrocytic stage (Fig. 33.1, site C). The drugs used for this purpose are mainly those listed under stage 1 (see above); they are often used in combinations.

Some drugs have the additional action of destroying the gametocytes (Fig. 31.1, site D) and thus preventing transmission by the mosquito, but they are rarely used for this action alone.

4-AMINOQUINOLINES

This group includes **chloroquine, hydroxychloroquine** and **amodiaquine**. Chloroquine is the most extensively used 4-aminoquinoline, and will be the one described here. Some structural formulae are given in Figure 33.3.

Chloroquine has a complex mechanism of action which requires functional glycolytic metabolism in the protozoon. It causes fragmentation of the parasite RNA, an effect associated with coarse clumping of pigment within the organism. The ability of the drug to intercalate in the DNA may also be involved in its antimalarial action. It is thought that there is a mechanism for selective uptake of chloroquine into infected red cells and that there are high affinity binding sites for chloroquine in the parasite.

(In other mammalian cells, such as macrophages, chloroquine and other weak bases are lysosomotropic, being sequestered in these organelles and raising their pH; p. 215).

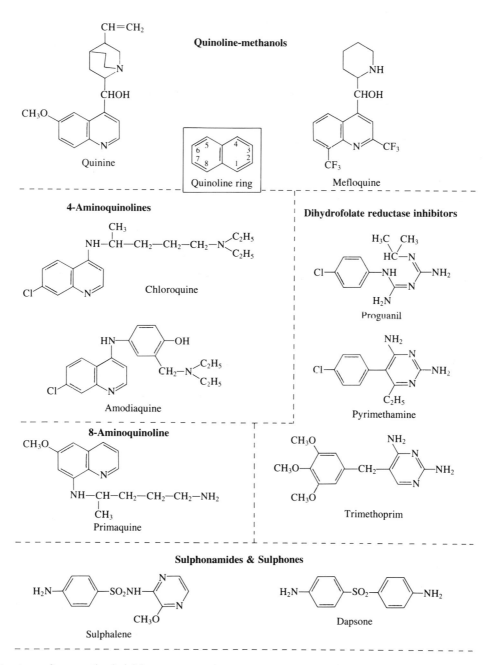

Fig. 33.3 Structures of some antimalarial drugs.

Chemotherapeutic action against malaria

Chloroquine is a very potent blood schizonticidal drug, effective against the erythrocytic forms of all four plasmodial species, but it does not have any effect on sporozoites or hypnozoites. Used to treat the clinical attack of malaria, it reduces the fever and clears the blood of parasites within about 24 hours. With *P. falciparum* strains which are sensitive to its action this results in radical cure since this parasite has no exoerythrocytic cycle. However, the gametocytes are not affected and may remain in the circulation for months. Thus the patient, though cured, may be a potential source for infection of mosquitoes and thus for transmission of malaria.

Chloroquine is an effective *prophylactic drug* against sensitive strains of *P. falciparum* and will prevent any clinical manifestations of malaria if continued for 2 weeks after the individual has left the malarious area. With vivax and ovale malaria, a clinical attack may occur later because of the hypnozoites which may be present in the liver. It is recommended that when chloroquine is used for prophylaxis it should be combined with other drugs to decrease the possibility of development of resistance.

Resistance to chloroquine in *P. falciparum* is a major problem and appears to be due to the loss of the high affinity binding sites for chloroquine, which, consequently, is no longer concentrated in parasite-infected red cells. The resistance appears to be due to a drug-selected chromosomal mutation.

Pharmacological actions

Chloroquine has a fairly marked anti-inflammatory action (p. 215) and also some quinidine-like actions on the heart.

Pharmacokinetic aspects

The drug is given orally, is completely absorbed, and is extensively distributed throughout the tissues, concentrations in the liver, the spleen and the central nervous system being several times higher than in the plasma. As explained above, chloroquine concentrates particularly in parasitized red cells. It is released slowly from the tissues and metabolized in the liver. It is excreted in the urine—70% as unchanged drug and 30% as metabolites. There are several phases of clearance—an initial, major phase with a half-time of 50 hours, a second phase with a half-time of 6–7 days, and a third phase with a half-time of 17 days.

Unwanted effects

Chloroquine has few side effects when given for prophylaxis. With the larger doses used to treat the clinical attack of malaria, nausea and vomiting, dizziness and blurring of vision, and urticarial symptoms may occasionally occur. Long-term malaria prophylaxis has sometimes resulted in retinopathies.

Quinoline-methanols

The two main agents in this group are **quinine** and **mefloquine** (Fig. 33.3). The latter is a new drug which shows great promise (see below) but quinine is the main quinoline-methanol currently in use and will be described here.

Quinine is an alkaloid derived from Cinchona bark. (Quinidine, the D-isomer of quinine also has some antimalarial activity but is used mainly for its antidysrhythmic effects on the heart; p. 246). Its mechanism of action as an antimalarial agent is not understood, but it is known to intercalate in the DNA.

Chemotherapeutic action against malaria

Quinine was relegated to a drug of second choice when chloroquine was introduced, but with the emergence and spread of chloroquine resistance, quinine has again assumed therapeutic importance. It is effective against the erythrocytic forms of all four species of plasmodia, but has no effect on exoerythrocytic forms or on the gametocytes of *P. falciparum*.

It is the drug of choice for controlling the acute clinical attack with *P. falciparum* resistant to chloroquine.

Pharmacological actions

These include a quinidine-like action on the heart, a mild oxytocic effect in the uterus in pregnancy, a slight blocking action on the neuromuscular junction and a weak antipyretic effect.

Pharmacokinetic aspects

Quinine is usually given orally but may be given intravenously for severe *P. falciparum* infections. It is well absorbed from the gastrointestinal tract and 80% is bound to plasma protein. It is metabolized in the liver, the metabolites being excreted in the urine within about 24 hours.

Unwanted effects

Quinine is irritant to the gastric mucosa and oral doses may cause nausea and vomiting. If the concentration in the plasma exceeds $30–60\,\mu M$ the syndrome of 'cinchonism' is likely to occur. This consists of nausea, dizziness, tinnitus, headache and blurring of vision. The skin may be hot, flushed and sweaty. In severe forms of cinchonism, more marked disturbances of vision and hearing occur, thought to be due to both direct neural damage and indirect effects due to vascular spasm.

'Blackwater fever', a severe and often fatal condition in which acute haemolytic anaemia is associated with renal failure, has occurred in malaria patients treated with quinine and was at one time thought to be due to the therapy. However, the consensus now appears to be that it is due to the malaria.

8-AMINOQUINOLINES

The main 8-aminoquinoline used is **primaquine** (see Fig. 33.3). This drug has been shown in tissue culture studies to affect the mitochondria of the exocythrocytic forms of an avian form of *P. falciparum*, but the details of its mechanism of action are not really known. It does not affect DNA transcription or replication.

Its antimalarial action is exerted against the liver hypnozoites. It does not affect sporozoites and has little if any action against the erythrocytic stage of the parasite. However, it has a gametocidal action and is the most effective antimalarial drug for stopping transmission of the disease in all four species of plasmodia. It is virtually the only drug which can effect a radical cure of those forms of malaria in which the parasites have a dormant stage in the liver—*P. vivax* and *P. ovale*. It is almost invariably used in combination with another drug, usually chloroquine. Resistance to primaquine is rare, though evidence of a decreased sensitivity of some vivax strains has been reported.

Pharmacokinetic aspects

Primaquine is given orally and is well absorbed. Its metabolism is rapid and very little drug is present in the body after 10–12 hours.

Unwanted effects

Primaquine has few unwanted effects when used in normal therapeutic dosage for most Caucasian patients. Dose-related gastrointestinal symptoms may occur and large doses may cause methaemoglobinaemia with cyanosis.

A particular side effect which is seen with primaquine is related to an X chromosome-linked genetic metabolic condition—a deficiency of glucose-6-phosphate dehydrogenase in the red cells (see Chapter 4). This means that the cells are not able to regenerate NADPH, the concentration of which is reduced by the oxidant metabolic derivatives of primaquine and other drugs. As a consequence, the general metabolic functions of the red cells are impaired and haemolysis occurs. The deficiency of the enzyme is found in some black males and some Caucasian groups, and in these individuals primaquine must be used with great care.

DRUGS AFFECTING THE SYNTHESIS OR UTILIZATION OF FOLATE

This group includes both folate antagonists, and agents which inhibit the synthesis of folate. The former group acts by inhibiting dihydrofolate reductase and includes pyrimethamine, proguanil and trimethoprim; the latter group acts by competing with para-aminobenzoic acid and includes the sulphonamides and sulphones (see Chapters 28 & 30).

Pyrimethamine is a 2,4,diaminopyrimidine (see Fig. 33.3) and is very similar in structure to **trimethoprim** (see Fig. 30.3). The structure of **proguanil** is different (see Fig. 33.3), but it can assume a configuration similar to that of pyrimethamine. These compounds, by inhibiting dihydrofolate reductase, inhibit the formation of tetrahydrofolate with the consequences for DNA synthesis outlined in Chapter 29. As explained in Chapter 28, some agents (pyrimethamine, proguanil) have a greater affinity for the plasmodial enzyme than for the human enzyme. Trimethoprim has greater affinity for the bacterial than the plasmodial enzyme but is effective in malaria if combined with a sulphonamide.

The main sulphonamides used in malaria are **sulphadoxine**, **sulphalene**, and **sulphamethoxazole**. The only sulphone used is **dapsone** (see Fig. 33.3). Details of these groups of drugs are given in Chapter 30. They are active against the erythrocytic forms of plasmodia but not against the sporozoite or hypnozoite forms. They are never used alone, but only in combination with pyrimethamine or proguanil.

Antimalarial actions

The three folate antagonists are usually used with a sulphonamide or with dapsone. They have a slow action against the erythrocytic forms of the parasite and they are used to treat the acute attack of malaria only if the plasmodium is resistant to chloroquine, in which case they may be combined with quinine therapy. They are used particularly for suppressive prophylaxis in vivax and ovale infections but, since dormant hyponozoites are likely to be present in the liver, therapy with these agents should continue for at least 10 weeks after the individual leaves the malarious area. All three folate antagonists are effective in interrupting transmission of malaria because, although not gametocytocidal, they prevent the development of the parasite in the mosquito.

The commonest combinations are: pyrimethamine with sulphadoxine, pyrimethamine with dapsone and pyrimethamine with sulphalene. The first of these combinations is particularly useful for suppressive prophylaxis since the half-life of sulphadoxine is 10 days.

Pharmacokinetic aspects

Both pyrimethamine and proguanil are given orally and are well absorbed, though the process is slow. Pyrimethamine has a plasma half-life of 4 days and effective 'suppressive' plasma concentrations may last for 14 days. With proguanil the plasma concentration falls to zero by 24 hours. It is a pro-drug, metabolized in the liver to its active form—a triazine metabolite—which is excreted mainly in the urine. It must be taken daily.

Unwanted effects

These drugs have virtually no untoward effects if used in therapeutic doses. In toxic doses, pyrimethamine may affect mammalian dihydrofolate reductase and cause a megaloblastic anaemia (see Chapter 18).

POTENTIAL NEW ANTIMALARIAL DRUGS

Mefloquine is a schizonticidal quinoline–methanol compound, with a very long plasma half-life (more than 30 days) which may be due to an active metabolite. It was discovered in the course of a programme in which over 250 000 compounds were evaluated. It is related to quinine, but unlike quinine it does not intercalate in the DNA. Resistance can be produced in laboratory experiments but there may not be cross-resistance with quinine or with chloroquine. Unwanted actions are reported to include skin photosensitivity in some individuals. It may be a valuable drug for the treatment of multi-resistance falciparum malaria, particularly if combined with sulphadoxine and pyrimethamine. Because of its long half-life it can be given once every 2 weeks for suppressive prophylaxis and it may be the mainstay of chemotherapy against malaria in the immediate future.

Qinghaosin is derived from a traditional Chinese herbal remedy for malaria. It is a shizonticide and has been effective in some cases of chloroquine-resistant malaria. Synthetic analogues are being developed and one such agent, **artesunate**, is undergoing trials.

Other approaches include the development of new folate antagonists and the possibility of administering antimalarial drugs in biodegradable polymer matrices for slow-release and thus long action.

AMOEBIASIS

Amoebiasis is an infection with *Entamoeba histolytica* produced by the ingestion of cysts of this organism. The cysts develop into trophozoites which may invade the submucosa of the gastrointestinal tract, causing ulceration. Dysentery is a frequent result but there may be a chronic intestinal infection without dysentery. An amoebic granuloma in the intestinal wall (an 'amoeboma') occurs, infrequently, and can be confused with a neoplasm. In 0.1% of cases the parasite invades the liver and establishes itself in the parenchyma, leading to the development of liver abscesses. In very rare instances, other tissues may also be parasitized. Some individuals are 'carriers'—they harbour the parasite without developing overt disease, but the cysts are present in their faeces and may infect other individuals. The cysts can survive outside the body for about a week in a moist and cool environment.

The use of drugs in this condition depends largely on the site and type of infection, and different drugs may be effective in acute amoebic dysentery, in chronic intestinal amoebiasis, in extraintestinal infection and in the carrier state.

The main drugs currently used are: imidazoles, (e.g. metronidazole), dichloracetamides (e.g. diloxanide), chloroquine, and halogenated hydroxyquinolines (e.g. di-iodohydroxyquinoline). Emetine was the first effective drug in amoebiasis. It has been used for 70 years and may still be used in some circumstances. The agents may be used in combination.

The treatment of choice for the various forms of amoebiasis is as follows:

1. For invasive intestinal amoebiasis resulting in acute severe amoebic dysentery, or chronic intestinal infection: metronidazole plus diloxanide or di-iodohydroxyquinoline
2. For hepatic amoebiasis: metronidazole followed by chloroquine plus diloxanide
3. For the carrier state: diloxanide.

Metronidazole

Metronidazole (Fig. 33.4) was originally developed during a programme of search for antitrichomonad drugs. It is the most effective drug available for invasive amoebiasis involving the intestine or the liver, but it is less effective against organisms in the lumen of the gut. Its action is attributed to the generation in the parasite of reduced intermediates

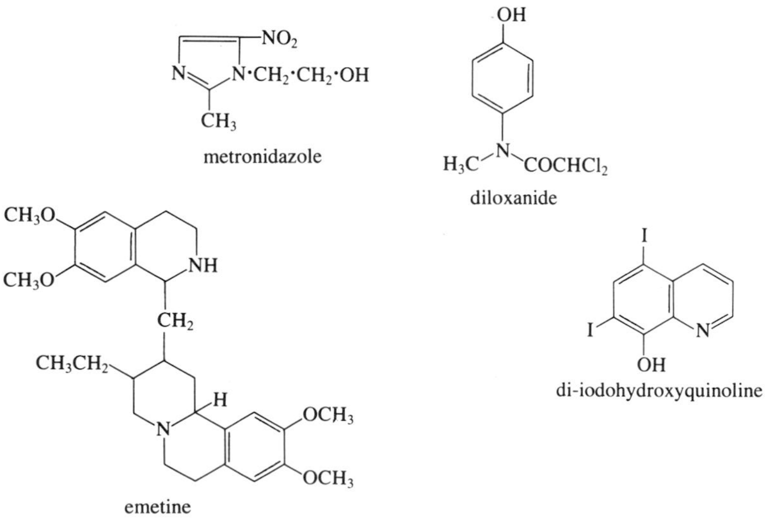

Fig. 33.4 Structures of some drugs used in amoebiasis.

of the drug which are oxidised, to produce super-oxide anions (O_2^-) and other toxic oxygen products such as hydroxyl radicals (OH^-).

It is usually given orally and is rapidly and completely absorbed, giving peak plasma concentration in 1–3 hours. It has a short plasma half-life of about 7 hours and needs to be given 8-hourly. Preparations for intravenous use are also available. There is little protein binding and it is distributed rapidly throughout the tissues, reaching high concentrations in the body fluids, including the cerebrospinal fluid. Some is metabolized but most is excreted in urine, though a small proportion is eliminated in the faeces.

Unwanted effects are few and in general metronidazole is considered to be a safe drug in therapeutic doses. Minor gastrointestinal side effects have been reported occasionally as have symptoms referable to the central nervous system (dizziness, headache). The drug interferes with alcohol metabolism. On the basis of tests on rodents there was thought to be a potential for teratogenicity but prolonged and extensive use in pregnant women has not resulted in foetal deformities.

Diloxanide

Both diloxanide itself (Fig. 33.4) and more particularly, an insoluble ester, diloxanide furoate are effective against the non-invasive parasite. The drugs have a direct amoebicidal action, affecting the amoebae before encystment, the effective concentration of the furoate being less than 100 nM in *in vitro* tests. It is given orally for 3–10 days, is partially absorbed, metabolized in the liver and excreted in the urine within 48 hours, mostly as the glucuronide. There are no serious unwanted effects.

Chloroquine

Chloroquine is a 4-aminoquinoline. It has little effect on intestinal amoebiasis but is effective in amoebic liver abscess. It is used in malaria and details of its pharmacokinetics and unwanted effects are given in the earlier section of this chapter. Its use as an anti-inflammatory drug in arthritis is described in Chapter 9. For amoebiasis it is given orally for 5–25 days, is well absorbed and reaches a high concentration in the liver. It can be used to prevent hepatic amoebiasis. It is sometimes combined with emetine in the treatment of hepatic amoebiasis which fails to respond to metronidazole.

Halogenated hydroxyquinolines

The member of this group which has been most widely used in amoebiasis is di-iodohydroxyquinoline. It has a direct amoebicidal action on luminal parasites. It is given orally and only 10% is absorbed; this is metabolized and secreted in the form of sulfates and glucuronides.

Prolonged use of halogenated hydroxyquinolines has been associated with a serious immunological disorder—subacute myelo-optic neuropathy (SMON) characterized by polyneuritis and optic atrophy. The compound which was implicated was clioquinol (iodochlorhydroxyquin). The syndrome occurred originally in Japan and later in the USA and Europe and was the result of the wide-spread use of this compound for non-specific diarrhoea. The compounds have been withdrawn from the market in many parts of the world but di-iodohydroxyquinoline is still available in some areas.

Emetine

Emetine is an alkaloid of ipecachuana and preparations for clinical use can be extracted from natural sources or synthesized. It has a direct amoebicidal action, acting mainly on the invasive parasites in the tissues. Its mechanism of action is partly by irreversible inhibition of parasite protein synthesis. Both emetine and the more potent derivative dehydroemetine are highly irritant and are given intramuscularly. Unwanted effects are likely to occur, especially if the drug is given for prolonged periods. Gastrointestinal, neuromuscular and cardiovascular toxic effects are seen. About 30% of patients experience nausea, and diarrhoea and vomiting also occur. Neuromuscular effects reported are muscle weakness and myalgia. The cardiovascular effects are more serious and consist of dysrhythmias, precordial pain and congestive cardiac failure. Because of the unwanted effects, emetine should only be given to patients under careful supervision in hospital.

In general this drug has been superseded in amoebiasis therapy by metronidazole.

LEISHMANIASIS

There are a variety of *Leishmania* organisms which cause disease, mainly in tropical and subtropical regions.

The parasite exists in two forms—an amastigote in the mammalian host, and a flagellated promastigote in the insect vector, which is a flesh-eating sandfly. The amastigote is taken up by the mononuclear phagocyte system and remains alive and viable within the host cells.

There are several clinical types of leishmaniasis—a simple skin infection which may heal spontaneously, a muco-cutaneous form (in which there may be large ulcers of the mucous membranes) and a visceral form ('Kala-Azar'). In this last form, the parasite spreads through the blood stream and causes hepato- and spleno-megaly, anaemia and intermittent fever.

The main drug used in visceral leishmaniasis is **sodium stibogluconate**, an organic pentavalent antimony compound, which is a complex of two molecules of gluconate with two atoms of antimony. It is given intramuscularly or by slow intravenous injection in a 10-day course. More than one course may be required. Unwanted effects are anorexia, vomiting, bradycardia and hypotension. Coughing and substernal pain may occur during intravenous infusion.

Other drugs used in leishmaniasis are **amphotericin** (also used as an antifungal agent, p. 653) and **metronidazole** (see above) which is effective against cutaneous lesions.

Allopurinol is reported to be converted to toxic metabolites in the amastigote and since this does not happen in the host cells some selective toxicity may be achieved. It may be combined with sodium stibogluconate. This compound is considered in Chapter 9 (p. 217).

TRYPANOSOMIASIS

There are three main species of trypanosomes which cause disease in man—*T. gambiense* and *T. rhodesiense* which cause sleeping sickness in Africa, and *T. cruzi* which causes Chagas' disease in South America.

The main drugs used for African sleeping sickness are **suramin** and **pentamidine**. Drugs used in Chagas' disease include **primaquine** (see above), **puromycin** (see Chapter 28) and **nitrofurantoin derivatives** (p. 642), but there is, in essence, no really effective treatment for this disease.

Suramin

This drug is a naphthylamine-sulphonic acid derivative which was introduced into the therapy of trypanosomiasis in 1920. It does not kill the parasites immediately but induces biochemical changes which result in the organisms being cleared from the circulation after an interval of 24 hours.

The drug binds firmly to host plasma proteins and in this form enters the trypanosome by endocytosis. It is then liberated by lysosomal proteases. It has a selective action on trypanosomal enzymes as compared to those in man.

It is given by slow intravenous injection. The blood concentration drops rapidly during the first few hours and then more slowly over the succeeding days. A low concentration remains for 3–4 months. It tends to accumulate in the mononuclear phagocyte system and is also found in the cells of the proximal tubule in the kidney.

This drug is relatively toxic, particularly in a malnourished patient—the main toxic effect being on the kidney. Other slowly developing unwanted effects which have been reported include optic atrophy, adrenal insufficiency, skin rashes, haemolytic anaemia and agranulocytosis.

A small proportion of individuals (0.1–0.3%) have an immediate idiosyncratic reaction to suramin injection—nausea, vomiting, shock, seizures, and loss of consciousness.

Pentamidine

This agent (Fig. 33.5) has a direct trypanocidal action *in vitro*. It is rapidly taken up in the parasites

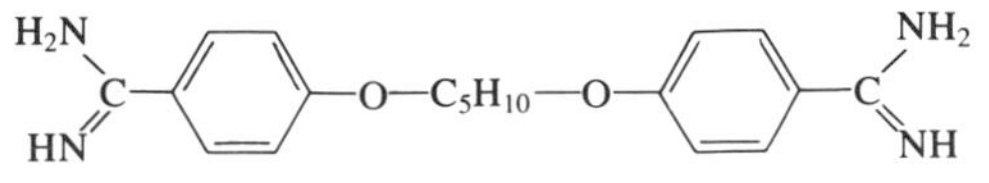

Fig. 33.5 Pentamidine

by a high-affinity energy-dependent carrier and is thought to interact with the DNA.

Pentamidine is given intramuscularly, usually daily for 10–15 days and, after absorption from the injection site, soon leaves the circulation. Fairly high concentrations of the drug persist in the kidney, the liver and the spleen for several months.

The most serious unwanted effect is nephrotoxicity. Neurotoxicity has also been reported. The most frequently seen side effect is an immediate decrease in blood pressure with tachycardia, breathlessness and vomiting. Histamine release may explain these latter effects.

TRICHOMONIASIS

The principal trichomonas organisms which produces disease in humans is *T. vaginalis*. Virulent strains cause inflammation of the vagina in females and sometimes of the urethra in males.

The main drug used in therapy is **metronidazole** (p. 665).

REFERENCES AND FURTHER READING

Howells R E 1982 Advances in chemotherapy in Malaria. Br Med Bull 38 (2): 193–199

James Dinah M, Gilles H M 1985 Human antiparasite drugs: pharmacology and usage. John Wiley, Chichester
Chapter 4: The Trypanosomiases 72–91
Chapter 5: The Leishmaniases 92–104
Chapter 6: Amoebiasis 105–119
Chapter 7: Malaria 120–164
Chapter 8: Trichomoniasis 180–182

Knight R 1980 The chemotherapy of amoebiasis. J Antimicrob Chemother 6: 577–593

Mansfield J M (ed) 1984 Parasitic diseases; Vol 2: The chemotherapy. Marcel Dekker, New York
Desjardins R E, Trenholme G M Antimalarial chemotherapy, p1–71

Marr J J The chemotherapy of Leishmaniasis, p201–227

Meshmick S R The chemotherapy of African Trypanosomiasis, p165–199

Kierszenbaum F The chemotherapy of *Tryptanosoma cruzi* infections, p133–163

Powell S J 1972 Latest development in the treatment of amoebiasis. Adv Pharmacol Chemother 10: 91–103

Vakil B J, Dala N J 1974 Comparative evaluation of amoebicidal drugs. Progress in Drug Research 18: 353–364

WHO Report of the Steering committees of the Scientific Working groups on Malaria 1980–1983

Wyler D J 1983 Malaria: resurgence, resistance and research. N Eng J Med 308: part 1 p875–878; part 2 p934–940.

34

Anthelminthic drugs

A large proportion of mankind harbours worms of one species or another. In some cases these infections result mainly in discomfort and do not cause substantial ill health (an example being threadworms in children). Other worm infections, such as bilharziasis and hookworm disease, produce very serious morbidity. In many countries, particularly those in tropical and subtropical regions, almost all the indigenous population is infected with hookworm and the problem of the treatment of helminthiasis is, therefore, one of very great practical importance.

There are two types of worm infections—those in which the worm lives in the host's alimentary canal, and those in which the worm lives in other tissues of the host's body.

The principal worms which live in the host's alimentary canal are:

1. Tapeworms (Cestodes): *Taenia saginata*, *Taenia solium*, *Hymenolepis nana*, *Diphyllobothrium latum* (only the former two are likely to be seen in the United Kingdom).

   The usual intermediate hosts for the larval stages of the two most common tapeworms—*Taenia saginata* and *Taenia solium* are cattle and pigs respectively. Man becomes infected by eating raw or undercooked meat containing the infective larvae, which have encysted in the muscle tissue. (In some circumstances, the larval stage of *Taenia solium* can develop in man, resulting in *cysticercosis*, a condition characterized by encysted larvae in muscle and viscera or, more seriously, in the eye or the brain.)

   Hymenolepis nana can have both the adult stage (the intestinal worm) and the larval stage in the same host, which can be man or rodent, though some insects (fleas, grain beetles) can also serve as intermediate hosts.

   Diphyllobothrium latum has two sequential intermediate hosts—a fresh water crustacean and a fresh water fish. Man becomes infected by eating raw or incompletely cooked fish containing the infective larvae.

2. Roundworms (Nematodes): *Ascaris lumbricoides*; *Enterobius vermicularis* (threadworm); *Trichuris trichiuria* (whipworm). *Strongyloides stercoralis*. *Necator americanus*, *Ankylostoma duodenale* (hookworm).

The principal worms which live in the tissues of the host are:

1. Schistosomes (these are trematodes or flukes which cause bilharzia). The adult worms of both sexes live in the veins or venules of the gut wall or the bladder. The female lays eggs which pass into the bladder or the gut and produce inflammation of these organs, resulting in haematuria in the former case and loss of blood in the faeces in the latter. The eggs hatch in water after discharge from the body and give rise to *miracidia* which enter the secondary host— a particular species of snail. After a period of development in this host, free-swimming *cerceriae* emerge. These are capable of infecting man by penetration of the skin.

2. Filaria. The filariae are long thread-like nematodes. The adult worms live in the lymphatics, connective tissues or mesentery of the host and produce live embryos or microfilariae which find their way into the blood stream. They may be ingested by mosquitoes or similar biting insects when these take up blood. After a period of development within this secondary host, the

larvae pass to the mouthparts of the insect and are re-injected into man. The chief filarial disease is filariasis due to *Wuchereria* and *Brugia* which cause obstruction of lymphatic vessels producing elephantiasis; other related diseases are onchocerciasis, loaiasis and dracontiasis.

3. Hydatid tapeworm: *Echinococcus* species. These are cestodes for which canines are the primary hosts and sheep the intermediate hosts. The primary, intestinal stage does not occur in man, but under some circumstances man can function as the intermediate host, in which case the larvae develop into *hydatid cysts* within the tissues.

Details of the life cycles of the worms and the diseases caused in man should be obtained from textbooks on parasitology and medicine.

ACTIONS OF ANTHELMINTHIC DRUGS

To be an effective anthelminthic, a drug must be able to penetrate the cuticle of the worm or gain access to its alimentary tract.

An anthelminthic drug may act by causing narcosis or paralysis of the worm, or by damaging the cuticle, leading to partial digestion or to rejection by immune mechanisms. Anthelminthic drugs may also interfere with the metabolism of the worm, and since the metabolic requirements of these parasites vary greatly from one species to another, this may be the reason why drugs which are highly effective against one type of worm are ineffective against others.

The use of *in vitro* tests to asses the efficacy of an anthelminthic agent is generally unsatisfactory since the effect of the drug *in vivo* may depend on its conversion by the host into a more active compound. Conversely a drug which is active by *in vitro* tests, may be inactivated by secretions in the alimentary tract of the host. For these reasons anthelminthic drugs usually have to be tested by measuring their ability to eliminate worms from infected animals. The clinical evaluation of drugs in

Table 34.1 Drugs used in helminth infestations

Helminth	Drug
Threadworm (pinworm) (*Enterobius vermicularis*)	piperazine, thiabendazole, mebendazole, pyrantel
Strongyloides stercoralis (called threadworm in USA)	thiabendazole
Common Roundworm (*Ascasis lumbricoides*)	piperazine,* pyrantel,* thiabendazole, mebendazole, levamisole, bephenium
Other roundworms (*Wucheria bancrofti, Loa loa, Oncocerca volvulus*)	diethylcarbamazine
Tapeworm (*Taenia saginata, Taenia solium*)	niclosamide,* praziquantel
Cysticercosis (infection with larval *T. solium*)	praziquantel
Hydatid disease (*Echinococcus granulosus*)	mebendazole
Hookworm (*Ankylostoma duodenale, Necator americanus*)	Pyrantel,* mebendazole,* bephenium, thiabendazole
Whipworm (*Trichuris trichiura*)	mebendazole
Blood flukes (Schistosomes) S. haematobium S. mansomi S. japonicum	praziquantel,* metriphonate praziquantel,* oxamniquine praziquantel*

* Indicates drugs of first choice

intestinal helminth infections is usually based on the effect of the drug in reducing the number of eggs or worms in the faeces. Control observations are concurrently made on untreated patients in order to take into account the occurrence of spontaneous cures.

Individual drugs are described briefly below, their structures are given in Figure 34.1, and the indications for their use are given in Table 34.1.

Piperazine

Piperazine (Fig. 34.1) is a basic compound, which reversibly inhibits neuromuscular transmission in the worm. The paralysed worms are expelled alive.

It is given orally and some, but not all of a dose is absorbed. It is partly metabolized and the remainder is eliminated, unchanged, via the kidney. The drug has singularly little pharmacological action in the host.

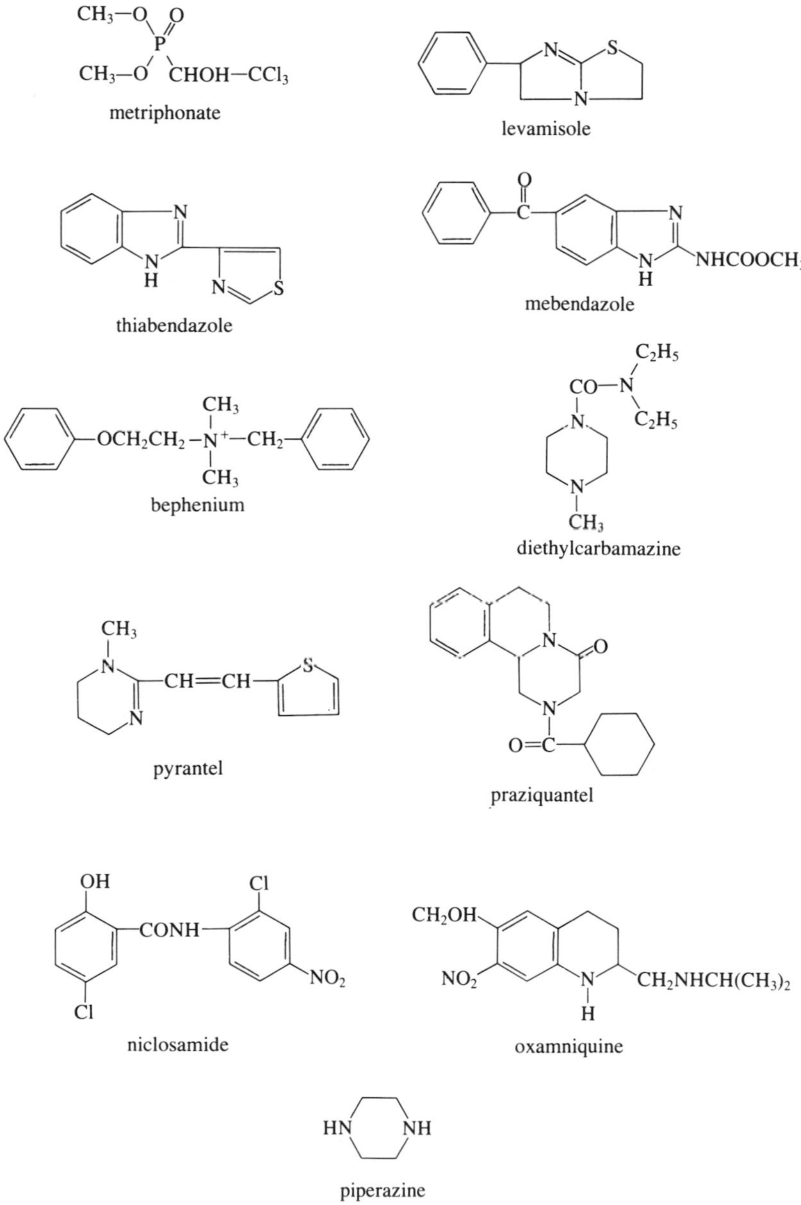

Fig. 34.1 Structures of some antithelminthic drugs

Unwanted effects

These are uncommon but gastrointestinal disturbances occur occasionally and some patients report neurotoxic side effects—dizziness, parasthaesias, vertigo, incoordination.

Used to treat roundworm, piperazine is highly effective in a single dose. For threadworm a longer course (7 days) in lower dosage is necessary.

Benzimidazoles

The two benzimidazoles anthelminthics are **mebendazole** and **thiabendazole** (Fig. 34.1). Thiabendazole forms complexes with various metals but does not chelate calcium. These compounds have a selective inhibitory action on helminth microtubular function—being 250–400 times more potent in helminth than in mammalian tissue (e.g. on bovine brain tubulin), in inhibiting colchicine binding. The effect takes time to develop and the worms may not be expelled for several days. Mebendazole is pharmacologically inert in man but thiabendazole is reported to have some effect in restoring immune deficiency.

Only 10% of mebendazole is absorbed after oral administration though if it is taken during a fatty meal, more is likely to be absorbed. It is rapidly metabolized, the products being excreted in the urine and the bile within 24–28 hours. It is given as a single dose for threadworm and twice daily for 3 days for roundworm infestations. Thiabendazole is rapidly absorbed from the gastrointestinal tract, very rapidly metabolized and excreted in the urine in conjugated form. It is given in 3 doses at weekly intervals for threadworm and twice daily for 3 days for roundworm.

Unwanted effects are few with mebendazole though gastrointestinal upsets may occasionally occur. Unwanted effects with thiabendazole are more frequent but are usually transient. The commonest side effects are gastrointestinal disturbances, but headache, dizziness and drowsiness may occur. Allergic reactions (fever, rashes) are reported. More serious toxic effects (such as parenchymal liver damage) have occurred in a few cases.

Bephenium

Bephenium is a quaternary ammonium compound (Fig. 34.1) and is poorly absorbed from the gut. It has nicotinic-like actions in both helminths and man but is considerably more potent on helminths, causing initial excitation at the neuromuscular junction followed by paralysis. (If given intravenously in mammals it has effects on autonomic ganglia.)

Unwanted effects include nausea vomiting, diarrhoea, abdominal cramps and dizziness.

Pyrantel

Pyrantel is a derivative of tetrahydro-pyrimidine (Fig. 34.1) which is thought to act by depolarizing the helminth neuromuscular junction, causing spasm and paralysis. It also has some anticholinesterase activity. There is poor absorption from the gastrointestinal tract after oral dosing—more than 50% of the drug being eliminated in the faeces.

It is generally regarded as a safe drug. Unwanted effects are mild and transitory and involve mostly gastrointestinal upsets. Dizziness and fever have been reported but no serious effects on blood, kidney or liver.

Niclosamide

Niclosamide is a derivative of salicylamide (Fig. 34.1) and is the drug of choice for tapeworm infestations. The scolex and a proximal segment are irreversibly damaged by the drug, and the worm separates from the intestinal wall and is expelled. The ova are not affected. It is given as chewable tablets in 2 doses separated by a 1 hour interval followed by a purgative 2 hours later. There is negligible absorption from the gastrointestinal tract.

Unwanted effects are few, infrequent and transient. Nausea and vomiting may occur. Since the damaged tapeworm segments may release ova, and as the ova are not affected by the drug, there is a theoretical possibility that cysticercosis may develop when niclosamide is used to treat pork tapeworm (*Taenia solium*).

Praziquantel

This is a new broadspectrum anthelminthic drug.

It is the drug of choice for all species of schistosomes and has been reported to be effective in cysticercosis—for which there was previously no effective therapy.

It is an isoquinoline-pyrazine derivative (Fig. 34.1) and it acts by increasing the calcium permeability of the plasma membrane of helminth cells. This results in spasm of the musculature and eventually paralysis and death of the worm. The drug affects not only the adult schistosomes but also the immature forms and the cercariae—the form of the parasite which infects man by burrowing into the skin.

Praziquantel has no pharmacological effects in man in therapeutic dosage. Given orally it is rapidly absorbed: much of the drug is rapidly metabolized to inactive metabolites on first passage through the liver and the metabolites are excreted in the urine. The plasma half-life of the parent compound is 60–90 mins. Mild unwanted effects are fairly frequent but are usually transitory. They include gastrointestinal upsets, dizziness, aching in muscles and joints, skin eruptions and low grade fever. Some effects are more marked in patients with a heavy worm load and may be due to products released from the dead worms. The therapeutic index is high—in experimental animals serious toxicity requires doses 2 orders of magnitude higher than those used for clinical treatment.

Oxamniquine

Oxamniquine is a tetrahydroquinoline derivative (Fig. 34.1) used for schistosomiasis, and is related chemically to the thioxanthone drugs, hycanthone and lucanthone, previously used against these blood flukes. Oxamniquine is effective only against *Schistosoma mansoni*, affecting both mature and immature forms. Its mechanisms of action may involve intercalation in the DNA and its selective action may be related to the ability of the parasite to concentrate the drug. There is experimental evidence showing that resistance can occur. It is given orally, is well absorbed, and is metabolized in the gut wall and in the liver to inactive metabolites which are excreted in the urine. It has a short half-life of 1–2 hours and is eliminated from the plasma by 10–12 hours. Transient dizziness and headache

are reported in 30–95% of patients in various studies, and gastrointestinal disturbances in 10–20% of patients. Symptoms caused by CNS stimulation may occur and include hallucinations and convulsive episodes. Allergic manifestations and other symptoms, which appear several days after treatment has stopped, may be related to the release of products from the dead fluke.

Metriphonate

Metriphonate is an organophosphate anticholinesterase which was originally used as an insecticide. It was subsequently found to be effective against *Schistosoma haematobium* and is now the drug of choice for treatment of infestations with this blood fluke. It is a pro-drug, giving rise spontaneously to the active drug, dichlorvos *in vivo*. Its action is thought to be due to an inhibitory effect on cholinesterases in the helminth, causing paralysis. The ova of the fluke are not affected. Given orally it is absorbed rapidly and the parent compound is cleared from the plasma within 8 hours. The serum concentration of active metabolite constitutes about 1% of that of the parent compound and both are cleared from the tissues within 1–2 days.

Effects on the host enzymes occur but do not usually result in serious physiological changes. Plasma cholinesterase activity is totally inhibited and there is a marked decrease in red cell acetylcholinesterase activity. Recovery from these effects takes 4–15 weeks, the plasma enzyme recovering more rapidly.

Unwanted effects occur in some patients (gastrointestinal disturbances, bronchospasm, dizziness) but usually last less than a day.

Diethylcarbamazine

Diethylcarbamazine is a piperazine derivative (Fig. 34.1) which is active in filarial infections caused by *Wuchereria bancrofti* and *Loa loa*, against which piperazine itself is ineffective. Diethylcarbamazine rapidly removes the microfilariae from the blood circulation and may also kill the adult worms in the lymphatics, but it has little action on microfilariae *in vitro*. It has been suggested that it modifies the parasite so that it becomes susceptible to the host's normal immune responses.

The drug is given orally, is absorbed and is distributed throughout the cells and tissues of the body, excepting adipose tissue. It is partly metabolized and both the parent drug and its metabolites are excreted in the urine, being cleared from the body within about 48 hours.

Unwanted effects are common but transient, subsiding within a day or so even if the drug is continued. Side effects due to the drug itself are gastrointestinal disturbances, arthralgias, headache and a general feeling of weakness. Allergic side effects referable to the filariae are common and vary with the species of worm. In general these start during the first day's treatment and last 3–7 days and include skin reactions, enlargement of lymph glands, dizziness, tachycardia and gastrointestinal and respiratory disturbances. When these symptoms disappear larger doses of the drug can be given without further problem.

Levamisole

Levamisole is the *laevo* isomer of tetramisole, a racemic imidazothiazole derivative. In roundworms it has a nicotine-like action, stimulating and subsequently blocking the neuromuscular junctions. The paralysed parasites are then passed in the faeces. Ova are not killed.

An immunomodulating effect in man has been claimed for this drug but has been difficult to prove, High concentrations may have nicotinic actions on autonomic ganglia in the mammalian host.

The drug is given orally, is rapidly absorbed, and is widely distributed (crossing the blood-brain-barrier). It is metabolized in the liver to inactive metabolites which are excreted via the kidney. Its plasma half-life is 4 hours. When single-dose therapy is used, unwanted effects are few and soon subside. They include gastrointestinal disturbances, dizziness and skin eruptions.

New drugs reported to be of use in schistosomiasis are **oltipraz** and **amoscanate**.

REFERENCES AND FURTHER READING

Bennett J L, Depenbusch J W 1984 The chemotherapy of schistosomiasis. In: Mansfield J M (ed) Parasitic Diseases: the Chemotherapy, Vol 2. Marcel Dekker, Basle, p 73–131
Calvier R 1973 Chemotherapy of intestinal nematodes. International Encyclopaedia of Pharmacology and Therapeutics. Pergamon Press, London, Vol 1, p 215–436
Friedhelm E 1973 Chemotherapy of schistosomiasis. In: Chemotherapy of helminthiasis. International Encyclopaedia of Pharmacology and Therapeutics. Pergamon Press, London, Vol 1, p 29–144
James Dinah H, Gilles H M 1985 Human antiparasitic drugs: Pharmacology and usage. John Wiley, Chichester, Section C: Anthelminthic drugs, p 189–268

General topics

35

Non-therapeutic drugs: nicotine, alcohol and cannabis

There are many drugs that human beings consume because they choose to and not because they are advised to by doctors. Society in general disapproves, because in most cases there is a recognizable social cost; in the more highly ordered societies this is considered to outweigh the individual benefit, and certain types of drug usage have been declared illegal. In Western societies the three most commonly used non-therapeutic drugs are caffeine, nicotine and alcohol, all of which are legally and freely available. There is a much larger number of drugs which are widely used, though their manufacture, sale and consumption has been declared illegal in most Western countries, except when it is under the control of the medical profession. A list of the more important ones is given in Table 35.1. The reasons why a particular group of drugs should come to be used in a way that constitutes a problem to society are obviously extremely complex and outside the scope of this book. The drug and its pharmacological activity are only the starting point, for drug-taking is clearly seen by society in a quite different light from other forms of self-gratification, such as opera-going or sex or even alcohol consumption. Furthermore, the 'drugs of abuse' form an extremely heterogenous pharmacological group—we can find little in common between, say morphine, cocaine and barbiturates. What links them together is that people enjoy the sensation that they produce and tend to want to repeat it. It becomes a problem when (a) the want becomes so insistent that it dominates the life-style of the individual and prevents him from living in a way that the rest of society can accept; and (b) when the habit itself causes actual harm to the individual.

Examples of the latter kind of problem are the

Table 35.1 The main drugs of abuse

Type	Examples	Dependence liability	Discussed in
Narcotic analgesics	Morphine	V. Strong	Chapter 25
	Heroin	V. strong	Chapter 25
General CNS depressants	Ethanol	Strong	This chapter
	Barbiturates	Strong	Chapter 21
	Methaqualone	Moderate	Chapter 21
	Glutethimide	Moderate	Chapter 21
	Anaesthetics	Moderate	Chapter 20
	Solvents	Strong	—
Anxiolytic drugs	Benzodiazepines	Moderate	Chapter 21
Psychomotor stimulants	Amphetamines	Strong	Chapter 26
	Cocaine	Strong	Chapter 26
	Caffeine	Weak	Chapter 26
	Nicotine	V. Strong	This chapter
Psychotomimetic agents	LSD	Weak or Absent	Chapter 26
	Mescaline	Weak or Absent	Chapter 26
	Phencyclidine	Moderate	Chapter 26
	Cannabis	Weak or Absent	This chapter

mental incapacity and eventual liver damage caused by alcohol, the host of diseases associated with smoking, or the serious danger of overdosage with most narcotics.

In this chapter we discuss the pharmacology of three important drugs which have no place in therapy but are consumed in large amounts, namely nicotine, ethanol and cannabis. Other drugs of this type are described elsewhere in this book (Table 35.1). For further information, including discussion of non-pharmacological aspects of drug abuse, many texts are available (e.g. Hofmann, 1983; Martin, 1977; Ashton & Stepney, 1982; Goldstein, 1983) including excellent chapters in two standard pharmacology textbooks (Gilman et al, 1985; Bowman & Rand, 1980).

NICOTINE AND TOBACCO

Tobacco growing, chewing and smoking was indigenous throughout the American sub-continent and Australia at the time that European explorers first visited these places and smoking spread through Europe during the 16th century, coming to England mainly as a result of its enthusiastic espousal by Raleigh in the court of Elizabeth I. James I strongly disapproved of both Raleigh and tobacco, and initiated the first anti-smoking campaign in the early 17th century with the support of the Royal College of Physicians. Parliament responded by imposing a substantial duty on tobacco, thereby setting up the dilemma, from which we show no sign of being able to escape, of giving the state an economic interest in the continuation of smoking at the same time that its official expert advisers are issuing emphatic warnings about its dangers.

Nowadays tobacco is grown commercially in many countries, the largest producers being USA, China, India and USSR.

Until the latter half of the 19th century, tobacco was smoked in pipes, and by men. Cigarette manufacture began at the end of the 19th century and

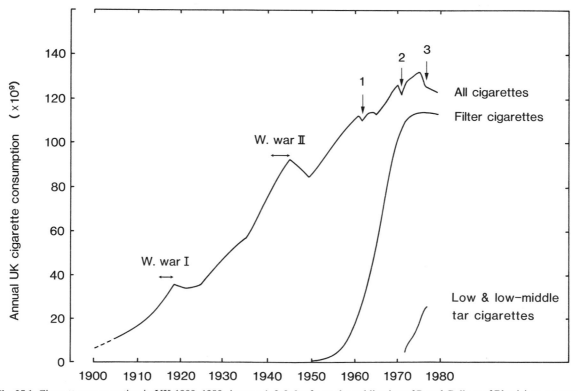

Fig. 35.1 Cigarette consumption in UK 1900–1980. Arrows 1, 2 & 3 refer to the publication of Royal College of Physicians reports on smoking and health. (From: Ashton & Stepney, 1982)

now cigarettes account for more than 90% of tobacco consumption. Cigarette smoking by women only began after the first World War; the prevalence is now about equal in men and women. Cigarette sales have now more or less levelled off (Fig. 35.1) possibly as a result of increasing adverse publicity, restrictions on advertising and the compulsory publication of health warnings. It is significant that filter cigarettes (which give a somewhat lower delivery of tar and nicotine than standard cigarettes) and low-tar cigarettes (which are also low in nicotine) constitute an increasing proportion of the total. What is concealed by figures of total cigarette sales is a substantial change in individual smoking habits. Concurrently with the increase in cigarette sales over the last 30 years, the number of smokers has actually gone down, so per capita consumption has increased substantially (from 14 to 22 per day among male smokers and from 7 to 17 per day among female smokers in the period 1949–78). This may be related to the reduction of nicotine yields, which has caused habitual smokers to smoke more heavily. Some figures, dating from 1980, are given in Table 35.2.

Table 35.2 Tobacco consumption (UK 1980)

Total tobacco sales (kg)	1.1×10^8
Percentage of total tobacco consumption:	
Cigarettes	93%
Pipe tobacco	4%
Cigars	3%
Number of cigarettes sold	1.24×10^{11}
Number of smokers	1.8×10^7
Average consumption among smokers	19 cigarettes/day
% of smokers in adult population	42 (male); 39 (female)
Average nicotine delivery	1.5 mg/cigarette

(Data from: Ashton & Stepney, 1982)

Absorption of nicotine

An average cigarette contains about 0.8 g of tobacco and 9–17 mg of nicotine, of which about 10% is normally absorbed by the smoker. This fraction varies greatly with the habits of the smoker and the type of cigarette. Nicotine (see Table 26.3 for structure) is the only pharmacologically active constituent of tobacco smoke that is present in sufficient quantity to produce systemic effects. In heavy smokers, carbon monoxide may also be important.

Nicotine in cigarette smoke is rapidly absorbed from the lungs, but poorly from the mouth and nasopharynx. Thus, inhalation is required to give appreciable absorption of nicotine. Pipe or cigar smoke is less acidic than cigarette smoke, and nicotine is more readily absorbed from the mouth and nasopharynx than with cigarette smoke, presumably because the drug is less fully ionized. Absorption is considerably slower than from inhaled cigarette smoke, and a later and longer-lasting peak in the plasma nicotine concentration occurs with pipe or cigar smoking than with cigarette smoking (Fig. 35.2).

An average cigarette, smoked over 10 minutes, causes the plasma nicotine concentrations to rise to 20–30 ng/ml (130–200 nM). It falls to about half within 10 minutes and then more slowly over the next 1–2 hours. The rapid decline results mainly from redistribution between the blood and other tissues, the slower decline being due to hepatic metabolism, mainly by oxidation to an inactive ketone metabolite.

Pharmacological effects of smoking

Nicotine appears to be the only pharmacologically active substance in tobacco smoke apart from carcinogenic tars; the acute effects of smoking can be mimicked by injection of nicotine, and are blocked by **mecamylamine**, an antagonist at nicotinic acetylcholine receptors (see Chapter 6).

Effects on the central nervous system

The central effects of nicotine are complex and cannot be summed up simply in terms of stimulation or inhibition. At the spinal level an inhibition of spinal reflexes occurs, and this produces skeletal muscle relaxation which can be measured by electromyography. It is probably due to stimulation of the Renshaw cells in the ventral horn of the spinal cord (see Chapter 19); these cells receive a cholinergic innervation from motoneuron collaterals and exert an inhibitory effect on the motoneurons. The higher level functioning of the brain, as reflected in the subjective sense of alertness, or the EEG pattern, can be affected in either direction by nicotine, according to dose and circumstances. Smokers report that smoking wakes them up when they are

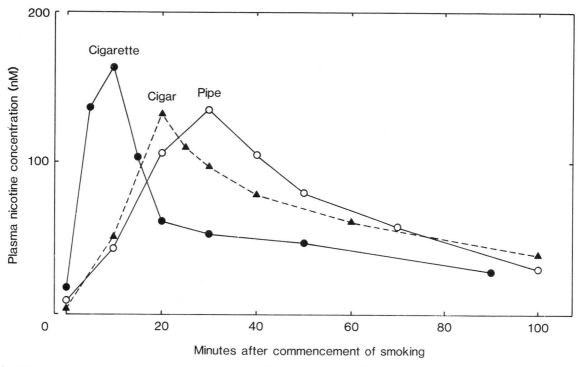

Fig. 35.2 Nicotine concentration in plasma during smoking. The subjects were habitual smokers, who smoked a single cigarette, pipe or cigar according to their usual habit, starting at time zero. (From: Bowman & Rand, 1980)

drowsy and calms them down when they are tense, and EEG recordings broadly bear this out. It also seems that small doses of nicotine tend to cause arousal whereas large doses do the reverse. Tests of motor and sensory performance (e.g. reaction time measurements or vigilance tests) in humans have generally shown improvement after smoking, but the studies are difficult to interpret because no satisfactory placebo, in the form of a nicotine-free smoking medium that the subject cannot distinguish from tobacco, is available, so the subjects were necessarily aware when they were receiving the drug.

Measures of learning and retention in rats (for example, in a maze-running test) have generally shown improvement in response to nicotine. Some extremely elaborate tests have been conducted to see, for example, whether the effect of nicotine on performance and aggression varies according to the amount of stress. Some border on nasty-mindedness. In one, the subject first has to name the colours of a series of squares (low stress), and then

has to name the colours of the print in which the names of other colours are written (high stress). The difference between the scores reflecting the extent by which performance is affected by stress, was diminished by smoking. In another, subjects played a complicated logical game with a computer which initially played fair and then began to cheat randomly, causing stress and aggression in the subjects, and a decline in their performance. Smoking, it was reported, did not reduce the anger, but did reduce the decline in performance.

Peripheral effects

The peripheral effects of small doses of nicotine result from stimulation of autonomic ganglia (see Chapter 6) and of peripheral sensory receptors, mainly in the heart and lungs. Stimulation of these receptors elicits various autonomic reflex responses, causing tachycardia, vasoconstriction, increased cardiac output and increased arterial pressure, reduction of gastrointestinal motility and sweating. Smoking by neophytes usually causes nausea and sometimes vomiting, partly because of stimulation of sensory receptors in the stomach. All of these effects decline with repeated dosage, though the central effects remain.

Secretion of antidiuretic hormone from the posterior pituitary is increased, causing a decrease in urine flow. The plasma concentration of free fatty acids is increased, probably due to sympathetic stimulation and adrenaline secretion.

Tolerance and dependence

The effects of nicotine associated with peripheral ganglionic stimulation show rapid tachyphylaxis, perhaps as a result of desensitization of nicotinic acetylcholine receptors by nicotine. With large doses of nicotine this desensitization produces a block of ganglionic transmission rather than stimulation (see Chapter 6). Some degree of tolerance to the central effects of nicotine can be demonstrated (e.g. in the arousal response) but it is much less than in the periphery.

There is good evidence that the addictive nature of tobacco smoking is associated with the intake of nicotine (see review: Griffiths & Henningfield, 1982). Nicotine-free cigarettes have been found not to provide an acceptable alternative for habitual smokers. Various animal experiments confirm that nicotine is addictive. Thus, rats choose to drink dilute nicotine solution in preference to water if given a choice, and will perform various tasks to obtain nicotine-containing water as a reward. In a situation in which lever-pressing causes an injection of nicotine to be delivered, rats do not spontaneously learn to self-administer the drug, but if they have previously been injected with nicotine for a few days, they quickly learn to self-administer it. Similarly, monkeys who have been trained to smoke, by providing a reward in response to smoking behaviour, will continue to do so spontaneously (i.e. unrewarded) if the smoking medium contains nicotine, but not if nicotine-free tobacco is offered instead. Studies such as these show that nicotine has inherent 'reward' qualities. It has also been shown in several tests that mecamylamine, a centrally-acting antagonist at nicotinic acetylcholine receptors (see Chapter 6) reduces the rewarding effect of nicotine. Thus, if monkeys are

habituated to tobacco smoking, so that they choose to puff tobacco smoke in preference to warm air, administration of mecamylamine causes them to switch to puffing air instead of tobacco smoke.

Attempts to substitute nicotine administration for smoking in humans have had mixed success. Under laboratory conditions, intravenous injections of nicotine, adjusted to give plasma concentrations equivalent to those achieved during smoking, did not reduce cigarette consumption by habitual smokers. It seems clear, therefore, that the reward properties of nicotine itself are only a part of the reason why humans smoke cigarettes.

A physical withdrawal syndrome occurs in both humans and experimental animals accustomed to regular nicotine administration. Its main features are increased irritability, impaired performance of psychomotor tasks, aggressiveness and sleep disturbance. The withdrawal syndrome is much less severe than that produced by opiates, and it can be alleviated not only by nicotine, but also by amphetamine. This is interesting as it suggests that the effect of nicotine may be partly due to catecholamine release in the brain, an hypothesis for which other pharmacological evidence exists. This withdrawal syndrome is probably important in the short-term maintenance of the smoking habit, but it disappears in 2–3 weeks; however, the craving for cigarettes persists for much longer than this, and relapses during attempts to give up cigarette smoking occur most commonly at a time when the physical withdrawal syndrome has long since subsided.

Pharmacological approaches to helping habitual smokers to give up have been only partially successful. The use of mecamylamine, which antagonizes the effects of nicotine, is not promising. Small doses actually increase smoking, presumably because the nicotine effect can break through the antagonism if the amount of nicotine is increased. Larger doses of mecamylamine, which abolish the effects of nicotine more effectively, have so many autonomic side effects (see Chapter 6) that subjects are unwilling to comply.

The use of nicotine chewing gum (Jarvis et al, 1982) seems to be partially successful. In this double blind study, subjects were given nicotine chewing gum or a placebo, plus plenty of encouragement. In the placebo group 22% of the subjects were still not smoking after 1 year compared with 47% of the nicotine group. The use of nicotine has disadvantages in that it produces side effects such as nausea and hiccups, and is in any case not a completely satisfactory solution to the problem, since some of the adverse effects of smoking on the cardiovascular system (see below) are probably caused by nicotine itself. For more general accounts of procedures for helping smokers to give up, see the Report of the Royal College of Physicians (1977) and Ashton & Stepney (1983).

Harmful effects of smoking

It is well established that the life expectation of smokers is shorter than that of non-smokers. For example, in a study of British doctors (see Report of Royal College of Physicians, 1971) the proportion of heavy smokers dying between the ages of 35 and 65 was estimated to be 40%, compared with 15% for non-smokers. Though it has been strenuously argued (Eysenck & Eaves, 1980) that the association is not necessarily a causal one, most of the many studies on this topic have concluded that smoking constitutes a major risk to health (Report of Royal College of Physicians, 1977; US Public Health Service Reports 1981, 1982, 1983).

The main health risks are:

1. Cancer, particularly of the lung, but also of the mouth, throat and oesophagus. Smoking 20 cigarettes per day is estimated to increase the risk of lung cancer about 10-fold. Lung cancer accounts for about half of the total cancer deaths in men; and about 90% is estimated to be caused by smoking. Pipe and cigar smoking carry much less risk than cigarette smoking, though it is still appreciable.
2. Coronary heart disease, and other forms of peripheral vascular disease. The mortality among men aged 55–64 from coronary thrombosis is about 60% greater in men who smoke 20 cigarettes per day compared with non-smokers. Even though the effect of smoking is less striking than with lung cancer, the actual number of excess deaths associated with smoking is larger, because coronary heart disease is so common.

    Other kinds of peripheral vascular disease (e.g. intermittent claudication, diabetic gangrene) are also strongly smoking-related.

It is interesting that there is no clear increase in coronary disease in pipe and cigar smokers. This suggests that nicotine may not be the causative factor, since the arterial blood nicotine concentration is not much less in pipe or cigar smokers than in cigarette smokers.

3. Chronic bronchitis. Many studies have shown a much higher incidence of chronic bronchitis in smokers than non-smokers. Nonetheless, in contrast to lung cancer, chronic bronchitis has declined in prevalence over the past 50 years. This is generally attributed to cleaner air and other social changes, and smoking now appears to be the most important remaining cause.
4. Effects in pregnancy. Smoking, particularly during the latter half of pregnancy, significantly reduces birth weight and increases perinatal mortality (estimated to be 30% higher among babies born to mothers who smoke in the last half of pregnancy). There is evidence that children born to smoking mothers remain backward, in both physical and mental development, for at least 7 years. By 11 years of age, the difference has ceased to be significant. These effects of smoking, though measurable, are much smaller than the effects of other factors, such as social class and birth order.

    Various other complications of pregnancy are also more common in women who smoke, including spontaneous abortion (increased 30–70% by smoking), premature delivery (increased about 40%) and placenta praevia (increased 25–90%).

    Nicotine is excreted in breast milk in sufficient amounts to cause tachycardia in the infant.

The causative agents that are probably responsible for these effects are:

1. Tar and irritants, such as NO_2, formaldehyde, etc. Cigarette smoke tar contains many known carcinogenic hydrocarbons (e.g. benzpyrene, nitrosamines; see Chapter 36), which account for the high cancer risk. It is likely that the various irritant substances are also responsible for the increase in bronchitis and emphysema.
2. Nicotine. There is no evidence that nicotine contributes to the cancer risk (indeed the lower cancer risk in pipe or cigar smokers suggests that it does not). It is an obvious candidate for

causing peripheral vascular disease and retarding fetal development, because of its vasoconstrictor properties, that there is no clear evidence implicating it.

3. Carbon monoxide. The average carbon monoxide content of cigarette smoke is about 3%. Carbon monoxide has a high affinity for haemoglobin and the average carboxyhaemoglobin content in the blood of cigarette smokers has been estimated at about 2.5% (mean for non-smoking urban dwellers is 0.4%). In very heavy smokers up to 15% of haemoglobin may be complexed with carbon monoxide, a level which has been shown to cause retardation of fetal development in rats. It is possible that this factor also contributes to the increased incidence of heart and vascular disease. Fetal haemoglobin has a higher affinity for carbon monoxide than adult haemoglobin, and the proportion of carboxy-haemoglobin is higher in fetal than maternal blood. 'Low tar' cigarettes give a lower yield of both tar and nicotine than standard cigarettes. It has, however, been shown that smokers puff harder, inhale more, and smoke more cigarettes when low tar brands are substituted for standard brands. The end result is a reduced intake of tar and nicotine, but an increase in carbon monoxide intake. Many studies have confirmed a reduced lung cancer risk with low tar cigarettes, but the risk of coronary heart disease is unchanged or even increased compared with that associated with standard cigarettes, suggesting that carbon monoxide may be important.

ALCOHOL

Judged on a molar basis, the consumption of ethanol far exceeds that of any other drug. The ethanol content of various drinks ranges from about 2.5% (weak beer) to about 55% (strong spirits), and the size of the normal measure is such that a single drink usually contains about 8–12 g (0.17–0.26 moles) of ethanol, and it is by no means unusual to consume 1–2 moles at a sitting, equivalent to about 0.5 kg of most other drugs. Its low pharmacological potency is reflected in the range of plasma concentrations needed to produce pharmacological effects: minimal effects occur at about 10 mM (46 mg/100 ml), and ten times this concentration may be lethal.

Pharmacological effects

Effects on the central nervous system

The main effects of ethanol are on the central nervous system, where it acts as a depressant in a manner very similar to volatile anaesthetics (see Chapter 20). There is biophysical evidence suggesting that ethanol, at pharmacologically effective concentrations, produces a measurable increase in the structural disorder (i.e. increased fluidity) of lipid membranes, similar to the effect of volatile anaesthetics. At a cellular level, the effect of ethanol is purely depressant. Like volatile anaesthetics, ethanol appears to act mainly by inhibiting transmitter release, and it affects impulse conduction and the post-synaptic actions of most neurotransmitters only at higher concentrations than are likely to be achieved *in vivo*. Ethanol inhibits transmitter release in response to nerve terminal depolarization, without affecting release evoked by calcium ionophores (Littleton, 1984). Thus it is likely that the primary effect is to inhibit the opening of voltage-sensitive Ca^{++}-channels in the nerve terminal membrane.

The effects of acute ethanol intoxication in man are well-known, and include slurred speech, motor inco-ordination, increased self-confidence and euphoria. The effect on mood varies among individuals, most becoming louder and more out-going, but some becoming morose and withdrawn. At higher levels of intoxication, the mood tends to become highly labile, with euphoria and melancholy, aggression and submission, often occurring successively.

Intellectual and motor performance and sensory discrimination, which can be measured in many different ways, show uniform impairment by ethanol, but subjects are generally unable to judge this for themselves. In tests on bus drivers, for example, in which subjects were asked to drive through a gap which they considered to be the minimum for their bus to go through, ethanol caused them not only to hit the barriers more often at any given gap setting, but also to set the gap to a narrower dimension.

Much effort has gone into measuring the effect of

ethanol on driving performance in real life, as opposed to artificial tests under experimental conditions. In one American study, large numbers of city drivers were tested for plasma ethanol concentration, including drivers who had been involved in an accident and those that had not. This allowed the relative probability of being involved in an accident to be calculated as a function of ethanol concentration. It was found that no significant change occurred up to 50 mg/100 ml (10.9 mM); by 80 mg/100 ml (17.4 mM) the probability was increased about 4-fold and by 150 mg/100 ml (32.6 mM) about 25-fold. In the UK, driving with a blood ethanol concentration greater than 80 mg/100 ml constitutes a legal offence.

The relationship between plasma ethanol concentration and effect is highly variable. A given concentration produces a larger effect when the concentration is rising than when it is steady or falling. A substantial degree of tissue tolerance develops in habitual drinkers with the result that a higher plasma ethanol concentration is needed to produce a given effect (see below). In a large American study, 'gross intoxication' (assessed by a battery of tests that measured speech, gait, etc) occurred in 30% of subjects between 50 and 100 mg/100 ml and 90% of subjects with more than 150 mg/100 ml. Coma generally occurs at about 300 mg/ml and death from respiratory failure is likely at 400–500 mg/ml.

Other effects

The main cardiovascular effect of ethanol is to produce cutaneous vasodilatation, central in origin, which causes a warm feeling but actually increases heat loss.

Ethanol increases salivary and gastric secretion. This is partly a reflex effect produced by the taste and irritant action of ethanol, but heavy consumption of spirits causes damage directly to the gastric mucosa, causing chronic gastritis. Both this and the increased acid secretion are factors in the high incidence of gastric bleeding in alcoholics.

Ethanol produces a variety of endocrine effects. It increases the output of adrenal steroid hormones, by stimulating the anterior pituitary gland to secrete ACTH. Plasma cortisol is usually raised in human alcoholics, but this may be due partly to inhibition by ethanol of cortisol metabolism in the liver. On the other hand, the rate of ethanol metabolism is increased by corticosteroids, and this effect may be a factor in the development of tolerance.

Diuresis is a familiar effect of ethanol; it is caused by inhibition of ADH secretion, and tolerance develops rapidly, so that the diuresis is not sustained. There is a similar inhibition of oxytocin secretion, which can cause postponement of parturition at term. Attempts have been made to use this effect to delay premature labour, but the dose needed is large enough to cause obvious drunkenness in the mother. If the baby is born prematurely in spite of the ethanol, it too may be intoxicated at birth, sufficiently for respiration to be depressed. The procedure evidently has serious disadvantages.

Chronic male alcoholics often show signs of feminization, which is associated with a decrease of plasma testosterone rather than increased oestrogen. The decrease is thought to be caused mainly by impaired testicular steroid synthesis, but induction of hepatic microsomal enzymes by ethanol, and hence an increased rate of testosterone inactivation, may also contribute.

Effects of ethanol on the liver

Liver damage is the most serious long-term consequence of excessive ethanol consumption. The sequence of effects is that increased fat accumulation (fatty liver) progresses to hepatitis (i.e. inflammation of the liver) and eventually to irreversible hepatic necrosis and fibrosis. Increased fat accumulation in the liver occurs, in rats or in man, after a single large dose of ethanol. The mechanism is complex, the main factors being (a) increased release of fatty acids from adipose tissue, which is the result of increased stress, causing sympathetic discharge; and (b) impaired fatty acid oxidation, because of the metabolic load imposed by the ethanol itself.

With chronic ethanol consumption, many other factors contribute to liver damage. One is malnutrition, for an alcoholic may satisfy much of his calorie requirement from ethanol itself. 200 g of ethanol, which is approximately the content of one bottle of whisky, provides about 1400 kCal, but, unlike a normal diet, it provides no vitamins, amino-acids or fatty acids. The hepatic changes occurring in alcoholics closely resemble the effects of chronic malnutrition. Another factor is the cellular toxicity of ethanol, which promotes inflammatory changes in the liver.

The overall incidence of chronic liver disease seems to be a function of cumulative ethanol consumption over many years. Thus, overall consumption, expressed as g/kg body weight per day multiplied by years of drinking, provides an accurate predictor of the incidence of cirrhosis.

Effects on lipid metabolism, platelet function and atherosclerosis

There is evidence that drinking has the effect of reducing the incidence of coronary heart disease (Fig. 35.3). Two mechanisms have been proposed. The first involves the effect of ethanol on plasma lipoprotein concentrations. These lipoproteins are the carrier molecules for cholesterol and other lipids in the bloodstream (see Chapter 15, and review by Brown et al, 1981). The delivery of cholesterol to the vascular endothelial cells, where it can form atheromatous plaques, depends mainly on the presence of **low density lipoprotein (LDL)** and there is a strong positive correlation between LDL concentration, cholesterol concentration and the incidence of coronary disease. **High-density lipoprotein (HDL)** is involved in the esterification of cholesterol in the plasma, and is thought to exert a protective effect against atheroma formation. Various epidemiological studies, and also some experimental studies on volunteers, have shown that alcohol increases plasma HDL concentration. In one experimental study (Belfrage et al, 1977), a very small daily dose of ethanol, well below the threshold for intoxication, caused a 30% rise in plasma HDL within 5 weeks.

The other mechanism whereby alcohol may protect against coronary disease involves its recently-discovered effect of inhibiting platelet aggregation. This occurs at ethanol concentrations in the range achieved by normal drinking in man (10–20 mM) and probably results from inhibition of arachidonic acid formation from phospholipid. In man, the magnitude of the effect depends critically on dietary fat intake (Fenn & Littleton, 1984), and it is not yet clear how important it is clinically.

The effect of ethanol on fetal development

It was demonstrated convincingly in the early 1970s that ethanol consumption during pregnancy has an adverse effect on fetal development. **Fetal alcohol syndrome (FAS)** is the term used to describe the effects commonly seen in the children of mothers who drink heavily in pregnancy (see reviews: Clarren & Smith, 1978; Streissguth et al, 1980; Ciba Foundation Symposium, 1984). This full-blown picture is relatively uncommon, but it is estimated that lesser degrees of ethanol-related abnormality may occur very frequently. Indeed one survey suggests that ethanol is responsible for about 8% of cases of mild mental retardation.

The characteristic features of the fetal alcohol syndrome are:

1. Abnormal facial development, with wide-set eyes, short palpebral fissures and small cheek bones
2. Reduced cranial circumference
3. Retarded growth
4. Mental retardation and behavioural abnormalities, often taking the form of hyperactivity and difficulty with social integration

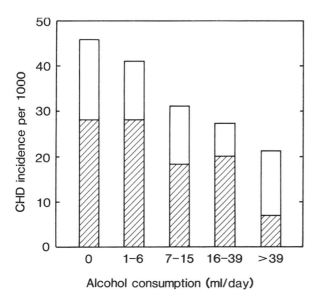

Fig. 35.3 Relationship between ethanol consumption and the incidence of coronary heart disease (CHD). Hatched bars show incidence of myocardial infarction, including coronary deaths. Open bars show incidence of angina pectoris and coronary insufficiency. The data were obtained from the male Japanese population in Hawaii. (From: Yano et al, 1977)

5. Other anatomical abnormalities, which may be major or minor (e.g. congenital cardiac abnormalities, malformation of the eyes and ears).

The overall incidence of FAS is estimated at 1–2 per 1000 live births. The incidence correlates strongly with maternal ethanol consumption during pregnancy, being about 19% in mothers who drink, on average, at least 4 drinks per day during pregnancy.

There is no clearly-defined threshold of ethanol consumption, below which the risk of FAS disappears (Streissguth et al, 1984). It is unknown whether FAS is associated with steady ethanol consumption, or with 'binge' drinking. It is also uncertain whether there is a critical period during pregnancy when ethanol consumption is likely to lead to FAS. One study (Hanson et al, 1978) suggests that FAS incidence correlates most strongly with ethanol consumption very early in pregnancy, even before pregnancy is recognized. If this is corroborated it means that not only pregnant women, but also women who are likely to become pregnant, must be advised not to drink.

The mechanism by which ethanol produces these effects is unknown. Both ethanol and its metabolite, acetaldehyde, inhibit cell division and migration in culture, so it is possible that the same mechanism operates *in vivo*. From experiments on rats and mice it is suggested that the effect on facial development may be produced very early in pregnancy (up to 4 weeks in man), while the effect on brain development is produced rather later (up to 10 weeks).

Tolerance and dependence

Tolerance to the effects of ethanol can be demonstrated in both man and experimental animals, to the extent of a 2–3-fold reduction in potency occurring over 1–3 weeks of chronic ethanol administration. A small component of this (up to about 30% decrease in potency) is due to pharmacokinetic tolerance resulting from more rapid elimination of ethanol. The major component is tissue tolerance, which accounts for a roughly 2-fold decrease in potency, and which can be observed *in vitro* (e.g. by measuring the inhibitory effect of ethanol on transmitter release from synaptosomes) as well as *in vivo*.

The mechanism of this tolerance is not known for certain (Littleton, 1984), but has been postulated to involve a change in the membrane lipid content (an increase in the cholesterol:phospholipid ratio), such that the lipid (in which ethanol causes an increase in fluidity similar to the effect of volatile anaesthetic drugs; see Chapter 20) becomes less fluid, and thus less susceptible to alteration of its properties by ethanol (Elingboe & Mendelson, 1981). A similar adaptive change in membrane lipid composition occurs in response to changes in body temperature in poikilothermic or hibernating animals. In support of this idea, it is known that ethanol tolerance is associated with tolerance to many anaesthetic agents, and alcoholics are often difficult to anaesthetize with drugs such as halothane. The process that triggers off the change is not known.

Studies on brain synaptosomes from ethanol-tolerant rats have demonstrated various changes (Littleton, 1984). The ability of ethanol to inhibit depolarization-induced Ca^{++} entry and transmitter release is reduced compared with normal. At the same time, transmitter release in response to a calcium ionophore is *increased*, suggesting that the release mechanism somehow adapts to the continuous presence of ethanol by requiring less Ca^{++} to enter the nerve terminal in order to evoke release.

In summary, chronic ethanol administration (a) produces changes in membrane lipids that cause the functioning of ionic channels to become less sensitive to ethanol; and (b) causes the transmitter release mechanism to operate at lower levels of Ca^{++} entry. The latter process may well be a factor in the production of the alcohol abstinence syndrome.

A well-defined physical abstinence syndrome develops in response to ethanol withdrawal. As with most other dependence-producing drugs, this is probably important as a short-term factor in sustaining the drug habit, but other (mainly psychological) factors are more important in the longer term. The physical abstinence syndrome usually subsides in a few days, but the craving for ethanol, and the tendency to relapse, last for very much longer.

The physical abstinence syndrome in man, in severe form, develops after about 8 hours. In the first stage the main symptom is severe tremor, and sometimes hallucinations, which last for about 24 hours. This phase may be followed by tonic-clonic convulsions, indistinguishable from grand mal epilepsy. Over the next few days, the condition of '*delirium tremens*' develops, in which the patient becomes confused and agitated, and may suffer much more severe hallucinations. Aggressive behaviour is common, and a variety of autonomic responses develop, including nausea and vomiting, sweating and fever. A similar syndrome of central and autonomic hyperactivity can be produced in experimental animals by terminating ethanol treatment. The most effective treatment in man is the use of benzodiazepines (see Chapter 21).

Pharmacokinetic aspects

Ethanol, being uncharged and highly lipid soluble, is rapidly absorbed, an appreciable amount being absorbed from the stomach. A substantial fraction is removed from the portal vein blood by first-pass hepatic metabolism. Because the rate of hepatic metabolism of ethanol shows the property of saturation at quite low ethanol concentrations, the frac-tion of ethanol removed is greatest when the concentration is low, and decreases as the concentration increases. Thus, if ethanol absorption is rapid, so that the concentration in the portal vein is high, most of the ethanol escapes into the systemic circulation, whereas with slow absorption, more is removed by first-pass metabolism. This is one reason why drinking ethanol on an empty stomach produces a much greater pharmacological effect. Ethanol is quickly distributed throughout the body water, the rate of its redistribution depending mainly on the blood flow to individual tissues, as with volatile anaesthetics (see Chapter 20).

Ethanol is about 90% metabolized in the body, 5–10% being excreted unchanged in expired air and in urine. This fraction is not pharmacokinetically significant, but provides the basis for estimating blood ethanol concentration from measurements on breath or urine. The ratio of ethanol concentrations in blood and alveolar air is taken to be 2100:1 (i.e. 1 ml of blood contains as much ethanol as 2.1 litres of alveolar air). The concentration in urine is more variable and provides a less good measure of blood concentration.

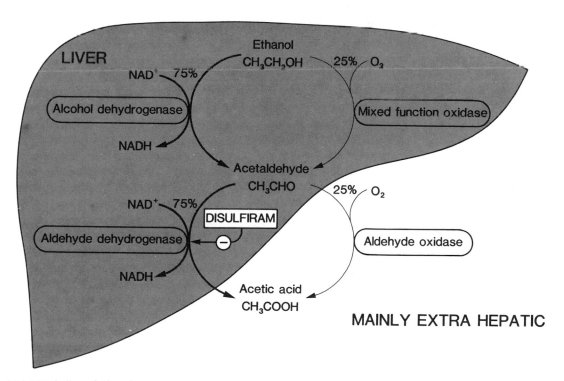

Fig. 35.4 Metabolism of ethanol.

Ethanol metabolism occurs almost entirely in the liver, and mainly by a pathway involving successive oxidations, first to acetaldehyde and then to acetic acid. Since ethanol is often consumed in large quantities (compared with most drugs), 1–2 moles daily being by no means unusual, it constitutes a substantial load on the hepatic oxidative systems. As Goldstein (1983) points out, the oxidation of 2 moles of ethanol consumes about 1.5 kg of the co-factor NAD^+. This means that ethanol oxidation can only proceed at a limited rate, irrespective of the concentration that is presented to the liver (i.e. it shows zero-order, or saturating, kinetics; see Chapter 3). It also means that competition occurs between the ethanol and other metabolic substrates for the available NAD^+ supplies, which may be a factor in ethanol-induced liver damage (see Chapter 36). The intermediate metabolite, acetaldehyde, is a reactive and toxic compound and this may also contribute to the hepatotoxicity.

Alcohol dehydrogenase is a soluble cytoplasmic enzyme confined mainly to liver cells, which oxidizes ethanol at the same time as reducing NAD^+ to NADH (Fig. 35.4). It has a relatively low affinity for ethanol (apparent $K_m \sim 1.6$ mM), and the plasma ethanol concentration after even a small intake of ethanol is such that the enzyme is fully saturated and ethanol elimination takes place at a rate that is virtually independent of the plasma concentration (Fig. 35.5) corresponding in man to about 2 mmol/kg body weight/hour, or about 10 ml/hour in a normal subject. This rate is actually limited by NAD^+ availability rather than by substrate saturation. Ethanol metabolism causes the ratio of NAD^+:NADH to fall, and this has other metabolic consequences (e.g. increased lactate, and slowing down of the Krebs cycle). The limitation on ethanol metabolism imposed by the limited rate of NAD^+ regeneration has led to attempts to find a 'sobering-up' agent that works by regenerating NAD^+ from NADH. One such agent is **fructose**, which is reduced by an NADH-requiring system. In large doses it causes a small, but measurable, increase in the rate of ethanol metabolism, but the effect is not large enough to cause a significant increase in the rate of return to sobriety.

Some ethanol (about 25%) is metabolized by the microsomal mixed function oxidase system (see Chapter 3). This may be responsible for some

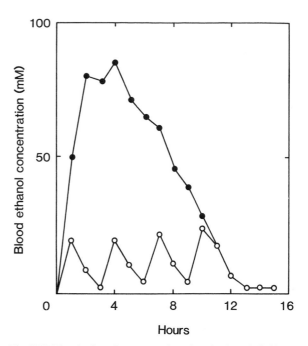

Fig. 35.5 Blood ethanol concentration after single and divided doses. Data were obtained in rats given oral doses of ethanol. A single dose (104 mmol/kg) produces a much higher and more sustained blood concentration than four divided doses. Note that the rate of decline of the blood concentration is approximately the same after a large or small dose, because of the saturation phenomenon. (From: Kalant et al, 1975)

reported drug interactions involving ethanol. Ethanol often seems to produce a dual effect on the metabolism of the many other drugs that are metabolized by the mixed function oxidase system (e.g. phenobarbitone, warfarin, steroids), with an initial inhibitory effect produced by competition, followed by enhancement of the rate of drug metabolism due to enzyme induction.

Nearly all of the acetaldehyde produced is converted to acetate in the liver, by **aldehyde dehydrogenase** (see Fig. 35.4). Normally, only a little acetaldehyde escapes from the liver, giving a blood acetaldehyde concentration of 20–50 µM after an intoxicating dose of ethanol in man. This circulating acetaldehyde is oxidized by a non-specific and widely distributed oxidase. It usually has little or no effect, but the concentration may become much larger under certain circumstances, and produce toxic effects. This occurs if aldehyde dehydrogenase is inhibited by drugs such as **disulfiram**. In the presence of disulfiram, which produces no marked effect when given alone, ethanol consumption is followed by a severe and distressing reaction comprising flushing, tachycardia, hyperventilation and nausea, which is due to excessive acetaldehyde accumulation in the bloodstream. This reaction is extremely unpleasant, but not dangerous, and disulfiram can be used as aversion therapy to discourage people from taking ethanol. Some other drugs, notably oral hypoglycaemic agents of the sulphonylurea class (e.g. chlorpropamide; see Chapter 17) and certain antibacterial drugs (e.g. nitrofurantoin; see Chapter 30), also occasionally produce similar reactions to ethanol.

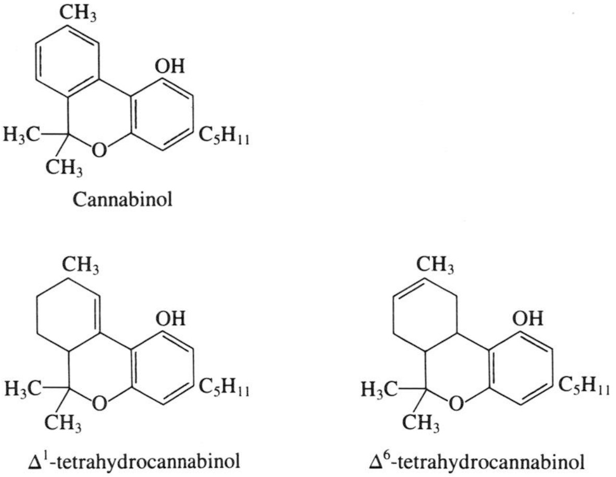

Methanol is metabolized in the same way as ethanol, but produces formaldehyde instead of acetaldehyde from the first oxidation step. Formaldehyde is more reactive than acetaldehyde, and reacts rapidly with proteins, causing the inactivation of enzymes involved in the tricarboxylic acid cycle. It is converted to another toxic metabolite, formic acid. This, unlike acetic acid, cannot be utilized in the tricarboxylic acid cycle, and is liable to cause tissue damage. Conversion of alcohols to aldehydes occurs not only in the liver, but also in the retina, where the dehydrogenase responsible for the retinol/retinal conversion also oxidizes exogenous alcohols. Formation of formaldehyde in the retina accounts for one of the main toxic effects of methanol, namely blindness, which can occur after ingestion of as little as 10 g. The other main toxic effect is damage to peripheral nerves (neuropathy), causing weakness and sensory loss. Formic acid production, and derangement of the tricarboxylic acid cycle, also produce severe acidosis.

Methanol is used as an industrial solvent, and is also used to adulterate industrial ethanol in order to make it unfit to drink. Methanol poisoning is nonetheless quite common. The effects of chronic methanol consumption are irreversible, but acute poisoning may be treated by administration of large doses of ethanol, which acts to retard methanol metabolism by competition for alcohol dehydrogenase.

CANNABIS

Extracts of the hemp plant, *Cannabis sativa*, which grows freely in temperate and tropical regions, contain the active substance Δ^1-**tetrahydrocan-**

Fig. 35.6 Structure of cannabinoids.

nabinol (**THC**; Fig. 35.6). **Marijuana** is the name given to the dried leaves and flower heads, prepared as a smoking mixture, while **hashish** is the extracted resin. These substances have been used for various medicinal purposes, and as intoxicant preparations, for centuries. Marijuana was brought to North America by immigrants, mainly in the 19th century and began to be regarded as a social problem in the early years of this century, becoming legally banned during the 1930s. Its use increased dramatically in the 1960s and recent figures suggest that about 15% of the adult population in America and Western Europe have taken cannabis at some time, with a much higher proportion, close to 50%, among teenagers and young adults.

Chemical aspects

Cannabis extracts contain numerous related compounds, called **cannabinoids**, most of which are insoluble in water. The most abundant cannabinoids are Δ^1-**THC** (which is often called Δ^9-THC, according to a different ring-numbering system); Δ^6-**THC**, which is more weakly active than Δ^1-THC; and **cannabinol**, which is formed by spontaneous decomposition of Δ^1-THC. Δ^1-THC is the most important from a biological point of view, and constitutes roughly 1–10% by weight of marijuana and hashish preparations. Various radio-immunoassays have been developed for cannabinoids, but they lack sufficient chemical specificity to be able to distinguish Δ^1-THC from the numerous other cannabinoids found in crude extracts, and from the various metabolites that are formed *in vivo*, so the assay of pharmacologically active Δ^1-THC in biological fluids still presents a problem.

Pharmacological effects

The actions of Δ^1-THC cannot be categorized simply in terms of stimulant or depressant activity on the central nervous system, but can best be described as a mixture of mild psychotomimetic actions and sedative actions, together with various peripheral autonomic effects (see reviews: Harris et al, 1977; Coper, 1981).

The main subjective effects in man consists of (a) a feeling of relaxation and well-being, not unlike that produced by alcohol; and (b) a feeling of sharpened sensory awareness, with sounds and sights seeming more intense and fantastic, these effects being similar to, but usually less pronounced than, those produced by psychotomimetic drugs such as LSD. Subjects report that time passes extremely slowly. The alarming sensations and paranoid delusions that often occur with LSD are seldom experienced after cannabis. Cannabis also increases appetite, an effect seen in experimental animals as well as human subjects. Objective tests of psychomotor performance show general impairment after cannabis. This includes simple learning and memory tasks, as well as more complex tests of motor coordination, such as driving. The subjective feelings of confidence and heightened creativity are not reflected in actual performance. Aggressive behaviour is not enhanced after cannabis, nor is sexual activity, contrary to popular belief. Other effects that have been demonstrated include analgesia (which is demonstrable in hot-plate tests on experimental animals but is not clear-cut in man) and a state of catalepsy (the adoption of a fixed immobile posture) which occurs in rats and mice.

The main peripheral effects of cannabis are: (a) tachycardia, which can be prevented by drugs that block sympathetic transmission; (b) vasodilatation, which is particularly marked on the scleral and conjunctival vessels, producing a characteristic blood-shot appearance; (c) reduction of intraocular pressure; (d) inhibition of nausea and vomiting; and (e) bronchodilatation.

The mechanism of action of cannabinoids at a cellular level are not at all well understood. They have some characteristics in common with lipid-soluble anaesthetic substances, but this cannot account for many of their central and peripheral actions. Furthermore, even in large doses, cannabis does not produce a state of profound CNS depression, as would occur with a conventional anaesthetic agent.

The effects of cannabis on intraocular pressure, bronchial smooth muscle and the vomiting reflex are of potential therapeutic value, but have not so far been exploited, partly because of the legal difficulties, and partly because the extremely low water solubility of cannabinoids makes it difficult to produce a satisfactory formulation for oral use.

Tolerance to cannabis occurs only to a minor degree and physical dependence has not been clearly demonstrated, though it appears that habitual cannabis users experience feelings of anxiety, depression and irritability when the drug is suddenly withdrawn.

Pharmacokinetic aspects

The effect of cannabis, taken by smoking or by intravenous injection, takes about 1 hour to develop fully, and lasts for several hours. Cannabinoids bind strongly to plasma protein and most of the drug remains in the plasma for this reason. If radioactive Δ^1-THC is given, the half-life of radioactivity in the plasma is very long (2–3 days), but conversion to inactive metabolites means that the pharmacological effect is much briefer. Most of the radioactivity is excreted in the faeces, and only about 25% appears in the urine. The products that are excreted are mainly conjugates formed after hydroxylation of the five-carbon side chain, and there appears to be a considerable enterohepatic circulation, involving biliary excretion of the conjugate followed by hydrolysis and reabsorption in the intestine.

Adverse effects

Δ^1-THC has been shown to produce a teratogenic and mutagenic effect in rodents, and an increased incidence of chromosome breaks in circulating white cells has been reported in humans. Such breaks are, however, by no means unique to cannabis, and epidemiological studies have not shown any increased risk of fetal malformation or cancer among cannabis users.

Certain endocrine effects occur in man, notably a decrease in plasma testosterone, and a reduction of sperm count. One study (Kolodny et al, 1974) showed a reduction of more than 50% in both plasma testosterone and sperm count in subjects smoking 10 or more marijuana cigarettes per week.

It is very difficult to assess the evidence that cannabis causes long-term psychological changes. It has been suggested that it can cause schizo-phrenia, and that it leads to a gradually developing state of apathy and under-achievement.

The long-running argument over the legalization of cannabis centres mainly on the seriousness of these adverse effects. Opponents of legalization argue that it would be folly to change the law in favour of the use by the public at large of a substance which could turn out to have serious toxic effects. Proponents of a change argue that the present law is clearly ineffective and encourages crime, and that cannabis is undoubtedly safer than either alcohol or tobacco.

REFERENCES AND FURTHER READING

Ashton H, Stepney R 1982 Smoking. Psychology and pharmacology. Tavistock, London

Belfrage P, Berg B, Hagerstrand I, Nilsson-Ehle P, Tornqvist H, Wiebe T 1977 Alterations of lipid metabolism in healthy volunteers during long-term ethanol intake. Eur J Clin Invest 7: 127–131

Bowman W C, Rand M J 1980 Textbook of Pharmacology. Blackwell, Oxford, ch 42

Brown M S, Kovanen P T, Goldstein J L 1981 Regulation of plasma cholesterol by lipoprotein receptors. Science 212: 628–635

Ciba Foundation Symposium 1984 Mechanisms of alcohol damage in utero. Pitman, London

Clarren S K, Smith D W 1978 The fetal alcohol syndrome. New Eng J Med 298: 1063–1067

Coper H 1981 Pharmacology and toxicology of cannabis. In: Hoffmeister F, Stille G (eds) Psychotropic agents, Part III. Handbook of Experimental Pharmacology 55 (iii): 135–160

Elingboe J, Mendelson J H (1981) Biochemical pharmacology of ethanol. In: Hofmeister F, Stille G (eds) Psychotropic agents. Handbook of Experimental Pharmacology 55 (iii): 209–238

Eysenck H J, Eaves L J 1980 The causes and effects of smoking. Maurice Temple Smith, London

Fenn C G, Littleton J M 1984 Interactions between ethanol and dietary fat in determining human platelet function. Thrombosis and Haemostasis 51: 50–53

Gilman A G, Goodman L S, Rall T W, Murad F 1985 The pharmacological basis of therapeutics. Macmillan, New York, ch 23

Goldstein D B 1983 Pharmacology of alcohol. Oxford University Press, New York

Griffiths R R, Henningfield J E 1982 Pharmacology of cigarette smoking behaviour. Trends in Pharmacological Sciences 3: 260–263

Hanson J W, Streissguth A P, Smith D W 1978 The effects of moderate alcohol consumption during pregnancy of fetal growth and morphogenesis. J Paediatrics 92: 457–460

Harris L S, Dewey W L, Razdan R K 1977 Cannabis: its chemistry, pharmacology and toxicology. In: Martin W R (ed) Drug addiction Part II. Handbook of Experimental Pharmacology 45 (ii): 331–430

Hofmann F 1983 A handbook on drug and alcohol abuse. Oxford University Press, New York

Horak J K, Brandon T A, Ribeiro L G T, Ware J A, Miller R R, Solis R T 1982 Effects of ethanol and haemolysis on in vivo and in vitro platelet aggregation. J Cardiovasc Pharmacol 4: 1037–1041

Jarvis M J, Raw M, Russell M A H, Feyerabend C 1982 Randomized controlled trial of nicotine chewing-gum. Br Med J 285: 537–540

Kolodny R C, Masters W H, Kolodner R M, Toro G 1974 Depression of plasma testosterone levels after chronic intensive marijuana use. New Eng J Med 290: 872–874

Littleton J M 1984 Biochemical pharmacology of ethanol tolerance and dependence. In: Pharmacological treatments for alcoholism. Edwards G, Littleton J M (eds). Croom-Helm, London

Martin W R (ed) 1977 Drug addiction. Handbook of Experimental Pharmacology, 45

Royal College of Physicians Report 1977 Smoking or Health. Pitman, London

Streissguth A P, Landesman-Dwyer S, Martin J C, Smith D W 1980 Teratogenic effects of alcohol in humans and laboratory animals. Science 209: 353–361

Streissguth A P, Barr H M, Martin D C 1984 Alcohol exposure in utero and functional deficits in children during the first four years of life. Ciba Foundation Symposium on Mechanisms of Alcohol Damage in utero. Pitman, New York

US Department of Health & Human Services Reports 1981, 1982, 1983 The health consequences of smoking. US Government Publication, Washington

36

Harmful effects of drugs

TYPES OF DRUG TOXICITY

All drugs are capable of producing harmful as well as beneficial effects. The nature of these harmful effects falls into two mechanistic categories*:

1. Effects related to the principal pharmacological action of the drug.
2. Effects unrelated to the principal pharmacological action of the drug.

It is also important to categorize harmful effects in terms of their severity, and to distinguish between those that cause a temporary inconvenience or discomfort, and those that can lead to permanent disability or even death.

Many of the unwanted effects in the first category are readily predictable from knowledge of the mode of action of the drug, and have been discussed in previous chapters. For example, postural hypotension occurs with some antihypertensive drugs, bleeding with anticoagulants, bronchoconstriction with β-adrenoceptor blocking drugs, cardiac dys-rhythmias with glycosides or tricyclic antidepressants; these effects are closely associated with the pharmacodynamic action for which the drug is being used. There are also examples in which the unwanted effect appears at first sight to be unrelated to the basic pharmacological action of the drug (e.g. drowsiness with antihistamines, gastric bleeding with aspirin-like drugs), but the strong association of particular unwanted effects with particular types of drug makes it very likely that closely related mechanisms are involved in producing both the desired and the unwanted effects. In most cases, these unwanted effects are reversible, and the problem can often be coped with by reducing the dose or changing to a different drug. Sometimes, however, such effects are not easily reversible, for example in the case of tardive dyskinesia produced by neuroleptic drugs (see Chapter 22) or the syndrome of drug dependence produced by opiate analgesics, alcohol, nicotine and many other drugs.

In contrast to this category, where the unwanted effect represents an extension of the underlying pharmacological action of the drug, the second category of adverse reactions arises by an unrelated biochemical mechanism, often involving a chemically reactive metabolite of the drug rather than the parent compound. Effects of this kind are often much more serious than unwanted effects in the first category, and include such reactions as liver or kidney damage, bone marrow suppression, carcinogenesis and disordered fetal development. Such effects are by no means confined to drugs, but are liable to occur with any kind of chemical, and conventionally fall into the area of toxicology rather than pharmacology.

Because of the importance of chemically reactive metabolites which cause cellular damage in the

---

* An alternative classification was proposed by Rawlins & Thompson (1981), who divide adverse effects into **Type A** and **Type B**. Type A reactions result from an excessive, though qualitatively normal pharmacodynamic effect of the drug, and occur in any subject given a sufficiently large dose. Type B reactions (also known as **idiosyncratic reactions**) are aberrant effects unrelated to the normal action of the drug, which occur unpredictably in a small proportion of subjects. This seems an unsatisfactory classification, since there are many examples of toxicity which is unrelated to the major pharmacodynamic effect of the drug (e.g. paracetamol hepatotoxicity, aspirin-induced tinnitus, streptomycin-induced ototoxicity, thalidomide teratogenesis), but which still occur predictably when the drug is given in too large a dose. It is preferable to classify adverse reactions on the basis of mechanism rather than pattern of incidence.

production of this type of toxic reaction, there tends to be a wide variation in the susceptibility of different individuals. Thus, any genetic or external influence on drug metabolism is likely to affect the probability of a toxic reaction occurring. This means that the relationship between dose and toxicity can be highly variable, to the extent that some individuals may develop a fatal reaction after a small dose of the drug, whereas others show no toxicity even after much larger doses. There are also wide interspecies variations in the incidence and pattern of toxic reactions, so that toxicity testing in animals may give little guidance to hazards in man.

In this chapter some important types of harmful drug effects belonging to the second (toxicological), rather than the first (pharmacodynamic), category are discussed, effects of the former type being mentioned in appropriate chapters on systemic pharmacology earlier in the book.

The types of toxic effect discussed in this chapter are:

1. Hepatotoxicity
2. Mutagenesis and carcinogenesis
3. Teratogenesis
4. Allergic reactions to drugs.

For fuller accounts of these and other types of drug toxicity see Loomis (1978), Gorrod (1981), Timbrell (1982), Davies (1981) and Hathway (1984). The first three categories on this list have a good deal in common, for they all involve biochemical damage to cellular constituents (proteins, membrane lipids or DNA) resulting principally from covalent reactions with metabolic products of the parent compound. If the affected biological molecules are lipid or protein the effect is often to change the metabolism of the cell, or to kill it; if the target is DNA, the result may be carcinogenesis, mutagenesis or teratogenesis. Some examples of drugs which cause these effects are given in Table 36.1.

HEPATOTOXICITY

Various drugs are able to produce liver damage of essentially the same pattern, consisting initially of

Table 36.1 Examples of toxic metabolites

Starting compound			Reactive metabolite	
CCl_4	Carbon tetrachloride	$\longrightarrow$	$CCl_3^{\cdot}$	Trichloromethyl radical
HO—⬡—NHCOCH$_3$	Paracetamol	$\longrightarrow$	HO—⬡—N(OH)COCH$_3$	Hydroxylamine derivative
⬡N—CONH·NH$_2$	Isoniazid			
⬡N—CONH·NHCOCH$_3$	Acetyl-isoniazid	$\longrightarrow$	NH$_2$NHCOCH$_3$	Acetylhydrazine
(CH$_3$)$_2$N—N=O	Dimethyl nitrosamine	$\longrightarrow$	CH$_3$NHN=O	Monomethyl nitrosamine
Benzpyrene structure	Benzpyrene	$\longrightarrow$	Benzpyrene-diolepoxide structure	Benzpyrene-diolepoxide

centri-lobular necrosis, in which the hepatocytes bordering on the bile canaliculi are killed. This is followed by **fatty degeneration** and eventually **hepatic cirrhosis**, with which is associated a high incidence of hepatic carcinoma. These effects are caused by various clinically used drugs (e.g. paracetamol, isoniazid, iproniazid, halothane) and also by many other substances which may be present in the environment (e.g. carbon tetrachloride, benzene derivatives such as bromobenzene and toluene, nitrosamines and aflatoxins). Ethanol also has similar effects. Hepatotoxicity of a rather different kind occurs with chlorpromazine (see Chapter 22), and a number of other drugs (e.g. androgens, sulphonamides) which produce a reversible obstructive jaundice; this is apparently due to precipitation of bile salts in the biliary canaliculi as a complex with the drug, which is present in the bile in high concentration.

Many of the drugs that cause hepatic necrosis are believed to do so by forming highly reactive free radicals, or other unstable intermediaries, in the process of metabolic degradation within the liver cells. This has been investigated in considerable detail for **carbon tetrachloride** (Rechnagel & Glende, 1973). This substance, which is highly lipid soluble and therefore widely distributed in the body, produces toxic effects that are largely con-fined to the liver. In common with many other hepatotoxic agents, its toxicity is increased by agents (e.g. phenobarbitone) which induce microsomal drug metabolizing enzymes (see Chapter 4) and reduced by inhibitors of these enzymes. The sequence of events is shown in Figure 36.1. The microsomal mixed function oxidase system withdraws an electron from carbon tetrachloride leaving the reactive trichloromethyl radical CCl_3'. This free radical has a lifetime of only about $100\,\mu\text{sec}$, and so has time to diffuse for only a short distance within the liver cell before undergoing secondary reactions. These secondary reactions, which are responsible for the biochemical damage, may be of various kinds (Fig. 36.1): (a) oxidation of thiols to disulphide bonds; (b) saturation of double bonds in lipids, proteins or nucleotides, resulting in covalent attachment of the free radical group at those sites; and (c) lipid peroxidation reactions, in which polyunsaturated membrane lipids are converted to peroxide derivatives, and eventually to aldehydes and other products, leading to a further cascade of reactions that result in irreversible membrane damage (Fig. 36.1.).

Another important example is **paracetamol** (see Chapter 9), a drug which causes no hepatotoxicity in normal clinical doses, but is fatal in overdose. It is oxidized by the P450 system to a reactive quin-

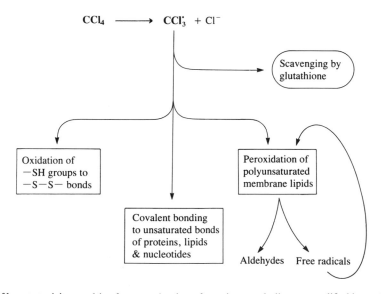

Fig. 36.1 Mechanism of hepatotoxicity resulting from production of reactive metabolites, exemplified by carbon tetrachloride.

one, which is removed by reaction with glutathione. If the dose of paracetamol is large, or glutathione is deficient, the quinone binds covalently to proteins of the hepatocytes, causing irreversible cellular damage. Administration of sulphydryl compounds, such as N-acetyl-cysteamine, which replenish hepatic glutathione, gives useful protection against paracetamol toxicity.

Many of the agents that cause hepatoxicity are also liable to damage the kidney, most commonly by producing necrosis of renal tubular cells. Because of the high concentration of solutes in the renal papilla, this region is preferentially affected, producing the syndrome known as acute papillary necrosis. The mechanisms involved seem to be generally similar to those operating in the liver, with metabolism to a reactive intermediate, which causes membrane and enzymic effects that are damaging to the cells. Among drugs in common use, **phenacetin** is the most important compound that causes renal toxicity, though non-steroidal anti-inflammatory drugs (see Chapter 9) have also been implicated. **Cyclosporin**, used to prevent transplant rejection (see Chapter 29) can also cause renal damage. In routine toxicity testing of potential new drugs on experimental animals, the occurrence of renal and/or hepatic damage is a very common reason for abandoning a compound.

As well as causing biochemical damage to macromolecules by reacting with them directly, reactive metabolic intermediates can cause indirect immunologically mediated toxic effects. This occurs when the intermediate forms a complex with a soluble protein, which is thereby rendered antigenic, producing various types of hypersensitivity or autoimmune response. Reactions of this kind sometimes affect the liver. This is believed to account for the occasional hepatotoxicity that occurs when halothane is administered repeatedly (see Chapter 20).

MUTAGENESIS AND CARCINOGENICITY

Mutation occurs through a change in the genotype of a cell which is passed on when the cell divides. It occurs when the structure of the DNA is changed by a covalent modification. Mutations occur in the absence of any external predisposing factor, but the probability of mutation is greatly increased by ionizing radiation or by various kinds of chemical. Changing a single base in DNA may produce effects on the cell ranging from none at all to rapid death, depending on whether the gene sequence affected is undergoing transcription and translation, and if so, whether the resulting change in the peptide sequence for which it codes is functionally important or trivial. Certain kinds of mutation result in carcinogenesis because, it is generally assumed, the affected protein is somehow involved in growth regulation. The current view is that cancer arises when the function of 'proto-oncogenes' (which are probably normal growth-regulator genes) is altered by mutation. This can result in the expression of a protein that is not normally formed by the cell or of a modified version of a normally expressed protein (see Chapter 29). It usually requires more than one such mutation in a cell to produce malignancy. It may at first sight seem vanishingly improbable that random changes among the thousands of base pairs in a DNA strand will hit on the right combination to alter a particular proto-oncogene without irreparably damaging the genome. Since it has to occur in only one of millions of cells, however, to produce a tumour, the probability is much higher than it appears. The nature of these oncogene products which transform cells from a normal to a malignant growth pattern is currently under very energetic study. Some oncogenes have been found to code for growth factors or growth factor receptors or for elements of the intracellular transduction mechanism by which growth factors regulate cell proliferation (see Chapter 29). Growth factors are polypeptide mediators, many of which are structurally related to insulin, which stimulate division of certain types of cell; examples are **epidermal growth factor** (EGF) and **platelet derived growth factor** (PDGF). The receptors for these growth factors have protein kinase activity and they catalyse the phosphorylation of various target proteins, and thus regulate a number of cellular processes. Other oncogenes code for kinases that are involved in the formation of polyphosphoinositides (Berridge & Irvine, 1984). Though there are many details to be filled in, and doubtless many more oncogenes than have yet been identified, the complex connection between the introduction of a mutagenic chemical and the development of a cancer is now beginning to be understood.

Biochemical mechanisms of mutagenesis

The translation of genetic information built into DNA involves the recognition of patterns of triplets of base pairs. Each 3-base sequence either codes for a particular amino-acid or serves as a stop-start signal. The base pairs in double-stranded DNA each consist of a purine-pyrimidine pair, either adenine-thymine (A-T) or guanine-cytosine (G-C) and it is by chemical modification of these bases, particularly guanine, that most chemical carcinogens act. There are two sites on the guanine molecule to which groups can easily be covalently attached in the presence of reactive metabolites of chemical carcinogens namely the O^6 and N^7 positions (Fig. 29.3). Substitution at the O^6 position of guanine is the most likely to produce a permanent mutagenic effect, since N^7 substitutions are usually quickly repaired by cellular mechanisms involving excision and replacement of the altered base. Substitution at O^6 is more likely to produce a stable misreading of the code which is perpetuated when the DNA is replicated. It is important to realise that spontaneous chemical reactions involving the genetic material occur all the time (e.g. deamination reactions) but are prevented from irretrievably corrupting the genome by the existence of different types of DNA repair mechanism. Crucial to this stability is the fact that DNA exists as a double strand, so that each strand can serve as a template for rebuilding the other if either is damaged.

The accessibility of bases in DNA to chemical attack is greatest when the DNA is in the process of replication (i.e. during cell division), so most mutagens act preferentially on rapidly dividing cell populations. This is important in relation to mutagenesis of germ cells, particularly in the female, because in humans the production of primary oocytes occurs early in embryogenesis by a rapid succession of mitotic divisions. Each of these primary oocytes then undergoes only two further divisions at the time of ovulation. It is thus during early pregnancy that female germ cells in the embryo are most likely to undergo mutagenesis; this will not affect the developing embryo itself but is likely to become manifest in successive generations. In the male, germ cell divisions occur throughout life, and sensitivity to mutagens is continuously present. It must be stressed that some mutagens (e.g. ionizing radiations) can affect DNA whether or not it is replicating, so that even the female germ cells are sensitive throughout reproductive life. Chemical mutagens are only one of many types of agent responsible for germ cell mutation, and its effects range from infertility, if the mutation is incompatible with life, to effects that actually confer a biological advantage. Between these extremes lie many forms of inherited disease.

The dependence of genetic damage by many mutagens on the frequency of cell division means that, in general, the developing fetus is particularly susceptible. It is for this reason that many mutagens and carcinogens are also teratogenic (see later section).

The importance of drugs, as opposed to other chemicals, such as pollutants and food additives, as a causative factor in mutagenesis has not been established, and such epidemiological evidence as exists does not suggest that they are of major significance in causing cancer.

Even if chemical modification of a base does persist in the form of a mutation, this may have no discernible effect on the organism. Thus, it may be on a part of the genome that is not expressed, or it may cause a single amino-acid substitution in a region of a protein molecule that has no effect on the function of the protein. It may, on the other hand, have a drastic effect by affecting an enzyme or other functional protein in a major way (e.g. in the thalassaemic or sickle cell traits, which lead to the production of abnormal haemoglobins and result in serious illness).

Types of carcinogenesis

Not all carcinogens act directly on DNA. Various substances act at a later stage to increase the likelihood that mutagenesis will result in the production of a tumour (Fig. 36.2). According to one recent classification (Weisburger & Williams, 1984) carcinogens can be divided into:

1. Genotoxic carcinogens (i.e. mutagens, as discussed above), which can be further divided into:

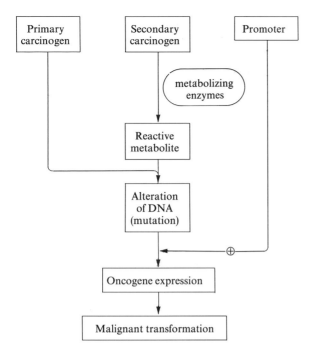

Fig. 36.2 Sequence of events in mutagenesis and carcinogenesis.

   a. Primary carcinogens, which attract DNA directly.
   b. Secondary carcinogens, which must be converted to a reactive metabolite before they affect the DNA. They are more numerous and important than primary carcinogens.
2. Epigenetic carcinogens (i.e. agents that do not themselves cause genetic damage, but increase the likelihood that such damage will cause cancer).

There are several different types of epigenetic carcinogen, the most important being:

   a. Co-carcinogens (substances which are not carcinogenic by themselves but enhance the effect of genotoxic agents when given simultaneously; examples are **phorbol esters**, various aromatic and aliphatic hydrocarbons, etc).
   b. Promotors (substances which are not carcinogenic by themselves, but increase the likelihood of tumour development from genetically damaged cells; they can thus produce cancers when given *after* the genotoxic agent). Examples include phorbol esters, bile acids, saccharin, etc).
   c. Hormones. Tumours may be hormone-dependent (see Chapter 29), the most im-

portant example being oestrogen-dependent breast cancers and androgen-dependent prostatic cancers. In humans, endometrial hyperplasia induced by excessive oestrogen can give rise to cancer. This is probably due to a change in the DNA which is given expression when the cells proliferate.

Measurement of mutagenicity and carcinogenicity

Mutagenesis by drugs and other chemicals to which human beings are exposed is a matter of great public concern because of the serious long-term consequences that it may produce—particularly cancer and teratogenesis. A great deal of effort has therefore gone into developing test procedures for detecting mutagenicity and carcinogenicity.

   Available test procedures can be broadly divided into:

1. *In vitro* tests for mutagenicity and tendency to induce malignant transformation. These tests are generally quite quick, and suitable for screening a large number of compounds, but they have a tendency to give positive results on compounds which are not subsequently shown to be carcinogenic in tests on whole animals.
2. Whole animal tests for carcinogenicity and teratogenesis. Such tests are expensive and time-consuming, but are required by most drug regulatory authorities to be carried out before a new drug can be registered for use in man. The main limitation of this kind of study is that there are important species differences, mainly to do with the metabolism of the foreign compound and the formation of reactive products.
3. Epidemiological studies in man.

In vitro tests for carcinogenicity

Bacteria have great advantages as a test system for measuring mutagenicity, because of their high replication rate. One of the most widely used is the **Ames test**, which measures the rate of back-mutation (i.e. reversion from mutant to wild-type form) in a culture of *Salmonella typhimurium*. The normal wild-type strain grows in a medium containing no added amino-acids because it can synthesize all amino-acids from carbon and nitrogen sources. A common mutant occurs which requires added histidine. The tests involves growing a culture of the mutant form in a medium containing a small amount of histidine. After several divisions, the histidine becomes depleted, and the only cells which continue dividing are those which have back-mutated to the wild-type. A count of the surviving colonies after 2–3 days gives a measure of the mutation rate. Most drugs and chemicals tested on their own as primary carcinogens give a negative result, but the test becomes highly sensitive when a microsomal preparation of liver cells is incorporated so that metabolic degradation of the test substance occurs, enabling secondary carcinogens to be detected. Some of the many variants of the Ames test are described by Venitt (1981) and Styles (1981).

Other *in vitro* mutogenicity tests (Styles, 1981) include measurement of chromosomal damage in cells in culture, measurement of the rate of mutation or neoplastic transformation in mammalian cell cultures, and measurement of changes in the physical characteristics of DNA, indicative of breakage or cross-linking of DNA strands.

In vivo tests for carcinogenicity

In vivo tests for carcinogenicity range from measurements of chromosomal abnormalities in lymphocytes, bone marrow cells or germ cells removed from animals to which the drug has been adminstered, to detection of tumours in groups of test animals. These latter tests are very slow, since there is usually a latency of months or years before tumours develop. Some of these tests are discussed further by Brusick (1983).

It is important to realize that none of the tests for mutagenicity so far described can detect epigenetic carcinogenesis. To do this it is generally necessary to use an assay system that measures a proliferative cellular response rather than effects on DNA, and to combine the test substance with a known genotoxic carcinogen. Such tests are being developed but have not yet become routinely applicable in toxicity testing.

The number of drugs known to be associated with increased cancer risk in man is small (Table 36.2), the most important group being those that are known to act on DNA, i.e. cytotoxic and immunosuppressant drugs, and which are rarely used except in life-threatening situations.

TERATOGENESIS

This term is usually used to mean the production of gross structural malformations during fetal development, to distinguish it from other kinds of drug-induced fetal damage such as the fetal alcohol syndrome (see Chapter 35), impairment of fetal development by nicotine (Chapter 35), impaired bone development by tetracyclines (Chapter 30) or the effects of antithyroid drugs (Chapter 16).

It has been known that external agents can affect

Table 36.2 Examples of drug toxicity

	Hepatotoxicity	Carcinogenesis/mutagenesis	Teratogenesis
Drugs	Paracetamol Hydrazines (e.g. iproniazid) Indomethacin Halothane Trichloroethylene Tetracycline Phenylbutazone	Cytotoxic drugs and immunosuppressants (e.g. methotrexate) Oestrogens Pyrimethanine Tetracycline Phenylbutazone	Cytotoxic drugs and immunosuppressants (e.g. methotrexate) Androgens Oestrogens Thalidomide Cortisone (not in man) ? Phenytoin ? Warfarin ? Anaesthetics ? Antiemetic phenothiazines
Poisons	Aromatic hydrocarbons (e.g. benzpyrene) Carbon tetrachloride Aflatoxin Nitrosamines	Aromatic hydrocarbons Carbon tetrachloride Aflatoxin Nitrosamines	Heavy metals (Pb, Cd, Hg)

Table 36.3 Adverse effects of drugs on human foetal development

Agent	Effects in man
Definite	
Cytotoxic drugs (esp folate antagonists)	Hydrocephalus, cleft palate. Neural tube defects. Rib and limb defects.
Steroid hormones (oestrogens, progestogens, androgens)	Masculinization of female. Testicular atrophy and reduced sperm count in male.
Heavy metals (esp mercury)	Impaired brain development. Neural tube defects.
Anticonvulsant drugs	
Phenytoin	Cleft lip/palate microcephaly mental retardation.
Trimethadione	Facial abnormalities, high-arched palate. Delayed growth.
Ethanol	Facial abnormalities, mental retardation, cardiac defects (see Chapter 35).
Thalidomide	Phocomelia, gut atresia, cardiac defects.
Tetracycline	Staining of bones and teeth. Thin tooth enamel and impaired bone growth.
Antithyroid drugs	Hypothyroidism, goitre.
Coumarin anticoagulants	Various effects including retarded growth and defects of limbs, eyes and central nervous system.
Possible	
General anaesthetics (esp halothane)	
Antimetics (meclozine, cyclizine)	
Antidepressants (imipramine)	

fetal development since about 1920, when it was discovered that X-irradiation during pregnancy can cause fetal malformation or death. 20 years later the importance of *Rubella* infection as a causative factor was recognized, but it was not until 1960, when thalidomide was introduced, that drugs were implicated. The shocking experience with thalidomide led to a widespread reappraisal of many other drugs in clinical use, and the discovery of other agents with appreciable teratogenicity in man (Table 36.3), though none approached thalidomide in frequency and severity. It needs to be stressed that the majority of birth defects (about 70%) occur with no recognizable causative factor. Of the remainder, two-thirds represent an inherited abnormality, since they show a strong familial pattern; this leaves about 10% that can be ascribed to some environmental factor, such as radiation, maternal infection or other disease, and drugs administered during pregnancy. The latter factor is believed to

account for only about 1% of all congenital defects (Wilson, 1973), but could also be involved in the much larger group of defects whose cause is at present undetermined.

Mechanisms of teratogenesis

The timing of the teratogenic insult in relation to the stage of fetal development is critical in determining the type and extent of damage produced. In the mammal, fetal development passes through three major phases (Table 36.4)

1. Blastocyst formation
2. Organogenesis
3. Histogenesis and maturation of function.

During **blastocyst formation**, the main process is that of cell division. This phase continues until the primitive streak (i.e. the group of cells from which the embryo later develops) appears as a distinct

Table 36.4 The nature of drug effects of fetal development

Stage	Gestation period in man	Main cellular processes	Affected by
Blastocyst formation	0–16 days	Cell division	Cytotoxic drugs
Organogenesis	17–60 days approx	Division Migration Differentiation Death	Teratogens
Histogenesis and functional maturation	60 days–term	As above	Miscellaneous drugs e.g. alcohol, nicotine, antithyroid drugs, steroids

structure. During this phase, drugs can cause death of the embryo by inhibiting cell division, but provided the embryo survives, its subsequent development does not seem to be compromised. There is very little evidence that environmental agents acting at this stage can cause maldevelopment, though the epidemiological study of Hanson et al (1978) on the incidence of fetal alcohol syndrome (see Chapter 35) suggested that this drug may affect development at this very early stage.

It is during **organogenesis**, covering roughly the first trimester of pregnancy, that drugs can cause gross malformations. The structural organization of the embryo occurs in a well-defined sequence: eye and brain, skeleton and limbs, heart and major vessels, palate, genitourinary system. The type of malformation produced thus depends on the time of exposure to the teratogen.

In the final stage of **histogenesis and functional maturation**, gross structural malformations no longer occur. The fetus is dependent on an adequate supply of nutrients, and development is regulated by a variety of hormones.

The cellular mechanisms by which teratogenic substances produce their effects are not at all well understood. In the case of thalidomide, which is exceptional in its ability to cause abnormalities in virtually 100% of fetuses under certain experimental conditions, and has been studied more intensively than any other teratogen, it is possible that a reactive metabolite is responsible. None of the known metabolic products of thalidomide is teratogenic, however, suggesting that a short-lived intermediate may be involved. Covalent binding of labelled thalidomide to various cell constituents, including DNA, has been demonstrated (Hathway, 1984), but only in intact cells, suggesting the need

for prior metabolism of the drug. In this regard, thalidomide closely resembles a mutagen, though it has not been reported to show a mutagenic effect. A large survey (Schreiner & Holden, 1983) showed a considerable overlap between drugs shown to be teratogenic in various species, and those with mutagenic activity. Among 78 compounds, 34 were both teratogenic and mutagenic, 19 were negative in both tests and 25 (among them thalidomide) were positive in one but not the other. It therefore seems that damage to DNA may be important, but it is certainly not the only factor. Consistent with the theory that damage to DNA is important is the fact that known teratogens include a number of drugs (e.g. methadone, phenytoin) which do not react directly with DNA, but inhibit its synthesis by their effects on folate metabolism. It has also been reported that administration of folate during pregnancy reduces the frequency of both spontaneous and drug-induced malformations.

Testing for teratogenicity

The thalidomide disaster in 1960 suddenly brought home the need for routine teratogenicity studies on potential new drugs. It quickly became clear that there are major differences in susceptibility to various teratogens between different species, and even between strains of a species. Most regulatory authorities require negative results of teratogenicity testing in one rodent (usually rat or mouse) and one non-rodent (usually rabbit) species. Pregnant females are dosed at various levels during the critical period of organogenesis, and the fetuses are examined prior to parturition for structural abnormalities. The poor cross-species correlation means that tests of this kind are not reliably predictive in man. New drugs are therefore normally introduced with the caution that they should not be used in pregnancy unless it is essential.

In vitro methods, based on the culture of cells, organs or whole embryos, have not so far been developed to a level where they satisfactorily predict teratogenesis *in vivo*.

Assessment of teratogenicity in man is a particularly difficult problem, for various reasons. One is that the 'spontaneous' malformation rate is high (3–10%, depending on the definition of a significant malformation) and highly variable between different regions, age groups and social classes. Unless the 'test' and 'control' groups of patients turn out to be well-matched in these respects, the trial will be very hard to interpret. Large scale retrospective studies are therefore required, which take many years and much money to perform, and usually give suggestive, rather than conclusive results.

Some definite and probable teratogens in man (see Table 36.3)

Though many drugs have been found to be teratogenic in varying degrees in experimental animals, only a few are known to be, or suspected of being, teratogenic in man (see review: Beckman & Brent, 1984). Some of the more important ones that are not presented elsewhere are discussed below.

Thalidomide

This drug is virtually unique in producing, at modest clinical dosage, virtually 100% malformed infants when taken in the first 3–6 weeks of gestation. It was introduced in 1957 as a hypnotic and sedative with the special feature that it was extremely safe in overdosage, and it was even recommended specifically for use in pregnancy. As was then normal, it had been subjected only to acute toxicity testing, and not the chronic toxicity* or teratogen-

icity testing. Thalidomide was marketed energetically and successfully, and the first suspicion of its teratogenicity arose early in 1961 when reports of a sudden increase in the incidence of *phocomelia* (an absence of development of the long bones of the arms and legs) which had hitherto been virtually unknown, came simultaneously from Hamburg and Sydney, and the connection with thalidomide was made. The drug was withdrawn late in 1961, by which time an estimated 10 000 malformed babies had been born (Fig. 36.3). In spite of intensive study, its mechanism of action remains very poorly understood. Study of the many cases of thalidomide teratogenesis in man showed very clearly the correlation between the time of exposure and the type of malfunction produced (Table 36.5).

Cytotoxic drugs (see Chapter 29)

Many alkylating agents (e.g. chlorambucil, cyclophosphamide) and antimetabolites (e.g. azathioprine, mercaptopurine) can cause malformations when used in early pregnancy, but much more often lead to abortion. Folate antagonists (e.g. methotrexate, aminopterin) produce a much higher incidence of major malformations, evident in both live-born and still-born fetuses.

Heavy metals

Lead, cadmium and mercury have all been found to cause fetal malformations in man. The main evidence comes from Minamata disease, named after the locality in Japan where an epidemic occurred when the local population ate fish that had been heavily contaminated with methylmercury that had been used as an agricultural fungicide.

The effect was to produce impaired brain development, resulting in cerebral palsy and mental retardation, often with microcephaly. Mercury, like other heavy metals, is known to inactivate many enzymes by forming covalent bonds with sulphydryl and other groups, and this is presumed to be responsible for the developmental abnormality.

Anticonvulsant drugs (see Chapter 24)

Congenital malformations are 2–3 times as frequent in babies born to epileptic mothers compared

---

* A severe peripheral neuropathy, leading to irreversible paralysis and sensory loss, was reported within a year of the drug's introduction and subsequently confirmed in many reports. The drug company responsible was less than punctilious in acting on these reports (see Sjostrom & Nilsson, 1972), which were soon eclipsed by the discovery of teratogenic effects, but the neurotoxic effect was severe enough in its own right to necessitate prompt withdrawal of the drug.

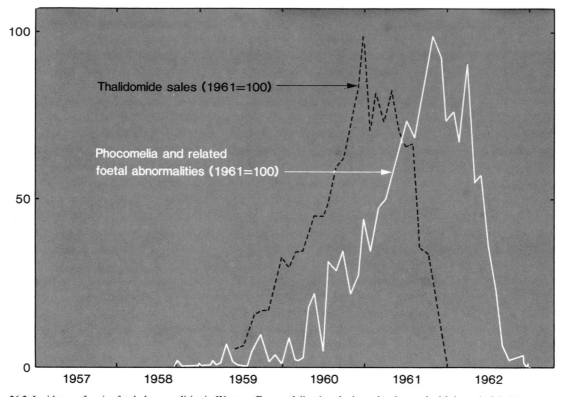

Fig. 36.3 Incidence of major fetal abnormalities in Western Europe following the introduction and withdrawal of thalidomide.

with normal mothers, and there is some evidence that this is associated with the use of anticonvulsant drugs rather than with the epilepsy itself. The drugs that are probably implicated are phenytoin and trimethadione. With phenytoin the syndrome includes a variety of abnormalities, notably cleft palate, facial abnormalities and cardiac defects. The incidence of some degree of abnormality is estimated at 10–30%. With trimethadione, the incidence is higher, but the syndrome is less severe.

Warfarin (see Chapter 12)

Administration of warfarin in the first trimester is

Table 36.5 Thalidomide teratogenesis

Day of gestation	Type of deformity
21–22	Malformation of ears Cranial nerve defects
24–27	Phocomelia of arms
28–29	Phocomelia of arms and legs
30–36	Malformation of hands Anorectal stenosis

associated with nasal hypoplasia and various central nervous system abnormalities, affecting roughly 25% of babies. The effect is due to warfarin itself, and is not due to local bleeding.

Anti-emetics

These drugs are particularly important, as they have been widely used in treating morning sickness in early pregnancy. Many such drugs are teratogenic in animals, but the results of surveys in human beings are inconclusive, providing no clear evidence of teratogenicity. It is obviously prudent, however, to avoid the use of these drugs if possible.

The situation is similar (i.e. positive evidence of teratogenicity in animals without clear evidence in man) with many other drugs, some of which are listed in Table 36.3.

ALLERGIC REACTIONS TO DRUGS

Allergic reactions of various kinds are a very common form of adverse response to drugs (see review: De Weck, 1983). Most drugs, being low molecular weight substances, are not immunogenic in themselves. They can, however, form stable conjugates with proteins and thereby produce an immunogen. Repeated administration of the drug can then evoke a variety of immune responses, just as injection of a foreign protein may. In some instances, the immunological basis for such responses has been well worked out. Very often, however, it is inferred from the general clinical characteristics of the reaction, and direct evidence of an immunological mechanism is lacking. The main criteria that are suggestive of an immune-type response are:

1. The reaction is either delayed in onset, occurring a few days after the drug, or occurs only with repeated exposure to the drug.
2. The reaction may occur with very small doses of the drug, too small to elicit its own pharmacodynamic effects.
3. The reaction conforms to one of the clinical syndromes associated with allergy (see later), and is unrelated to the pharmacodynamic effect of the drug.

The overall incidence of allergic drug reactions is probably about 2%. The great majority are relatively harmless skin eruptions. Serious reactions (e.g. anaphylaxis, haemolysis, bone marrow depression) which may be life-threatening, are rare. The incidence of death from allergic reactions among hospital patients is estimated at 1:10 000. Penicillin, which is by far the commonest cause of drug-induced anaphylaxis, produces this response in an estimated 1 in 50 000 patients given the drug.

Immunological mechanisms

The formation of an immunogenic conjugate between a small molecule and an endogenous macromolecule requires covalent bonding. Ionic and van der Waals bonding of the sort responsible for the reversible binding of drugs to plasma proteins (see Chapter 3) does not produce an immunogenic complex, though the formation of coordination complexes between metals, such as nickel and chromium, and cell surface proteins can do so. Thus, the tendency of a drug to evoke this type of response depends, as with mutagenicity, carcinogenicity and many forms of teratogenicity, on the ability of it or its metabolites to attach covalently to macromolecules; the difference is that immunogenecity depends nearly always on binding to protein, whereas the other types of toxicity involve binding to DNA. The mechanism for covalent coupling of benzylphenicillin to protein is shown in Figure 36.4.

The types of allergic response that drugs can produce conform broadly to Types I, II, III and IV of the Gell–Coombs classification (see Chapter 8).

In nearly all of these reactions, conjugation to protein appears to be essential, not only for the

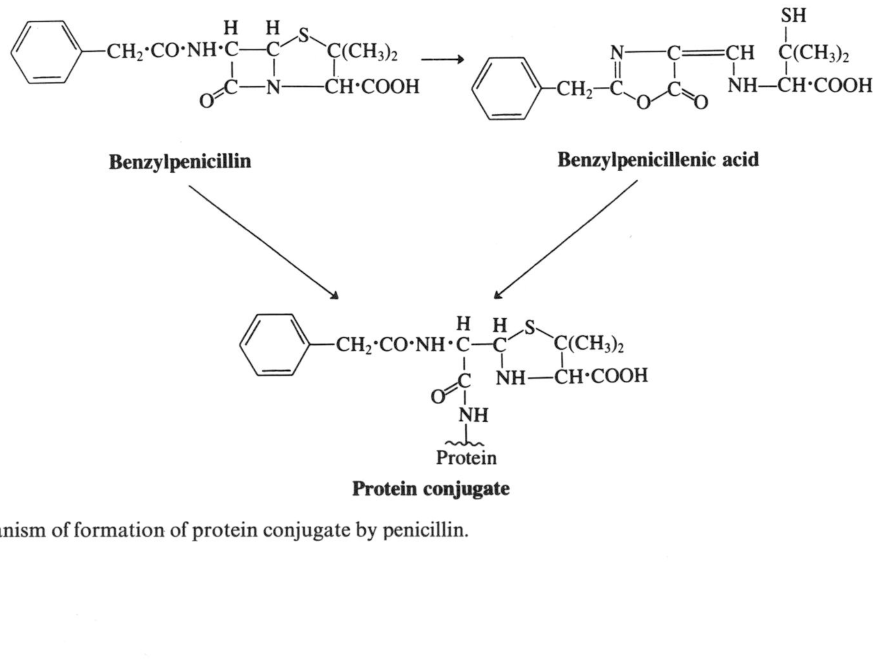

Fig. 36.4 Mechanism of formation of protein conjugate by penicillin.

primary sensitization process, but also for the secondary response. A possible exception is penicillin, which can form dimers and polymers in solution, forming sufficiently large conglomerates of antigenic determinants to elicit an anaphylactic response in a sensitized individual without conjugation to protein (De Weck, 1983).

Though these mechanisms provide a good framework for explaining immune responses to drugs, there are many examples for which the mechanism has not been fully elucidated. The most highly immunogenic drugs (e.g. penicillins) can produce a variety of syndromes involving more than one of these mechanisms (see reviews: De Weck, 1983; Assem, 1981). In a few instances impurities in the preparation, rather than the drug itself, may be responsible.

Clinical types of allergic response to drugs

Anaphylactic shock (see Chapter 8)

Anaphylactic shock is a sudden and life-threatening reaction which results from the release of histamine from mast cells in various regions of the body. The main symptoms, whose pattern and severity varies greatly, are urticarial rash, swelling of soft tissues, bronchoconstriction and hypotension. Most of the deaths from anaphylactic shock are the result of respiratory tract obstruction, partly due to intense oedema of the tongue and upper respiratory tract and partly due to bronchoconstriction. Cardiovascular collapse may also be life-threatening.

The agents most likely to cause anaphylactic reactions under clinical conditions are foreign proteins and other macromolecules. These include various enzymes (e.g. streptokinase, asparaginase), hormones (e.g. ACTH, insulin preparations), vaccines and serological products, heparin and dextrans. Some of these agents carry fairly high risk, but about 75% of anaphylactic deaths result from the use of penicillin, reflecting its very frequent clinical use. Other commonly used drugs that can cause anaphylactic shock, though they do so only very rarely, are local anaesthetics, cromoglycate, neuromuscular blocking drugs (e.g. gallamine, suxamethonium, tubocurarine), thiopentone, and a variety of antibiotics.

Acute anaphylactic attacks are treated, if severe, by injection of adrenaline, corticosteroids and antihistamines. It may be feasible to carry out a skin test, by injecting a minute dose of the drug intradermally, for the presence of anaphylactic hypersensitivity. This may be done if a patient reports that he or she is allergic to a particular drug, but the test is not completely reliable. False negative results are not uncommon, and occasionally the test dose itself elicits a severe reaction. The use of penicilloyl-polylysine as a skin test reagent for penicillin allergy appears to be an improvement over the use of penicillin itself, because it by-passes the need for conjugation of the test substance, thereby reducing the likelihood of a false negative. Other tests are available to detect the presence of specific IgE in the plasma, or to measure histamine release from basophils, but these are not used routinely.

Haematological reactions

Type II cytotoxic reactions to drugs can affect any or all of the formed elements of the blood, which may be destroyed by toxic effects either on the blood cells themselves or on their progenitors in the bone marrow. Haemolytic anaemia can occur with many drugs, but has been most commonly reported with sulphonamides and related drugs and with the antihypertensive drug, methyldopa (see Chapters 7 & 11). With methyldopa, significant haemolysis occurs in less than 1% of patients, but the appearance of antibodies directed against the surface of red cells is detectable in 15% by the Coombs test. The antibodies are directed against Rh antigens, but it is not known how methyldopa produces this effect.

Drug-induced agranulocytosis is usually delayed in onset (2–12 weeks after beginning drug treatment) and may then be sudden in onset. The condition often presents as a severe sore throat or other infection, and fever due to the products of leukocyte lysis. Serum from the patient will cause leukocyte death in blood samples from other individuals, and circulating anti-leukocyte antibodies can be detected immunologically. The main group of drugs associated with agranulocytosis are non-steroidal anti-inflammatory drugs (e.g. aminopyrine, phenylbutazone; see Chapter 9), sulphonamides and related drugs (e.g. chlorpropamide) and chloramphenicol. It is a rare, but highly dangerous condition, because recovery when the drug is stopped is often absent or incomplete. This type of antibody-mediated leukocyte destruction must be distinguished from the direct effect of cytotoxic drugs (see Chapter 29), most of which cause granulocytopenia. With these drugs, however, the effect is rapid in onset, predictably related to dose and readily reversible. Thrombocytopenia, rather than granulocytopenia, tends to occur with quinidine or digoxin.

The distinction between Type III and Type IV hypersensitivity reactions in the causation of haematological reactions is not clear-cut, and it is likely that either or both mechanisms are often involved.

Other hypersensitivity reactions

The clinical manifestations of Type IV hypersensitivity reactions are many and varied, ranging from minor skin rashes to generalized autoimmune disease. Fever may accompany these reactions.

Skin rashes range from very mild eruptions to extensive exfoliative lesions which can be life-threatening. In some cases the lesions are photosensitive, probably because of degradation of the drug to reactive substances in the presence of UV light.

Some drugs (particularly hydralazine) can produce an autoimmune syndrome resembling systemic lupus erythematosus.

REFERENCES AND FURTHER READING

Assem E S K 1981 Drug allergy. In: Davies D M (ed) Textbook of adverse drug reactions. Oxford University Press, Oxford

Beckman D A, Brent R L 1984 Mechanisms of teratogenesis. Ann Rev Pharmacol Toxicol 24: 483–500

Berridge M J, Irvine R F 1984 Inositol triphosphate, a novel second messenger in cellular signal transduction. Nature 312: 315–321

Brusick D J 1983 The future of short-term testing for mutagens and carcinogens. Trends in Pharmacological Sciences 4: 111–115

Davies D M (ed) 1981 Textbook of adverse drug reactions. Oxford University Press, Oxford

De Weck A L 1983 Immunopathological mechanisms and clinical aspects of allergic reactions to drugs. In: De Weck A L, Bundgaard H (eds) Allergic responses to drugs. Handbook of Experimental Pharmacology 63: 75–135

Gorrod J W (ed) 1981 Testing for toxicity. Taylor & Francis, London

Hanson J W, Streissguth A P, Smith D W 1978 The effects of moderate alcohol consumption during pregnancy of fetal growth and morphogenesis. J Paediatr 92: 457–460

Hathway D E 1984 Molecular aspects of toxicology. Royal Society of Chemistry, London

Loomis T A 1978 Essentials of toxicology, 3rd Edn. Lea & Febiger, Philadelphia

Rawlins M D, Thomson J W 1981 In: Davies D M (ed) Textbook of adverse drug reactions. Oxford University Press, Oxford

Rechnagel R O, Glende E A 1973 Carbon tetrachloride hepatotoxiticity; an example of lethal degree. CRC Critical Reviews in Toxicology 2: 263–297

Schreiner C A, Holden H E 1983 Mutagens as teratogens: a correlative approach. In: Johnson E M, Kochhar D M (eds) Teratogenesis and reproductive toxicology. Handbook of Experimental Pharmacology 65: 135–170

Sjostrom H, Nilsson R 1972 Thalidomide and the power of the drug companies. Penguin Books, London

Styles J A 1981 Other short-term tests in carcinogenesis studies. In: Gorrod J W Testing for toxicity. Taylor & Francis, London

Timbrell J A 1982 Principles of biochemical toxicology. Taylor & Francis, London

Venitt S 1981 Microbial tests in carcinogenesis studies. In: Gorrod J W 1981 Testing for toxicity. Taylor & Francis, London

Weinberg R A 1984 Cellular oncogenes. Trends in Biochemical Sciences 9: 131–133

Weisburger J H, Williams G M 1984 New, efficient approaches to tests for carcinogenicity of chemicals based on their mechanisms of action. In: Zbinden et al (eds) Current problems in drug toxicology. Libbey, Paris

Wilson J G 1973 Present status of drugs as teratogens in man. Teratology 7: 3–15

Figure acknowledgement references

CHAPTER 1

Abramson S N, Molinoff P B 1984 In vitro interactions of agonists and antagonists with beta-adrenergic receptors. Biochem Pharmacol 33: 869

Anderson C R, Stevens C F 1973 Voltage clamp analysis of acetylcholine produced end-plate current fluctuations at frog neuromuscular junction. J Physiol 235: 655

Birdsall N J M, Burgen A S V, Hulme E C et al 1978 The binding of agonists to brain muscarinic receptors. Mol Pharmacol 14: 723

Frankhuijsen A L, Bonta I L 1974 Receptors involved in the action of 5-HT and tryptamine on the isolated rat stomach fundus preparation. Eur J Pharmacol 26: 220

Furchgott R F 1965 The use of beta-haloalkylamines in the differentiation of receptors and in the determination of dissociation constants of receptor–agonist complexes. Advances in Drug Research 3: 21

Hirata F, Axelrod J 1980 Phospholipid methylation and biological signal transmission. Science 209: 1082

Katz B, Thesleff S 1957 A study of the desensitization produced by acetylcholine or the motor end-plate. J Physiol 138: 63

Kistler J, Stroud R M 1981 Crystalline arrays of membrane-bound acetylcholine receptor. Proc Natl Acad Sci USA 78: 3678

Nestler E J, Walaas S I, Greengard P 1984 Neuronal phosphoproteins; physiological and clinical implications. Science 225: 1357

Ogden D C, Colquhoun D, Siegelbaum S A et al 1981 Block of acetylcholine-activated ion channels by an uncharged local anaesthetic. Nature 289: 596

Olsen R, Meunier J-C, Changeux J-P et al 1972 Progress in the purification of the cholinergic receptor protein from 'electrophorus electricus' by affinity chromatography. FEBS Lett 28: 96

Perkins J P 1981 Catecholamine-induced modification of the functional state of beta-adrenergic receptors. Trends in Pharmacol Sci 2: 326

Potter L T 1967 Uptake of propranolol by isolated guinea-pig atria. J Pharmacol 155: 91

Schramm M, Orly J, Eimerl S, Korner M 1977 Coupling of hormone receptors to adenylate cyclase of different cells by cell fusion. Nature 268: 310

Van Rossum J M 1958 Pharmacodynamics of cholinometic and cholinolytic drugs. St Catherine's Press, Bruges

CHAPTER 2

Beyer K H 1978 Discovery, development and delivery of new drugs. Spectrum Publications, Jamaica, ch10, p112

Capella P, Horning E C 1966 Separation and identification of derivatives of biologic amines by gas–liquid chromatography. Anal Chem 38: 316

Colquhoun D 1971 Lecture notes on biostatistics. Oxford University Press, Oxford

Holton P 1948 A modification of the method of Dale and Laidlaw for standardization of posterior pituitary extract. Br J Pharmacol 3: 278

Houde R W, Wallenstein S L, Beaver W T 1965 In: de Stevens (ed) Clinical measurement of pain in analgesics. Academic Press, New York

Paxton J W, Rowell F J, Cree G M 1978 Comparison of three radiologists in the radioimmunoassay of methotrexate. Clin Chem 24: 1534

Polak R L, Molenaar P C 1979 A method for determination of acetylcholine by slow pyrolysis combined with mass fragmentography on a packed capillary column. J Neurochem 32: 407

Snell E S, Armitage P 1957 cited in Armitage P 1975 Sequential medical trials, 2nd edn. Blackwell, Oxford

Vane J R 1969 The release and fate of vaso-active hormones in the circulation. Br J Pharmacol 35: 209

CHAPTER 3

Brodie B B, Hogben C A M 1957 Some physico-chemical factors in drug action. J Pharm Pharmacol 9: 345

Conney A H, Miller E C, Miller J A 1957 Substrate-induced synthesis and other properties of benzpyrene/hydroxylase in the rat liver. J Biol Chem 228: 753

Crammer J L, Scott B, Rolfe B 1969 Metabolism of 14C-imipramine. Psychopharmacology 15: 207

Curry S H 1980 Drug disposition and pharmacokinetics. Blackwell, Oxford

Drew G C, Colquhoun W P, Long H A 1958 Effect of small doses of alcohol on a skill resembling driving. Brit Med J 2: 5103

Gunne, Anggard 1974 In: Teorell T et al (eds) Pharmacology and pharmacokinetics. Plenum, New York

Lindenbaum J, Mellow M H, Blackstone M O 1971 Variation in biologic availability of digoxin from four preparations. New Engl J Med 285: 1344

Prescott L F, Steel R F, Ferrier W R et al 1970 The effects of particle size on the absorption of phenacetin in man. Clin Pharmacol Ther 11: 496

Schanker L S, Shore P A, Brodie B B, Hogben C A M 1957 Absorption of drugs from the stomach. The Rat. J Pharmacol 120: 528

Swintowsky J V 1956 Illustrations and pharmaceutical interpretations of first order drug elimination rate from bloodstream. J Am Pharmacol Assoc 45: 395

CHAPTER 4

Curry S H 1980 Drug disposition and pharmacokinetics. Blackwell, Oxford

Ewy G A, Kapadia G C, Yao et al 1969 Digoxin metabolism in the elderly. Circulation 34: 449

Kalow W 1962 Pharmacogenetics. Saunders, Philadelphia

Klotz U, Avant G R, Hoyumpa A et al 1975 The effects of age and liver disease on the disposition and elimination of diazepam in adult man. J Clin Invest 55: 347

Mitchell J R, Cavanaugh J H, Arias L, Oates J A 1970 Guanethidine and related agents: antagonism by drugs which inhibit the norepinephrine pump in man. J Clin Invest 49(2): 1596

Price-Evans D A 1963 Pharmacogenetics. Am J Med 34: 639

Sellers E M, Koch-Weser J 1970 Potentiation of warfarin-induced hypoprothrombinemia by chloral hydrate. New England J Med 283: 827

CHAPTER 5

Dale H H, Feldberg W 1934 Chemical transmitter of vagus effects to stomach. J Physiol 81: 329

Feldberg W, Krayer O 1933 Das Auftreten eines azetylcholinartigen stoffes in Herzvenenblut von Warmblutern bei Reizung der Nervi vagi. Arch exp Path Pharmak 172: 179

Vizi E S 1979 Presynaptic modulation of neurochemical transmission. Prog Neurobiol 12: 181

CHAPTER 6

Blackman J G, Crowcroft P J, Devine C E 1969 Transmission from preganglionic fibres in the hypogastric nerve to peripheral ganglia of male guinea-pigs. J Physiol 201: 723

Bowman W C 1980 Pharmacology of neuromuscular function. Wright, Bristol

Burn J H 1963 Autonomic pharmacology. Blackwell, Oxford

Desmedt J E 1962 Recent data on the pathogenesis of myasthenia gravis. Bull Acad Roy Med Belg VII 2: 213

Ginsborg B L, Guerrero S 1964 On the action of depolarizing drugs on sympathetic ganglion cells of the frog. J Physiol 172: 189

Paton W D M, Zaimis E 1949 The pharmacological actions of polymethylene bistrimethylammonium salts. Br J Pharmacol 4: 381

Payne J P, Hughes R 1981 Evaluation of atracurium in anaesthetized man. Br J Anaesth 53: 45

Sim V M 1965 Diagnosis and therapy for anticholinesterase poisoning. JAMA 192: 403

Tobey R E, Jacobsen P M, Kahle C T et al 1972 The serum potassium response to muscle relaxants in neural injury. Anaesthesiology 37: 322

CHAPTER 7

Burnstock G 1970 In: Bulbring et al (eds) Smooth muscle. Edward Arnold, London

Cavero I, Dennis T, Lefevre-Borg F et al 1979 Effects of clonidine prazosin, and phentolamine on heart rate and coronary sinus catecholamine concentration during cardioaccelerator nerve stimulation in spinal dogs. Br J Pharmacol 67: 283

Furness J B, Campbell G R, Gillard S M et al 1970 Cellular studies of sympathetic denervation produced by 6-hydroxydopamine in the vas deferens. J Pharmacol exp Ther 174: 111

Sandler M, Ruthven 1960 Adrenergic mechanisms. Churchill, London

Taylor S H, Meeran M K 1973 In: Burley et al (eds) New perspectives in beta-blockade. CIBA Laboratories, Horsham

CHAPTER 10

Allen D G, Blinks J R 1978 Calcium transients in aequorin-injected frog cardiac muscle. Nature 273: 509

Giles W R, Noble S J 1976 Changes in membrane currents in bullfrog atrium produced by acetylcholine. J Physiol 261: 103

Hutter O F, Trautwein W 1956 Vagal and sympathetic effects on pacemaker fibres in sinus venosus of heart. J Gen Physiol 39: 715

Noble D 1975 The initiation of the heart beat. Oxford University Press, Oxford

Reuter H 1974 Localization of BETA adrenergic receptors, and effects of noradrenaline and cyclic nucleotides on action potentials, ionic currents and tension in mammalian cardiac muscle. J Physiol 242: 429

Sarnoff S J, Brockman S K, Gilmore J P et al 1960 Regulation of ventricular contraction. Circ Res 8: 1108

Wit A K, Cranefield P F 1975 Triggered and automatic activity in the canine coronary sinus. Circul Res 41: 435

CHAPTER 11

Van Neuten J M, Janssen P A J, Van Beek J et al 1981 Vascular effects of Ketanserin (R41468), A novel antagonist of 5-HT$_2$ serotonergic receptors. J Pharmacol Exp Ther 218: 217

Wolff H G 1948 Headache and other head pain, Oxford University Press, cited by Clark B J et al 1978 In: Ergot alkaloids and related compounds. Handbook Exp Pharmacol 49

CHAPTER 12

Jackson C M 1978 The biochemistry of prothrombin activation. Brit J Haematol 39: 1

Ogston D 1983 The physiology of haemostasis. Croom Helm, London

CHAPTER 13

Cockroft D W 1983 Mechanism of perennial allergic asthma. Lancet i: 253

Kay A B 1986 Mediators and inflammatory cells in asthmas. In: Kay A B (ed) Asthma: clinical pharmacology and therapeutic progress. Blackwell Scientific Publications, Oxford 1

CHAPTER 14

Sullivan L P, Grantham J J 1982 Physiology of the kidney 2E. Lea & Febiger, Philadelphia

Timmerman R J, Springmann F R, Thoms R K et al 1964 Evaluation of frusemide, a new diuretic agent. Current Ther Res 6: 88

CHAPTER 15

Borison H L, Borison R, McCarthy L E 1981 Phylogenic and neurologic aspects of the vomitting process. J Clin Pharmacol 21: 235

Parsons L M 1977 Cimetidine. Excerpta Medica, Amsterdam

CHAPTER 16

Baxter J D, Rousseau G G 1979 Glucocorticoid Hormone Action. Springer Verlag, Berlin

Blackburn C M, McConahey W M, Raymond F et al 1954 Calorigenic effects of single intravenous doses of α-triiodothyronine and α-thyroxine in myxedematous persons. J Clin Invest 33: 819

Furth E D, Becker O V, Schwartz M S 1963 Significance of rate of response of basal metabolic rate and serum cholesterol in hyperthyroid patients receiving neomercazole and other antithyroid agents. J Clin Endocrinol Metab 23: 1130

Pfeifer M A, Halter J B, Porte D 1981 Insulin secretion in diabetus mellitus. Am J Med 70: 579

Taurog A 1976 The mechanism of action of the thioureylene antithyroid drugs. Endocrinology 98: 1031

CHAPTER 17

Fuchs R 1966 The physiological note of oxytocin in the regulation of myometrial activity in the rabbit. In: Pickles, Fitzpatrick (eds) Endogenous substances affecting the myometrium. Cambridge University Press, London

Hollenberg M D, Goren H J, Hanif K et al 1983 Oxytocin, its receptor and its insulin-like activity: a new look at an old hormone. TIPS 4: 310

Moir C 1935 Proc Roy Soc (See Br Med J 1964(ii): 102)

Moir C 1944 Oxytoxic drugs and their use. J Obstet Gynaecol 51: 247

Ruis H, Rolland R, Doesburg W et al 1981 Oxytocin enhances onset of lactation among mothers delivering prematurely. Brit Med J 283: 341

Van de Wiele R L, Dyrenfurth I 1974 Pharmacological reviews. Williams & Wilkins, Baltimore, Vol 25, p 189–207

CHAPTER 18

Ganong W F 1983 Review of medical physiology, 11th ed. Lange Medical Publications, California

Jacobs A, Worwood M 1982 Iron metabolism, iron deficiency and overload. In: Hardisty R M, Weatherall D J (eds) Blood and its disorders. Blackwell Scientific Publications, Oxford, p149

Thomson R B, Proctor S J 1984 A short textbook of haematology. Pitman, Melbourne, p190

CHAPTER 19

Bradley P B, Elkes J 1957 The effects of some drugs on the electrical activity of the brain. Brain 80: 77

Garnett E S, Firnau G, Nahmias C 1983 Dopamine visualised in the basal ganglia of living man. Nature 305: 137

CHAPTER 20

Brodie B B, Mark L C, Papper E M et al 1950 The fate of

thiopental in man and a method for its estimation in biological material. J Pharmacol Exp Ther 98: 85

Eger E I, Lundgren C, Miller S L, Stevens W C 1969 Anaesthetic potencies of sulfur hexafluoride, carbon tetrafluoride, chloroform and ethrane in dogs. Anaesthesiology 30: 129

Papper E M, Kitz R (eds) 1963 Uptake and distribution of anaesthetic agents. McGraw Hill, New York

CHAPTER 21

Braestrup C, Squires R F 1978 Pharmacological characterization of benzodiazepine receptors in the brain. Eur J Pharmacol 78: 263

Kaplan S A, Jack M L, Alexander K et al 1973 Pharmacokinetic profile of diazepam in man following single intravenous and oral and chronic oral administrations. J Pharmaceutical Sciences 62: 1789

Kelleher R T, Morse W H 1964 Escape behaviour and punished behaviour. Fed Proc 23: 808

MacDonald R, Barker J L 1978 Benzodiazepines specifically modulate GABA-mediated postsynaptic inhibition in cultured mammalian neurones. Nature 271: 563

Oswald I, French C, Adam K et al 1982 Benzodiazepine hypnotics remain effective for 24 weeks. Br Med J 284: 860

Schallek W 1981 Handbook Exp Pharmacol 5(II): 330

CHAPTER 22

Bassuk E L, Gerson S 1978 Deinstitutionalization and mental health services. Scientific American 238: 46

Curry S H, Marshall J H L, Davis J M ct al 1970 Chlorpromazine plasma levels and effects. Arch Gen Psychiat 22: 289

Meltzer H Y et al 1978 In: Lipton et al (eds) Psychopharmacology: a generation of progress. Raven Press, New York, p509

NIMH Collaborative Study 1964 Phenothiazine treatment in acute schizophrenia. Arch Gen Psychiat 10: 246

Reynolds G P 1983 Increased concentrations and lateral asymmetry of amygdala dopamine in schizophrenia. Nature 305: 527

Seeman P, Lee T, Chau-Wong M, Wong K 1976 Antipsychotic drug doses and neuroleptic dopamine receptors. Nature 261: 717

White F J, Wang R Y 1983 Comparison of the effects of chronic haloperidol treatment on A9 and A10 dopamine neurons in the rat. Life Sci 32: 983

CHAPTER 23

Asberg M, Cronholm B, Sjoquist F et al 1971 Relationship between plasma level and therapeutic effect of nortriptyline. Br Med J 3: 331

Iversen L L, Mackay A V P 1979 Pharmacodynamics of antidepressants and antimanic drugs. In: Paykal E S, Coppen A (eds) Psychopharmacology of affective disorders. Oxford University Press, Oxford

MRC Trial 1965 Clinical trial of the treatment of depressive illness. Br Med J 1: 881

CHAPTER 24

Eliasson S G et al 1978 Neurological pathophysiology, 2nd edn. Oxford University Press, New York

Herrling P L, Morris R, Salt T E 1983 Effects of excitatory amino acids and their antagonists on membrane and action potentials of cat caudate neurones. J Physiol 339: 207

Matsumoto H, Marsan C A 1964 Cortical cellular phenomena in experimental epilepsy: interictal manifestations. Exp Neurol 9: 286

Richens A, Dunlop A 1975 Serum phenytoin levels in management of epilepsy. Lancet ii: 247

CHAPTER 25

Melzack R, Wall P D 1982 The challenge of pain. Penguin, London

Mense S 1981 Sensitization of group IV muscle receptors to bradykinin by 5-hydroxytroptamine and prostalglandin E_2. Brain Res 225: 95

Sharma S K, Klee W A, Nirenberg M 1975 Dual regulation of adenylate cyclase accounts for narcotic dependence and tolerance. Proc Nat Acad Sci 72: 3092

Way E L, Lok H H, Shen F-H 1969 Simultaneous quantitative assessment of morphine tolerance and physical dependence. J Pharmacol Exp Ther 167: 1

Yaksh T L, Jessell T M, Gamse R et al 1980 Intrathecal morphine inhibits substance P release from mammalian spinal cord in vivo. Nature 286: 155

CHAPTER 27

Hille B 1970 Ionic channels in nerve membranes. Prog Biophys 21: 1

Molgo J, Lemeignan M, Lechat P 1977 Effects of 4-amonopyridine at the frog neuromuscular junction. J Pharmacol Exp Ther 203: 653

Schmitt O, Schmidt H 1972 Influence of calcium ions on the ionic currents of nodes of Ranvier treated with scorpion venom. Pflug Arch 333: 51

Tasaki I, Hagiwara S 1957 Demonstration of two stable potential states in the squid giant axon under tetraethylammonium chloride. J Gen Physiol 40: 859

CHAPTER 28

Mandelstam J, McQuillen K, Dawes I (eds) 1982

Biochemistry of bacterial growth, 3E. Blackwell Scientific, Oxford

CHAPTER 29

Calabresi P, Parks R E 1980 In: Gilman A G, Goodman L S, Gilman A (eds) The pharmacological basis of therapeutics, 6E. Macmillan, New York, ch 54, p1249

CHAPTER 33

Bray R S, Garnham P C C 1982 The life cycle of primate malaria parasites. Brit Med Bull 38: 117

CHAPTER 35

Ashton H, Stepney R 1982 Smoking psychology and pharmacology. Tavistock, London

Bowman W C, Rand M J 1980 Textbook of pharmacology. Blackwell, Oxford, ch 42

Kalant H, Khanna J M, Seymour F et al 1975 Acute alcoholic fatty liver metabolism or stress. Biochem Pharmacol 24: 431

Yano K, Rhoads G G, Kagan A 1977 Coffee, alcohol and risk of coronary heart disease amongst Japanese men living in Hawaii. New Eng J Med 297: 405

Index

Abortifacients
  combined, sulprostone, 421
  progestogens, 421
  prostaglandins, 197–198, 421, 431
Absorption of drugs, 57–71
  alimentary canal, 59, 66–69
    sub-lingual, 66
  cutaneous, 69
  delaying absorption, 70–71
  by eyedrops, 69–70
  by inhalation, 66, 70
  by injection, 70
  movement across cell barriers, 58–63
  rectal, 69
  particle size, 67
  plasma proteins, binding, 63–65
  spectrophotometry, 55
  translocation, 57–58
Acceptor proteins, 26–27
  exocytosis, 26
  see also Protein kinases
Acebutolol
  antidysrhythmia, 247
  and metoprolol, 165
Acetaminophen see Paracetamol
Acetazolamide
  action as diuretic, 312, 320, 326
  in glaucoma, 326
  structure, 319
Acetohexamide, 390–392
Acetomenaphthone, vitamin K, 284–285
Acetyl group, conjugation, 74, 76
Acetyl transferase in neonates, 91
Acetylation, 'fast' and 'slow' acetylators, 92–93
Acetylcholine
  action, 16–17
  binding site, 14–15
  bioassay, 36, 102
  in central nervous system, 457–460
  channel conductance, 18
  chemical assay, 54
  denervation supersensitivity, 106
  distribution, brain, 458–459
  effect of drugs, 118–144
    anticholinesterases, 137–144
    ganglion blocking, 125–129
    ganglion stimulating, 124–125

  hyoscine, 460
  muscarinic agonists, 119–121
  muscarinic antagonists, 121–124
  neuromuscular blocking drugs, 129–137
  physostigmine and atropine, 459–460
  in gastric secretion, 333–335
  historical notes, 102, 113
  inhibition by adrenaline, 108
  magnocellar forebrain nuclei, 458
  muscarinic and nicotinic actions, 113–114, 459
  noise analysis, 16, 18
  -operated ion channels, 19
  receptors, 8, 113–115
    affinity chromatography, 15
    nicotinic processes, 17
    reconstruction, 16
  Renshaw cell, spinal cord, 459
  in senile dementia, 460
  structure, 119
  synapses, cholinergic, 115–118
  synthesis and release, 116
  transmitter role, 104–105, 457–460
Acetylcholinesterase
  active site, 138–140
  distribution, 137–138
  duration, 138–141
  effects, 141–142
  histochemistry, 137
  in Huntington's chorea, 460
  hydrolysis mechanism, 138
  in myasthenia gravis, 143–144
  reactivation, 142–143
  uses, 142
Acetylcysteine, acute paracetamol poisoning, 212
Acetylsalicylic acid (aspirin), 204–213
  see also Aspirin
Acetyltriethylcholine (false transmitter), 130
Achlorhydria in pernicious anaemia, 336
Acidosis, metabolic/respiratory, 298
Acne and oral contraceptives, 426
Aconitine, 590
Acrolein, 612, 614

Acromegaly, 362–363
  and dopamine, 455
ACTH see Corticotrophin
Actinomysin D, 603, 618
Acyclovir
  action, 603, 649–650
  structure, 648
Addison's disease, 394, 404
Adenine arabinoside, 648–649
  action, 603
Adenohypophysis, 359–366
Adenosine
  compounds, effects, 266
  as transmitters, 265
  in coronary flow, 235
  in heart, 254–255
Adenosine diphosphate, in haemostasis, 281
Adenosine monophosphate see Cyclic adenosine monophosphate
Adenosine triphosphate
  as CNS transmitter, 468
  in NANC nerve transmission, 110
  potential transmitter, 552–553
Adenylate cyclase
  calmodulin activation, 6, 26–27
  dopamine activation, 267
  inhibition, 22
  membrane coupling, 14
  receptor regulation, 22
  synthesis of cAMP, 20–21
Administration of drugs see Absorption
Adrenal insufficiency, acute, 402
Adrenal medulla, innervation, 103
Adrenal steroids, 393–405
  comparison, corticosteroids, 393
  conjugation, 77
  glucocorticoids, 394–395
  immunosuppressive effect, 397–398
  mechanism, 398–401
  metabolic and systemic effects, 397
  mineralocorticoids, 404–405
  therapeutic uses, 401
  unwanted effects, 401–402
Adrenal virilism, 394
Adrenaline
  action, 8
  anaesthetic, local, 161
  biosynthesis, 150

Adrenaline (*contd*)
  cardiovascular effects, 159
  definition, 175
  historical note, 101
  inhibitory effect on acetylcholine, 108
  lipolytic effect, effect of insulin, 382
  receptor specificity, 148
  reversal, ergotamine, 162
  structure, 146
  structure-activity, 156–158
  summary, 164
  uterus, inhibition, 428
  vasoconstriction, 258, 259
  vasoconstrictor effect, 95–96
Adrenergic transmission, 146–176
  adrenergic neurons, drugs acting on,
      169–176
  adrenoceptors, drugs acting on,
      156–175
    agonists, 158–161
    blocking drugs, 161–169
  catecholamine uptake and
      degradation, 153–156
  classification of receptors, 146–149
  noradrenaline, 150–153
    release, 151–153
      drugs acting on, 170–171
    storage, 151
      drugs acting on, 170
    synthesis, 150–151
      drugs acting on, 170
  physiology, 149–156
Adrenoceptors *see* Alpha-receptors:
      Beta-receptors
Adrenocortical steroids *see* Adrenal
      steroids: Glucocorticoids:
      Mineralocorticoids
Adrenocorticotrophic hormone *see*
      Corticotrophin
Adriamycin, 51
Affective disorders, 513–529
  antidepressants, 517–529
  nature, 513–517
Affinity constant, definition, 34
Agar, 347
Age, effects, 90–92
  drug metabolism, 91–92
  renal excretion, 90–91
Aglycones, 239
Agonists
  α_1-agonists, 19
  α_2-agonists, 19
  definition, 33
  partial agonist effect, 11, 148–149
Agonists and antagonists, 6
  competitive antagonism, 9, 12
  efficacy, 12, 33
  partial and full agonists, 10, 12
  receptor reserve, 12
Agranulocytosis
  drug-induced, 186, 704–705
  in hyperthyroidism, 377
ALA *see* δ-Amino laevulinic acid
β-Alanine, amino acid transmitter?, 461
Alcohol, 683–689

and coronary heart disease, 685
  dehydrogenase, 688–689
    and NAD$^+$, 87
  -induced flushing, 94, 392
  pharmacokinetics, 687–689
  pharmacological effects, 683–686
  tolerance and dependence, 686–687
Alcoholism, hyperlipoproteinaemia,
      355
Aldosterone, 393–394, 404–405
  action, 314
  comparison, corticosteroids, 393
  role in blood pressure, 272
  structure, 396
Alfacalcidiol, 408–409
Alkalosis
  and aldosterone, 404
  hypokalaemic, 322, 324, 327
  metabolic/respiratory, 298
Alkylating agents, cancer therapy,
      611–614
Allergic reactions, 702–705
  loop diuretics, 322–323
  types I-IV, 186–187
Allopathy, 3
Allopurinol
  anticancer action, 618
  enzyme inhibition, 97
  in gout, 217
  in Leishmaniasis, 667
Allosteric regulatory site, 6
Alpha-blockers, blood pressure
      regulation, 272
Alpha-receptors
  agonists, list, 148
  antagonists, list, 148
  classification, 146–149
  effects mediated, 147
Alphadolone, 485
Alphaxolone (althesin), 483–485
Alprenolol
  action, 167
  antidysrhythmia, 247
  plasma albumin, 63
  side effects, 169
  summary, 165
Alprostodil (prostaglandin E$_1$), 198
Aluminium hydroxide gel, 338
Alzheimer's disease, 460
Amantadine, 647–648
  in Parkinsonism, 543
Amenorrhea and prolactin, 365–366
Ames test, mutagenicity, 697–698
Amethocaine
  pharmacokinetics, 587
  structure, 583
Amikacin, 638–639
Amiloride
  action, 315, 323–325
  structure, 320
Amine-precursor-uptake-
      decarboxylation cells, 111
Amine transmitters, synthesis, storage
      and release, 111
Amino acid transmitters, 460–463

β-alanine, 463
  γ-aminobutyric acid, 461–462
  aspartate, 461
  cysteine, 461
  excitatory amino acids, 463–464
  glutamate, 461
  glycine, 462
α-Aminoadipic acid, 533
p-Aminobenzoic acid *see* Para-
      aminobenzoic acid
γ-Aminobutyric acid, 460
  action, benzediazepine, 6
  and benzodiazepines, 490–493
  metabolism in brain, 463
  occurrence, 461
  receptor classification, 462
  structure, 461
Aminocaproic acid, 294–295
Aminoglutethimide, 395
Aminoglycoside antibiotics, 626–627,
      638–640
  absorption, 67
  acetylcholine release, blockage, 119
  calcium entry, inhibition, 130
  see also Spectinomycin: Streptomycin
p-Aminohippuric acid clearance, 80
δ-Aminolaevulinic acid
  and hepatic porphyria, 94
  synthetase, 497
Aminophosphonovaleric acid, 533
Aminophylline, 326
  in asthma, 304–305
Aminopyridines, 590
  action, 144, 582
  depolarizing shift, 532
  K$^+$ channels, blocking, 582
  function, 579, 590
  structure, 144, 583
Aminoquinolines in malaria, 660–663
4-Aminoquinoline, 215–216
Amiodarone, antidysrhythmia, 247–248
Amiphenazole, 568, 570
Amitryptiline, 519–522
  antidepressant, 346
  antiemetic, 343
  atropine-like effects, 520
  and imipramine, 166
  in plasma albumin, 63
  transmitter uptake, 526
Ammonium chloride
  diuresis, 326
  urine, pH, 328
Amodiaquine, 660–661
Amoebiasis, 665–666
Amoscanate, 674
Amoxycillin, 632–633
c-AMP *see* Cyclic adenosine
      monophosphate
Amphetamine, 568–573
  dependence and tolerance, 573
  in hyperactive children, 92, 573
  monoamine oxidase inhibitors, 523,
      524
  motor activity, dopaminergic, 454
  and related compounds, 571–573

Amphetamine (*contd*)
  renal clearance, 80
  structure-activity, 157, 172–173,
    571–572
  summary, 165, 569
Amphotericin
  action, 603
  with flucytosine, 653
  in Leishmaniasis, 667
  with rifampicin, 653
  structure, 653
  unwanted effects, 654
  uses, 652
Ampicillin, 626–627, 632–633
  plasma half-life, 90
Amrinone, action, on heart, 255
Amyl nitrite, 251
Anabolic steroids, 423
Anaemias, 433–434
  pernicious, 438
Anaesthetics, 471–485
  blood:gas partition coefficient, 476,
    477
  effects, on cardiovascular system,
    475–476
    on CNS, 474
  inhalation, 476–483
  intravenous, 483–485
  local, 579 590
    bioassay, 35
    cell interactions, 5
    inhalation, adrenaline, addition, 70
      bronchoscopy, 70
  oil:gas coefficient, 473, 476
  physicochemical theories, 472–474
  toxicity to theatre staff, 480
    nitrous oxide, 482
Analeptics, 299
Analgesics, 547–566
  measurement, 42
  morphine-like, receptor sites, 6
Anaphylactic reactions, acute,
    catecholamines, 161
Anaphylactic shock, 704
Ancrod, 289
Androgens
  antiandrogens, 423
  male reproductive system, 421–423
  and pregnancy, 415
  structures, 420
  teratogenicity, 698
Androstenedione
  biosynthesis, 396
  from testosterone, liver, 423
  precursor, testosterone, 422
  structure, 416
Angina, 236
  antianginal drugs, 251–254
  β-receptor antagonists, 167–169, 254
  organic nitrates, 251–254
  treatments compared, 250
  variant angina, 236, 250, 253
Angiotensin I and II
  biosynthesis, glucocorticoids, 396
  -converting enzyme inhibitors, 270

lungs, 299
  renin activity, 269–271
  uterine action, 429
Angiotensin-converting enzyme
    (kininase II), 199–200
Angiotensinogen, 269
Animal tests
  anxiolytic drugs, 486–487
  carcinogenicity, 697
  LD50, 46–47
  whole animal, 700–701
  see also Tests
Antacids, 338–339
Antagonists, 6, 10
  chemical, 28
  competitive antagonism, 9, 33
    irreversible, 28–29, 30–31, 33
    potency (pA$_2$ value), 10
    reversible, 28
  definition, 33
  irreversible competitive, 28–31, 163
  non-competitive, 31
  pharmacokinetic, 28
  physiological, 31
  by receptor block, 28
Antiandrogens, 423
Antibiotics, 626–646
  and micro-organisms, 626–627
  and resistance, 604 607
  see also specific names
Antibodies
  and B lymphocytes, 184
  classification, 184
  and complement sequence, 184
  ingestion of bacteria, 185
  mast cells and basophils, 185
Antibody-drug conjugates, experimental
    animals, 89
Anticancer drugs, 609–625
Anticholinesterases, 137–144
  enzyme inhibition, 97
Anticonvulsants, 490, 533–539
  teratogenesis, 701–702
Antidepressants, 469
  guanethidine uptake, 95
  monoamine oxidase, inhibition, 95
  tricyclic, 517–522, 524–528
Antidiabetic drugs, 388–393
Antidiuretic hormone, 259–260,
    366–369
  action, 314–316
Antidysrhythmic drugs, 247
  cardiac effects, 249–250
  list, 148
Antiemetic drugs, 342–346
Antiepileptic drugs, 533–539
Antifungal drugs, 652–656
Antigen presenting cells, 183
  see also Immune response
Antihelminth drugs, 669–674
Antihistamines, 188–192, 218–221
Anti-hypertensive drugs, 274–275
  see also Individual drugs
Anti-inflammatory drugs, action, sites,
    191

Antilymphocyte immunoglobulin, 223
Anti-metabolites, cancer therapy, 610,
    614–618
Antimony compounds, 667
Antioestrogens, 419
Antipsychotic drugs, bioassay, 35
Antiprogestogens, 421
Antiprotozoal drugs, 657–668
Antipyretic analgesics, 204–206
Antipyrine, plasma half life, and age,
    91–92
Antirheumatoid drugs, 213–216
Antithrombin III, in coagulation
    cascade, 288
Antiviral drugs, 647–651
Anxiolytics, 469, 486–496
  classification, 488
  tests, animals, 486–487
    man, 487–488
Apomorphine
  dopamine, antagonist, 454
    receptors, 267–268
  emetic action, 268, 340–341
  prolactin release, 365
APUD *see* Amine-precursor
APV (aminophosphonovaleric acid), 533
Arachidonate, 181, 192–193
  cascade, in intestinal secretion, 350
  cyclo-oxygenase, inhibition,
    NSAIDs, 207
  platelet metabolism, 292–293
  and renal function, 318
  from phosphatidyl choline, 25, 27
'Area under the curve', 85
Arecoline, effect on learning, 460
Arginine
  vasopressin (ADH), 366–369
  -vasotocin, 367
Artesunate, 664
Atenolol
  action, 167
  in hypertension, 274–275
  and metoprolol, 165
  receptor specificity, 148
Arthus reaction, 186
Ascorbic acid, iron absorption, 435
L-Asparaginase
  anticancer action, 611, 620
  resistance, 621
Asparate
  amino acid transmitter, 461
  excitatory function, 463–464
Aspergillosis, 652
Aspirin, 204, 205, 207
  action, 5
  antidiarrhoeal action, 351
  assay, 56
  as displacing agent, 96
  gastric effects, 210
  inhibition, renal tubular secretion, 98
  interactions, 211–212
  local toxic effects, 210
  and oral anticoagulants, 287
  oral dose and plasma concentration, 61
  plasma albumin, 63

Aspirin (*contd*)
  platelet aggregation, 210, 287
  radiation-induced diarrhoea, 213
  structure, 209
  systemic toxic effect, 210–211
  theoretical partition in body, 60
  thrombo-embolic disease, 293
Astemizole, 218–220
Asthma, 301–307
  isoprenaline, 161
  propanolol, bronchoconstrictive
    effects, 168–169
  salbutamol, 161
Assay *see* Bioassay: Chemical assay
Association, dissociation constants,
  definition, 34
Atherosclerosis, 280
  cholesterol metabolism, 354
Atracurium
  absorption, oral and placental, 131
  pharmacokinetic aspects, 136–137
  structure, 127
Atrial peptides, 268–269
Atrial tachycardias, muscarinic,
  agonists, 121
  antagonists, 123
Atriopeptins, 269
Atrioventricular block, 240, 242–244
Atropine
  acetylcholine receptors, action, 118
    142, 459–460
  anaesthesia, premedication, 123
  gastric motility, inhibition, 123
  and gastric secretion, 337
  gastrointestinal absorption, 95
  historical note, 101
  -methonitrate, structure, 122
    uses, 123
  poisoning, 122–123
  sphincter of Oddi, effect, 354
  structure, 122
AUC *see* Area under the curve
Aurothioglucose, rheumatoid arthritis,
  213–214
Autonomic nervous system, 101–112
  anatomy and physiology, 103–106
  chemical transmission, 106–108
    peripheral neurotransmitters,
      110–111
    presynaptic interactions, 108–110
  receptors, 105
  sites of drug action, 111–112
Autonomic transmitters, 236–239
  heart, parasympathetic system,
    238–239
  sympathetic system, 237–238
Azapropazone, 205
  structure, 208
Azathioprine, 222–223
  allopurinol, effect, 97
  anticancer action, 618
  metabolite, 78
  in myasthenia gravis, 144
Aziridinium ion, spontaneous
  formation, 30

Babies, drug metabolism, 91
Bacitracin, 642
Baclofen, muscle tone, control, 545
Bacteria
  antibiotic resistance, 604
  antibody resistance, 604
  biochemical reactions, 597–603
    Class I, 597
    Class II, 597
    Class III, 598–603
  Gram negative, 626–627
    ampicillin resistance, 607
    β-lactamases, 606
    cell wall, 599, 628
    chloramphenicol inactivation, 606,
      637
    outer membrane, 596–597, 628
  Gram positive, 626–627
    cell wall, 599, 628
    conjugation, 605
    plasmids, 605
    resistance genes, 605–606
    structure, 595–597
Bactericidal drugs, and bacteriostatic
  drugs, 95
Barbiturates, 496–498
  and age, variations, 92
  cell interactions, 5
  and oral anticoagulants, 287
  renal clearance, 80
  see also Pentabarbitone:
    Phenobarbitone
Basophils, 180
  histamine, 188
  IgE receptors, 185
Batrachotoxin, 582, 590
BAY K 8644, 249
  structure, 248
Beclomethasone
  in asthma, 307
  comparison, corticosteroids, 393
  pharmacokinetics, 402
Bendrofluazide
  action, 329, 323–324
  structure, 319
Benorylate, 212
Benperidol, 501
Benzamides, neuroleptic drugs,
  502–505
Benzhexol, binding curve, 14
Benzocaine, structure, 583
Benzodiazepines, 488–496
  action, 489–494
  in acute overdose, 494
  adverse effects, 494–496
  and age, 92
  agonists, 493
  antagonists, 491–493
  characteristics, 494
  disulfiram, inhibition, 97
  in epilepsy, 534, 539
  in ethanol withdrawal, 687
  metabolites, 78, 494
  muscle tone, control, 545
  onset of confusion, 494

  pharmacokinetics, 493
  pharmacological effects, 488–489
  and sleep, 489
  specific receptor sites, 5–6
  structure and classification, 488
Benzoylcholine hydrolysis, 137
Benzpyrene
  hepatotoxicity, 698
  microsome activity, 77
Benztropine, in Parkinsonism, 543–544
Benzylpenicillin, 632–633
  salts, 633
Bephenium, 670–672
Beta-blockers, 247, 250
  and blood pressure regulation, 272
  see also Beta-receptors, antagonists
Beta-receptors
  and adenylate cyclase, 22–23, 32
  agonists, list, 148
    in asthma, 302–304
  antagonists, 247, 250
    in angina, 254
    and bronchodilators, 94
    cardiovascular system, 167–169
    comparison, nitrates and calcium
      antagonists, 250
    effects, 167–168
    list, 148
    uses, 168–169
    see also Adrenergic receptors:
      specific Beta-blockers
β_1 and β_2, distinction, 147–148
  effects mediated, 147
  heart, 236–238
    antagonists, in angina, 255
    class II antidysrhythmic drugs,
      247, 250
    in lung, 301
Betahistine
  potency, 189
  structure, 190
Betamethasone
  in asthma, 307
  comparison, corticosteroids, 393
  pharmacokinetics, 402
Betazole
  acid secretion, test, 336
  potency, 189
  structure, 190
Bethanechol
  gastrointestinal motility, 349
  muscarinic agonist, 119–121
Bethanidine
  action, 171–172
  and guanethidine, 166
  in hypertension, 274–275
  structure, 171
Bezafibrate, 356
Bicuculline, 569–571
  structure, 570
Biguanides, 392–393
Bile (biliary)
  carrier mediated transport, 62
  constituents, 353
  duct, spasm, 354

Bile (biliary) (contd)
  gallstones, 353–356
Bilirubin, conjugation, 77
Binding see Receptors, drug-binding
Bioassay, 35–50
  biological standards, 37–38
  decision, 38–41
  direct/indirect, 38–41
  general principles, 37–46
  graded responses, 41–42
  in man, 42–46
  matching assays, 40
  measurement of toxicity, 46–48
  parallel assays, 36, 40
  quantal response, 41–42
  therapeutic index, 48–50
  2 + 2 assay, 41–42
  variation, biological, 38–39
Bioavailability, measurement, 68–69, 85
Biological standards, bioassays, 37–38
Bisacodyl, 348
Bishydroxycoumarin, 286
Bismuth subsalicylate, 351
Blackwater fever, 663
Blastomycosis, 652
Bleomycin, 51
  anti-cancer action, 604, 611, 618
Blood loss
  gastrointestinal tract, 436
  menstruation, 436
  pregnancy, 437
Blood pressure
  action of acetylcholine, 113–114
  action of atropine, 113–114
  regulation, 450–451
  see also Hypertension
Bombesin, 331–332
  from lung cancers, monoclonal
    antibodies, 624
Bone marrow anaemias, 433
Bone structure, 405
Botulinum toxin
  acetylcholine release, blockage, 119
  potency, 130–131
Bradycardia, muscarinic action,
    suxamethonium, 135
Bradykinin, 198–201
  and pain, 551
  and prostaglandins, vasodilation, 197
Brain
  blood-brain barrier, 72, 346
    anticholinesterase drugs, 142
    transport, 72
  cerebral oedema, diuretics, 325–326
  chemoreceptor trigger zone, 340–346
  rat, cholinergic pathways, 458
    dopaminergic pathways, 452
    noradrenergic pathways, 449
    serotinin pathways, 456
  see also Central nervous system
Breast
  carcinoma, anabolic steroids, 423
    testosterone, 423
  cystic disease, Danazol in, 424–425
  oxytocin, effect, 429

Bretylium, effect, 171
Bromocriptine
  action, 155, 365
  in acromegaly, 363
  lactation, inhibition, 425
  in Parkinsonism, 268, 543
  prolactin, inhibition, 268, 365–366,
    425, 454
    dopamine receptors, 267
  structure, 162
  unwanted effects, 366
Bronchial asthma, 301–308
  drugs used, 304–307
  immediate and late response,
    302–304
  inflammatory changes, 302
  platelets, in hyper-reactivity, 302
  status asthmaticus, 304, 307
Bronchial system, smooth muscle β-
    receptor antagonists, 167–169
Bronchoconstriction, β-receptor
    antagonists, 304
  propranolol, 247, 304
Bronchoconstrictors, leukotrienes, C_4,
    D_4, E_4, 191
Bronchus(i)
  constriction, 330–301
  dilatation, 300–301, 302
  hyper-reactivity, in asthma, 302
Bumetanide, action, 320–322
α-Bungarotoxin, 14
  action, 31
  autonomic and neuromuscular
    action, 114
β-Bungarotoxin, 130, 131
Bupivacaine, 583, 587
Busulphan, in granulocytic leukemia,
    614
Butoxamine
  receptor specificity, 148
  summary, 165
Butyrophenones
  characteristics, 504
  dopamine receptor, action, 268
  neuroleptic drugs, 502–505
  serotonin antagonist, 265
Butyrylcholinesterase, 137–138

Caffeine, 5, 574–575
  bronchodilation, 304–305
  psychomotor action, 569, 574
  side effects, 575
Calcifediol, 408–409
Calciferol (vitamin D_2), 406, 408
  clinical use, 409
  ergocalciferol, 408
Calcitonin, 369
  action, 410
  and thyroid hormone, 373
Calcitriol
  clinical use, 408–409
  and parathormone, 405
  structure, 406

Calcium
  antagonists, 248–250, 258
    action, 249–250, 258
    adverse effects, 250
    in asthma, 307
    in hypertension, 274–275
    indications, 246
    reversal of paralysis, 130
  carbonate, antacid, 339
  cytosolic, neutrophils, 181
  depletion diuresis, 322
  distribution body, 405–407
    -gluconate, oral, 407
    -lactate, oral, 407
  excretion in loop diuresis, 327
  heart, antagonists, 248–250
    in myocardial infarction, 236
    in sympathetic activity, 238–239
  and histamine release, 189
  ions, calmodulin, 25–27
    regulation, 23–25
    second messenger, 19
  islets of Langerhans, insulin
    response, 380
Calmodulin
  action, 25–27
  inhibition, 27
  structure, 25
cAMP see Cyclic adenosine
    monophosphate
Cancer chemotherapy, 608–625
  cell cycle, 621
  drugs, 610–620
    resistance, 620–621
  future strategies, 622
  general principles, 608–610
  immune response, 622
  oncogene products, 623–625
  treatment, 621–622
  tumour promoters, 625
Candidiasis, 652
Cannabis, 689–691
  cannabinoids, anti-emetic, 343,
    346
  pharmacological effects, 690
  psychomimetic action, 569
  structures, 689
Canrenone, diuresis, 324
Cantharidin, in pain measurement,
    550–551
Capillaries, endothelium, 58
  see also Peripheral vascular disease
Capreomycin in tuberculosis, 645
Capsaicin, 464
  desensitization effect, 552
  pain production, 551–552
Captopril
  angiotensin, converting enzyme
    inhibitor, 270–272
    production, 259
  in hypertension, 274–275
Carbachol
  muscarinic agonist, 119–120
  structure, 119
  uterine contraction, 429

Carbamazepine in epilepsy, 534–535, 539
Carbenicillin, 627, 632–633
  distribution, 72
Carbenoxolone, 339
Carbidopa
  action, 170
  and levodopa, Parkinsonism, 543
  summary, 166
Carbimazole, 376–377
Carbon monoxide and smoking, 683
Carbon tetrachloride, toxic effects, 694, 698
Carbonic anhydrase inhibitors, 319
γ-Carboxy-glutamic acid in Factors II-X, 283
Carcinogenesis, 695–698
Carcinoid syndrome, 5-hydroxyindoleacetic acid, 263
Cardiac failure, 233–234, 273
  glycosides in, 240–241
  and diuretics, 94
  vasodilators, 273
  see also Heart
Cardiac inhibition, adenosine compounds, 266
Cardionatrins, 269
Cardiovascular function
  ganglion blocking drugs, effect, 128–129
  ganglion stimulating drugs, 125
  muscarinic agonists, 120
  antagonists, 122
  see also Heart
Cardiovascular system
  β-receptor antagonists, 167–169
    effects, 167–168
    side effects, 169
    uses, 168–169
  histamine, effects, 190–191
Carmustine, 613–614
Carrier mediated transport, 62
  competition, drugs, 79
  competitive inhibition, 62
  drug transport, sites, 62, 67
  facilitated diffusion, 62
  renal carrier systems, 78
Cascade superfusion, 36–37
Castor oil, 348
CAT see Choline acetyltransferase
Cataracts and glucocorticoids, 402
Catecholamines
  action, 158
  agonist potency, order, 146
  biosynthesis, 150
  in bronchial smooth muscle, 300–301
  definition, 175
  derivatives, assay, 52
  heart, effects on, 237–238
  hormones, effect of, 386
  inotropic and chronotropic effects, 147–148
  metabolic degradation, 154–156

catechol-O-methyl transferase, 154–156
  monoamine oxidase, 154–156
  receptor specificity, agonists and antagonists, 148
  uptake I and II, 154
  see also Adrenaline: Dopamine: Isoprenaline: Noradrenaline
Catechol-O-methyl transferase
  dopamine pathways, 451–452, 541
  occurrence and action, 154–156
CCK8 (Cholecystokinin octapeptide), 552
CDCA see Chenodeoxycholic acid
Cefoxitin, 626–627, 634–636
Cefuroxime, 634–636
Cell cycle, 609
  drug effects, 621
Cell membranes
  active transport, 62
  diffusion, characteristics, 57
    coefficient of, 57
  permeability coefficient P, 59
  movement of small molecules, 58–62
    carrier-mediated transport, 62
    lipid, diffusion through, 58–62
    pinocytosis, 58
  pH and ionization, 59–61
  partition and ion trapping, 61–62
Central nervous system
  effects of alcohol, 683
  effects of smoking, 679–681
  hallucinogens, 575–577
  neurotransmitters, 448–469
    see also specific names
  psychotropic drugs, 469–470
  stimulants, 568–575
  see also Brain
Cephalosporins, 626–627, 634–636
  action, 635–636
  inactivation, β-lactamases, 606
  structures, 635
Cephamycins, 634–636
Cerebral oedema, diuretics, 325–326
Cervix
  cancer and oral contraceptives, 426
  and prostaglandins, 431
Channels, blocking see Ionic channels
Charcoal, 351
'Cheese reaction', tyramine, 95, 524
Chemical assay, 49–56
  chromatography, 51–53
  enzyme linked immunoassay, 49–51
  fluorimetry, 55–56
  mass spectrometry, 53–55
  radioimmunoassay, 49
  spectrophotometry, 55–56
Chemotaxins
  inflammatory reaction, 180–191
  leukotrienes, 197
Chenodeoxycholic acid, 352, 354
Chloral hydrate, 498
  as 'displacing agent', 96
  and warfarin, action, 96, 287
Chlorambucil, 223, 612–614

Chloramphenicol, 626–627, 637–638
  and anticoagulants, 287
  bacterial protein synthesis, 601
  inactivation, 606, 607, 637
  enzyme inhibition, 97
  'grey baby' syndrome, 91
  reservoir effect, 81
  structure, 637
  unwanted effects, 638
Chlordiazepoxide
  characteristics, 494
  dosage, 495
  plasma albumin, 63
Chloroform, 5, 471–473
p-Chlorophenylalanine (PCPA)
  serotonin inhibition, 455
  sleep, abolishment, 457
  temperature response, 457
Chloroquine, 215–216
  in amoebiasis, 666
  assay, 56
  in malaria, 660–662
Chlorothiazide
  action, 329, 324
  structure, 319
Chlorotrianisene, 418
Chlorozotocin, 613–614
Chlorpheniramine, 220
Chlorpromazine
  anti-emetic, 343
  characteristics, 504
  clinical dose, 495, 501
  jaundice, 509
  leukopenia, 509
  measurement, 51
  plasma albumin, 63
  structure, 345, 503
Chlorpropamide
  and ADH, 368
  in diabetes, 390–391
  renal clearance, 78
  structure, 390
Chlorthalidone, 323
Cholecalciferol (vitamin D_3), 406
Cholecystokinin, 331
  octapeptide, 552
Cholelithiasis, 353–354
Cholera toxin, action, 22
Cholesterol
  and amphotericin, 653
  bile, formation, 352
  cholelithiasis, 353–354
  and cholestyramine, 356
  corticotrophin, effect, 403
  in glucocorticoid synthesis, 395–396
  lipoprotein transport, 354–355
    drugs in, 356
  metabolism and excretion, 354
  oestrogen synthesis, 416
  testosterone synthesis, 422
Cholestyramine, cholesterol reduction, 356
Choline
  and acetylcholine, 113
  acetyltransferase, 457

Choline (*contd*)
    in Huntington's chorea, 544
  in body fluids, 116
  in dementia, 460
  in Huntington's chorea, 460
  in Parkinsonism, 460
Cholinergic transmission, 113–144
  and arecoline, 460
  effect of drugs, 118–144
  and hyoscine, 460
  physiology, 115–118
  rat brain, 458
  short term memory, 460
  synapses, 115–116
  see also Acetylcholine:
      Acetylcholinesterase
Cholinesterase
  in cholinergic transmission, 113–118
  drug inactivation, 93
  hydrolysis of acetylcholine, 8
  see also Acetylcholinesterase
Chorionic gonadotrophin, 424
Chromaffin cells
  definition, 175
  noradrenaline storage, 151
  serotonin production, 262–263
Chromatographic techniques, gas
    chromatography-mass
    spectroscopy, 52–55
  high performance liquid, 53
Chromogranin A, 151–152
Chylomicrons, in
    hyperlipoproteinaemia, 355
Cigarettes and smoking, 678–683
  see also Nicotine: Smoking
Cimetidine
  H_2-receptor antagonist, 337
  and oral anticoagulants, 287
  vitamin B_{12} deficiency, 438
Cinchocaine, 583
Cinoxacin, 641–642
Circulation, drugs affecting, 256–278
  see also Cardiovascular system: Heart:
    Peripheral vascular system:
    and specific names
Circulatory shock, 161
Cirrhosis, 694
Cisplatin, 619
  action, 603, 611
  and anti-emetics, 344–345
  structure, 619
Citalopram, 525–526
Clindamycin, 627, 640–641
  bacterial protein synthesis, 601
Clinical trials, 43–46
  bias, 43
  double blind techniques, 43–44
  power, 44
  organization, 45–46
  randomization, 43
  sample size, 44
  sequential trials, 44–45
  Type I and II errors, 44
  see also Tests
Clofazimine, in leprosy, 646

Clofibrate, structure-activity, 356
Clomiphene, 419, 420
Clomipramine, 518–522
Clonazepam, 488
  in absence seizures, 539
  characteristics, 494
Clonidine
  action, 148, 173
  blood pressure regulation, 272, 450
  in hypertension, 161, 272–275
  in migraine, 278
  receptor specificity, 148
  summary, 164
Clorazepate, 488
Clorgyline, 522–523
Clotrimazole, 652, 656
  structure, 655
Cloxacillin, 632–633
Clozapine
  agranulocytosis, 509
  characteristics, 504
  clinical dose, 501
  structure, 503
Coagulation system, 179, 280–283
  defects, 283–285
  platelets, 289–296
    see also Platelets
  unwanted coagulation, 285–289
Cobalamins, 441
Cocaine, 573–574, 584–587
  action, 584–587
  psychomotor effect, 569, 574, 586
  structure, 583
  summary, 166
Coccidiomycosis, 652
Codeine, 564
  classification, 557
  cough suppressant, 307
  gastrointestinal motility, 351
  structure, 554
  $2+2$ assay, 42
Colchicine, 218
  and ADH, 368
  anticancer action, 604, 611
  diuretic effect, 316
  in gout, 619
  microtubules, 611
  structure, 217
  vitamin B_{12} deficiency, 438
Colistin, plasma half life, 90
Collagen
  diseases, and glucocorticoids, 401
  exposure and haemostasis, 281
  in platelet activation, 291
  synthesis, penicillamine, action, 214
Competitive drug antagonism, 5, 9
Complement system, 179
  and antibodies, 184–185
  alternate pathway, 179
  classical pathway, 184
  C3 enzymic splitting, 179
  C3a, anaphylatoxin, 184
    histamine, 186, 189
    inactivation, kininase I, 200
    mast cells, 180

C3b, opsonin, 181
  phagocytosis, 185
C4a inactivation, kininase, 200
C5 enzymic splitting, 179
C5a, chemotactic factor, 184
  histamine, 189
  inactivation, kininase, 200
  mast cells, 180
  neutrophil activation, 186, 193
  effect of glucocorticoids, 398
  kallikrein, activation, 199
COMT *see* Catechol-O-methyl
    transferase
Concentration-effect curves, 8
Conjugation, 73–77
  phase II reactions, glucuronide, 77
Contraceptives
  depot progestogen, 426
  oral *see* Oral contraceptives
  post-coital, 426
  spray, 424
Cooperativity, definition, 34
Coronary heart disease
  and alcohol, 685
  atherosclerosis, 235–236
  and smoking, 682
  see also Angina
Corpus striatum
  and cholinergic pathways, 458–460
  and dopaminergic pathways, 451–452
  Huntington's chorea, 539, 541
  Parkinsonism, 539–541
Corticosterone, 393
  biosynthesis, 390
  mechanism, 398–401
  metabolic and system effects, 397
  uses, unwanted effects, 401–402
  see also Glucocorticoids
Corticotrophin, 358–359, 366
  actions, 403
  and ADH, 368
  clinical use, 404
  'rate sensitive negative feedback
    response', 401
  -releasing factor, 359, 362, 366,
    403
  second messenger, 19
  structure, 403
  synthesis of glucocorticoids, 394–395
Cortisone, 393
  activation in liver, 78
  enzyme inhibition, 97
  pharmacokinetics, 402–403
Cotrimoxazole, 626–627
Cough, 307–308
  reflex, 559
  suppressants, sequential clinical trial,
    45
Coumarin anticoagulant
  and bacterial drugs, 95
  effect of disulfiram, 97
  genetic factors, plasma half life, 92
  and liquid paraffin, 95
  and vitamin K, 95
Cretinism, 369, 375

Cromoglycate
  in asthma, 303–304, 306–307
  biliary secretion, 73, 81
  inhalation, 70
Cryptococcosis, 652
Curare, 131
  see also Tubocurarine
Cushing's syndrome, 394, 402
  metyrapone in, 395
Cyanocobalamin, 441, 443
Cyclazocine, 555, 557
Cyclic adenosine monophosphate
  adenylate cyclase, 14, 20–22
  brain, accumulation, noradrenaline,
    449
  drugs increasing, 258
  effects, 265–266
  insulin-receptor interaction, 383
  nucleotide regulatory protein, 21
  protein kinases, 21–22, 25–27
  receptor, 21
    classification, 266
  regulation, 20–23
  second messenger, 19–20
Cyclic endoperoxides, 193
Cyclizine, 220–221
  antiemetic, 343
Cyclofenil, 419
Cyclo-oxygenase inhibition, by aspirin,
    293
Cyclopegia, muscarinic antagonists, 123
Cyclopenthiazide
  action, 320, 323–324
  structure, 319
Cyclopentolate
  ophthalmological use, 124
  structure, 122
Cyclophosphamide, 223, 612
  corticosteroids, effect, 97
  cytotoxicity, 89, 612
  metabolism, 89, 615
  nephrotoxicity, 78
  structure, 614
Cyclopropane, 476
  drawbacks, 482
  structure, 480
Cyclopropylamines, 523
Cycloserine, in tuberculosis, 645
Cyclosporin
  action, 221
  immune response, site, 182–183
  interleukin-2, 184
  renal toxicity, 695
  structure, 220
Cyproheptadine, 219, 265
Cyproterone, 420, 423
Cysteine, amino acid transmitter, 461
Cystinuria, penicillamine in, 214
Cytarabine
  anticancer action, 603, 611, 617–618
  resistance, 621
Cytochrome p450, 74
  inhibition, 337
Cytomegalovirus, 648
Cytosine arabinoside, 51

Cytotoxic antibodies, 610, 618–619
  drugs, 701

Dale's principle, nerve transmission,
    106–107, 187
Danazol, 420, 424–425
Danthron, 348
Dantrolene, muscle contraction, 136
Dapsone, 661, 664
  in leprosy, 646
Daunorubicin, 611, 618
  cell cycle, 621
DBH see Dopamine-β-hydroxylase
DDT, microsomal induction, 77
1-Deamino-oxytocin, 367
Debrisoquin
  action, 171–172
  genetic factors, 93
  and guanethidine, 166
  in hypertension, 274–275
  structure, 171
Decamethonium, 10
  action, 114
  disadvantages, 133
  fasciculation effect, 132–133
  neuromuscular blocking, 118, 127
  nicotinic agonists, 124–125
  structure, 124
Deep vein thrombosis, 295
Demeclocycline, action on ADH, 316,
    368
  structure-activity, 636–637
Dementia, 460
Denervation supersensitivity, 13
  and dopaminergic reception, 454
  increased postjunctional response,
    106
  loss of transmitter removal, 106
  proliferation of receptors, 106
Deoxycortone, 393
  absorption, 71
  in aldosterone replacement, 405
Deoxyuridylate monophosphate,
    439–440
Dependence, and tolerance, 560–563
Depolarizing blocking agents, 132–137
  comparison, non-depolarizing,
    133–135
  in myasthenia gravis, 133
  pharmacokinetic aspects, 136
  Phase I and Phase II, 135
  side effects and dangers, 135–136
Depot preparation, sustained release,
    89
Deprenyl (see Selegiline)
Depression
  animal models, 516–517
  antidepressants, 517–529
  bipolar and unipolar, 513
  hypothesis, 450
  monoamine theory, 513–517
  tryptophane in, 457
Dermatomycoses, 652

Dermatomyositis and lipocortin, 401
Desensitization, 31–33
Desferrioxamine in iron toxicity, 437
Desipramine, 518–522
  and imipramine, 166
Desmethylimipramine
  assay, 56
  binding to plasma albumin, 63
Desmopressin, 367–368
Dexamethasone, 346, 393, 402
Dexamphetamine, 569–573
Dextromethorphan, cough suppressant,
    308
Dextropropoxyphene, 555
Diabetes, 386–393
  β-receptor antagonists, effects,
    168–169
  drugs, 388–393
  drug interactions, 382
  hyperlipoproteinaemias, 355
  juvenile-onset, 387
  maturity-onset, 387
  oral contraceptives, 425
Diabetes insipidus, 367
  thiazides, antidiuresis, 324
Diacylglycerol, 23, 25
  lipase, 193
Diarrhoea, 350–352
  adsorbents in, 351
  antimotility agents, 350–351
Diazepam
  basal anaesthesia, 482–483
  benzodiazepines, 488–496
  characteristics, 494
  distribution volume, 72
  effective, and lethal dose, 495
  measurement, 51
  pharmacokinetics, 495
  plasma albumin, 63
  plasma half life, and age, 91
  saturation kinetics, 87
  status epilepticus, 539
  structure, 488
Diazoxide
  in hypertension, 261, 274–275, 320
  vasodilation, 324
Dibenzazepines, 518–522
Dibenzcycloheptenes, 518–522
Dibucaine (Cinchocaine)
  number, definition, 92
  pharmacokinetics, 587
  structure, 583
Dichloroisoprenaline, 167
Dichlorphenamide, 326
Dicloxacillin, 633
Dicoumarol, 284, 286
  inhibition, renal tubular secretion, 98
Dicyclomine, 337–338
Dienoestrol, 419
Diethylcarbamazine, 673–674
Diethyl ether, 5
Diflunisal, 205
  anti-inflammatory effects, 313
  control, severe pain, 206
  structure, 209

Digitoxin, 239–244
  drugs modifying action, 97
  indications, 243, 244
  measurement, 51
  plasma albumin, 63
Digoxin, 239–244
  distribution volume, 72
  formulation, 68
  indications, 243, 244
  loading dose, 84
  measurement, 51
  oral absorption, 68
  and renal function, 91
  'reservoir' effect, 81
Dihydrocodeine, 564
  structure, 554
Dihydroergotamine
  in migraine, 163
  partial agonist, 155
  receptor specificity, 148
  structure and action, 162
Dihydrofolate reductase
  action of folates, anticancer, 615–616
  inhibitors, 664
    structures, 661
  methotrexate receptor, 6
Dihydropyridines, 248–250
  structure, 248
Dihydrotachysterol, 408–409
Dihydroxymandelic acid (DOMA), 155–156
Dihydroxyphenylacetic acid (DOPAC), 451–452
Dihydroxyphenylalanine (DOPA), 150
Diiodohydroxyquinoline, 665
Diloxanide, 665–666
Diltiazem, 248–250
  structure, 248
Dimaprit
  potency, 189
  structure, 190
Dimenhydrinate, 220–221
  in motion sickness, 343
Dimercaprol, 28
Dimethylphenylpiperazinium (DMPP)
  ganglion stimulation, 124–125
  structure, 124
Dimethyltryptamine in schizophrenia, 500
Dinoprost (prostaglandins F_2, E_2), 198, 431
Dinoprostone, 431
Dioctyl sodium sulphosuccinate, 347–348
Diphenadione, 284, 286
Diphenhydramine, 218–220
  antiemetic, 343
Diphenoxylate, 351
Diphosphonates, calcium homeostasis, 410–411
Diphtheria toxin, 4
Dipyridamole
  action, 254, 255
  adenosine uptake, inhibition, 266
  antithrombotic action, 293

in coronary circulation, 253
Disodium etidronate, 410
Disopyramide, 246
Distribution, 71–73, 81–89
  antibody-drug conjugates, 89
  body fluid compartments, 71–72
  liposomes, packaging, 89
  removal from body, 72–73
  sustained release preparations, 89
  time course models, saturation
      kinetics, 87–89
    single compartment, 81–86
    two compartment, 86–87
  volumes, examples, 73
Disulfiram
  and alcohol, 688
  dopamine β-hydroxylase inhibition, 151
  enzyme inhibition, 97
Diuretics, 318–328
  acid-base balance, 327
  braking phenomenon, 326
  calcium balance, 327
  cerebral oedema, 325–326
  distal nephron, 323–325
  general aspects, 326–327
  and glycoside toxicity, 94
  in hypertension see Thiazide diuretics
  loop, 314, 321–323
  obsolete drugs, 326
  organic molecules, alterations in
      excretion, 318, 328
  osmotic, 319, 325–326
  potassium balance, 327
  pH alteration, 327–328
  sodium absorption, sites of drug
      action, 313
  uric acid excretion, 327
  see also Individual drugs
DMPP see Dimethylphenylpiperazinium
DNA
  alkylation and cross linking, 613
  cytotoxic agents, summary, 611
  folates, DNA synthesis, 615–616
  intrastrand linking, 612
  and mutagenesis, 695–696
    see also Cell cycle
  oncogenes, 623–625
  synthesis, in erythrocytes, 437–438
    folates, 439
  transcription, regulation, 27
Dobutamine receptor specificity, 148
DOMA see Dihydroxymandelic acid
Domperidone
  action, 345–346
  anti-emetic, 343
  as dopamine receptor, 268
  gastrointestinal motility, 349
  reduction, side effects, levadopa, 543
  structure, 345
DOPA see Dihydroxyphenylalanine
Dopa decarboxylase, 150, 541–543
DOPAC (Dihydroxyphenylacetic acid), 451–452
Dopamine, 451–455

action, 268
  β-hydroxylase, 151
  biosynthesis, 150
  definition, 175
  functional aspects, 453–455
  growth hormone, 455
  hypovolaemic shock, 275–277
  pathways, CNS, 451–453
  peripheral transmitters, 266–267
  pituitary gland mediators, 454–455
  and prolactin, 454
  receptors, CNS, 453, 505–507
    classification, 267–268, 453
  schizophrenia, theories, 500–501
  second messenger, 19
  structure-activity, 146, 157, 452
  sympathetic ganglia, 110
  as transmitter, 36
  turnover index, 451
  vomiting reflex, 341–342
    antiemetics, 343
Dosage
  'area under the curve', 85
  loading dose, 84
  varying absorption, 84–85
  varying schedules, 83–84
Dose ratio, 9–10, 33
Dose-response curve, 8
Doxapram, 299, 568–571
  structure, 570
Doxepin, 518
Doxorubicin
  anticancer action, 611, 618
  and anti-emetics, 344
  cell cycle, 621
Doxycycline, 636–637
Droperidol, anti-emetic, 344
  characteristics, 504
  clinical dose, 501
Drug-receptor complex, 6
  see also Receptors
Dyflos
  action, 139
  eyedrops, 69
  irreversibility, 141
  structure, 139
Dynorphin, 556

Ear, ototoxicity, aminoglycosides, 639
  loop diuretics, 322
Econazole, 652, 656
  structure, 654
Ecothiopate
  action, 139
  in glaucoma, 142
  interactions, 97
  'irreversibility', 141
  structure, 139
ED50 (median, individual effective
    doses), 38
  difficulty of definition, 48
Edrophonium
  anticholinesterase, 138
  structure, 139

Efficacy, definition, 34
Ehrlich, Paul, 4
Eicosanoids, 181, 192–199
    and chloroquine, 216
    see also Leukotrienes: Prostaglandins:
        Thromboxanes
Electroconvulsive therapy, 517, 526
Elimination, drug
    protein binding, 85–86
    rate constant, k_{el}, 82
    see also Excretion
Embolus, definition, 280
Emetics, 342
    anti-emetics, teratogenicity, 702
    cannabis, 690
Emetine, in amoebiasis, 665–666
EMIT (Enzyme multiplied
        immunoassay technique), 51
Endocrine system, 359–411
    adrenal steroids, 393–405
    pancreas, 369–393
    parathyroid, 405–411
    pituitary, anterior, 359–366
        posterior, 366–369
    thyroid, 369–378
Endometrium
    carcinoma, 421
    effect of danazol on, 425
    hyperplasia, oestrogen induced, 697
    in menstrual cycle, 413–414
    prostaglandin synthesis, 430
Endorphins, opioid peptides, 556
Enkephalin, and morphine, 465
Enkephalins, opioid peptides, 556
Enflurane, 476, 482
    structure, 480
Entero-oxyntin, 332
Enzyme induction, drug interactions,
        table, 96–97
Enzyme multiplied immunoassay
        technique, 51
Eosinophils
    anaphylactic hypersensitivity, 186
    parasites, reactions against, 185
Ephedrine
    in asthma, 304
    and monoamine oxidase inhibitors,
        94, 524
    structure-activity, 172–173
    tachycardia, 259
Epidermal growth factor, 695
    monoclonal antibodies, 624
Epstein-Barr virus, 648
Epilepsy, 530–539
    absences, 531
    anticonvulsant drugs, 533–539
    drugs used in, 533–539
    Jacksonian, 531
    mechanisms, 531–533
    psychomotor, 531
    tonic-clonic (grand mal), 531
Epsp *see* Excitatory post-synaptic
        potential
Equilibrium constant, definition, 33
Ergocalciferol (vitamin D_2), 408–409

Ergometrine, 429–430
    action, 155, 162, 430
    dopamine blocking, 267, 454
    structure, 162
    unwanted effects, 430
Ergosterol
    and amphotericin, 653
    structure, 406
Ergot alkaloids, 161–163
Ergotamine, 430
    in migraine, 162–163, 277–278
    receptor specificity, 148
    structure, 162
    summary, 165
Erythrocytes, 433
Erythromycin, 626–627, 640
    effect, 601
    structure, 640
Erythropoiesis, and vitamin B_{12} or
        folate, 437
Eserine
    eyedrops, 69
    see also Physostigmine
Estramine phosphate, 614
Ethacrynic acid, 320–322
    and organic nitrates, 251
Ethamarin, 299
Ethambutol, in tuberculosis, 644–645
Ethanol
    biological specificity, 4
    chemical specificity, 4–5
    distribution volume, 72
    enzyme induction, 97
    microsomal activity, 77
    potency, 4
    saturation kinetics, 87
    specific antagonists, 5
    see also Alcohol
Ether, 476, 481
    structure, 480
Ethinyloestradiol, 418
Ethoglucid, 614
Etomidate, 483
Etoposide, anticancer, 620
Ethosuximide
    in epilepsy, 533–535, 537–538
    measurement, 51
Ethoxzolamide, 326
Ethylbiscoumacetate, vitamin
        K antagonist, 284, 286
Ethyloestrenol, 423
Excitatory aminoacids, 463–464
    receptors, 464
Excitatory post-synaptic potential,
        116–117
    action, tubocurarine, 117
Excretion, of drugs
    biliary, 81
    renal, 78–81
Exophthalmia, 374
Extrinsic pathway, blood coagulation,
        282–283
Eye
    canal of Schlemm, 121
    ciliary muscle, innervation, 105

eyedrops, 69–70
    glaucoma, 121
    intraocular pressure, increase,
        suxamethonium, 135
    muscarinic agonists, effect, 120–122
        antagonists, 123–124
    oculomicocutaneous syndrome,
        practolol, 169
    oculomotor nerve, 103
    pupil, innervation, 105
    see also Ophthalmology

Factors II-X, and oestrogens, 417
Factors II-XII in blood coagulation
    coagulation cascade, 179, 288
    extrinsic pathway, 282–283
    intrinsic pathway, 281–282
    and oestrogens, 417
    vitamin K, 283–286
Factor VIII, and ADH, 368
Factor XII
    activation, 199
    coagulation cascade, 179
'False transmitter', 130
Fat, partition of drug molecules, 62–63
Fazadinium, muscle block, recovery
        rate, 136
Felypressin, 367
    in vasoconstriction, 260
Fenbufen, 205
    structure, 208
Fenclofenac, 205
Fenfluramine, 571–573
    anorexia, 572
    in obesity, 573
    structure, 570
Fenoprofen, 208
    analgesia, 212
Fentanyl, 555, 557
    in anaesthesia, 564
Ferritin, storage, 434–436
Ferrous iron salts, 437
Fetal development, 699–700
    and cannabis, 690
    effect of smoking, 682
    fetal alcohol syndrome, 685–686
    teratogenesis, definite and possible
        agents, 699
Fever, prostaglandin E_1, 198
Fibrin formation, in haemostasis,
        281
Fibrinolysis, 294–296
Fibroblasts, effects, glucocorticoids,
        398
Filaria, 669
First-order kinetics, 87
First pass metabolism, 77–78
    and alcohol absorption, 687
Flucloxacillin, 633
Flucytosine
    action, 603
    antifungal effect, 654
    and amphotericin, 653

Flucytosine (*contd*)
  resistance, development, 654
Fludrocortisone, 393
  adrenal replacement therapy, 405
Flufenamic acid, 213
Fluid compartments of body, 71–72
Flunitrezepam, 488
Fluorescence histochemistry, 150
Fluorimetry, 55–56
Fluorouracil
  absorption, 67
  action, 603, 611, 617
  structure, 617
Fluoxymesterone, 423
Flupenthixol
  characteristics, 504
  structure, 503
Fluphenazine
  anti-emetic action, 343
  characteristics, 504
  clinical dose, 501, 510
  structure, 345, 503
Fluphenazine undecanoate, sustained
    release, 89
Flurazepam, 488
Flurbiprofen, 205
  structure, 208
Folate antagonists
  anticancer drugs, 614–617
  bacterial, class II reactions, 603
  fetal malformations, 701
  see also Methotrexate
Folate synthesis, antimalarial drugs,
    663–664
Folic acid, 437–440
  deficiency, 440
Follicle stimulating hormone, 359,
    413–415
Framycetin, 638–639
Frusemide, 320–322
  excretion of indomethacin, 98
Fusidic acid, 601, 642

GABA *see* γ-Aminobutyric acid
Galactorrhea, 365–366
Gallamine
  absorption failure, oral and
      placental, 131–132
  excretion, 79, 80
  muscarinic receptors, 132
  pharmacokinetic aspects, 136–137
  structure, 126
Gallstones, 353–354
Galvanic skin response, 487
Gamma-aminobutyric acid (GABA) *see*
    γ-Aminobutyric acid
Gamma globulin, antiviral action, 648
Ganglia, autonomic nervous system,
    103–107
Ganglion blocking drugs, 125–129
  action, 125–128
  effects, 128–129
  uses, 129

Ganglion stimulating drugs, 125–129
Gastric function, histamine, 189, 191
  see also Stomach
Gastric inhibitory peptide, 331–332
  and growth hormone releasing factor,
      360
Gastrin activity, 333–334
Gastrointestinal disorder, bradykinin
    in, 200
Gastrointestinal tract, 330–356
  bile, 352–356
  ganglion stimulating drugs, 125
  gastric secretion, 332–339
  innervation and hormones, 330–332
  morphine, effects, 559–560
  motility, 346–352
  muscarinic agonists, 120
    antagonists, 122–124
  serotonin, effects, 263
  vomiting, 339–346
Gate control theory, 548–549
  gating behaviour, 579–582
  gating currents, 582
  potassium channels, drugs, 582–583
  gating, 589–590
  sodium channels, drugs, 590
  see also 4-Aminopyridine: Ionic
      channels:
      Tetraethylammonium
GDP *see* Guanosine diphosphate
Gel filtration chromatography, 52
Genetic factors, drug metabolism,
    92–94
  idiosyncratic reactions, 94
Genins, 239
Gentamycin, 638
  bacterial protein synthesis, 600
  extracellularity, 72
  plasma half life, 91
  in babies, 91
Glaucoma
  β-receptor antagonists, 169
  ecothiopate, 142
  eyedrops, 69
  and glucocorticoids, 402
  physostigmine, 142
  timolol, 165, 169
Glibenclamide, 390–392
Glibornuride, 390–392
Glicazide, 391–392
Glipizide, 390–392
β-Globulin, 63
Glossopharyngeal nerve, 103
Glucagon, 383–385
  action, on heart, 255
  blood glucose, effect on, 386, 387
  second messenger, 19
Glucocorticoids
  action, 193, 395–401
    drugs modifying, 97
  anti-inflammatory drugs, 223
    sites of action, 191
  in asthma, 307
  cell-mediated immune response,
      183

'counter regulatory hormones', 386
Cushing's syndrome, 394
effect of hormones, 386
endogenous and synthetic, 393–394
interactions, 398–401
pharmacokinetics, 402
synthesis and release, 394–395
therapeutic use, 401
unwanted effects, 401–402
Glucose, blood
  control, 385–386
  effect of hormones, 386
Glucose-6-phosphate dehydrogenase
    and primaquine, 94
Glucuronides
  conjugation, 77
  enterohepatic circulation, 81
Glucuronyl groups, conjugation, 74–76
Glucuronyl transferase in neonates, 91
Glutamate
  amino acid transmitter, 461
  'Chinese restaurant syndrome', 464
  excitatory transmitter, 463–464
Glutamic acid decarboxylase in
    Huntington's chorea, 544
Glutamyl group, conjugation, 76
Glutathione deficiency and
    paracetamol, 695
Glutethimide
  action, 498
  effective, and lethal dose, 495
  and oral anticoagulants, 287
  structure, 496
Glyceryl trinitrate, 251–254
  administration, cutaneous, 69
    oral, 66, 78
  biliary spasm, 354
Glycine, as amino acid transmitter,
    461–463
Glycogen synthase, inactivation, 27
Glycogenolysis, β-adrenoreceptor
    activation, 27
Glycoprotein, acid, in plasma, 63
Glycosuria, 386–387
Glycyl group, conjugation, 76
cGMP *see* Guanosine monophosphate
Goitre
  diffuse toxic, 374
  drugs in, 375–378
  exophthalmic, 334
  simple, 375, 377
  toxic nodular, 374–375
Gold, in rheumatoid arthritis, 213–214
Gonadorelin (gonadotrophic releasing
    hormone), 362, 424
Gonadotrophin releasing factor, 359,
    362, 424
  prolactin, effect, 365
Gonadotrophins
  clinical use, 424
  preparations, 424
  see also Follicle stimulating hormone:
      Luteinizing hormone
Gout, 216–217
  probenecid in, 79

Grand mal *see* Epilepsy
Graves disease, 374, 376
    and radio-iodine, 378
'Grey baby' syndrome, 91, 638
Griseofulvin, 652, 656
    action, 604
    enzyme induction, 97
    structure, 654
Growth hormone, 358, 362–363
    blood glucose, 386
    lipolytic action, effect of insulin, 382
    -release inhibiting factor
        (somatostatin), 359–363
    -releasing factor, 359–362
GTP *see* Guanosine triphosphate
Guanethidine
    absorption, 67
    action, 171–172
    in hypertension, 274–275
    structure, 171
    summary, 166
    uptake, and antidepressants, 95
Guanosine diphosphate (GDP),
    and adenylate cyclase, 21–23
Guanosine monophosphate (cGMP),
    and smooth muscle, 251, 258
Guanosine triphosphate (GTP),
    and adenylate cyclase, 21–23
Guanylate cyclase, 27
Gynaecomastia
    danazol in, 425
    and prolactin, 365–366

H_2 receptor antagonists, 336–337
Haematological reactions to drugs,
    704–705
Haemoglobin
    absorption in diet, 434–435
    structure, 434
Haemolytic anaemias, 433
Haemophilia, 283
Haemopoietic system, 433–443
Haemosiderin, 434–436
    storage, 434
Haemostasis, 281–296
Hageman factor (XII)
    coagulation cascade, 179
    fibrinolysis, 294
    intrinsic pathway, 281–282
    kininogen activation, 199
Hallucinogens, 470, 575–577
Haloalkylamines, 31, 163
Haloperidol
    action, rat brain, 506
    anti-emetic, 343–344
    characteristics, 504
    clinical dose, 501
    distribution volume, 72
    dopamine, blocking effect, 267
    structure, 503
Halothane, 5, 476
    hepatotoxicity, 698
    malignant hyperpyrexia, 94

metabolization, 480–481
    structure, 480
Hapten, definition, 186
Hashimoto's disease, 375
HDL *see* Lipoproteins, high density
Heart, 227–255
    atrioventricular block, 161, 242–244
    contraction, 231–234
        effect of autonomic transmitters,
            236–239
        effect of dopamine, 267
        effect of glycosides, 239–241
        effect of methylxanthines, 254
    coronary blood flow and oxygen
        consumption, 234–235
        effects of drugs, 250–254
    disturbances of rhythm, 229–231
    drugs acting on, 236–255
        antianginal, 250–254
        antidyrhythmias, 244–250
        autonomic transmitters, 236–239
        cardiac glycosides, 239–244
        endogenous substances, 254–255
        see also specific drugs
    failure, 233–234, 241
        drugs, used in, 273, 276
        pathogenesis, 276
    mutual presynaptic inhibition, 108
    rate and rhythm, 227–231
    see also Cardiovascular function
Heavy metals, teratogenicity, 701
Hemicholinium, 130
    acetylcholine inhibition, 119
Henderson-Hasselbalch equation, 60
Heparin
    anticoagulant, 285, 287–289
    clinical trial *vs* urokinase, 46
    cofactor, antithrombin III, 283
    distribution, 72
        by injection, 70
    from mast cells, 180
Hepatic metabolism
    clearance rate, 81
    enterohepatic circulation, 81
Hepatotoxicity, 693–695
Hering-Breuer reflex, 297
Heroin, 557, 563–564
    high performance chromatography,
        53
    sequential trial, 45
    structure, 554
    see also Morphine
Herpes viruses, and vidarabine,
    648–649
Hexamethonium
    action, 31, 127–128
    chain length, and activity, 125
    'hexamethonium man', 128
    structure, 126
Hexobarbitone, effective and lethal
    dose, 495
Hexoestrol, 419
5 HIAA *see* 5-Hydroxyindoleacetic acid
Hill plot
    coefficient, 34

definition, 34
Histamine, 187–192
    acid secretion test, 336
    action, 189–192
        heart, 255
    anaphylactic hypersensitivity, 186
    antagonists, 218–221
    antihistamines, 188
    biological specificity, 4
    chemical specificity, 4–5
    as CNS transmitter, 468–469
    competitive antagonists, 6
    gastric secretion, 191, 333–335
    H_1, H_2 effects, 6, 19, 218–221
    H_1 and H_2 agonists, action, 188–192
        structures, 190
    potency, 4
    and prostaglandins, vasodilatation,
        197
    receptors, 5, 188–189
    release, and catecholamines, 160
        morphine induced, 560, 563
    smooth muscle, 189
    specific antagonists, 5
    in stomach, 332, 335
    structure, 188
    'triple response', 190–191
Histoplasmosis, 652
'Hit and run' drugs, 57
Hodgkin's disease
    mustine in, 612
    procarbazine in, 620
Homatropine
    ophthalmological use, 124
    structure, 120
Homeopathy, 3
Homovanillic acid
    dopamine turnover, 451
    structure, 452
Hookworm infestation, iron loss,
    436–437
Human chorionic gonadotrophin, 424
Huntington's chorea, 544
    and acetylcholine release, 460
    cause, possible, 539
    dopamine excess, 454
    glutamate metabolism, 464
Hyaluronidase, and drug absorption, 70
Hydantoins *see* Phenytoin
Hydatid tapeworm, 670
Hydatidiform mole, prostaglandins,
    431
Hydrallazine
    acetylator status, 260
    in hypertension, 274–275
    plasma half-life, 63
    vasodilation, 260–261
Hydrazines, 523
    hepatotoxicity, 698
Hydrochlorothiazide
    action, 320, 323–324
    structure, 319
Hydrocortisone, 393, 401–403
    mechanism, 398–401
    metabolic effects, 397

Hydrocortisone (*contd*)
structure, 396
therapeutic uses and unwanted
effects, 401–402
Hydrolytic reactions, 76
Hydroquinone (vitamin K), 283–286
Hydroxocobalamin, 441, 443
Hydroxyapatite, in bone, 405
oral, 407
Hydroxychloroquine, 660–661
6-Hydroxydopamine, action, 170
5-Hydroxyindoleacetic acid
carcinoid syndrome, 263
monoamine theory of depression, 515
serotonin metabolism, 262–263
structure, 262
in suicide, 516
Hydroxyprogesterone hexanoate, 420
4-Hydroxypropanolol, 78
Hydroxyquinolines, amoebiasis, 666
5-Hydroxytryptamine *see* Serotonin
Hydroxyurea, 619, 620
Hyoscine
anaesthesia, premedication, 123
anti-emetic, 343–344
cutaneous administration, 69
in learning and memory, 460
in motion sickness, 124
structure, 122
Hyperaldosteronism, 394
Hypercalcaemia
glucocorticoids, 411
loop diuretics, 323
sodium cellulose phosphate, 411
vitamin D, 409–410
Hyperemesis gravidarum, 342, 344
Hyperglycaemia, 386, 390
Hyperkalaemia
and aldosterone, 404
and diuretics, 323, 324, 327
Hyperlipidaemia, 354–356
Hyperlipoproteinaemia, 354–356
Hyperprolactinaemia, 365
Hyperpyrexia, malignant, 94
Hypersensitivity reactions, 186–187
thiazides, 324
Hypertension
adrenergic blocking drugs, 172
antagonists, α-receptor, 167
α_2-receptors, 173
β-receptors, 167–169
clonidine, 161
mechanisms and drugs, 272
Hyperthermia, malignant, 136
Hyperthyroidism, 375–378
Hyperuricaemia, 327
Hypnotics, 495
see also Benzodiazepines: Chloral
hydrate: Glutethimide:
Methaqualone:
Trichlorethanol
Hypoglycaemic drugs, 388–393
Hypokalaemia, 327
and aldosterone, 404
Hypoparathyroidism, 410

Hypoprothrombinaemia, 285
Hypotension, 272–275
Hypotensive drugs, 274–275
see also Individual drugs
Hypothalamus, 358
hormones, 359–366
Hypothyroidism, 375, 378
hyperlipoproteinaemia, 355
Hypovolaemia, following diuresis, 322
HVA (Homovanillic acid), 451–452

Ibuprofen, 205
action, 207
analgesia, 212
structure, 208
Idiosyncratic reactions, 48, 90, 94
footnote, 692
and LD50, 46
Idoxuridine, 603, 648–649
Ifosfamide, 614
Imidazoles, 654–656
action, 604
arachidonate metabolites, platelets,
292
Imipramine
antischizophrenic action, 517
measurement, 51
metabolism, 74–75, 521
and oral anticoagulants, 287
plasma albumin, 63
structure, 519
summary, 166
Immune response, 178–203
antibody-mediated, drugs, sites, 182
augmentation, in cancer, 622–623
bradykinin, 198–201
cell-derived mediators, 181–182, 187
cell-mediated, drugs, sites, 183
cellular events, 180–181
chemical mediators, Dale's criteria,
106–107, 187
chronic inflammation, 187
effector phase, 184–185
eicosanoids, 181, 192–199
histamine, 187–192
induction and regulation, 183–184
interleukin, 202–203
lymphocytes, 182
outcome, 187
platelet activating factor, 182,
201–202
specific response, 182–187
unwanted responses, Types I-IV,
185–187
vascular events, 178–179
Immunoassay
enzyme-linked, 49–51
radio-, 49
Immunoglobulins *see* Antibodies
Immunological mechanisms, 703–704
Immunosuppressants, 221–223
antilymphocyte immunoglobulin, 223
and mycoses, 652
Implantation, subcutaneous, 71

Impotence, and prolactin, 365–366
Impromidine
potency, 189
structure, 190
Indapamide
action, 324
structure, 323
Indomethacin
acute and chronic toxicity, 46–47,
698
and ADH, 368
antidiarrhoeal action, 351
anti-inflammatory action, 205, 207
inhibition, renal tubular secretion, 98
LD50, 47
severe pain, 206
Indoramin
antagonists, α_1 receptors, 163
and prazosin, 165
receptor specificity, 148
Induction, microsomal activity, 77
Inflammatory reaction, 178
asthma, acute, 302–304
diagram, 180
effects, glucocorticoids, 397–398
see also Immune response
Infusion of drugs, continuous, 83
INH *see* Isoniazid
Inhalation anaesthetics, 476–483
action of ethanol, 5
Inhibitory post-synaptic potential, 117
Injection
intramuscular, 70
intrathecal, 71
intravenous, 70
subcutaneous, 70
Inositol triphosphate *see*
Triphosphoinositol
Insecticides
DDT, 590
neurotoxicity, 141–142
organophosphates, 69
parathion, 139–141
praloxidine, antidote, 142–143
pyrethrins, 590
Insulin, 379–383, 388–390
actions, 381–383
allergy, 390
blood glucose, summary, 386
'insulin-like' effect, growth hormone,
363
insulin-opposing hormones, 390
isophane, 388–389
lipodystrophy, 390
preparations, actions, 388–390
receptors, isolation, 16
summary diagram, 384
synthesis and secretion, 379–381
zinc suspensions, 71
Interactions of drugs, 94–98
effects, distribution, 96
excretion, 97–98
haemodynamic, 97
metabolic, 96–97
pharmaceutical, in vitro, 94

Interactions of drugs (*contd*)
  pharmacodynamic, 94–95
  pharmacokinetic, 95–96
Interferons, 203, 623
  mechanism, 650–651
  nomenclature, 650
  unwanted effects, 651
Interleukin-1
  'endogenous pyrogen', 198, 206
  gold salts, effect, 214
  release, 183
  structure-activity, 202–203
Interleukin-2
  proliferation of T-cells, 184
  recombinant, trials, 623
Interstitial cell stimulating hormone
        (luteinising hormone), 359,
        421
Intestine
  absorption, 59, 66–69
  carrier mediated transport, 62
Intravenous anaesthetics, 483–485
Intrinsic factor, 438
  action, 441
Intrinsic pathway, blood coagulation,
        281–282
Iodide, iodine, 377–378
  and perchlorate, 378
  see also Thyroid hormone
Ionic channels, 16–19
  acetylcholine patch clamp technique,
        19, 31
  agonist concentration, 31
  channel blocking, 127–128
  of excitable membranes, 579–583
        inactivation, 581
        potassium channels, 590
        sodium channels, 582–583
  noise analysis, 17–18
  receptor binding, 16–19
  single channel, current measurement,
        18–19
Ionization
  dissociation constant pKa, 60
        drug values, 61
  Henderson-Hasselbalch equation,
        60
  partition and ion trapping, 61–62
Ion-trapping effect, 61–62
  renal excretion, 79–80
Ipratropium bromide, antiasthmatic,
        306
Iprindole, 514, 525–526
Iproniazid, 517, 522–523
  hepatotoxicity, 524, 698
Ipsp *see* Inhibitory post-synaptic
        potential
IP₃ *see* Triphosphoinositol
Iron, 434–437
  absorption, 67
  clinical use, 437
  daily turnover, 436
  deficiency anaemia, 436–437
  requirements, 434
  toxicity, 437

Islets of Langerhans, 378–389
  α₁ (somatostatin-secreting) cells,
        378–379
  α₂ (glucagon-secreting) cells, 378–379
  β (insulin-secreting) cells, 378, 380
  streptozotocin, antitumour, 613–614
Isoniazid (INH)
  assay, 56
  genetic factors, 91–93
  hepatotoxicity in fast acetylators, 93
  neuropathy, 93
  structure, 643
  in tuberculosis, 643–644
Isonicotinic acid hydrazide *see* Isoniazid
Isophane insulin, 388–389
Isoprenaline
  adenylate cyclase response, 32
  aerosol use, 70
  in asthma, 161
  cardiovascular effects, 159
  definition, 175
  receptor specificity, 148
  structure, and activity, 146, 157
  summary, 164
Isosorbide, 325–326
  dinitrate, 251–254
Isoxsuprine, uterus, inhibition, 428
Ispaghula, 347

Juxtaglomerular apparatus, 310–311

Kainic acid (KAI receptor), 464
Kallidin, 198–200
  pain production, 551
Kallikrein, 198–201
Kanamycin, 600, 638
  plasma half life, 90
Kaolin, 351
Kernicterus, and bilirubin, 96
Ketaconazole, 652, 655
  structure, 655
Ketamine, 470
  basal anaesthesia, 483, 485
Ketanserin, and serotonin, 263, 456
Ketoprofen, 205
  structure, 208
Ketosis, diabetes mellitus, 387
Ketotifen
  in asthma, 307
  serotonin antagonist, 265
Khellin *see* Cromoglycate
Kidney, 309–328
  control of osmolarity, 315–318
  disease, complex-mediated
        hypersensitivity, 186
  drugs, action, 318–328
        oxytocin, antidiuresis, 429
        sodium excretion, aldosterone, 405
  function, 309–315
  oxytocin, antidiuresis, 429
  sodium excretion, aldosterone, 405

  structure, 309–315
  see also Renal
'Killer' cells, *see* Lymphocytes
Kinetic models *see* Pharmacokinetics
Kininogens, 198–200
Kinins, 179–180
  pain production, 551

Labetalol
  α and β receptor blocking, 163
  in hypertension, 274–275
  in phaeochromocytoma, 167
  receptor specificity, 148
  summary, 165
Lachesine, structure, 122
β-Lactamases, in inactivation of
        penicillins, 606, 632–633
Lactation
  and nicotine, 682
  prolactin, 365
Lactulose, 348
Langmuir equation, 7, 12–13
  definition, 34
Latamoxef, 635–636
LATS (long acting thyroid stimulants)
        see Hyperthyroidism
Law of Mass Action, 7
  equilibrium constant, 7
  occupancy, 7
Laxatives, 347–348
Lecithin, in dementia, 460
LD50 test, 46–47
Leech, dorsal muscle bioassay, 102
Leishmaniasis, 667
Leprosy, 645–646
  inflammatory response, 187
Leptazol, 299
  induced convulsions, 532, 568–571
  structure, 570
Leukotrienes
  action, 197
  anti-inflammatory drugs, 206
  in asthma, 303
  B4, 184
  classification, 195–197
  cysteinyl-leukotrienes, 198
  in inflammation, 197–198
Levallorphan, 554
Levamisole, 670–671, 674
  antihelminth action, 604
Levodopa
  absorption, 67
  in acromegaly, 363
  dopamine release, 455
        replacement, 541–543
  hypotension, 542
  nausea and anorexia, 542
  optimization of treatment, 542
  in Parkinsonism, 541–543
  'on-off' effect, 542
  plasma half-life, 541
  prolactin release, 365
  psychological effects, 542

Levodopa (*contd*)
  structure, 540
Levorphanol, 554–555
  cough suppressant, 308
LHRH *see* Luteinizing hormone
  releasing hormone
Lidocaine (Lignocaine), 583
Lie detector test, 487
Ligands
  binding curves, 14
  definition, 33
  and occupancy, 7
Lignocaine
  action, 584–586
  administration, 587–588
  injection, 70, 78
  liver metabolism, 97
  measurement, 51
  plasma albumin, 63
  structure, 583
  unwanted effects, 587
  ventricular dysrhythmia, 245–247
Limbic system
  dopamine, 451
  mesolimbic pathway, 452
Lincomycin, 640
  bacterial protein synthesis, 601
Liothyronine, 378
Lipid metabolism, effect of alcohol,
  685
Lipid solubility, renal excretion, 79
Lipolysis, β-adrenoreceptor activation,
  27
Lipocortin, 399
Lipodystrophy, 390
Lipomodulin, 399–401
Lipoproteins, 354–356
  high density, alcohol-induced
    increase, 685
  low density, 685
Liposomes, 'packaging' of drugs, 89
Lipoxygenase pathway, 195–197
Liquid paraffin, 347
  effect on drug absorption, 68, 95
Lithium
  and ADH, 368
  diuretic effect, 316
  in hyperthyroidism, 378
  in manic-depressive illness, 528–529
  in psychosis, 470
  toxic effects, 529
Liver disease, acquired clotting defects,
  283
Liver function
  ADH and glycogen breakdown, 368
  effects of ethanol, 684–685
  hepatotoxicity, 693–695
  metabolism of alcohol, 687–688
  and oral contraceptives, 426
Lobeline
  ganglion stimulation, 124
  structure, 124
Local anaesthetics, 583–588
  administration, 587–588
    epidural, 588

intravenous regional, 587
  nerve block, 588
  surface, 588
  comparison, 587
  mechanism, 584–586
  unwanted effects, 587
Lomustine, 613–614
Loperamide, gastrointestinal motility,
  351
Lorazepam, 488
LSD *see* Lysergic acid diethylamide
Lung
  airways, regulation, 299–301
  musculature, regulation, 299–301
  non-respiratory functions, 299
Luteinising hormone, 359, 413–415,
  421–422
  releasing hormone, 110–111
Lymphocytes, 180, 182–187
  antigen-sensitive 'memory' cells, 183
  catecholamines, 160
  glucocorticoids, effects, 398
  K (killer) cells, 185
  prostaglandins, neutrophils, 198
  T-cells, cytotoxic, 184
    lymphokines, 184–186
Lymphotoxin, recombinant cloning,
  623
Lypressin, 368 369
Lysergic acid, 161 163
Lysergic acid diethylamide
  psychomimetic action, 569, 576–577
  serotonin antagonist, 265, 455
  structure, 162, 575
Lyso-PAF *see* Platelet activating factor

M_1, M_2 receptors *see* Muscarinic
  receptors
Macrocortin, 399–401
  inflammatory inhibition, 181
Macrocytes, in megaloblastic anaemia,
  438
Macrolides (erythromycin), 640
Macrophages, 181
  Fc receptors, 185
  growth factor, suppression of
    leukaemia, 625
  interleukin-1, 202
    '-activating factor', 203
  phagocytosis, 185
  see also Complement system
Magnesium
  acetylcholine release, blockage, 119
  aluminium silicate, 351
  calcium entry, inhibition, 130
  depletion, in diuresis, 322
  hydroxide, 338
  salts, in purgation, 347–348
  trisilicate, 338
Malaria, 657–665
  antimalarial drugs, 3, 215, 660–665
  eradication programme, failure, 657
  glutathione deficiency, 94

immunity, 660
  life cycle, 657–659
  recombinant DNA techniques, 660
  species, 659–660
Malignant hyperthermia (hyperpyrexia,
  94, 136
Mammotrophin (prolactin), 363–366
Mania, hypothesis, 450
Mannitol, in diuresis, 325–326
MAO *see* Monoamine oxidase
MAOI *see* Monoamine oxidase
  inhibitors
Maprotiline, 525–526
Mast cells, 180
  and antibodies, 185
  heparin in, 288
  histamine, 187–192
  Type III hypersensitivity, 186
McNA343, M_1 agonist, 114
Mebendazole, 670–672
Mecamylamine
  action, 114
  ganglion blocking, 126–128
  nicotine blocking, 679
  structure, 125
Mechanisms, drug action, 3–34
  desensitization, 31–33
  drug antagonism, 28–31
  receptor binding, 4–6
    characterization, 14–16
    classification, 6
    -effector linkage, 16–27
    measurement, 12
  systems, 3
Mechloroethamine, and anti-emetics,
  344
Mecillinam, 633
Meclofenamic acid, 205
Meclozine, 219, 220
Medroxyprogesterone, 420
  contraceptive, intramuscular, 426
Medulla, blood pressure regulation, 451
Mefenamic acid, 205
  analgesia, 212
Mefloquine, 662, 664–665
  structure, 661
Megaloblastic anaemia, 433, 437
  dihydrofolate reductase inhibition,
    664
  vitamin B_{12} versus folate deficiency,
    440
Melanocyte stimulating hormone, 359,
  366
  -releasing factor, 359, 366
Melphalan, 612, 614
Membranes
  channels of excitable membranes *see*
    Channels
  see also Cell membranes
'Memory' cells, antigen-sensitive, 183
Menaphthone (vitamin K), 284–285
Meningitis, cryptococcal, 652
Menopause
  menotrophin, 424
  and oestrogens, 416

Menotrophin, 424
Menstruation, 413–415
  disorders, oestrogens, 419
    progestogens, 421
    prostaglandins, 430–431
  endometrial change, 414
  iron loss, 436–437
  uterine contraction, 427
Mephenesin, muscle tone, control, 545
Meprobamate, 497–498
  effective and lethal dose, 495
Mepyramine, 218–220
Mercaptopurine, 222, 618
  action, 603, 611
  allopurinol, effect, 97
  genetic factors, 93
  inactivation, 75
  metabolism, 78
  see also Azathioprine
Mercurial diuretics, 312, 314, 319
  nephrotoxicity, 326
Mescaline
  psychomimetic action, 569, 576–577
  structure, 575
Mesterolone, 423
Mestranol, 418
Metabolism, catecholamines, 159–160
Metabolism of drugs, 73–78
  first-pass effect, 66, 77–78
  pharmacologically active metabolites, 78
  Phase I reactions, 73–76
  Phase II reactions, 73, 76–77
Metabolites, pharmacological activity, 78
Metaraminol, structure-activity relationship, 157–158
Metformin, 393
Methacholine
  muscarinic agonist, 119–120
  structure, 119
Methacycline, 636–637
Methadone, 554–555
  in addiction, 565
  structure, 555
Methallenoestril, 419
Methanol, 689
Methaqualone, 496, 498
Methazolamide, 326
Methicillin, 632–633
  β-lactamase resistance, 606
  plasma half life, 90
Methimazole, 376–377
Methionine
  acute paracetamol poisoning, 212
  and nitrous oxide, 481–482
  synthesis, 442
Methonium compounds, activity, 127
Methotrexate, 614–617
  anticancer action, 611
  assay, method, 51
    sensitivity, 56
  clinical use, 617
  folate deficiency, 438, 615
  pharmacokinetics, 616

protein building, reduction, 96
  structure, 615
  thymidylate synthesis, action on, 616
Methoxamine, summary, 165
Methoxyflurane, 476, 482
  and ADH, 368
  metabolic inactivation, 480
  renal toxicity, 482
  structure, 480
3-Methoxy, 4-hydroxyphenylglycol, 515
  in brain, 156
5-Methoxytryptamine, serotonin metabolism, 263
Methylamphetamine, 569–573
Methylcellulose, 347, 351
N-Methyl-D-aspartate (NMDA), 463–464
  receptors, 464
Methyldopa
  action, 173, 174
  blood pressure regulation, 272, 450–451
  haemolysis, incidence, 704
    Coomb's test, 704
  in hypertension, 272–275
  noradrenaline synthesis, 170, 450
  summary, 166
Methyl group, conjugation, 76
2-Methylhistamine, 189–190
4-Methylhistamine, 5
α-Methylnoradrenaline
  action, 170, 173–174
  receptor specificity, 148
  structure-activity, 157
  summary, 164
Methylphenidate, 569–573
1-Methyl 4-phenyl tetrahydropyridine (MPTP), 541
Methylprednisolone, 393
Methyltestosterone, 422–423
Methyltransferases, 25
α-Methyltyrosine
  action, 174
  noradrenaline synthesis, blocking, 150, 170
  summary, 166
Methylxanthines, 574–575
  heart stimulation, 254
  psychomotor action, 569, 574
  purine receptors, interaction with, 266
  see also Caffeine: Theophylline
Methysergide
  action, 155, 162
  in migraine, 277–278
  serotonin antagonist, 265
  structure, 162
Metoclopramide
  anti-emetic, 343, 455
  gastric emptying, 68, 95, 349–350
  lactation, stimulation, 429
  structure, 345
Metoprolol, antidysrhythmia, 247
  action, 165
Metriphonate, 670–673

Metronidazole, 642
  in amoebiasis, 665–666
  in Leishmaniasis, 667
  and oral anticoagulants, 287
Metyrapone, 395
mHelen, definition, 37
MHPG (3-methoxy 4-hydroxyphenylglycol), 515
Mianserin, 525–526
Miconazole, 652, 655
  action, 604
Microsomal enzymes, induction, 77
Microsomal oxidase in neonates, 91
Microsomal oxidase system and carbon tetrachloride, 694
  and ethanol, 688
Microtubules and griseofulvin, 656
Migraine, 275–278
  clonidine in, 173
Milk *see* Lactation
Mineralocorticoids, 318, 404–405
  excess production, 394
Minocycline, 636–637
Mithramycin
  in hypocalcaemia, 411
  in Paget's disease, 411
Mitobronitol, 614
Mitomycin
  action, 603, 611
  myelosuppression, 618–619
Mitotane, 395
  anticancer action, 620
Molindone, clinical dose, 501
Monoamines
  theory of depression, 513–517
    biochemical studies, 515–517
Monoamine oxidase (MAO)
  inhibition, 171, 173
  noradrenaline and tyramine, inactivation, 75–76
  occurrence and action, 154–156
  phenelzine, inhibitor, 166
  serotonin degradation, 75–76, 263, 455
Monoamine oxidase inhibitors (MAOI)
  clinical effectiveness, 526–528
  comparison, tricyclic antidepressants, 522
  in depression, 514, 517–518
  hepatotoxicity, 524
  interactions, 524–525
  noradrenaline, adrenergic terminals, 75, 76, 94
  pharmacological effects, 523
  selegiline, 543
    with levodopa, 543
  side effects, 524
  structures, 523
  substrates, 522
Monocytes, 180–181
MOPEG *see* 3-Methoxy, 4-hydroxyphenylglycol
Moperone, clinical dose, 501
Morphine, 553–563

Morphine (*contd*)
  action, 557–558
  analogues, 554
  in body fat, 63
  conjugation, slow, 91
  distribution volume, 72
  effective dose, 495
  effects, 558–560
  first-pass effect, 78
  gastric motility, 350–351
  lethal dose, 495
  measurement, 51
  pharmacokinetic aspects, 563
  receptors, 555–557
  reservoir effect, 81
  sphincter of Oddi, effect, 354
  structure, 555
  synthetic derivatives, 555
  tolerance/dependence, 560–563
  in trauma, 70
  '2 + 2' assay, 42
  unwanted effects, 563
Motilin, 331
Motion sickness, 507
  hyoscine, 124
  see also Vomiting
Motoneuron excitability, 457
Motor disorders, 530–545
MPTP *see* 1-methyl 4-phenyl
    tetrahydropyridine
Mucormycosis, 652
Muscarine
  acetylcholine receptors, 118–120
  activity, 113–114
  historical note, 101
  partial agonist, 120
  structure, 119
Muscarinic receptors, 114–115
  acetylcholine, effect, 459–460
  activation, 104 105
  agonists, 119 121
  antagonists, in asthma, 306
    effects, 122–123
    second messenger, 19
    structure-activity, 121–122
    uses, 123–125
  isolation, 16
  M_1 and M_2 subtypes, 114
  spare receptor hypothesis, 13–14
Muscle
  cardiac, 227–234
  skeletal
    catecholamines, 159–160
    tone, effects of drugs, 544–545
    potassium release, 135
  smooth
    α receptors, 158–159
    vascular, 256–258
Mustine, 612, 614
Mutagenesis, 695–698
Myasthenia gravis, 143–144
  blocking agents, action, 133
Mycoses, 652–653
Myocardial depressant factor, 274
Myocardial infarction, 236

Myxoedema, 369, 375
  -coma, 378

Nabilone, anti-emetic, 346
NAD +, and alcohol dehydrogenase, 87
Nafcillin, 633
Nalidixic acid, 603, 642–643
Nalorphine, 557, 565
  receptor binding, 556
  structure, 554
Naloxone, 565–566
  analgesia prevention, 549
  receptor binding, 556
  structure, 554
Naltrexone, 566
NANC *see* Non-adrenergic, non-
    cholinergic transmission
Nandrolone, 420, 423
Naproxen, 205
  analgesia, 206, 213
  structure, 208
Narcolepsy, 573
Neomycin, 600, 638
  plasma half-life, 90
Neonates
  displacing drugs, contraindications,
    96
  drug metabolism, 91
Nephrotoxicity
  aminoglycosides, 639
  cyclosporin, 695
  lithium, 529
  methoxyflurane, 482
  phenacetin, 695
Neostigmine
  action, 138–140, 349
  autonomic effects, 141
  cholinesterase inhibition, 118
  eyedrops, 70
  in myasthenia gravis, 143–144
  structure, 139
Nervi erigentes, 104
Netilmycin, 638
Neurochemical transmission
  autonomic nervous system, 103–107
  central nervous system, 447–470
  chemically-transmitting synapses,
    111–112
  history, 101–103
  presynaptic interactions, 108–111
  recent developments, 107–108
Neurohypophysis, 366–369
Neuroleptic drugs, 469, 499, 502–511
  see also Schizophrenia
Neuromodulators, 108
  definition, 177, 448
Neuromuscular blocking, 129–137
  see also Acetylcholine
Neuromuscular blocking drugs,
    129–137
  acetylcholine release, 130
  acetylcholine synthesis, effect,
    129–130
  comparison, table, 129, 131

postsynaptic action, 131–137
  depolarizing, 132–137
  non-polarizing, 131–132
  see also Depolarizing blocking drugs
Neuromuscular junction, synaptic
    transmission, 116
  see also Depolarizing blocking drugs
Neurons
  adrenergic terminals, 108–110
    presynaptic regulation, 109
  autoinhibitory feedback, 108
  cholinergic terminals, 108–110
    presynaptic regulation, 109
  denervation supersensitivity, 106
  heterotropic and homotropic
    interactions, 108
  non-adrenergic, non-cholinergic
    transmission, 110
Neuropeptides, 464–468
  classification, 465
Neurotensin, 331
Neurotransmitters, 103–107, 177,
    447–448
  see also Individual transmitters
Neutrophils
  adhesion, and prostaglandins, 197
  C5a activation, 186
  Fc receptors, 185
  in lung, 299
  'marginated pool', 299
  slow reacting substance, of
    anaphylaxis, 197
  toxic oxygen metabolites, 198
Niclosamide, 670–672
Nicotine, 678–683
  absorption, 69, 679
  chewing gum, 680
  depolarization block, 117 118, 125
  effect of mecamylamine, 681
  ganglion stimulation effect, 124–125
  harmful effects, 682–683
  structure, 124
  tolerance and dependence, 681
Nicotinic acid, lipid lowering, 356
Nicotinic activity, 113–114
Nicotinic receptors, 114
  acetylcholine, action, 104
  radiolabelling, 14–15
Nicoumalone, vitamin K antagonist,
    284, 286
Nifedipine, 31, 248–250
  structure, 248
Nigrostriatal pathway, 451–453
  and dopamine, 452–454
Nikethamide, 299, 569–571
  structure, 570
Nisoxetine, 526
Nitrates, intrabiliary pressure, 354
Nitrazepam, 488
  characteristics, 494
  and confusion, 494
Nitrofurantoin, 642, 667
Nitrogen mustard derivatives
  action, 603, 612
  alkylation of DNA, 613

Nitrogen mustard derivatives (*contd*)
  structure, 614
Nitroprusside, in hypertension, 260,
    274–275
Nitrosoureas
  anticancer action, 603, 612–614
  structure, 614
Nitrous oxide, 476, 481
  structure, 480
  unwanted effects, 481
  vitamin B_{12} metabolism, 481
NMDA *see* N-methyl-D-aspartate
Nociception, 547–548, 553
  bradykinin, activation, 551
  substance P, release, inhibition by
      morphine, 558
Noise analysis, 18
Nomifensine, 525–526
Non-adrenergic, non-cholinergic
      transmission (NANC), 110
  gastrointestinal tract, 330
  in lungs, 301
Non-depolarizing neuromuscular
      blocking drugs, 131–132
  comparison, depolarizing, 133–135
  rate of recovery, 136
Non-steroidal anti-inflammatory drugs
      (NSAID)
  action, 191, 193, 204–207
    mechanism, 207–208
    unwanted action, 209–212
  clinical use, 212–213
  renal function, 318
Noradrenaline, 76, 146–156, 448–451
  action, 104
  α-receptor feedback, 152–153
  to adrenaline, glucocorticoids, 395
  arousal, 450
  biosynthesis, 150
  blood pressure, 450–451
  cardiovascular effects, 159
  central noradrenergic pathways,
      448–449
  definition, 175
  denervation supersensitivity, 106
  drugs affecting release, adrenergic
      blocking, 170–171
    indirect, sympathomimetic amines,
      171–173
    presynaptic receptors, 173
  functional aspects, 449–450
  historical note, 103
  in lung, 299
  metabolic pathways, 154–156
  N-methylation, 151
  monoamine oxidase inhibitors, 94
  overflow, 152–153
  receptor specificity, 148
  release, 151–153
    by postganglionic fibres, 104
  reward and mood, 450
  schizophrenia, theories, 500
  structure, 146
  summary, 164
  turnover, 151

uptake and degradation, 153–156
    uptake I and II characteristics, 154
  uptake by receptors, 8
  uterus, action, 427–428
Nordiazepam, 488
  duration of action, 493–494
Norethisterone, 420
Norgestrel, 426
Nortryptiline
  anti-emetic, 343, 346
  antidepressant, 518–522
  inhibition, noradrenaline uptake, 526
  measurement, 51
  in plasma albumin, 63
NRM *see* Raphe nucleus
NSAID *see* Non-steroidal anti-
    inflammatory drugs
Nucleotide regulatory protein, 21
Nystatin, 603, 652, 654

Occupancy
  definition, 33
  formula, 7
  rectangular hyperbola, 7
  and response, 8
Oestradiol, 415–419
  biosynthesis, 396
  implants, 71
  late responses, 417
  structure, 418
Oestriol, 415–419
  biosynthesis, 396
  and early responses, 417
  as 'impeded' oestrogen, 416
  structure, 418
Oestrogens, 415–419, 425–426
  action, 417
  androgens, 415
  anti-oestrogens, 419
  biosynthetic pathway, 416
  carcinogenesis, 698
  cholesterol, 354, 415
  degradation, rate, 419
  in menstrual cycle, 414
  and thyroid function, 374
  unwanted effects, 419
  uses, 419, 425–426
Oestrone, 415–419
  structure, 418
Oltipraz, 674
Oncogenes, 695–696
  products, modification, 623–624
Ondine's curse, 298
Ophthalmology, drugs, 124
Opiates, 553–565
  antimotility, 350
  gastrointestinal absorption, 95
  see also Opioids
Opioid peptides, 466–468
  list, 465
Opioids, 553–566
  affinity, binding sites, 556
  agonist-antagonist classification, 557

antagonists, 565–566
  definition, 553
  effects on central nervous system,
      558–560
  in pain transmission, 550
  receptors, 555
  second messenger, 19
  tolerance and dependence, 560–563
  see also specific names
Opium, 553–554
Opportunistic infections, 652
Opsonins, inflammatory reaction, 180
Oral contraceptives, 425–426
  and anticoagulants, 287
  beneficial effects, 426
  deficiency, folate, 438
    vitamin B_{12}, 438
  for males, 423
  metabolic changes, 97
  metabolization to androgens, 415
  post-coital, 426
  and thromboembolism, 417
  unwanted effects, 425–426
Orciprenaline, uterus, inhibition,
      428
Organic nitrates in angina, 251–254
  adverse effects, 253
  structure-activity, 252
  uses, 254
Organophosphates, 139–142
Osteomalacia
  mithramycin, 411
  vitamin D in, 410
Osteoporosis
  excessive vitamin D, 409
  glucocorticoids, 402, 411
  hydroxyapatite in, 407
  oestrogens, 411
  post-menopausal, 416
Ouabain, 239–244
  pharmacokinetics, 243–244
  uses and adverse effects, 244
Oxacillin, plasma half life, 90
Oxamniquine, 670–673
Oxazepam, 488
  characteristics, 494
Oxidative reactions, 74–76
  mixed function oxygenase system, 74
Oxolinic acid, action, 603
Oxotremorine
  binding curve, 14
  muscarinic agonist, 119–120
  structure, 119
Oxprenolol
  action, 167, 168
  in hypertension, 274–275
  receptor specificity, 148
  side effects, 169
  structure-activity, 157
Oxymetholone, 423
Oxytocic assay, 42
Oxytocic drugs *see* Ergometrine:
      Oxytocin: Prostaglandins E
      and F
Oxytocin, 366–367, 369, 428–429

PAF *see* Platelet activating factor
PAG (periaqueductal grey area),
        549–550
Paget's disease
    and calcitonin, 410
    disodium etridonate in, 411
Pain (footnote), 547
    measurement, 550–551
    and nociception, 553
    opioids, sites of action, 550
    skin, pain endings, stimulation,
        551–552
Pancuronium
    action, 132
    distribution, 131
    pharmacokinetic aspects, 136–137
    structure, 126
Pancreatic polypeptide, 331
Pancreatitis, in hyperlipidaemia, 354
Pancreozymin, 331
Papaverine, gastric motility, 261
    vascular smooth muscle, 258, 259
Para-amino-benzoic acid
    in folate metabolism, 438–439
    structure, 628
    and sulphonamides, 95, 628–630
Paracetamol, 204–207
    action, 211
    and ADH, 368
    and glutathione, 695
    hepatotoxicity, 694–695, 698
    metabolism, 74
        Phase I metabolites, 77
        and phenacetin, 78
    particle size, 67
    structure, 212
Paracrine secretions, 178
Paralysis, suxamethonium, 135–136
Paraoxon, genetic factors, 93
Parasympathetic nervous system
    anatomy and physiology, 103–107
        receptors and effects, 105
    muscarinic agonists
        (parasympathomimetic), 119
Parathion
    action, 139
    irreversibility, 141
    structure, 139
Parathyroid hormone, 405–408
    calcium, distribution in body, 405–407
    parathormone, 408
    phosphate, 407
    and thyroid hormone, 373
Pargyline, 522–523
Parkinsonism, 539–544
    acetylcholine release, 460
    and amantadine, 648
    causes, 539
    dopamine breakdown, 454, 539–541
    drugs in, 541–544
    neuroleptic-induced, 507–508
    and prolactin, 366
PCPA (p-chlorophenylalanine), 455,
        457
PDGF *see* Platelet-derived growth factor

Pempidine, 127, 128
Penicillamine, 214–215
Penicillin, 626–627, 631–634
    allergic reactions, 703
    and bacteriostatic drugs, 95
    broad spectrum types, 633–634
    formulation, 68
    penicilloyl-polylysine, skin test, 703
    procaine penicillin, 71
    properties, 632
    protein conjugate formation, 703
    renal clearance, 79, 80
    resistance, β-lactamases, 606,
        632–633
    structures, 631–632
    unwanted effects, 634
Pentaerythritol tetranitrate, 251–254
Pentagastrin, acid secretion test, 336
Pentamidine, 667–668
Pentazocine, 555, 557
    action, 565
    dependence, 565
Pentobarbitone, 496–497
    bioassay, ED50, 39
    distribution volume, 72
Peptides *see* Neuropeptides: Opioid
        peptides: and specific names
Peptidoglycan, bacterial, 599–600
Perchlorate, hyperthyroidism and
        aplastic anaemia, 378
Periaqueductal grey area (PAG),
        549–550
Peripheral vascular disease, 167
    and smoking, 682
Peripheral vascular system, 256–279
    capillaries, 58
    vascular smooth muscle, 256–258
    vasoconstrictors, 258–260
    vasodilators, 260–278
Pernicious anaemia, 438
    therapy, 443
Pethidine, 557, 564
    measurement, 51
    and monoamine oxidase inhibitors,
        97, 525
    receptor binding, 556
    sphincter of Oddi, effect, 354
    structure, 555
Phaeochromocytoma, 167
    diagnostic test, 156
Pharmacodynamics, 57, 90
    definition, 57
    interaction of drugs, 94–95
Pharmacokinetics, 57, 81–89, 90
    definition, 57
    drug characteristics, plasma half-life,
        83
    interaction of drugs, 94–96
    saturation kinetics, 87–89
    single compartment model, 81–86
    two compartment model, 86–87
Phase I and II reactions, 73–76
Phenacetin, 209
    metabolism, 74
    particle size, 67

renal toxicity, 695
    structure, 211
Phencyclidine
    analgesia, 557
    psychomimetic action, 569
    schizophrenia, 577
    structure, 575
Phenelzine, 166
    structure, 523
Phenformin, vitamin B_{12} deficiency, 438
Phenobarbitone, 496–497
    anticonvulsant, 496, 533–537
    effect on other drugs, 537
    effective, and lethal dose, 495
    measurement, 51
    microsomal enzyme induction, 77, 97
    overdose, 537
    renal clearance, 80
    side effects, 537
    structure, 496
    and vitamin D, 410
    and warfarin, 28, 97
Phenothiazines
    antidiarrhoeal action, 352
    anti-emetics, 344, 455
    antihistamines, 218–220
    blocking, mediators, 505, 508
    characteristics, 504
    dopamine receptor, action, 268
    in lactation, 429
    neuroleptic drugs, 502–505
    serotonin antagonist, 265
    side effects, 509
    structure, 345
    sustained release, 89
    in thyroid function, 374
Phenoxybenzamine
    action, 163, 165–167
    and phaeochromocytoma, 167
    receptor specificity, 148
    summary, 165
Phenprocoumon, vitamin K antagonist,
        284, 286
Phentolamine
    receptor specificity, 148
    reversible competitive antagonist,
        noradrenaline, 163
    summary, 165
Phenylbutazone, 205
    and aplastic anaemia, 47
    binding to plasma albumin, 63,
        64–65, 72, 78
    as displacing agent, 96
    enzyme induction, 97
    microsomal induction, 77
    plasma half life, 92
    renal tubule secretion, 98
    structure, 208
Phenylephrine
    bradycardia, 259
    nasal decongestion, 161
    receptor specificity, 148
    summary, 164
Phenylethanolamine, structure-activity,
        157

Phenylethanolamine N-methyl transferase
  baroreceptor reflex and hypertension, 451
  noradrenaline, N-methylation, 151
Phenylethylamine, structure-activity, 157
Phenylpiperidines, 555
Phenytoin
  atrial antidysrhythmia, 245–247
  chloramphenicol, effect, 97
  distribution volume, 72
  enzyme immunoassay, 51
    induction, 97
  in epilepsy, 533–536
  and folate deficiency, 438
  genetic factors, 93
  and H_2-receptor antagonists, 337
  hepatic clearance, with other drugs, 535
  plasma albumin, 63
  plasma half life, 535–536
  saturating kinetics, 88–89
  side effects, 536
  teratogenesis, 698, 702
  in thyroid function, 374
  and vitamin D, 410
Phorbol esters, cocarcinogenic activity, 697
Phosphate, function in body, 407
Phosphatidic acid, 23
Phosphatidylinositol, 23–25
  action of diacylglycerol, 25
  action of phospholipase C, 25
  biphosphate, in cell proliferation, 623–624
  and glucocorticoids, 400–401
  insulin secretion, 380
Phosphodiesterases, and cyclic AMP, 21, 23, 126–127
Phospholipase, 193
  A_2, effect of glucocorticoid lipocortin, 400
  action, leukotrienes, 197
    platelet stimulating factor, 202
  C, agonist activation, 23–25
Phospholipid
  'flip-flop', 25
  in haemostasis, 281
  in platelet activation, 291
  stimulus/activation coupling mechanisms, tumours, 623–624
  transmethylation pathway, 25
Phosphonoformic acid, 648, 650
Phosphoramide mustard
  cytotoxic effect, 612
  structure, 614
Phosphorylase kinase activation, energy stores, 27
Phosphorylase, phosphorylation, 20
Phthalysulphathiazole, 629
Physostigmine
  action, 138–140
  atropine, antidote to, 123

  autonomic effects, 141
  EEG activity, 459–460
  glaucoma, 412
  structure, 139
Phytomenadione (vitamin K), 283
Picrotoxin, 568–571
Picrotoxinin, 569–571
  structure, 570
Pilocarpine
  in glaucoma, 121
  structure, 119
Pilomotor muscles, innervation, 105
Pimozide, clinical dose, 501
Pindolol, 165
  antidysrhythmic action, 247
Pinocytosis, 58
Piperazine, 670–672
  anti-emetic, 343
  antihelminthic, 604
Piperidines, neuroleptic drugs, 504
Pirenzepine, 337–338
  M_1 receptors, 114
  peptic ulcer, tests, 124
  structure, 122
Piroxicam, 205
  action, 207
  structure, 208
Pizotifen, serotonin antagonist, 265
Pituitary gland
  anterior (adenohypophysis), 359–366
  glucocorticoids, effect, 401
  posterior (neurohypophysis), 366–369
  tumour suppression, bromocriptine, 454
pKa values, various drugs, 60–61
Placenta
  as barrier, 72
  gonadotrophins in, 424
  hormonal functions, 415
Plasma
  albumin, renal filtration, 78
  esterases in neonates, 91
    see also Cholinesterase
  half life, 82–83
    antibiotics, 90
    definition, 80
    diazepam, increase with age, 91
    pH, effect of increase, 62
  proteins, binding of drugs, 63–65
Plasmids, bacterial, 605
  porin synthesis, 607
  resistance to tetracyclines, 606–607
Plasminogen activation, 294
Platelet activating factor (PAF)
  action, 191, 201–202
  activation, 291
  effect of glucocorticoid lipocortins, 400
  in haemostasis, 281
  lyso-PAF, precursor, 193
  structure, 201
Platelet-derived growth factor (PDGF), 695
  in tumours, 624

Platelets, 181
  adhesion and activation, 289–292
  aggregation, agents impairing, 285
  effect of alcohol, 685
  platelet factor-3, 282
  platelet factor-4, 289
PNMT see Phenylethanolamine N-methyl transferase
Polydipsia, 387
Polyene antibiotics, 653
Polyenes, action, 603–604
Polymixins, 603, 641–642
  with trimethoprim, 642
Polymorphonuclear cells, 180–181
  'respiratory burst', 181
Polyphospholinositides
  neutrophils, turnover, 181, 314
  see also Phosphatidylinositol
Polyuria, 387
Porin synthesis, plasmid-determined inhibition, 607
Porphyria, acute, drug addiction, inherited, 94
Potassium, plasma, effect of suxamethonium, 135
Potassium balance, 317–318
  effect of diuretics, 323–325, 327
  hyperkalaemia, 323, 324
Potassium channel blocking, 590
  see also 4-Aminopyridine: Tetraethylammonium
Potassium chloride, oral and parenteral use, 327
Potency ratio, definition, 38–40
Practolol
  action, 167
  oculomucocutaneous syndrome, 169
  receptor specificity, 148
  summary, 165
Pralidoxime, cholinesterase reactivation, 142–143
Praziquantel, 670–673
Prazosin
  antagonists, α_1-receptors, 163
  in hypertension, 274–275
  receptor specificity, 148
  summary, 165
Prednisolone
  action, 393–403
  measurement, 51
  in myasthenia gravis, 144
Prednisone
  action, 393–403
  as pro-drug, 76
Pregnancy
  blood loss, 437
  effects of alcohol, 685–686
  effects of smoking, 682
  iron demand, 437
  teratogenesis, 699–702
Pregnenolone
  glucocorticoid synthesis, 395–396
  oestrogen synthesis, 416
  progesterone metabolite, 421

Prenylamine, 248–250
  structure, 248
Presynaptic receptors, auto-inhibitory
        feedback mechanism, 152–153
Prilocaine, 583, 587
Primaquine, 663
  in Chagas' disease, 667
  glucose-6-phosphate dehydrogenase
        deficiency, 94
  structure, 661
Primidone, in epilepsy, 534–535, 537
Probenecid
  and aspirin, 212
  inhibition, 5HIAA transport, 515
    penicillin secretion, 97–98
    uric acid, 79
  and penicillin, prolongation, 634
  structure, 217
  uricosuric action, 328
Probucol, lipid lowering, 356
Procainamide
  radioimmunoassay, 51
  spectrophotometric assay, 56
  ventricular dysrhythmia, 245–247
Procaine
  action, 586
  anticholinesterases, interaction with, 97
  hydrolysis, 137
  pharmacokinetics, 587
  structure, 583
  suxamethonium, action slowed, 136
Procaine penicillin, 632–633
Procarbazine
  anticancer action, 620
  structure, 619
Prochlorperazine
  anti-emetic, 343
  clinical dose, 501
  structure, 345
Prodrugs, definition, 78
  examples, 76
Prodynorphin, hypothalamus, 467
Proenkephalin, adrenal medulla, 467
Progesterone, 419–421
  biosynthesis, 396
  menstrual cycle, 414
  mRNA, activation, 27
  oestrogen biosynthesis, 416
  rectal administration, 69
  uses, 421
Proguanil, 661, 664
Prolactin, 358, 363–366
  dopamine inhibition, 454
  -release inhibiting factor, 359
  -releasing factor, 359, 364
Promazine, clinical dose, 501
Promethazine, 218–220
  anti-emetic, 343
Prontosil, 628–630
  structure, 628
Pro-opiomelanocortin, 467
Propanidid
  and anaesthesia, 483
  and anticholinesterases, 97
  hydrolysis, 137

suxamethonium, action slowed, 136
Propantheline, 337–338
  action, 167
  gastrointestinal motility, 123
  structure, 122
Propargylamines, 523
Propranolol
  antidysrhythmia, 247
  in asthma, 304
  first pass effect, 78
  in hypertension, 274–275
  in hyperthyroidism, 378
  liver metabolism, 97
  measurement, 51
  in migraine, 278
  and phaeochromocytoma, 167
  receptor specificity, 148
  side effects, 169
  structure-activity, 157
  summary, 165
Propylthiouracil, 376–377
Prostacyclin
  action, sites, 191, 196
  biosynthesis, 194
  metabolism, 193
  platelet metabolite, 292, 293
  uterine, 430
Prostaglandins
  abortifacients, 431
  action, 171, 196
  adenylate cyclase, action, 198
  biosynthesis, 194
  coronary blood flow, 235
  E and F, in obstetrics, 430
    ulcers, healing, 339
    in uterus, 430–431
  haemodynamics, influence, 318
  in inflammation, 197 198
  in lung, 299
  metabolism, 193, 197–198
  pain, enhancement, 197, 551
  platelet metabolites, 292
  second messenger, 19
  synthesis, 25, 27
  uterus, endogenous, 430
    exogenous, 431
Prostate carcinoma, cyproterone, 423
Protamine sulphate, heparin
        antagonist, 289
Protamine-zinc insulin, 388–389
Protein
  binding, effect on elimination, 85–86
  C, vitamin K dependence, 283
  kinases, 20
    calmodulin activation, 25–27
    cyclic AMP-dependent, 21–22
    membrane-bound, 25–27
    table, 21
  phosphorylation, regulation, 20
Prothrombin time, 287
Protirelin, 361
Pseudocholinesterase, 137–138
Psilocin, 576–577
  structure, 576
Psilocybin, 576–577

psychomimetic action, 569
Psychotomimetic drugs, 575–577
Psychotropic drugs, classification, 469
Pteroylglutamic acid (folic acid),
        438–440
Purgatives, 347–350
Purines, 265–266
  cardiac actions, 254–255
  as CNS transmitters, 468
  as peripheral transmitters, 110
  see also Adenosine compounds: Cyclic
        adenosine monophosphate
'Purity-in-heart index', 37
Puromycin, in Chagas' disease, 667
Pyrantel, 670–672
Pyrazinamide, in tuberculosis, 645
Pyrazolethylamine (betazole), 336
Pyridostigmine
  autonomic effects, 141
  medium duration cholinesterase,
        138–140
  in myasthenia gravis, 142
  structure, 139
2-Pyridylethylamine, 189–190
Pyrilamine see Mepyramine
Pyrimethamine
  action, in bacteria, 598
  antimalarial action, 660, 664
  carcinogenicity, 698
  and mefloquine, 664
  structure, 630, 661

Qinghaosin, 664
Quaternary ammonium compounds, 67
  absorption and excretion, 31
Quinacrine, affinity for cell nuclei, 63
Quinestradol, 419
Quinestrol, 419
Quinidine
  antimalarial activity, 662
  atrial dysrhythmia, 245–247
  measurement, 51
  plasma albumin, 63
  theoretical partition in body, 60
Quinine, 3, 662–663
  assay, 56
  structure, 661
Quinone (vitamin K), 283–286
Quisqualic acid (QUIS) receptor, 464

Radioactive isotopes, anticancer, 620
Radioimmunoassay, 50–51
Radioiodine, 378
Radioreceptor assay, 50
Ramus communicans, 103
Ranitidine, H_2-receptor antagonist, 337
Raphe nucleus, 549–550
  effect of morphine, 558
  serotonin, 455–457
Raynaud's disease, 167

Receptors
  acetylcholine, 114–115
  adrenoceptors, 146–149
    see also Alpha-receptors: Beta-
      receptors
  agonists and antagonists, 6, 10–12
  alkylation, 30
  bronchial, 300
    β-receptors, 301
    muscarinic, 300
  classification, 6
  definition, 6, 33
  denervation supersensitivity,
    proliferation, 106
  desensitization, 31–33, 118
    depolarizing drugs, 135
  drug binding, β-adrenoreceptors, 13
    direct measurement, 12–14
    muscarinic agonists, antagonists, 14
  -effector linkage, 16–27
  exhaustion of mediators, 32
  isolation and characterization, 14–16
  loss, 32
  muscarinic, 114–115
  nicotinic, 114
  proliferation, post-denervation, 106
    see also Alpha-receptors: Beta-
      receptors
  quantitative aspects, 7–12
    competitive antagonism, 9–10, 33
    concentration-effect curves, 8
    partial agonists, efficacy, 10–12, 34
  receptor-effector linkage, 16–27
    DNA transcription, regulation, 27
    ionic permeability, direct
      regulation, 16–19
    second messenger, mechanisms,
      19–27
  slow conformational change, 32
  spare, 29, 32
Rectum(al), drug administration, 69
Reductive reactions, 76
Renal
  carrier systems, 78
  clearance of drugs, 79–81
  excretion of drugs, 78–81
  failure
    acute, 325–326
    chronic hyperlipoproteinaemia, 355
  function, 78–81
    clearance, definition, 79–80
    glomerular filtration, 78
  plasma flow, 80
  proximal tubule, actively secreted
    drugs, 79
  tubule, diffusion and secretion, 78–80
    secretion, probenecid, inhibition
      by, 97–98
  toxicity, cyclosporin, 695
    lithium, 529
    methoxyflurane, 482
    phenacetin, 695
  tubule, carrier-mediated transport, 62
    juxta-glomerular cells, 269
  see also Kidney

Renin, action, 269
Renin-angiotensin and aldosterone, 404
Reproductive system, 413–431
  contraception, 425–426
  endocrine aspects, in female,
    413–421, 426–431
    in male, 421–423
  gonadotrophins, 424
Reserpine
  action, 170
  depressive effect, 170
  in hypertension, 274–275
  noradrenaline depletion, 151
  summary, 166
Respiratory depression, morphine-
  induced, 559, 563
Respiratory system, 297–308
  disorders, 301–308
  drugs affecting, 299
  regulation, 297–301
Retinoids, in premalignant conditions,
  625
Rheumatoid arthritis
  cell-mediated hypersensitivity, 186,
    187
  drugs, chloroquine, 215–216
    gold, 213–214
    penicillamine, 214–215
    sulphasalazine, 216
  interleukin-1, 203
  and lipocortin, 401–402
Rhinitis, allergic, 186, 192
Rickettsiae, 627
Rifampicin, 626–627
  action, 603
  antifungal effect, with amphotericin,
    653
  bacterial resistance, 606
  biliary secretion, 73, 81
  enzyme induction, 96, 97
  in leprosy, 645
  in tuberculosis, 644
Rifamycin, 603
Rimantadine, 647–648
Rimiterol, anti-asthma, 304
Ro 15–1788, benzodiazepine, 488, 491
Roundworms, 669

S-adenosylmethionine methyl
    transferases, 25
St Anthony's fire (ergot poisoning),
    161–162
Salbutamol
  as aerosol, 70
  in asthma, 161, 304, 306
  in bronchial tone, 301
  receptor specificity, 148
  structure-activity, 157
  summary, 164
  uterus, inhibition, 428
Salcatonin ('salmon' calcitonin), 410
Salicylates
  CNS, toxic effect, 210

plasma concentration, genetic
    variation, 92
  systemic toxic effect, 210–211
  in thyroid function, 374
  see also Aspirin
'Salicylism', 210
Salivary glands
  ganglion stimulating drugs, 125
  innervation, 105
  muscarinic agonists, 120
    antagonists, 122
  vasoactive intestinal polypeptide, 111
Saralasin
  angiotensin antagonist, 259
  in hypertension, 270–272, 274–275
Saturation kinetics
  comparison, non-saturating, 88
  elimination, alcohol, 87
    diazepam, 87
  model, 82
Saxitoxin (STX), 588–589
  sites of action, 582
  structure, 589
Scatchard plot, 13
  definition, 33
Schild equation, 9
Schild plot, 10, 28
Schistosomes, 669
Schizophrenia, 499–502
  antischizophrenic drugs
    (neuroleptics), 502–511
    action, 505–506
    behavioural effects, 506
    characteristics, 504
    dopamine antagonist effects,
      507–508
    pharmacokinetics, 509–511
    and placebos, 511
    potencies, 501
    side effects, 509
    tardive dyskinesia, 507, 509
  dopaminergic hyperactivity, 454
  theories, 499–502
Sclerosing peritonitis and practolol, 47
Scorpion toxin, 582, 589–590
Scurvy, 443
'Second messengers', intracellular,
    19–27
  definition, 19
  protein kinases, 26–27
    table, 21
  regulation of calcium ions, 23–25
  regulation of cyclic AMP, 20–23
  system of intracellular control, 20
Sedative drugs, 496–498
Seizures *see* Epilepsy
Selegiline, 522–523
  and levodopa, 543
  in Parkinsonism, 543
Senile dementia, 460
Serotonin, 261–265
  action, hypothalamus, 457
  antagonists, 265
  in chromaffin cells, 262–263
  CNS transmitter, 455–457

Serotonin (*contd*)
  in coagulation, haemostasis, 281
  degradation, monoamine oxidase,
      455
  distribution, 261–263
  functional aspects, 455–457
  inactivation, 76
  in lung, 299
  metabolites, affective disorders,
      515–516
  microvasculature, action, 264
  in migraine, 275–278
  neurons containing, 455
  pharmacological effects, 263–264
  in platelet activation, 291
  raphe nucleus, 454
  receptors, classification, 464
  schizophrenia, theories, 500
  second messenger, 19
  and sleep, 457
  transmitter substance, myenteric
      plexus, 110
Sex steroids
  androgens, 422–423
  behavioural effects, 415
  -binding globulin, 423
  biosynthesis, 396
  gonadotrophins, 424
  oestrogens, 415–419
  progestogens, 419–421
  related compounds, 420
Shock and hypotensive states, 273–275
Skin reactions, allergic, 705
  type IV hypersensitivity, 186
Sleep, and wakefulness, 489
  and serotonin, 457
Slow reacting substance of anaphylaxis,
      192, 197
Smoking, 678–683
  action of nicotine, 125
  and oral contraception, 425–426
Smooth muscle
  adenosine, compounds, effect, 266
  in airways, 299–303
  cyclic GMP and organic nitrates,
      252–253
  dopamine, effect, 267
  muscarinic agonists, 120
      antagonists, 123
  vascular, 256–258
Sodium bicarbonate, 338–339
Sodium cellulose phosphate, 411
Sodium citrate alkalinization, urine,
      328
Sodium excretion, 405
Sodium nitroprusside vasodilation, 260
Sodium stilbogluconate, 667
Sodium sulphate, 348
Somatomedins, 363
Somatostatin, 263, 331
  growth hormone release, inhibition,
      359, 361–363
  insulin, inhibition, 380, 385
  thyrotrophin release, 371
'Spare receptors', 29

definition, 34
  see also Receptors
Spasticity, 544–545
Specific immune response *see* Immune
      response
Spectinomycin, 626
  effect, 601, 639–640
Spectrophotometry
  absorption, 55
  fluorescence, 55–56
Spirochaetes, 627
Spironolactone
  action, 323–325
  and aldosterone, 405
  as diuretic, 314
  in hypertension, 272
  structure, 320
Spiroperidol, clinical dose, 501
Splanchnic drug flow, 68
Spleen, function, 433
Stanolone, 423
Stanozolol, 423
Status epilepticus, 539
  diazepam, 490
Steatorrhea, iron, malabsorption, 437
Sterculia, 347
Steroids
  delaying absorption, 71
  receptor for, 27
  topical application, 69
  see also Adrenal steroids:
      Corticotrophin:
      Mineralocorticoids: Sex
      steroids
Stilboestrol, 418
  and carcinoma, female offspring, 419
  reservoir effect, 81
Stomach, 332–346
  antacids, 338
  anticholinergic agents, 337–338
  gastric secretion, 332–335
    H$_2$-receptor agonists, 336
    regulation, 333
    stimulants, 336
  ulcers, 339
  vomiting, 339–346
  see also Gastric
Straub tail reaction, 560
Streptokinase, 295
Streptomycin, 627, 638–639
  excretion, 79
  plasma half life, 90
  protein synthesis, 600
  structure, 638
Streptozotocin, 613–614
Strophanthidin, bioassay, variation, 39
Strophanthin, 239
Strychnine, 568–570
  blocking of glycine, 463
  structure, 570
  and tetanus toxin, 570
STX *see* Saxitoxin
Substance P, 111, 263
  action, 331
  and histamine, 189

second messenger, 19
  transmitter, primary afferents, 552
Substantia gelatinosa, 548–549
Sucralfate, 339
Sulindac, 205, 207
  anti-inflammatory effects, 213
Sulphadoxine, and mefloquine, malaria,
      664
Sulphalene, 661, 664
Sulphanilamide diuretics, 319–320
Sulphasalazine, 216
Sulphate groups, conjugation, 74, 76
Sulphinpyrazone
  aspirin, interference, 212
  inhibition, platelet adhesion, 293–294
  and phenylbutazone, 328
  structure, 217
  in uricosuria, 328
Sulphisoxazole, 63
Sulphonamides, 597, 628–630
  antimalarial action, 660–661
  chemistry, 629
  class II reactions, 603
  as 'displacing' agents, 96
  inhibition of p-aminobenzoic acid, 95
  of renal tubular secretion, 98
  mechanism, 629–630
  pharmacokinetics, 630
  plasma protein binding, 64
  and sulphonylureas, 392
  trimethoprim, as synergist, 95
  unwanted effects, 630
Sulphones, 660–661
Sulphonylureas, 390–392
  alcohol-induced flushing, 94, 392
  in diabetes, 390–393
  effect on cardiovascular system, 392
  interactions, other drugs, 392
  unwanted effects, 392
Sulpiride
  characteristics, 504
  dopamine receptor, action, 268
  structure, 503
Suramin, trypanosomiasis, 667
Sustained release preparations, 89
Suxamethonium
  action, 133
  anticholinesterases, 97
  butyrylcholinesterase, action, 137
  failure to inactivate, 93
  genetic variation, 93
  hydrolysis, 135–136
  malignant hyperpyrexia,
      (hyperthermia), 94, 136
  metabolism, plasma, 74
  nicotinic agonists, effect, 125
  paralysis, 135–136
  pharmacokinetic aspects, 136
  post-operative muscle pain, 133
  side effects and dangers, 135–136
  structure, 124
  with tubocurarine, 133–135
Sweat glands
  ganglion stimulating drugs, 125
  innervation, 105

Sweat glands (*contd*)
 muscarinic agonists, 120
  antagonists, 122
Sympathetic nervous system
 anatomy and physiology, 103–107
  receptors and effects, 105
Sympathomimetic drugs, 258–259
 definition, 176
Synapses
 depolarization block, 117–118
  phase I and II, 118, 125
 effect of drugs, 118–144
 'margin of safety', 117
 mode of action, 111–112, 115–117
Syphilis, 187
Systemic lupus erythematosus and
  lipocortin, 401

Tachyphylaxis, 32–33
Talampicillin, 633
Tamoxifen, 419, 420
Tapeworms, 669
Tardive dyskinesia, 507–508
TCA *see* Tricyclic antidepressants
TEA *see* Tetraethylammonium
Temazepam, 488
 characteristics, 494
Teratogenesis, 698–702
 recognition, 47
Terbutaline
 anti-asthma, 304
 uterus, inhibition, 428
Terfenadine, 218–220
Testicular failure, replacement therapy,
  423
Testosterone, 421–423
 biosynthesis, 396
 and cannabis, 691
 implants, 61
 oestrogen synthesis, 416
 preparations, 422
 rectal dose, 69
 structure, 420
 unwanted effects, 423
 virilization of female offspring, 415
Tests, on drugs
 Ames, 697–698
 anxiolytic drugs
  animals, 486–487
  man, 487–488
 clinical trials, 43–46
 toxicity tests
  in man, 700
  in vitro, 697–698, 701
  in vivo, 698
 whole animal, 697, 700–701
 see also Assays
'Tetanic fade', and depolarizing drugs,
  133–135
Tetracaine (Amethocaine), 583
Tetracosactrin, 403
 see also Corticotrophin
Tetracyclines, 636–637

action, 636
affinity, for calcium, 63, 68
 and iron, 95
assay, 56
calcium chelation, 637
plasmid resistance, 606–607
structures, 636
vitamin K deficiency, 287
Tetraethylammonium (TEA)
 action, 584–586
 block, K^+ channel, 581–582
 cholinergic enhancement, 144
 ganglion blocking, 125–126
 structure, 126, 583
Tetrahydrocannabinol (THC), 689–690
 anti-emetic, 690
 measurement, 51
Tetrahydrofolates, 615–616
Tetrodotoxin (TTX), 588–589
 sites of action, 582
 structure, 589
Thalidomide, 47, 699, 701–702
THC (Tetrahydrocannabinol), 689–690
Theobromine, bronchodilation,
  304–305
Theophylline, 574–575
 bronchodilation, 302–305
 and H_2-receptor antagonists, 337
 effect on heart, 254
 interaction with purine receptors,
  266
 psychomotor action, 569, 574
Therapeutic index, 48–50
Thiabendazole, 670–672
Thiazide diuretics, 320, 323–325
 in hypertension, 274–275
 inhibition of renal tubular secretion,
  98, 315
2-Thiazolylethylamine
 potency, 189
 structure, 190
Thiethylperazine
 action, 344
 structure, 345
Thioguanine, 611, 618
 anticancer action, 603, 611, 618
Thiopentone, 483–484, 496
 in body fat, 63
 side effects, 484
Thioridazine
 clinical dose, 501
 structure, 503
Thiotepa, 614
Thioureylene drugs, in hyperthyroidism,
  375–376
Thioxanthines
 clinical dose, 501
 neuroleptic drugs, 503
Thrombocytes *see* Platelets
Thrombocytopenic purpura, 290
 cytotoxic hypersensitivity, 186
 danoxol, 425
Thrombo-embolism
 arterial, 295–296
 venous, 295

Thrombomodulin coagulation,
  inhibition, 290
Thrombosis, 281–296
 blood coagulation, 281–283
 defects in, 283–289
 fibrinolysis, 294–295
 platelet adhesion, 289
  antiplatelet agents, 293–294
  and arachidonates, 292–293
Thromboxane
 A_2, vasoconstriction, 258
 action sites, 191, 195
 biosynthesis, 194
 in haemostasis, 281, 291–293
 metabolism, 193
 second messenger, 19
Thymic hormones, immune response,
  623
Thymidylate monophosphate,
  439–440
Thymoleptics, 469
Thymoxamine, and tolazoline, 165
Thyroglobulin, 369–371
Thyroid disorders
 carcinoma, radioiodine, 378
 diagnosis, 361
Thyroid hormone, 369–378
 abnormalities, 374–378
 action, 373–374
 effect on insulin, 373, 387
 regulation, 371–373
 synthesis, storage, secretion, 369–371
 T_3 and T_4, 369, 378
 transport and metabolism, 374
Thyroid stimulating hormone *see*
  Thyrotrophin
Thyroliberin, 361
Thyrotrophin, 358, 361, 371–373
 -releasing factor, 359, 361
 and prolactin, 364
Thyroxine (T_4) *see* Thyroid hormone
Time-course, drug action, 81–85
 half life, $t_{\frac{1}{2}}$, 83
 variation, absorption rates, 84–85
  dosage schedules, 83–84
Timolol, and propanolol, 165
Tinea infections, 652
Tissue sensitivity and age, 90
Tobramycin, 638
Tolazamide, 390–392
Tolazoline, summary, 165
Tolbutamide
 in diabetes, 390–391
 drugs modifying action, 97
 plasma albumin, 63, 64
 protein building, reduction, 96
 structure, 390
Tolerance, 32–33
 see also specific names
Tolnafate, 656
Toxicity, 692–705
 measurements, 38, 46–48
  LD50 test, 46–47
 monitoring, 37, 48
 therapeutic index, 48

Toxicity (*contd*)
  see also Allergic reactions:
      Carcinogenesis:
      Hepatotoxicity: Mutagenesis:
      Teratogenesis
α-Toxins, radiolabelling, 14
Tranquillizers, minor *see*
      Benzediazepine
Transcobalamins, 441–442
Transferrin, iron carriage, 435
Translocation
  bulk flow, 57–58
  diffusional, 57–58
Transmethylation hypothesis, 25
Transmitter amino acids, 460–464
Transmitters *see* Adrenergic
      transmission: Cholinergic
      transmission: Presynaptic
      receptors
Transport of lipoproteins, 354–356
Tranylcypromine, 522–523
Trazodone, 501
Treosulfan, 614
Triamcinolone, 393
Triamterene
  action, 315, 323–325
  structure, 320
Trichlorethanol, 498
Trichomoniasis, 668
Tricyclic antidepressants (TCA),
      517–522, 524–528
  action, 519
  acute toxicity, 521
  clinical trials, 526–528
  comparison, monoamine oxidase
      inhibitors, 524
  pharmacokinetics, 521–522
  side effects, 520 522
Triethylcholine, 130
Trifluoperazine
  anti-emetic, 344
  clinical dose, 501
  inhibitor, calmodulin, 27
Trigeminal neuralgia, 553
  carbamazepine, 538
Triiodothyronine (T_3), 369, 378
  see also Thyroid hormone
Trimetaphan
  action, 128
  in hypertension, 274–275
  plasma half-life, shortness, 127
  structure, 126
  use in anaesthesia, 129
Trimethadione
  in epilepsy, 534–535, 538
  teratogenesis, 698, 702
Trimethoprim, 630–631
  antibacterial action, 598
  antimalarial action, 664
  and cotrimoxazole, 631
  and polymixins, 642
  structure, 630, 661
  and sulphonamide as synergist, 95
  see also Cotrimoxazole:
      Sulphonamides

Tripelennamine, 218–220
Triphosphoinositol (IP_3)
  and intracellular calcium, 24
  in platelet activation, 291–292
Tripotassium dicitratobismuthate,
      339
Tropicamide, ophthalmological use,
      124
Troponin C, 25–26
Trypanosomiasis, 667–668
Tryptophan
  antidepressant (L-), 517
  hydroxylase, 455
  serotonin precursor, 262, 455
TTX *see* Tetrodotoxin
Tuberculin reaction, 186
Tuberculosis, 643–645
  inflammatory reaction, 187
Tuberoinfundibular system, 452–453
  and arcuate nucleus, 452
  prolactin secretion, control, 454
Tubocurarine
  absorption, 131
  action, 31, 128, 131–132
  administration, 67
  distribution, 72
  effect on post-synaptic membrane,
      117
  pharmacokinetic aspects, 136
  structure, 126
  suxamethonium, antagonism, 133
Tumour necrosis factor recombinant
      cloning, 623
Tumour promoters, 625
TXA_2 *see* Thromboxane
Tyramine
  bronchial muscle, 301
  'cheese reaction', 524
  inactivation, 74, 76
  monoamine oxidase inhibitors, 94,
      524
  structure-activity, 172–173
  summary, 165
Tyrosine
  catecholamines, biosynthesis, 150
  iodination, in thyroid, 370–371

UDP-glucuronyl transferase, 77
Urea, in diuresis, 325–326
Uric acid
  reabsorption, inhibition, 79
  retention, 327–328
Uricosuric agents, 217–218
Urine
  acidification, 62
  alkalinization, 62
  diuresis, drug excretion, 98
  forced alkaline diuresis, 79
  pH changes in, 327–328
  pH in, 79
  unchanged drugs in, 81
Urokinase, 295
  clinical trial, *vs* heparin, 46

Ursodeoxycholic acid, 352, 354
Urticaria, anaphylactic hypersensitivity,
      186
USDA *see* Ursodeoxycholic acid
Uterus, 426–431
  motility and innervation, 426–428
  oxytocic drugs, 428–431

Vancomycin, 626–627, 641
Vagus nerve
  cranial outflow, 104, 107
  physiology, 101–103
  'Vagusstoff', 101–102
Valproate
  in epilepsy, 533–534, 538
  plasma albumin, 63
Variability, causes, 90–98
  age, effects, 90–92
  drug interactions, 94–98
  genetic factors, 92–94
Varicella zoster virus, 648–649
Vasoactive intestinal polypeptide (VIP),
      263, 331, 552
  and growth hormone releasing factor,
      360
  salivary gland release, 111
Vasoconstrictors, 258–260
  see also Thromboxane
Vasodilators, 260–278
  adenosine compounds, 266
  classification, 259
  dopamine, 267
  endothelium dependent, 190
  ethanol, 684
  glucocorticoids, 397–398
  oxytocin induced, 429
Vasopressin, 259–260
  action, 314 315
  'second messenger', 19
  uterine contraction, 429
Verapamil, 248–250
  action, 31
  structure, 248
Veratridine, 582, 590
Vidarabine, 648–649
Vinca alkaloids, 619
  and ADH, 368
  diuretic effect, 316
  and microtubules, 604, 611
  vinblastine, 604, 619
  vincristine, 604, 619
  vinedesine, 604, 619
VIP *see* Vasoactive intestinal
      polypeptide
Vitamin B_{12}, 437–438, 440–443
  action, 442
  deficiency, 440
  drug related, 438
  in folate synthesis, 442
  storage, 442
  structure, 441
Vitamin C, 443
Vitamin D_2 (calciferol), 406

Vitamin D$_3$ (Cholecalciferol)
  biosynthesis, 406
  interactions, anticonvulsants,
      410
  unwanted effects, 409–410
Vitamin K
  deficiency, 283
  synthesis of clotting factors, 283–286
Volume of distribution (V$_d$), 72–73,
      81–86
VMA *see* 3-methoxy-4-
      hydroxymandelic acid, 156
Vomiting, 339–346
  dopaminergic neurons, 455
  emetics and anti-emetics, 342–346
  reflex mechanism, 340–342
Von Willebrand's factor, 290

War gases, 139–142
Warfarin
  action, 28
  chloral hydrate, action, 96
  disulfiram, inhibition, 97
  effect of phenobarbitone, 28
  inactivation, 76
  plasma albumin, 63, 72, 96
  vitamin K antagonist, 284–286
Wintergreen, oil of (methylsalicylate),
      209

Xanthine oxidase, 75
  purines, analogues, 97

Xanthines, diuretics, 319
Xanthomas in hyperlipidaemia, 354
Xipamide, structure, 323

Yohimbine
  receptor specificity, 148, 163
  summary, 165

Zero-order kinetics, 87
Zimelidine, 525–526
Zollinger-Ellison syndrome, 334, 336